ZOO ANIMAL AND WILDLIFE IMMOBILIZATION AND ANESTHESIA

Second Edition

ZOO ANIMAL AND WILDLIFE IMMOBILIZATION AND ANESTHESIA

Second Edition

Edited by

Gary West, DVM, Dipl ACZM
Phoenix Zoo

Darryl Heard, BSc, BVMS, PhD, Dipl ACZM
College of Veterinary Medicine
University of Florida

Nigel Caulkett, DVM, MVetSc, Dipl ACVA
College of Veterinary Medicine
University of Calgary

WILEY Blackwell

Editorial offices: 1606 Golden Aspen Drive, Suites 103 and 104, Ames, Iowa 50014-8300, USA
The Atrium, Southern Gate, Chichester, West Sussex, PO19 8SQ, UK
9600 Garsington Road, Oxford, OX4 2DQ, UK

For details of our global editorial offices, for customer services and for information about how to apply for permission to reuse the copyright material in this book please see our website at www.wiley.com/wiley-blackwell.

Library of Congress Cataloging-in-Publication Data

Zoo animal and wildlife immobilization and anesthesia / [edited by] Gary West, Darryl Heard, Nigel Caulkett. – Second edition.
    p. ; cm.
  Includes bibliographical references and index.
  ISBN 978-0-8138-1183-3 (cloth)
  I. West, Gary (Gary Don), 1969– editor of compilation.   II. Heard, Darryl J., editor of compilation.   III. Caulkett, Nigel, editor of compilation.
  [DNLM: 1. Anesthesia–veterinary. 2. Animals, Wild. 3. Animals, Zoo. 4. Immobilization–veterinary. SF 914]
  SF914
  636.089'796–dc23
                              2014004707

A catalogue record for this book is available from the British Library.

Wiley also publishes its books in a variety of electronic formats. Some content that appears in print may not be available in electronic books.

Dedication

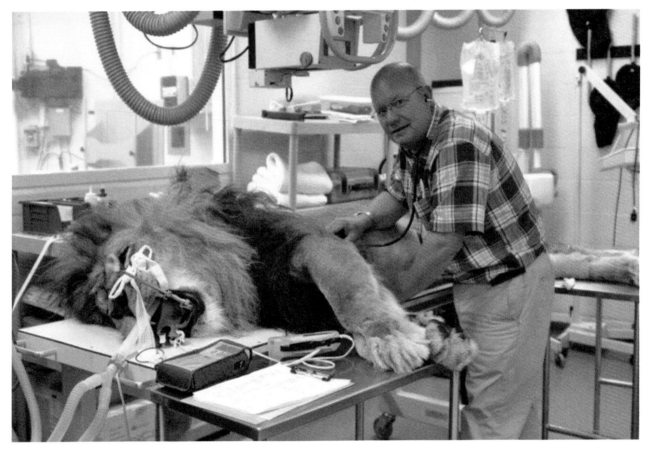

The second edition of *Zoo Animal and Wildlife Immobilization and Anesthesia* is dedicated to our dear friend and colleague, Dr. Greg Fleming (March 13, 1966–March 9, 2013).

How miserably things seem to be arranged in this world. If we have no friends, we have no pleasure; and if we have them, we are sure to lose them, and be doubly pained by the loss.

—Abraham Lincoln

(Photo credit: Department of Animal Health, Disney's Animals, Science, and Environment.)

Contents

Contributors

Noha Abou-Madi, DVM, Msc
Clinical Associate Professor, Section of Zoological Medicine
Department of Clinical Sciences
College of Veterinary Medicine
Cornell University
Ithaca, NY 14853-6401
Phone: 607-253-3371
E-mail: na24@cornell.edu

Frederick B. Antonio
Director
Orianne Center for Indigo Conservation
30931 Brantley Branch Road
Eustis, FL 32736
Phone: 407-516-7694
E-mail: fantonio@oriannesociety.org

Douglas L. Armstrong, DVM
Director of Animal Health
Omaha's Henry Doorly Zoo and Aquarium
3701 S. 10th St.
Omaha, NE 68107
Phone: 402-738-2044

Jon M. Arnemo, DVM, PhD, DECZM
Department of Forestry and Wildlife Management
Faculty of Applied Ecology and Agricultural Sciences
Hedmark University College, Campus Evenstad
NO-2418 Elverum
Norway
Department of Wildlife, Fish and Environmental Studies
Faculty of Forest Sciences, Swedish University of Agricultural Sciences
SE-901 83, Umeå
Sweden
Cell/work phone: +47 99585019
E-mail: jon.arnemo@hihm.no

James Bailey, DVM, MS, DACVAA
University of Florida
College of Veterinary Medicine
Service Chief
Anesthesia and Pain Management
P.O. Box 100136
Gainesville, FL 32610-0136
Phone: 352-258-6600
E-mail: baileyj@mail.vetmed.ufl.edu

Eric Baitchman, DVM, DACZM
Director of Veterinary Services
Zoo New England
1 Franklin Park Road
Boston, MA 02121
E-mail: ebaitchman@zoonewengland.com

Ray L. Ball, DVM
Senior Veterinarain, Director of Medical Sciences
Tampa's Lowry Park Zoo
1101 W. Sligh Avenue
Tampa, FL 33604
Phone: 813-935-8552 ext. 349
E-mail: Ray.Ball@LowryParkZoo.com

Mads F. Bertelsen, DVM, DVSc, DECZM (Zoo Health Management), DACZM
Staff Veterinarian
Centre for Zoo and Wild Animal Health
Copenhagen Zoo
Roskildevej 38
DK-2000 Frederiksberg
Denmark
Phone: +45 72200227
E-mail: mfb@zoo.dk

Kate Bodley, BSc (Vet), BVSc (Hons), MVS
Melbourne Zoo
Elliott Ave.
Parkville, VIC
Australia

Søren Boysen, DVM, DACVECC
Department of Veterinary Clinical and Diagnostic Sciences
Faculty of Veterinary Medicine
University of Calgary
3330 Hospital Drive NW
Calgary, AB
T2N 4N1
Phone: +403 210-8129
Fax: +403 220-3929
E-mail: srboysen@ucalgary.ca

David B. Brunson, DVM, MS, DACVAA
Senior Veterinary Specialist
Companion Animal Division, Zoetis
Adjunct Associate Professor
Department of Surgical Sciences in the School of Veterinary
Medicine
University of Wisconsin
Madison, WI 53706
2780 Waubesa Ave.
Madison, WI 53711
E-mail: david.brunson@zoetis.com

Mitchell Bush, DVM, DACZM
Senior Veterinarian Emeritius
Smithsonian Conservation Biology Institute
Front Royal, VA

Tracy Carter, BS, MS, PhD
Adjunct Professor
Oklahoma State University
Department of Zoology
415 LSW
Stillwater, OK 74078
Phone: 405-744-9675
Fax: 405-744-7824
E-mail: tracy.carter@okstate.edu

Nigel Caulkett, DVM, MVetSc, DACVAA
Department of Veterinary Clinical and Diagnostic Science
3280 Hospital Drive NW
Calgary, AB
Canada T2N 1N4
Phone: 403 220 8224
E-mail: nacaulke@ucalgary.ca

Shannon Cerveny, DVM, DACZM
Oklahoma City Zoo
2101 NE 50th St.
Oklahoma City, OK 73111

Scott B. Citino, DVM, DACZM
Staff Veterinarian
White Oak Conservation Center
Yulee, FL

Tonya M. Clauss, DVM, MS
Georgia Aquarium
Atlanta, GA
E-mail: tclauss@georgiaaquarium.org

Jonathan Cracknell, BVMS, CertVA, CertZooMed, MRCVS
Director of Animal Operations
Longleat Safari and Adventure Park
Safari Park Office
Longleat, Wiltshire
England BA12 7NJ
Phone: +44 (0) 1985 845 413
Mobile: +44 (0) 7855 763319
E-mail: jon.cracknell@longleat.co.uk

Christopher Dold, DVM
Vice President of Veterinary Services
SeaWorld Parks & Entertainment
E-mail: christopher.dold@seaworld.com

Alina L. Evans, DVM, MPH
Department of Forestry and Wildlife Management
Faculty of Applied Ecology and Agricultural Sciences
Hedmark University College
Campus Evenstad
NO-2418 Elverum
Norway
E-mail: alina.evans@hihm.no

Åsa Fahlman, DVM, VetMedLic, PhD, DECZM
Department of Clinical Sciences
Faculty of Veterinary Medicine and Animal Science,
Swedish University of Agricultural Sciences,
P.O. Box 7054
SE-750 07 Uppsala
Sweden
Phone: +46 70 6106388
E-mail: asa_fahlman@hotmail.com

Gregory J. Fleming, DVM, DACZM
Disney's Animals, Science, and Environment
P.O. Box 10000
Lake Buena Vista, FL 32830

Kurt A. Grimm, DVM, MS, PhD, DACVAA, DACVCP
Owner Veterinary Specialist Services, PC
P.O. Box 504
Conifer, CO 80433
Phone: (303) 918 1321
E-mail: grimm.dvm@gmail.com

Nina Hahn, DVM, PhD, DACLAM
Attending Veterinarian
Lawrence Berkeley National Laboratory
Berkeley, CA

Michelle G. Hawkins, BS, VMD, DABVP (Avian Practice)
Associate Professor, Companion Avian and Exotic Animal
Medicine and Surgery
Department of Medicine and Epidemiology
University of California-Davis
School of Veterinary Medicine
Davis, CA

Martin Haulena, DVM, MSc, DACZM
Vancouver Aquarium
PO Box 3232
Vancouver, BC
Canada V6B 3X8
604-659-3468
E-mail: Martin.Haulena@vanaqua.org

Darryl Heard, BSc, BVMS, PhD, DACZM
Associate Professor Zoological Medicine
Department of Small Animal Clinical Sciences
College of Veterinary Medicine
University of Florida
Gainesville, FL 32610-0126
E-mail: heardd@ufl.edu

Sonia M. Hernandez, DVM, DACZM, PhD
Assistant Professor
Warnell School of Forestry and Natural Resources and the
Southeastern Cooperative Wildlife Disease Study
University of Georgia
Athens, GA 30602

Markus Hofmeyr, BVSc, MRCVS, MDP
Principal Scientist, Veterinary Services
South African National Parks
P.O. Box 122
Skukuza, Mpumalanga
South Africa 1350
Phone: 27-84-7001355 or 27-13-7354239
Fax: 27-13-735-4057
E-mail: markush@parks-sa.co.za

Peter Holz, BVSc, DVSc, MACVSc, DACZM
Tidbinbilla Nature Reserve
RMB 141
Via Tharwa, ACT 2620
Australia
E-mail: holz@megalink.com.au.

William A. Horne, DVM, PhD, DACVAA
Chairperson
Department of Small Animal Clinical Sciences
Michigan State University
Room D208
Veterinary Medical Center
736 Wilson Rd.
East Lansing, MI 48824

Ramiro Isaza, DVM, MS, MPH, DACZM
Associate Professor of Zoological medicine
Department of Clinical Sciences
Cornell University College of Veterinary medicine
University of Florida
Gainesville, FL 32610-0126
Phone: (352) 392 4700
E-mail: isazar@mail.vetmed.ufl.edu

Randall E. Junge, MS, DVM, DACZM
Vice President for Animal Health
Columbus Zoo and the Wilds
Cumberland, OH

Jeff C. Ko, DVM, MS, DACVAA
Professor, Anesthesiology
Department of Veterinary Clinical Sciences
College of Veterinary Medicine
Purdue University
625 Harrison Street
West Lafayette, IN 47907-2026
Phone: (765) 496 9329
E-mail: jcko@purdue.edu

George V. Kollias, DVM, PhD, DACZM
J. Hyman Professor of Wildlife Medicine
Department of Clinical Sciences and
Janet L. Swanson Wildlife Health Center
College of Veterinary Medicine
Cornell University
Ithaca, NY 14853-6401
Email: gvk2@cornell.edu

Terry J. Kreeger, MS, DVM, PhD
State Wildlife Veterinarian
Wyoming Game and Fish Department
2362 Highway 34
Wheatland, WY 82201
E-mail: tkreeg@gmail.com

Rebecca A. Krimins, DVM, MS
Medical Director
Veterinary Imaging of the Chesapeake
808 Bestgate Rd.
Annapolis, MD 21401
Phone: (410) 224 0121
E-mail: rkrimins@vetimagingchesapeake.com

Leigh A. Lamont, DVM, MS, DACVAA
Associate Dean, Academic and Student Affairs
Atlantic Veterinary College
University of Prince Edward Island
550 University Avenue
Charlottetown, PE
Canada C1A 4P3
Phone: (902) 566 0374
E-mail: llamont@upei.ca

Jennifer N. Langan, DVM, DACZM
Clinical Associate Professor
University of Illinois
College of Veterinary Medicine
Associate Veterinarian
Chicago Zoological Society
Brookfield Zoo
8400 W 31st St.
Brookfield, IL 60513

R. Scott Larsen, DVM, MS, DACZM
Vice President of Veterinary Medicine
Denver Zoo
2300 Steele St.
Denver, CO 80205
E-mail: slarsen@denverzoo.org

Gregory A. Lewbart, MS, VMD, DACZM
NCSU-CVM
1060 William Moore Drive
Raleigh, NC 27607
Email: galewbar@ncsu.edu

Michael R. Loomis, DVM, MA, DACZM
Chief Veterinarian
North Carolina Zoological Park
4401 Zoo Parkway
Asheboro, NC 27205

Michael Lynch, BVSc, PhD, MANZCVSc (Epi)
Melbourne Zoo
Parkville, VIC
Australia

Khursheed R. Mama, DVM, DACVAA
Professor, Anesthesiology
Department of Clinical Sciences
Colorado State University
Fort Collins, CO 80526
Phone: 970 297 4124
Email: kmama@colostate.edu

Michele Miller, DVM, MS, MPH, PhD
Professor, South African Research Chair in Animal
Tuberculosis
Division of Molecular Biology and Human Genetics
Faculty of Medicine and Health Sciences
Tygerberg, South Africa

Anneke Moresco, DVM, MS, PhD
Research Associate
Denver Zoo
2300 Steele St.
Denver, CO 80205
Phone: 720 337 1590
E-mail: anneke_moresco@hotmail.com

Peter vdB. Morkel, BVSc
Private Consultant
P.O. Box 260
Kakamas 8870
South Africa

Cornelia I. Mosley, Dr Med Vet, DACVAA
Assistant Professor
Ontario Veterinary College
University of Guelph
Guelph, ON
Canada

Daniel M. Mulcahy, PhD, DVM, DACZM
Wildlife Veterinarian
U.S. Geological Survey
Alaska Science Center
4210 University Drive
Anchorage, AK 99508

Natalie D. Mylniczenko, DVM, MS, DACZM
Disney's Animals, Science, and Environment
P.O. Box 10000
Lake Buena Vista, FL 32830
Phone (office): 407-938-3277
Cell phone: 321-299-4079
Fax: 407-938-3266
Email: Natalie.Mylniczenko@Disney.com

Julie Napier, DVM
Senior Veterinarian
Omaha's Henry Doorly Zoo and Aquarium
3701 S. 10th St.
Omaha, NE 68107

Donald L. Neiffer, VMD, DACZM
Veterinary Operations Manager
Disney's Animal Programs
P.O. Box 10,000
Lake Buena Vista, FL 32830
Phone: 407-938-2719
Fax: 407-939-6391

Elizabeth C. Nolan, DVM, MS, DACZM
Disney's Animals, Science, and Environment,
P.O. Box 10,000,
Lake Buena Vista, FL 32830
Email: elizabeth.c.nolan@disney.com.

Rolf-Arne Ølberg, DVM, DVSc
Director of Animal Care
Kristiansand Dyrepark
4609 Kardemomme By
Norway
Phone: +47 97059860
Email: rolfarne@dyreparken.no

Larissa Ozeki, DVM, MSc
Department of Veterinary Clinical and Diagnostic Science
3280 Hospital Drive NW
Calgary, AB
Canada T2N 1N4
Phone: (403) 466 0115
E-mail: lmozeki@ucalgary.ca

Luis R. Padilla, DVM, DACZM
Director of Animal Health
St. Louis Zoo
1 Government Drive
St. Louis, MO 63110

John M. Parker, DVM
Campus Veterinarian
Laboratory Animal Resource Center
University of California San Francisco

An Pas, DVM
Breeding Center for Endangered Arabian Wildlife
P.O. Box 29922
Sharjah
United Arab Emirates

Peter J. Pascoe, BVSc
Professor
Surgical and Radiological Sciences
University of California Davis
Davis, CA 95616

Jessica Paterson, BSc (Hons), DVM, MVetSc
Department of Veterinary Clinical and Diagnostic Science
3280 Hospital Drive NW
Calgary, AB
Canada T2N 1N4
E-mail: paterson_jessica@hotmail.com

Julia Ponder, DVM
Executive Director
The Raptor Center
College of Veterinary Medicine
University of Minnesota
St. Paul, MN 55108

Robin W. Radcliffe, DVM, DACZM
Director Cornell Conservation Medicine Program
Adjunct Assistant Professor of Wildlife and Conservation Medicine
College of Veterinary Medicine
Cornell University
Ithaca, NY

Edward C. Ramsay, DVM, DACZM
Professor, Zoological Medicine
The University of Tennessee
Department of Small Animal Clinical Sciences
C247 Veterinary Teaching Hospital
Knoxville, TN 37996-4544
Ph 865-755-8219
FAX 865-974-5554
E-mail: eramsay@utk.edu

Patrick T. Redig, DVM, PhD
Professor of Avian Medicine and Surgery
Co-Founder and Director Emeritus
The Raptor Center
College of Veterinary Medicine
University of Minnesota
St. Paul, MN 55108

Sam Ridgway, DVM, PhD, DACZM
National Marine Mammal Foundation
2240 Shelter Island Drive Ste 200
San Diego, CA 92106
Phone: 619-553-1374
E-mail: sridgway@UCSD.edu

Todd L. Schmitt, DVM
SeaWorld San Diego
500 SeaWorld Dr.
San Diego, CA 92109
E-mail: todd.schmitt@seaworld.com

Jim Shaw, BS, MS, PhD
Professor, Oklahoma State University
Department of Natural Resources, Ecology and Management
008 Ag Hall
Stillwater, OK 74078
Phone: 405-744-9842
Fax: 405-744-3530
E-mail: jim.shaw@okstate.edu

Todd Shury, DVM
Wildlife Health Specialist|Spécialiste en santé de la faune
Office of the Chief Ecosystem Scientist|Bureau de Scientifique en chef des écosystèmes
Protected Area Establishment and Conservation|Établissement et conservation des aires protégées
Parks Canada Agency|Agence Parcs Canada
Saskatoon, SK
Canada S7N 5B4
Phone: (306) 966 2930
E-mail: Todd.Shury@pc.gc.ca

Jessica Siegal-Willott, DVM, DACZM
Center for Animal Care Sciences
Smithsonian's National Zoological Park
Smithsonian Conservation Biology Institute
P.O. Box 37012, MRC 5502
Washington, DC 20013-7012

Melissa Sinclair, DVM, DVSc, DACVAA
Associate Professor in Anesthesiology
Ontario Veterinary College
University of Guelph
Department of Clinical Studies
University of Guelph
Guelph, Ontario
Canada
N1G 2W1
Phone: 519 824-4120 EXT 54450
Email: msinclai@ovc.uoguelph.ca

Jonathan Sleeman, MA, VetMB, DACZM, DECZM, MRCVS
Center Director
USGS, National Wildlife Health Center
6006 Schroeder Road
Madison, WI 53711
Tel: (608) 270 2401
Fax: (608) 270 2415
Email: jsleeman@usgs.gov

M. Andrew Stamper, DVM, DACZM
Research Biologist/Clinical Veterinarian
The Seas, Disney's Animal Programs
Walt Disney World Resorts
EC Trl. W-251
2020 North Avenue of the Stars
Lake Buena Vista, FL 32830-1000
Phone: 407-560-5576
Fax: 407-560-5750

Mark Stetter, DVM, DACZM
Dean
College of Veterinary Medicine and Biomedical Sciences
Colorado State University
Fort Collins, CO
Phone (office): (970) 491-7051
Email: mark.stetter@colostate.edu

Wm. Kirk Suedmeyer, DVM, DACZM
Director of Animal Health
The Kansas City Zoo
6800 Zoo Drive
Kansas City, MO 64132

Gregory Timmel, DVM, MS, DACLAM
Attending Veterinarian
Legacy Research
Portland, OR

Alessio Vigani, DVM, PhD, DACVAA
University of Florida
Gainesville, FL
E-mail: alessio.vigani@gmail.com

Kent A. Vliet, PhD
Coordinator of Laboratories
University of Florida
Department of Biology
208 Carr Hall
P.O. Box 118525
Gainesville, FL 32611-8525

Michael T. Walsh, DVM
Aquatic Animal Health Program
Large Animal Clinical Sciences
College of Veterinary Medicine
University of Florida
2015 SW 16th Ave.
Gainesville, FL 34787
E-mail: walshm@ufl.edu

Chris Walzer, DECZM, Dr Med Vet, DECZM
University Professor
Research Institute of Wildlife Ecology
Department of Integrative Biology and Evolution
University of Veterinary Medicine
Savoyenstrasse 1, A-1160
Vienna, Austria
E-mail: Chris.Walzer@vetmeduni.ac.at

Mary L. Weldele, BA
Associate Research Specialist
Department of Psychology
University of California Berkeley
Berkeley, CA

Gary West, DVM, DACZM
Executive Vice President
Animal Health and Collections
Phoenix Zoo
455 North Galvin Parkway
Phoenix, AZ 85008

Douglas P. Whiteside, DVM, DVSc, DACZM
Senior Staff Veterinarian
Calgary Zoo Animal Health Centre
Clinical Associate Professor
University of Calgary Faculty of Veterinary Medicine
1625 Centre Ave East
Calgary, AB
Canada T2E 9K2
Phone: (403) 232 9390
E-mail: dougw@calgaryzoo.com

Michelle Willette, DVM
Staff Veterinarian
The Raptor Center
College of Veterinary Medicine
University of Minnesota
St. Paul, MN 55108

Cathy V. Williams, DVM
Senior Veterinarian
Duke Lemur Center
Duke University
Durham, NC
Adjunct Assistant
Professor of Zoological Medicine
College of Veterinary Medicine
North Carolina State University
Raleigh, NC

Murray Woodbury, DVM, MSc
Associate Professor and Research Chair,
Specialized Livestock Health and Production,
Western College of Veterinary Medicine
52 Campus Drive
Saskatoon, SK
Canada S7N 5B4
Phone: 306 966 7170
E-mail: murray.woodbury@usask.ca

Ashley M. Zehnder, DVM, ABVP (Avian)
Postdoctoral Fellow
Department of Dermatology
CCSR Bldg., 2150
269 Campus Drive
Stanford University
Stanford, CA 94305-5168
E-mail: azehnder.dvm@gmail.com

Preface

Welcome to the second edition of *Zoo Animal and Wildlife Immobilization and Anesthesia*. The publication of this edition occurs at a time when continual advances in wildlife anesthesia are being made. Increasingly, veterinarians, biologists, veterinary technicians, and others are challenged to provide exemplary care to threatened or endangered species. To meet these challenges, we continually strive to ensure the highest level of patient safety. The goal of this book is to provide an efficient method to access knowledge about wildlife anesthesia.

We wish to express our appreciation to all of our contributing authors. Their hard work, willingness to share their expertise, and their dedication to this field allow us to produce a high quality and clinically useful publication.

There is still much to learn about the anesthetic and analgesic management of our wildlife patients. We hope that this book can help augment educational experiences for veterinarians and veterinary students and provide important information about anesthesia in some of the most challenging species that veterinarians work with.

We recognize the monumental effort of Susan Engelken at Wiley for helping us organize the production of this book. Without her extraordinary effort and guidance, this book would not be possible.

We are very proud of our final product and feel that we have produced another excellent piece of work.

Gary West, Darryl Heard, and Nigel Caulkett

ZOO ANIMAL AND WILDLIFE IMMOBILIZATION AND ANESTHESIA

Second Edition

Section I
General

1 Clinical Pharmacology

Leigh A. Lamont and Kurt A. Grimm

INTRODUCTION

Pharmacology is the study of drugs and their interactions with organisms (Page & Maddison 2002). Pharmacology incorporates aspects of statistics, biochemistry, biology, pathology, and medicine. Failure to interpret the description of drugs' pharmacological properties in the context of the clinical picture (i.e., clinical pharmacology) can result in unintended outcomes.

The pharmacological data available for most drugs are mean values derived from a relatively small number of individuals (usually healthy individuals). While this approach provides a starting point for clinical use of drugs, individual responses can vary greatly due to disease states, body condition, environment, genetics, coadministered drugs, and many other factors. When the toxic dose is close to the therapeutic dose (as is often the case with drugs used for immobilization and anesthesia), careful titration of dose and patient monitoring are required. However, the nature of working with wildlife and captive nondomestic species often precludes baseline health assessment, individualization of dosing, and intensive patient monitoring. This is one factor associated with increased risk of adverse outcomes when capturing or anesthetizing nondomestic species. It should also be appreciated that advances in drug safety will likely result in only limited improvement of the safety of anesthesia and immobilization. Management of other risk factors through airway management, reduction of stress, and improvements in supportive care will also be beneficial.

PHARMACOKINETICS

Pharmacokinetics (PK) can be generally defined as what an organism does to a drug. Absorption, distribution, biotransformation, and elimination are processes that determine the concentration of the drug at the site of action (i.e., biophase). Pharmacokinetic parameters are estimates of these processes in the group of animals studied. These estimates can be used to predict or understand the way a drug interacts with an organism. It is important to understand that pharmacokinetic parameters can vary between individual animals and can be influenced by many different drug- and organism-related factors. Additionally, pharmacokinetic parameters are derived using mathematical models selected by the investigator. There is usually no correlation between model components and anatomical structures.

PHARMACODYNAMICS

Pharmacodynamics (PD) can be generally defined as what a drug does to an organism. PD includes intended drug effects, as well as adverse drug actions. Drugs such as opioids, alpha-2 adrenergic agonists, and antimuscarinics act by binding to relatively well-characterized receptor complexes located on cellular membranes. Nonsteroidal anti-inflammatory drugs (NSAIDs) inhibit prostaglandin production by binding to cyclooxygenase enzyme isoforms. Relating plasma drug concentrations to observed NSAIDs actions can be complex in comparison with other drugs (e.g., opioids) due to the different nature of their action. Preexisting progstaglandins, as well as their slower process of inhibiting an enzyme system, confound the relationship between drug concentration and effect. The molecular actions of inhalant anesthetics have not been completely characterized, even though their clinical use has been well described (Steffey & Mama 2007).

Pharmacodynamic effects are predictable for most clinically used drugs. However, individual animal

Zoo Animal and Wildlife Immobilization and Anesthesia, Second Edition. Edited by Gary West, Darryl Heard, and Nigel Caulkett.

responses can vary considerably. Additionally, the nature of capture of free-ranging and captive wildlife often makes accurate dosing and drug delivery difficult or impossible. Therefore, close monitoring of patient response and preparation for supportive care are paramount to safe immobilization and anesthesia.

INHALANT ANESTHETICS

Inhalant anesthetics are commonly used in companion animal veterinary practice. Their use under field conditions is limited due to the requirement for specialized delivery devices and a supply of delivery gas (e.g., oxygen). However, inhalant anesthetics are used commonly in controlled settings, such as zoological parks and research laboratories, because of the ease of titration of anesthetic depth and rapidity of recovery. Inhalant anesthetics should be delivered by a well-maintained anesthetic machine and properly trained individuals. While inhalant anesthetics are relatively safe, their low therapeutic index mandates frequent and careful monitoring of anesthetic depth.

Physics of Gases and Vapors

An understanding of the processes that influence the uptake and delivery of inhalant anesthetics allows the anesthetist to predict and respond to individual circumstances.

Brief Review of Molecular Theory Molecules in a liquid state have more vibrational energy than when in a solid state, and each molecule can move through the liquid. If heat is added to a liquid, each molecule gains more kinetic energy and eventually some overcome the forces exerted by their neighbors and are able to escape into the space above the liquid. This state is that of a gas or a vapor. A gas is a phase of matter that expands indefinitely to fill a containment vessel. A vapor is the gaseous state of a material below its boiling point.

A vapor is in equilibrium with the liquid beneath it. Because both gaseous and liquid molecules have kinetic energy, they are in constant motion. The molecules in the vapor phase are striking the liquid–gas interface and returning to the liquid while liquid molecules are leaving the interface to become vapor. The relationship between these two phases depends mainly on the physicochemical properties of the molecules and the temperature of the system.

Vapor Pressure Molecules in a gaseous state possess kinetic energy and collide with the walls of the containment vessel. These collisions produce a force on the walls. This force is spread over a surface area and therefore is a pressure (Pressure = Force/Area). This pressure is called the vapor pressure. Since kinetic energy increases directly with temperature, vapor pressure must always be given with reference to the temperature

Table 1.1.   Anesthetic agent vapor pressures at 20 and 24°C

Anesthetic Agent	Vapor Pressure at 20°C in mmHg	Vapor Pressure at 24°C in mmHg
Methoxyflurane	23	28
Sevoflurane	160	
Enflurane	172	207
Isoflurane	240	286
Halothane	243	288
Nitrous oxide	Gas	Gas

Source: Adapted from Steffey EP, Mama RM. 2007. Inhalation anesthetics. In: *Lumb and Jones' Veterinary Anesthesia*, 4th ed. (WJ Tranquilli, JT Thurmon, KA Grimm, eds.). Ames: Blackwell.

it was measured at (e.g., vapor pressure of water is 47 mmHg at 37°C).

When many gases are present in a mixture, such as with atmospheric air or during delivery of inhalant anesthetics, each gas has a vapor pressure that is independent of the other gases (Dalton's law of partial pressures). It is convention to refer to vapor pressure as partial pressure under these conditions. Partial pressure of an anesthetic agent is analogous to the concept of "free drug" and is important for determining the effect of the anesthetic (e.g., the level of CNS depression correlates directly with the partial pressure of isoflurane within the brain) (see Table 1.1) (Steffey & Mama 2007).

Vapor Concentration Vapor (i.e., partial) pressure is important for the observed pharmacological effect of inhalant anesthetics. However, almost all anesthesiologists refer to the amount of anesthetic delivered in units of volumes % (said as volumes-percent), or just percent, which is a concentration. The fundamental difference between anesthetic partial pressure and anesthetic concentration is partial pressure relates to the absolute number of molecules and their kinetic energy whereas concentration refers to the number of molecules of anesthetic relative to the total number of molecules present.

Critical Temperature The critical temperature is the temperature above which a substance cannot be liquefied no matter how much pressure is applied. The critical temperature of nitrous oxide is 36.5°C. Consequently, nitrous oxide can be (and is) a liquid below this temperature, but is a gas at greater temperatures. Placing a nitrous oxide tank near a heat source will result in volatilization of liquid nitrous oxide, resulting in a high tank pressure and danger of explosion or tank venting.

The critical temperature of oxygen is −119°C. Therefore, at room temperature, oxygen cannot be liquefied. All compressed cylinders of medical oxygen contain only gas. There are liquid oxygen tanks, but the internal tank temperature is below −119°C.

Table 1.2. Selected partition coefficients of commonly used anesthetic agents

Anesthetic	Blood:Gas Partition Coefficient	Brain:Blood Partition Coefficient
Nitrous oxide	0.47	1.1
Desflurane	0.42	1.3
Enflurane	1.4	1.4
Sevoflurane	0.69	1.7
Methoxyflurane	12.0	2.0
Isoflurane	2.6	2.7
Halothane	2.9	2.9

Source: Adapted from Steffey EP, Mama RM. 2007. Inhalation anesthetics. In: *Lumb and Jones' Veterinary Anesthesia*, 4th ed. (WJ Tranquilli, JT Thurmon, KA Grimm, eds.). Ames: Blackwell.

Henry's Law Henry's law states the solubility of a gas in a liquid is proportional to the pressure of the gas over the solution. It describes the solubility of an anesthetic in body fluids or other liquids. From it you can derive the following formula: $c = k \cdot P$; where c is the molar concentration (mol/L) of the dissolved gas and P is the pressure (in atmospheres) of the gas over the solution. For a given gas, k is the Henry's law constant and is dependent on temperature.

Partition Coefficient A partition coefficient is the ratio of the concentration of a substance in one medium relative to another at equilibrium. It is related to the solubility of an agent. At equilibrium, the partial pressure is the same throughout the body, including the alveolar gas, but the concentration of total drug may be very different due to partitioning into tissues or body fluids (Table 1.2) (Steffey & Mama 2007). Partition coefficients are not absolute constants for an anesthetic agent. Tissue composition may change as a function of age, sex, body condition, and so on, and these changes may influence partitioning.

Mechanism of Action of Inhaled Anesthetics The specific mechanism of action of most anesthetics remains unknown. Volatile anesthetics appear to share some common cellular actions with other sedative, hypnotic, or analgesic drugs. A sound theory of anesthetic action should provide an explanation for the observed correlation of potency with the oil/gas partition coefficient, the observation that a large number of diverse chemical structures can cause anesthesia, and explain why the agents produce side effects. Experimental work has implicated a protein "target" on a diverse population of ionophores that is required for anesthetic action (Franks & Lieb 2004). The alteration in ionophore conductance may be related to direct action of the anesthetic at a two amino acid sequence within the transmembrane spanning domains.

The protein receptor hypothesis postulates that protein receptors in the central nervous system are responsible for the mechanism of action of inhaled anesthetics. This theory is supported by the steep dose–response curve for inhaled anesthetics. However, it remains unclear if inhaled agents disrupt ion flow through membrane channels by an indirect action on the lipid membrane, via a second messenger, or by direct and specific binding to channel proteins. Another theory describes the activation of gamma-aminobutyric acid (GABA) receptors by the inhalation anesthetics. Volatile agents may activate or facilitate GABA channels, resulting in hyperpolarized cell membranes. In addition, they may inhibit certain calcium channels, preventing the release of neurotransmitters and inhibit glutamate channels.

Evidence for the protein receptor theory includes the observation made by Franks and Lieb that a broad range of inhalant anesthetics inhibited the water-soluble enzyme firefly luciferase (Franks & Lieb 1984). This enzyme hydrolyzes luciferin to create light and is often a model for anesthetic action because the rank orders of potency of the anesthetics in animals parallels that of luciferase inhibition. Franks and Lieb studied the enzyme in a lipid free environment, with only the enzyme present, and observed the enzyme could be completely inhibited. This suggests the site of action is within the protein structure and is not strictly dependent on lipid. Franks and Lieb also noted that some anesthetics exist as stereoisomers and that the effects of these isomers can differ. However, when the stereoisomers are introduced into a lipid substrate, the physical effects on the lipid are identical. This is further evidence that the anesthetic is acting at a stereoselective "receptor" and would implicate a protein as the site of action.

Following up on the work by Franks and Lieb, Harrison, Harris, Mihic, and colleagues attempted to reconcile the apparent problem of the nonspecific action of anesthetics on a wide range of protein channels including glycine, glutamate, GABA, and other neurotransmitter activated channels (Mihic et al. 1997). For the anesthetic to act on all of these channels, one would expect a target amino acid sequence would be conserved among all channels or the anesthetic would be altering receptor function by distorting the surrounding environment. In their experiments, this group began making chimeric DNA encoding the c-terminal human GABA rho receptor subunit, which is an anesthetic insensitive receptor, and the N-terminal glycine-binding part of the human glycine alpha-receptor subunit that is situated in the transmembrane spanning domain. They expressed the cDNA in *Xenopus* oocytes and measured resulting chloride conductance. They determined the site of anesthetic action was within the N-terminal sequence of the third transmembrane spanning domain. The researchers then began to construct cDNA containing point mutations within this region and created receptors that were insensitive to enflurane. They ultimately found two amino acids in the glycine receptor that abolished enflurane sensitivity when mutated. Changing the corresponding amino acids on the GABA receptor also abolished enflurane sensitivity. However, these mutations did not reduce the receptor's sensitivity to the injectable anesthetic propofol.

Inhalant Anesthetic Pharmacokinetics

Anesthetic Uptake and Distribution A series of partial pressure gradients, beginning at the vaporizer, continuing in the anesthetic breathing circuit, the airways, alveoli, blood, and ending in the tissues, will drive the movement of an anesthetic gas. The movement of that gas will continue until equal partial pressures are present throughout the system. Since the lung is the point of entry and exit to the body, the alveolar partial pressure governs the partial pressure of the anesthetic in all body tissues. Therefore, it is most important to understand how to influence the alveolar partial pressure. Increasing alveolar minute ventilation, flow rates at the level of the vaporizer, and inspired anesthetic concentration, can speed the delivery of anesthetic and increase the rate of rise of alveolar anesthetic partial pressure. Solubility, cardiac output, and the alveolar-to-venous anesthetic gradient are factors that determine the uptake of the anesthetic from the alveoli into the blood. Solubility describes the affinity of the gas for a medium such as blood or adipose tissue and is reported as a partition coefficient. The blood/gas partition coefficient describes how the gas will partition itself between the two phases (blood and alveolar gas) after equilibrium has been reached. Isoflurane for example has a blood/gas partition coefficient of approximately 1.4 (Steffey & Mama 2007). This means that if the gas partial pressures are in equilibrium, the concentration in blood will be 1.4 times greater than the concentration in the alveoli. A higher blood/gas partition coefficient means a greater uptake of the gas into the blood, therefore, a slower rate of rise of alveolar and blood partial pressure. Since the blood partial pressure rise is slower, it takes longer for the brain partial pressure of the gas to increase resulting in a longer induction time.

Increased cardiac output exposes the alveoli to more blood per unit time. The greater volume of blood removes more inhalant anesthetic from the alveoli, therefore lowering the alveolar partial pressure. The agent might be distributed faster within the body, but the partial pressure in the arterial blood is lower. It will take longer for the gas to reach equilibrium between the alveoli and the brain. Therefore, a high cardiac output usually prolongs induction time. The alveolar to venous partial pressure difference reflects tissue uptake of the inhaled anesthetic. A large difference is caused by increased uptake of the gas by the tissues during the induction phase.

Transfer of the gas from the arterial blood into tissues such as the brain will depend on perfusion and the relative solubility of the gas in the different tissues. The brain/blood coefficient describes how the gas will partition itself between the two phases after equilibrium has been reached. Isoflurane has a brain/blood coefficient of 2.7; therefore, when the system is at equilibrium the concentration in the brain will be 2.7 times greater than the concentration in the blood (Steffey & Mama 2007). All contemporary inhalation anesthetics have high adipose/blood partition coefficients. This means that most of the gas will accumulate in adipose tissue as times goes by. The partial pressure of the gas in adipose tissue will rise very slowly since this tissue has a high capacity (as indicated by the high adipose/blood partition coefficient). Inhalation anesthetics stored in obese patients may delay awakening at the end of long periods of anesthesia. Fortunately, adipose tissue has a relatively low blood flow and does not accumulate significant amounts of anesthetic during the short periods of anesthesia commonly encountered in veterinary medicine.

Elimination of Inhaled Anesthetics The rate of induction and recovery from anesthesia with inhalant anesthetics differs between agents due to differences in tissue solubility; however, general statements can be made. During induction, all tissue partial pressures are zero. During recovery, different tissues in the body have different partial pressures of anesthetic which is governed by the tissue anesthetic content and not the alveolar partial pressure. Recovery is not as controllable as induction of anesthesia. During recovery from anesthesia, elimination occurs due to exhalation and biotransformation.

Enzymes responsible for inhalant anesthetic metabolism are mainly located in liver and kidneys. Anesthetic elimination via metabolism is approximately 50% for methoxyflurane, 10–20% for halothane, 5–8% for sevoflurane, 2.5% for enflurane, about 0.2% for isoflurane, 0.001% for desflurane, and nearly zero for nitrous oxide (Steffey & Mama 2007). The amount of anesthetic eliminated from the body during anesthesia due to metabolism is small compared with the amount exhaled. However, anesthetic metabolism accounts for a larger proportion of the anesthetic clearance after anesthetic delivery ceases. The low, but prolonged, blood partial pressure of the anesthetic found after terminating delivery is no longer overwhelming the enzyme systems (enzymes become saturated above ~1 MAC), so metabolism accounts for a larger proportion of clearance than it did during exposure to high partial pressures.

Elimination of the anesthetic via the lungs can be complex. The first point to consider is what effect an increase in alveolar minute ventilation will have on recovery. During recovery, increasing minute ventilation will decrease alveolar anesthetic partial pressure and increase the gradient for diffusion from the blood to the alveoli. This increases elimination, especially for most anesthetic agents with high blood/gas partition coefficients.

Another situation to consider is what effect a change in cardiac output will have on the rate of decrease of partial pressure of the inhalant anesthetic. During induction, high cardiac output will increase the rate at which anesthetic is removed from the lung, slowing the rate of rise of anesthetic partial pressure, slowing induction. When cardiac output is reduced (e.g., cardiogenic shock), there is a slower removal of anesthetic and subsequently a faster rate of rise of alveolar partial pressure and induction occurs. During recovery, a high cardiac output will increase the rate at which anesthetic is returned to the lung for excretion. Since the partial pressure of anesthetic in the blood is determined by the tissues, the higher blood flow will shorten recovery. During low cardiac output situations, there will be a slower recovery due to the decreased rate at which tissue anesthetic partial pressure decreases.

The last major influence on the rate of induction and recovery is the solubility of the anesthetic agent. Agents with high blood/gas solubility will be partitioned into the blood to a greater extent than agents with low blood/gas solubility. The blood acts as a depot for agent maintaining anesthetic partial pressure. Agents with low blood/gas solubility do not partition into the blood to the extent of highly soluble agents, thus the decrease in partial pressure is faster and recovery time is reduced. Highly soluble agents have high blood concentrations, and it will take longer for the partial pressure to decrease if all other factors are equal. In summary, elimination of a volatile anesthetic depends on ventilation, cardiac output, and solubility of the gas in blood and tissue.

Control of the Partial Pressure of Delivered Anesthetic
Inhalant anesthetics can be classified as either gaseous (nitrous oxide and xenon) or volatile (isoflurane, sevoflurane, halothane, methoxyflurane, and desflurane). Gaseous anesthetics are usually delivered to the anesthesia machine under pressure, and their rate of delivery to the breathing circuit is controlled by a flow meter. Volatile anesthetics are liquids at room temperature and pressure, and are usually delivered by a specialized apparatus that controls the volatilization of the liquid, and proportioning of the vapor in the fresh gas delivered to the patient. A vaporizer can be as simple as a piece of cotton soaked with agent held near the nose (not recommended), or can be as complex as the Tec 6 vaporizer for desflurane.

The Breathing System With most modern anesthetic machines, the outflow gas from the vaporizer will be delivered to the patient through a set of tubes and machinery collectively called a breathing system. There are many styles of breathing systems, each with a multitude of uses. It is important that the anesthetist understands how the type of breathing circuit used will impact the rate at which the anesthetic concentration can be changed and the relationship between the vaporizer setting and inspired concentration.

Waste Anesthetic Gases The health effects of chronic exposure to waste anesthetic gases are not completely known. The frequency of inhalant anesthetic use and the lack of significant associations between exposure, and most types of chronic toxicities (e.g., cancer, infertility, birth defects, etc.) would suggest there is only a very low risk (if any) associated with chronic exposure. However, certain individuals are highly susceptible to potentially life-threatening reactions, even with trace level exposure (e.g., malignant hyperthermia). In light of this, and with the admission that we do not completely understand all the risks associated with chronic exposure, it is generally agreed that the exposure of personnel be kept as low as reasonably acceptable (ALARA). In the United States, the Occupational Safety and Health Administration (OSHA) requires veterinary hospitals to maintain a system to prevent waste gases from building up in the area of use and can enforce exposure limits that are consistent with recommendations offered by the National Institute of Occupational Safety and Health (NIOSH). The NIOSH recommends that the maximum time-weighted average concentration of volatile halogenated anesthetics should not exceed 2 ppm when used alone or 0.5 ppm when used with nitrous oxide, and that nitrous oxide concentration should not exceed 25 ppm (American College of Veterinary Anesthesiologists 1996).

Minimum Alveolar Concentration (MAC)
The measurement of the dose of an inhalant anesthetic is the minimum alveolar concentration (MAC) multiple. It is defined as the minimum alveolar concentration at 1 atm, required to prevent gross purposeful movement in 50% of the subjects tested, following a 60-second application of a supramaximal stimulus (Steffey & Mama 2007). One MAC is by definition the EC_{50} (i.e., effective concentration in 50% of patients) for that agent. Animals awaken from anesthesia at approximately 0.5 MAC, surgical anesthesia occurs at approximately 1.3 MAC, and severe autonomic nervous system depression occurs around 2 MAC. Birds and many reptiles do not have true alveoli so the concept of MAC has been modified or redefined to be the minimum anesthetic concentration. It is not identical to MAC from other species, but closely approximates it in many ways.

Physiological and Pharmacological Factors that Alter MAC Minimum alveolar concentration is age dependent, being lowest in newborns, reaching a peak in infants, and then decreasing progressively with increasing age (Lerman et al. 1983, 1994; Taylor & Lerman 1991). Increases in MAC can also occur from hyperthermia and hypernatremia, and decreases in MAC can result from hypothermia, hyponatremia, pregnancy, hypotension, and drugs, such as lithium, lidocaine, opioids, and α_2-adrenergic agonists.

General Pharmacological Actions of Inhalant Anesthetics

Inhalant anesthetic agents have more similarities than differences with respect to their effects on vital organ systems. The differences are primarily related to the speed and magnitude with which the changes occur. There are a few classic differences that have been included in the following synopsis.

Central Nervous System All inhalant general anesthetics alter consciousness, memory, and pain perception by acting on the central nervous system. Most inhalant anesthetics cause a mild to moderate decrease in the cerebral metabolic requirement for oxygen ($CMRO_2$), and they usually have minimal effects on cerebral blood flow autoregulation at low MAC multiples (Mielck et al. 1998, 1999). Patients with intracranial hypertension should not be anesthetized, with nitrous oxide because it may cause an increase in $CMRO_2$ (Algotsson et al. 1992; Hoffman et al. 1995; Roald et al. 1991). Halothane is also a poor choice because of its significant effects on cerebral blood flow autoregulation (Steffey & Mama 2007). Isoflurane, sevoflurane, and desflurane are the inhalants of choice at this time.

Cardiovascular System Most inhalant anesthetic agents cause direct myocardial depression. Halothane is the most depressant on contractility; however, it generally has the fewest effects on vascular resistance (Steffey & Mama 2007). Isoflurane, enflurane, sevoflurane, and desflurane cause some degree of vasodilatation, which tends to improve forward blood flow and maintain tissue perfusion. The reduction in afterload also tends to offset some of the direct myocardial depressant effects and may result in a net improvement in cardiac output. Nitrous oxide is a sympathomimetic and can improve contractility, blood pressure, and heart rate at light levels of anesthesia. Rapid changes in anesthetic concentration (especially with desflurane) may result in a sympathetic response and temporarily increase cardiac work.

Respiratory System All anesthetics tend to depress the chemoreceptor response to carbon dioxide leading to an accumulation of carbon dioxide and a respiratory acidosis unless ventilation is assisted or controlled. The ether derivatives tend to be the most depressant; however, all agents may cause significant depression.

Most inhalant agents may interfere with hypoxic pulmonary vasoconstriction and may worsen ventilation–perfusion matching in the lung. This is most dramatic in larger animals where significant pulmonary shunting is often observed.

Genital–Renal Systems Most anesthetics cause a decrease in renal perfusion and an increase in antidiuretic hormone (ADH) secretion. Inhalant anesthetics may be the safest anesthetic techniques in anuric renal failure since pulmonary excretion is not dependent upon renal function.

Inhalant anesthetics may cause an increase in postpartum uterine bleeding. This is a bigger consideration in primate anesthesia due to placentation characteristics. Isoflurane, sevoflurane, desflurane, and nitrous oxide have been advocated for use during Caesarian section because of the rapid onset and termination of effect, and the transient effects on the delivered fetuses. Methoxyflurane and halothane are less desirable due to their greater solubility and slower elimination.

Clinically Useful Inhalant Anesthetics

Nitrous Oxide Nitrous oxide is commonly used in combination with a primary inhalant or injectable anesthetic drug. The reason it is not useful in veterinary anesthesia as a solo anesthetic is because of its low potency. Nitrous oxide's MAC value has been estimated to be near 100% for humans and closer to 200% for veterinary patients. It is obvious that 200% nitrous oxide cannot be delivered; in fact, no more than 79% nitrous oxide can be safely delivered without creating a hypoxic gas mixture. In practice, it is common to use a 50% nitrous oxide mixture with the balance of the mix being oxygen. If 50% nitrous oxide is delivered to an animal, it is only providing approximately 0.25 MAC of anesthesia. A potent volatile anesthetic, injectable agent, or other sedative/analgesic drug must supply the remaining 0.75 MAC. Because of this limited anesthetic effect, nitrous oxide use for anesthetic maintenance is not widespread in veterinary medicine. Nitrous oxide is used by some anesthetists during induction of anesthesia for the *second gas effect*. Since nitrous oxide is present in the inspired gas mixture in a relatively high concentration and it rapidly diffuses into the body from the alveoli, the rate of rise of partial pressure of a second coadministered inhalant anesthetic is increased, and induction time can be shortened.

Nitrous oxide has a low blood/gas partition coefficient and has a rapid onset and recovery. The gas can diffuse out of the blood so rapidly that if nitrous oxide delivery is suddenly halted and supplemental oxygen is not administered, a situation known as *diffusion hypoxia* may result. Diffusion hypoxia happens when the mass movement of nitrous oxide down its partial pressure gradient results in high alveolar nitrous oxide partial pressure at the expense of oxygen and nitrogen partial pressures. Since breathing room air will result in an alveolar oxygen partial pressure of approximately 100 mmHg under ideal circumstances, any displacement of oxygen by nitrous oxide will result in alveolar hypoxia. Diffusion hypoxia can be minimized or prevented by continuing the administration of oxygen enriched gas for 5–10 minutes following the discontinuation of nitrous oxide. This helps because during normal breathing, 100% oxygen should result in an alveolar oxygen partial pressure close to 500 mmHg. The partial pressure of oxygen can drop a lot further before hypoxia develops.

Nitrous oxide is contraindicated in animals with pneumothorax, gastric dilatation/rumen tympany, gas embolism, and other conditions that are exacerbated by accumulation of gas inside a closed space. This effect is caused by diffusion of nitrous oxide out of the blood into the preexisting gas space in an attempt to establish equilibrium. Nitrous oxide is also contraindicated in animals with gas diffusion impairment, such as interstitial pneumonia. These animals typically have low arterial oxygen partial pressure when breathing oxygen-rich mixtures. The dilution of oxygen by nitrous oxide will lower the inspired oxygen partial pressure and may worsen hypoxemia.

Halothane Halothane was a major advancement in inhalant anesthesia in its day. It was introduced in the late 1950s and was potent, nonirritating, and nonflammable. Chemically, it is classified as a halogenated hydrocarbon, and it is not chemically related to the ethers. Halothane was used widely in human anesthesia until it became apparent there were potentially fatal adverse effects associated with its use. Human patients developed a syndrome known as *halothane hepatitis* (Daghfous et al. 2003; Neuberger 1998). This rare, but life-threatening, complication is still somewhat of a mystery, although an immunological etiology is implicated. The disease appears as a fulminant hepatitis, similar to that seen with viral hepatitis, which develops after a short period of apparent recovery. A second more common form of hepatitis is less severe and is characterized by a reversible elevation in liver enzymes. The etiology of this second form is thought to be anesthetic related hepatic hypoxia and does not appear to be immune related. Diagnosis of the correct form is important since a repeated exposure to halothane, or any of the volatile agents producing trifluoroacetic acid, is more likely to trigger the immunologically mediated form and result in high morbidity and mortality. Both forms are not commonly documented in veterinary patients; however, transient elevation of liver enzymes may occur postoperatively in some patients. A thorough diagnostic workup is required due to the nonspecific and multifactorial etiology of elevated liver enzymes.

A second complication associated with halothane anesthesia is the development of arrhythmias. Halogenated hydrocarbon anesthetics, especially halothane, can sensitize the myocardium to the arrythmogenic effects of epinephrine. Halothane is generally contraindicated in patients that are predisposed to ventricular arrhythmias (e.g., hypoxia, trauma, or myocardial disease) (Steffey & Mama 2007). Arrhythmias that develop during halothane anesthesia may resolve when the anesthetic agent is switched to isoflurane or sevoflurane. Other causes of perianesthetic arrhythmias should also be ruled out.

Halothane undergoes extensive hepatic metabolism (~20%) and is not chemically stable (Steffey & Mama 2007). Commercially available halothane contains thymol, a preservative, that does not volatilize to the same degree as halothane. This results in a sticky residue inside the vaporizer that should be cleaned out during periodic maintenance. Veterinary use of halothane is declining due to the increasing popularity of isoflurane, and sevoflurane and its limited availability worldwide.

Isoflurane Isoflurane is arguably the most widely used veterinary inhalant anesthetic in the world today. Isoflurane is stable, potent, and undergoes little metabolism. Isoflurane can be irritating to airway tissues at high inspired concentrations and its use for induction in people has been limited because of patient complaints and complications. However, in veterinary medicine, isoflurane mask induction is still common. Isoflurane is a potent agent (MAC ~1.3% in dogs) and has a high saturated vapor pressure (~240 mmHg at room temperature) (Steffey & Mama 2007). These characteristics, coupled with the fact that it is possible to cause rapid partial pressure changes in the brain, would suggest that only precision vaporizers located outside the circuit (VOC) should be used to deliver the agent. However, several reports of the use of modified VIC vaporizers suggest that this type of anesthetic system can be used to safely administer the agent (Bednarski et al. 1993; Laredo et al. 1998).

Isoflurane metabolism is minimal (less than 1%) and fluoride induced nephrotoxicity is uncommon. Isoflurane and many of the ether-derivative volatile agents are excellent vasodilators and can cause or worsen hypotension. Administration of fluids and/or sympathomimetic agents can usually counteract the observed hypotension. Likewise, administering preanesthetic drugs (e.g., opioids) that reduce the amount of inhalant required will also reduce the degree of vasodilation.

Desflurane Desfluane use in veterinary medicine is limited to academic institutions and a very limited number of private practices. The main disadvantage to desflurane use is cost associated with the agent and the cost associated with a specialized vaporizer that is required to deliver the drug. Desflurane is extremely insoluable and is capable of producing extremely rapid inductions and recoveries (Barter et al. 2004; Clarke 1999). Its main market is for human outpatient anesthesia where rapid recovery is a large cost savings. It is highly fluorinated, has a very low potency (MAC ~ 9%), and has a high saturated vapor pressure (~670 mmHg at room temperature) (Steffey & Mama 2007). Desflurane boils at 23°C and must be handled using a specialized apparatus for vaporizer filling. The vaporizer is specific for desflurane and is electrically heated to boil the desflurane so that a reliable vapor pressure will be produced. Then, sophisticated differential pressure transducers and electronic circuits calculate an injection ratio for delivery of the desired anesthetic concentration. Desflurane is very stable and undergoes almost no metabolism.

Sevoflurane Sevoflurane is the newest volatile inhalant anesthetic approved for veterinary use. Sevoflurane has a low blood/gas partition coefficient (~0.7) that is greater than desflurane and nitrous oxide, but about half of that of isoflurane. Extensive pulmonary elimination of sevoflurane minimizes the amount available for metabolism. Up to 3–8% of the sevoflurane dose is metabolized and appears in the urine as inorganic fluoride (Steffey & Mama 2007). This fluoride exposure doesnot appear to be clinically significant, although serum levels of fluoride can approach those previously reported to be nephrotoxic for methoxyflurane. Factors other than peak serum fluoride concentrations appear important for predicting the incidence of nephrotoxicity (Driessen et al. 2002).

Sevoflurane represents a deviation from the methyl ethyl ether structural theme present in other contemporary volatile anesthetics. Sevoflurane is chemically related to methyl-isopropyl ethers. The structure is significant because an important metabolite of most methyl-ethyl ether volatile anesthetic agents (trifluoroacetic acid) is a suspected trigger of halothane hepatitis. Sevoflurane cannot be metabolized to form this compound. This is not a major consideration in veterinary medicine, but is important in human anesthesia. Sevoflurane is also pleasant and non-irritating when used for mask induction and many pediatric anesthesiologists suggest this agent is the drug of choice for pediatric induction via mask. Sevoflurane is less potent than isoflurane (MAC ~2.3% for dogs and horses). When used for induction of anesthesia it is common to use 7–9% sevoflurane.

An early subject of controversy surrounding sevoflurane anesthesia was the production of compound A. Compound A is a degradation product produced when sevoflurane reacts with the carbon dioxide absorbent. Early toxicology studies performed in rats suggested that proximal tubular renal damage could result from

Table 1.3. Structure and characteristics of inhalation anesthetics

Agent	Year Introduced	Structure	Type
Halothane	1956	CF_3–CHClBr	Alkane
Isoflurane	1981	CF_3CHCl–O–CHF_2	Ether
Enflurane	1972	CHClF–CF_2–O–CHF_2	Ether
Methoxyflurane	1960	$CHCl_2$–CF_2–O–CH_3	Ether
Desflurane	1992	CF_3CHF–O–CHF_2	Ether

clinically relevant exposure to compound A. This led to the suggestion that sevoflurane should not be used in closed circuit anesthesia or with fresh gas flow rates lower than 2 L per min. However, since that time, little clinical evidence of renal damage in humans and dogs has emerged, even with very low fresh gas flows. Some have suggested that rats have a 10–100 times higher level of the enzyme beta-lyase that is believed to convert the intermediate compounds of Compound A metabolism to a nephrotoxic molecule (Kharasch et al. 2005; Sheffels et al. 2004). Humans and dogs do not appear to have the same level of enzyme conversion and are therefore less susceptible to Compound A toxicity. Safety studies in most other rodents and exotic animals are not published and caution should be used when administering sevoflurane via a breathing system using a carbon dioxide absorbant until further safety data is available (Table 1.3).

INJECTABLE ANESTHETICS

Injectable anesthetics are an important family of compounds used for immobilization and anesthesia of wildlife. The dissociative anesthetics in particular are commonly combined with other adjunctive drugs, such as alpha-2 adrenergic agonists and opioids, to improve reliability and speed of onset of action.

Barbiturates

Barbiturates can be classified in several ways. One is by chemical structure. Oxybarbiturates are historically important, but not commonly used today due to their slower onset of action, long recovery characteristics, and relatively small margin of safety. Pentobarbital is the protypical oxybarbiturate. It has been combined with several adjunctive drugs for anesthesia. The thio (i.e., sulfur substituted) analog of pentobarbital, thiopental, is still used by intravenous administration for induction of anesthesia in domestic animals. However, perivascular injection can result in tissue necrosis, and its use in nondomestic species is limited due to the inability to obtain reliable intravenous access prior to anesthetic induction and current availability problems.

Barbiturates cause anesthesia through global depression of CNS activity. This is accomplished through interference with nervous system impulse conduction. Like many other anesthetics, other excitable tissues can be affected, resulting in commonly encountered side effects, including depression of cardiorespiratory function. Barbiturates decrease cerebral blood flow (CBF) and cerebral metabolic requirement for oxygen ($CMRO_2$). Cerebral metabolic requirement for oxygen decreases progressively until electroencephalographic activity becomes isoelectric (Branson 2007).

Propofol

Propofol (2,6-diisopropylphenol) is commonly used for sedation, induction, and maintenance of anesthesia in humans and domestic species. Propofol is supplied as a milky white liquid for intravenous injection. It is insoluble in aqueous solution; therefore, it is usually formulated as an emulsion of 10% soybean oil, 2.25% glycerol, and 1.2% egg phosphatide. Some formulations of propofol (e.g., Diprivan®, Propoflo™) do not contain preservative and will support bacterial and fungal growth should the drug become contaminated. This has led to the label recommendation of discarding unused drug at the end of the procedure or within 6 hours of opening a vial. A newer formulation has been available in some European contries (PropoClear®) which uses a different carrier solution than the traditional soybean emulsion. The inhibition of bacterial growth allowed a 28-day shelf life. However, there have been reports of tissue irritation following injection, and the product is being reevalutaed. Some formulations have additives, such as benzyl alcohol (e.g., Propo-Flo28®), to improve stability or reduce the potential of contamination with storage. Species-sensitivities to these additives should be investigated before their use (Davidson 2001).

Propofol is classified as an ultrashort-acting injectable anesthetic agent. Duration of effect is typically 5–10 minutes in dogs and 5–20 minutes in cats. Its rapid recovery characteristics are maintained in most species following prolonged infusions. Recovery times may be prolonged in the cat (and other species that have reduced capacity for glucuronidation of drugs) following repeated doses or continuous rate infusions.

Propofol has been used in dogs, cats, horses, pigs, goats, sheep, and even birds. Wild turkeys, mallard ducks, pigeons, and chickens have been anesthetized with propofol, but there is significant cardiorespiratory depression in ducks and chickens, indicating birds may need ventilatory support during anesthesia (Machin & Caulkett 1998). Apnea and respiratory depression are the best known side effects of propofol administration. The incidence of apnea may be reduced by administering the drug over 60–90 seconds (Muir & Gadawski 1998). It would be prudent to be prepared to intubate and support ventilation if apnea occurs. Pain is reported on propofol injection by some people. Muscle fasciculations and spontaneous twitching can occur in some animals.

Dissociative Anesthetics

Ketamine Most veterinary formulations of ketamine are a racemic mixture consisting of two optical enantiomers. However, in many countries, (S)-ketamine is available as a human or veterinary product. The S enantiomer is less cardiodepressant and has a fourfold greater affinity for the phencyclidine site in the NMDA (N-methyl-D-aspartate) receptor. Serotonin transport is inhibited twofold by the R form. Some of ketamine's effects are not stereoselective. Norepinephrine release is equivalent from the S and R forms (Kohrs & Durieux 1998).

Ketamine can be administered intramuscularly to anesthetize animals which are not easily given drugs intravenously. Intramuscular administration will produce a longer duration of anesthesia than intravenous administration, but the recovery is usually longer and can be accompanied by more dysphoria. Recovery from ketamine appears to be due to redistribution and metabolism similar to the thiobarbiturates. Hepatic biotransformation to norketamine (a.k.a. metabolite I) and dehydronorketamine (aka metabolite II) is the major route of metabolism in most species studied. It was thought ketamine was excreted unchanged in the urine of cats, however this originated from one paper published in 1978 by Gaskell et al. and since that time it has been shown by Waterman that biotransformation is an important route of elimination in domestic cats (Waterman 1983). Norketamine is about one-third to one-fifth as potent as the parent compound but may contribute to the prolonged analgesic effects of ketamine (Kohrs & Durieux 1998).

Ketamine produces a form of anesthesia that is different from other hypnotic drugs. In general terms, ketamine induces anesthesia and amnesia by functional disruption (dissociation) of the CNS through marked CNS stimulation resulting in catalepsy, immobility, amnesia, and marked analgesia. Electroencephalographic analysis indicates that depression of the thalamoneocortical system occurs in conjunction with activation of the limbic system. Awakening from ketamine anesthesia in people is frequently characterized by disagreeable dreams and hallucinations. Sometimes, these unpleasant occurrences may recur days or weeks later. Almost half of adults over the age 30 exhibit delirium or excitement, or experience visual disturbances. The occurrence of adverse psychological experiences is much lower in children. The incidence of adverse psychological experiences in animals is unknown; however, a significant number of animals transiently vocalize and have motor disturbances during recovery.

Ketamine's neuropharmacology is complex. The compound interacts with N-methyl-D-aspartate and non-NMDA glutamate receptors, nicotinic, muscarinic cholinergic, monoaminergic, and opioid receptors. In addition, there are interactions with voltage-dependent ion channels, such as Na^+ and L-type Ca^{2+} channels. It is believed that the NMDA receptor antagonism accounts for most of the analgesic, amnestic, psychomimetic, and neuroprotective effects of the compound, but the exact mechanism of its anesthetic action is not known. NMDA receptor activation is believed to play a role in the "memory" of the central nervous system, which is involved in the "wind-up," hyperalgesia, and allodynia seen in certain pain syndromes (Kohrs & Durieux 1998).

Ketamine can increase the $CMRO_2$ due to increased metabolic activity associated with increased activity in certain areas of the brain. Intracranial pressure (ICP) also increases, possibly because of two mechanisms: (1) Ketamine can increase mean arterial blood pressure so cerebral blood flow (CBF) can increase and ICP passively increase in patients with altered autoregulation, and (2) Ketamine can depress respiration increasing P_aCO_2. The brain responds to elevations in P_aCO_2 by increasing CBF which will increase ICP. Ventilation may reduce the increase in CBF. Current clinical dogma dictates avoiding ketamine in patients with suspected head trauma.

Ketamine causes a characteristic breathing pattern termed *apneustic breathing*, characterized by prolonged inspiratory duration and relatively short expiratory time. When ketamine is administered by itself, it typically causes minimal respiratory depression that is short-lived. Hypoxic and hypercapnic respiratory regulation appears to remain intact. Howevere, ketamine is seldom given alone. It is often combined with benzodiazepines, acepromazine, opioids, or alpha-2 adrenergic agonists. The combined effect of these drugs is usually decreased minute ventilation, increased P_aCO_2, and mild respiratory acidosis.

Ketamine, when given to animals with functioning sympathetic nervous systems, generally increases heart rate and arterial blood pressure. Cardiac output will usually stay the same or slightly increase. Ketamine is seldom given alone to healthy animals. The use of adjunctive drugs, such as benzodiazepines, acepromazine, or alpha-2 adrenergic agonists, tends to blunt the sympathomimetic effect of ketamine and will tend to decrease cardiac function and decrease arterial blood pressure.

Tiletamine/Zolazepam Tiletamine/zolazapam combinations are available in a fixed ratio. Telazol® is a nonnarcotic, nonbarbiturate, injectable anesthetic agent. Chemically, Telazol® is a combination of equal parts by weight of tiletamine hydrochloride (2-[ethylamino]-2-[2-thienyl]-cyclohexanone hydrochloride), an aryl-aminocycloalkanone dissociative anesthetic, and zolazepam hydrochloride (4-[o-fluorophenyl]-6,8-dihydro-1,3,8-trimethylpyazolo[3,4-e][1,4]diazepin-7[1H]-1-hydrochloride), a benzodiazepine having minor tranquilizing properties. The product is supplied sterile in vials, each containing a total of 500 mg of active drug as free base equivalents and 288.5 mg mannitol. The addition of 5-mL diluent produces a solution containing the equivalent of 50-mg tiletamine base, 50-mg zolazepam base, and 57.7-mg mannitol per milliliter. The resulting solution has a pH of 2–3.5. Zoletil® is available in many countries outside North America and is commonly marketed as a mixture containing 25 mg/mL each of zolazepam and tiletamine (Zoletil 50) or 50 mg/mL each (Zoletil 100).

Duration of effect is dependent upon route of administration and amount of drug given. When used intravenously, it lasts approximately 15–20 minutes. When given intramuscularly, it may last 30–45 minutes. It is commonly used in place of ketamine and its duration is typically longer.

Tiletamine induces dissociative anesthesia similar to ketamine. It has the potential to cause seizure activity; however when combined with zolazepam, the incidence of seizures is greatly reduced. Its effects on CBF and ICP are similar to those of ketamine. Nephrotoxicity in New Zealand white rabbits has been reported following Telazol administration (Doerning et al. 1992). Anecdotally, tigers do not appear to recover well after Tiletamine/zolazepam, therefore its use is generally contraindicated. Tiletamine/zolazepam can be combined with other drugs to improve its analgesic and recovery characteristics.

Miscellaneous Anesthetics

Etomidate Etomidate has been used extensively as a hypnotic agent for the induction of anesthesia in man, but less commonly in other species. Etomidate is a rapidly acting, ultrashort acting imidazole derivative. The duration of effect following intravenous bolus administration is typically 5–10 minutes. Etomidate causes dose dependent CNS depression, leading to sedation, hypnosis, and finally an isoelectric electroencephalogram.

Etomidate, in contrast to almost all other induction agents, does not seem to cause significant depression of cardiac contractility and has minimal effects on heart rate, cardiac output, and arterial blood pressure. Elimination of etomidate occurs by ester-hydrolysis in plasma and in the liver at approximately equal rates. Metabolism of etomidate in the liver is a capacity-limited Michaelis–Menten process. Hepatic hydrolysis results in the corresponding inactive carboxylic acid. Etomidate will temporarily reduce steroidogenesis (Boidin 1985; Moon 1997). Steroid synthesis usually increases with the stress of anesthesia so the net effect may be little or no change (Dodam et al. 1990). It is not a clinical contraindication except for animals with hypoadrenocorticism (Addison's disease.) Intravenous administration of etomidate may induce excitement, myoclonus, pain on injection, vomiting, and apnea during induction of anesthesia. Some animals may have purposeless myoclonic muscle movements during recovery from anesthesia. The frequency and severity of the side effects can be attenuated or eliminated by the administration adjunctive drugs, such as diazepam, acepromazine, or opioids prior to etomidate administration. A constant rate infusion of etomidate may result in hemolysis (Moon 1994; Van de Wiele et al. 1995). This is thought to be due to the propylene glycol carrier and the very high osmolality of available products (Doenicke et al. 1997).

Alphaxalone/Alphadolone
Saffan® Alphaxalone is a steroid anesthetic with a relatively wide margin of safety, little cardiovascular or respiratory depression, and minimal induction and recovery excitement. Alphaxalone is poorly soluble in water so to improve solubility, it is formulated with another steroid, alphadolone acetate, which also has anesthetic activity. The addition of alphadolone increases the water solubility of alphaxalone by threefold. One commercially available formulation, Saffan®, is a mixture of alphadolone, alphaxalone, and cremophor EL®. The cremophor is a nonionic surfactant, which makes the aqueous solution possible; however, cremaphor can cause histamine release and severe cardiovascular adverse events in some species (e.g., domestic dog). The main route of elimination is by biotransformation in the liver and secretion in the bile.

Alfaxan CD® Alphaxalone is available as a novel formulation that uses cyclodextran in water as a solvent rather than cremophor EL. The resulting compound lacks the histamine-releasing properties of Saffan, yet retains the therapeutic index and efficacy of alphaxalone.

OPIOIDS

All drugs classified as "opioids" are chemically related to a group of compounds that have been purified from the juice of a particular species of poppy, *Papaverum somniferum*. The unrefined extract from the poppy is called opium and contains approximately 20 naturally occurring pharmacologically active compounds, including morphine and codeine. In addition, numerous semisynthetic and synthetic analogs of these natural compounds have been developed for clinical use. The word opioid is typically used to encompass all chemical derivatives of the compounds purified from opium and will be the term used to describe this class of analgesics throughout this section.

The opioids are a versatile group of drugs with extensive applications related to the management of pain in companion animal veterinary medicine. In the past, their use in wild and exotic species has been largely limited to the ultra-potent agents utilized in remote capture techniques. However, with the rapid evolution of zoo animal medicine and surgery, the opioids are being used increasingly as analgesics for the management of surgical pain in a wide variety of species. Though there are few pharmacokinetic or pharmacodynamic studies involving opioids in wild and exotic animals, a general discussion of opioid pharmacology is relevant and may facilitate extrapolation from companion animal species.

Opioid Receptors
It is well known that exogenously administered opioids, such as morphine or heroin, exert their effects by interacting with specific opioid receptors and mimicking naturally occurring molecules known as endogenous opioid peptides. Based on work carried out over the past 20 years, it is now accepted that there are three well-defined types of opioid receptors, most commonly known by their Greek letter designations as μ (mu), δ (delta), and κ (kappa) (Harrison et al. 1998; Inturrisi 2002; Janecka et al. 2004; Kieffer 1999). This classic system of nomenclature has been under reconsideration for a number of years and during this time several alternative naming systems have been proposed leading to considerable confusion. In addition, a fourth type of opioid receptor, the nociceptin receptor (also known as the orphanin FQ receptor) has been characterized (Moran et al. 2000; Smith & Moran 2001). According to the most recent recommendations of the International Union of Pharmacology subcommittee on nomenclature, variations based on the Greek letters remain acceptable. Thus, mu, μ or MOP (for "mu opioid peptide"); delta, δ or DOP (for "delta opioid peptide"); kappa, κ or KOP (for "kappa opioid peptide"); and NOP (for "nociceptin opioid peptide") are considered interchangeable abbreviations. Distinct cDNA sequences have been cloned for all four opioid receptor types, and each type appears to have a unique distribution in the brain, spinal cord, and periphery (Smith & Lee 2003).

The diversity of opioid receptors is further extended by the existence of several subtypes of μ, δ, and κ receptors. Based on pharmacologic studies, there are thought to be at least three μ receptor subtypes, μ_1, μ_2, and μ_3; two δ receptor subtypes, δ_1, and δ_2; and perhaps as many as four κ receptor subtypes, κ_{1a}, κ_{1b}, κ_2, and κ_3 (Smith & Lee 2003). The discovery of opioid receptor subtypes generated great enthusiasm among researchers and introduced the possibility of developing subtype-specific therapeutic agents with favorable side effect profiles. At this point, however, the functional significance of these receptor subtypes remains unclear, and distinct cDNA sequences corresponding to these subtypes have not yet been identified (Smith & Lee 2003).

In general, it appears that the μ receptor mediates most of the clinically relevant analgesic effects, as well as most of the adverse side effects associated with opioid administration (Kieffer 1999). Drugs acting at the δ receptor tend to be poor analgesics, but may modify μ receptor-mediated antinociception under certain circumstances and mediate opioid receptor "cross-talk." The κ receptor mediates analgesia in several specific locations in the central nervous system and the periphery; however, distinguishing μ- and κ-mediated analgesic effects has proven to be difficult (Kieffer 1999; Smith & Lee 2003). In contrast to the classic opioid receptors, the nociceptin receptor does not mediate typical opioid analgesia, but instead produces antiopioid (pronociceptive) effects (Inturrisi 2002; Janecka et al. 2004; Moran et al. 2000; Smith & Moran 2001). Due to the considerable structural homology between the three classically described opioid receptors, it is likely that there are significant interactions between these receptors in different tissues, and the loosely defined physiologic roles ascribed to each receptor type still require further clarification.

Endogenous Opioid Receptor Ligands

The opioid receptors discussed earlier are part of an extensive opioid system that includes a large number of endogenous opioid peptide ligands. Endogenous opioid peptides are small molecules that are naturally produced in the central nervous system and in various glands throughout the body, such as the pituitary and the adrenal (Janecka et al. 2004). Three classical families of endogenous opioid peptides have been identified: the enkephalins, the dynorphins, and β-endorphin. Each of these is derived from a distinct precursor polypeptide, pro-enkephalin, pro-dynorphin, and pro-opiomelanocortin, respectively (Janecka et al. 2004). These classical endogenous opioid peptides are expressed throughout the central nervous system, and their presence has more recently been confirmed in peripheral tissues as well (Janecka et al. 2004). There are considerable structural similarities between these three groups of peptides, and each family demonstrates variable affinities for μ, δ, and κ receptors. None of them bind exclusively to a single opioid receptor and none of them have any significant affinity for the nociceptin receptor. The physiological roles of these peptides are not completely understood at this time. They appear to function as neurotransmitters, neuromodulators and, in some cases, as neurohormones. They mediate some forms of stress-induced analgesia and also play a role in analgesia induced by electrical stimulation of discrete regions in the brain, such as the periaqueductal gray of the mesencephalon (Inturrisi 2002).

Nociceptin (also known as orphanin FQ) is the endogenous ligand for the more recently discovered nociceptin receptor. Nociceptin is derived from pronociceptin, and its amino acid sequence is closely related to that of the classical endogenous opioid peptides discussed earlier (Janecka et al. 2004; Moran et al. 2000). Despite this homology, nociceptin binding is specific for the nociceptin-receptor and the peptide does not appear to interact with μ, δ, or κ receptors. Furthermore, the physiologic effects of nociceptin are in direct contrast to the actions of the classical endogenous opioid peptides, with nociceptin producing a distinctly pro-nociceptive effect (Janecka et al. 2004; Moran et al. 2000; Smith & Moran 2001). The functional significance of nociceptin and its receptor remain to be elucidated, but additional insight into this novel opioid peptide may have substantial implications in future therapeutic drug development.

In addition to the enkephalins, dynorphins, β-endorphin, and nociceptin, there are now two other recently discovered endogenous opioid peptides called endomorphin-1 and endomorphin-2 (Zadina et al. 1999). These peptides are putative products of an, as yet, unidentified precursor, and have been proposed to be the highly selective endogenous ligands for the μ receptor (Janecka et al. 2004; Zadina et al. 1999). The endomorphins are small tetrapeptides that are structurally unrelated to the classical endogenous opioid peptides (Zadina et al. 1999). Their identification has heralded a new era in research of the μ opioid system, which may contribute to our understanding of the neurobiology of opioids, and provide new avenues for therapeutic interventions.

Opioid Receptor Signaling and Mechanisms of Analgesia

Binding of an opioid agonist to a neuronal opioid receptor, regardless of whether the agonist is endogenous or exogenous, typically leads to several events that serve to inhibit the activation of the neuron. Opioid receptors are part of a large superfamily of membrane-bound receptors that are coupled to G-proteins (Smith & Lee 2003). As such, they are structurally and functionally related to receptors for many neurotransmitters and other neuropeptides ,which act to modulate the activity of nerve cells. Opioid receptor binding, via activation of various types of G-proteins, may lead to inhibition of adenylyl cyclase (cAMP) activity, activation of receptor-operated K^+ currents, and suppression of voltage-gated Ca^{2+} currents (Inturrisi 2002).

At the presynaptic level, decreased Ca^{2+} influx will result in reduced release of transmitter substances, such as substance P, from primary afferent fibers in the spinal cord dorsal horn, thereby inhibiting synaptic transmission of nociceptive input (Inturrisi 2002). Postsynaptically, enhanced K^+ efflux will result in neuronal hyperpolarization of spinal cord projection neurons and inhibition of ascending nociceptive pathways. A third potential mode of opioid action involves upregulation of supraspinal descending antinociceptive pathways in the periaqueductal gray. It is now known that this system is subject to tonic inhibition mediated by GABAergic neurons, and opioid receptor activation has been shown to suppress this inhibitory influence and augment descending antinociceptive transmission (Christie et al. 2000; Inturrisi 2002). The proposed cellular basis for this involves μ receptors present on presynaptic GABAergic nerve terminals, which activate voltage-dependent K$^+$ currents and thereby inhibit GABA release into the synaptic cleft (Christie et al. 2000). It is important to note that while our collective understanding of opioid receptor-mediated signaling has increased dramatically in recent years, the relationship of such subcellular events to clinical analgesia at the level of the organism requires further clarification.

Opioid Receptor Distribution and Therapeutic Implications

While cellular and molecular studies of opioid receptors and ligands are invaluable in understanding their function, it is critical to place them in their anatomical and physiological context to fully appreciate the opioid system and its relevance to pain management. It has long been a principle tenet of opioid analgesia that these agents are centrally acting, and this understanding has shaped the way we use opioid analgesics clinically. It has been well established that the analgesic effects of opioids arise from their ability to directly inhibit the ascending transmission of nociceptive information from the spinal cord dorsal horn, and to activate pain control circuits that descend from the midbrain via the rostral ventromedial medulla to the spinal cord. Within the central nervous system, evidence of μ, δ, and κ opioid receptor mRNA and/or opioid peptide binding has been demonstrated in supraspinal sites including the mesencephalic periaqueductal gray, the mesencephalic reticular formation, various nuclei of the rostral ventromedial medulla, forebrain regions including the nucleus accumbens, as well as spinally within the dorsal horn (Gutstein & Akil 2001; Yaksh 1998). The interactions between groups of opioid receptors at various spinal and supraspinal locations, as well as interactions between different receptor types within a given location, are complex and incompletely understood at this time.

Systemic administration of opioid analgesics via intravenous, intramuscular, or subcutaneous injection will result in a relatively rapid onset of action via interaction with these central nervous system receptors. Oral, transdermal, rectal, or buccal mucosal administration of opioids will result in variable systemic absorption, depending on the characteristics of the particular

agent, with analgesic effects being mediated largely by the same receptors within the central nervous system. In addition, neuraxial administration, either into the subarachnoid or epidural space, is a particularly efficacious route of administration. Small doses of opioids introduced via these routes readily penetrate the spinal cord and interact with spinal and/or supraspinal opioid receptors to produce profound and potentially long-lasting analgesia, the characteristics of which will depend on the particular drug utilized.

Despite the fact that opioids have long been considered the prototype of centrally acting analgesics, a body of evidence has emerged over the past decade, which clearly indicates that opioids can produce potent and clinically measurable analgesia by activation of opioid receptors in the peripheral nervous system (Stein et al. 2001). Opioid receptors of all three major types have been identified on the processes of sensory neurons, and they respond to peripherally applied opioids and locally released endogenous opioid peptides when upregulated during inflammatory pain states (Fields et al. 1980; Stein 1993; Stein et al. 1993, 2001, 2003). Furthermore, sympathetic neurons and immune cells have also been shown to express opioid receptors, but their functional role remains unclear (Stein et al. 2003). While the binding characteristics of peripheral and central opioid receptors are similar, the molecular mass of peripheral and central μ opioid receptors appears to be different, suggesting that selective ligands for these peripheral receptors could be developed, which would produce opioid analgesia without the potential to induce centrally mediated adverse side effects (Stein 1995; Stein & Yassouridis 1997; Stein et al. 1996, 2001, 2003).

Adverse Effects of Clinically Used Opioids

While opioids are used clinically primarily for their pain relieving properties, they also produce a host of other effects on a variety of body systems. This is not surprising in light of the wide distribution of endogenous opioid peptides and their receptors in supraspinal, spinal and peripheral locations. Since information regarding opioid side effects in most wild and exotic animals is lacking, reference is made to common domestic species, where appropriate.

Central Nervous System

Level of Arousal There are considerable species differences in the central nervous system response to opioid analgesics that cannot be attributed to pharmacokinetic variations alone. Central nervous system depression (i.e., sedation) is typically seen in the dog, monkey, and human, while central nervous system stimulation (i.e., excitement and/or spontaneous locomotor activity) may be elicited in the cat, horse, goat, sheep, pig, and cow following systemic administration of various opioids, most notably morphine (Branson et al. 2001).

Reasons for these different responses are not entirely clear at this time, but are presumably related to differing concentrations and distributions of μ, δ, and κ receptors in various regions of the brain in these species (Hellyer et al. 2003). Details regarding the central nervous system responses of specific wild and exotic species to opioids are not known at this time. Regardless of the species, however, there are numerous factors which may play a role, including the temperament or condition of the animal, the presence or absence of pain in the animal, the dose, route and timing of drug administration, and the specific opioid administered.

Thermoregulatory Center The hypothalamic thermoregulatory system is also affected by opioid administration. Hypothermia tends to be the most common response, particularly when opioids are used during the perioperative period in the presence of other central nervous system depressant drugs (Branson et al. 2001; Gutstein & Akil 2001). Under some clinical circumstances, however, hyperthermia is observed in cats, horses, swine, and ruminants following opioid administration (Niedfeldt & Robertson 2006; Posner et al. 2007, 2010). Part of this increase in body temperature may be attributed to an increase in muscle activity associated with central nervous system excitation in these species; however, a specific central hypothalamic mechanism has also been implicated but remains poorly understood (Branson et al. 2001).

Emetic Center Nausea and vomiting associated with opioid administration are a result of direct stimulation of the chemoreceptor trigger zone for emesis located in the area postrema of the medulla (Gutstein & Akil 2001; Stoelting 1999). As with the other centrally mediated side effects, species plays a role in determining an individual's tendency to vomit after an opioid is administered. Horses, rabbits, ruminants, and swine do not vomit with opioid administration. Cats may vomit, but usually at doses that are greater than those which stimulate vomiting in dogs. Dogs will commonly vomit following opioid administration, especially with morphine.

Cough Center Opioids have variable efficacy in depressing the cough reflex, at least in part by a direct effect on a cough center located in the medulla (Gutstein & Akil 2001). Certain opioids are more effective antitussives than others, including drugs such as codeine, hydrocodone, and butorphanol.

Pupillary Diameter As a general rule, opioids tend to produce mydriasis in those species that exhibit central nervous system excitation, and miosis in those that become sedated following opioid administration (Branson et al. 2001; Stephan et al. 2003; Lee & Wang 1975; Wallenstein & Wang 1979). Miosis is due to an excitatory action of opioids on neuronal firing in the oculomotor nucleus (Lee & Wang 1975; Stoelting 1999; Wallenstein & Wang 1979). In the cat, and presumably in other species that exhibit mydriasis, this increase in activity in the oculomotor nuclear complex still occurs, but the miotic effect is masked by increased release of catecholamines, which results in mydriasis (Wallenstein & Wang 1979).

Respiratory System Opioids produce dose-dependent depression of ventilation, primarily mediated by μ_2 receptors leading to a direct depressant effect on brainstem respiratory centers (Gutstein & Akil 2001; Stoelting 1999). This effect is characterized by decreased responsiveness of these centers to carbon dioxide and is reflected in an increased resting $PaCO_2$ and displacement of the carbon dioxide response curve to the right. This effect is compounded by the coadministration of sedative and/or anesthetic agents, meaning that significant respiratory depression and hypercapnia are much more likely to occur in anesthetized patients that receive opioids versus those that are conscious. It should be noted that, in general, humans tend to be more sensitive to the respiratory depressant effects of opioids when compared with most veterinary species. However, respiratory support and/or specific opioid antagonists should be immediately available anytime very high doses, or very potent opioids, are used.

Cardiovascular System Most opioids have minimal effects on cardiac output, cardiac rhythm, and arterial blood pressure when clinically relevant analgesic doses are administered. Bradycardia may occur as a result of opioid-induced medullary vagal stimulation and will respond readily to anticholinergic treatment if warranted. Particular opioids (morphine and merperidine) can cause release of histamine, especially after rapid intravenous administration, which may lead to vasodilation and hypotension (Branson et al. 2001; Smith et al. 2001). Due to their relatively benign effects on cardiovascular function, opioids commonly form the basis of anesthetic protocols for human patients or animals with preexisting cardiovascular disease.

Gastrointestinal System The gastrointestinal effects of the opioids are mediated by μ and δ receptors located in the myenteric plexus of the gastrointestinal tract (Branson et al. 2001; Gutstein & Akil 2001). Opioid administration may stimulate defecation in certain species. Following this initial response, spasm of gastrointestinal smooth muscle predisposes to ileus and constipation. Horses and ruminants in particular may be predisposed to gastrointestinal complications associated with opioid administration, such as colic and ruminal tympany, respectively. Chronic opioid use may predispose to gastrointestinal stasis in other species.

In human patients, opioids (most notably fentanyl and morphine) have been shown to increase bile duct pressure through constriction of the sphincter of Oddi (Radnay et al. 1984). The incidence of this side effect in humans is, however, quite low (Jones et al. 1981). The incidence of increased bile duct pressure secondary to opioid administration in various animal species, and its potential clinical significance, is unknown at this time.

Genitourinary System Opioids, particularly when administered neuraxially, may cause urinary retention through dose-dependent suppression of detrusor contractility and decreased sensation of urge (el Bindary & Abu el-Nasr 2001; Kuipers et al. 2004). Urine volume may also be affected by opioids, and the mechanism of this effect appears to be multifactorial. Mu agonists tend to produce oliguria in the clinical setting, and this is in part a result of increased antidiuretic hormone release, leading to altered renal tubular function (Mercadante & Arcuri 2004; Stoelting 1999). Elevations in circulating plasma atrial natriuretic peptide may also play a role in morphine-induced antidiuresis (Mercadante & Arcuri 2004). Conversely, κ agonists tend to produce a diuretic effect, possibly through inhibition of antidiuretic hormone secretion (Mercadante & Arcuri 2004; Stoelting 1999). Other peripheral mechanisms involving stimulation of renal alpha-2 adrenergic receptors may also contribute to this κ agonist effect (Mercadante & Arcuri 2004).

Opioid Agonists

Almost all clinically useful opioids exert their analgesic and immobilizing effects by acting as agonists at μ receptors. While there are a few opioids that act as κ agonists, these drugs also tend to have antagonist or partial agonist effects at μ and/or δ receptors and are thus not classified as *pure* agonists. Pure or full opioid agonists are capable of eliciting maximal activation of the receptor when they bind it and the subsequent downstream processes result in a maximal analgesic effect (Fig. 1.1). Clinically, the full μ agonists are superior analgesics, and they are the drugs of choice for pain of moderate to severe intensity in many veterinary species. The following section contains brief descriptions of full μ agonists currently used in veterinary medicine. Specific details regarding μ agonist clinical pharmacology in various wild and exotic species is lacking.

Morphine (Morphine Sulfate) Morphine is the prototypical opioid analgesic and acts as a full agonist not only at μ receptors, but also at δ and κ receptors (Gutstein & Akil 2001). Despite the development of numerous synthetic opioids, many of which are more potent than morphine and may have other characteristics that make them desirable alternatives to morphine in

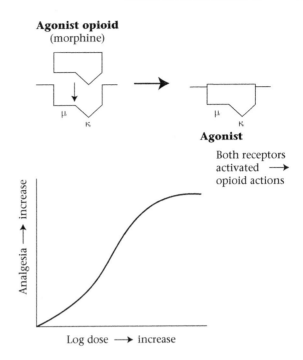

Figure 1.1. Effects of opioid agonists.

certain circumstances, it is worth noting that no other drug has been shown to be more efficacious than morphine at relieving pain in humans. Compared with the synthetic opioid agonists, morphine is relatively hydrophilic in nature and crosses the blood–brain barrier more slowly than fentanyl or oxymorphone, thereby delaying the peak effect somewhat even after intravenous administration (Gutstein & Akil 2001; Stoelting 1999). Clinically, this lag is not likely to be significant under most circumstances, with the onset of analgesia occurring reasonably promptly after a single dose of morphine and typically lasting 3–4 hours (Barnhart et al. 2000; Taylor et al. 2001). Morphine's poor lipid solubility means that it can produce long-lasting analgesia when administered into the epidural or subarachnoid space, with effects persisting for 12–24 hours. The first-pass effect is significant after oral administration and the bioavailability of oral morphine preparations is only in the range of 25%.

In most species, the primary metabolic pathway for morphine involves conjugation with glucuronic acid leading to the formation of two major metabolites, morphine-6-glucuronide and morphine-3-glucuronide (Faura et al. 1998; Gutstein & Akil 2001). Despite the low levels of glucuronyl transferase in the cat, the PK of morphine in this species seem to be broadly comparable with the dog and human, though clearance rates may be marginally slower (Barnhart et al. 2000; Faura et al. 1998; Taylor et al. 2001). This suggests that morphine must undergo a different type of conjugation reaction in this species. Morphine-6-glucuronide has pharmacological activities that are indistinguishable from those of morphine in animal models and in human beings, while morphine-3-glucuronide appears to have little affinity for opioid receptors, but may contribute to the excitatory effects of morphine in some situations (Gutstein & Akil 2001; Smith 2000). With chronic morphine administration, it is likely that the active metabolite, morphine-6-glucuronide, contributes significantly to clinical analgesia.

Very little morphine is excreted unchanged in the urine. The major metabolites, morphine-3-glucuronide and, to a lesser extent, morphine-6-glucuronide, are eliminated almost entirely via glomerular filtration. In human patients, renal failure may lead to accumulation of morphine-6-glucuronide and persistent clinical effects, while liver dysfunction seems to have minimal impact on morphine clearance (Gutstein & Akil 2001; Stoelting 1999).

The side effects associated with morphine administration are typical of most opioid agonists and have been discussed previously in this chapter. In particular, the increased incidence of vomiting after morphine administration, as well as its potential to cause histamine release after intravenous administration, distinguish morphine from other full opioid agonists.

Oxymorphone Oxymorphone is a synthetic opioid that acts as a full agonist at μ receptors and is comparable with morphine in its analgesic efficacy and duration of action. It is a more lipid-soluble drug than morphine and is readily absorbed after intramuscular or subcutaneous administration. Oxymorphone is not available as an oral formulation.

When compared with morphine, oxymorphone may be less likely to cause vomiting and tends to produce more sedation when administered to domestic species. Its respiratory depressant effects are similar to those induced by morphine, but oxymorphone seems more likely to cause panting in dogs. It does not produce histamine release, even when administered intravenously (Smith et al. 2001). Oxymorphone's other side effects are typical of other full μ agonist opioids and have been discussed previously.

Hydromorphone Hydromorphone is a synthetic opioid that acts as a full agonist at μ receptors and is used in both human and veterinary medicine. Clinically, hydromorphone and oxymorphone have similar efficacy, potency, duration of analgesic action, and side effect profiles, but hydromorphone remains significantly less expensive. Like oxymorphone, hydromorphone is not associated with histamine release so bolus intravenous administration is considered safe (Smith et al. 2001).

Meperidine Meperidine is a synthetic opioid that exerts its analgesic effects through agonism at μ receptors. Interestingly, it also appears able to bind other types of

receptors, which may contribute to some of its clinical effects other than analgesia. Meperidine is capable of blocking sodium channels and inhibiting activity in dorsal horn neurons in a manner analogous to local anesthetics (Wagner et al. 1999; Wolff et al. 2004). It has also recently been shown that meperidine exerts agonist activity at alpha-2 receptors, specifically the alpha$_{2B}$ subtype, suggesting that it may possess some alpha-2 agonist-like properties (Takada et al. 1999, 2002).

Meperidine has a considerably shorter duration of analgesic action compared to morphine, oxymorphone, or hydromorphone, typically not extending beyond 1 hour (Branson et al. 2001). Metabolic pathways vary among different species but, in general, most of the drug is demethylated to normeperidine in the liver and then undergoes further hydrolysis and ultimately renal excretion (Branson et al. 2001; Taylor et al. 2001; Yeh et al. 1981). Normeperidine is an active metabolite and possesses approximately one-half the analgesic efficacy of meperidine (Branson et al. 2001; Gutstein & Akil 2001). Normeperidine has produced toxic neurologic side effects in human patients receiving meperidine for prolonged periods of time, especially in the presence of impaired renal function (Stoelting 1999; Stone et al. 1993).

Unlike most of the other opioids in clinical use, meperidine has been shown to produce significant negative inotropic effects when administered alone to conscious dogs (Priano & Vatner 1981). Also, due to its modest atropine-like effects, meperidine tends to increase heart rate rather than predispose to bradycardia, as is often seen with other opioids (Branson et al. 2001; Stoelting 1999). The clinical significance of these cardiovascular effects in the perianesthetic period has never been clearly ascertained. Like morphine, meperidine also causes histamine release when administered intravenously (Branson et al. 2001).

A rare but life-threatening drug interaction has been reported in human patients receiving meperidine that may have relevance in veterinary medicine. The combination of meperidine (and perhaps other opioids) with a monoamine oxidase inhibitor may lead to "serotonin syndrome," which is characterized by a constellation of symptoms, including confusion, fever, shivering, diaphoresis, ataxia, hyperreflexia, myoclonus, and diarrhea (Bowdle 1998; Heinonen & Myllyla 1998; Sporer 1995; Tissot 2003). A monoamine oxidase inhibitor, selegiline (Deprenyl®), has been used in dogs to treat pituitary-dependent hyperadrenocorticism or to modify behavior in patients with canine cognitive dysfunction. Though there have not, to date, been any reports of adverse meperidine-selegiline interactions in dogs, the veterinarian must be aware of the potential for complications if analgesia is required in patients receiving monoamine oxidase inhibitors. A recent study has evaluated the effects of other opioids (oxymorphone and butorphanol) in selegiline-treated dogs and did not identify any specific adverse drug interactions in these animals (Dodam et al. 2004).

Fentanyl Fentanyl is a highly lipid soluble, short-acting synthetic μ opioid agonist. A single dose of fentanyl administered intravenously has a more rapid onset and a shorter duration of action than morphine. Peak analgesic effects occur in about 5 minutes and last approximately 30 minutes (Gutstein & Akil 2001; Stoelting 1999). Rapid redistribution of the drug to inactive tissue sites, such as fat and skeletal muscle, leads to a decrease in plasma concentration and is responsible for the prompt termination of clinical effects. In most veterinary species the elimination half-time after a single bolus or a brief infusion is in the range of 2–3 hours (Carroll et al. 1999; Lee et al. 2000; Maxwell et al. 2003). Administration of very large doses or prolonged infusions may result in saturation of inactive tissues with termination of clinical effects becoming dependent on hepatic metabolism and renal excretion (Gutstein & Akil 2001; Stoelting 1999). Thus, the context-sensitive half-time of fentanyl increases significantly with the duration of the infusion, and clinical effects may persist for an extended period following termination of a long-term intravenous infusion.

Side effects associated with fentanyl administration are similar to those of the other full μ agonist opioids. In general, cardiovascular stability is excellent with fentanyl, and intravenous administration is not associated with histamine release (Gutstein & Akil 2001; Stoelting 1999). Bradycardia may be significant with bolus doses but readily responds to anticholinergics if treatment is warranted (Branson et al. 2001; Gutstein & Akil 2001). In human patients, muscle rigidity, especially of the chest wall, has been noted after administration of fentanyl or one of its congeners (Bowdle 1998; Fahnenstich et al. 2000; Muller & Vogtman 2000). The potential significance of this adverse effect in animal patients is not clear at this time, and the risk is considered minimal if large rapid bolus administrations are avoided.

Clinically, fentanyl is used most frequently in dogs and cats, but it is also a potentially useful analgesic in other species, including the horse, cow, sheep, goat, and pig. Historically, fentanyl was available in combination with the butyrophenone tranquilizer, droperidol, in a product called Innovar-Vet, which was typically administered in the preanesthetic period to provide sedation and analgesia. This product is no longer available, and systemic administration of fentanyl today is usually via the intravenous route.

The development of novel less invasive routes of opioid administration for use in human patients led to the marketing of transdermal fentanyl patches (Duragesic®). The patches are designed to release a constant amount of fentanyl per hour, which is then absorbed across the skin and taken up systemically. Fentanyl

patches are designed for human skin and body temperature, however, their use has been evaluated in a number of domestic veterinary species (Carroll et al. 1999; Egger et al. 1998, 2003; Franks et al. 2000; Gellasch et al. 2002; Gilberto et al. 2003; Maxwell et al. 2003; Robinson et al. 1999; Wilkinson et al. 2001). Substantial variations in plasma drug concentrations have been documented, and significant lag times after patch placement are common prior to onset of analgesia (Carroll et al. 1999; Egger et al. 1998, 2003; Lee et al. 2000). Furthermore, changes in body temperature have been shown to significantly affect fentanyl absorption in anesthetized cats, and it is likely that other factors associated with skin preparation and patch placement have the potential to substantially alter plasma fentanyl levels and analgesic efficacy (Pettifer & Hosgood 2003). Fentanyl patch safety and efficacy in most species is unknown at this time.

Alfentanil, Sufentanil, and Remifentanil Alfentanil, sufentanil, and remifentanil are all structural analogues of fentanyl that were developed for use in humans in an effort to create analgesics with a more rapid onset of action and predictable termination of opioid effects. All three are similar with regard to onset, and all have context-sensitive half-times that are shorter than that of fentanyl after prolonged infusions (Stoelting 1999) Remifentanil is unique among opioids because it is metabolized by nonspecific plasma esterases to inactive metabolites (Chism & Rickert 1996; Hoke et al. 1997). Thus, hepatic or renal dysfunction will have little impact on drug clearance and this, in combination with the robust nature of the esterase metabolic system, contributes to the predictability associated with infusion of remifentanil (Gutstein & Akil 2001; Stoelting 1999).

All three of these drugs are used during general anesthesia for procedures requiring intense analgesia and/or blunting of the sympathetic nervous system response to noxious stimulation. As yet, they have limited applications for postoperative or chronic pain management. Like fentanyl, they can be administered at relatively low infusion rates as adjuncts to general anesthetic protocols based on volatile inhalant or other injectable agents, or they can be administered at higher rates as the primary agent for total intravenous anesthesia. The minimum alveolar anesthetic concentration-sparing properties of these agents have been demonstrated in both the dog and cat (Hoke et al. 1997; Ilkiw et al. 1997; Mendes & Selmi 2003; Michelsen et al. 1996; Pascoe et al. 1997). In the horse, systemic infusions of alfentanil did not have significant effects on minimum alveolar concentrations of inhalant anesthetics and when administered to conscious horses were associated with increases in locomotor activity (Pascoe & Taylor 2003; Pascoe et al. 1991, 1993). There is little evidence to suggest that any of the fentanyl analogues offer advantages over morphine when administered into the epidural space for analgesia (Natalini & Robinson 2000).

Methadone Methadone is a synthetic μ opioid agonist with pharmacologic properties qualitatively similar to those of morphine, but possessing additional affinity for N-methyl-D-aspartate receptors (Gorman et al. 1997; Ripamonti & Dickerson 2001). Methadone's unique clinical characteristics include excellent absorption following oral administration, no known active metabolites, high potency, and an extended duration of action (Branson et al. 2001; Gutstein & Akil 2001; Ripamonti & Dickerson 2001). In human patients, the drug has been used primarily in the treatment of opioid abstinence syndromes, but is being used increasingly for the management of chronic pain. Though there are reports of intramuscular or intravenous administration of methadone in the perioperative period in dogs, cats, and horses, the drug is not commonly used in this setting in North America at this time (Dobromylskyj 1996; Fisher 1984; Kramer et al. 1996).

Codeine Codeine is the result of substitution of a methyl group onto morphine, which acts to limit first-pass hepatic metabolism and accounts for codeine's high oral bioavailability (Gutstein & Akil 2001; Stoelting 1999). Codeine is well known for its excellent antitussive properties and is often combined in an oral formulation with a non-opioid analgesic, such as acetaminophen (Tylenol 3®), for the management of mild to moderate pain in human patients.

Oxycodone and Hydrocodone Oxycodone and hydrocodone are opioids that are typically administered orally for the treatment of pain in human patients. Though oxycodone is available as a single-drug continuous-release formulation (Oxycontin®), these drugs are most often prepared in combination with nonopioid analgesics, such as aspirin and acetaminophen (Percocet®, Percodan®, Lorcet®, Vicodan®, etc.). Little has been published regarding the use of these opioids in veterinary species.

Etorphine and Carfentanil (M-99® and Wildnil®, Respectively) These two opioids are discussed together because they are both used exclusively for the restraint and capture of wild animals, rather than as analgesic agents. They are extremely potent opioids, and the immediate availability of a suitable antagonist is mandatory before these drugs are to be used, not only to reverse drug effects in animal patients, but also as a safety precaution in the event of accidental human injection. Though etorphine and carfentanil are most often injected intramuscularly (usually using a remote drug delivery technique), recent studies suggest that carfentanil is useful when administered orally in a

variety of species, including the brown bear, the Brazilian tapir, and the chimpanzee (Kearns et al. 2000; Mama et al. 2000; Mortenson & Bechert 2001; Pollock & Ramsay 2003). A number of different drugs have been used in combination with etorphine or carfentanil to enhance muscle relaxation, including acepromazine, xylazine, and medetomidine (Caulkett et al. 2000; Miller et al. 2003; Ramdohr et al. 2001; Roffe et al. 2001).

Thiafentanil Thiafentanil is an opioid agonist that has been utilized to facilitate capture of several species of birds and mammals (Borkowski et al. 2009; Cushing & McClean 2010; Grobler et al. 2001; Kilgallon et al. 2010). It is pharmacologically classified as a synthetic opioid that has a relatively short duration of action. The shorter duration of action in combination with its reversibility with the opioid antagonist naltrexone make it an attractive agent when long periods of narcotization are not desirable.

Opioid Agonist–Antagonists and Partial Agonists

This group includes drugs that have varying opioid receptor binding profiles, but which have one thing in common: they all occupy μ opioid receptors, but do not initiate a maximal clinical response. Drugs such as butorphanol and nalbuphine are classified as agonist–antagonists. They are competitive μ receptor antagonists, but exert their analgesic actions by acting as agonists at κ receptors (Fig. 1.2). Buprenorphine, on the other hand, is classified as a partial agonist and binds

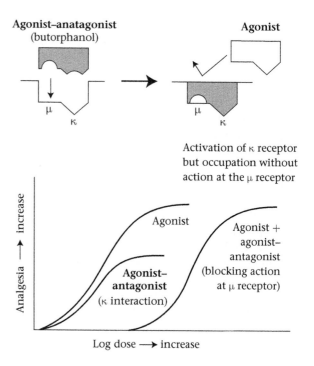

Figure 1.2. Activation of κ receptor, but occupation without action at the μ receptor.

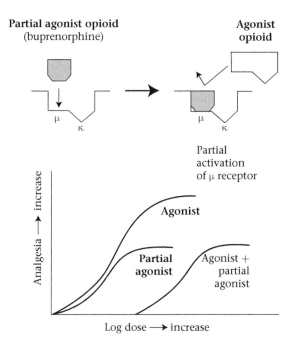

Partial agonist opioid
(buprenorphine)

Agonist
opioid

Partial
activation
of μ receptor

Figure 1.3. Partial activation of μ receptor.

μ receptors but produces only a limited clinical effect (Fig. 1.3). These mixed agonist–antagonist drugs were developed for the human market in an attempt to create analgesics with less respiratory depression and addictive potential. Due to their opioid receptor-binding affinities, the side effects associated with these drugs demonstrate a so-called ceiling effect, whereby increasing doses do not produce additional adverse responses. Unfortunately, the benefits of this ceiling effect on ventilatory depression come at the expense of limited analgesic efficacy and only a modest ability to decrease anesthetic requirements.

The coadministration of opioids with differing receptor binding profiles is currently an active area of research that deserves further attention. The interactions in this setting are complex and it appears that opioid coadministration has the potential to produce additive, synergistic, or antagonistic analgesic effects depending on the particular species, dosage, drugs, and pain model being evaluated. The following section contains brief descriptions of opioid agonist–antagonists and partial agonists that are currently used in veterinary medicine.

Butorphanol Butorphanol is a synthetic agonist–antagonist opioid and has been used extensively in a wide variety of veterinary species. The drug was originally labeled as an antitussive agent in dogs and, even now, is approved as an analgesic in the cat and horse only (Branson et al. 2001). Butorphanol exerts its relevant clinical effects through its interactions at κ receptors and acts as an antagonist at μ receptors. The duration of butorphanol's analgesic effects remains somewhat debatable and likely varies with species, type and intensity of pain, dosage, and route of administration (Sawyer et al. 1991; Robertson et al. 2003a; Sellon et al. 2001). In general, its effects are shorter lived than those of morphine and are probably in the range of 1–3 hours. Butorphanol does not induce histamine release when administered intravenously and has minimal effects on cardiopulmonary function. There is conflicting evidence regarding the effects of butorphanol on inhalant anesthetic requirements in the dog, cat, and horse. Earlier studies failed to demonstrate a significant sparing effect on minimum alveolar concentration when butorphanol was co-administered with halothane in dogs and ponies (Doherty et al. 1997; Matthews & Lindsay 1990; Quandt et al. 1994). More recently, isoflurane MAC reductions have been documented after administration of clinically relevant doses of butorphanol in both dogs and cats (Ilkiw et al. 2002; Ko et al. 2000). Reasons for these discrepancies are probably related to differences in study techniques and, in the dog and cat specifically, it seems that butorphanol is capable of inducing at least modest reductions in inhalant anesthetic requirements.

Traditionally, it was thought that the simultaneous or sequential administration of butorphanol with a pure μ opioid agonist, such as morphine or hydromorphone, would be counterproductive from an analgesic standpoint because butorphanol's ability to antagonize μ receptors could inhibit or even reverse the effects of the agonist drug. Certainly, it has been clearly demonstrated that excessive sedation associated with a pure μ agonist can be partially reversed by the administration of low doses of butorphanol, and it was presumed that butorphanol would similarly reverse the μ-mediated analgesic effects as well. It would now appear that the potential interactions between butorphanol and full μ opioid agonists are more complex than originally believed. One study demonstrated that coadministration of butorphanol and oxymorphone to cats subjected to a visceral noxious stimulus resulted in enhanced analgesic effects (Briggs et al. 1998). A more recent feline study, however, evaluated the combination of butorphanol and hydromorphone in a thermal threshold pain model and failed to demonstrate enhanced analgesia and suggested that butorphanol did, in fact, inhibit hydromorphone's analgesic effects (Lascelles & Robertson 2004). These contradictory findings illustrate that we still have much to learn about coadministration of opioid agents with differing receptor-binding profiles and the clinical effects produced by such co-administration likely depend on many factors, including species, type of pain, dose, and the specific drugs involved.

Nalbuphine and Pentazocine Nalbuphine and pentazocine are classified as agonist–antagonist opioids and are clinically similar to butorphanol. They induce mild analgesia accompanied by minimal sedation, respiratory depression, or adverse cardiovascular effects. Like butorphanol, nalbuphine is occasionally used to partially reverse the effects of a full μ agonist opioid while maintaining some residual analgesia.

Buprenorphine Buprenorphine is a semisynthetic, highly lipophilic opioid derived from thebaine. Unlike other opioids in this category, buprenorphine is considered to be a partial agonist at μ opioid receptors. The drug binds avidly to and dissociates slowly from μ receptors, but is not capable of eliciting a maximal clinical response. Due to its receptor-binding characteristics, buprenorphine has a delayed onset of action and takes at least 60 minutes to attain peak effect after intramuscular administration. It also has a relatively long duration of action with clinical analgesic effects persisting for 6–12 hours in most species. Also, its high affinity for the μ receptor means that it may be difficult to antagonize its effects with a drug, such as naloxone. Buprenorphine has most often been administered intravenously or intramuscularly; however, due to the long lag time before clinical effects are achieved after intramuscular administration, the intravenous route is preferred. Comparable plasma drug levels and analgesic efficacy with oral transmucosal administration versus intravenous administration has been demonstrated in cats (Robertson et al. 2003b). Compounded versions of buprenorphine are widely available and include higher concentrations for convenient dosing to larger animals and sustained release formulations for increased duration of action. If sustained release preparations are used, there should be a plan for supportive care should significant adverse effects occur since complete reversal of buprenorphine with conventional antagonists is often unsuccessful.

Opioid Antagonists

These drugs have high affinities for the opioid receptors and are able to displace opioid agonists from μ and κ receptors. After this displacement, the pure antagonists bind to and occupy opioid receptors, but do not activate them (Fig. 1.4). Under ordinary circumstances, in patients that have not received exogenous agonist opioids, the opioid antagonists have few clinical effects when administered at clinically relevant dosages (Gutstein & Akil 2001). It is important to recognize that these drugs will rapidly reverse all opioid-induced clinical effects including analgesia.

Naloxone This pure opioid antagonist is capable of reversing all opioid agonist effects, producing increased alertness, responsiveness, coordination and, potentially, increased perception of pain. Naloxone's duration of action is shorter than many of the opioid agonists, with recommended intravenous doses lasting between 30 and 60 minutes. Consequently, animals

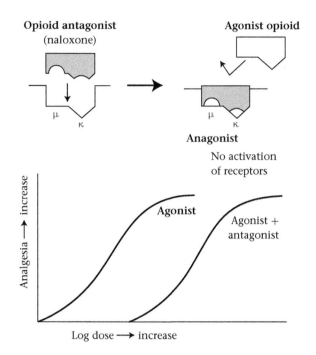

Figure 1.4. No activation of receptors.

need to be closely monitored for renarcotization after a dose of naloxone. Occasionally, excitement or anxiety may be seen after naloxone reversal of an opioid agonist. Premature ventricular contractions have also been documented after reversal, but are not a common occurrence and seem to be more likely if there are high levels of circulating catecholamines. This drug is sometimes administered sublingually to neonatal patients exhibiting respiratory depression that have been delivered by cesarean section after maternal administration of an opioid agonist.

Nalmefene and Naltrexone Both of these drugs are pure opioid antagonists with clinical effects that last approximately twice as long as naloxone (Veng-Pedersen et al. 1995). Though little is published about the use of these drugs in veterinary patients, they may be advantageous in preventing renarcotization when used to antagonize the effects of a long-acting opioid.

NONSTEROIDAL ANTI-INFLAMMATORIES

The nonsteroidal antiinflammatory drugs (NSAIDs) relieve mild to moderately severe pain and have been used extensively in a wide variety of domestic animals for many years. While pharmacokinetic and pharmacodynamic studies involving NSAIDs in wild and exotic animals are lacking, their use in such species continues to increase.

This class of drugs dates back thousands of years with the salicylates being among the oldest and still most commonly used analgesics (Vane & Botting 2003). Salicylate is a naturally occurring substance found in willow bark and was used for centuries to manage pain associated with rheumatism prior to production of the synthetic compound. In 1878, Felix Hoffman working at the Bayer company in Germany made the acetylated form of salicylic acid which has come to be known as aspirin (Vane & Botting 2003). While aspirin (acetylsalicylic acid or ASA) has been found to be effective in the management of acute and chronic mild discomfort, the newer injectable NSAIDs appear to have comparable efficacy to the pure μ agonist opioids in controlling moderate to severe soft tissue and orthopedic pain. The NSAIDs appear to confer synergism when used in combination with opioids and may demonstrate an opioid sparing effect should lower dosages of opioid be required. Their extended duration of action, in addition to their analgesic efficacy make the NSAIDs ideal for treating acute and chronic pain in veterinary species. Careful patient and drug selection is critical, however, due to their potential for harmful side effects.

The Cyclooxygenases and Prostaglandin Synthesis

In 1971, Vane discovered the mechanism by which aspirin exerts its antiinflammatory, analgesic and antipyretic actions. He proved that aspirin and other NSAIDs inhibited the activity of a cyclooxygenase (COX) enzyme, which produced prostaglandins (PGs) involved in the pathogenesis of inflammation, swelling, pain, and fever (Vane 1971). Twenty years later, the discovery of a second COX enzyme was made, and more recently, a newly identified COX-3 (Botting 2000, 2003; Chandrasekharan et al. 2002). Cyclooxygenase (previously termed prostaglandin synthase) oxidizes arachidonic acid (previously termed eicosatetraenoic acid) to various eicosanoids (including PGs and other related compounds) (Fig. 1.5) (Livingston 2000). Oxidation of arachidonic acid by 5-lipoxygenase (5-LOX), the most biologically important of the mammalian oxygenases, results in the series of eicosanoids termed leukotrienes (Fig. 1.5). The release of arachidonic acid from membrane phospholipid is catalyzed by the

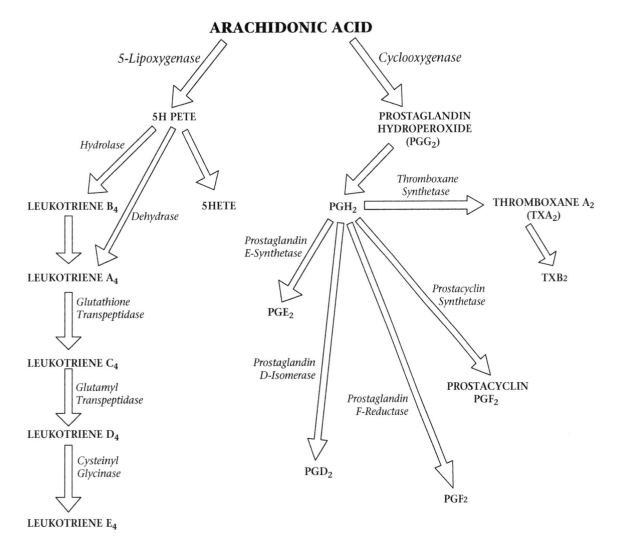

Figure 1.5. Eicosanoid synthesis.

enzyme phospholipase A_2 and is the rate-limiting step in PG and leukotriene synthesis. Prostaglandin G_2 is the initial prostenoid formed, followed by prostaglandin H_2, which serves as a substrate for prostaglandin E-synthetase, prostaglandin D-isomerase, prostaglandin F-reductase, prostacyclin synthetase, and thromboxane synthetase for conversion to a variety of other prostenoids ubiquitous throughout cells and tissues in the body (Livingston 2000). These include the PGs PGE_2, PGD_2, PGF_2, and PGI_2 (prostacyclin), and the thromboxanes TXA_2 and TXB_2, all with diverse functions (Vane & Botting 1995). The PGs are not stored but are synthesized at a constant rate. They have short half-lives of 4–6 minutes at 37°C, and act locally at the site of production.

The PGs produced by both COX-1 and COX-2 are ubiquitous throughout the body and serve to facilitate many normal physiologic functions during both health and illness. Consequently, the clinical use of NSAIDs has the potential to disrupt these functions with the possibility of significant organ dysfunction. Thus, in addition to their role as analgesics, the effects of NSAIDs on the constitutive functions of the PGs must always be considered. There are several key points to note: (1) COX-1 generates PGs that are responsible for "mucosal defense" (i.e., secretion of bicarbonate and mucus, mucosal blood vessel attenuation of constriction, and mucosal epithelial regeneration), as well as thromboxane A_2, which is necessary for platelet function; (2) COX-2 produces PGs, which function in the prevention and promotion of healing of mucosal erosions, exert antiinflammatory effects by inhibiting leukocyte adherence, as well as play a role in renal protection and maturation; and (3) COX-3 produces PGs, which exert a protective function by initiating fever (Botting 2003; Vane & Botting 1995).

Thus, depending on the NSAID selected, primary plug formation of platelets, modulation of vascular tone in the kidney and gastric mucosa, cytoprotective functions within the gastric mucosa, smooth muscle contraction, and regulation of body temperature will all be affected (Vane & Botting 1995). However, in this regard, not all NSAIDs are created equal. As noted above, the COX-1, COX-2, and COX-3 enzymes make variable contributions to these functions, and individual NSAIDs inhibit each of these enzymes differently. Some NSAIDs inhibit both COX-1 and COX-2, (i.e., aspirin, phenylbutazone, ketoprofen/Anafen®, ketorolac/Toradol®, and flunixin meglumine/Banamine®); other NSAIDs preferentially inhibit COX-2 with only weak inhibition of COX-1 (i.e.. meloxicam/Metacam®, carprofen/Rimadyl®, etodolac/Etogesic®, vedaprofen/Quadrisol-5®, and tolfenamic acid/Tolfedine®); others inhibit COX-2 exclusively (i.e.. deracoxib/Deramax®, firacoxib/Prevacox®, Robenacoxib/Onsior®, and mavicoxib/Trocoxcil®); while still another drug, acetaminophen, only weakly inhibits both COX-1

and COX-2, but is able to inhibit COX-3 activity preferentially (Botting 2000).

Several *in vitro* studies investigating NSAID selective inhibition of the COX-1 and COX-2 isoenzymes have been published; however, these are very difficult to interpret due to inconsistencies in the assays used (Kay-Mugford et al. 2000). Clinically, this information is confusing as it does not consider the PK of particular drugs and their concentrations in various tissues (Bertolini et al. 2001). Most NSAIDs that inhibit COX have been shown to result in diversion of arachidonate to the 5-LOX pathway. The 5-LOX is principally found in polymorphonuclear cells, mast cells, monocytes, basophils, and B lymphocytes that are recruited during inflammatory and immune reactions (Bertolini et al. 2001). This enzyme catalyzes the initial step in leukotriene biosynthesis, which subsequently produces various eicosanoids, with LTB_4 being the most notable potent mediator of inflammation. The excessive production of leukotrienes has been implicated in the creation of NSAID-induced ulcers (Hudson et al. 1993; Rainsford 1992). As always, however, the biological system is not clear-cut. While the LOX pathway is pro-inflammatory, there is also an anti-inflammatory pathway, which is discussed in more detail later (Serhan & Chiang 2004).

The contribution of the leukotrienes to the inflammatory process would seem to suggest that inhibition of both the COX and 5-LOX pathways by a therapeutic agent would result in an enhanced safety profile and may confer even greater analgesic efficacy due to broader anti-inflammatory and anti-nociceptive effects (Kirchner et al. 1997b). Data available show that dual-acting compounds are effective in arthritic models, where they also retain anti-thrombotic activity, produce little or no gastrointestinal damage, and do not adversely affect the asthmatic state (Bertolini et al. 2001). A recently approved dual COX/5-LOX inhibitor (tepoxalin/Zubrin®) has undergone clinical trials and is now approved for veterinary use (Kirchner et al. 1997b; Argentieri et al. 1994). Tepoxalin has demonstrated gastrointestinal antiinflammatory activity in mice, supporting the theory that 5-LOX inhibition has the potential to play a vital role in the prevention of NSAID-induced gastric inflammation (Kirchner et al. 1997a).

The NSAIDs and Mechanisms of Analgesia

Prostaglandins, notably PGE_2 and prostacyclin, are potent mediators of inflammation and pain. These molecules exert hyperalgesic effects and enhance nociception produced by other mediators, such as bradykinin. The NSAIDs' analgesic mechanism of action is through inhibition of COX-1, COX-2, and COX-3, activity with subsequent prevention of PG synthesis.

The antinociceptive effects of the NSAIDs are exerted both peripherally and centrally (Chopra et al. 2000).

The NSAIDs penetrate inflamed tissues where they have a local effect, which makes them excellent analgesic choices for injuries with associated inflammation, as well as conditions such as synovitis, arthritis, cystitis, and dermatitis (Chopra et al. 2000). The central action is at both the spinal and supraspinal levels, with contributions from both COX-1 and COX-2 (Chopra et al. 2000; McCormack 1994; Malmberg & Yaksh 1992; Yaksh et al. 1998). This central effect may account for the overall well-being and improved appetite that is often observed in patients receiving parenterally administered NSAIDs for relief of acute pain.

The rational use of NSAIDs as analgesics should be based on an understanding of pain physiology and pathophysiology. Nociceptive pathways may involve either the COX-1 or COX-2 gene, and these genes are expressed in different locations and under different circumstances. The COX-2 isoenzyme is known as the inducible isoform because it is upregulated in inflammatory states and is known to play a key role in nociception. While the COX-1 gene has traditionally been thought of as being expressed constitutively, this isoenzyme also plays an integral role in the pain experience (Chandrasekharan et al. 2002). The COX-1 selective NSAIDs are superior to COX-2 selective NSAIDs at inhibiting visceronociception caused by chemical pain stimulators in a mouse peritoneal model (Ochi et al. 2000). This has been confirmed by visceronociception being greatly reduced in COX-1 but not COX-2 knockout mice (Ballou et al. 2000). These studies concluded that peripheral COX-1 mediates nociception in slowly developing pain in mice, such as in visceral pain, and central COX-1 may be involved in rapidly transmitted, nonvisceral pain, such as that caused by thermal stimulation (Ballou et al. 2000). Visceral pain may be mediated, at least in part, by stimulation of intraperitoneal receptors located on sensory fibers by COX-1-produced prostacyclin (Botting 2003). Interestingly, there may be gender differences, as in Ballou's mouse model, which demonstrated that spinal COX-2 did in fact contribute to visceral nociception, but only in female mice (Ballou et al. 2000). The analgesic potency of a range of NSAIDs in relieving tooth extraction pain in humans correlates closely with increasing selectivity toward COX-1 rather than COX-2. These findings highlight the importance of both COX-1 and COX-2 contributions to pain and the selective efficacy of the NSAIDs in treating various painful conditions.

The COX-2 or inducible isoenzyme can potentially increase by 20-fold over baseline in the presence of tissue injury and inflammation (Malmberg & Yaksh 1992). Pro-inflammatory cytokines and mitogens, such as interleukin-1-beta, (IL-β), interferon gamma, and tumor necrosis factor-alpha (TNF-α), induce COX-2 expression in macrophages, as can platelet-activating factor (PAF), and PGE$_2$ (Bertolini et al. 2001). These events may also occur in chondrocytes, osteoblasts and synovial microvessel endothelial cells. The higher COX levels increase prostenoid production, where these compounds serve as amplifiers of nociceptive input and transmission in both the peripheral and central nervous systems (Malmberg & Yaksh 1992). The COX-2 selective NSAIDs have been shown to be clinically useful in managing inflammatory pain in humans and animals. This has been a focus of the pharmaceutical industry, as a selective COX-2 inhibitor may potentially show efficacy in alleviating pain and hyperalgesia while sparing COX-1 constitutive activity and potential adverse effects associated with NSAID administration. Unfortunately, the biological system is not as simple as first envisioned. While COX-2 is induced during inflammation, it has also been shown to be induced during resolution of the inflammatory response where the antiinflammatory PGs (PGD$_2$ and PGF$_2\alpha$), but not pro-inflammatory PGE$_2$, are produced. Potentially, inhibition of COX-2 during this phase may actually prolong inflammation (Bertolini et al. 2001). As is the case for COX-1, it now appears that the COX-2 isoenzyme also has important constitutive functions. Studies indicate there may be a protective role for COX-2 in maintenance of gastrointestinal integrity, ulcer healing, and in experimental colitis in rats (DuBois et al. 1998; Reuter et al. 1996; Schmassmann et al. 1998). In addition, the COX-2 isoenzyme appears to have constitutive functions associated with nerve, brain, ovarian and uterine function, and bone metabolism (DuBois et al. 1998). Therefore, the potential for NSAID associated side effects with these systems is of concern. Of major importance are the COX-2 constitutive functions within the kidney which differ from those of COX-1 in hypotensive and hypovolemic states (Imig 2000). Also, COX-2 appears to be important in nephron maturation (Harris 2000). The canine kidney is not fully mature until three weeks after birth, and administration of a NSAID during this time, or to the bitch prior to birth, may cause a permanent nephropathy (Horster et al. 1971). In fact, in COX-2 null mice which lack the gene for COX-2, all animals die before 8 weeks of age from renal failure (Morham et al. 1995). This does not occur in COX-1 null mice, and interestingly, these mice did not develop gastric pathology (Morham et al. 1995).

When considering the COX selectivity of a particular NSAID, the concentration (i.e., dose) of the NSAID may also influence its actions. A drug may function as a competitive, nonpreferential ,or selective COX inhibitor (COX-1 or COX-2) at higher concentrations, and as a COX-2 selective inhibitor at lower concentrations (Lipsky et al. 2000). The significance of this is the potential for inhibition of COX-1 with administration of an allegedly COX-2 selective NSAID. The COX selectivity may be present *in vitro*, however, at the dosing required to achieve analgesia, such selectivity may be lost. Cloning studies comparing canine COX isoenzymes with human COX isoenzymes found that they are highly homologous (Gierse et al. 2002). Canine COX-1 and COX-2 had a 96% and 93% DNA sequence homology, respectively, with their human counterparts. This suggests that they would be similarly affected by pharmaceuticals, such as NSAIDs designed to inhibit their function. However, the distribution of the COX enzymes may differ among species. When summarizing the common adverse effects noted in veterinary patients following administration of NSAIDs (ie. gastrointestinal ulceration, renal perturbations, and hemorrhage), hemorrhage is the only one that appears to be spared with COX-2 selective NSAIDs in animals with normal platelet numbers and function.

Cyclooxygenase-2 is reduced following administration of glucocorticoids, which may partially explain the antiinflammatory and analgesic effects of this class of medications. Of interest, in addition to the COX-2 role in inflammation, aberrantly upregulated COX-2 expression is increasingly implicated in the pathogenesis of a number of epithelial cell-origin carcinomas, including colon, esophagus, breast, and skin, and in Alzheimer's disease and other neurological conditions (Fosslien 2000; Lipsky 1999; Smalley & DuBois 1997). The COX-2 inhibitors are being researched as potential anti-carcinogenic agents (FitzGerald & Patrono 2001).

Dissecting out the details of the derivation and specific actions of COX-1 and COX-2 continues to provide important insight into the management of pain with NSAIDs. The picture, however, remains incomplete, as some NSAIDS do not significantly inhibit these enzymes. This finding stimulated the search for a potential COX-3 isoenzyme. Based on studies using canine cortex, a COX-3 isoenzyme was discovered that was derived from the same gene as COX-1 (Chandrasekharan et al. 2002). The COX-3 isoenzyme is also present in human brain and heart tissues. It is distinct from COX-1 and -2, as demonstrated in studies using common analgesic/antipyretic NSAIDS in suppressing COX production. Acetaminophen inhibited COX-3 activity, but not COX-1 and -2, as did dipyrone (Chandrasekharan et al. 2002). Both of these agents are frequently used to reduce fever in animals. Other analgesic/antipyretic NSAIDs found to be effective COX-3 inhibitors are diclofenac (the most potent), and aspirin and ibuprofen (which preferentially inhibit COX-3 over COX-1 and -2). The overall conclusion of this particular study was that COX-3 possesses COX activity that differs pharmacologically from both COX-1 and -2, but is more similar to COX-1 (Chandrasekharan et al. 2002). This study also reported that the COX-3 isoenzyme is more susceptible to inhibition by drugs that are analgesic and antipyretic but which lack anti-inflammatory activity. This observation again emphasizes the potential utility of administering NSAIDs with different COX selectivities for managing pain of different etiologies. As the COX-3 isoenzyme

genetic profile is derived from the COX-1 gene, it appears that the COX-1 gene plays an integral role in pain and/or fever, depending on the physiologic context (Chandrasekharan et al. 2002). This has been confirmed by the studies mentioned earlier (Ballou et al. 2000; Botting 2003; Ochi et al. 2000). The COX-1 selective NSAIDs used in veterinary and human patients with poor central nervous system penetration (i.e., ketoprofen and ketorolac) may, in fact, reach sufficient concentrations in the brain to inhibit COX-3 (Warner et al. 1999). It is also recognized that the analgesic effects of these NSAIDs frequently occur at lower dosages than those required to inhibit inflammation.

The NSAIDs and Fever

Just as the relationship between pain and the various activities of the COX system is complex, so too is the association between fever and the COX isoenzymes. The mechanisms leading to the generation of fever vary depending on the inciting factor that may be peripheral (i.e., endotoxin) or central (i.e., endogenous pyrogens, such as IL-1). Interspecies variation is also substantial, and the definitive role of the COXs in pyresis remains to be clearly elucidated. Evidence suggests that COX-2 plays a role in endotoxin pyrexia while, based on the antipyretic effects of acetaminophen and aspirin, COX-1 and COX-3 appear to function in endogenous pyrexia (Botting 2000, 2003; Chandrasekharan et al. 2002).

The NSAIDs and Endogenous Antiinflammatory Mechanisms

Endogenously generated small chemical mediators, or autacoids, play a key role in controlling inflammation by inhibiting polymorphonuclear cell recruitment and enhancing monocyte activity in a nonphlogistic manner (Rainsford 1992). Arachadonic acid-derived lipoxins (LX), particularly LXA4, have been identified as anti-inflammatory mediators, indicating that the LOX pathway has a dual proinflammatory and anti-inflammatory function.

The NSAIDs may amplify or decrease this endogenous anti-inflammatory system. Aspirin is more COX-1 selective and can impair many components of mucosal defense and enhance leukocyte adherence within the gastric and mesenteric microcirculation (Wallace & Fiorucci 2003). However, with chronic use of aspirin, there is an adaptation of the gastric mucosa that is associated with a marked upregulation of COX-2 expression and lipoxin production. This lipoxin is specifically termed aspirin-triggered lipoxin (ATL). Aspirin is unique among current therapies because it acetylates COX-2, thereby enabling the biosynthesis of 15(R)-hydroxyeicosatetraenoic acid (15(R)-HETE) from arachidonic acid, which is subsequently converted to ATL by 5-LOX. Inhibition of either the COX-2 or 5-LOX enzymes results in blockade of ATL synthesis (Wallace

& Fiorucci 2003). Lipoxin A4 and ATL (a carbon-15 epimer of LX) attenuate aspirin-induced leukocyte adherence, whereas administration of selective COX-2 inhibitors blocks ATL synthesis and has been shown to augment aspirin-induced damage and leukocyte adherence to the endothelium of mesenteric venules in rats (Wallace & Fiorucci 2003).

In addition to the lipoxins, aspirin-induced COX-2 acetylation results in the generation of numerous other endogenous autacoids derived from dietary omega-3 fatty acids (Serhan et al. 2002). Some of these local autacoids are potent inhibitors of neutrophil recruitment, thereby limiting the role of these cells during the resolution phase of inflammation, and thus are referred to as "resolvins" (Serhan et al. 2002). The identification of both the lipoxins and the resolvins has introduced new potential therapeutic avenues for the treatment of inflammation, cardiovascular disease, and cancer.

Other Pharmacologic Considerations for NSAID Use

Because of their high protein binding, NSAIDs can displace other drugs from their plasma protein binding sites and potentially increase their plasma concentration. This is rarely a concern unless administered to animals with organ dysfunction or in those receiving other highly protein bound medications with a narrow therapeutic index. Interference with the metabolism and excretion of certain coadministered drugs may occur; therefore, verifying the safety of combination therapy is always mandatory.

Some NSAIDs may induce the syndrome of inappropriate secretion of antidiuretic hormone (ADH). Renal water reabsorption depends on the action of ADH mediated by cyclic adenosine monophosphate (cAMP). As PGs exert a controlled negative feedback action on cAMP production, inhibition of PG synthesis results in above-normal levels of cAMP with potential for enhanced ADH activity. In addition, the administration of a COX-2 selective NSAID may enhance sodium and water reabsorption. Clinically, both mechanisms may result in high specific gravity urine with dilutional hyponatremia. Urine volume may be decreased through this mechanism but without renal injury (Dunn & Buckley 1986; Petersson et al. 1987).

Contraindications for NSAIDs

NSAIDs should not be administered to animals with acute renal insufficiency, hepatic insufficiency, dehydration, hypotension, conditions associated with low "effective circulating volume" (i.e., congestive heart failure and ascites), coagulopathies (i.e., factor deficiencies, thrombocytopenia, and von Willebrand's disease), or evidence of gastric ulceration (i.e., vomiting with or without the presence of "coffee ground material," and melena). Administration of NSAIDs following gastrointestinal surgery must be determined by the health of

this organ at the time of surgery. As the COX-2 isoenzyme is important for healing, intuitively, NSAIDs would be contraindicated where compromised bowel is noted. Concurrent use of other NSAIDs (i.e., aspirin) or corticosteroids is not recommended. The COX-1 preferential NSAIDs are contraindicated in animals with spinal injury (including herniated intervertebral disc) due to the potential for hemorrhage and neurologic deterioration, and due to excessive bleeding at the surgical site should surgical treatment be pursued. The NSAIDs should never be administered to animals in shock, trauma cases at the time of presentation, or animals with evidence of hemorrhage (i.e., epistaxis, hemangiosarcoma, and head trauma). Animals with severe or poorly controlled asthma, or other types of moderate to severe pulmonary disease, may deteriorate with NSAID administration. Aspirin has been documented to exacerbate asthma in human patients; however, COX-2 specific NSAIDs did not result in worsening of clinical signs (West & Fernandez 2003). It is not known whether animals may be affected in this way. Although administration of NSAIDs in head trauma, pulmonary diseases, or thrombocytopenia is generally contraindicated, COX-2 preferential NSAIDs (i.e., meloxicam, etodolac, carprofen, tolfenamic acid, and deracoxib) may prove to be safe with further study. Due to inhibition of PG activity, the NSAIDs may be detrimental to reproductive function. Indomethacin may block prostaglandin activity in pregnant women, resulting in cessation of labor, premature closure of the ductus arteriosus in the fetus, and disruption of fetal circulation (DuBois et al. 1998). These effects may occur in animals; therefore, NSAIDs should not be administered during pregnancy. As COX-2 induction is necessary for ovulation and subsequent implantation of the embryo (DuBois et al. 1998), NSAIDs should also be avoided in breeding females during this stage of the reproductive cycle. As previously mentioned, the COX-2 isoenzyme is required for maturation of the embryological kidney so administration to lactating mothers should be avoided.

NSAIDs used in Veterinary Medicine

There is little data regarding clinical pharmacology of NSAIDs in exotic species, thus care must be taken when extrapolating from common domestic species.

Meloxicam Meloxicam is a COX-2 preferential NSAID approved for use in dogs in Australasia, Europe, and North America. The parenteral formulation is approved for cats in the United States and Australasia. Its use in cats in Canada is under investigation with completed studies indicating safety and efficacy. Its use in horses is also under investigation, with pharmacokinetic studies indicating that the half-life is shorter and clearance greater than in the dog, suggesting that dosing more than once a day may be necessary (Sinclair et al. 2003).

Studies indicate no renal or hepatic abnormalities with acute administration and minimal to no anti-thromboxane activity, suggesting hemostasis in normal animals may not be a problem (Mathews et al. 1999; Poulsen Nautrep & Justus 1999). Few adverse reactions have been documented, and most involve the gastro-intestinal tract. A recent study showed no difference in gastric erosions over saline placebo when meloxicam was administered at 0.1 mg/kg for 3 days postelectrical stimulation (i.e., surgical simulation) under anesthesia. However, corticosteroids plus meloxicam in this study resulted in significant gastric erosions (Boston et al. 2003). A case report of combination aspirin and meloxi-cam in a dog resulted in duodenal perforation (Reed 2002). This case illustrates the importance of COX-2 in intestinal protection when aspirin is coadministered, and reinforces that different NSAIDs should not be administered concurrently. Analgesia is excellent when meloxicam is combined with an opioid.

Carprofen Although classified as a NSAID, carprofen administration to beagle dogs did not inhibit PGE_2, 12-hydroxyeicosatetrenoic acid or thromboxane B_2 synthesis in an experimental study utilizing subcutane-ous tissue cage fluids (McKellar et al. 1994a). It was concluded that the principle mode of action of carpro-fen must be by mechanisms other than cyclooxygenase or 12-lipoxygenase inhibition. However, more recent studies indicate that it is a COX-2 preferential NSAID (Kay-Mugford et al. 2000; Ricketts et al. 1998). Carpro-fen is approved for perioperative and chronic pain management in dogs in Australasia, Europe, and North America. Carprofen is approved for single dose, periop-erative use in cats in Europe, and is licensed for use in horses in the United Kingdom. In sheep, carprofen (0.7 mg/kg, IV) resulted in plasma concentrations of 1.5 μg/mL, similar to those required to confer analgesia in horses, for up to 48 hours (Welsh et al. 1992). However, analgesia was not assessed in this sheep study (Welsh et al. 1992). Antithromboxane activity is minimal, suggesting that induced coagulopathy may not be a problem in animals with intact hemostatic mechanisms (McKellar et al. 1990; Poulsen Nautrep & Justus 1999).

Ketoprofen Ketoprofen is approved for postoperative and chronic pain in both dogs and cats in Europe and Canada. Ketoprofen is also approved for use in horses and ruminants. As ketoprofen is an inhibitor of both COX-1 and COX-2, adverse effects are a potential problem requiring careful patient selection. Although several studies using ketoprofen preoperatively indicate its effectiveness in controlling postoperative pain, a general consensus among veterinarians has restricted its use primarily to the postoperative period to reduce the potential for hemorrhage (Lobetti & Joubert 2000; Mathews et al. 1999; Pibarot et al. 1997). Ketoprofen

should not be administered to patients with risk factors for hemorrhage. It is often administered to animals immediately after orthopedic procedures (i.e., fracture repair, cruciate repair, and onychectomy).

Etodolac Etodolac is COX-2 preferential and is approved in the United States for use in dogs for the management of pain and inflammation associated with osteoarthri-tis, but is also useful in other painful conditions (Buds-berg et al. 1999; Glaser et al. 1995). The adverse effects appear to be restricted to the gastrointestinal tract.

Deracoxib Deracoxib is a COX-2 specific inhibitor. Deracoxib is approved in the United States and Canada for control of postoperative pain and inflammation associated with orthopedic surgery in dogs. The inci-dence of vomiting and diarrhea were similar in dogs receiving deracoxib compared with dogs receiving placebo in a perioperative field trial, and overall the drug was well tolerated and effective (Novartis Animal Health USA 2004). It was also shown to be effective in attenuating lameness in dogs with urate crystal-induced synovitis after prophylactic and therapeutic adminis-tration (McCann et al. 2004; Millis et al. 2002). This group of NSAIDs appeared to be gastroprotective in human patients when compared with the less COX-2 specific NSAIDs, when used for 8 days to 3 months (Silverstein et al. 2000). However, more recent studies in humans indicate these NSAIDs cannot guarantee gastroprotection with chronic use. Furthermore, in a recent canine study comparing the gastrointestinal safety profile of licofelone (a dual inhibitor) to rofe-coxib (another specific COX-2 inhibitor), rofecoxib, was found to induce significant gastric and gastroduo-denal lesions (Moreau et al. 2005).

Diclofenac Diclofenac is available worldwide as several different human and veterinary formulations. It is a useful antiinflamatory and analgesic drug and has been studied for antimicrobial activity (Dutta et al. 2007). Diclofenac has been observed to cause severe hepatic and nephrotoxicity in many species of birds and its use, or accidentally ingestion from carcasses should be avoided (Hussain et al. 2008; Jain et al. 2009; Jayaku-mar et al. 2010; Naidoo et al. 2009; Oaks et al. 2004; Taggart et al. 2007).

Firocoxib Firocoxib is available as an oral paste and injectable for horses and as an oral formulation for dogs. The efficacy and adverse events appear similar to other coxib-class NSAIDs (Food and Drug Adminis-tration: Center for Veterinary Medicine [FDA-CVM], 2011).

Robenacoxib Robenacoxib is available (currently outside the United States) as an oral and injectable formulation for treatment of pain and inflammation in both dogs and cats. The efficacy and adverse events appear similar to other coxib-class NSAIDs.

Mavicoxib Mavicoxib is a long-acting NSAID approved outside the United States for use in dogs. The dosing interval is usually 2 weeks between doses 1 and 2, the 4 weeks between subsequent doses. The elimination half-life in healthy dogs is approximately 2 weeks (range 7.9–38.8 days) (Cox et al. 2010). Significant individual and breed associated differences have been observed, but effects on drug safety and effectiveness have yet to be determined (Cox et al. 2011).

Tepoxalin Tepoxalin is a COX-1, COX-2, and LOX inhibitor of varying degrees with efficacy comparable with meloxicam or carprofen and safety comparable with placebo (FDA-CVM 2005). Tepoxalin has been approved for management of osteoarthritic pain in dogs. The safety profile of tepoxalin showed no difference from placebo when administered prior to a 30-minute anesthesia period and a minor surgical procedure in dogs (Kay-Mugford et al. 2004).

Tolfenamic Acid Tolfenamic acid is approved for use in cats and dogs in Europe and Canada for controlling acute postoperative and chronic pain. The dosing schedule is 3 days on and 4 days off that must be strictly adhered to. Reported adverse effects are diarrhea and occasional vomiting. Tolfenamic acid has significant anti-inflammatory and antithromboxane activity; therefore, posttraumatic and surgical hemostasis may be compromised during active bleeding after administration of this NSAID (McKellar et al. 1994b).

Flunixin Meglumine Flunixin meglumine is a COX-1 and COX-2 inhibitor and is approved for use in dogs in Europe but not North America. It is also approved for use in ruminants and horses and is commonly used for equine colic pain.

Phenylbutazone Phenylbutazone is approved for use in horses, cattle, and dogs in North America. Since safer NSAIDs are approved for dogs, phenylbutazone is not recommended for this species. In horses, there is high risk of gastric ulceration and nephrotoxicity, where signs of toxicity may progress from inappetence and depression to colic, gastrointestinal ulceration, and weight loss (Collins & Tyler 1984; MacAllister et al. 1993; Snow et al. 1981). Phenylbutazone has a prolonged elimination half-live in cattle, ranging from 30 to 82 hours (Arifah & Lees 2002; DeBacker et al. 1980).

Aspirin Aspirin is primarily a COX-1 inhibitor. It has been most commonly used as an analgesic for osteoarthritic pain in dogs. It is also available in proprietary combinations with various opioids (aspirin plus codeine or aspirin plus oxycodone) to achieve a synergistic effect for the treatment of moderate pain. It is also used as an antipyretic and anticoagulant in dogs and cats. Aspirin has also been recommended in cattle (Gingerich et al. 1975).

NSAIDs Not Approved for Use in Veterinary Medicine (Off-Label Use)

Ketorolac Ketorolac is a COX-1 and COX-2 inhibitor and is included for the benefit of those working in the research setting associated with human hospitals where the availability of ketorolac is more likely than other NSAIDs. Adverse gastrointestinal effects are common.

Acetaminophen Acetaminophen is a COX-3 inhibitor with minimal COX-1 and COX-2 effects. It should not be administered to feline species due to deficient glucuronidation of acetaminophen in these species (Court & Greenblatt 1997).

Dipyrone Dipyrone is a COX-3 inhibitor and is approved for use in cats and dogs in Europe and Canada. Dipyrone should be given intravenously to avoid the irritation experienced when given intramuscularly. The analgesia produced is not usually adequate for moderate to severe postoperative pain, and dipyrone is reserved for use as an antipyretic in cases where other NSAIDs are contraindicated. Dipyrone induces blood dyscrasias in humans; however, this has not been reported in animals.

ALPHA-2 ADRENERGIC RECEPTOR AGONISTS AND ANTAGONISTS

Introduction

The use of alpha-2 adrenergic agonists in veterinary medicine began following the synthesis of xyalazine in 1962. Early reports of the sedative and anesthetic sparing qualities of xylazine predated the elucidation of its mechanism of action in 1981. Alpha-2 adrenoreceptors have been identified in the CNS, cardiovascular, respiratory, renal, endocrine, gastrointestinal, and hemotologic systems, resulting in widespread drug effects (Aantaa et al. 1995). Most FDA-CVM approved alpha-2 agonists carry label indications as sedatives and analgesics.

Alpha-2 adrenoceptors are linked to Gi-protein second messengers (Aantaa et al. 1995). These are similar to those used by many opioid receptor subtypes and in fact, opioid and alpha-2 agonists usually have additive or synergistic effects (Maze & Tranquilli 1991). Alpha-2 adrenoreceptors are classically described as being located presynaptically at noradrenergic neurons exerting an inhibitory feed-back role on the release of subsequent norepinephrine (NE) (Maze & Tranquilli 1991). This results in decreased sympathetic nervous system efferent activity and probably is related to the decreased vigilance, decreased anesthetic requirements, and decreased heart rate and blood pressure observed following administration of these drugs to most species. Alpha-2 adrenoreceptors are also found in the vascular smooth muscle (a nonpresynaptic site) and when activated result in vasoconstriction. This results in increased vascular resistance and will result in increased baroreceptor-mediated vagal tone. The result is slowing of heart rate and decreasing cardiac output, but blood pressure remains within physiologic normal values. Confusion often exists about the clinical effect of alpha-2 agonist administration (e.g., hypertension [postsynaptic] vs. hypotension [presynaptic]) expected in a patient. The net clinical result will vary with route of administration, dose, species, and the duration of time following the administration.

Alpha-2 agonist doses vary at least 10-fold across species. Pigs tend to have the highest requirements, followed by cats, dogs, horses, and finally ruminants. Breed and sex differences also exist within cattle that should be appreciated.

Alpha-2 Adrenergic Agonist Effects

Central Nervous System Alpha-2 adrenergic agonists exert many of their inhibitory effects on central nervous system (CNS) function through inhibiting NE release from sympathetic neurons (Maze & Tranquilli 1991). Inhibition of intraneuronal transmission is also responsible for muscle relaxation observed following alpha-2 adrenergic agonist administration. Analgesia is mediated by spinal and supraspinal alpha-2 adrenergic receptors. Agonist binding modulates afferent activity at a spinal level and increases the diffuse noxious inhibitory control system activity. The net result is sedation, reduced anesthetic requirements, reduced stress responses, and analgesia. It should be noted that alpha-2 agonists, like all sedatives and tranquilizers, are not anesthetics. Although animals can appear in a sleep-like state, they may become aroused by noxious stimulation and may become defensive. Additionally, on rare occasions, paradoxical behavior (aggression rather than sedation) may be noted. Accidental intracarotid injection of alpha-2 adrenergic agonists will induce seizure-like activity and must be avoided.

Emetic Center Alpha-2 agonists are predictable emetics in cats and dogs, especially at high doses. This is due to activation of the chemoreceptor trigger zone of the area postrema (Hikasa et al. 1992). Dopaminergic blocking agents do not prevent alpha-2-induced emesis.

Thermoregulation Alpha-2 agonists will often cause changes in thermoregulation. The effect is usually a decrease; however, increases can be seen when animals are placed in warm environments. This is especially a concern when alpha-2 agonists are used for capture of cattle or other hoof-stock. If possible, body temperature should be monitored for 12–24 hours following

sedation or administration of an alpha-2 adrenergic antagonist should be considered. In smaller animals, hypothermia is more common and may be due to decreased metabolic activity accompanying sedation as well as decreased thermoregulatory control. It is usually not a life-threatening problem if managed appropriately.

Eye Alpha-2 agonists generally cause mild miosis to little change in pupil diameter and a mild decrease in intraocular pressure (IOP) (Verbruggen et al. 2000). The class of drugs is relatively contraindicated with increases in intraocular pressure or corneal lacerations because of the probability of inducing vomiting (which causes further increases in IOP) in those species that can vomit.

Respiratory System Most alpha-2 adrenergic receptor agonists can cause decreased responsiveness to CO_2, especially in higher doses. This effect is compounded by the coadministration of opioids or anesthetic agents and is of concern during anesthesia. In some species, alpha-2 agonists do not normally depress respiration to the point of creating hypoxia and cyanosis. In fact, arterial blood gas values for PaO_2 are usually normal. The bluish color of the mucous membranes that may be noticed on occasion is usually due to slowed venous blood flow accompanying vasoconstriction. As the capillary transit time increase, oxygen extraction increases, and notable hemoglobin desaturation will appear as a blue(ish) color. Oxygen therapy will often resolve this condition. However, in sheep and possibly some other species, xylazine administration has been shown to result in central hypoxemia related to pulmonary changes (Celly et al. 1997, 1999).

Cardiovascular System Intravenous administration of alpha-2 adrenergic agonists typically results in rapid and pronounced vasoconstriction (Pypendop & Verstegen 1998). If heart rate and cardiac output do not decrease (as can be seen with atropine administration), blood pressure would increase impressively (Alibhai et al. 1996; Short 1991). However, normal baroreceptor reflexes attempt to maintain blood pressure within physiologic limits by increasing vagal tone and slowing heart rate. Heart rate may decrease by 50–75% in some individuals. The cardiac rhythm is often a slow sinus rhythm characterized by two or three sequential beats followed by a long sinus pause. Occasionally, second-degree atrioventricular blockade will be seen. Both rhythms are often responsive to antimuscarinic administration (block the vagal reflex) and high heart rates (and blood pressures) will result. Intramuscular or oral administration tends to decrease the incidence of profound bradycardia.

After the initial direct vasoconstriction occurs, vasodilation and reduction in blood pressure may be seen.

This is more prominent in primate species. The alpha-2 adrenergic receptor agonists decrease sympathetic nervous system efferent activity, which results in decreased vasomotor tone and heart rate. Alpha-2 adrenergic agonists have historically been used in humans as antihypertensive agents because they reduce vasomotor tone and block the reflex increase in heart rate that can accompany alpha-1 antagonists.

Most of the contraindications to alpha-2 adrenergic receptor agonist administration are related to their cardiovascular side effects. As a general rule, this class of drugs should not be administered to animals that do not have normal healthy cardiovascular systems and/ or are exercise intolerant. There are some exceptions, but a thorough understanding of the underlying disease is required and appropriate monitoring necessary.

Urinary Tract Alpha-2 adrenergic receptor agonists increase urine output by increasing production of dilute urine (Grimm et al. 2001; Saleh et al. 2005). This is primarily related to inhibition of antiduretic hormone (ADH) release and/or synthesis, as well as changes in renal hemodynamics (Saleh et al. 2005).

Gastrointestinal Tract Animals may have complications associated with decreased propulsive activity, including colic and bloat, although this is unusual in most species (Thompson et al. 1991). Longer-acting drugs are more likely to result in a problem. Patients should be observed following alpha-2 adrenergic receptor agonist administration for signs of abdominal distension.

Endocrine A classic neroendocrine response is hyperglycemia following alpha-2 agonist administration (Abdel el Motal & Sharp 1985; Osman & Nicholson 1991). This is due to a decrease in insulin release. It is usually transient and not clinically significant, although alpha-2 agonists should not be used to sedate animals for glucose curves.

Since alpha-2 agonists reduce sympathetic activity and inhibit the stress response, neuroendocrine markers of the stress response should be affected. Cortisol levels are usually decreased following alpha-2 agonist administration and may not be reliable as indicators of stress or pain (Brearley et al. 1990; Sanhouri et al. 1992).

Specific Drugs

Several alpha-2 adrenergic receptor agonists are approved for veterinary use. Generally, their pharmacologic actions will be similar, but the duration of action and species compatibility will vary. All alpha-2 agonists are potent and potentially dangerous following accidental human ingestion or injection. Care should be taken when handling syringes loaded with these drugs and medical help should be sought immediately if exposure occurs.

Xylazine Xylazine is the prototypical veterinary alpha-2 adrenergic receptor agonist. Another alpha-2 agonist, clonidine, has been used in humans as an antihypertensive agent and is often used as the prototypical drug in research applications. Xylazine has been administered to many different species, both domestic and exotic. It is readily available and relatively inexpensive.

Xylazine has a shorter duration of action than many of the other drugs. Typical doses will result in muscle relaxation and sedation of horses for 45–60 minutes. This can be advantageous when performing field anesthesia/sedation when a rapid recovery is desired. Xylazine is often combined with opioids like butorphanol to enhance sedative and analgesic qualities.

Detomidine Detomidine is a longer acting alpha-2 agonist approved for use in horses as a sedative. It is commonly administered when profound, long-lasting sedation is needed. When used in high doses as a preanesthetic, low respiratory rates may accompany induction. Detomidine is not used in small animals and has not been widely evaluated in exotic species.

Medetomidine Medetomidine is approved for use as a sedative/analgesic in dogs. The drug has also been extensively evaluated in all domestic species and many exotic and zoological species. It is extremely selective for the alpha-2 receptor and binds it avidly. Atipamezole was developed as the specific antagonist for medetomidine for this reason.

Romifidine Romifidine is an alpha-2 adrenergic receptor agonist that is approved for use in horses. It has been evaluated in other species and appears to be relatively safe, but offers few advantages over other approved products. Some equine clinicians believe is it is a good sedative without causing excessive ataxia.

Dexmedetomidine Dexmedetomidine is the newest of the alpha-2 adrenergic agonists to be marketed to veterinarians. Unlike medetomidine, which is a racemic mixture of two stereoisomers, dexmedetomidine contains only the pure dextrorotatory enantiomer, which appears to be responsible for all of the clinically relevant properties of the drug. Due to the absence of the inactive levorotatory enantiomer, dexmedetomidine is twice as potent as medetomidine. It is currently marketed as a solution with half the strength of medetomidine, meaning that equivalent doses of dexmedetomidine and medetomidine have the same volume. The sedative, analgesic, and anesthetic-sparing effects of both drugs appear to be similar when administered at equivalent doses in dogs and cats (Ansah et al. 1998; Granholm et al. 2006, 2007; Kuusela et al. 2000). Hemodynamic side effects also appear similar. While it has been proposed that recoveries from dexmedetomidine may be faster compared with medetomidine due to the additional metabolic burden imposed by levome-detomidine, there is no current evidence to support this claim.

Alpha-2 Adrenergic Receptor Antagonists

One big advantage alpha-2 adrenoreceptor agonists have over other sedative/tranquilizers like acepromazine is reversibility. It is possible to administer an antagonist and within minutes animals will regain function and be able to be released. Antagonist administration will usually result in opposite hemodynamic effects (e.g., acute vasodilation and tachycardia), and they should not be administered in a cavalier fashion. Many of the difficulties (including some deaths) occur with reversal. Also, alpha-2 agonist-mediated analgesia is reversed, necessitating administration of other analgesic classes to animals in pain. Some species (e.g., domestic horses) are not routinely reversed because of the potential for uncontrollable activity and possible self-trauma.

Yohimbine Yohimbine is a plant-derived compound that has been used by humans for centuries because of its performance enhancing properties. It is relatively effective for reversing xylazine in horses, dogs, and cats, but is less effective in ruminants. Additionally, yohimbine has some stimulant actions that may result in excitation upon recovery. Yohimbine has not been effective at reversing newer agents like medetomidine.

Tolazoline Tolazoline was originally used as a therapy for human infants suffering from pulmonary hypertension. It is a relatively nonselective alpha-receptor blocker and is useful for reducing pulmonary vascular resistance. It is also effective at antagonizing xylazine sedation. It is most commonly used for equine and ruminant species. It appears more effective in ruminant species than yohimbine.

Atipamezole Atipamezole is the marketed antagonist for medetomidine and dexmedetomidine. It is effective at reversing all available alpha-2 adrenoreceptor agonists and its use is limited only by cost. It is relatively selective for alpha-2 adrenergic receptors and usually does not cause excessive stimulation, although excitation may occur. Atipamezole is approved for use in dogs; however, it is used in other species commonly. Under most circumstances, it is best given by the IM route except in emergency situations.

PHENOTHIAZINES AND BUTYROPHENONES

Introduction

The phenothiazines and butyrophenones produce an array of behavioral, autonomic, and endocrine effects and have been used clinically in numerous domestic and wild species. Their tranquilizing effects are mediated by antagonism of dopamine receptors (primarily the D2 subtype) located in the cerebral cortex, basal ganglia, and limbic system. In addition, other antidopamine effects are noted in the hypothalamus (increased prolactin secretion and impaired thermoregulation), brainstem (impaired vasomotor reflexes), and chemoreceptor trigger zone of the medulla (antiemesis). Both drug classes also have varying antagonistic effects at adrenergic (alpha-1 and alpha-2), serotonergic (5HT), muscarinic (M1), and histaminergic (H1) receptor systems. It is important to note that they do not possess any inherent analgesic properties and their effects are not reversible.

Acepromazine Acepromazine is the most widely used phenothiazine tranquilizer in veterinary medicine. In dogs and cats it is commonly combined with an opioid to produce a state historically referred to as "neuroleptanalgesia." Such combinations are suitable to provide chemical restraint for short, noninvasive procedures or as preanesthetic medication prior to induction of general anesthesia. Acepromazine administration in the preanesthetic period will cause dose-dependent reductions in both injectable and inhalant anesthetic requirements in these species. In horses and cattle, the drug is used primarily for its antianxiety effects. In susceptible pigs, acepromazine has been shown to prevent or reduce the onset of halothane-induced malignant hyperthermia. In certain wild and exotic species, the combination of acepromazine and the potent opioid etorphine (Large Animal Immobilon) has been used for immobilization and anesthesia.

Cardiovascular effects of acepromazine include decreases in mean arterial blood pressure in the range of 20–30% accompanied by dose-dependent reductions in stroke volume and cardiac output. Isoflurane, due to its potent vasodilatory effects, appears to potentiate acepromazine-induced hypotension. At clinically relevant doses, heart rate may not change appreciably or may increase slightly. At very high doses, bradycardia and sinoatrial block may occur. Acepromazine has also been shown to reduce the arrhythmogenic effects of epinephrine and halothane.

In general, effects on pulmonary function (i.e., oxygenation and ventilation) tend to be minimal in conscious animals, though respiratory rate may decrease somewhat. Acepromazine has been shown to dose-dependently decrease hematocrit by as much as 20–50% in dogs and horses due to splenic sequestration. This effect occurs within 30 minutes and appears to persist for at least 2 hours. The drug also decreases platelet aggregation but the clinical hemostatic significance of this appears minimal.

Regarding the gastrointestinal system, acepromazine has been shown to have antiemetic effects when administered 15 minutes prior to morphine, hydromorphone, or oxymorphone. Lower esophageal sphincter tone is reduced, which may lead to an increased risk of gastric reflux, though this has not been proven. Decreased gastrointestinal motility and delayed gastric emptying have been demonstrated in horses.

Renal blood flow and glomerular filtration rate appear to be well maintained in dogs receiving acepromazine and isoflurane. In cats under halothane anesthesia, urethral pressure has been shown to decrease by 20% with acepromazine administration. There are anecdotal reports of penile prolapse/priapism in stallions. The magnitude and duration of the protrusion appear to be dose-dependent, and this side effect appears to be mediated by alpha adrenergic antagonism. Also, because of its antihistaminergic effects, acepromazine is not suitable for allergic skin-testing.

Azaperone Azaperone is classified as a butyrophenone and its only approved indication is for control of aggression associated with mixing or regrouping of swine. It is also used as a preanesthetic agent in pigs and has clinical properties and side effects similar to acepromazine. In various wild and exotic species, azaperone is used in combination with potent opioids, such as etorphine or carfentanil, to produce immobilization or anesthesia.

REFERENCES

Aantaa R, Marjamaki A, Scheinin M. 1995. Molecular pharmacology of alpha 2-adrenoceptor subtypes. *Annals of Medicine* 27(4): 439–449.

Abdel el Motal SM, Sharp GW. 1985. Inhibition of glucose-induced insulin release by xylazine. *Endocrinology* 116(6): 2337–2340.

Algotsson L, Messeter K, Rosen I, et al. 1992. Effects of nitrous oxide on cerebral haemodynamics and metabolism during isoflurane anaesthesia in man. *Acta Anaesthesiologica Scandinavica* 36(1):46–52.

Alibhai HI, Clarke KW, Lee YH, et al. 1996. Cardiopulmonary effects of combinations of medetomidine hydrochloride and atropine sulphate in dogs. *The Veterinary Record* 138(1):11–13.

American College of Veterinary Anesthesiologists. 1996. Commentary and recommendations on control of waste anesthetic gases in the workplace. *Journal of the American Veterinary Medical Association* 209(1):75–77.

Ansah OB, Raekallio M, Vainio O. 1998. Comparison of three doses of dexmedetomidine with medetomidine in cats following intramuscular administration. *Journal of Veterinary Pharmacology and Therapeutics* 21:380–387.

Argentieri DC, Ritchie DM, Ferro MP, et al. 1994. Tepoxalin: a dual cyclooxygenase/5-lipoxygenase inhibitor of arachidonic acid metabolism with potent anti-inflammatory activity and a favorable gastrointestinal profile. *The Journal of Pharmacology and Experimental Therapeutics* 271:1399–1408.

Arifah AK, Lees P. 2002. Pharmacodynamics and pharmacokinetics of phenylbutazone in calves. *Journal of Veterinary Pharmacology and Therapeutics* 25:299–309.

Ballou LR, Botting RM, Goorha S, et al. 2000. Nociception in cyclooxygenase isozyme-deficient mice. *Proceedings of the National Academy of Sciences of the United States of America* 97: 10272–10276.

Barnhart MD, Hubbell JAE, Muir WW, et al. 2000. Pharmacokinetics, pharmacodynamics, and analgesic effects of morphine after rectal, intramuscular, and intravenous administration in dogs. *American Journal of Veterinary Research* 61:24–28.

Barter LS, Ilkiw JE, Pypendop BH, et al. 2004. Evaluation of the induction and recovery characteristics of anesthesia with desflurane in cats. *American Journal of Veterinary Research* 65(6): 748–751.

Bednarski RM, Gaynor JS, Muir WW 3rd. 1993. Vaporizer in circle for delivery of isoflurane to dogs. *Journal of the American Veterinary Medical Association* 202(6):943–948.

Bertolini A, Ottani A, Sandrini M. 2001. Dual acting anti-inflammatory drugs: a reappraisal. *Pharmacological Research* 44: 437–450.

Boidin MP. 1985. Serum levels of cortisol in man during etomidate, fentanyl and air anesthesia, compared with neurolept anesthesia. *Acta Anaesthesiologica Belgica* 36(2):79–87.

Borkowski R, Citino S, Bush M, et al. 2009. Surgical castration of subadult giraffe (Giraffa camelopardalis). *Journal of Zoo and Wildlife Medicine* 40(4):786–790.

Boston SE, Moens NM, Kruth SA, et al. 2003. Endoscopic evaluation of the gastroduodenal mucosa to determine the safety of short-term concurrent administration of meloxicam and dexamethasone in healthy dogs. *American Journal of Veterinary Research* 64:1369–1375.

Botting R. 2003. COX-1 and COX-3 inhibitors. *Thrombosis Research* 110:269–272.

Botting RM. 2000. Mechanism of action of acetaminophen: is there a cyclooxygenase 3? *Clinical Infectious Diseases: An Official Publication of the Infectious Diseases Society of America* 31(Suppl. 5):S202–S210.

Bowdle TA. 1998. Adverse effects of opioid agonists and agonist-antagonists in anaesthesia. *Drug Safety: An International Journal of Medical Toxicology and Drug Experience* 19:173–189.

Branson K. 2007. Injectable and alternative anesthetic techniques. In: *Lumb and Jones' Veterinary Anesthesia and Analgesia*, 4th ed. (WJ Tranquilli, JC Thurmon, KA Grimm, eds.), pp. 273–299. Ames: Blackwell Publishing.

Branson KR, Gross ME, Booth NH. 2001. Opioid agonists and antagonists. In: *Veterinary Pharmacology and Therapeutics* (HR Adams, ed.), p. 274. Ames: Iowa State Press.

Brearley JC, Dobson H, Jones RS. 1990. Investigations into the effect of two sedatives on the stress response in cattle. *Journal of Veterinary Pharmacology and Therapeutics* 13(4):367–377.

Briggs SL, Sneed K, Sawyer DC. 1998. Antinociceptive effects of oxymorphone-butorphanol-acepromazine combination in cats. *Veterinary Surgery* 27:466–472.

Budsberg SC, Johnston SA, Schwarz PD, et al. 1999. Efficacy of etodolac for the treatment of osteoarthritis of the hip joints in dogs. *Journal of the American Veterinary Medical Association* 214:206–210.

Carroll GL, Hooper RN, Boothe DM, et al. 1999. Pharmacokinetics of fentanyl after intravenous and transdermal administration in goats. *American Journal of Veterinary Research* 60:986–991.

Caulkett NA, Cribb PH, Haigh JC. 2000. Comparative cardiopulmonary effects of carfentanil-xylazine and medetomidine-ketamine used for immobilization of mule deer and mule deer/white-tailed deer hybrids. *Canadian Journal of Veterinary Research* 64:64–68.

Celly CS, McDonell WN, Young SS, et al. 1997. The comparative hypoxaemic effect of four alpha 2 adrenoceptor agonists (xylazine, romifidine, detomidine and medetomidine) in sheep. *Journal of Veterinary Pharmacology and Therapeutics* 20(6): 464–471.

Celly CS, Atwal OS, McDonell WN, et al. 1999. Histopathologic alterations induced in the lungs of sheep by use of alpha2-adrenergic receptor agonists. *American Journal of Veterinary Research* 60(2):154–161.

Chandrasekharan NV, Dai H, Roos KL, et al. 2002. COX-3, a cyclooxygenase-1 variant inhibited by acetaminophen and other analgesic/antipyretic drugs: cloning, structure, and expression. *Proceedings of the National Academy of Sciences of the United States of America* 99:13926–13931.

Chism JP, Rickert DE. 1996. The pharmacokinetics and extra-hepatic clearance of remifentanil, a short acting opioid agonist, in male beagle dogs during constant rate infusions. *Drug Metabolism and Disposition: The Biological Fate of Chemicals* 24: 34–40.

Chopra B, Giblett S, Little JG, et al. 2000. Cyclooxygenase-1 is a marker for a subpopulation of putative nociceptive neurons in rat dorsal root ganglia. *The European Journal of Neuroscience* 12: 911–920.

Christie MJ, Connor M, Vaughan CW, et al. 2000. Cellular actions of opioids and other analgesics: implications for synergism in pain relief. *Clinical and Experimental Pharmacology and Physiology* 27:520–523.

Clarke KW. 1999. Desflurane and sevoflurane. New volatile anesthetic agents. *The Veterinary Clinics of North America. Small Animal Practice* 29(3):793–810.

Collins LG, Tyler DE. 1984. Phenylbutazone toxicosis in the horse: a clinical study. *Journal of the American Veterinary Medical Association* 184:699–703.

Court MH, Greenblatt DJ. 1997. Molecular basis for deficient acetaminophen glucuronidation in cats. An interspecies comparison of enzyme kinetics in liver microsomes. *Biochemical Pharmacology* 53:1041–1047.

Cox SR, Lesman SP, Boucher JF, et al. 2010. The pharmacokinetics of mavacoxib, a long-acting COX-2 inhibitor, in young adult laboratory dogs. *Journal of Veterinary Pharmacology and Therapeutics* 33(5):461–470.

Cox SR, Liao S, Payne-Johnson M, et al. 2011. Population pharmacokinetics of mavacoxib in osteoarthritic dogs. *Journal of Veterinary Pharmacology and Therapeutics* 34(1):1–11.

Cushing A, McClean M. 2010. Use of thiafentanil-medetomidine for the induction of anesthesia in emus (*Dromaius novaehollandiae*) within a wild animal park. *Journal of Zoo and Wildlife Medicine* 41(2):234–241.

Daghfous R, el Aidli S, Sfaxi M, et al. 2003. Halothane-induced hepatitis. 8 case reports. *La Tunisie Medicale* 81(11):874–878.

Davidson G. 2001. To benzoate or not to benzoate: cats are the question. *International Journal of Pharmaceutical Compounding* 5(2):89–90.

DeBacker P, Braeckman R, Belpaire F. 1980. Bioavailability and pharmacokinetics of phenylbutazone in the cow. *Journal of Veterinary Pharmacology and Therapeutics* 3:29–33.

Dobromylskyj P. 1996. Cardiovascular changes associated with anaesthesia induced by medetomidine combined with ketamine in cats. *The Journal of Small Animal Practice* 37: 169–172.

Dodam JR, Kruse-Elliott KT, Aucoin DP, et al. 1990. Duration of etomidate-induced adrenocortical suppression during surgery in dogs. *American Journal of Veterinary Research* 51(5): 786–788.

Dodam JR, Cohn LA, Durham HE, et al. 2004. Cardiopulmonary effects of medetomidine, oxymorphone, or butorphanol in selegiline-treated dogs. *Veterinary Anaesthesia and Analgesia* 31:129–137.

Doenicke A, Roizen MF, Hoernecke R, et al. 1997. Haemolysis after etomidate: comparison of propylene glycol and lipid formulations. *British Journal of Anaesthesia* 79(3):386–388.

Doerning BJ, Brammer DW, Chrisp CE, et al. 1992. Nephrotoxicity of tiletamine in New Zealand white rabbits. *Laboratory Animal Science* 42(3):267–269.

Doherty TJ, Geiser DR, Rohrbach BW. 1997. Effect of acepromazine and butorphanol on halothane minimum alveolar concentration in ponies. *Equine Veterinary Journal* 29:374–376.

Driessen B, Zarucco L, Steffey EP, et al. 2002. Serum fluoride concentrations, biochemical and histopathological changes associated with prolonged sevoflurane anaesthesia in horses. *Journal of Veterinary Medicine. A, Physiology, Pathology, Clinical Medicine* 49(7):337–347.

DuBois RN, Abramson SB, Crofford L, et al. 1998. Cyclooxygenase in biology and disease. *The FASEB Journal* 12:1063–1073.

Dunn AM, Buckley BM. 1986. Non-steroidal anti-inflammatory drugs and the kidney. *British Medical Journal* 293:202–203.

Dutta NK, Annadurai S, Mazumdar K, et al. 2007. Potential management of resistant microbial infections with a novel non-antibiotic: the anti-inflammatory drug diclofenac sodium. *International Journal of Antimicrobial Agents* 30(3):242–249.

Egger CM, Duke T, Archer J, et al. 1998. Comparison of plasma fentanyl concentrations by using three transdermal fentanyl patch sizes in dogs. *Veterinary Surgery* 27:159–166.

Egger CM, Glerum LE, Allen SW, et al. 2003. Plasma fentanyl concentrations in awake cats and cats undergoing anesthesia and ovariohysterectomy using transdermal administration. *Veterinary Anaesthesia and Analgesia* 30:229–236.

el Bindary EM, Abu el-Nasr LM. 2001. Urodynamic changes following intrathecal administration of morphine and fentanyl to dogs. *Eastern Mediterranean Health Journal* 7:189–196.

Fahnenstich H, Steffan J, Kau N, et al. 2000. Fentanyl-induced chest wall rigidity and laryngospasm in preterm and term infants. *Critical Care Medicine* 28:836–839.

Faura CC, Collins SL, Moore RA, et al. 1998. Systematic review of factors affecting the ratios of morphine and its major metabolites. *Pain* 74:43–53.

Fields HL, Emson PC, Leigh BK, et al. 1980. Multiple opiate receptor sites on primary afferent fibres. *Nature* 284:351–353.

Fisher RJ. 1984. A field trial of ketamine anaesthesia in the horse. *Equine Veterinary Journal* 16:176–179.

FitzGerald GA, Patrono C. 2001. The coxibs, selective inhibitors of cyclooxygenase-2. *The New England Journal of Medicine* 345:433–442.

Food and Drug Administration: Center for Veterinary Medicine (FDA-CVM). 2005. Zubrin (Tepoxalin) Freedom of Information (FOI) Summary.

Food and Drug Administration: Center for Veterinary Medicine (FDA-CVM). 2011. Freedom of Information Summary for Firocoxib. http://www.fda.gov (accessed February 10, 2014).

Fosslien E. 2000. Molecular pathology of cyclooxygenase-2 in neoplasia. *Annals of Clinical and Laboratory Science* 30:3–21.

Franks NP, Lieb WR. 1984. Do general anaesthetics act by competitive binding to specific receptors? *Nature* 310 (5978):599–601.

Franks NP, Lieb WR. 2004. Seeing the light: protein theories of general anesthesia. 1984. *Anesthesiology* 101(1):235–237.

Franks JN, Boothe HW, Taylor L, et al. 2000. Evaluation of transdermal fentanyl patches for analgesia in cats undergoing onychectomy. *Journal of the American Veterinary Medical Association* 217:1013–1020.

Gellasch KL, Kruse-Elliott KT, Osmond CS, et al. 2002. Comparison of transdermal administration of fentanyl versus intramuscular administration of butorphanol for analgesia after onychectomy in cats. *Journal of the American Veterinary Medical Association* 220:1020–1024.

Gierse JK, Staten NR, Casperson GF, et al. 2002. Cloning, expression, and selective inhibition of canine cyclooxygenase-1 and cyclooxygenase-2. *Veterinary Therapeutics: Research in Applied Veterinary Medicine* 3:270–280.

Gilberto DB, Motzel SL, Das SR. 2003. Postoperative pain management using fentanyl patches in dogs. *Contemporary Topics in Laboratory Animal Science* 42:21–26.

Gingerich DA, Baggot JD, Yeary RA. 1975. Pharmacokinetics and dosage of aspirin in cattle. *Journal of the American Veterinary Medical Association* 167:945–948.

Glaser K, Sung ML, O'Neill K, et al. 1995. Etodolac selectively inhibits human prostaglandin G/H synthase 2 (PGHS-2) versus human PGHS-1. *European Journal of Pharmacology* 281: 107–111.

Gorman AL, Elliott KJ, Inturrisi CE. 1997. The d- and l-isomers of methadone bind to the non-competitive site on the N-methyl-D-aspartate (NMDA) receptor in rat forebrain and spinal cord. *Neuroscience Letters* 223:5–8.

Granholm M, McKusick BC, Westerholm FC, et al. 2006. Evaluation of the clinical efficacy and safety of dexmedetomidine or medetomidine in cats and their reversal with atipamazole. *Veterinary Anaesthesia and Analgesia* 33:214–223.

Granholm M, McKusick BC, Westerholm FC, et al. 2007. Evaluation of the clinical efficacy and safety of intramuscular and intravenous doses of dexmedetomidine and medetomidine in dogs and their reversal with atipamezole. *The Veterinary Record* 160:891–897.

Grimm JB, Grimm KA, Kneller SK, et al. 2001. The effect of a combination of medetomidine-butorphanol and medetomidine, butorphanol, atropine on glomerular filtration rate in dogs. *Veterinary Radiology and Ultrasound* 42(5):458–462.

Grobler D, Bush M, Jessup D, et al. 2001. Anaesthesia of gemsbok (Oryx gazella) with a combination of A3080, medetomidine and ketamine. *Journal of the South African Veterinary Association* 72(2):81–83.

Gutstein HB, Akil H. 2001. Opioid analgesics. In: *Goodman and Gilman's: The Pharmacological Basis of Therapeutics* (JG Harman, LE Limbird, A Goodman Gilman, eds.), p. 569. New York: McGraw-Hill.

Harris RC. 2000. Cyclooxygenase-2 in the kidney. *Journal of the American Society of Nephrology* 11:2387–2394.

Harrison LM, Kastin AJ, Zadina JE. 1998. Opiate tolerance and dependence: receptors, G-proteins, and antiopiates. *Peptides* 19:1603–1630.

Heinonen EH, Myllyla V. 1998. Safety of selegiline (deprenyl) in the treatment of Parkinson's disease. *Drug Safety: An International Journal of Medical Toxicology and Drug Experience* 19: 11–22.

Hellyer PW, Bai L, Supon J, et al. 2003. Comparison of opioid and alpha-2 adrenergic receptor binding in horse and dog brain using radioligand autoradiography. *Veterinary Anaesthesia and Analgesia* 30:172–182.

Hikasa Y, Akiba T, Iino Y, et al. 1992. Central alpha-adrenoceptor subtypes involved in the emetic pathway in cats. *European Journal of Pharmacology* 229(2–3):241–251.

Hoffman WE, Charbel FT, Edelman G, et al. 1995. Nitrous oxide added to isoflurane increases brain artery blood flow and low frequency brain electrical activity. *Journal of Neurosurgical Anesthesiology* 7(2):82–88.

Hoke JF, Cunningham F, James MK, et al. 1997. Comparative pharmacokinetics and pharmacodynamics of remifentanil, its principle metabolite (GR90291) and alfentanil in dogs. *The Journal of Pharmacology and Experimental Therapeutics* 281: 226–232.

Horster M, Kemler BJ, Valtin H. 1971. Intracortical distribution of number and volume of glomeruli during postnatal maturation in the dog. *The Journal of Clinical Investigation* 50:796–800.

Hudson N, Balsitis M, Everitt S, et al. 1993. Enhanced gastric mucosal leukotriene B4 synthesis in patients taking nonsteroidal anti-inflammatory drugs. *Gut* 34:742–747.

Hussain I, Khan MZ, Khan A, et al. 2008. Toxicological effects of diclofenac in four avian species. *Avian Pathology: Journal of the W.V.P.A* 37(3):315–321.

Ilkiw JE, Pascoe PJ, Fisher LD. 1997. Effect of alfentanil on the minimum alveolar concentration of isoflurane in cats. *American Journal of Veterinary Research* 58:1274–1279.

Ilkiw JE, Pascoe PJ, Tripp LD. 2002. Effects of morphine, butorphanol, buprenorphine, and U50488H on the minimum alveolar concentration of isoflurane in cats. *American Journal of Veterinary Research* 63:1198–202.

Imig JD. 2000. Eicosanoid regulation of the renal vasculature. *American Journal of Physiology—Renal Physiology* 279:F965–F981.

Inturrisi CE. 2002. Clinical pharmacology of opioids for pain. *The Clinical Journal of Pain* 18:S3–S13.

Jain T, Koley KM, Vadlamudi VP, et al. 2009. Diclofenac-induced biochemical and histopathological changes in white leghorn birds (Gallus domesticus). *Indian Journal of Pharmacology* 41(5): 237–241.

Janecka A, Fichna J, Janecki T. 2004. Opioid receptors and their ligands. *Current Topics in Medicinal Chemistry* 4:1–17.

Jayakumar K, Mohan K, Swamy HD, et al. 2010. Study of nephrotoxic potential of acetaminophen in birds. *Toxicology International* 17(2):86–89.

Jones RM, Detmer M, Hill AB, et al. 1981. Incidence of choledochoduodenal sphincter spasm during fentanyl-supplemented anesthesia. *Anesthesia and Analgesia* 60:638–640.

Kay-Mugford P, Benn SJ, LaMarre J, et al. 2000. In vitro effects of nonsteroidal anti-inflammatory drugs on cyclooxygenase activity in dogs. *American Journal of Veterinary Research* 61:802–810.

Kay-Mugford PA, Grimm KA, Weingarten AJ, et al. 2004. Effect of preoperative administration of tepoxalin on hemostasis, hepatic and renal function in dogs. *Veterinary Therapeutics: Research in Applied Veterinary Medicine* 5:120–127.

Kearns KS, Swenson B, Ramsay EC. 2000. Oral induction of anesthesia with droperidol and transmucosal carfentanil citrate in chimpanzees (Pan troglodytes). *Journal of Zoo and Wildlife Medicine* 31:185–189.

Kharasch ED, Schroeder JL, Sheffels P, et al. 2005. Influence of sevoflurane on the metabolism and renal effects of compound A in rats. *Anesthesiology* 103(6):1183–1188.

Kieffer BL. 1999. Opioids: first lessons from knockout mice. *Trends in Pharmacological Sciences* 20:19–26.

Kilgallon CP, Lamberski N, Larsen RS. 2010. Comparison of thiafenantil-xylazine and carfentanil-xylazine for immobilization of gemsbok (Oryx gazella). *Journal of Zoo and Wildlife Medicine* 41(3):567–571.

Kirchner T, Aparicio B, Argentieri DC, et al. 1997a. Effects of tepoxalin, a dual inhibitor of cyclooxygenase/5-lipoxygenase, on events associated with NSAID-induced gastrointestinal inflammation. *Prostaglandins, Leukotrienes, and Essential Fatty Acids* 56:417–423.

Kirchner T, Argentieri DC, Barbone AG, et al. 1997b. Evaluation of the antiinflammatory activity of a dual cyclooxygenase-2 selective/5-lipoxygenase inhibitor, RWJ 63556, in a canine model of inflammation. *The Journal of Pharmacology and Experimental Therapeutics* 282:1094–1101.

Ko JCH, Lange DN, Mandsager RE, et al. 2000. Effects of butorphanol and carprofen on the minimal alveolar concentration of isoflurane in dogs. *Journal of the American Veterinary Medical Association*;217:1025–1028.

Kohrs R, Durieux ME. 1998. New uses for ketamine. *Anesthesia and Analgesia* 87:1186–1193.

Kramer S, Nolte I, Jochle W. 1996. Clinical comparison of medetomidine with xylazine/l-methadone in dogs. *The Veterinary Record* 138:128–133.

Kuipers PW, Kamphuis ET, van Venrooij GE, et al. 2004. Intrathecal opioids and lower urinary tract function: a urodynamic evaluation. *Anesthesiology* 100:1497–1503.

Kuusela E, Raekallio M, Anttila M, et al. 2000. Clinical effects and pharmacokinetics of medetomidine and its enantiomers in dogs. *Journal of Veterinary Pharmacology and Therapeutics* 23: 15–20.

Laredo FG, Sanchez-Valverde MA, Cantalapiedra AG, et al. 1998. Efficacy of the Komesaroff anaesthetic machine for delivering isoflurane to dogs. *The Veterinary Record* 143(16):437–440.

Lascelles BD, Robertson SA. 2004. Antinociceptive effects of hydromorphone, butorphanol, or the combination in cats. *Journal of Veterinary Internal Medicine* 18:190–195.

Lee DD, Papich MG, Hardie EM. 2000. Comparison of pharmacokinetics of fentanyl after intravenous and transdermal administration in cats. *American Journal of Veterinary Research* 61:672–677.

Lee HK, Wang SC. 1975. Mechanism of morphine-induced miosis in the dog. *The Journal of Pharmacology and Experimental Therapeutics* 192:415–431.

Lerman J, Robinson S, Willis MM, et al. 1983. Anesthetic requirements for halothane in young children 0–1 month and 1–6 months of age. *Anesthesiology* 59(5):421–424.

Lerman J, Sikich N, Kleinman S, et al. 1994. The pharmacology of sevoflurane in infants and children. *Anesthesiology* 80(4):814–824.

Lipsky PE. 1999. Specific COX-2 inhibitors in arthritis, oncology, and beyond: where is the science headed? *The Journal of Rheumatology* 26(Suppl. 56):25–30.

Lipsky PE, Brooks P, Crofford LJ, et al. 2000. Unresolved issues in the role of cyclooxygenase-2 in normal physiologic processes and disease. *Archives of Internal Medicine* 160:913–920.

Livingston A. 2000. Mechanism of action of nonsteroidal anti-inflammatory drugs. *The Veterinary Clinics of North America. Small Animal Practice* 30:773–781, vi.

Lobetti RG, Joubert KE. 2000. Effect of administration of nonsteroidal anti-inflammatory drugs before surgery on renal function in clinically normal dogs. *American Journal of Veterinary Research* 61:1501–1507.

MacAllister CG, Morgan SJ, Borne AT, et al. 1993. Comparison of adverse effects of phenylbutazone, flunixin meglumine, and ketoprofen in horses. *Journal of the American Veterinary Medical Association* 202:71–77.

Machin KL, Caulkett NA. 1998. Cardiopulmonary effects of propofol and a medetomidine-midazolam-ketamine combination in mallard ducks. *American Journal of Veterinary Research* 59(5):598–602.

Malmberg AB, Yaksh TL. 1992. Antinociceptive actions of spinal nonsteroidal anti-inflammatory agents on the formalin test in the rat. *The Journal of Pharmacology and Experimental Therapeutics* 263:136–146.

Mama KR, Steffey EP, Withrow SJ. 2000. Use of orally administered carfentanil prior to isoflurane-induced anesthesia in a Kodiak brown bear. *Journal of the American Veterinary Medical Association* 217:546–549, 503.

Mathews KA, Pettifer G, Foster RF. 1999. A comparison of the safety and efficacy of meloxicam to ketoprofen and butorphanol for control of post-operative pain associated with soft tissue surgery in dogs. Proceedings of the Symposium on Recent Advances in Non-Steroidal Anti-Inflammatory Therapy in Small Animals, p. 67. Paris.

Matthews NS, Lindsay SL. 1990. Effect of low-dose butorphanol on halothane minimum alveolar concentration in ponies. *Equine Veterinary Journal* 22:325–327.

Maxwell LK, Thomasy SM, Slovis N, et al. 2003. Pharmacokinetics of fentanyl following intravenous and transdermal administration in horses. *Equine Veterinary Journal* 35:484–490.

Maze M, Tranquilli W. 1991. Alpha-2 adrenoceptor agonists: defining the role in clinical anesthesia. *Anesthesiology* 74(3):581–605.

McCann ME, Andersen DR, Zhang D, et al. 2004. In vitro effects and in vivo efficacy of a novel cyclooxygenase-2 inhibitor in dogs with experimentally induced synovitis. *American Journal of Veterinary Research* 65:503–512.

McCormack K. 1994. Non-steroidal anti-inflammatory drugs and spinal nociceptive processing. *Pain* 59:9–43.

McKellar QA, Pearson T, Bogan JA. 1990. Pharmacokinetics, tolerance and serum thromboxane inhibition of carprofen in the dog. *The Journal of Small Animal Practice* 31:443–448.

McKellar QA, Delatour P, Lees P. 1994a. Stereospecific pharmacodynamics and pharmacokinetics of carprofen in the dog. *Journal of Veterinary Pharmacology and Therapeutics* 17:447–454.

McKellar QA, Lees P, Gettinby G. 1994b. Pharmacodynamics of tolfenamic acid in dogs. Evaluation of dose response relationships. *European Journal of Pharmacology* 253:191–200.

Mendes GM, Selmi AL. 2003. Use of a combination of propofol and fentanyl, alfentanil, or sufentanil for total intravenous anesthesia in cats. *Journal of the American Veterinary Medical Association* 223:1608–1613.

Mercadante S, Arcuri E. 2004. Opioids and renal function. *The Journal of Pain* 5:2–19.

Michelsen LG, Salmenpera M, Hug CC Jr, et al. 1996. Anesthetic potency of remifentanil in dogs. *Anesthesiology* 84:865–872.

Mielck F, Stephan H, Buhre W, et al. 1998. Effects of 1 MAC desflurane on cerebral metabolism, blood flow and carbon dioxide reactivity in humans. *British Journal of Anaesthesia* 81(2):155–160.

Mielck F, Stephan H, Weyland A, Sonntag H. 1999. Effects of one minimum alveolar anesthetic concentration sevoflurane on cerebral metabolism, blood flow, and CO2 reactivity in cardiac patients. *Anesthesia and Analgesia* 89(2):364–369.

Mihic SJ, Ye Q, Wick MJ, et al. 1997. Sites of alcohol and volatile anaesthetic action on GABA(A) and glycine receptors. *Nature* 389(6649):385–389.

Miller BF, Muller LI, Storms TN, et al. 2003. A comparison of carfentanil/xylazine and Telazol (R)/xylazine for immobilization of white-tailed deer. *Journal of Wildlife Diseases* 39:851–858.

Millis DL, Weigel JP, Moyers T, et al. 2002. Effect of deracoxib, a new COX-2 inhibitor, on the prevention of lameness induced by chemical synovitis in dogs. *Veterinary Therapeutics: Research in Applied Veterinary Medicine* 3:453–464.

Moon PF. 1994. Acute toxicosis in two dogs associated with etomidate-propylene glycol infusion. *Laboratory Animal Science* 44(6):590–594.

Moon PF. 1997. Cortisol suppression in cats after induction of anesthesia with etomidate, compared with ketamine-diazepam combination. *American Journal of Veterinary Research* 58(8):868–871.

Moran TD, Abdulla FA, Smith PA. 2000. Cellular neurophysiological actions of nociceptin/orphanin FQ. *Peptides* 21:969–976.

Moreau M, Daminet S, Martel-Pelletier J, et al. 2005. Superiority of the gastroduodenal safety profile of licofelone over rofecoxib, a COX-2 selective inhibitor, in dogs. *Journal of Veterinary Pharmacology and Therapeutics* 28:81–86.

Morham SG, Langenbach R, Loftin CD, et al. 1995. Prostaglandin synthase 2 gene disruption causes severe renal pathology in the mouse. *Cell* 83:473–482.

Mortenson J, Bechert U. 2001. Carfentanil citrate used as an oral anesthetic agent for brown bears (*Ursus arctos*). *Journal of Zoo and Wildlife Medicine* 32:217–221.

Muir WW 3rd, Gadawski JE. 1998. Respiratory depression and apnea induced by propofol in dogs. *American Journal of Veterinary Research* 59(2):157–161.

Muller P, Vogtmann C. 2000. Three cases with different presentation of fentanyl-induced muscle rigidity: a rare problem in intensive care of neonates. *American Journal of Perinatology* 17:23–26.

Naidoo V, Wolter K, Cuthbert R, et al. 2009. Veterinary diclofenac threatens Africa's endangered vulture species. *Regulatory Toxicology and Pharmacology* 53(3):205–208.

Natalini CC, Robinson EP. 2000. Evaluation of the analgesic effects of epidurally administered morphine, alfentanil, butorphanol, tramadol, and U50488H in horses. *American Journal of Veterinary Research* 61:1579–1586.

Neuberger J. 1998. Halothane hepatitis. *European Journal of Gastroenterology and Hepatology* 10(8):631–633.

Niedfeldt RL, Robertson SA. 2006. Postanesthetic hyperthermia in cats: a retrospective comparison between hydromorphone and buprenorphine. *Veterinary Anaesthesia and Analgesia* 33(6): 381–389.

Novartis Animal Health USA. 2004. Deracoxib Pakage Insert.

Oaks JL, Gilbert M, Virani MZ, et al. 2004. Diclofenac residues as the cause of vulture population decline in Pakistan. *Nature* 427(6975):630–633.

Ochi T, Motoyama Y, Goto T. 2000. The analgesic effect profile of FR122047, a selective cyclooxygenase-1 inhibitor, in chemical nociceptive models. *European Journal of Pharmacology* 391: 49–54.

Osman TE, Nicholson T. 1991. Alpha-2 adrenoreceptors mediate clonidine-induced hypoinsulinaemia in sheep. *Journal of Veterinary Pharmacology and Therapeutics* 14(3):293–299.

Page SW, Maddison JE. 2002. Principles of clinical pharmacology. In: *Small Animal Clinical Pharmacology* (J Maddison, S Page, D Church, eds.), pp. 1–26. London: W.B. Saunders.

Pascoe PJ, Taylor PM. 2003. Effects of dopamine antagonists on alfentanil-induced locomotor activity in horses. *Veterinary Anaesthesia and Analgesia* 30:165–171.

Pascoe PJ, Black WD, Claxton JM, et al. 1991. The pharmacokinetics and locomotor activity of alfentanil in the horse. *Journal of Veterinary Pharmacology and Therapeutics* 14:317–325.

Pascoe PJ, Steffey EP, Black WD, et al. 1993. Evaluation of the effect of alfentanil on the minimum alveolar concentration of halothane in horses. *American Journal of Veterinary Research* 54: 1327–1332.

Pascoe PJ, Ilkiw JE, Fisher LD. 1997. Cardiovascular effects of equipotent isoflurane and alfentanil/isoflurane minimum alveolar concentration multiple in cats. *American Journal of Veterinary Research* 58:1267–1273.

Petersson I, Nilsson G, Hansson BG, et al. 1987. Water intoxication associated with non-steroidal anti-inflammatory drug therapy. *Acta Medica Scandinavica* 221:221–223.

Pettifer GR, Hosgood G. 2003. The effect of rectal temperature on perianesthetic serum concentrations of transdermally administered fentanyl in cats anesthetized with isoflurane. *American Journal of Veterinary Research* 64:1557–1561.

Pibarot P, Dupuis J, Grisneaux E, et al. 1997. Comparison of ketoprofen, oxymorphone hydrochloride, and butorphanol in the treatment of postoperative pain in dogs. *Journal of the American Veterinary Medical Association* 211:438–444.

Pollock CG, Ramsay EC. 2003. Serial immobilization of a Brazilian tapir (Tapirus terrestrus) with oral detomidine and oral carfentanil. *Journal of Zoo and Wildlife Medicine* 34:408–410.

Posner LP, Gleed RD, Erb HN, et al. 2007. Post-anesthetic hyperthermia in cats. *Veterinary Anaesthesia and Analgesia* 34(1): 40–47.

Posner LP, Pavuk AA, Rokshar JL, et al. 2010. Effects of opioids and anesthetic drugs on body temperature in cats. *Veterinary Anaesthesia and Analgesia* 37(1):35–43.

Poulsen Nautrep B, Justus C. 1999. Effects of some veterinary NSAIDs on ex vivo thromboxane production and in vivo urine output in the dog. Proceedings of the Symposium on Recent Advances in Non-Steroidal Anti-Inflammatory Therapy in Small Animals, p. 25. Paris.

Priano LL, Vatner SF. 1981. Generalized cardiovascular and regional hemodynamic effects of meperidine in conscious dogs. *Anesthesia and Analgesia* 60:649–654.

Pypendop BH, Verstegen JP. 1998. Hemodynamic effects of medetomidine in the dog: a dose titration study. *Veterinary Surgery* 27(6):612–622.

Quandt JE, Raffe MR, Robinson EP. 1994. Butorphanol does not reduce the minimum alveolar concentration of halothane in dogs. *Veterinary Surgery* 23:156–159.

Radnay PA, Duncalf D, Novakovic M, et al. 1984. Common bile duct pressure changes after fentanyl, morphine, meperidine, butorphanol, and naloxone. *Anesthesia and Analgesia* 63:441–444.

Rainsford KD. 1992. Mechanisms of NSAID-induced ulcerogenesis: structural properties of drugs, focus on the microvascular factors, and novel approaches for gastro-intestinal protection. *Acta Physiologica Hungarica* 80:23–38.

Ramdohr S, Bornemann H, Plotz J, et al. 2001. Immobilization of free-ranging adult male southern elephant seals with Immobilon (TM) (etorphine/acepromacine) and ketamine. *South African Journal of Wildlife Research* 31:135–140.

Reed S. 2002. Nonsteroidal anti-inflammatory drug-induced duodenal ulceration and perforation in a mature rottweiler. *The Canadian Veterinary Journal. la Revue Veterinaire Canadienne* 43: 971–972.

Reuter BK, Asfaha S, Buret A, et al. 1996. Exacerbation of inflammation-associated colonic injury in rat through inhibition of cyclooxygenase-2. *The Journal of Clinical Investigation* 98:2076–2085.

Ricketts AP, Lundy KM, Seibel SB. 1998. Evaluation of selective inhibition of canine cyclooxygenase 1 and 2 by carprofen and other nonsteroidal anti-inflammatory drugs. *American Journal of Veterinary Research* 59:1441–1446.

Ripamonti C, Dickerson ED. 2001. Strategies for the treatment of cancer pain in the new millennium. *Drugs* 61:955–977.

Roald OK, Forsman M, Heier MS, et al. 1991. Cerebral effects of nitrous oxide when added to low and high concentrations of isoflurane in the dog. *Anesthesia and Analgesia* 72(1):75–79.

Robertson SA, Taylor PM, Lascelles BDX, et al. 2003a. Changes in thermal threshold response in eight cats after administration of buprenorphine, butorphanol and morphine. *The Veterinary Record* 153:462–465.

Robertson SA, Taylor PM, Sear JW. 2003b. Systemic uptake of buprenorphine by cats after oral mucosal administration. *The Veterinary Record* 152:675–678.

Robinson TM, Kruse-Elliott KT, Markel MD, et al. 1999. A comparison of transdermal fentanyl versus epidural morphine for analgesia in dogs undergoing major orthopedic surgery. *Journal of the American Animal Hospital Association* 35:95–100.

Roffe TJ, Coffin K, Berger J. 2001. Survival and immobilizing moose with carfentanil and xylazine. *Wildlife Society Bulletin* 29:1140–1146.

Saleh N, Aoki M, Shimada T, et al. 2005. Renal effects of medetomidine in isoflurane-anesthetized dogs with special reference to its diuretic action. *The Journal of Veterinary Medical Science* 67(5):461–465.

Sanhouri AA, Jones RS, Dobson H. 1992. Effects of xylazine on the stress response to transport in male goats. *The British Veterinary Journal* 148(2):119–128.

Sawyer DC, Rech RH, Durham RA, et al. 1991. Dose response to butorphanol administered subcutaneously to increase visceral nociceptive threshold in dogs. *American Journal of Veterinary Research* 52:1826–1830.

Schmassmann A, Peskar BM, Stettler C, et al. 1998. Effects of inhibition of prostaglandin endoperoxide synthase-2 in chronic gastro-intestinal ulcer models in rats. *British Journal of Pharmacology* 123:795–804.

Sellon DC, Monroe VL, Roberts MC, et al. 2001. Pharmacokinetics and adverse effects of butorphanol administered by single intravenous injection or continuous intravenous infusion in horses. *American Journal of Veterinary Research* 62:183–189.

Serhan CN, Chiang N. 2004. Novel endogenous small molecules as the checkpoint controllers in inflammation and resolution: entree for resoleomics. *Rheumatic Diseases Clinics of North America* 30:69–95.

Serhan CN, Hong S, Gronert K, et al. 2002. Resolvins: a family of bioactive products of omega-3 fatty acid transformation circuits initiated by aspirin treatment that counter proinflammation signals. *The Journal of Experimental Medicine* 196:1025–1037.

Sheffels P, Schroeder JL, Altuntas TG, et al. 2004. Role of cytochrome P4503A in cysteine S-conjugates sulfoxidation and the nephrotoxicity of the sevoflurane degradation product fluoromethyl-2,2-difluoro-1-(trifluoromethyl)vinyl ether (compound A) in rats. *Chemical Research in Toxicology* 17(9): 1177–1189.

Short CE. 1991. Effects of anticholinergic treatment on the cardiac and respiratory systems in dogs sedated with medetomidine. *The Veterinary Record* 129(14):310–313.

Silverstein FE, Faich G, Goldstein JL, et al. 2000. Gastrointestinal toxicity with celecoxib vs nonsteroidal anti-inflammatory drugs for osteoarthritis and rheumatoid arthritis: the CLASS study: a randomized controlled trial. Celecoxib Long-term Arthritis Safety Study. *JAMA: The Journal of the American Medical Association* 284:1247–1255.

Sinclair M, Mealey KL, Mathews NS, et al. 2003. The pharmacokinetics of meloxicam in horses. Proceedings of the 8th World Congress of Veterinary Anesthesia, p. 112. Knoxville, TN.

Smalley WE, DuBois RN. 1997. Colorectal cancer and nonsteroidal anti-inflammatory drugs. *Advances in Pharmacology* 39: 1–20.

Smith AP, Lee NM. 2003. Opioid receptor interactions: local and nonlocal, symmetric and asymmetric, physical and functional. *Life Sciences* 73:1873–1893.

Smith LJ, Yu JKA, Bjorling DE, et al. 2001. Effects of hydromorphone or oxymorphone, with or without acepromazine, on preanesthetic sedation, physiologic values, and histamine release in dogs. *Journal of the American Veterinary Medical Association* 218:1101–1105.

Smith MT. 2000. Neuroexcitatory effects of morphine and hydromorphone: evidence implicating the 3-glucuronide metabolites. *Clinical and Experimental Pharmacology and Physiology* 27:524–528.

Smith PA, Moran TD. 2001. The nociceptin receptor as a potential target in drug design. *Drug News & Perspectives* 14: 335–345.

Snow DH, Douglas TA, Thompson H, et al. 1981. Phenylbutazone toxicosis in equidae: a biochemical and pathophysiological study. *American Journal of Veterinary Research* 42:1754–1759.

Sporer KA. 1995. The serotonin syndrome. Implicated drugs, pathophysiology and management. *Drug Safety: An International Journal of Medical Toxicology and Drug Experience* 13: 94–104.

Steffey EP, Mama RM. 2007. Inhalation anesthetics. In: *Lumb and Jones' Veterinary Anesthesia and Analgesia*, 4th ed. (WJ Tranquilli, JT Thurmon, KA Grimm, eds.), pp. 355–394. Ames: Blackwell.

Stein C. 1993. Peripheral mechanisms of opioid analgesia. *Anesthesia and Analgesia* 76:182–191.

Stein C. 1995. The control of pain in peripheral tissue by opioids. *The New England Journal of Medicine* 332:1685–1690.

Stein C, Yassouridis A. 1997. Peripheral morphine analgesia. *Pain* 71:119–121.

Stein C, Hassan AH, Lehrberger K, et al. 1993. Local analgesic effect of endogenous opioid peptides. *Lancet* 342:321–324.

Stein C, Pfluger M, Yassouridis A, et al. 1996. No tolerance to peripheral morphine analgesia in presence of opioid expression in inflamed synovia. *The Journal of Clinical Investigation* 98: 793–799.

Stein C, Machelska H, Schafer M. 2001. Peripheral analgesic and antiinflammatory effects of opioids. *Zeitschrift fur Rheumatologie* 60:416–424.

Stein C, Schafer M, Machelska H. 2003. Attacking pain at its source: new perspectives on opioids. *Nature Medicine* 9: 1003–1008.

Stephan DD, Vestre WA, Stiles J, et al. 2003. Changes in intraocular pressure and pupil size following intramuscular administration of hydromorphone hydrochloride and acepromazine in clinically normal dogs. *Veterinary Ophthalmology* 6:73–76.

Stoelting RK. 1999. Opioid agonists and antagonists. In: *Pharmacology and Physiology in Anesthetic Practice* (RK Stoelting, ed.), p. 77. Philadelphia: Lippincott Williams and Wilkins.

Stone PA, Macintyre PE, Jarvis DA. 1993. Norpethidine toxicity and patient controlled analgesia. *British Journal of Anaesthesia* 71:738–740.

Taggart MA, Senacha KR, Green RE, et al. 2007. Diclofenac residues in carcasses of domestic ungulates available to vultures in India. *Environment International* 33(6):759–765.

Takada K, Tonner PH, Maze M. 1999. Meperidine functions as an alpha2B adrenoceptor agonist. *Anesthesiology* 91:U363.

Takada K, Clark DJ, Davies MF, et al. 2002. Meperidine exerts agonist activity at the alpha(2B)-adrenoceptor subtype. *Anesthesiology* 96:1420–1426.

Taylor PM, Robertson SA, Dixon MJ, et al. 2001. Morphine, pethidine and buprenorphine disposition in the cat. *Journal of Veterinary Pharmacology and Therapeutics* 24:391–398.

Taylor RH, Lerman J. 1991. Minimum alveolar concentration of desflurane and hemodynamic responses in neonates, infants, and children. *Anesthesiology* 75(6):975–979.

Thompson JR, Kersting KW, Hsu WH. 1991. Antagonistic effect of atipamezole on xylazine-induced sedation, bradycardia, and ruminal atony in calves. *American Journal of Veterinary Research* 52(8):1265–1268.

Tissot TA. 2003. Probable meperidine-induced serotonin syndrome in a patient with a history of fluoxetine use. *Anesthesiology* 98:1511–1512.

Van de Wiele B, Rubinstein E, et al. 1995. Propylene glycol toxicity caused by prolonged infusion of etomidate. *Journal of Neurosurgical Anesthesiology* 7(4):259–262.

Vane JR. 1971. Inhibition of prostaglandin synthesis as a mechanism of action for aspirin-like drugs. *Nature: New Biology* 231:232–235.

Vane JR, Botting RM. 1995. New insights into the mode of action of anti-inflammatory drugs. *Inflammation Research* 44: 1–10.

Vane JR, Botting RM. 2003. The mechanism of action of aspirin. *Thrombosis Research* 110:255–258.

Veng-Pedersen P, Wilhelm JA, Zakszewski TB, et al. 1995. Duration of opioid antagonism by nalmefene and naloxone in the dog: an integrated pharmacokinetic/pharmacodynamic comparison. *Journal of Pharmaceutical Sciences* 84:1101–1106.

Verbruggen AM, Akkerdaas LC, Hellebrekers LJ, et al. 2000. The effect of intravenous medetomidine on pupil size and intraocular pressure in normotensive dogs. *The Veterinary Quarterly* 22(3):179–180.

Wagner LE, Eaton M, Sabnis SS, et al. 1999. Meperidine and lidocaine block of recombinant voltage-dependent Na+ channels: evidence that meperidine is a local anesthetic. *Anesthesiology* 91:1481–1490.

Wallace JL, Fiorucci S. 2003. A magic bullet for mucosal protection. . .and aspirin is the trigger! *Trends in Pharmacological Sciences* 24:323–326.

Wallenstein MC, Wang SC. 1979. Mechanism of morphine-induced mydriasis in the cat. *The American Journal of Physiology* 236:R292–R296.

Warner TD, Giuliano F, Vojnovic I, et al. 1999. Nonsteroid drug selectivities for cyclo-oxygenase-1 rather than cyclo-oxygenase-2 are associated with human gastrointestinal toxicity: a full in vitro analysis. *Proceedings of the National Academy of Sciences of the United States of America* 96:7563–7568.

Waterman AE. 1983. Influence of premedication with xylazine on the distribution and metabolism of intramuscularly administered ketamine in cats. *Research in Veterinary Science* 35(3): 285–290.

Welsh EM, Baxter P, Nolan AM. 1992. Pharmacokinetics of carprofen administered intravenously to sheep. *Research in Veterinary Science* 53:264–266.

West PM, Fernandez C. 2003. Safety of COX-2 inhibitors in asthma patients with aspirin hypersensitivity. *The Annals of Pharmacotherapy* 37:1497–1501.

Wilkinson AC, Thomas ML, Morse BC. 2001. Evaluation of a transdermal fentanyl system in yucatan miniature pigs. *Contemporary Topics in Laboratory Animal Science* 40:12–16.

Wolff M, Olschewski A, Vogel W, et al. 2004. Meperidine suppresses the excitability of spinal dorsal horn neurons. *Anesthesiology* 100:947–955.

Yaksh TL. 1998. Pharmacology and mechanisms of opioid analgesic activity. In: *Anesthesia: Biologic Foundations* (TL Yaksh, C Lynch III, WM Zapol, eds.), p. 921. Philadelphia: Lippincott-Raven.

Yaksh TL, Dirig DM, Malmberg AB. 1998. Mechanism of action of nonsteroidal anti-inflammatory drugs. *Cancer Investigation* 16:509–527.

Yeh SY, Krebs HA, Changchit A. 1981. Urinary excretion of meperidine and its metabolites. *Journal of Pharmaceutical Sciences* 70:867–870.

Zadina JE, Martin-Schild S, Gerall AA, et al. 1999. Endomorphins: novel endogenous mu-opiate receptor agonists in regions of high mu-opiate receptor density. *Neuropeptides: Structure and Function in Biology and Behavior* 897:136–144.

2 Monitoring

Larissa Ozeki and Nigel Caulkett

INTRODUCTION

The anesthetist must serve as the patient's advocate from the time of induction until it is fully recovered. To serve in this role, it is vital that the anesthetist is constantly aware of the patient's physiological status. There have been many advances in monitoring technology over the past 20 years, and portable, sturdy monitors are available for use in the field and remote situations. Zoo and wild animals can be particularly challenging to monitor as their diversity in physiology may result in a lack of normal values for commonly monitored parameters. Much of the monitoring equipment we use was designed for human patients, and diversity in size can introduce a challenge when these monitors are applied to very large or very small patients.

As with any patient, it is important to monitor cardiovascular and respiratory function; ideally, there should be constant monitoring of these systems. It is also vital to monitor thermoregulation. Hyperthermia is a common complication during wildlife capture that may lead to acute death or possibly contribute to capture myopathy. Since animals are often anesthetized outdoors, hypothermia may occur more rapidly in small patients. Body temperature should be monitored frequently in anesthetized wildlife.

This chapter will discuss an approach to monitoring anesthetized zoo and wild animals. It will discuss the utility of commonly used monitoring techniques and their application in a variety of species. The chapter will start with the basic requirements of monitoring and will be expanded to discuss monitoring by body system. The focus will be on the monitoring technology with specific normals and application of these techniques being discussed in the species-specific chapters.

MONITORING BASICS

Before any anesthetic procedure, it is important to devise an anesthetic and a monitoring plan. The monitoring plan must take into account the anesthetic risk, the procedure the patient is about to undergo, the environment where the procedure will take place, and any anticipated complications. With anesthesia of free-ranging wildlife, there are often limitations in the amount of equipment that can be carried or the number of personnel available to monitor the patient, as even if a veterinarian is present, they may often be involved in sampling or surgical procedures.

Frequency of monitoring is an important consideration. Ideally, cardiovascular and respiratory function should be monitored continuously, with depth of anesthesia and body temperature being monitored intermittently. If continuous monitoring is not available, frequency of monitoring will probably be dependent on the availability of personnel who can devote their time to monitoring. Ideally, monitoring should be performed continuously with specific values recorded every 5–10 minutes.

Appropriate monitoring always requires an anesthetic record. During anesthesia, trends in physiological status are as important as absolute values. A well-designed record allows for the visual observation of trends. The record should contain patient information, including age, species, sex, and temperament. It should contain any hematological information and physical condition. It should include information regarding the procedures being performed and the ambient conditions (with field procedures). The record should contain information regarding capture technique and drugs administered (including number of darts). Typically, a time to sternal recumbancy and

Zoo Animal and Wildlife Immobilization and Anesthesia, Second Edition. Edited by Gary West, Darryl Heard, and Nigel Caulkett.
© 2014 John Wiley & Sons, Inc. Published 2014 by John Wiley & Sons, Inc.

head down is also recorded. Any therapeutic interventions should be recorded, for example, oxygen therapy, and monitoring modalities should also be recorded. A section is devoted to a record of physiological values over time. The record should include dose and administration time of any antagonist drugs and time to head up and walking. A section should also be included for comments to include any additional information that may be pertinent to the procedure.

Why Is Monitoring Important?

There have been many improvements in wildlife capture and handling over the years, and the efficacy and safety of anesthetic techniques has increased greatly, but we still encounter many complications, even in healthy animals. Some of these complications, such as hypoxemia in ungulates, are predictable, but others, such as hyperthermia, acidosis, and capture myopathy, may result from the capture event itself. With capture of free-ranging wildlife or dangerous zoo animals we cannot perform a pre-anesthetic exam and although we often assume that we are dealing with healthy animals we cannot determine the health status until the animal is under anesthesia. In some situations, anesthesia can result in decompensation and emergent situations. With anesthesia of domestic animals, it is often possible to titrate induction drugs to minimize side effects. During anesthesia of wildlife, we will often deliver drugs at the higher end of the dose range in an attempt to induce anesthesia rapidly, without repeated dart administration and prolonged pursuit. Anesthesia of zoo and wild animals is further complicated by the massive variety of species and varied physiology between species. There is often a paucity of information in the scientific literature concerning anesthetic techniques of many of these species, and we are often forced to extrapolate from other closely related species. Free-ranging wildlife are subject to the environmental conditions in which they live, and may be exposed to extremes of temperature and physical hazards during induction and recovery. Anesthesia of zoo and wildlife patients is arguably one of the most challenging aspects of veterinary anesthesia. Given the potential risks involved, it is vital to initiate monitoring procedures as soon as the animal has been approached and to continue monitoring throughout the procedure.

What Should be Monitored?

Neglecting to monitor depth of anesthesia can have very adverse consequences for capture personnel during anesthesia of potentially dangerous wildlife. It is vital to take the time to monitor anesthetic depth on a routine basis. Anesthetic drugs have many side effects and the choice of monitoring techniques will often depend on the drugs that are being used, the species being anesthetized, and the availability of equipment.

In an ideal world, it would be best to use a monitor that would ensure that blood flow is preserved to vital organs and that oxygen delivery to the tissues is adequate to meet the tissue oxygen demand. Monitors are available to provide this information, but unfortunately they are not practical in routine clinical situations. For this reason, we typically use monitors that will indirectly allow us to determine that we are adequately perfusing organs and meeting the body's oxygen demand.

Global oxygen delivery (DO_2) is the product of cardiac output × arterial oxygen content (CaO_2) and is represented by the following equation:

$$DO_2 = \text{Cardiac output} \times 0.003\,(PaO_2) + 1.39\,(SaO_2 \times Hb).$$

From the above equation, it is apparent that to maximize global oxygen delivery, it is important to ensure an adequate cardiac output, maximize percent hemoglobin saturation, and ensure an adequate hemoglobin concentration (or hematocrit). We have the ability to measure PaO_2, SaO_2, and Hb concentration, it is difficult to measure cardiac output under field conditions; therefore we must rely on indirect measurements such as blood pressure and heart rate. It is also apparent that appropriate monitoring should evaluate cardiovascular and respiratory function. Hyperthermia will increase metabolic oxygen demand, necessitating an increase in oxygen delivery to meet the increased oxygen demand. If this increased demand is not met, tissue hypoxia may result. Frequent measurement of body temperature is vital during wildlife capture and handling.

MONITORING THE RESPIRATORY SYSTEM

The most basic monitoring of the respiratory system consists of visualization of chest excursions to determine rate and subjectively determine depth of respiration. Respiratory rate should be monitored every 5 minutes at minimum. To effectively monitor the respiratory system, it is important to determine oxygenation, and ventilation. A crude method to determine oxygenation is to visualize mucous membranes, and determine if cyanosis is present. This can be extremely subjective. The pulse oximeter can be used to determine percent hemoglobin concentration, which will assist with a diagnosis of hypoxemia. The pulse oximeter will not determine if ventilation is adequate. Capnography can be used to assess the adequacy of ventilation in field situations; it will quantify end-tidal carbon dioxide, and this value can be analyzed to determine if hypoventilation or hyperventilation is present. Both of these techniques will provide an indirect measure of respiratory function and are very useful tools, but both techniques are subject to considerable error during wildlife anesthesia. Arterial blood gas analysis is the gold standard to determine oxygenation and ventilation; it will provide a direct measurement of PaO_2 and $PaCO_2$, which can be used to effectively diagnose hypoxemia, hypoventilation, or hyperventilation. These techniques are discussed below.

Pulse Oximetry

The pulse oximeter is a simple, noninvasive monitor that provides real-time values of hemoglobin saturation and pulse rate; therefore, it enables the anesthetist to detect hypoxemia in the patient before other clinical signs develop (Dorsch & Dorsch 2008; Sinex 1999). It is ideal for perioperative monitoring because it is an automatic, continuous, and audible monitor. The pulse oximeter's portability, ease of operation, and wide availability make it a useful tool to monitor anesthesia in field situations.

The pulse oximeter estimates the oxygen percentage linked to hemoglobin in arterial blood by measuring light absorption characteristics. The main principle of this spectral analysis is the Beer–Lambert law, which states that an absorbing substance's concentration can be determined by the intensity of light transmitted through it, given the transmission path length, the absorbance characteristic of that substance at that specific wavelength, and the intensity and wavelength of incident light (Sinex 1999).

Two light-emitting diodes (LEDs) in the pulse oximeter's probe emit two wavelengths (660 nm—red and 940 nm—infrared) through the vascular bed of a tissue, such as the tongue (Fig. 2.1). Opposite the LED, a pho-

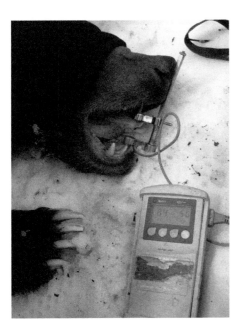

Figure 2.1. Pulse oximeter placement on the tongue of a brown bear.

todiode detects the intensity of the transmitted light and converts it into an electrical signal (Sinex 1999). The two different wavelengths allow the differentiation between reduced hemoglobin and oxyhemoglobin, due to the fact that the reduced hemoglobin absorbs more light in the red band and the oxyhemoglobin in the infrared band (Dorsch & Dorsch 2008). A ratio between these two signals is calculated and related to the arterial O_2 saturation (SaO_2) via an empiric algorithm. The algorithm was created by measuring the ratio in volunteers and comparing it with simultaneous blood gas analysis (Sinex 1999).

To determine the value of the oxygen saturation (SpO_2) correctly, the equipment must isolate absorbance of arterial hemoglobin from other absorbents such as venous blood, connective tissues, non-pulsatile arterial blood and skin pigment (Haskins 2007). To isolate these confounders, the pulse oximeter exploits the pulsatile nature of arterial blood (Dorsch & Dorsch 2008; Sinex 1999). Vender and Hand (Vender et al. 1995) evaluated the reliability of the pulse oximetry comparing it to blood gas analysis in rats. They concluded that the device could predict the SaO_2 93–98% of the time. However, the accuracy and reliability of the pulse oximetry can be affected by hemoglobin concentration, placement of the probe close to large vessels, motion artifacts, ambient light, vasoconstriction, and vasodilation (Barton et al. 1996; McEwen et al. 2010). In white-tailed deer, SpO_2 generally overestimated the SaO_2, and with $SaO_2 < 80\%$, the agreement between pulse oximetry and blood gas analysis could not be considered sufficient (Muller et al. 2012). This is especially important to be considered in species that are more susceptible to develop hypoxemia, as ungulates.

Correlation (and not the agreement) between SaO_2 and SpO_2 was calculated for rabbits, dogs, sheep, goats and pigs (Erhardt et al. 1990). The results demonstrated that in all species, SpO_2 was always higher; and the lower the SaO_2 was, the greater was the difference between them.

Vasoconstriction and vasodilation cause inaccurate SpO_2 readings (McEwen et al. 2010). In wild animals, vasoconstriction is commonly associated with use of alpha-2 agonists in immobilization protocols for either captive or free-ranging animals (Arnemo 2010; Fenati et al. 2008; King et al. 2010; Shilo et al. 2010; Sontakke et al. 2009; Wolfe et al. 2008). Patients presenting with low blood pressure may also have a less accurate pulse oximetry reading, as the animal may respond to the low pressure by redirecting the blood flow to vital organs via peripheral vasoconstriction (Barton et al. 1996).

Knowing that so many factors can influence the reliability of the pulse oximeter readings, the anesthetist should verify the quality of the pletysmographic waveform and/or the signal strength indicator (which should reach at least three-quarters of the total length). It is also important to compare the heart rate shown by the oximeter and that produced by the electrocardiograph or auscultation (Dorsch & Dorsch 2008). Evaluation of the quality of the information produced by the device associated with clinical observations and knowledge of pharmacodynamics can insure a better interpretation of the values displayed by the pulse oximeter.

It is worth mentioning that these devices are calibrated for mammals and do not have the same consistency in avian species or reptiles as their hemoglobin has different absorption characteristics and SpO_2 values may not accurately reflect SaO_2 (Longley 2008; Schmitt et al. 1998).

Capnography

Capnometry is a noninvasive method of monitoring the partial pressure of CO_2 from airway gasses. The device displays the value of $ETCO_2$ (end tidal CO_2), which is the maximum value of carbon dioxide obtained at the end of the expiration (Dorsch & Dorsch 2008; Nagler & Krauss 2008). Analysis of the capnograph waveform is a useful method to evaluate the animal's respiratory status. The "capnogram" enables the anesthetist to verify the validity of the measured $ETCO_2$ and provides more detailed information regarding physiological and pathological conditions (Dorsch & Dorsch 2008). The capnogram also provides the respiratory rate, and permits the anesthetist to evaluate the adequacy of ventilation, correct placement of the endotracheal tube, and airway patency by utilization of waveform analysis. Capnography was shown to recognize changes in 70% of human patients who had an acute respiratory event, 4 minutes before any unusual clinical observations, or an observable decrease in pulse oximetry values (Burton et al. 2006).

Capnography is based on infrared spectroscopy. A beam of infrared radiation is sent, through an air sample, from a light source to a photometer. CO_2 absorbs at a wavelength of 4.26 μm; the amount transmitted is measured by the photometer and CO_2 concentration is calculated (Nagler & Krauss 2008). There are two main types of capnograph, the *mainstream* and the *sidestream* analyzer. This classification depends on the location of the sensor. The mainstream has the sensor directly on the hub of the endotracheal tube and the sidestream aspirates airway gas continuously, via a section of microtubing, to a sensor located inside the monitor (Fig. 2.2) (Nagler & Krauss 2008).

The mainstream capnograph should be used only in intubated patients, and the sidestream may be used in both intubated and nonintubated patients. The sidestream analyzer is not reliable with small respiratory volumes; it has a slower response time and the sample line can be contaminated or blocked by mucous or moisture. Standard flow sidestream capnographs can be

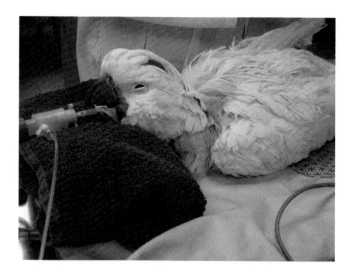

Figure 2.2. Sidestream capnography on a cockatoo.

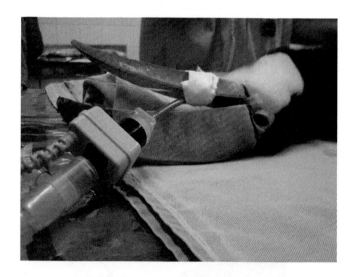

Figure 2.3. Mainstream capnograph placed between the anesthetic circuit and the endotracheal tube of a toucan.

inaccurate for $ETCO_2$ monitoring in animals with small tidal volumes and high respiratory rates, such as birds and small rodents. To help alleviate this problem, low aspiration flow rate sidestream capnographs have been developed (Desmarchelier et al. 2007). Mainstream monitors may have the sensor contaminated by mucous or moisture. They function better than sidestream with smaller volumes, and have a faster response time, but they are also heavy and can dislodge the endotracheal tube (Fox et al. 2009). Mainstream capnographs typically provide more accurate readings; however, in species that have small tidal volumes, such as birds and small rodents, the dead space added by its sensor makes the use of this device problematic (Fig. 2.3).

$ETCO_2$ reflects $PaCO_2$ values but usually underestimates $PaCO_2$ by 2–5 mmHg (Nagler & Krauss 2008).

There are some important situations where the difference between $ETCO_2$ and $PaCO_2$ can increase. The most important one is immediately prior to systemic circulatory collapse or cardiac arrest. As cardiac output drops, so will pulmonary blood flow and CO_2 elimination will be impaired. Typically, a large acute drop in the $ETCO_2$ value is observed, while arterial CO_2 increases. This may be observed before any change in blood pressure values. The capnograph is a useful monitor to predict circulatory collapse (Dorsch & Dorsch 2008; Fox et al. 2009).

MONITORING THE CARDIOVASCULAR SYSTEM

The simplest method of monitoring the cardiovascular system consists of determination of heart rate and rhythm. This can be determined by auscultation with a stethoscope or by palpation of a pulse. Ideally, heart rate should be monitored continuously, and many modern monitors will enable this. If intermittent monitoring is the only technique available, it should be performed every 5–10 minutes at minimum. In an ideal world, it would be useful to be able to measure cardiac output continuously. There have been major advances in the measurement of cardiac output, but monitors are still not available in a form that would prove useful for field situations. Blood pressure is dependent on cardiac output and systemic vascular resistance. An increase in blood pressure may result from an increase in cardiac output or an increase in systemic vascular resistance. Hypertension is commonly encountered in wildlife anesthetized with high dosages of alpha-2 agonists. This increase in blood pressure results from vasoconstriction, and cardiac output may decrease considerably from baseline values (Caulkett et al. 1996). It is always important to consider the cardiovascular effects of the anesthetic technique when blood pressure values are interpreted.

Blood Pressure

Blood pressure is an important determinant of the heart's work and is commonly performed to assess cardiovascular performance. By itself, it is not the best indicator of tissue perfusion, but a low blood pressure can lead to a blood flow decrease and impaired oxygenation of major organs (Shih et al. 2010). Anesthesia, especially inhalant anesthesia, can cause a significant decrease in blood pressure. Hypotension is usually diagnosed at a mean arterial pressure (MAP) lower than 60 mmHg in small animals (Shih et al. 2010). There are several ways to measure blood pressure. They can be divided into *invasive*, or *direct*, and *noninvasive*, or *indirect*.

Invasive Blood Pressure Direct blood pressure measurement is accepted as the gold standard for determin-

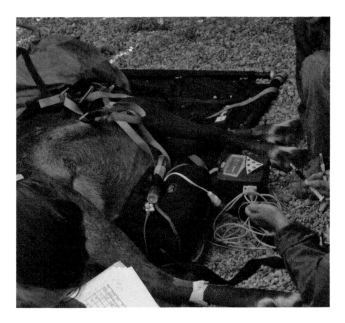

Figure 2.4. Invasive blood pressure measurement in a reindeer.

ing the systolic (SAP), diastolic (DAP), and mean arterial pressures (MAP). It requires an arterial catheter placement, which can be challenging in small or hypovolemic patients. Typical locations for catheter placement are the auricular artery in ungulgates, or the femoral or pedal artery in carnivores (Fig. 2.4). The artery is connected to a transducer, via noncompliant, fluid-filled tubing. The transducer connects to the monitor and translates the mechanical signal into an electrical signal. This technique is considered to be the most accurate method of measuring blood pressure, and it should be the technique of choice in research procedures.

Noninvasive Blood Pressure Monitors Noninvasive methods (NIBP) simplify monitoring and do not require special skills for their placement. The two most common NIBP devices are the *Oscillometric* and the *Doppler ultrasound*. The most clinically important blood pressure is the mean, because it represents the mean driving pressure for organ perfusion. The systolic pressure has a variable relationship with the mean so the anesthetist should be aware of it when measuring only systolic pressure (Haskins 2007). To decrease this margin of error with NIBP methods is important to maintain the cuff width: limb circumference ratio at approximately 40% (Haskins 2007).

The oscillometric monitor utilizes an automatically inflating blood pressure cuff to detect oscillations produced by blood flow and uses these oscillations to determine arterial pressure (Dorsch & Dorsch 2008).(Fig. 2.5) The Doppler also utilizes a cuff, but the operator must

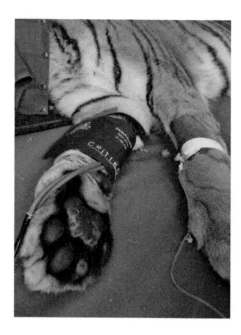

Figure 2.5. Oscillometric cuff placed over the distal limb of a tiger.

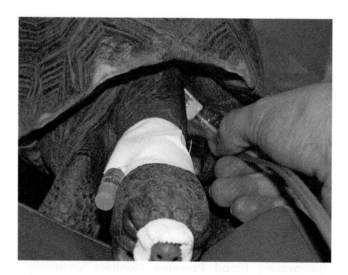

Figure 2.6. Ultrasonic Doppler flow probe being used to monitor heart rate.

inflate it, and determine the systolic arterial pressure (SAP) by listening for the return of the pulse signal on deflation of the cuff.

A major advantage of the ultrasonic Doppler is the ability to continuously monitor heart rate. This is especially important in species with small body size, such as rodents, birds, and reptiles. In these animals, the doppler probe can be placed over an artery or the heart, and the blood flow will generate a sound that allows real-time monitoring of heart rate (Fig. 2.6). However, noninvasive techniques have been shown to be unreliable in some avian species, such as parrots and ducks (Acierno et al. 2008; Lichtenberger 2005).

A high rate of error has been observed when oscillometric monitors were assessed in red-tailed hawks. In the same study, the Doppler NIPB measurement tended to underestimate the SAP at all sites of cuff placement, but doppler was a good predictor of the MAP (Zehnder et al. 2009). Many factors can affect the accuracy of NIBP measurements, including the monitor itself, the site of the cuff placement, the cuff size, and the blood pressure itself (Dorsch & Dorsch 2008).

Electrocardiography Electrocardiography can be used to assess heart rate, and to diagnose arrhythmias and some electrolyte disorders. It is not a first-line monitor, but it can be used to provide important additional information required to diagnose and treat cardiac complications. Drugs used in wildlife capture can often induce arrhythmias. Bradyarrhythmias are common with alpha-2 agonists. Ventricular ectopic arrhythmias have been noted during immobilization with potent narcotics. Hypoxemia, hypercarbia, and catecholamine release can also been associated with arrhythmias. Since the treatment of arrhythmias varies greatly, it is important to make an accurate diagnosis of the rhythm prior to treatment.

Blood Gas Analysis Blood gas analyses is an important part of anesthetic monitoring in wild and zoo animal medicine (Kilgallon et al. 2008). When the results are correctly interpreted, they can show an overview of the respiratory and metabolic status in the anesthetized patient (Proulx 1999).

The blood gas analyzer is the only monitor that provides real values of pH, partial pressure of oxygen, and carbon dioxide in arterial or venous blood. Another advantage of the blood gas analyzer is the fact that it utilizes whole blood and the results can be provided in few minutes (Fauquier et al. 2004).

Free-ranging or captive wild hoof stock occasionally develop acute or delayed capture myopathy associated with lactic acidosis, electrolyte imbalance, circulatory compromise, hyperthermia, and free-radical production. This syndrome can be compounded by drug-induced respiratory depression and a negative balance in ventilation-perfusion ratio; only blood–gas and acid–base analysis enables early detection and constant monitoring of these derangements (Kilgallon et al. 2008).

Large animals such as rhinoceros can regularly develop hypoxemia and hypercapnia especially when they are immobilized with protocols that utilize very potent opioids, such as etorphine. This depression is dose-dependent and can be made worse due to the rigidity of the thoracic musculature of these species (Wenger et al. 2007).

Oxygenation is best assessed with arterial samples. It is crucial to preheparinize the syringe and the needle to avoid blood coagulation (Proulx 1999). It is also important to avoid air bubbles in the syringe, as they interfere with the analysis. Ambient air PO_2 is 160 mmHg at sea level; if the arterial blood has a PaO_2 higher than ambient air, a bubble will cause it to drop over time, and the opposite will occur if the PaO_2 in the blood is lower than 160 mmHg (Hasan 2008). The PCO_2 in the ambient air is virtually zero so no matter which $PaCO_2$ the blood has, it will change towards zero; and as the $PaCO_2$ falls, the pH will rise (Hasan 2008).

The blood gas analyzer has electrodes comprised of two half-cells each. Each half-cell is immersed in an electrolyte solution and an external ammeter completes the circuit (Hasan 2008). Blood gas analyzers usually contain at least three electrodes: O_2, CO_2, and *pH*. The O_2 electrode works through polarography. A silver anode and a platinum cathode are immersed in a KCl solution and a semipermeable membrane separates it from the blood sample. When the O_2 molecules in the sample diffuses into the half-cell and react with the cathode, this reaction produces an amount of electrons that is proportional to the PaO_2 (Hasan 2008). The CO_2 electrode is immersed in a bicarbonate buffer solution, which is separated from the blood sample also by a membrane. Similarly, the CO_2 diffuses through the membrane and changes the buffer's pH. The concentration of H^+ is measured by a modified pH cell and the difference in the electrical potential creates a current (Hasan 2008). The pH electrode is the most complex of the three and has a special hygroscopic membrane that separates the blood from the electrolyte solution. In contact with the blood, the hydrogen ions dissociate from the membrane producing a flow of electrons and creating a current depending upon the difference in the electrical charges on either side (Hasan 2008). After obtaining the results, the first parameter to be interpreted is the pH and the nature of the imbalance should be defined as metabolic, respiratory, or mixed. After this, the treatment can be defined (Muir & de Morais 2007). Portable clinical blood–gas and acid–base analyzers have allowed the anesthetist to perform this type of monitoring in settings where it was previously impossible (Fauquier et al. 2004).

Body Temperature Hypothermia during anesthesia can be related to drug-induced depression of muscular activity, metabolism, or hypothalamic thermostatic mechanisms (Haskins 2007). During wildlife capture, *hyperthermia* is commonly observed. Root causes are high ambient temperature, increased muscular activity during pursuit, and alpha-2 agonist-induced impairment of thermoregulation (Caulkett & Arnemo 2007).

Hyperthermia can be treated with cold water enemas or cold intravenous crystalloids. Reversal of alpha-2 agonist drugs may also be considered (Caulkett & Arnemo 2007; Haskins 2007). Hyperthemic animals may benefit from supplemental oxygen as increased metabolism increases the oxygen demand for major organs.

Hypothermia can be treated by passive or active rewarming. Passive rewarming involves minimizing heat loss and enabling the patient to warm themselves metabolically, it can only be performed in animals with core temperatures between 36 and 34°C. Active rewarming is achieved by providing a source of heat to the patient. Convective warming works particularly well in these situations.

The most common devices used for temperature monitoring are esophageal or rectal thermistors attached to a thermometer, or handheld digital thermometers (Spelman et al. 1997). Telemetric temperature monitoring devices have been recently developed and show promise in this area.

Anesthetic Depth Monitoring the anesthetic depth during wildlife capture is fundamental for the safety of the animals and also of the staff. A light plane of anesthesia represents a threat for the people involved in the procedure and a very deep plane represents a risk for the animal, since vital organ functions may be compromised.

Parameters most commonly monitored are: *palpebral reflex* (lateral and medial), *corneal reflex, jaw tone, and ocular globe positioning*. The palpebral reflexes can be present or absent depending on the protocol used. The corneal reflex should be present in most species, as its loss characterizes a very deep anesthetic plan. Jaw tone varies depending on the anesthetic protocol used, as some drugs promote better muscle relaxation than others.

The ocular globe position varies among species. Mammals, in general, rotate the globe medially and ventrally in a surgical plane of volatile anesthesia. A centralized globe may represent a shallow plane when palpebral reflexes are present; or a very deep plane, when the palpebral reflexes are absent. Avian species and reptiles do not rotate the ocular globe, but they do generally prolapse the nictitating membrane during a surgical plane.

Dissociative drugs, when used alone, maintain all reflexes and increase muscular tone (Ramsden et al. 1976). Most protocols combine dissociative drugs with agents that induce muscle relaxation, such as alpha-2 agonists or benzodiazepines (Atkinson et al. 2002; Citino et al. 2001; Jalanka 1989; Smith et al. 2006). It is crucial to know what to expect in a given species when using these combinations, as combinations of dissociatives and sedatives are arguably the most utilized drug combinations to immobilize wildlife.

When anesthetized with combinations of dissociative drugs and benzodiazepines, especially tiletamine and zolazepam, some animals can demonstrate some somatic movement during the procedure, even when well immobilized. When these drugs are used at lower doses and combined with alpha-2 agonists, head movement is a sign of very light anesthesia, and the potential for sudden arousal.

Heart rate, respiratory rate, and arterial blood pressure should be evaluated and interpreted along with reflexes, degree of muscle relaxation, and eye position. Typically, the lighter the anesthetic plan, the higher the sympathetic activity. Clinically, this presents as: increases heart rate, respiratory rate, and arterial blood pressure. Assessment of anesthetic depth has always been a challenge for the anesthetist; given the breadth of species covered in this text, it is important to consult individual chapters and experts in the field to determine how to appropriately monitor depth of anesthesia in a given species, with a particular anesthetic protocol.

REFERENCES

Acierno MJ, da Cunha A, Smith J, Tully TN Jr, Guzman DSM, Serra V, et al. 2008. Agreement between direct and indirect blood pressure measurements obtained from anesthetized Hispaniolan Amazon parrots. *Journal of the American Veterinary Medical Association* 233(10):1587–1590.

Arnemo JM. 2010. Immobilization of free-ranging moose (*Alces alces*) with medetomidine-ketamine and remobilization with atipamezole. *Rangifer* 15(1):19–25.

Atkinson MW, Hull B, Gandolf AR, Blumer ES. 2002. Repeated chemical immobilization of a captive greater one-horned rhinoceros (*Rhinoceros unicornis*), using combinations of etorphine, detomidine, and ketamine. *Journal of Zoo and Wildlife Medicine* 33(2):157–162.

Barton LJ, Devey JJ, Gorski S, Mainiero L, DeBehnke D. 1996. Evaluation of transmittance and reflectance pulse oximetry in a canine model of hypotension and desaturation. *Journal of Veterinary Emergency and Critical Care* 6(1):21–28.

Burton JH, Harrah JD, Germann CA, Dillon DC. 2006. Does end-tidal carbon dioxide monitoring detect respiratory events prior to current sedation monitoring practices? *Academic Emergency Medicine* 13(5):500–504.

Caulkett NA, Arnemo JM. 2007. Chemical immobilization of free-ranging terrestrial mammals. In: *Lumb & Jones' Veterinary Anesthesia and Analgesia* (WJ Tranquilli, JC Thurmon, KA Grimm, eds.), pp. 807–832. Ames: Blackwell Publishing.

Caulkett NA, Duke T, Cribb PH. 1996. Cardiopulmonary effects of medetomidine: Ketamine in domestic sheep (*Ovis ovis*) maintained in sternal recumbency. *Journal of Zoo and Wildlife Medicine* 27:217–226.

Citino S, Bush M, Grobler D, Lance W. 2001. Anaesthesia of roan antelope (Hippotragus equinus) with a combination of A3080, medetomidine and ketamine. *Journal of the South African Veterinary Association* 72(1):29–32.

Desmarchelier M, Rondenay Y, Fitzgerald G, Lair S. 2007. Monitoring of the ventilatory status of anesthetized birds of prey by using end-tidal carbon dioxide measured with a microstream capnometer. *Journal of Zoo and Wildlife Medicine* 38(1):1–6.

Dorsch JA, Dorsch SE. 2008. *Understanding Anesthesia Equipment*, 5th ed. Philadelphia: Wolters Kluwer Health/Lippincott Williams & Wilkins. 1056 p.

Erhardt W, Lendl C, Hipp R, ·Hegel G, Wiesner G, Wiesner H. 1990. The use of pulse oximetry in clinical veterinary anaesthesia. *Veterinary Anaesthesia and Analgesia* 17(1):30–31.

Fauquier D, Harr K, Murphy D, Bonde R, Rommel S, Haubold E, eds. 2004. Preliminary evaluation of a portable clinical analyzer to determine blood gas and acid-base parameters in manatees (*Trichechus manatus*). AAZV, AAWV, WDA Joint Conference.

Fenati M, Monaco A, Guberti V. 2008. Efficiency and safety of xylazine and tiletamine/zolazepam to immobilize captured wild boars (*Sus scrofa* L. 1758): analysis of field results. *European Journal of Wildlife Research* 54(2):269–274.

Fox LK, Flegal MC, Kuhlman SM. 2009. Principles of anesthesia monitoring–capnography. *Journal of Investigative Surgery* 22(6):452–454.

Hasan A. 2008. *Handbook of Blood Gas/Acid-Base Interpretation*. London: Springer Verlag.

Haskins SC. 2007. Monitoring anesthetized patients. In: *Lumb & Jones' Veterinary Anesthesia and Analgesia* (W Tranquilli, J Thurmon, K Grimm, eds.), pp. 533–560. Ames: Blackwell Publishing.

Jalanka HH. 1989. Evaluation and comparison of two ketamine-based immobilization techniques in snow leopards (*Panthera uncia*). *Journal of Zoo and Wildlife Medicine* 20:163–169.

Kilgallon C, Bailey T, Arca-Ruibal B, Misheff M, O'Donovan D. 2008. Blood-gas and acid-base parameters in nontranquilized Arabian oryx (*Oryx leucoryx*) in the United Arab Emirates. *Journal of Zoo and Wildlife Medicine* 39(1):6–12.

King JD, Congdon E, Tosta C. 2010. Evaluation of three immobilization combinations in the capybara (*Hydrochoerus hydrochaeris*). *Zoo Biology* 29(1):59–67.

Lichtenberger M. 2005. Determination of indirect blood pressure in the companion bird. *Seminars in Avian and Exotic Pet Medicine* 14(2):149–152.

Longley L. 2008. Reptile anesthesia. In: *Anaesthesia of Exotic Pets*, pp. 185–241. Edinburgh: Saunders.

McEwen M, Bull G, Reynolds K. 2010. Vessel calibre and haemoglobin effects on pulse oximetry. *Physiological Measurement* 31:727.

Muir WW, de Morais HAS. 2007. Acid-base physiology. In: *Lumb and Jones' Veterinary Anesthesia and Analgesia* (WJ Tranquilli, JC Thurmon, KA Grimm, eds.), pp.169–182. Ames: Blackwell Publishing.

Muller LI, Osborn DA, Doherty T, Keel MK, Miller BF, Warren RJ, et al. 2012. A comparison of oxygen saturation in white-tailed deer estimated by pulse oximetry and from arterial blood gases. *Journal of Wildlife Diseases* 48(2):458–461.

Nagler J, Krauss B. 2008. Capnography: a valuable tool for airway management. *Emergency Medicine Clinics of North America* 26(4):881–897.

Proulx J. 1999. Respiratory monitoring: arterial blood gas analysis, pulse oximetry, and end-tidal carbon dioxide analysis. *Clinical Techniques in Small Animal Practice* 14(4):227–230.

Ramsden RO, Coppin PF, Johnston DH. 1976. Clinical observations on the use of ketamine hydrochloride in wild carnivores. *Journal of Wildlife Diseases* 12(2):221–225.

Schmitt PM, Göbel T, Trautvetter E. 1998. Evaluation of pulse oximetry as a monitoring method in avian anesthesia. *Journal of Avian Medicine and Surgery* 12:91–99.

Shih A, Robertson S, Vigani A, Da Cunha A, Pablo L, Bandt C. 2010. Evaluation of an indirect oscillometric blood pressure monitor in normotensive and hypotensive anesthetized dogs. *Journal of Veterinary Emergency and Critical Care* 20(3):313–318.

Shilo Y, Lapid R, King R, Bdolah-Abram T, Epstein A. 2010. Immobilization of red fox (*Vulpes vulpes*) with medetomidine-ketamine or medetomidine-midazolam and antagonism with atipamezole. *Journal of Zoo and Wildlife Medicine* 41(1):28–34.

Sinex JE. 1999. Pulse oximetry: principles and limitations. *The American Journal of Emergency Medicine* 17(1):59–66.

Smith KM, Powell DM, James SB, Calle PP, Moore RP, Zurawka HS, et al. 2006. Anesthesia of male axis deer (*Axis axis*): evaluation of thiafentanil, medetomidine, and ketamine versus medetomidine and ketamine. *Journal of Zoo and Wildlife Medicine* 37(4): 513–517.

Sontakke SD, Umapathy G, Shivaji S. 2009. Yohimbine antagonizes the anaesthetic effects of ketamine–xylazine in captive Indian wild felids. *Veterinary Anaesthesia and Analgesia* 36(1): 34–41.

Spelman LH, Jochem WJ, Sumner PW, Redmond DP, Stoskopf MK. 1997. Postanesthetic monitoring of core body temperature using telemetry in North American river otters (*Lutra canadensis*). *Journal of Zoo and Wildlife Medicine* 28:413–417.

Vender JR, Hand CM, Sedor D, Tabor SL, Black P. 1995. Oxygen saturation monitoring in experimental surgery: a comparison of pulse oximetry and arterial blood gas measurement. *Laboratory Animal Science* 45(2):211.

Wenger S, Boardman W, Buss P, Govender D, Foggin C. 2007. The cardiopulmonary effects of etorphine, azaperone, detomidine, and butorphanol in field-anesthetized white rhinoceroses (*Ceratotherium simum*). *Journal of Zoo and Wildlife Medicine* 38(3): 380–387.

Wolfe LL, Goshorn CT, Baruch-Mordo S. 2008. Immobilization of black bears (*Ursus americanus*) with a combination of butorphanol, azaperone, and medetomidine. *Journal of Wildlife Diseases* 44(3):748–752.

Zehnder AM, Hawkins MG, Pascoe PJ, Kass PH. 2009. Evaluation of indirect blood pressure monitoring in awake and anesthetized red-tailed hawks (*Buteo jamaicensis*): effects of cuff size, cuff placement, and monitoring equipment. *Veterinary Anaesthesia and Analgesia* 36(5):464–479.

3 Airway Management

Jonathan Cracknell

INTRODUCTION

Induction of general anesthesia or sedation tends to result in hypoxia as a result of airway obstruction, respiratory depression, and decreased cardiac output. Airway management consists of the management of a patent airway, the effective delivery of oxygen rich anesthetic gases, and the safe elimination of waste gases, such as carbon dioxide, from the patient. Often, this is the management of gases in the case of the terrestrial species but can also be considered to be water management in the aquatic species.

The upper airway represents an area where patency can be reduced through obstruction by normal anatomical features, pathology, or foreign bodies. During anesthesia, normal anatomical structures can reduce, or even obstruct, the passage of oxygen, air, or anesthetic gases on inspiration or the loss of waste gasses on expiration. Suitable positioning, preferably combined with airway management devices, is essential for optimal homeostasis during anesthesia and the prevention of hypoxia and hypercapnoea. In some cases, respiration ceases and the anesthetist must maintain a patent airway and ensure adequate ventilation occurs. This is only possible with the placement of a suitable airway device. It is essential to ensure that the airway remains patent and is managed appropriately: serious problems are rare if suitable planning and preparation is taken for each individual anesthetic.

GENERAL PRINCIPLES OF AIRWAY MANAGEMENT

While there is a considerable variety of patient size, anatomy, respiratory physiology, and environmental requirements, there are general principles that can be followed when approaching any airway management case. Calder and Pearce (2007) highlights these general principles to airway management as follows: Preparation is paramount including selection of suitable equipment, resources, and staffing for the procedure. Preoxygenation gives valuable time for establishment of a patent airway.

Good monitoring equipment certainly reduces the frequency of complications.

Signs of Airway Obstruction

- An obstructed upper airway results in an increase in negative intrathoracic pressure during inspiration, this is noted as the thorax sinking and the abdomen rising (the opposite of normal) (Cook 2007). Turbulent flow may occur in the upper airway, resulting in noise that is worse on inspiration. Auscultation of the larynx and trachea is useful to assess airway patency. It should be noted that lack of sounds can occur with narrowed or obstructed airways. Secretions or foreign bodies may cause obstruction; this includes the anesthetic circuits and airway devices. Normal values of pulse oximetry or PaO_2 are not reliable indicators of airway patency. The airway should be expected to become less patent when the consciousness level declines. Capnometery is extremely useful for assessing airway patency and changes that may occur during anesthesia. In general, there are fewer problems with the airway when an animal is deeply anesthetized, but aspiration of material into lungs becomes a possibility as the conscious level declines

APPROACHES TO AIRWAY MANAGEMENT

There are a variety of different methods in managing the airway:

Zoo Animal and Wildlife Immobilization and Anesthesia, Second Edition. Edited by Gary West, Darryl Heard, and Nigel Caulkett.

- *Airway Unsupported:* This is commonly practiced, especially in the field. An animal spontaneously ventilates through an unaltered airway. Often, this is the only viable option; however, it is associated with an increased risk of obstruction or aspiration, and as such, positioning and continual assessment is essential.
- *Supraglottic Airway Devices (SAD):* Airway management is achieved with a variety of devices that sit at the level of the glottis or above. This allows supplementation with oxygen or volatile agents and, depending on the system employed, ventilation to occur. While aspiration and obstruction are possible, this method of airway management has a lower risk of these occurring when compared with unsupported airways, depending on the device employed.
- *Tracheal Intubation:* Considered by many to be the gold standard of airway management, this method employs the use of a tube inserted directly into the trachea, often with an inflated cuff. This offers the greatest degree of protection against aspiration and allows optimal airway management and control of respiration.

Unsupported Airway

Following induction, there is a period where an animal relies on the patency of its own airway. In some cases, an animal may not be intubated for a procedure and the anesthetist must maintain a patent airway using that animal's own anatomical features. Often not a problem on expiration, airway patency can be compromised on inspiration due to critical instability of oral structures, such as partial posterior displacement of the tongue, soft palate, pharyngeal fat, pharyngeal neoplasia, or foreign bodies (Farmery 2007). The neck should be extended, the tongue pulled forward and laterally, and patency assessed through either physical assessment of airway movement on respiration or on auscultation of the laryngeal or thoracic area. If any concerns are noted, then the animal should be repositioned or the anesthetist intervenes with an airway device, such as a tracheal tube or supraglottic device.

Consideration should be given to aspiration. While the airway should never be considered protected with any method of airway device, having no airway management in place poses the highest risk of aspiration. This is especially so in ruminants but can occur in any animals, especially if the procedure requires dental or oral surgery. The rostrum should be positioned lower than the larynx, reducing gastrointestinal fluids passing up the esophagus but also allowing passive drainage from the oral cavity. Suction is useful in reducing any fluids found within the oral or pharyngeal cavity during or at the end of surgery. Manual and active suction systems are available and should be considered as part of the basic anesthetic kit.

The position of the animal must be considered, for instance, large mammals in dorsal recumbency are likely to have abdominal viscera pressing on the diaphragm resulting in a reduction in ventilation. Equally, animals that are being moved in stretchers or have their neck flexed for cerebrospinal fluid taps may be at risk of decreased airway patency, and intubation or armored tubes should be considered. It is essential that airway patency is monitored and maintained throughout a procedure, whether intubated or not.

Awake Intubation

"Awake" intubation is relatively common in human anesthesia. The logistical challenges in zoo and wildlife anesthesia make this unsuitable for most patients; however, it is a useful technique in reptiles and avian patients with existing airsac cannulae. It is described in sedated foals (Bednarski 2009) and could potentially be employed under sedation, if indicated.

Snakes, where intravenous or intramuscular inductions are contraindicated or simply not preferred due to the nature of the procedure, may be restrained and intubated consciously with or without sedation (Redrobe 2004). The animal must often be ventilated and can be induced using a volatile agent, leaving the tracheal tube in place for management throughout anesthesia (Fig. 3.1).

Avian patients with previously placed airsac cannulae can be connected to the anesthetic machine while gently restrained and induced via the caudal airsacs (Hawkins & Pascoe 2007).

Intubation Following Induction

Intubation following induction is the most common route for intubation in both domestic and wildlife patients. Induction can be achieved through the use of inhalation, intramuscular, or intravenous agents depending on the species and the choice of anesthetic

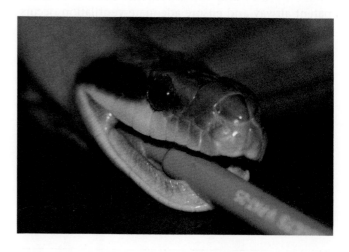

Figure 3.1. Cave racer (*Elaphe taeniura ridleyi*) consciously intubated with a Cole tube prior to being induced with isoflurane.

agent. Inhalation induction can be achieved with the direct application of a facemask, the use of an induction chamber, or through conscious intubation. Muscle relaxants are not often employed in veterinary medicine yet are a useful aid to augment intubation; these do require the use of manual or mechanical ventilation, and rapid intubation must be ensured to prevent hypoxia. Once the patient is anesthetized, the oral cavity can be opened and intubation should be relatively straightforward, depending on the species and the implementation of the airway management plan (Hartsfield 2007).

Planning Airway Management

The American Society of Anesthesiologists (Hasan 2010) has five basic steps in airway management (Calder & Pearce 2007):

- Evaluation of the airway
- Preparation of the airway
- Airway strategy at the start of anesthesia
- Airway management at the end of anesthesia
- Follow-up.

The same principles apply to airway management in zoo animals and wildlife. Evaluation of the airway seeks to establish which airway device will provide the appropriate level of protection and maintenance for the proposed procedure. It requires a basic level of knowledge regarding the patient's anatomy, physiology, and any risks that may occur during anesthesia. In some cases, airway devices maybe ruled out due to being incompatible with the species, for example, cuffed tubes must be used with care in species with complete tracheal rings, or is the tracheal tube selected long enough to reach the thoracic larynx of the giant anteater (*Myrmecophaga tridactyla*) The inherent risk of each device must also be considered, especially when utilizing a new technique for the first time.

Selection is based upon:

- Species suitability
- Experience of the anesthetist
- Size of the patient
- Perceived risk of aspiration
- The nature of the surgery
- Whether positive pressure ventilation is required
- Requirement for surgical access to the head or neck
- Whether the surgery is likely to interfere with the airway
- Availability.

Evaluation is often difficult, especially when anesthetizing a new species for the first time. Anatomical variation is considerable across the taxonomic groups and as such the clinician should endeavor to gain as much insight into the idiosyncrasies of their patient's anatomy prior to induction, or at a minimum have a wide variety of options available when planning and implementing the airway strategy.

An airway strategy simply considers the default plan for intubation and having a plan B if plan A fails, and potentially a plan C if plan B fails (Calder & Pearce 2007). It is important to consider common eventualities and have support through colleagues and alternative airway management devices during intubation. Intubation is often a simple, hassle free exercise but when it goes wrong it can be extremely stressful and have a major impact on the patient. Difficulty in intubation can occur in a variety of causes depending on who you are, where you are, what equipment and drugs you have, who you have to help you, and what the patient is like. Patient causes of difficult airway management include normal but poorly assessed anatomy, poorly positioned patient, unwanted reflexes, stiffness or deformity of the head or peripharyngeal anatomy, swelling, foreign bodies, and airway pathology. It can be extremely useful to have a difficult airway algorithm. Examples can be found on the ASA and Difficult Airway Society (DAS) websites (http://www.asahq.org or http://www.das.uk.com, respectively).

It is important that the process of the airway strategy is documented on the anesthetic chart and in the subsequent medical records. This should include, as a basic minimum, any specific notes on the anatomy that pertain to intubation, the airway device used, the size of the device and any problems noted during anesthesia, and any comments on the act of intubation itself. This information is useful for follow-up audits or subsequent anesthetics for that individual or the species as a whole, which may benefit the anesthetist and their colleagues.

MAINTENANCE OF THE AIRWAY DURING ANESTHESIA

Patient Positioning

The position of the patient is often dictated by the needs of the surgery but must take into consideration the impact on ventilation and subsequent alteration of respiratory mechanics and physiology.

The upper airway should remain patent prior to intubation or during the procedure if intubation is not performed. For most species, this simply consists of extending the neck, pulling the tongue rostrolaterally, and placing the head with the rostrum lower than the larynx to protect against aspiration: this applies to obligate nasal breathers and oral breathers. It is important to make sure that no environmental structures can obstruct the nares or mouth during anesthesia, for example, if an animal is anesthetized in a deep straw bed.

Positioning of the body is extremely variable depending on the individual species and the need of the procedure. In general terms, sternal recumbency is preferred but often impractical; lateral recumbency is most common and for short periods has minimal impact on respiratory function; with dorsal often having the greatest impact on respiratory function due to the abdominal viscera pressing on the diaphragm, airsacs or lungs. It should be noted though that species variation is considerable and positioning needs to take into account the anatomy of the species concerned for example, sternal recumbency is considered to be contraindicated, except in extreme circumstances, in elephants due to their unique pulmonary anatomy (Steffey 2006).

Supraglottic Airway Devices

The term *supraglottic* refers to the area situated or occurring above the glottis, this encompasses the epiglottis and anything rostral to the vocal cords. As soon as an airway device enters the larynx, passing the vocal cords, it is classed as an *infraglottic* device or simply endotracheal. Some authors utilize an alternative classification with the supraglottic airway devices (SAD) separated into simple airway adjuncts and SAD, which includes the various laryngeal mask airways only (Cook 2012). The former classification will be used here. Subglottic devices are found below the larynx, for example, tracheostomy tubes.

There are many supraglottic airway devices and these include:

• Oropharyngeal airway
• Nasopharyngeal airway
• Facemasks
• Laryngeal mask airway (LMA).

Oropharyngeal (Guedel) Airways This is a simple device that ensures patency of the supraglottic airway by pushing the tongue and epiglottis from the posterior pharyngeal wall. Commonly used in human anesthesia, their use is limited in zoo and wildlife species due to more useful alternatives such as tracheal intubation. Their use in zoo and wildlife medicine is questionable, but homemade variants can be used as bite blocks or to augment preoxygenation following induction, in an emergency prior to intubation proper.

Nasopharyngeal Airways These are passed through the nares, along the ventral nasal meatus to sit in the oropharynx above the epiglottis. They are useful as they can bypass nasal, soft palate and tongue obstructions and allow delivery of oxygen and volatile agents (Fig. 3.2). Nasopharyngeal airways are commonly used in equine anesthesia during recovery, especially when the horse has been in dorsal recumbency for a prolonged period (Taylor & Clarke 2008). If there are any concerns regarding airway patency, then nasopharyngeal tubes are a simple preventative method that can

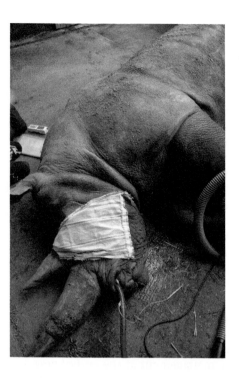

Figure 3.2. White rhinoceros (*Ceratotherium simum*) with a nasopharyngeal tube in place that was later used as a nasotracheal tube. Nasopharyngeal tubes can be useful in recovery where nasal edema may lead to obstruction or restricted upper airways in nasal obligate breathers.

easily be passed by most species soon after recovery. Placement of nasopharyngeal tubes can be extended to nasotracheal intubation simply by advancing the tube through the glottis (Bednarski 2009).

Facemasks Face masks are designed to fit over the nose and mouth of patients with a low pressure seal. The facemask consists of three parts: the mount, the body, and the edge. Facemasks are commonly used in zoo and wildlife medicine for induction of smaller, manually restrained mammals or birds. Larger animals require sedation prior to facemask induction. In some cases, they are used for maintenance as well, although this is not recommended for anything more than the shortest of procedures or where intubation is impossible or contraindicated. Facemasks can be a useful tool for augmenting or preoxygenating patients. In some cases, intermittent positive pressure ventilation is possible but carries the risk of gastric tympany.

Facemasks are either opaque or transparent. Opaque masks are useful during induction as they eliminate any visual stimulation to the animal. However, transparent masks have an advantage during maintenance as signs of regurgitation and expiration fogging can be seen through the mask's body. Choice is down to the individual anesthetist.

When selecting the facemask size, consideration must be given to the volume of the mask. Large volumes result in increased apparatus dead space, which can have considerable impact on smaller patients due to rebreathing expired gases. It is preferable to have the smallest volume within the mask possible: this can be achieved with snug fitting masks or by reducing the space by packing the mask with cotton wool or similar materials. Placing the whole head in the mask reduces this space, also but care must be taken to ensure that the edge does not compress the skin of the muzzle, trachea or even the thorax (Dorsch & Dorsch 2008a). In practice, increased flow rates of carrier gas can eliminate the risk of rebreathing, and clinicians are more likely to have flow rates that exceed the requirement intended for selected patient-circuit combinations.

Facemasks can be commercially produced or homemade. Often, commercially made masks do not meet the variety of our patient head and nares sizes. Homemade masks are often easy to produce, can be made cheaply and even disposable depending on the type. This author often uses the neoprene from old wet suits for the edge and a variety of tubs and drain pipes as the body of his facemasks, using standard endotracheal tube mounts attached at the circuit end. Latex gloves can also be used as an effective edge, requiring disposal afterwards. These homemade masks are safe and often very effective. Consideration should be given to the type of facemask used, a small mask is just as effective and may have smaller apparatus dead space then a larger one (Fig. 3.3).

Facemasks do not prevent supraglottic obstruction, and the patient must always be monitored for signs of airway obstruction. Equally, they do not provide any protection against aspiration. While commonly used on their own, this cannot be recommended due to their inability to ensure a patent airway (Bateman et al. 2005).

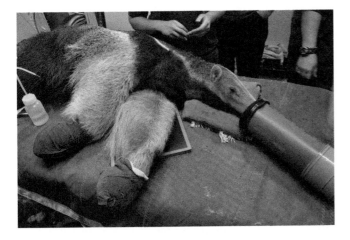

Figure 3.3. A homemade facemask being used for maintenance in a giant anteater (*Myrmecophaga tridacytyla*): such a large apparatus dead space requires high flow rates to prevent rebreathing when compared to a smaller facemask.

Laryngeal Mask Airways (LMA) These are a relatively new method of airway management introduced in the late 1980s in human anesthesia, with subsequent trials in the 1990s in veterinary patients and the first commercial veterinary LMAs becoming available in 2010 (Dorsch & Dorsch 2008b). They have been used in a variety of species, varying from great apes to swine to small mammals including rabbits (Bateman et al. 2005; Cassu et al. 2004; Fulkerson & Gustafson 2007). Currently, commercial LMAs are only available for rabbits and cats, with six sizes being available for each species (Crotaz 2010). LMAs can be considered as a bridge between the ease of use of simple airway adjuncts and the technical and sometimes challenging aspects of tracheal intubation. The LMA consists of an inflatable cuff that sits over or above the level of the larynx, overlying a bowl, similar to a small facemask, joined to a stem that extends out of the oral cavity where it is attached to the anesthetic circuit. The LMA sits over the larynx, directly above the glottis in most cases: the limitation being quality of the seal is dependent on the variation in laryngeal anatomy across the species and the requirement for the LMA to be compatible with species-specific anatomical variation. This major limitation has been overcome with the development of the commercial veterinary LMAs.

LMAs are fitted in a variety of methods depending on the type (there are currently more then 40). In general, the LMA is a reusable device and must undergo sufficient checks prior to use, including: does the cuff leak, is there eccentric inflation of the cuff, or failure of the inflation valve, is the lumen clear? The cuff is then deflated, with the cuff retracting behind the level of the bowl. This is then lubricated with a water-based gel. The LMA is typically advanced along the hard palate, then the soft palate to be guided into place until resistance is felt. The cuff is then inflated with air. Each has a maximum volume and inflation should be achieved with a lower, optimal volume; overinflation can increase cuff pressures, reduce the seal and increase the risk of aspiration. In humans the success rate using the blind technique is extremely high (>95%) (Cook 2012). Checks for correct placement are described as follows: on inflation, the mask tip rises 0.5–2 cm, the anterior neck of the patient is seen to slightly fill and the midline on the tube should remain anatomically in midline: if any of these do not occur then the LMA should be refitted. In the case of the commercial veterinary LMAs, the devices have a shoulder that catches on the palatine arch providing confirmation of correct placement. These lack an inflatable cuff and rely on a tight fit locally to effect the seal and have features specific to the individual species that ensure the seal occurs.

The advantage of the LMAs include the maintenance of a patent upper airway, improved airway maintenance compared with other supraglottic devices, they are useful in species that are difficult to intubate, reduce risk of endotracheal or laryngeal damage, ease of application, and they are well tolerated by patients, especially in recovery. However, they do not guarantee tracheal isolation from aspiration; ventilation is dependent on a tight seal, which is species-LMA brand dependent, and gastric tympany is possible if the seal is not tight or ventilation pressures are high. In humans, complications include failures, displacements, airway obstruction, sore throats, pharyngeal trauma and nerve injuries from pressure effects: with the main concern being that of aspiration (Cook 2012). A similar picture is likely in animals. There are several different LMAs and readers are advised to utilize species-specific veterinary LMAs or alternatively follow manufacturer's guidelines and seek advice for individual species prior to the use of human LMAs in wild animal patients.

Infraglottic Devices

Tracheal Tubes Tracheal, orotracheal, or endotracheal tubes are considered to provide the highest level of airway maintenance and protection as well as providing the most suitable route for airway ventilation. They are unlikely to be dislodged, provide protection from inhalation of foreign material, glottis reflexes are bypassed, and they allow good intraoral surgical access, which is needed in zoo and wildlife patients with dental work being a part of standard health checks. This is a common method of airway maintenance and is familiar to most veterinarians. However, it is not a benign methodology, and an understanding of the anatomy of the endotracheal tube is essential.

The generic tracheal tube consists of a beveled end, often with a murphy eye, a cuff, the tube itself, a self-sealing valve, and a 15-mm connector (with larger ones found on large animal tubes). Additional features include markings for the length of the tube, a radio-opaque line, and the internal diameter of the tube in millimetres (Cook 2012). Tracheal tubes can be straight but are usually curved with some, such as RAE tubes, having a 180° curve in them. The bevel assists in insertion through the glottis, with the murphy eye preventing obstruction if the bevel were to become occluded against the tracheal wall or blocked with foreign material. The tracheal tube is often made of either transparent soft silicone or more rigid plastics, such as PVC or polyurethane. Older, but still available, "red rubber" tubes may also be seen, which are made of mineralized rubber. The "red rubber" tube's disadvantage being that they are opaque and risk not being adequately cleaned, and the rubber tends to crack over time leading to further hygiene concerns. Armoured tubes are also available, which have a steel spiral running the length of the tube: these are kink resistant but not kink proof. They are particularly useful if moving animals in stretchers where the neck may become kinked

leading to airway obstruction. Tracheal tubes come in a large variety of sizes and shapes that meet the need of most of the species that may be met in a zoo or wild setting.

When choosing the type of tracheal tube, the cuff design is an important consideration. There are two basic types: low volume–high pressure (LVHP) and high volume–low pressure (HVLP) (Mitchell & Patel 2007). LVHP cuffs are uncommon but can still be seen on the "red rubber" type tracheal tubes. They have several disadvantages when compared with the HVLP types: the high pressure needed to inflate the cuff can result in excessive transluminal pressures resulting in tracheal ischemia, scarring, and stenosis; the cuff inflates in a circular manner and does not conform to the tracheal shape: and as the rubber cuff ages, it has the potential to deteriorate with weaknesses appearing, resulting in balloons forming that could herniate over the end of the tube leading to obstruction. The HVLP cuffs in comparison have a much larger volume and a lower pressure is required to effect a seal of the airway. This minimizes the transluminal pressures and reduces the impact on the tracheal mucosa; however, the cuff does develop folds through which liquids can pass and be aspirated (Cook 2012). Therefore, the concept of tracheal tubes protecting the airway should be challenged as this protection is incomplete. In practice, however, the benefits of the HVLP may be theoretical as their contact is over a larger area then the LVHP with the potential for low level damage to the tracheal mucosa over a larger area, as such the cost–benefit is likely to be similar when all aspects are considered.

All cuffs should be inflated to the pressure needed to create a seal, not to a predetermined volume. Excessive pressures can lead to tracheal pathology as noted previously. Cuff pressure always exceeds lateral wall pressure and it is advisable, although rarely performed, to measure cuff pressures with an intracuff pressure monitor (Mitchell & Patel 2007). Cuff pressures vary throughout a procedure: in the case of nitrous oxide, the gas can diffuse into the cuff and inflate the cuff, or in the case of positive pressure ventilation, as airway pressure increases the cuff becomes compressed, raising the internal cuff pressure. Cuff pressures are also not uniform within the same cuff, with variation across a cuff being considerable. Tracheal tubes close to tracheal lumen diameter will have a greater tracheal mucosal pressure if a similar volume is used for insufflation of a smaller diameter tube. This may seem obvious, but often clinicians insufflate with a standard volume, whatever the size of the patient. The recommended insufflation pressure is 20–34 cm H_2O, any higher then 40 cm H_2O will potentially result in tracheal ischemia and its subsequent sequelae (Dorsch & Dorsch 2008c; Hartsfield 2007). Any lower then the risk of aspiration is increased. Overinflation can also result in occlusion of the tracheal tube itself. The use of an intracuff pres-

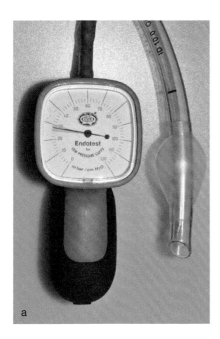 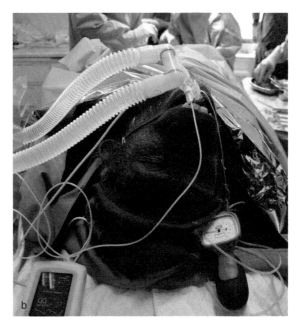

Figure 3.4. An intracuff pressure monitoring device allows accurate selection of cuff pressure and a reduction in risks associated with excessive cuff pressures.

sure monitor device is strongly recommended but these are rarely seen in clinical practice (Fig. 3.4).

Some tracheal tubes do not have a cuff. There is a variety of choices, the most common being the uncuffed tube and the Cole tube. The Cole tube has a patient end that is smaller than the rest of the shaft. This is commonly used in avian and reptilian patients with the shoulder placed against the larynx to form a seal. This is a misuse of this type of tube and the shoulder should not come into contact with the laryngeal structures as it may result in their damage. The Cole tube is designed to have less resistance to flow then a tube with a narrower consistent internal diameter for its entire length (Dorsch & Dorsch 2008c).

Selection of tube length and diameter is an important factor in tube choice. The length of the tube should be taken from the level of the incisors/tip of beak to a distance safely past the larynx. In mammals, this is often reported to be just cranial to the thoracic inlet but 1/3 distance from the larynx is fine. In other species, knowledge of the tracheal anatomy is essential. In the case of penguins, the trachea bifurcates between 1 and 5 cm from the glottis depending on the species. Tracheal bifurcation is also seen in amphibians and chelonia. Often the bifurcation can be seen at intubation but radiography can be useful in assessing tube placement if unsure. Length is directly proportional to resistance and the shortest length of tracheal tube should be used; often this requires cutting down the tube. The tube should be cut off at the level of the incisors/beak tip to reduce apparatus dead space and resistance. Another challenge is seen in some avian species that have a dorsal oriented projection of the

ventral cricoid cartilage into the glottis called the crista ventralis (McLelland 1989); this reduces the diameter of the tube that can be safely placed (Fig. 3.5a,b). Diameter selection is often down to the individual's choice and the need of the procedure. It is recommended to use the widest diameter tube that will easily pass through the vocal cords or the cricoid ring (or equivalent structure). The tracheal tube offers the narrowest point in the anesthetic circuit and, apart from possible valves in a circle, offers the greatest resistance, and therefore work of breathing, on expiration for the patient (Mitchell & Patel 2007). Smaller diameter tubes are easier to insert, cause less laryngeal damage, and have a lower incidence of tracheal irritation. However, smaller diameters increase airway resistance, have excessive cuff volumes, are difficult to use suction with in the airway, and are difficult to use with fibreoptic endoscopy. Larger tube diameters conversely have a lower work of breathing in spontaneously breathing patients, and tracheal suction is easier. They are harder to insert, have greater potential for laryngeal trauma, infolding of the cuff may lead to leakage around the cuff, and risk of excessive insufflation volumes can result in greater tracheal damage. Resistance is inversely proportional to the radius to the power of four; in practical terms, this means doubling the tube radius decreases the resistance by a factor of 16 (Middleton et al. 2012). While doubling the radius seems excessive, this is equivalent to moving to a 5-mm from a 2.5-mm internal diameter tube, which this author has noted with students using a laryngoscope (clear visualization) or not for feline intubation (limited visualization), this also holds for many zoo and wildlife species. The

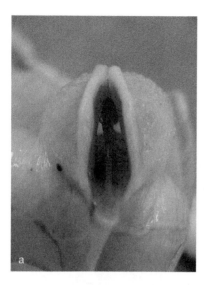
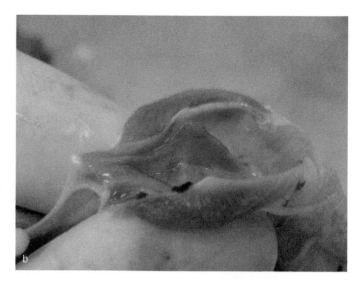

Figure 3.5. (a and b) The crista ventralis is a projection from the ventral aspect of the cricoid cartilage found in a variety of avian species (a). This reduces the size of tracheal tube that can be used. This is not a bifurcation as can be aseen when the dorsal larynx is removed (b) (Eastern white pelican, *Pelecanus onocrotalus*).

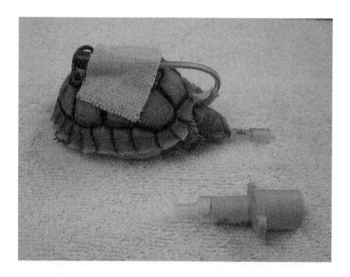

Figure 3.6. Intravenous cannulae can be used as tracheal tubes in extremely small patients. To attach to the anesthetic circuit a cut down 2.5-mL syringe and a standard 7.5 15-mm connector can be used as an adapter (African spurred tortoise, *Geochelone sulcata*).

number on the outside of a tube determines the internal diameter. Depending on the brand or type of tube used, there can be considerable variation on the external diameter. It is essential that the type and brand of tube used is recorded on the anesthetic sheet, not just the size of tube.

In extremely small patients, intravenous cannulae can be utilized as tracheal tubes. Care must be taken in ensuring the material (rigid to prevent collapse) and the length is suitable. Cannulae will attach to the end of a cut down 2.5-mL syringe barrel with a 7.5-mm tracheal tube connector inserted in the syringe lumen (Fig. 3.6), allowing connection to an anesthetic circuit. It should be noted that with such small tracheal tubes,

when using pressure cycled ventilators, the resistance to ventilation is not simply overcome by increasing flow rate and airway pressure as most ventilators measure the pressure at the connector end of the tube and not the lung pressure. Clinicians are advised to calibrate flow and pressure settings to individual cannulae if using them in this way.

Subglottic Devices

Tracheostomy Tubes Tracheostomy tubes are rarely used in zoo and wildlife patients. They are indicated in cases where intubation with supraglottic devices or tracheal tubes is impossible or where longer term airway management is required. The techniques used are similar to that described in the domestic species and their use has been described in various wildlife species (Brainard et al. 2008).

Avian Air Sac Cannulae Due to the unique anatomical and physiological adaptations of the avian respiratory system, airsac cannulae can be employed for management of upper airway obstruction or longer term respiratory support (Hawkins & Pascoe 2007).

Intrapneumonic Cannulae These have been reported in reptiles for intrapneumonic therapy. If already surgically placed, then these have the potential to be used for respiratory support or even induction if required; however, the author is unaware of them being used in this fashion (Wilkinson 2004).

AIDS TO TRACHEAL INTUBATION

Tracheal intubation is the most challenging airway management technique, yet is one that is considered basic and part of daily routines. Some species are easy and offer no challenge while others are extremely difficult due to anatomical features and lack of species-specific equipment. There are many tools and techniques available that can increase our success of a rapid, safe, and effective intubation.

Laryngoscope

The laryngoscope should be considered a basic part of the anesthetic equipment. A laryngoscope consists of a light source, a handle, and a blade. The blade is designed to sit in the vallecula, just rostral to the epiglottis. A slight tilt of the blade drops the epiglottis and depresses the tongue providing improved visualization of the glottis. There are two basic types of light source: a screw on bulb at the end of the blade or a fibreoptic blade. Blades come in a variety of shapes, lengths, and sizes. Choice is down to the individual; this author prefers the macintosh (curved) and miller (straight with a slight curve at the end) blades and a custom-built 35-cm long miller blade. Laryngoscopes are relatively cheap, improve visualization, and can also be used to improve oral and dental visualization during health checks (Cook 2012).

Optical laryngoscopes have become available in the last decade that have the added advantage of a video monitor built into the handle which is linked to the tip of the blade, allowing accurate tube placement. One such device uses a series of mirrors similar to a periscope to achieve a similar result without the need for video or fibreoptic technology (Cook 2012). Some brands come with a built-in guide for the tracheal tube. While potentially useful, they are limited due to their expense, size (designed for humans) and limited use in the field.

Optical Stylets

Optical stylets are rigid or malleable laparoscopes or dedicated laryngoscopes used as stylets with the tracheal tube placed over the scope. The scope is used to identify the glottis and direct the tube into the glottis or place the scope in the glottis and slide the tube down into the trachea. These are often used elsewhere in the clinic for laparoscopy and their use is limited to a veterinary clinic due to the need for power and their general bulk.

Flexible Endoscopes

Flexible endoscopes are commonplace in large veterinary clinics and can be used in a similar manner to optical stylets. Dedicated flexible fibreoptic endoscopes for intubation are commercially available, but are often designed for humans and as such do not have the length often required for some of the larger patients seen in zoo practices. Cystoscopes and bronchoscopes are useful and of suitable size for most patients. They offer unparalled flexibility and the ability to be used for nasal or oral intubation; however, they are expensive when compared with other techniques and are not often seen in zoo animal or wildlife practice nor can they be used in the field. They also allow the direct visualization of tracheal and lower airway structures, which can be useful in certain cases.

Bougies and Stylets

Bougies or stylets are malleable, plastic-coated stylets that are passed through a partially visible glottis and then the tracheal tube is passed over the top. These are especially useful with soft, flexible tubes. Light wands are available and are similar to stylets with a light on the end: this allows transillumination of the neck and assessment of the level of tube placement.

Gags and Ropes

The use of ropes or bandage allow controlled opening of the oral cavity to facilitate intubation without the operator's fingers being placed between the teeth, and being put at risk of being bitten, or obscuring the view for the anesthetist intubating.

Gags are available as either wooden or plastic devices that can be placed on one side of the dental arcade or across both, the latter often having a hole to allow the tracheal tube to be passed through into the glottis. In the megafauna, large wooden bite blocks have been used to obtain safe access for intubation (Steffey 2006).

METHODS OF TRACHEAL INTUBATION

Tracheal intubation is relatively straightforward in most of the patients encountered in zoo and wildlife anesthesia. The mnemonic PEACH is extremely useful: Position, Equipment, Attach oxygen and equipment, Checks on patient, and Help if required (Maran et al. 2008). Assuming equipment selection is appropriate for the species and that all standard safety checks have been completed, the main factor for successful intubation to occur is the positioning of the patient. There is considerable variation between the species, but general comments hold true for most patients (Hartsfield 2007):

- Check the mouth for food or foreign material and wash out if required
- Open the oral cavity as wide as possible to facilitate passage of the tracheal tube
- Ensure the oral and laryngeal axis are as close together as possible by extending the neck and pulling the head rostrally
- Ensure the larynx is in midline: this is usually the case in sternal or dorsal recumbency intubation but it can drop down if intubating in lateral recumbency and may need to be manipulated into place
- Pull the tongue forwards and laterally
- Use aids to visualize the larynx when appropriate (unless undertaking blind intubation)

- Use appropriate tube diameter for the patient: be prepared to step down or up depending on findings at visual inspection
- Use topical local anesthetic spray depending on the need: in some species, laryngospasm can hinder the passage of a tracheal tube, and if unsure, then often better to use then not. Wait 30 seconds for this to take effect.
- Pass the tube into the glottis and into the trachea, ensuring the larynx is passed but the tube remains cranial to the bifurcation
- Confirm tube placement
- Secure the tube in place
- Attach to the anesthetic circuit
- Inflate the cuff to 25–34 cm H_2O

Direct Visualization
This is the preferred method of intubation. In animals with large oral cavities, this is relatively straightforward, and a clear view of the larynx can often be achieved. Using laryngoscopes or other aids can facilitate intubation and allow the use of large diameter tubes.

Blind Intubation
This technique requires the anesthetist to guide the tube into the glottis without being able to visualize the glottis. Blind intubation is possible, and is commonly practiced in a large proportion of the patients seen, for example, lagomorphs, artiodactylids, and perissodactylids. This technique requires knowledge of the anatomical features of that patient. Depending on the animal, this is often performed in lateral recumbency for large animals or sternal for smaller animals. In larger animals, the tracheal tube is measured against the outside of the animal to estimate the length required to reach the larynx; the tracheal tube is passed through the oral cavity, and the respiratory sounds are listened to. Once the larynx is reached, the sounds change, the animal may swallow, and the tube is passed gently into the glottis, and secured in the usual fashion. In smaller animals, a similar technique is used, but the anesthetist can listen through the tube as it is inserted. A single person can do this in both cases.

Palpation Intubation
This technique is used in large mammals where the anesthetist passes their hand through the oral cavity, into the pharynx, and feels for the glottis, passing the tube alongside their arm. This is quick and effective and often used in artiodactylids; however, care must be taken as if prolonged it can lead to hypoxemia (Riebold et al. 1995; Steffey 2006).

Retrograde Intubation
This is a technique where a hypodermic needle is placed into the trachea at the level of the second and third tracheal cartilages and a guide wire passed out through the larynx and oral cavity, a tube then being passed over the guide wire and into the trachea. This technique is frequently used in rodents and smaller animals but can be used where direct visualization or blind techniques have failed. The cuff should be placed caudal to the needle insertion site to prevent leakage of anesthetic gases into the surrounding tissues, which could lead to subcutaneous emphysema or even pneumothorax (Hartsfield 2007; Pearce 2007).

Confirmation of Tracheal Intubation
Misplacement of the tracheal tube is the most common complication of intubation, especially when using blind techniques. The tube may be placed in the esophagus or a bronchi and it is important that confirmation of correct placement is obtained immediately after intubation takes place. Oesophageal tube placement can lead to insufflation of the stomach, increased risk of regurgitation, hypoxia, and potentially death. Bronchial intubation can lead to hypoxemia, lung or lobar collapse, and increased risk of barotrauma to the intubated lung. Methods to assess correct placement include (Sanehi 2007):

- Visual confirmation that the tracheal tube has passed through the glottis and is in the trachea.
- Palpation of the trachea on intubation: the anesthetists can feel the tube pass over the tracheal rings; this is not felt if the tube is in the esophagus
- Confirmation of respiratory gases passing through the tracheal tube on expiration. A quick fur pluck can be useful: this is held at the end of the tracheal tube, and on expiration, they bend away from the tube; if nothing happens, then either the fur is too stiff or the tube is in the esophagus. Note the anesthetist should not press on the thorax to elicit expiration; this can lead to regurgitation. An alternative is to put a hand close to the end of the tube and feel for the gas passing through.
- Attach the tube to the circuit and monitor the reservoir bag movement on expiration and inspiration
- Gentle pressure on the reservoir bag should result in the thorax expanding. However, this can on occasion also appear to happen with insufflation of the stomach. It also allows assessment of whether the tracheal tube is in a bronchi: the compliance decreases and unequal insufflation of the thorax may occur.
- Capnography is extremely useful and a normal capnogram for six breaths suggests tracheal intubation. False negatives can occur with large gas leaks, cardiac arrest, and severe bronchospasm where no trace would appear on the capnogram
- Auscultation of both sides of the chest suggest tracheal placement and not bronchial
- Radiography: often the tracheal tube appears on any thoracic radiographs and can be assessed for posi-

tion. Due to the 2D nature of this technique, it cannot be used alone for assessment.

Extubation

Extubation should occur at the time that a patient has the ability to swallow and protect their airway. If extubation is too early, then there is risk of aspiration and loss of airway; if too late, then it can lead to irritation and potential laryngospasm and sympathetic stimulation. In some cases, suction of the oral cavity is essential to prevent any aspiration at extubation. There are no rules on the best time to extubate, and the timing has to be assessed depending on the species, the ease of removal, the risk to the animal and the clinician, the procedure, and the ease of maintaining the airway if reintubation is required (Dugdale 2010; Gray 2007; Hartsfield 2007). Extubation should include:

- Administer 100% oxygen or air depending on the species
- Assessment followed by suction of the oropharynx and oral cavity under direct vision if required
- Untie the tube
- Deflate the tracheal tube cuff
- Apply positive pressure to the reservoir bag, immediately followed by removal of the tube (expiration immediately follows clearing any supraglottic secretions)
- Confirm airway patency and position of animal
- Supplementary 100% oxygen or air depending on the species
- (Placement of a nasal tube if required).

The anesthetist must be prepared for postextubation obstruction: edema of the upper airway, laryngeal spasm, soft palate or tongue obstruction, and laryngeal paralysis have all been reported (Rex 1971; Taylor & Clarke 2008). The airway must be maintained during recovery in a similar fashion to that outlined at induction.

Airway Idiopathic Trauma

Intubation is not entirely benign. The incidence of intubation-related trauma leading to the need for clinical intervention is low though. If care and consideration is taken during intubation, combined with suitable use of airway devices, then airway trauma can be minimized. Anesthetic trauma includes (Calder 2007):

- Dental damage can occur with inappropriate use of laryngoscopes, gags or ropes at the time of intubation.
- Nasopharyngeal damage can occur during nasopharyngeal intubation; accurate placement and knowledge of species anatomy can avoid this relatively easily.

- Oesophageal perforation while uncommon has been reported.
- Pharyngeal edema or trauma with excessive force at the time of intubation has been reported.
- Glottic damage: animal coughing or dyspneic postrecovery. This can occur with tubes of too large diameter or rough intubations, often passing after 1–2 days. If it persists or is considered severe, then examination under anesthesia is indicated.
- Tracheal damage can be acute or chronic. Acute rupture or perforation has occurred with excessive cuff pressure or through intubation itself: subcutaneous air is often apparent. Granulation tissue and edema can form, especially in excessively long procedures or animals that maybe being ventilated for a long time, for example, barbiturate poisoning in large felids (Saulez et al. 2009).

Cleaning and Disinfection

Most airway devices are reusable or clinics reuse systems that are designed to be disposable. It is essential that airway devices are appropriately decontaminated, cleaned, and sterilized before they are reused to prevent cross infection. Heat sterilization is preferred, with cold chemical sterilization used for some of the nonautoclavable tubes. If prion disease is considered a risk, then the equipment should be disposed of following a procedure.

REFERENCES

Bateman L, Ludders JW, Gleed RD, Erb HN. 2005. Comparison between facemask and laryngeal mask airway in rabbits during isoflurane anesthesia. *Veterinary Anaesthesia and Analgesia* 32(5):280–288.

Bednarski RM. 2009. Tracheal and nasal intubation. In: *Equine Anesthesia* (WW Muir, JAE Hubbell, eds.), pp. 277–287. Missouri: Saunders Elsevier.

Brainard BM, Newton A, Hinshaw KC, Klide AM. 2008. Tracheostomy in the giant anteater (*Myrmecophaga tridactyla*). *Journal of Zoo and Wildlife Medicine: Official Publication of the American Association of Zoo Veterinarians* 39(4):655–658.

Calder I. 2007. Trauma to the airway. In: *Core Topics in Airway Management* (I Calder, A Pearce, eds.), pp. 169–172. Cambridge: Cambridge University Press.

Calder I, Pearce A. 2007. General principles. In: *Core Topics in Airway Management* (I Calder, A Pearce, eds.), pp. 35–42. Cambridge: Cambridge University Press.

Cassu RN, Luna SP, Teixeira Neto FJ, Braz JR, Gasparini SS, Crocci AJ. 2004. Evaluation of laryngeal mask as an alternative to endotracheal intubation in cats anesthetized under spontaneous or controlled ventilation. *Veterinary Anaesthesia and Analgesia* 31(3):213–221.

Cook T. 2007. Maintenance of the airway during anaesthesia: supra-glottic devices. In: *Core Topics in Airway Management* (I Calder, A Pearce, eds.), pp. 43–56. Cambridge: Cambridge University Press.

Cook T. 2012. Airway management equipment. In: *Ward's Anaesthetic Equipment* (AJ Davey, A Diba, eds.), pp. 139–205. Edinburgh: Saunders Elsevier.

Crotaz IR. 2010. Initial feasibility investigation of the v-gel airway: an anatomically designed supraglottic airway device for use in companion animal veterinary anaesthesia. *Veterinary Anaesthesia and Analgesia* 37(6):579–580. doi: 10.1111/j.1467-2995.2010.00566.x.

Dorsch JA, Dorsch SE. 2008a. Face masks and airways. In: *Understanding Anesthesia Equipment* (JA Dorsch, SE Dorsch, eds.), pp. 443–460. Philadelphia: Lippincott, Williams & Wilkins.

Dorsch JA, Dorsch SE. 2008b. Supraglottic airway devices. In: *Understanding Anesthesia Equipment* (JA Dorsch, SE Dorsch, eds.), pp. 461–519. Philadelphia: Lippincott, Williams & Wilkins.

Dorsch JA, Dorsch SE. 2008c. Tracheal tubes and associated equipment. In: *Understanding Anesthesia Equipment.* (JA Dorsch, SE Dorsch, eds.), pp. 561–628. Philadelphia: Lippincott, Williams & Wilkins.

Dugdale A. 2010. Anaesthetic breathing systems. In: *Veterinary Anaesthesia Principles to Practice* (A Dugdale, ed.), pp. 76–92. Chichester: Wiley-Blackwell.

Farmery AD. 2007. Physics and physiology. In: *Core Topics in Airway Management* (I Calder, A Pearce, eds.), pp. 21–29. Cambridge: Cambridge University Press.

Fulkerson PJ, Gustafson SB. 2007. Use of laryngeal mask airway compared to endotracheal tube with positive-pressure ventilation in anesthetized swine. *Veterinary Anaesthesia and Analgesia* 34(4):284–288.

Gray H. 2007. Extubation. In: *Core Topics in Airway Management* (I Calder, A Pearce, eds.), pp. 87–92. Cambridge: Cambridge University Press.

Hartsfield SM. 2007. Airway management and ventialtion. In: *Lumb and Jones' Veterinary Anesthesia and Analgesia* (WJ Tranquilli, JC Thurmon, KA Grimm, eds.), pp. 495–531. Iowa: Blackwell Publishing.

Hasan A. 2010. The conventional modes of mechanical ventilation. In: *Understanding Mechanical Ventilation: A Practical Handbook* (A Hasan, ed.), pp. 71–113. London: Springer-Verlag London.

Hawkins MG, Pascoe PJ. 2007. Cagebirds. In: *Zoo Animal and Wildlife Immobilization and Anesthesia* (G West, D Heard, N Caulkett, eds.), pp. 269–297. Iowa: Blackwell Publishing.

McLelland J. 1989. Larynx and trachea. In: *Form and function in birds.* (AS King, J McLelland, eds.), pp. 69–103. London: Academic Press Ltd.

Maran N, Nichol N, Leigh-Smith S. 2008. Preparation for rapid sequence induction and tracheal intubation. In: *Emergency Airway Management* (J Benger, J Nolan, M Clancy, eds.), pp. 59–66. Cambridge: Cambridge University Press.

Middleton B, Phillips J, Thomas R, Stacey S. 2012. Measurement of gas flow. In: *Physics in Anaesthesia* (B Middleton, J Phillips, R Thomas, S Stacey, eds.), pp. 91–108. Banbury: Scion Publishing.

Mitchell V, Patel A. 2007. Tracheal tubes. In: *Core Topics in Airway Management* (I Calder, A Pearce, eds.), pp. 56–67. Cambridge: Cambridge University Press.

Pearce A. 2007. Retrograde intubation. In: *Core Topics in Airway Management* (I Calder, A Pearce, eds.), pp. 105–107. Cambridge: Cambridge University Press.

Redrobe S. 2004. Anaesthesia and analgesia. In: *BSAVA Manual of Reptiles* (SJ Girling, P Raiti, eds.), pp. 131–146. Gloucester: BSAVA.

Rex MA. 1971. Laryngospasm and respiratory changes in the cat produced by mechanical stimulation of the pharynx and respiratory tract: problems of intubation in the cat. *British Journal of Anaesthesia* 43(1):54–57.

Riebold TW, Geiser DR, Goble DO. 1995. Clinical techniques for food animal anesthesia. In: *Large Animal Anesthesia* (TW Riebold, DR Geiser, DO Goble, eds.), pp. 140–173. Ames: Iowa State University Press.

Sanehi O. 2007. Confirmation of tracheal intubation. In: *Core Topics in Airway Management* (I Calder, A Pearce, eds.), pp. 81–85. Cambridge: Cambridge University Press.

Saulez MN, Dzikiti B, Voigt A. 2009. Traumatic perforation of the trachea in two horses caused by orotracheal intubation. *The Veterinary Record* 164(23):719–722.

Steffey EP. 2006. Section II: general anesthesia. In: *Biology, Medicine, and Surgery of Elephants* (ME Fowler, SK Mikota, eds.), pp. 110–118. Ames: Blackwell Publishing.

Taylor PM, Clarke KW. 2008. Anaesthetic problems. In: *Handbook of equine anaesthesia* (PM Taylor, KW Clarke, eds.), pp. 123–175. Edinburgh: Saunders Elsevier.

Wilkinson R. 2004. Therapeutics. In: *Medicine and Surgery of Tortoises and Turtles* (S McArthur, R Wilkinson, J Meyer, eds.), pp. 465–485. Oxford: Blackwell Publishing.

4 Thermoregulation

Jeff C. Ko and Rebecca A. Krimins

MONITORING BODY TEMPERATURE

Body temperature is controlled by the hypothalamus; therefore, it is important to measure core body temperature that is in close approximation to the hypothalamus. A temperature sensor placed on the tympanic membrane theoretically monitors the blood flow in the branches of the internal carotid artery. The internal carotid artery supplies the hypothalamus, and thus reflects core body temperature. A sensor placed in the lower one-third of the esophagus can measure the temperature of aortic blood. If the sensor is placed in the proximal or middle third of the esophagus, it can be influenced by cool anesthetic gases in the endotracheal tube and give a falsely lower reading. Rectal temperature readings measure local changes in temperature and may depend on regional blood flow and other factors. Rectal temperatures may be somewhat different from core body temperature, but are often a useful way of monitoring relative changes in body temperature.

It is important to monitor body temperature during the perioperative period. The authors recommend monitoring body temperature every 5 minutes. The frequency of monitoring may be reduced for animals that are stressed by manipulation.

HYPOTHERMIA

It is estimated that 60–80% of all postoperative patients experience hypothermia. Hypothermia occurs when heat loss is greater than heat production. Hypothermia can be classified into primary or secondary based on the cause of the hypothermia (Oncken et al. 2001). Primary hypothermia results from a patient's exposure to a cold environment. Secondary hypothermia may result from the effects of anesthetic drugs or from illness, which alters heat production and effects thermoregulation.

Based on a retrospective study using 55 dogs and 77 cats, hypothermia was defined as mild (98–99.9°F [36.7–37.7°C]), moderate (96–98°F [35.6–36.7°C]), severe (92–96°F [33.3–35.6°C]), or critical (less than 92°F [33.3°C]). Hypothermia correlates with clinical signs of mental dullness, decreased heart and respiratory rates, decreased mean arterial blood pressure, central nervous system depression, and increased mortality rates.

Many small animal patients suffer hypothermia during thoracic or abdominal surgical procedures. A study in rabbits revealed that external heating devices are necessary for maintenance of normal body temperature during general anesthesia (Sikoski et al. 2007). Heat loss can also be dramatic in large animals when no steps are taken to prevent or treat hypothermia (Tomasic 1999). Avian species are homeothermic, with normal temperatures ranging from 98.6 (37°C) to 107.6°F (42°C). Heat dissipation is accomplished through panting and gular fluttering. Heat loss in birds during anesthesia can be rapid and dramatic. Hypothermia in avian patients can lead to decreased heart rates and cardiac instability. Reptilian species are heterothermic and require external thermal support during anesthesia. Reptiles do not have the ability to regulate body temperature perianesthetically and require thermal support until they are fully recovered (Heard 2001). Reptiles should be maintained near their preferred optimum temperature range. Also, reptiles should be monitored closely postoperatively to prevent hyperthermia and/or burns. Thermal burns can occur more easily in reptiles that are dehydrated with poor peripheral perfusion (Heard 2001).

PERIOPERATIVE HEAT LOSS

Patient heat loss during the perioperative period can be classified into four types: evaporative, conductive, convective, and radiant. Evaporative heat loss stems mainly from airway and respiration. Conductive heat loss is due to a direct transfer of body heat to a cold surface (i.e., surgery table or floor). Convective heat loss is due to direct transfer of heat to ambient air. Radiant heat loss is due to the animal's body temperature being warmer than the environment; consequently, the body heat of the animal radiates to the surrounding. This is especially true when the skin of the animal is not covered; the heat is radiated through the skin to the cold environment. Animals being prepped for surgical procedures have their hair clipped or feathers plucked. These patients are then scrubbed with disinfectants and alcohol, which further enhances evaporative heat losses. Animals with wet hair may then be exposed to metal or uninsulated surgery tables and further heat loss occurs through conduction on the cold surfaces. Intraoperatively, dry and cold inhalant anesthetic gases and oxygen in the patient's airway increase evaporative heat and moisture losses. Appropriate oxygen flow rates are an important consideration in order to prevent excessive cooling in the operating room. Inhalant anesthetics also lower the patient's threshold response to hypothermia. A study by Tan et al. demonstrated that large dogs undergo significant reduction in core body temperature especially during the first two hours of anesthesia and surgery (Tan et al. 2004). The same hypothermic responses are anticipated in wildlife species undergoing anesthesia and surgery. Abdominal surgery induces radiant, convective and evaporative heat losses. Intravenous fluids or lavaging fluids should be prewarmed before using them because cold fluids can further increase body heat loss.

Postoperatively, transportation of the patient from the operating room to the recovery area is an additional source of heat loss. Often, the warming devices used in the operating room are discontinued and the recovery area may not have warming equipment or may not have the equipment prewarmed for the patient. Wet hair or feathers can become an additional cause of heat loss in the recovery area. This is especially vital when recovering wildlife species in its environment during cold weather. Even large animals must have their body temperatures monitored and these patients should continue to receive thermal support during anesthesia and recovery (Tomasic 1999).

Horses and other large animal patients that are recovered on cool, dry surfaces without supplemental heating sources can lose body heat rapidly and may have prolonged anesthetic recoveries (Tomasic 1999). Anesthesia induces hypothermia by inhibiting the patient's ability to thermoregulate. This inhibition reduces metabolic heat production, and inhibits the patient's ability to shiver. Some anesthetics, such as acepromazine, propofol, and inhalant anesthetics, tend to induce peripheral vasodilation, which can worsen

radiant heat loss. Anesthesia and surgery represent a scenario that often encompasses a combination of heat loss and decreased heat production.

Consequences of Hypothermia

Hypothermia may affect the central nervous, cardiovascular, respiratory, gastrointestinal, and metabolic systems of the animal. Conscious or sedated animals vasoconstrict their peripheral vasculature, shiver, exhibit piloerection, or puff their feathers in the early stages of hypothermia during the perioperative period. Perioperative mortality and morbidity are increased when hypothermia occurs. When core body temperature falls below 94°F (34.4°C), the animal's ability to thermoregulate is diminished and the animal loses the ability to shiver. Prolonged recoveries are the most commonly seen central nervous system sign associated with perioperative hypothermia. Anesthetic drug metabolism and ensuing recoveries are significantly prolonged when the animal is hypothermic. Shivering often occurs in response to hypothermia as the animal attempts to thermoregulate its body temperature. Shivering is due to striated muscle contractions attempting to produce heat. Through shivering, the body can increase the rate of heat production by two to five times. In cases of extreme hypothermia, the shivering response is abolished. However, when exogenous heat sources are provided to rewarm hypothermic patients, shivering response may resume. Shivering may be one of the most severe consequences of hypothermia during rewarming processes. Shivering increases myocardial oxygen consumption and can lead to complete cardiac arrest. It has been shown that shivering increases myocardial oxygen consumption 400–500%. Hypoxemia is a common consequence of hypothermia induced shivering. Hypothermia also shifts the oxygen dissociation curve to the left and decreases the downloading of oxygen from hemoglobin to tissues. This may further prolong anesthetic recoveries and increase the chance for complications.

Hypothermia affects myocardial conduction and can cause myocardial irritability and arrhythmias. Hypothermia also decreases cardiac output and blood pressure. During hypothermia, bradycardia may develop and it may not respond to anticholinergics. This is because hypothermia reduces depolarization of cardiac pacemaker cells thus resulting in bradycardia (Polderman 2009). This hypothermia-induced bradycardia is not vagally mediated, therefore it is often refractory to atropine or glycopyrrolate treatment. Under general anesthesia, hypothermia-induced bradycardia, coupled with anesthetic-drug-induced vagally mediated bradycardia, can put the animal in severe danger. Clinically, when bradycardia is nonresponsive to an anticholinergic treatment, it is important to double check whether hypothermia plays a role; the treatment of the bradycardia should be directed toward the underlying cause. Ventricular arrhythmias, including ventricular fibrillation, can also occur during severe hypothermia. Hypoventilation, respiratory acidosis, and apnea may be sequelae of hypothermia during and after anesthesia. Hypothermia can also lead to clotting abnormalities and thrombosis. Gastrointestinal ileus may occur as a result of hypothermia. Decreased immune function may occur after prolonged hypothermia (Oncken et al. 2001).

Perioperative Hypothermia: Prevention and Treatment

Frequently, rewarming of hypothermic patients becomes necessary if preventative measures fail to prevent hypothermia. It has been suggested that a hypothermic patient should be actively rewarmed until a rectal temperature of 98.5°F (36.9°C) is reached. Reptiles should be maintained near their preferred optimum temperature range during the perioperative period. During rewarming procedures, coagulation parameters, the cardiorespiratory system, electrolytes, acid-base status, and mental alertness should be monitored.

The use of heating devices or methods of providing heat can be classified as warming from body surface to the core (externally supplied) and from the core to the body surface (internally supplied). Circulating heated water blankets and forced hot air warmers are typical warming devices that heat patients externally. Recently, a new device using an electric heat current with a reusable resistive polymer blanket covered by a polypropylene sheet (Hot Dog®) has been developed for human and veterinary use. Potential advantages of the resistive heating unit over forced-air warming include easy cleaning with a thin reusable blanket and silent operation (Kimberger et al. 2008). Using warm intravenous fluids, warm saline lavages, or warm water enemas are methods of warming a patient internally. All these methods have been shown to successfully decrease heat loss.

In avian patients, radiant energy heat sources were found to be effective in preventing hypothermia in doves (Phalen et al. 1996). In a study with Amazon parrots, a forced air warmer was superior in maintaining body temperature when compared with infrared heater or circulating water blanket (Rembert et al. 2001). Heat loss still occurred in birds anesthetized for greater than 30 minutes, but temperatures were maintained in acceptable ranges (Rembert et al. 2001).

Commercially available fluid warmers can be used to warm fluids or blood immediately prior to infusion. This includes incubating fluids prior to intravenous use on a patient as well as using in-line fluid warmers placed close to the patient. Operating room temperature should be maintained at 71–73°F or slightly higher. Some devices take time to reach desired temperature (up to 30 minutes), therefore heating water circulating blankets and pumps should be turned on and their temperatures maintained at appropriate ranges (around

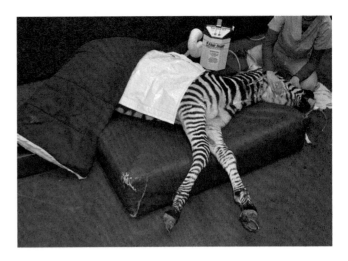

Figure 4.1. Even large animals can become hypothermic while under general anesthesia. A zebra is covered with a forced hot air warmer and a large blanket to prevent radiant heat loss. In addition, the zebra is placed on an insulated pad to prevent conductive heat loss through the concrete floor.

104°F [40°C]) prior to the patient being anesthetized. The patient should be kept covered with towels or forced hot air quilt blankets during the perioperative period (Figure 4.1). Results from a study in dogs showed that using heated water blankets around the feet and legs was the preferable method of preventing heat loss (Cabell et al. 1997). This was compared with a heating blanket applied on the trunk of the anesthetized dogs. Forced hot air warmers can be effectively used to provide heat before, during, and after surgery. Forced hot air is filtered and delivered to the patient's skin through a convective quilt. The quilts have several configurations to accommodate incision site exposure and various patient positioning. The quilts can be placed under or on top of the patient. Most of the quilts are durable and can withstand extensive use, although they are designed to be disposable.

Anesthesia and surgery predispose patients to hypothermia. Management of perioperative hypothermia includes properly monitoring the animal's body temperature, preventing heat loss, and providing heat supplementation. This reduces the morbidity and mortality of the patient during the perioperative period.

HYPERTHERMIA

Hyperthermia can also occur in anesthetized patients. Hyperthermia may occur with prolonged, stressful inductions during high ambient temperatures. This is a common occurrence during wildlife capture. Pursuit of an animal for capture may lead to excessive stress, exertion and trauma. These can all contribute to hyperthermia in immobilized wildlife. Also animals with thick hair coats are prone to being overheated with warming devices. Some mammals, including carnivores, lose heat through panting. Although advantages of using rebreathing (circle) systems include retaining and reusing expired heat from the patients, these system can also result in inadvertent hyperthermia. In addition, during hyperthermia, there is increased production of carbon dioxide. Carbon dioxide will interact with soda lime and generate additional heat through a chemical reaction (Thurmon et al. 1996). Malignant hyperthermia is a disease that can occur in pigs, dogs, cats, and horses. Malignant hyperthermia is characterized by increased aerobic and anaerobic metabolism in patients. Patients produce abnormal amounts of heat, carbon dioxide, and lactate, resulting in severe acid-base abnormalities. Hypercapnia may be the first sign of impending malignant hyperthermia in susceptible species. Certain anesthetic agents, including inhalants, contribute to the development of malignant hyperthermia. Expired carbon dioxide concentration and body temperature must be closely monitored during anesthesia.

If capture-related hyperthermia occurs in an immobilized animal, then immediate supportive measures should be used to lower the body temperature. Treating hyperthermia includes moving the animal to a cooler location, the use of cold water or ice topically, and administering cool intravenous fluids or cold water enemas. Supportive measures may also include the treatment of shock and the administration of nonsteroidal anti-inflammatory agents. Animals should be cooled gradually down to 103°F (39.4°C), and then cooling measures should stop. If cooling occurs too rapidly, coagulation disturbances, such as disseminated intravascular coagulation, may occur.

Immobilizing animals on warm days should be avoided whenever possible. Minimizing pursuit and capture times helps decrease stress-associated hyperthermia. Ventilation should be monitored closely and supported in hyperthermic animals.

A serious sequela of hyperthermia and capture is exertional rhabdomyolysis or capture myopathy. The reader should refer to Chapter 10 for more specific information about this potential complication.

REFERENCES

Cabell LW, Perkowski SZ, Greogor T, et al. 1997. The effect of active peripheral skin warming on perioperative hypothermia in dogs. *Veterinary Surgery* 26:79–85.

Heard D. 2001. Reptile anesthesia. *The Veterinary Clinics of North America* 14:83–119.

Kimberger O, Held C, Stadelmann K, et al. 2008. Resistive polymer versus forced-air warming: comparable heat transfer and core rewarming rates in volunteers. *Anesthesia and Analgesia* 107:1621–1626.

Oncken A, Kirby R, Rudloff E. 2001. Hypothermia in critically ill dogs and cats. *Compendium on Continuing Education for the Practicing Veterinarian* 23:506–520.

Phalen D, Mitchell ME, Cavazos-Martinez MI. 1996. Evaluation of three heat sources for their ability to maintain core body temperature in the anesthetized avian patient. *Journal of Avian Medicine and Surgery* 10:174–178.

Polderman KH. 2009. Mechanisms of action, physiological effects, and complications of hypothermia. *Critical Care Medicine* 37(7 Suppl.):S186–S202.

Rembert MS, Smith JA, Hosgood G, et al. 2001. Comparision of traditional thermal support devices with the forced-air warmer system in anesthetized Hispaniolan Amazon parrots (*Amazona ventralis*). *J Avian Med Surg* 15:187–193.

Sikoski P, Young R, Lockard M. 2007. Comparison of heating devices for maintaining body temperature in anesthetized laboratory rabbits (*Oryctolagus cuniculus*). *Journal of the American Association for Laboratory Animal Science* 46(3):61–63.

Tan C, Govendir M, Zaki S, et al. 2004. Evaluation of four warming procedures to minimize heat loss induced by anaesthesia and surgery in dogs. *Australian Veterinary Journal* 82(1&2):65–68.

Thurmon JC, Tranquili WJ, Benson GJ. 1996. *Lumb and Jones' Veterinary Anesthesia*, 3rd ed. p. 858. Baltimore: Lippincott Williams and Wilkins.

Tomasic M. 1999. Temporal changes in core body temperature in anesthetized adult horses. *American Journal of Veterinary Research* 60(5):648–651.

5 Oxygen Therapy

Åsa Fahlman

WHY O₂?

Oxygen is essential for life. Cellular function is dependent on adequate oxygenation and acid–base balance. Low levels of oxygen in the blood (hypoxemia) can lead to inadequate oxygen levels in the body (hypoxia). Brain cell death can occur within minutes and tissue necrosis can result in multi-organ failure. Even short periods of severe hypoxemia can result in irreversible damage. It is best to prevent it! In humans, hypoxemia can lead to cognitive impairment, such as learning and memory deficits. Although difficult to show in animals, it may also happens to them.

Hypoxemia frequently occurs in anesthetized wildlife with the drugs and doses used in the wild as well as in captivity (Read 2003). Hypoxemia during anesthesia can cause significant morbidity and mortality both during as well as after the anesthetic event. Although not always detected, hypoxemia can readily be prevented or treated with oxygen therapy. Since the consequences of hypoxemia may be difficult to measure, a negative impact on an organ system does not need to be proven before oxygen therapy can be initiated. Oxygen therapy is often life saving and there are simple, safe, effective, and inexpensive methods of oxygen administration that can easily be performed during field conditions.

Oxygen therapy increases safety during lung and heart disease, elevated body temperature (increased metabolism), and apnea. Since it is not possible to closely examine the physical status of free-ranging wildlife before capture, oxygen supplementation throughout anesthesia will improve safety for the animal in case of pneumonia or heart problems. Wild animals darted from helicopters commonly develop hyperthermia, which increases oxygen consumption

(Hurst et al. 1982). Intranasal oxygen supplementation will meet the increased oxygen requirements and protects the brain against hyperthermic damage (Einer-Jensen et al. 2002). In case of apnea or airway obstruction, supplemental oxygen is beneficial since it increases oxygen concentration in the functional residual capacity and will delay the onset of hypoxemia. Oxygen will provide additional working time to correct the problem (Becker & Casabianca 2009). During anesthesia, hypoxemia due to drug-induced respiratory depression (hypoventilation) and recumbency-induced ventilation–perfusion mismatch respond well to treatment with oxygen. Oxygen therapy should be provided to all anesthetized animals. The vast majority of physiological studies in anesthetized wildlife demonstrate the presence of hypoxemia. Hypoxemia should be anticipated and prevented.

HYPOXEMIA AND HYPOXIA

Hypoxemia is defined as an arterial oxygen tension (partial pressure of oxygen; PaO_2) in the blood below the expected normal level. Hypoxemia and hypoxia are not synonymous, and may or may not occur together. Hypoxia implies inadequate oxygen levels in the whole body, or a specific region (tissue hypoxia). Tissue hypoxia rapidly leads to cell damage in the most sensitive organs; the brain, heart, kidney and liver.

What Causes Hypoxemia?
Hypoxemia can develop due a low inspired oxygen concentration (high altitude, low barometric pressure), hypoventilation, or due to intrapulmonary causes, that is, ventilation–perfusion mismatch, shunt, or diffusion impairment.

Zoo Animal and Wildlife Immobilization and Anesthesia, Second Edition. Edited by Gary West, Darryl Heard, and Nigel Caulkett.
© 2014 John Wiley & Sons, Inc. Published 2014 by John Wiley & Sons, Inc.

What Causes Hypoxia?

The most common cause of hypoxia is hypoxemia, although it may not lead to hypoxia if oxygen delivery can be improved. This can be achieved by increasing cardiac output or decreasing tissue oxygen consumption. Hypoxia may also result from poor perfusion, low levels of hemoglobin, inability of hemoglobin to carry oxygen, or if tissues are unable to use oxygen effectively.

OXYGEN SOURCES

Oxygen can be stored and delivered as compressed gas or in cryogenic liquid form, or it can be produced on site by oxygen concentrators that extract nitrogen from the air.

High Pressure Oxygen Cylinders

The most common source of oxygen are cylinders with compressed gas under high pressure (~2000 psi; pound-force per square inch). Oxygen cylinders are constructed from steel or aluminum and should be equipped with a pressure regulator, a flow meter, and a manometer. Using oxygen from cylinders without a regulator is extremely dangerous. The pressure regulator is necessary to provide oxygen at a safe working pressure. The flow meter measures and indicates the flow rate of oxygen in L/min or mL/min. The amount of compressed oxygen in the cylinder can be measured by the manometer, since the pressure declines proportionately as the as the contents are used.

Medical oxygen has a higher purity than industrial oxygen, which can contain high levels of impurities. If industrial oxygen is being used for oxygen therapy, it should be checked for purity before use.

Small light-weight aluminum cylinders are easy to carry during fieldwork. Administration of the minimum effective flow rate is desirable to prolong the life of the oxygen cylinders. Refilling cylinders may entail complex logistics in remote areas.

Safety Gaseous oxygen is nonflammable but strongly supports combustion and may present a fire hazard. Materials that normally would not burn in air could ignite in oxygen-enriched atmospheres. Filled oxygen tanks (liquid or compressed gas) must not come in contact with grease, oil, or other combustible material. There are restrictions for transportation aboard aircraft, including helicopters.

Prevent oxygen cylinders form falling over by properly securing them at all times. If the cylinder or its valve is damaged, it can become a missile and shoot off at a high velocity. This can cause serious injury to animals, people, and equipment.

Portable Oxygen Concentrators

Portable battery-driven oxygen concentrators are an extra useful source of oxygen in the field when logistics and flight restrictions may limit the use of oxygen cylinders. Their advantages include a small size, low weight, easy to operate, rechargeable batteries, and cost-effective oxygen therapy. Fire and explosion hazards are less than with other oxygen sources. Oxygen concentrators do not store oxygen, it is produced on site. Maintenance consists of regular cleaning of the air inlet filter.

Portable oxygen concentrators were initially developed for home treatment of people and for travel applications (Chatburn & Williams 2010). They are also being used in human hospitals and field situations in developing countries, where oxygen cylinders pose considerable logistics and financial problems (Dobson 2001; Shrestha et al. 2002).

Depending on the device an oxygen concentration up to 96% can be produced by concentrating the oxygen in the air and separating it from the nitrogen through a series of filters. The current portable concentrators can provide oxygen by continuous flow up to 3 L/min, by pulse dose delivery, or both. With pulse dose technology, the negative pressure of the patient's inspiration triggers oxygen delivery. Thus, oxygen is provided only during the inspiratory phase, which is the crucial time for participation of gas exchange in the lungs. In comparison, oxygen delivered during exhalation is wasteful, as occurs during continuous flow of oxygen. It is important to note that the setting on an oxygen concentrator with pulse dose delivery is *not* equivalent to a continuous flow of oxygen. The pulse volume (in mL/breath) that corresponds to a setting and the maximum oxygen production per minute vary with different devices (Anonymous 2007; Bliss et al. 2004; Chatburn & Williams 2010). With a *fixed pulse volume*, the concentrator delivers a constant pulse volume of oxygen independent of respiratory rate. With *fixed oxygen minute volume*, a constant volume of oxygen is delivered per minute, so the pulse volume per breath decreases as respiratory rate increases. In addition, the variability in the patients' breathing pattern influences the fraction of inspired oxygen (FIO_2) delivered. The portable oxygen concentrators available on the market have all been produced for human use. Bench testing has only been performed at respiratory rates between 10 and 35 breaths/min. As a consequence, physiological differences between animals and humans may influence the efficacy when used in animals.

Stationary oxygen concentrators are being used in animal hospitals, but the use of portable concentrators has not yet been reported in domestic animals. The use of portable oxygen concentrators in wildlife is described later in this chapter.

Liquid Oxygen Containers

When oxygen is cooled below −119°C it becomes a liquid that can be stored under low pressure in insu-

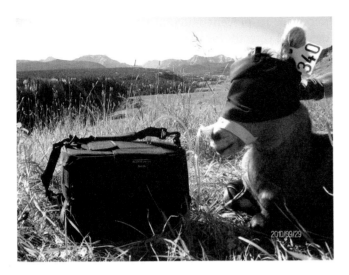

Figure 5.1. Intranasal oxygen supplementation from a portable battery-driven oxygen concentrator to a bighorn sheep in Alberta, Canada.

lated containers. It converts to a breathable gas when warmed. Portable units for liquid oxygen can be filled up from a stationary source and must be kept upright at all times. Liquid oxygen can cause severe cold burn injuries, is not allowed on aircrafts, and is very costly (Fig. 5.1).

METHODS OF ADMINISTERING OXYGEN

Oxygen can be administered to anesthetized animals intranasally, via face mask, endotracheal tube, tracheal catheter, or with flow-by technique. In conscious animals, oxygen cages and Elizabethan collar canopies can also be used. Noninvasive oxygen therapy is simple, quick, safe, and requires minimal training.

Intranasal Oxygen

Intranasal oxygen supplementation (insufflation) is a practical, simple, and effective method for increasing arterial oxygenation. The FIO_2 will vary according to the oxygen flow rate, the minute ventilation, the breathing pattern, the size of the anatomic reservoir (i.e., the nasopharynx), and the depth of anesthesia (Loukopoulus & Reynolds 1996; Yam 1993). Variations within and between subjects should be considered.

Nasal insufflation with oxygen is a safe and simple method to protect the brain against hyperthermic damage (Einer-Jensen et al. 2002). In anesthetized pigs and rats, brain temperature decreases when the nasal cavities are flushed with oxygen. Intubated animals have no airflow through the nasal cavities, and if oxygen is provided via the endotracheal tube only, this cooling mechanism is bypassed.

Placement Intranasal oxygen supplementation can be administered by unilateral or bilateral placement of a

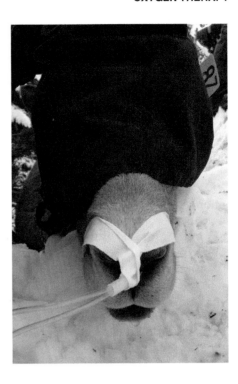

Figure 5.2. Oxygen supplementation administered to a bighorn sheep via two nasal lines secured with tape.

lubricated nasal line into the nasal cavity. The nasal line can be inserted a short bit into the nostril, or premeasured and marked before advanced through the ventral meatus to the level of the medial canthus of the eye. If advanced further, oxygen will be delivered in the caudal nasopharynx, and may enter into the esophagus, which increases the risk of gastric distention. Insertion of a single nasal line $\sim 2\,cm$ into the nasal cavity in brown bears effectively treats hypoxemia with low flow oxygen therapy (Fahlman et al. 2010). The nasal line should be secured as close to the nares as possible to prevent displacement. It can be secured by tape, sutures, or staples (Fig. 5.2).

Nasal Lines Nasal lines, also called cannulas or catheters, can be made up of various types of soft flexible plastic or rubber tubing, including feeding tubes and urinary catheters. Nasal cannulas with short prongs designed for people can be used in animals. The device consists of a plastic cannula, which can be put around the ears or neck, and single or double prongs, which are placed in the nostril(s). An inexpensive nasal line can be made from a fluid extension set, but the end must be smoothened to avoid damage of the nasal mucosa. Multiple fenestrations at the distal end reduce the risk of mucosal jet lesions.

Unilateral or Bilateral Nasal Oxygen Supplementation A unilateral catheter is as effective as bilateral catheters for oxygen supplementation of the same total flow rate. When comparing a specific flow rate administered to dogs via one nasal catheter to that same flow rate divided between two catheters, there was no difference in PaO_2 and FIO_2 (Dunphy et al. 2002). High flow rates administered through a single nasal catheter may cause jet lesions in the nasal mucosa and discomfort in conscious patients. Bilateral catheters are useful if high flow rates are necessary, but can result in a FIO_2 that could produce oxygen toxicity if provided for a prolonged period.

Complications Oxygen may not be properly delivered if the nasal line becomes kinked, blocked with secretions, dislodged from the nostrils, or disconnected from the oxygen source. Complications reported with the use of intranasal catheters in dogs include nasal discharge, coughing, and mild epistaxis upon insertion due to inappropriate dorsal passage (Fitzpatrick & Crowe 1986; Loukopoulus & Reynolds 1996). Gastric distention may occur if incorrectly positioned in the nasopharynx or esophagus, or at high flow rates (5 L/min to a 10 kg dog = 500 mL/kg/min) (Fitzpatrick & Crowe 1986).

Flow-by Oxygen

The flow-by technique includes holding an oxygen line as close as possible to the nose of the animal. Advantages include that is very simple, well tolerated, and has no complications. A short distance between the end of the oxygen line and animal's nose is important to enable treatment of hypoxemia. In dogs, when the line was held 2 cm from the nose and a flow rate of 2 L/min was used, the mean FIO_2 value increased to 37%, whereas from 4 cm, the technique was unreliable to use (Loukopoulus & Reynolds 1997). Disadvantages of the flow-by technique include that it requires constant supervision, it is wasteful of oxygen, and it is not as effective as other ways of oxygen administration.

Intra/Transtracheal Oxygen

Oxygen can be administered into the trachea through a nasal line inserted via the nasopharynx (nasotracheal insufflation), through an endotracheal tube, or through a transtracheal catheter. The anatomical dead space is bypassed when delivering oxygen directly into the trachea. A transtracheal catheter can be placed percutaneously into the cervical trachea after aseptically preparing the area. Tracheal gas samples can be collected from the catheter, or it can be connected to a gas analyzer for continuous measurement of the FIO_2 and end-tidal carbon dioxide ($EtCO_2$).

Humidification or Not?

The normal mechanism of the upper respiratory tract usually provide adequate humidification when oxygen is delivered intranasally, by face mask, or with flow-by technique at a low flow rate. Humidification may be necessary to prevent mucosal drying when oxygen is delivered directly into the trachea, at high flow rates, or during prolonged supplementation.

DETECTION OF HYPOXEMIA AND MONITORING THE EFFECTS OF OXYGEN THERAPY

Oxygen is a drug. When oxygen is used, a dose should be prescribed and response to treatment should be monitored and therapy adjusted accordingly. The lowest possible oxygen flow needed to maintain normoxia should be used.

Monitoring is essential to detect physiological alterations and to evaluate the effect of therapy. In humans, continuous monitoring of oxygenation and ventilation during and after anesthesia is mandatory.

Clinical Signs of Hypoxemia and Efficacy of Oxygen Therapy

Hypoxemia, like hypercapnia and acidosis, is often clinically silent and not easily detectable without specific monitoring devices and measurement of arterial blood gases and pH. Clinical signs that can be suggestive of hypoxemia include dyspnea, cyanosis, tachypnea, tachycardia, elevated blood pressure, and restlessness. Severe hypoxemia is associated with bradycardia, arrhythmias, and impaired myocardial contractility. Cyanosis may not be visible if hypoxemia is associated with peripheral vasoconstriction or anemia. Clinical signs are nonspecific and not sensitive enough to ensure recognition of hypoxemia.

Patients that respond favorably to oxygen therapy may show improved mucus membrane color, decreased respiratory rate and effort, decreased heart rate, and reduced anxiety (Fitzpatrick & Crowe 1986). In immobilized North American elk (*Cervus elaphus*), the frequency of body and limb rigidity decreased in animals as PaO_2 increased during oxygen supplementation. The lowest frequency of muscle rigidity, head, neck, and limb movements were observed when PaO_2 was ≥70 mmHg (Paterson et al. 2009).

Pulse Oximetry

Pulse oximeters provide continuous noninvasive assessment of hemoglobin oxygen saturation in arterial blood (SpO_2). The SpO_2 values should be >95%; lower values indicate hypoxemia. Pulse oximetry is a valuable tool for measurement of SpO_2, but it is important to be aware of the limitations with the technique. Pulse oximetry is less sensitive than arterial blood gas analysis (PaO_2) for detection of hypoxemia. The tendency for pulse oximetry to underestimate saturation at high oxygen tensions and to overestimate saturation at low oxygen tensions can lead to a significant risk of undiagnosed hypoxemia and makes it unsuitable as the sole monitor of oxygenation. In brown bears (*Ursus arctos*), hypoxemia can be missed if arterial oxygenation is evaluated based on pulse oximetry only and not arterial blood gases (Fahlman et al. 2010).

During oxygen therapy, pulse oximetry may not accurately reflect the effect of treatment. In brown bears supplemented with intranasal oxygen, despite a PaO_2 >100 mmHg and calculated hemoglobin oxygen saturation values (SaO_2) ≥96%, pulse oximetry-derived measurements of SpO_2 were <90% (Fahlman et al. 2010). Similar inconsistent pulse oximetry values have been reported during oxygen therapy of white-tailed deer (*Odocoileus virginianus*) and bongo antelopes (*Tragelaphus eurycerus isaaci*) (Mich et al. 2008; Schumacher et al. 1997). In wolverines (*Gulo gulo*), the SpO_2 values measured prior to intranasal oxygen supplementation increased from 50–74% to 90–100% when oxygen was provided (Inman et al. 2009).

Arterial Blood Gas Analysis

Blood gas analysis is considered gold standard for measurement of arterial oxygenation. Arterial blood samples can be used to evaluate the adequacy of oxygenation (PaO_2 and SaO_2), ventilation ($PaCO_2$), acid–base status (pH and $PaCO_2$), and the oxygen-carrying capacity of blood (PaO_2, HbO_2, Hb total, and dyshemoglobins).

Collection of Arterial Blood Samples Arterial blood can be collected percutaneously from palpable arteries, such as the femoral, auricular, radial, or brachial artery, depending on species. Arterial blood should be confirmed by the use of self-filling syringes (arterial pressure should cause the blood to flow into the syringe), or by visualizing a pulsed flow from an open needle stick. Firm pressure should be applied postsampling at the puncture site for a minimum of 2 minutes to avoid development of a hematoma. For multiple samples, an arterial catheter can be placed.

Arterial samples should be collected anaerobically for analysis of blood gases (PaO_2 and $PaCO_2$), pH, and lactate. Any air bubbles should immediately be expelled and the syringe capped. Immediate analysis is necessary to minimize the risk of affected values. Syringe material, storage temperature, and time before analysis can significantly affect the blood gas and pH results, depending on species (Deane et al. 2004). Storage in plastic syringes in room temperature should be avoided, and even if stored in glass syringes in iced water, changes will occur with time.

Field Analysis Battery-driven portable clinical analyzers enable blood analysis in remote settings where this previously was not possible. Analysis can be challenging during field conditions since portable analyzers are made for indoor laboratory settings. The i-STAT®1 Portable Clinical Analyzer (Abbott Laboratories, Abbott Park, IL, USA) is sensitive to extreme ambient temperatures and high humidity. The analyzer operates only

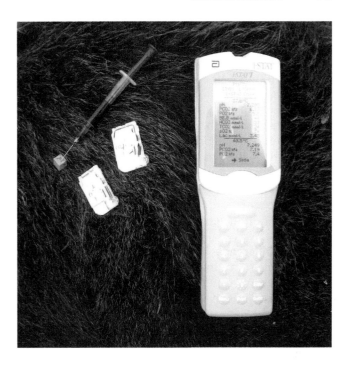

Figure 5.3. The i-STAT®1 Portable Clinical Analyzer and cartridges used for field analysis.

within +16 to 30°C and does not allowing testing outside this temperature range. In hot climate, it can be stored with ice packs in a polystyrene box in an insulated cooler bag. In cold climate, a hot water bottle placed in the box will prevent cooling of the analyzer. Thermoses with hot water can be brought to the field to refill the hot water bottle. The i-STAT® cartridges must be stored in a refrigerator. The cartridges may be stored at room temperature for 2 weeks or 2 months, depending on cartridge type, and they should not be returned to the refrigerator once they have been at room temperature. Do not allow cartridges to freeze (Fig. 5.3).

The i-STAT®1 analyzer has been validated with good accuracy and precision for humans, dogs, and horses (Sediame et al. 1999; Silverman & Birks 2002; Verwaerde et al. 2002). Although widely used in wild animals, validation remains to be performed for wildlife species. The oxygen dissociation curve and the p50 value varies between humans, domestic, and wildlife species (Clerbaux et al. 1993).

What Do Arterial Blood Gases Tell You?

Arterial blood gas analysis detects the presence and severity of hypoxemia and is the best way to evaluate the effect of oxygen therapy.

PaO_2 The arterial oxygen tension reflects the *oxygen uptake in the lungs*. The oxygen tension (partial pressure of arterial oxygen; PaO_2), is measured in mmHg or kPa

(1 mmHg = 0.133 kPa). The PaO_2 reflects only free oxygen molecules dissolved in plasma, and not those bound to hemoglobin. Low values indicate hypoxemia.

It is important to note that a normal PaO_2 does not equal adequate tissue oxygenation, which also depends on oxygen transport (hemoglobin concentration) and oxygen release (p50). The p50 value is the PaO_2 at which the hemoglobin is 50% saturated with oxygen and describes the position of the oxygen dissociation curve, which is essential for the oxygen release to the tissues. However, oxygen delivery can be compromised by poor circulation, which may be improved with administration of intravenous fluids.

P(A-a)O₂ Difference In order to evaluate adequacy of gas exchange within the lungs, the alveolar-arterial oxygen tension difference [$P(A-a)O_2$], also called the "A-a gradient", can be determined. The alveolar oxygen tension (PAO_2) is calculated by using the alveolar gas equation:

$$PAO_2 = FIO_2 \times (P_B - P_{H2O}) - (PACO_2/RQ),$$

where FIO_2 is the fraction of inspired oxygen (0.21), P_B is the barometric pressure (760 mmHg at sea level), and P_{H2O} is the saturated water vapor pressure at 37°C (47 mmHg), and RQ is the respiratory quotient. The RQ is determined by dividing CO_2 production in the body by its O_2 consumption, which varies with diet, health status, stress, and other factors. An RQ of 0.8 can be used for carnivores and omnivores (high protein or fat diet), and 1.0 can be used for herbivores (high carbohydrate diet). An elevated A-a gradient (>15 mmHg at FIO_2 0.21) indicates an impaired oxygen exchange, that the lungs are not transferring oxygen properly from the atmosphere to the pulmonary circulation.

SaO₂/SpO₂ Arterial oxygen saturation is the percentage of oxygenated hemoglobin in relation to the amount of hemoglobin capable of carrying oxygen. Hemoglobin oxygen saturation determined by pulse oximetry is abbreviated SpO_2 to distinguish it from saturation determined by arterial blood sampling (SaO_2). Portable blood gas analyzers, such as the i-STAT®1, calculate SaO_2 from measured PaO_2, pH, and $PaCO_2$ on the basis of standard oxygen dissociation curves in humans. Co-oximeters measure SaO_2, which is gold standard for determination of oxygen saturation.

PaCO₂ The arterial carbon dioxide tension (partial pressure of arterial carbon dioxide ($PaCO_2$)) reflects alveolar ventilation. Elevated $PaCO_2$ values (hypercapnia) indicate hypoventilation. Mild to moderate hypercapnia may be beneficial because it stimulates the sympathetic nervous system and supports cardiovascular function by positive inotropic effects and vasoconstriction, and enhances the release of oxygen from hemoglobin into the tissues. Severe hypercapnia can result in hemodynamic instability, tachyarrhythmia, impaired myocardial contractility, narcosis, and coma (Johnson & Autran de Morais 2006). Hypercapnia can be treated with tracheal intubation and mechanical ventilation. Oxygen therapy does not treat hypercapnia.

Temperature Corrected or Not? Body temperature has an important impact on measurements of blood gases (Bisson & Younker 2006). Blood gas analyzers measures the pH and blood gas partial pressures in blood at 37°C (uncorrected values). By entering body temperature, the analyzer will calculate temperature corrected values using certain algorithms. During hyperthermia, the uncorrected PaO_2 and $PaCO_2$ values will be lower and the pH will be higher than temperature corrected values would indicate. In case of hypothermia, an uncorrected PaO_2 may overlook a significant hypoxemia. When arterial blood gas values and pH are interpreted and reported, always report if the values are temperature corrected or not, and report body temperature.

Venous Blood Gases There is a large difference between arterial and venous oxygen values. Peripheral venous blood can never be used to assess oxygenation (lung function) or ventilation. Venous blood gases reflect the adequacy of tissue oxygenation and tissue carbon dioxide clearance.

Blood Gas Reference Values

In normally ventilating, conscious domestic mammals breathing air at sea level, the PaO_2 usually range between 80 and 100 mmHg and the $PaCO_2$ range between 35 and 45 mmHg. In awake animals at higher altitude, the PaO_2 will be lower due to a lower barometric pressure. The $PaCO_2$ can be lower as a result of altitude-associated compensatory hyperventilation.

Blood gas reference values for nonanesthetized wildlife are seldom available, but have been documented in some species. In unrestrained standing white rhinoceros, a mean $\pm$ SE (range) PaO_2 of 98 ± 1 (90–109) mmHg and a $PaCO_2$ of 49 ± 1 (44–54) mmHg were reported (Citino & Bush 2007). In unsedated standing and laterally recumbent African (*Loxodonta africana*) and Asian (*Elephas maximus*) elephants, blood gas values did not differ between the species. The mean $\pm$ SD PaO_2 values decreased from 96 ± 2 mmHg while standing to 84 ± 3 mmHg during lateral recumbency, whereas the $PaCO_2$ value stayed the same (44 ± 1 mmHg) (Honeyman et al. 1992). Remarkably low PaO_2 values of 56 ± 9 (52–60) mmHg were reported in unsedated Arabian oryx (*Oryx leucoryx*) restrained in a drop-floor crate, but the presented values were not temperature corrected and rectal temperature was not reported (Kilgallon et al. 2008). If the animals were hyperthermic, temperature corrected values would be higher than the presented uncorrected values. In unsedated North American elk habituated to chute restraint, a mean $\pm$ SD (range) PaO_2 of 100 ± 12

(87–121) mmHg and a $PaCO_2$ of 39 ± 4 (33–42) mmHg were documented during intranasal administration of medical air (Paterson et al. 2009).

Target PaO₂

Arterial oxygenation during anesthesia should be maintained within normal physiological limits. The goal with oxygen therapy in hypoxemic animals is to improve the animal's arterial oxygenation to reach a minimum target PaO_2 that could be expected in a normal awake animal. Arterial oxygenation varies with altitude according to the alveolar gas equation. The target PaO_2 can be calculated using the local barometric pressure for the altitude where anesthesia takes place. For example, the PaO_2 expected for conscious bighorn sheep at an altitude of 1500 m above sea level is approximately 73 mmHg, calculated using the local P_B and assuming a $PaCO_2$ of 35 mmHg, P_{H2O} of 47 mmHg, an RQ of 1.0, and a P(A-a)O_2 difference of 15 mmHg. In comparison, the expected PaO_2 at 2200 m above sea level would be 62 mmHg (Fahlman et al. 2012).

Discontinuing Oxygen Therapy

Oxygen should be supplemented continuously throughout anesthesia. If discontinued, the beneficial increases in arterial oxygenation associated with oxygen administration diminish rapidly (Dunphy et al. 2002; Fahlman et al. 2010). This has been shown in a wide variety of species, such as rhinoceros, brown bears, white-tailed deer, and bongo antelopes. Arterial oxygenation can fall to baseline values within 10 seconds if oxygen therapy is interrupted (Fitzpatrick & Crowe 1986). This indicates the necessity to provide oxygen throughout handling of anesthetized wildlife, also when moving the animals (Fig. 5.4). Intermittent oxygen therapy has been compared with bringing a drowning person to the surface—occasionally! (West 2003).

What If Oxygen Therapy Fails?

If hypoxemia persists despite oxygen therapy, physiological alterations should be considered and the oxygen delivery equipment should be inspected. Check the following:

- Does the animal have a patent airway? Is the animal apneic? Is intubation and manual ventilation needed?
- How is the animal's breathing pattern? Rapid shallow breathing increases dead space ventilation.
- Can the animal be repositioned from dorsal or lateral to sternal recumbency to reduce the degree of ventilation/perfusion mismatch? Is there a pneumothorax?
- Is there severe ruminal tympany? Is the nasal line kinked, blocked, or dislodged from the nostril? Is it incorrectly placed in the esophagus? Is the oxygen cylinder empty? Is the flow rate too low? Is the correct pulse dose setting chosen on the oxygen concentrator? Is the maximum oxygen production of the

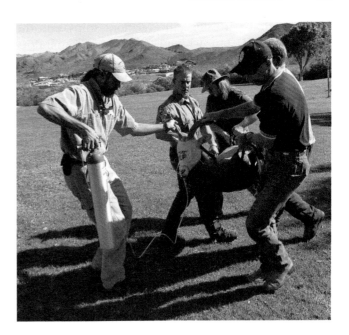

Figure 5.4. Oxygen therapy provided when moving an immobilized desert bighorn sheep in Nevada.

device adequate for the size of the animal? Is the ambient temperature, relative humidity, and altitude within its operating conditions? Is shunting present? Severe hypoxemia that is unresponsive to oxygen supplementation may be due to high shunt fractions.

Common Misconceptions

Hypercapnia can be treated with oxygen.

Oxygen therapy does not treat hypercapnia. Carbon dioxide elimination depends on alveolar ventilation. Alveolar ventilation = respiratory rate × (tidal volume—dead space).

An increase in respiratory rate improves ventilation.

Rapid shallow breathing mainly ventilates dead space. An increase in respiratory rate and/or tidal volume may improve ventilation.

Oxygen therapy causes respiratory depression (hypoventilation) by abolishing the hypoxic respiratory drive.

This is a theory that is still under debate and the mechanism for the elevated $PaCO_2$ is not fully understood. In human patients receiving oxygen therapy, some actually experienced an increase in ventilation, in some it was unchanged, and in some ventilation decreased (Schmidt & Hall 1989). Suggested reasons for elevations in $PaCO_2$ included the release of hypoxic vasoconstriction with an increase in alveolar dead space, changes in ventilation–perfusion ratio relations ships, and the Haldane effect, but without changes in respiratory drive (Benditt 2000). Withholding oxygen therapy in an attempt to maintain ventilatory drive may be harmful and is not advisable; treatment of hypercapnia consists of mechanical ventilation. During anesthesia of wildlife, hypercapnia is a common side effect, also when oxygen therapy is not provided. For example, a mild hypercapnia ($PaCO_2$ <55 mmHg) has been documented in brown bears during low oxygen flows (0.5–3 L/min), as well as in unsupplemented bears (Fahlman et al. 2010, 2011a). When similar flow rates were supplemented to white-tailed deer, a marked hypercapnia ($PaCO_2$ >60 mmHg) developed in some animals (Fahlman et al. 2011b). Elk anesthetized with xylazine-carfentanil developed severe hypercapnia ($PaCO_2$ >80 mmHg) during intranasal oxygen supplementation at 10 L/min (Paterson et al. 2009).

OXYGEN CYLINDER USE IN WILDLIFE

In the literature, specific oxygen flow rates are sometimes recommended for treatment of hypoxemia without experimental evidence that supports the statements. In the following section, the effect of oxygen therapy has been evaluated by blood gas analysis, unless stated otherwise. When interpreting data and publishing research results, it is imperative to not focus only on mean values since for the individual animal it may be critical to detect and correct hypoxemia.

Ungulates

Hypoxemia in white-tailed deer immobilized with butorphanol-azaperone-medetomidine (BAM) can be corrected with intranasal oxygen at a relatively low flow rate of 3 L/min (Mich et al. 2008). The efficacy of even lower flow rates have been evaluated in white-tailed deer anesthetized with medetomidine-ketamine (Fahlman et al. 2011b). A flow rate as low as 1 L/min (14–18 mL/kg/min) effectively treats hypoxemia in white-tailed deer. During field work, use of the minimum effective flow rate extends the life of the oxygen cylinder. A D-cylinder containing 425 L oxygen will last over 7 hours at a flow rate of 1 L/min, compared with only 2.4 hours if using a flow rate of 3 L/min.

Intranasal oxygen at 2.5 L/min effectively treats hypoxemia in adult rhebok (*Pelea capreolus*) immobilized with carfentanil-xylazine or etorphine-xylazine (Howard et al. 2004). In adult guanacos (*Lama guanicoe*), an intranasal flow rate of 4 L/min is sufficient for treatment of hypoxemia during anesthesia with medetomidine-ketamine-butorphanol (Georoff et al. 2010).

An intranasal flow rate of 5 L/min is sufficient for treatment of hypoxemia in immobilized bongo antelopes (Schumacher et al. 1997). Intranasal oxygen at 3–5 L/min has been evaluated in bongo and eland antelopes (*Tragelaphus oryx*) during three different circumstances: manual restraint in a drop floor chute, manual restraint following sedation, and chemical immobilization (Boyd et al. 2000). The *mean* PaO_2 values increased >100 mmHg in all groups, although some chemically immobilized animals remained hypoxemic despite oxygen therapy.

In North American elk, an intranasal flow rate of 10 L/min treated hypoxemia during immobilization with xylazine-tiletamine-zolazepam (Read et al. 2001). In another study on elk, intranasal oxygen was administered at 10 L/min prior to induction and during immobilization with carfentanil-xylazine (Paterson et al. 2009). The arterial oxygenation improved, but individual animals remained hypoxemic despite oxygen therapy, and severe hypercapnia with $PaCO_2$ values up to 100 mmHg was reported.

In desert bighorn sheep immobilized with butorphanol-azaperone-medetomidine, hypoxemia has been treated successfully with intranasal oxygen at 6 L/min (Fahlman et al., unpubl. data). Preoxygen PaO_2 values of 45–54 mmHg increased to 144–210 mmHg during oxygen therapy.

In a crossover study in immobilized reindeer with hypoxemia, animals that received intranasal oxygen at 6 L/min had significantly higher PaO_2 values (range 95–313 mmHg) compared with unsupplemented animals (26–70 mmHg) (Risling et al. 2011).

Based on pulse oximetry, in immobilized takin (*Budocas taxicolor*) (body weight ~200 kg) receiving intranasal oxygen at 4–6 L/min, the mean SpO_2 value increased above 90% (Morris et al. 2000). Anesthetized Przewalki's horses (*Equus ferus prezwalski*) were hypoxemic despite intratranasal oxygen at 10 L/min, according to pulse oximetry and arterial blood gas analysis (Walzer et al. 2009) (Table 5.1).

Rhinoceros Immobilized rhinoceros commonly develop hypoxemia, which can be more severe during lateral than sternal recumbency (Fahlman et al. 2004; Morkel et al. 2010; Wenger et al. 2007). Intranasal oxygen at a flow rate of 5–10 L/min rapidly increases the PaO_2 to >150 mmHg in black rhinoceros calves in sternal recumbency, and to >90 mmHg in white rhinoceros calves, irrespective of their body position (Fahlman et al. 2004). In adult white rhinoceros with severe hypoxemia during lateral recumbency, an intranasal flow rate of 15 L/min increases the PaO_2 to a less critical level. Oxygen should routinely be supplemented throughout the immobilization period, since hypoxemia in rhinoceros quickly resumes if oxygen is discontinued (Fahlman et al. 2004).

Tracheal insufflation of oxygen has been evaluated for treatment of severe hypoxemia (PaO_2 35 ± 9 mmHg) in adult and subadult white rhinoceros in sternal

Table 5.1. The effect on arterial oxygen tension by intranasal oxygen supplementation from portable oxygen cylinders at different flow rates in various ungulate species immobilized with various drug combinations

Species	Number of Animals (n), Body Mass, Body Position	Drug Combination	Intranasal Oxygen Flow Rate	PaO$_2$ (mmHg)		Reference
Bongo antelope (*Tragelaphus eurycerus isaaci*)	n = 8 264 ± 19 kg Sternal	Carfentanil xylaine	5 L/min	Pre-O$_2$ 15 minutes of O$_2$	71 ± 8 >180	Schumacher et al. (1997)
Rhebok (*Pelea capreolus*)	n = 12 13–25 kg Lateral	Carfentanil + xylazine, n = 6	2.5 L/min	Pre-O$_2$ 15 minutes of O$_2$	36 ± 23 (10–74) 120 ± 46 (71–174)	Howard et al. (2004)
		Etorphine + xylazine, n = 6	2.5 L/min	Pre-O$_2$ 15 minutes of O$_2$	38 ± 11 (20–55) 157 ± 65 (90–243)	
Guanaco (*Lama guanicoe*)	n = 7 98–127 kg Lateral	Medetomidine + ketamine + butorphanol	4 L/min	Pre-O$_2$ 20 minutes of O$_2$	66 ± 15 (50–96) 128 ± 32 (91–170)	Georoff et al. (2010)
North American elk (*Cervus elaphus*)	n = 8 245 ± 20 kg Lateral	Carfentanil + xylazine	10 L/min	Control group on medical air 9 minutes of O$_2$	47 ± 12 (31–66) 75 ± 40 (44–156)	Paterson et al. (2009)
	n = 9 Estimated 75–400 kg Lateral	Xylazine tiletamine + zolazepam	10 L/min	Pre-O$_2$ 5 minutes of O$_2$	43 ± 12 (27–65) 207 ± 60 (103–284)	Read et al. (2001)
White-tailed deer (*Odocoileus virginianus*)	n = 6 59–95 kg Lateral	Butorphanol + azaperone + medetomidine	3 L/min	Pre-O$_2$ 15 minutes of O$_2$	42 ± 4 (37–49) 125 ± 36 (88–183)	Mich et al. (2008)
	n = 9 56–72 kg Lateral	Medetomidine + ketamine	2 L/min	Pre-O$_2$ 10 minutes of O$_2$	67 ± 9 (56–77) 201 ± 41 (130–262)	Fahlman et al. (2011b)
			1 L/min	Pre-O$_2$ 10 minutes of O$_2$	55 ± 10 (38–71) 138 ± 21 (106–173)	Fahlman et al. (2011b)
Reindeer (*Rangifer tarandus*)	n = 6 97 ± 6 kg Lateral	Xylazine + etorphine	6 L/min	Unsupplemented O$_2$-supplemented	43 ± 13 175 ± 66	Risling et al. (2011)

Note: Mean ± SD and/or range is presented.

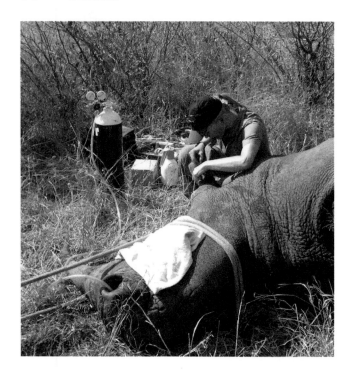

Figure 5.5.   Arterial blood sampling from an auricular artery during intranasal oxygen therapy to a white rhinoceros in Kruger National Park, South Africa.

Table 5.2.   Recommended flow rates of intranasal oxygen to anesthetized brown bears in relation to their body mass

Body Mass (kg)	Flow Rate (L/min)
10–25	0.5
25–100	1
100–200	2
200–250	3

recumbency (Bush et al. 2004). After nasotracheal intubation, oxygen supplementation was provided at a flow rate of 15–30 L/min, depending on the size of the animal. Although the mean PaO_2 increased (PaO_2 96 ± 59 mmHg), the high standard deviation shows that some rhinoceros remained severely hypoxemic.

With severe ventilation perfusion mismatch, poorly ventilated areas of the lung may become physiologic shunt. Oxygen therapy becomes less effective in the presence of intrapulmonary shunting, and insufficient at shunt fractions over 50%.

Hyperthermia is common when helicopter-darting free-ranging rhinoceros, and muscle tremors are frequently seen during opioid immobilization. Since hyperthermia and muscle tremors increase the oxygen consumption, these are additional reasons to provide oxygen therapy to immobilized rhinoceros (Fig. 5.5).

Elephants   Both African and Asian elephants are prone to develop severe hypoxemia during immobilization. Oxygen insufflation at 15–20 L/min in the trunk of an adult Asian elephant, or into endotracheal tubes in juvenile African elephants in lateral recumbency initially increased PaO_2 to >100 mmHg (Fowler & Hart 1973; Heard et al. 1986). The PaO_2 decreased progressively during immobilization, and hypoxemia resumed in some animals. Oxygen was also supplemented to intubated African elephants at 15 L/min via a Hudson demand valve attached to the end of the endotracheal tube. The PaO_2 increased up to 516 mmHg, followed by

a progressive decrease. A simple and effective portable ventilator have been developed to provide oxygen and intermittent positive pressure ventilation during immobilization of intubated elephants (Horne et al. 2001). When oxygen is delivered in synchrony with the elephants breathing pattern, PaO_2 values over 400 mmHg has been recorded. Both oxygenation and ventilation can be readily controlled even under remote field conditions by the use of this device.

Carnivores

Bears   Hypoxemia occurs during anesthesia of brown bears, black bears (*Ursus americanus*), and polar bears (Caulkett & Cattet 1997; Caulkett et al. 1999; Fahlman et al. 2011a). Low flow rates of intranasal oxygen is sufficient for treatment of hypoxemia in brown bears anesthetized with medetomidine-zolazepam-tiletamine, based on arterial blood gas studies (Fahlman et al. 2010). The minimum effective oxygen flow rates were determined to improve safety for the bears and to reduce the number of oxygen cylinders needed during remote field work. Flow rates from 0.5 to 3 L/min markedly improve arterial oxygenation in brown bears weighing up to 250 kg (Table 5.2). Oxygen should be provided throughout anesthesia since hypoxemia can occur at any time during anesthesia of bears and recur if oxygen supplementation is discontinued.

Brown bears anesthetized with carfentanil citrate given p.o. in honey were supplemented with intranasal oxygen at 6 L/min. Relatively low values of partial pressure of oxygen of 64 ± 10 (51–86) mmHg might be explained by low body temperatures (34.0–36.7°C) or the possibility of mixed venous-arterial samples when sampling sublingual vessels (Mortenson & Bechert 1996).

Wolverines   Free-ranging wolverines anesthetized with medetomidine-ketamine at 500–1300 m above sea level in Sweden develop impaired arterial oxygenation, based on arterial blood gas analysis and pulse oximetry (Fahlman et al. 2008). Altitude was responsible for approximately 30% of the reduction in PaO_2, while ventilation–perfusion mismatch probably was the major cause. Intranasal oxygen supplementation at a flow rate of 0.5–1.5 L/min improves oxygenation, as shown with pulse oximetry in wolverines anesthetized with the same drug combination in Montana at 2500 m elevation. Oxygen therapy is considered essential for safe handling of anesthetized wolverines (Inman et al. 2009).

Tigers Oxygen supplementation to Siberian tigers (*Panthera tigris altaica*) anesthetized with xylazine or medetomidine in combination with midazolam-ketamine has been described. Intranasal oxygen was administered at 6 L/min if the SpO$_2$ was below 80%, based on pulse oximetry. Arterial blood gas analysis did not indicate hypoxemia, since all tigers had PaO$_2$ values ≥89 mmHg whether or not receiving oxygen (Curro et al. 2004).

Cheetah Adult cheetahs (*Acinonyx jubatus*) anesthetized with tiletamine-zolazepam-medetomidine in captivity were intubated and administered oxygen at 2 L/min by the use of a semiclosed circle anesthetic machine. Although PaO$_2$ values were over 500 mmHg, their mucous membranes were pale to cyanotic, which probably was attributed to medetomidine-induced peripheral vasoconstriction (Deem et al. 1998).

PORTABLE OXYGEN CONCENTRATOR USE IN WILDLIFE

The efficacy of a portable oxygen concentrator with pulsed delivery has been evaluated for treatment of hypoxemia during anesthesia of selected wildlife species (Fahlman et al. 2011b, 2012). Arterial blood samples were collected before (pre-O$_2$), during, and after oxygen supplementation in brown bears, bighorn sheep (*Ovis canadensis*), reindeer (*Rangifer tarandus*), and white-tailed deer. The tested device weighed 4.5 kg and the rechargeable batteries could provide power for up to 8 hours (EverGo™Portable Oxygen Concentrator, Respironics®). It delivered oxygen in a pulsed flow with pulse volumes from 12 to 70 mL, up to a maximum capacity of 1.05 L/min. Oxygen was delivered intranasally, and the pulse dose setting was adjusted according to the animal's respiratory rate.

In brown bears, the arterial oxygenation improved significantly from mean ± SD (range) pre-O$_2$ PaO$_2$ values of 73 ± 11 (49–93) mmHg to 134 ± 29 (90–185) mmHg during supplementation (Fahlman et al. 2012). All bighorn sheep and reindeer were markedly hypoxemic with pre-O$_2$ PaO$_2$ values of 40 ± 9 (28–55) mmHg and 45 ± 13 (31–56) mmHg, respectively. Following successful oxygen delivery from the concentrator, arterial oxygenation improved in all reindeer and most bighorn sheep, although target PaO$_2$ was not reached in all animals. The limited response in bighorn sheep may have been due to tachypnea, high shunt fractions, as well as limited capacity of the evaluated device. At cold temperature and high altitude, a decreased oxygen concentration may be delivered.

In hypoxemic white-tailed deer, pulsed delivery of oxygen from the concentrator was equally effective to a continuous flow of 1 L/min from an oxygen cylinder. The FiO$_2$ was measured via a tracheal catheter. During supplementation from the concentrator, the PaO$_2$ was 115 ± 31 mmHg. With cylinder oxygen at 1 L/min, the PaO$_2$ was 138 ± 21 mmHg (Fahlman et al. 2011b).

Oxygen therapy from portable oxygen concentrators have great potential for use in animals and during field anesthesia. The efficacy may be influenced by the animals' respiratory rate and the pulse dose setting on the concentrator, and species-related differences in physiology during anesthesia, such as the degree of intrapulmonary shunting. Further research is needed to evaluate available devices in various species and under different conditions.

POSTANESTHETIC EFFECTS OF HYPOXEMIA

There are few reports on the actual effects of hypoxemia during and after anesthesia in wildlife, but since the consequences of hypoxemia are difficult to measure, a negative impact does not have to be proven before oxygen therapy should be initiated.

Immobilization-Induced Hypoxemia and Recovery

Reindeer that were severely hypoxemic during immobilization took a longer time to recover to standing than animals supplemented with oxygen during immobilization (Risling et al. 2011). In North American elk, recovery time was significantly shorter in animals receiving nasal oxygen during immobilization than in animals receiving medical air (Paterson et al. 2009). In white-tailed deer that received oxygen during immobilization, there was a trend toward more rapid recovery than in unsupplemented hypoxemic deer (Mich et al. 2008).

Oxygen Therapy during Recovery

Although difficult to evaluate in wildlife, hypoxemia during the immediate postanesthetic recovery period is common in domestic animals such as dogs and horses (Jackson & Murison 2010; McMurphy & Cribb 1989). Oxygen supplementation is often provided to horses in the recovery room after anesthesia. Wild animals may also benefit from oxygen therapy during the recovery period. Routine oxygen supplementation throughout anesthesia and the recovery period has been recommended for hypoxemic white-tailed deer, since full reversal to standing required 5–20 minutes (Mich et al. 2008). Hypothermic animals will benefit from oxygen supplementation during recovery from anesthesia because shivering increases oxygen consumption.

OXYGEN TOXICITY

Prolonged exposure to high oxygen concentrations should be avoided since oxygen toxicity depends on the duration of treatment and the concentration delivered (FIO$_2$). A general rule is to not administer an FIO$_2$ higher than 60% for more than 24 hours, and an FIO$_2$ of 100% for maximum 12 hours to prevent pulmonary changes associated with oxygen toxicity. Intubation is required to for administration of 100% oxygen (FIO$_2$ 1.0). The lowest FIO$_2$ possible should be used to achieve normoxemia and thus reduce the risk for oxygen toxicity. Wild animals are seldom anesthetized for prolonged periods, and with intranasal oxygen supplementation, the FIO$_2$ does not reach possible toxicity levels.

Oxygen toxicity should be prevented since there is no therapy for the toxic pulmonary changes. Cellular oxygen injury by toxic free radicals lead to cellular death. Accumulation of toxic oxygen metabolites acutely causes endothelial cell damage, resulting in alveolar edema, hemorrhage, and congestion. In the late stages of oxygen toxicity, fibrosis will develop (Mensack & Murtaugh 1999).

REFERENCES

Anonymous. 2007. *Your 2007 Guide to Understanding Oxygen Conserving Devices*. Apple Valley: Valley Inspired Products.

Becker DE, Casabianca AB. 2009. Respiratory monitoring: physiological and technical considerations. *Anesthesia Progress* 56:14–22.

Benditt JO. 2000. Adverse effects of low-flow oxygen therapy. *Respiratory Care* 45:54–64.

Bisson J, Younker J. 2006. Correcting arterial blood gases for temperature: (when) is it clinically significant? *Nursing in Critical Care* 11:232–238.

Bliss PL, McCoy RW, Adams AB. 2004. Characteristics of demand oxygen delivery systems: maximum output and settings recommendations. *Respiratory Care* 49:160–165.

Boyd EH, Mikota SK, Smith J, et al. 2000. Blood gas analysis in bongo (*Tragelaphus eurycerus*) and eland (*Tragelaphus oryx*) antelope. Proceedings of the American Association of Zoo Veterinarians/International Association of Aquatic Animal Medicine Joint Conference, New Orleans, LA, pp. 106–110.

Bush M, Raath JP, Grobler D, et al. 2004. Severe hypoxemia in field-anesthetised white rhinoceros (*Ceratotherium simum*) and effects of using tracheal insufflation of oxygen. *Journal of the South African Veterinary Association* 75:79–84.

Caulkett NA, Cattet MR. 1997. Physiological effects of medetomidine-zolazepam-tiletamine immobilization in black bears. *Journal of Wildlife Diseases* 33:618–622.

Caulkett NA, Cattet MR, Caulkett JM, et al. 1999. Comparative physiologic effects of Telazol, medetomidine-ketamine, and medetomidine-Telazol in captive polar bears (*Ursus maritimus*). *Journal of Zoo and Wildlife Medicine* 30:504–509.

Chatburn RL, Williams TJ. 2010. Performance comparison of 4 portable oxygen concentrators. *Respiratory Care* 55:433–442.

Citino SB, Bush M. 2007. Reference cardiopulmonary physiologic parameters for standing, unrestrained white rhinoceros (*Ceratotherium simum*). *Journal of Zoo and Wildlife Medicine* 38:375–379.

Clerbaux TH, Gustin P, Detry B, et al. 1993. Comparative study of the oxyhaemoglobin dissociation curve of four mammals: man, dog, horse and cattle. *Comparative Biochemistry and Physiology* 106A:687–694.

Curro TG, Okeson D, Zimmerman D, et al. 2004. Xylazine-midazolam-ketamine versus medetomidine-midazolam-ket-

amine anesthesia in captive Siberian tigers (*Panthera tigris altaica*). *Journal of Zoo and Wildlife Medicine* 35:320–327.

Deane JC, Dagleish MP, Benamou AEM, et al. 2004. Effects of syringe material and temperature and duration of storage on the stability of equine arterial blood gas variables. *Veterinary Anaesthesia and Analgesia* 31:250–257.

Deem SL, Ko JCH, Citino SB. 1998. Anesthetic and cardiorespiratory effects of tiletamine-zolazepam-medetomidine in cheetahs. *Journal of the American Veterinary Medical Association* 213:1022–1026.

Dobson MB. 2001. Oxygen concentrators and cylinders. *The International Journal of Tuberculosis and Lung Disease* 5:520–523.

Dunphy ED, Mann FA, Dodam JR, et al. 2002. Comparison of unilateral versus bilateral nasal catheters for oxygen administration in dogs. *Journal of Veterinary Emergency and Critical Care* 12:245–251.

Einer-Jensen N, Baptiste KE, Madsen F, et al. 2002. Can intubation harm the brain in critical care situations? A new simple technique may provide a method for controlling brain temperature. *Medical Hypotheses* 58:229–231.

Fahlman Å, Foggin C, Nyman G. 2004. Pulmonary gas exchange and acid-base status in immobilized black rhinoceros (*Diceros bicornis*) and white rhinceros (*Ceratotherium simum*) in Zimbabwe. Proceedings of the American Association of Zoo Veterinarians/American Association of Wildlife Veteterinarians/Wildlife Disease Association Joint Conference, San Diego, CA, p. 519.

Fahlman Å, Arnemo JM, Persson J, et al. 2008. Capture and medetomidine-ketamine anesthesia of free-ranging wolverines (*Gulo gulo*). *Journal of Wildlife Diseases* 44:133–142.

Fahlman Å, Pringle J, Arnemo JM, et al. 2010. Treatment of hypoxemia during anesthesia of brown bears (*Ursus arctos*). *Journal of Zoo and Wildlife Medicine* 41:161–164.

Fahlman Å, Arnemo JM, Swenson JE, et al. 2011a. Physiologic evaluation of capture and anesthesia with medetomidine-zolazepam-tiletamine in brown bears (*Ursus arctos*). *Journal of Zoo and Wildlife Medicine* 42:1–11.

Fahlman Å, Caulkett N, Woodbury M, et al. 2011b. Low flow oxygen therapy effectively treats hypoxaemia in anaesthetized white-tailed deer. Proceedings of the European Veteterinary Emergency and Critical Care Society, Utrecht, The Netherlands, p. 206.

Fahlman Å, Caulkett N, Arnemo JM, et al. 2012. Efficacy of a portable oxygen concentrator with pulsed delivery for treatment of hypoxemia during anesthesia of wildlife. *Journal of Zoo and Wildlife Medicine* 43:67–76.

Fitzpatrick RK, Crowe DT. 1986. Nasal oxygen administration in dogs and cats: experimental and clinical investigations. *Journal of the American Animal Hospital Association* 22:293–300.

Fowler ME, Hart R. 1973. Castration of an Asian elephant, using etorphine anesthesia. *Journal of the American Veterinary Medical Association* 163:539–543.

Georoff TA, James SB, Kalk P, et al. 2010. Evaluation of medetomidine-ketamine-butorphanol anesthesia with atipamezole-naltrexone antagonism in captive male guanacos (*Lama guanicoe*). *Journal of Zoo and Wildlife Medicine* 41:255–262.

Heard DJ, Jacobson ER, Brock KA. 1986. Effects of oxygen supplementation on blood gas values in chemically restrained juvenile African elephants. *Journal of the American Veterinary Medical Association* 189:1071–1074.

Honeyman VL, Pettifer GR, Dyson DH. 1992. Arterial blood pressure and blood gas values in normal standing and laterally recumbent African (*Loxodonta africana*) and Asian (*Elephas maximus*) elephants. *Journal of Zoo and Wildlife Medicine* 23:205–210.

Horne WA, Tchamba MN, Loomis MR. 2001. A simple method of providing intermittent positive-pressure ventilation to etorphine-immobilized elephants (*Loxodonta africana*). *Journal of Zoo and Wildlife Medicine* 32:519–522.

Howard LL, Kearns KS, Clippinger TL, et al. 2004. Chemical immobilization of rhebok (*Pelea capreolus*) with carfentanil-xylazine or etorphine-xylazine. *Journal of Zoo and Wildlife Medicine* 35:312–319.

Hurst RJ, Oritsland NA, Watts PD. 1982. Body mass, temperature and cost of walking in polar bears. *Acta Physiologica Scandinavica* 115:391–395.

Inman R, Packila M, Inman K, et al. 2009. Wildlife Conservation Society Greater Yellowstone Wolverine Program: progress report 2009. http://www.wcsnorthamerica.org (accessed January 19, 2013).

Jackson ZE, Murison PJ. 2010. Influence of oxygen supplementation on hypoxaemia during recovery from anaesthesia in dogs. *The Veterinary Record* 166:142–143.

Johnson RA, Autran de Morais H. 2006. Respiratory and acid-base disorders. In *Fluid, Electrolyte and Acid-Base Disorders in Small Animal Practice*, 3rd ed. (SP DiBartola, ed.), p. 291. St. Louis: Elsevier.

Kilgallon C, Bailey TB, Arca-Ruibal B, et al. 2008. Blood-gas and acid-base parameters in nontranquilized Arabian oryx (*Oryx leucoryx*) in the United Arab Emirates. *Journal of Zoo and Wildlife Medicine* 39:6–12.

Loukopoulus P, Reynolds W. 1996. Comparative evaluation of oxygen therapy techniques in anaesthetised dogs: intranasal catheter and Elizabethan collar canopy. *Australian Veterinary Practitioner* 26:199–205.

Loukopoulus P, Reynolds W. 1997. Comparative evaluation of oxygen therapy techniques in anaesthetised dogs: face mask and flow-by technique. *Australian Veterinary Practitioner* 27:34–39.

McMurphy RM, Cribb PH. 1989. Alleviation of postanesthetic hypoxemia in the horse. *The Canadian Veterinary Journal. la Revue Veterinaire Canadienne* 30:37–41.

Mensack S, Murtaugh R. 1999. Oxygen toxicity. *Compendium on Continuing Education for the Practicing Veterinarian* 21:341–351.

Mich PM, Wolfe LL, Sirochman TM, et al. 2008. Evaluation of intramuscular butorphanol, azaperone, and medetomidine and nasal oxygen insufflation for the chemical immobilization of white-tailed deer, *Odocoileus virginianus*. *Journal of Zoo and Wildlife Medicine* 39:480–487.

Morkel P, Radcliffe RW, Jago M, et al. 2010. Acid-base balance and ventilation during sternal and lateral recumbency in field immobilized black rhinoceros (*Diceros bicornis*) receiving oxygen insufflation: a preliminary report. *Journal of Zoo and Wildlife Medicine* 46:236–245.

Morris PJ, Bicknese E, Janssen D, et al. 2000. Chemical immobilization of takin (*Budorcas taxicolor*) at the San Diego Zoo. Proceedings of the American Association of Zoo Veterinarians/Internationall Association of Aquatic Animal Medicine Joint Conference, New Orleans, LA, pp. 102–105.

Mortenson J, Bechert U. 1996. Carfentanil citrate as an oral anesthetic agent for brown bears (*Ursus arctos*). Proceedings of the American Association of Zoo Veterinarians Annual Conference, Puerto Vallarta, Mexico, 518–527.

Paterson JM, Caulkett NA, Woodbury MR. 2009. Physiologic effects of nasal oxygen or medical air administered prior to and during carfentanil–xylazine anesthesia in North American elk (*Cervus canadensis manitobensis*). *Journal of Wildlife Diseases* 40:39–50.

Read MR. 2003. A review of alpha$_2$ adrenoceptor agonists and the development of hypoxemia in domestic and wild ruminants. *Journal of Zoo and Wildlife Medicine* 43:134–138.

Read MR, Caulkett NA, Symington A, et al. 2001. Treatment of hypoxemia during xylazine-tiletamine-zolazepam immobilization of wapiti. *The Canadian Veterinary Journal. la Revue Veterinaire Canadienne* 42:861–864.

Risling TE, Fahlman Å, Caulkett NA, et al. 2011. Physiological and behavioural effects of hypoxia in reindeer (*Rangifer tarandus*) immobilised with xylzine-etorphine. *Animal Production Science* 51:355–358.

Schmidt GA, Hall JB. 1989. Oxygen therapy and hypoxic drive to breathe: is there danger in the patient with COPD? *Critical Care Digest* 8:52–53.

Schumacher J, Citino SB, Dawson R. 1997. Effects of carfentanil-xylazine combination on cardiopulmonary function and plasma catecholamine concentrations in female bongo antelopes. *American Journal of Veterinary Research* 58:157–161.

Sediame S, Zerah-Lancner F, d'Ortho MP, et al. 1999. Accuracy of the i-STAT™ bedside blood gas analyser. *The European Respiratory Journal* 14:214–217.

Shrestha BM, Singh BB, Gautam MP, et al. 2002. The oxygen concentrator is a suitable alternative to oxygen cylinders in Nepal. *Canadian Journal of Anaesthesia* 49:8–12.

Silverman SC, Birks EK. 2002. Evaluation of the i-STAT hand-held chemical analyser during treadmill and endurance exercise. *Equine Veterinary Journal. Supplement* 34:551–554.

Verwaerde P, Malet C, Lagente M, et al. 2002. The accuracy of the i-STAT portable analyser for measuring blood gases and pH in whole-blood samples from dogs. *Research in Veterinary Science* 73:71–75.

Walzer C, Stadler G, Petit T, et al. 2009. Surgical field anesthesia in Prezwalski's horses (*Equus ferus prezwalski*) in Hortobágy National Park, Hungary. Proceedings of the American Association of Zoo Veterinarians/American Association of Wildlife Veterinarians Joint Meeting, Tulsa, OK, pp. 98–99.

Wenger S, Boardman W, Buss P, et al. 2007. The cardiopulmonary effects of etorphine, azaperone, detomidine and butorphanol in field-anesthetized white rhinoceros (*Ceratotherium simum*). *Journal of Zoo and Wildlife Medicine* 38:380–387.

West JB. 2003. *Pulmonary Pathophysiology the Essentials*, 6th ed. Philadelphia: Lippincott Williams & Wilkins.

Yam LYC. 1993. Clinical applications of oxygen therapy in hospitals and techniques of oxygen administration: a review. *Journal of the Hong Kong Medical Association* 45:318–325.

6 Analgesia

Douglas P. Whiteside

INTRODUCTION

Over the past decade, pain management has emerged as an important discipline in veterinary medicine, with significant growth of scientific knowledge in neuro-anatomy and neurophysiology across the vertebrate taxa. Pain is often now referred to as the fifth vital sign. Optimal management of pain, and the development of future analgesic strategies, requires a lucid understanding of the pathophysiology of pain across taxa, and of the basic pharmacology of the analgesic drugs used to treat it. While pain can be a protective mechanism against acute injury, it also can be a chronic, nonrelenting, and crippling sensory experience that leads to severe stress, with profound changes in normal behavior and in neuroendocrine, metabolic, and immune responses (Kehlet 1997; Kehlet & Wilmore 2002; Lemke & Creighton 2010).

Many myths have been associated with pain management in captive and free-ranging wildlife species, and this has led to poor analgesia use in the past. New understandings and techniques have allowed us to develop improved strategies for analgesia and to promote education in their use. Adequate pain relief is not only humane but improves recovery. Understanding that pain is a continuum across species allows for more effective treatment.

Zoo and wildlife clinicians face a number of unknown variables compared with their companion animal counterparts, due to the tremendous diversity of species they are presented with, marked differences in physiology across the vertebrate taxa, lack of diagnostic techniques and pain scoring systems to adequately evaluate pain, and the paucity of pharmacokinetic or clinical studies for free-ranging and captive wildlife species. However, the physiological, behavioral, and ethical consequences of inadequate pain management behoove us as responsible clinicians to make every effort possible to prevent or control pain in the animals under our care (Hess 2010).

Numerous barriers exist to appropriately managing pain in wildlife species, these include: lack of familiarity with current therapeutic modalities and techniques, concerns regarding drug induced adverse effects or toxicity, inadequate species-specific pharmacokinetic and clinical efficacy data, economic considerations, poor assessment of pain, and personal views on pain perception. However, studies of behavior demonstrate that animals not only experience pain, but remember the experience and try to avoid it in the future. No longer should the question be asked "does the animal experience pain?", but rather "what kind of pain can the animal experience?" Species variability in the expression in pain can occur due to a failure to recognize species-specific pain behaviors, difference in pain sensitivity, and the conscious response of a species. Pain does not always lend itself to objective measures, so the art of medicine should not be overlooked in favor of the science (Hawkins 2006; Nolen 2001; Paul-Murphy et al. 2004b).

This chapter is an overview of analgesia across vertebrates and invertebrates, and readers are encouraged to refer to other chapters for references on pharmacology and for more species-specific information.

PHYSIOLOGY OF PAIN

Pain is a complex sensation that requires integration of nociceptive and other sensory input at the cortical level, while nociception is the neural response to a noxious stimulus. The International Association for the Study of Pain defines pain as an unpleasant sensory and emotional experience associated with actual or

Zoo Animal and Wildlife Immobilization and Anesthesia, Second Edition. Edited by Gary West, Darryl Heard, and Nigel Caulkett.
© 2014 John Wiley & Sons, Inc. Published 2014 by John Wiley & Sons, Inc.

potential tissue damage. The inability to communicate pain, and the lack of understanding whether the vast captive and free-ranging species that are worked with actually experience the emotional experience of pain, does not negate the fact that all potential or actual tissue damages in animals should be considered painful. In addition, it must be recognized that neonates are capable of experiencing pain; in mammals, the pain pathways necessary for pain perception are well developed in late gestation, and in humans, the spinal cord sensory nerve cells are more excitable in infants with an amplified, prolonged response and larger receptive field to pain. As a result, painful experiences in early life may produce long-term alterations in sensory processing and pain sensitivity (Anand & Hickey 1987; Fitzgerald & McIntosh 1989; Walker 2008).

Our understanding of pain is based primarily on mammalian studies, although the recognition of pain and its treatment is receiving much more attention now in nonmammalian species. An understanding of the pathophysiology of pain is important to enable more effective management and target future research. Pain can be classified anatomically as somatic or visceral pain, or temporally as acute or chronic. While a significant amount of research has been carried out with acute pain, there is still a paucity of information regarding chronic pain. Pain also is commonly categorized as physiologic or clinical (inflammatory or neuropathic in origin). Physiological pain is protective in nature, well localized, proportionate to the peripheral stimulus, and subsides once the inflammatory process resolves. Clinical pain occurs with significant tissue trauma and inflammation and is pathological or debilitating in nature. It is diffuse, disproportionate to the peripheral stimulus, and can continue beyond the resolution of the inflammatory process. Clinical pain can take on a disease character in pathological states, such as inflammation, neuropathy, cancer, viral infections, chemotherapy, and diabetes. This state is manifested as an increased sensitivity to painful stimuli (hyperalgesia) or withdrawal behavioral responses to innocuous stimuli (tactile allodynia). Furthermore, individuals with chronic pain often show maladaptive, disease-induced, therapy-resistant deviations from normal tactile sensation, such as paraethesias and dysesthesias (Kuner 2010; Lemke & Creighton 2010; Truini & Cruccu 2006).

Ascending Nociceptive Pathways

Most tissues are rich in afferent nociceptors, the free nerve ending receptors that are responsible for the detection of thermal, mechanical, or chemical noxious stimuli. Most of these receptors are nonselective cation channels that are gated by temperature, chemical ligands, or mechanical shearing forces. Activation of these channels increases inward conduction of sodium and calcium ions, which ultimately depolarizes the membrane and generates a burst of action potentials. Tissue trauma leads to the release of inflammatory mediators from damaged cells (H+, K+, and prostaglandins), plasma (bradykinin), platelets (serotonin), mast cells (histamine), and macrophages (cytokines). Some of these inflammatory mediators activate nociceptors directly (bradykinin), whereas others sensitize nociceptors (prostaglandins). Release of neuropeptides, such as substance P, leads to vasodilation and edema, resulting in further activation and sensitization of nociceptors. Ultimately, tissue trauma and inflammation produce a "sensitizing soup" of chemical mediators that convert high threshold nociceptors to low threshold nociceptors. This is known as peripheral sensitization (Lemke & Creighton 2010; Muir & Woolf 2001).

Somatic tissues have a higher density of nociceptive nerve fibers and smaller receptive fields, whereas visceral tissues have a lower density of nociceptive nerve fibers and larger receptive fields. These anatomical differences may account for some of the qualitative differences between somatic (discrete) and visceral (diffuse) pain. The stimuli are converted to an electrical signal (transduction), which is then transferred via myelinated A β and Aδ fibers (sharp pain, rapid transmission) or unmyelinated C fibers (dull burning pain, slow transmission) to the spinal cord dorsal horn cells (nerve conduction), where they synapse with second-order neurons. Visceral pain, in contrast to somatic pain, lacks the fast and slow components (Julius & Basbaum 2001; Woolf & Ma 2007; Yaksh 2009). Polymodal C fibers can adapt to a variety of physiologic changes with responses to hypoxia, hypercapnea, hyperthermia, hypothermia, hypoglycemia, hyperosmolarity, hypoosmolarity, and lactic acidosis (Craig 2003).

Second-order projection neurons in the spinal cord are responsible for transmission of signals (projection) to the thalamus, hypothalamus, medulla, pons, and midbrain. Spinal inhibitory and excitatory interneurons are responsible for gating and modulating nociceptive input from the periphery. The spinothalamic tract is the major ascending nociceptive pathway. Additionally, propriospinal neurons that project across several dermatomes are present in the dorsal horn and are responsible for segmental reflexes associated with nociception. Glutamate is the primary excitatory neurotransmitter in the dorsal horn of the spinal cord. Nociceptive as well as non-nociceptive fibers corelease glutamate and neuropeptides, such as substance P and neurokinin A. Activation of a specific type of glutamate receptor, the NMDA receptor, plays a key role in the development of central sensitization, known as "wind up" (Lemke & Creighton 2010; Muir & Woolf 2001; Woolf & Chong 1993).

Third-order supraspinal neurons integrate the input from spinal neurons, thalamus, hypothalamus, medulla, pons, and midbrain and project to the somatosensory and insular (interoceptive) cortex where the pain is perceived (perception), and there are linkages with the autonomic nervous system. Projection from neurons in the lateral thalamus to neurons in the insular and secondary somatosensory cortex appears to be responsible for the sensory-discriminative aspects of pain. Projection from neurons in the medial thalamus to neurons in the anterior cingulate cortex appears to be responsible for the motivational-affective (emotional) aspects of pain. Projection from neurons in the motor thalamus to neurons in the primary somatosensory cortex appears to be responsible for sensory and motor integration. Once received by the conscious brain, the brain interprets and gives cognition to nociceptive signals, giving rise to a state of pain-induced distress (Kuner 2010; Lemke & Creighton 2010).

Antinociceptive Descending Pathways

Modulation or inhibition of nociceptive input at the spinal and supraspinal levels is the basis for descending antinociceptive pathways. This modulation leads to hyposensibility or a lack of pain in spite of inputs coming in from the periphery. The antinociceptive pathways begin at the supraspinal level (thalamus, hypothalamus, midbrain, medulla, and pons) with indirect input from the insular cortex and the anterior cingulate cortex. Release of norepinephrine, endogenous opioids (endorphins, enkephalins, and dynorphins), and gamma-aminobutyric acid (GABA) inhibits synaptic transmission between primary afferent neurons and projection neurons by inhibiting neurotransmitter release and hyperpolarizing the postsynaptic membrane, which effectively shuts down the key synapse in the dorsal horn. This has evolutionary value because they can enable the organism to ignore pain in critical situations, such as flight or fight, and may contribute to analgesia produced by a variety of nonpharmacological pain control approaches, such as transcutaneous electrical nerve stimulation and acupuncture (Kuner 2010; Lemke & Creighton 2010; Muir & Woolf 2001).

PRINCIPLES OF PAIN MANAGEMENT

Effective analgesic therapy blunts the neuroendocrine response, reduces major complications, produces discernible changes in posture and behavior, and improves outcome (Carli & Schricker 2009; Mosley 2011; Wu & Liu 2009). The World Health Organization outlines a three-step analgesic ladder for the control of cancer pain in people, which has been well received and adapted by the veterinary community for managing pain. Nonopioids, generally nonsteroidal anti-inflammatory drugs (NSAIDs), are used for mild pain. If the pain persists, or is of moderate intensity, it is treated with the combination of a nonopioid and a "weak" opioid. More severe pain dictates that a "strong"

opioid replace the "weak" opioid, often at higher doses or titrated to the degree of pain. At any of these levels, adjunctive analgesia (e.g., local anesthetics, α-2 agonists, NMDA antagonists, tricyclic antidepressants, anticonvulsants, corticosteroids, and nutraceuticals), can be used to augment analgesia, taking into consideration the potential interactions and side effects.

Pain management should not just revolve around drugs, and whenever possible, a more holistic, multimodal approach should be taken. Environmental conditions should be optimized for the species. Weight loss and adjunctive therapies, such as chondroprotectants, physical therapy and rehabilitation, acupuncture, dietary manipulations, and even surgery, also play an important role in the multimodal approach to pain (Koski 2011; Rychel et al. 2011; Truini & Cruccu 2006; Whiteside et al. 2006). Atraumatic surgical technique is always the most effective method to prevent peripheral and central sensitization and the development of pain postoperatively (Lemke & Creighton 2010).

There are five major classes of analgesic drugs, and each class blocks or modulates nociceptive input at one or more sites of action (Fig. 6.1). Alpha-2 agonists and opioids alter the central perception of pain. Activation of supraspinal and spinal alpha-2 receptors and opioid receptors also inhibits synaptic transmission in the dorsal horn of the spinal cord. Peripheral and central neural blockade with local anesthetics inhibits the development of central sensitization, as does administration of dissociative anesthetics, such as ketamine, which block NMDA receptors on projection neurons. COX inhibitors such as NSAIDs reduce the synthesis of prostaglandins, which reduces inflammation and limits the development of both peripheral and central sensitization (Grimm & Lamont 2007; Lemke & Creighton 2010).

Trauma and inflammation sensitize the peripheral nervous system, and the subsequent barrage of nociceptive input produces sensitization of neurons in the dorsal horn of the spinal cord. Peripheral and central sensitization of nociceptive pathways plays a central role in the development of pathological pain (Woolf & Chong 1993). Blockade or attenuation of ascending nociceptive pathways or activation of descending antinociceptive pathways by different classes of analgesic drugs usually provides better analgesia with fewer side effects than unimodal therapy with a single class of analgesic drugs. Because peripheral and central neural blockade with local anesthetics are the only analgesic techniques that can produce complete blockade of peripheral nociceptive input, these techniques are the most effective way to attenuate sensitization of the central nervous system and the development of pathological pain (Carli & Schricker 2009; Lemke & Creighton 2010; Lemke & Dawson 2000).

Behavioral responses are one of the first observable signs that an animal is reacting to a stimulus. Whenever

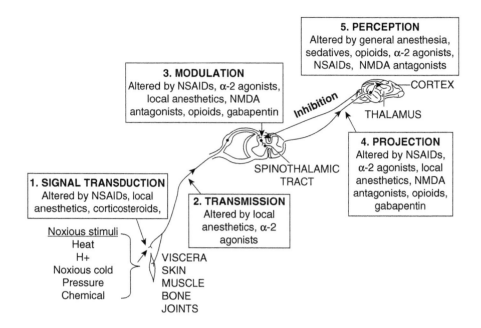

Figure 6.1. The pain pathway.

possible, species-specific pain scores should be developed that incorporates established normal behaviors and alterations associated with pain. However, using a consistent generic scale (e.g., 1–10 scale) can also be of great value to evaluate pain and response to therapy (Hawkins 2002; Paul-Murphy & Hawkins 2012; Sneddon 2009).

PAIN AND ITS MANAGEMENT IN VERTEBRATE SPECIES

Historically, it was a commonly held belief that mammals had a higher neurological capacity to experience pain compared with other nonmammalian species, and that this capacity was directly related to the phylogenetic hierarchy. However, biochemical, anatomical, and physiological studies convincingly show the transmission, mediation, and central processing and modulation of painful stimuli in the lower vertebrates is analogous to mammals (Chandroo et al. 2004). Neuroanatomy is largely conserved among vertebrate animals within the peripheral nervous system and CNS (Brenner et al. 1994; Chandroo et al. 2004). While mammals, birds, and reptiles, have more highly developed specialized sensory cortical regions of thickened gray matter covering the telencephalon known as the neopallium or neocortex, the relative lack of pallial development in amphibians and fish unfortunately has formed the basis for biases that the latter do not experience pain but rather only nociception (Striedter 1997). However, fundamental features that have been conserved throughout pallial evolution. The less evolved pallium still can execute similar physiological functions in fish and amphibians as higher vertebrates, as

the neural basis for consciousness involves widespread integration of differentiated neurons in the pallial and subpallial regions of the brain (Chandroo et al. 2004; Davis & Kassel 1983; Echteler & Saidel 1981; Northcutt 1981; Saidel et al. 2001; Wullimann & Rink 2002). A summary of commonly used analgesics in nonmammalian vertebrates and in mammals is provided in Table 6.1 and Table 6.2, respectively.

Fish

Fish nociceptors are physiologically identical to higher vertebrates, responding to mechanical pressure, heat, and noxious chemical stimuli (Ashley et al. 2007; Sneddon 2004; Sneddon 2009). Of the three major classes of fish, Osteichthyes (bony fishes) have both types of polymodal fibers (Aδ and C fibers), with Aδ fibers being the predominant type (Ashley et al. 2007; Chandroo et al. 2004; Sneddon et al. 2003b; Webber 2011). In Chrondrichthyes (elasmobranchs), only Aδ fibers have been identified (Chandroo et al. 2004; Coggeshall et al. 1978) while the Agnatha (hagfishes and lamprey) primarily have C-type fibers (Matthews & Wickelgren 1978).

Fish also show similar organization of their major spinal pathways (spinothalamic tract and trigeminal tract) as to other tetrapods, and analogous biochemical mediation of nociception (Ronan & Northcutt 1990; Sneddon 2009; Webber 2011). In teleosts, several peptides may transmit and modulate nociceptive signals (e.g., substance P), and the behavioral and autonomic nervous system responses to noxious stimuli are specifically indicative of detection (Chandroo et al. 2004; Ide & Hoffmann 2002; Ostlund & Von Euler 1956; Weld & Maler 1992). Electrical activity during noxious

Table 6.1. Commonly used analgesics in nonmammalian vertebrates

Analgesic	Avian	Reptiles	Amphibians	Fish
Opioids				
Buprenorphine	0.25–0.5 mg/kg IM (pigeons) (Gaggermeier et al. 2003) No evidence of analgesic efficacy in studied psittacines (Paul-Murphy et al. 2004a)	No evidence of analgesic efficacy	46–100 mg/kg SC, IC q 24h (Koeller 2009; Stevens 2004)	No evidence of analgesic efficacy
Butorphanol	1.0–5.0 mg/kg IM q 3–24h (Hawkins 2006; Hawkins & Paul-Murphy 2011; Klaphake et al. 2006; Paul-Murphy et al. 1999; Sanchez-Migallon Guzman et al. 2011a; Sladky et al. 2006)	1.5–8.0 mg/kg SC, IM UID-BID (Greenacre et al. 2008) Questionable efficacy in some studied species. Respiratory depression and profound sedation at >10 mg/kg	25–33 mg/kg SC q 8–12h (Stevens 2011) 0.5 mg/L continuous bath q 24h (Koeller 2009)	0.25–0.5 mg/kg IM q 24h (Davis et al. 2006; Harms et al. 2005) No efficacy in studied elasmobranch (dogfish)
Fentanyl	0.02 mg/kg IV (raptors) (Pavez et al. 2011)	2.5 mcg/h patch q 72h (Gamble 2009)	0.8 mg/kg SC q 24h (Stevens 2004, 2011)	No data available
Hydromorphone	Not recommended	0.1–1.0 mg/kg SC, IM q 24h (Mans et al. 2011) Watch for sedation and respiratory depression >0.5 mg/kg	No data available	0.25–0.5 mg/kg IM
Morphine	Not recommended	Saurians, Chelonians: 1–5 mg/kg SC, IM, IT q 24h (Hawkins 2006; Mans et al. 2011; Mauk et al. 1981; Crocodilians: 0.3 mg/kg q 24h (Kanui & Hole 1992)	114 mg/kg SC q 12h (Stevens 2004, 2011)	5–40 mg/kg IM, IP q 24–48h (Baker et al., 2010; Newby, Wilkie, and Stevens, 2009; Nordgreen et al., 2009)
Nalbuphine	12.5 mg/kg IM (Sanchez-Migallon Guzman et al. 2011b)	No data available	No data available	No data available
Remifentanil	No data available	No data available	2.8 mg/kg SQ (Mohan & Stevens 2006)	No data available
Tramadol	5–30 mg/kg PO q 6h (Black et al. 2010; Souza et al. 2009, 2010)	5.0–25 mg/kg PO q 4–72h (Greenacre et al. 2008; Baker et al. 2011)	25 mg/kg PO q 24–48h	0.26–2 mg/kg IM (Chervova & Lapshin 2000)

(Continued)

Table 6.1. (Continued)

Analgesic	Avian	Reptiles	Amphibians	Fish
NSAIDS				
Carprofen	2.0–4.0 mg/kg SC, IM q 12h (Oaks & Meteyer 2012; Paul-Murphy et al. 2009b)	2.0–4.0 mg/kg IM q 24h (Greenacre et al. 2008)	2.0–4.0 mg/kg IM q 24h	2–3 mg/kg IM (Mettam et al. 2011)
Flunixin	3.0–5.5 mg/kg IM Watch for renal lesions and muscle necrosis (Baert & DeBacker 2003; Machin et al. 2001)	0.1–2.0 mg/kg SQ, IM q 24–48h (Mosely 2011)	25 mg/kg SC q 24h (Coble et al. 2011; Terril-Robb et al. 1996)	No data available
Ketoprofen	2.0–5.0 mg/kg IM, PO q 8–12h (Graham et al. 2005; Machin et al. 2001; Oaks & Meteyer, 2012)	2.0 mg/kg SC, IM >q 31h (Greenacre et al. 2008; Tuttle et al. 2006)	No data available	No evidence of analgesic efficacy
Meloxicam	0.2–1 mg/kg SC, IM, PO q 12h (Baert & De Backer 2003; Paul-Murphy & Hawkins 2012; Wilson et al. 2005)	0.1–0.4 mg/kg SC, IM, PO q 24–48h (Greenacre et al. 2008; Divers et al. 2010)	0.2–0.3 mg/kg SC, IM q 24h (Coble et al. 2011; Minter et al. 2011)	0.2–0.3 mg/kg SC, IM q 24–48h
Piroxicam	0.5–0.8 mg/kg PO q 12h (Paul-Murphy and Hawkins 2012)	No data available	No data available	No data available
Local anesthetics				
Bupivicaine	1–5 mg/kg SC, IM	1.0–<2.0 mg/kg SC, IM, IT (Mans et al. 2011)	0.5–2.0 mg/kg SQ, TO	1.0 mg/kg SC, IM
Lidocaine	1–5 mg/kg SC, IM	1–4 mg/kg SC, IM, IT (Mans et al. 2011; Mosley 2011)	1–5 mg/kg SQ, TO	1–16 mg/kg SC, IM (Mettam et al. 2011)
Mepivicaine	No data available	1.0 mg/kg SC (Wellehan et al. 2006)	No data available	No data available
Alpha 2 agonists/other analgesics				
Medetomidine (Dex)	No data available	0.05–0.15 mg/kg SC, IM. (Mosley 2011) Not evaluated as an analgesic	0.6 mg/kg SQ, IM (Stevens 2011)	No data available
Gabapentin	10–82.5 mg/kg PO q 12h (Doneley 2007; Shaver et al. 2009; Siperstein 2007)	No data available	No data available	No data available

Source: Adapted from the literature and the author's experience.

IV, intravenous; PO, per os; IM, intramuscular; TO, topical; ED, epidural; IT, intrathecal; SC, subcutaneous; h, hour(s).

Table 6.2. Commonly used analgesics in mammals

Analgesic	Carnivores	Primates	Perissodactylids	Artiodactylids	Rodents/Lagomorphs	Marine Mammals	Other Mammals
Opioids							
Buprenorphine	0.01–0.02 mg/kg q 6–12h IV, IM (all), PO (felids, mustelids; viverrids) (Kolata 2002; Velguth et al. 2009)	0.01–0.05 mg/kg IV, IM q 8–12h	No data available	0.01–0.03 mg/kg IV, IM q 12h (Minter et al. 2010)	0.01–0.05 mg/kg SC, IM, IV, IP q 6–12h—rabbits 0.01–0.1 mg/kg SC, IV q 6–12h—rodents (Wenger 2012)	1–2 μg/kg (walrus) 9–10 μg/kg (California sea lion) 3–20 μg/kg (Northern fur seal) IM, PO q 12–24h (Moore et al. 2010)	0.028–0.042 mg/kg SC—sugar gliders (Morges et al. 2009) 0.01 mg/kg IM—edentates
Butorphanol	0.1–0.4 mg/kg IV, IM q 2–12h (Velguth et al. 2009) 0.4–1.5 mg/kg q 8h PO (Kolata 2002)	0.05–0.1 mg/kg IM q 6–8h	0.015–0.027 mg/kg IV, IM q 12–24h—Asian elephants (Abou-Madi et al. 2004; Tana et al. 2010) 0.02–0.05 mg/kg IV, IM—equids	0.1–0.2 mg/kg IM, SC q 6–12h (Carroll et al. 2001; Howard & Richardson 2005; MacLean et al. 2006)	0.1–0.5 mg/kg SC, IM, IV q 4h—rabbits 0.2–2.0 mg/kg SC, IM q 2–4h—rodents (Wenger 2012)	0.05–0.2 mg/kg PO, IM, IV q 6h—pinnipeds (Haulena 2007)	0.2–0.4 mg/kg IM—bats (Clarke & DeVoe 2011; Lafortune et al. 2004; Wellehan et al. 2001) 0.4 mg/kg q 12h—hedgehog (Done et al. 2007)
Fentanyl	2–4 μg/kg IV (Spriggs et al. 2007) 2–4 μg/kg/h patch q 72h (McNulty et al. 2000) 5–15 μg/kg/h CRI (Schroeder et al. 2010; Spriggs et al. 2007)	5–10 μg/kg/h IV CRI 2–5 μg/kg/h patch q 72h	No data available	1.5–2 μg/kg/h patch q 72h (Grubb et al. 2005; Howard & Richardson 2005)	2–4 μg/kg/h patch q 72h—rabbits, rodents (Wenger 2012)	No data available	No data available
Hydromorphone	0.04–0.2 mg/kg IM, IV q 6–12h (Spriggs et al. 2007)	0.02–0.05 mg/kg IM	0.05–0.1 mg/kg IM	0.025–0.1 mg/kg IM	0.05–0.2 mg/kg SC, IM, q 8–12h—rabbits, rodents	No data available	0.05–0.1 mg/kg IM—bats, marsupials
Morphine	0.05–0.5 mg/kg IV, IM, ED (McNulty et al. 2000; Mylniczenko et al. 2005)	0.1–2.0 mg/kg IV, IM, SC, ED (Pollock et al. 2008)	No data available	0.24–0.5 mg/kg IV, IM q 8–12h (Uhrig et al. 2007; Minter et al. 2010)	2.0–5.0 mg/kg IM, SC q 4h—rabbits 0.5–5.0 mg/kg SC, IM q 4–6h—rodents (Wenger 2012)	No data available	No data available
Oxymorphone	0.05–0.2 mg/kg IM, SC q 2–6h (Ketz et al. 2001)	0.02–0.04 mg/kg IV, IM, SC q 4–6h	0.02–0.03 mg/kg IM—equids	No data available	0.05–0.2 mg/kg IM SC q 8–12h—rabbits 0.2–0.5 mg/kg SC, IM q 6–12h—rodents (Wenger 2012)	No data available	No data available

(Continued)

Table 6.2. (Continued)

Analgesic	Carnivores	Primates	Perissodactylids	Artiodactylids	Rodents/Lagomorphs	Marine Mammals	Other Mammals
Tramadol	1–5 mg/kg PO, IM q 8–24h (McCain et al. 2009; Spriggs et al. 2007)	1–5 mg/kg PO, IM q 12–24h	No data available	No data available	2.5–5 mg/kg q 12–24h PO, IM—rodents (Wenger 2012)	0.8 mg/kg PO—dolphin (Schmitt & Sur 2012) 0.5–3.6 mg/kg PO q 12–24h—pinnipeds (Moore et al. 2010)	No data available
NSAIDs							
Carprofen	2.0–4.0 mg/kg PO, IM q 12–24h Avoid use in felids	2–4 mg/kg PO, SC q 12–24h (Okeson et al. 2010)	No data available	1.90 mg/kg PO q 24h (Dutton et al. 2002)	1.5–4.0 mg/kg PO, SC q 12h—rabbits 0.2–0.5 mg/kg SC, IM q 6–12h—rodents (Wenger 2012)	2.0–4.4 mg/kg PO q 24h—pinnipeds (Haulena 2007; Walker et al. 2011)	1.5–2.0 mg/kg PO q 24h—edentates
Flunixin meglumine	0.5–1.5 mg/kg PO, IM, SC q 12–24h Avoid use in felids	0.3–2.0 mg/kg IM, SC q 12–24 h	0.2–1.1 mg/kg IM, IV, PO q 12–24h	0.5–2.2 mg/kg IV, IM, PO q 12–24h (Borkowski et al. 2009; Gyimesi et al. 2008, 2011; Howard & Richardson 2005; James et al. 2000; Minter et al. 2010) 1.1 mg/kg IM q 12–24h—camel (Oukessou 1994)	1.0–2.0 mg/kg SC, IM q 12h—rabbits 0.5–2.5 mg/kg SC, IM q 12h—rodents (Wenger 2012)	1 mg/kg IM q 24h (Haulena 2007)	0.25–1.0 mg/kg SC, IM, q 12–24h
Ibuprofen	Not recommended in carnivores	2–8 mg/kg PO q 6–12h (Bronson et al. 2005; Wellehan et al. 2004)	6 mg/kg PO q 12h—Asian elephants 7 mg/kg PO q 12h—African elephants (Bechert & Christensen 2007) 1.8 mg/kg PO q 12h—Indian rhinoceros (Bertelsen et al. 2004)	No data available	No data available	No data available	No data available
Ketoprofen	0.5–2.2 mg/kg IM, SC, PO q 24h (Mylniczenko et al. 2005; Pye et al. 2010)	1–5 mg/kg PO, IM, SC q 24h (Bronson et al. 2005; Wellehan et al. 2004)	1–2 mg/kg IV, IM, PO q 24h (Wack et al. 2010)	1–4 mg/kg IM, SC q 24h (Dutton et al. 2002; Gyimesi et al. 2008, 2011; Howard & Richardson 2005)	2.0–3.0 mg/kg SC, IM q 12h—rabbits 1.0–3.0 mg/kg SC, IM q 12h—rodents (Heard, 2007a,b)	1–1.2 mg/kg IM, PO q 24h—pinnipeds (Dennison et al. 2007; Haulena 2007; Rush et al. 2012)	1.0 mg/kg IM—macropods

Meloxicam	0.2 mg/kg loading dose, then 0.1–0.2 mg/kg SC, PO q 24h (nonfelids) 0.2 mg/kg loading dose then 0.025–0.1 mg/kg q 24–48h (felids) (McCain et al. 2009; Pye et al. 2010; Whiteside & Black 2004; Whiteside et al. 2006)	0.1–0.2 mg/kg SC, PO, IV q 24h (Okeson et al. 2010; Pollock et al. 2008)	0.3–0.5 mg/kg PO q 24h—equids SC, IM,	0.25–0.5 mg/kg SC, PO q 24h	0.2–2.0 mg/kg q 12–24h SC, PO—rodents 0.1–0.3 mg/kg q24h PO, SC, IM—rabbits (Carpenter et al. 2009; Dadone et al. 2011; Wenger 2012)	0.1 mg/kg PO, SC q 24h—pinnepeds (Rush et al. 2012)	0.1–0.2 mg/kg SC, PO q 24h—marsupials, most mammals (Okeson et al. 2009; Pye et al. 2008; Whiteside & Black 2004) 0.2–0.5 mg/kg SC, PO q 24h—bats (Clarke & DeVoe 2011)
Phenylbutazone	Not recommended	Not recommended	3 mg/kg PO q 48h—Asian elephants 2 mg/kg PO q 24h—African elephants (Bechert et al. 2008) 2.5–3.5 mg/kg PO q 48h—rhinoceros (Harrison et al. 2011) 2.2–4.4 mg/kg P q12–24h—equids	1–6 mg/kg PO q 24–48h (Howard & Richardson 2005; James et al. 2000; Kadir et al. 1997; Larsen et al. 2000)	No data available	No data available	No data available
Local anesthetics							
Bupivacaine	0.25–2.0 mg/kg SC, IM (Schroeder et al. 2010) Do not exceed 1.5mg/kg	Do not exceed 1.5mg/kg	Do not exceed 1.5mg/kg	Do not exceed 1.5mg/kg	0.5–1.0 mg/kg SC, IM (Dadone et al. 2011)	Do not exceed 1.5 mg/kg	Do not exceed 1.5 mg/kg
Lidocaine	Do not exceed 4mg/kg	0.5–2.0 mg/kg SQ	Do not exceed 4mg/kg	Do not exceed 4mg/kg	Do not exceed 4mg/kg	Do not exceed 4mg/kg	1.8–3.7 mg/kg SC—sugar gliders (Morges et al. 2009)
Alpha 2 agonists/other analgesics							
Medetomidine	No data available	No data available	0.01–0.02 mg/kg IM—equids	No data available	No data available	0.01–0.04 mg/kg IM—pinnipeds (Haulena 2007; Moore et al. 2010)	No data available
Gabapentin	2–5 mg/kg PO q 12h (Adkesson 2006)	4–5 mg/kg PO q 12h (Adkesson 2006)	2.5 mg/kg PO q 12h—equids (Bronson et al. 2008)	5–15 mg/kg PO q 12h	No data available	1.1 mg/kg (walrus) 2.3–7.4 mg/kg (California Sea lion) 4.3–12.0 mg/kg (Northern fur seal) 4.5–8.2 mg/kg (sea otter) PO q 8–12h (Moore et al. 2010)	No data available

Source: Adapted from the literature and the author's experience.

IV, intravenous; PO, per os; IM, intramuscular; TO, topical; ED, epidural; IT, intrathecal; SC, subcutaneous; h, hour(s).

stimulation has been recorded in the forebrain and midbrain of rainbow trout, goldfish, and Atlantic salmon (Dunlop & Laming 2005; Nordgreen et al. 2007), and this electrical activity differed according to stimulus type (e.g., simple touch vs. noxious, potentially painful stimuli). In addition, rainbow trout and carp exposed to noxious stimuli underwent global gene expression changes to their brains, particularly the forebrains, which mirrors the importance of the forebrain in mammalian pain processing (Reilly et al. 2008; Sneedon 2009).

Opioid receptors and endogenous substances (e.g., enkephalin-like) are present in the brain and spinal cord of studied fish species, and often demonstrated a similar distribution pattern to that of higher vertebrates (Alvarez et al. 2006; Buatti & Pasternak 1981; Li et al. 1996; Porteros et al. 1999; Rosenblum & Callard 1988; Sneedon 2009). Administration of morphine can blunt physiological and behavioral changes associated with noxious stimuli in fish species (Ehrensing et al. 1982; Nordgreen et al. 2009; Sneddon 2003b). COX enzymes also have been identified in a zebrafish (Grosser et al. 2002; Teraoka et al. 2009).

Recognition of Pain in Fish Current behavioral studies of pain in fish are restricted to a very small number of species (rainbow trout, common carp, and zebrafish) and two models of pain (subcutaneous injection of noxious substances such as acetic acid and bee venom, and thermonociception). As fish are one of the most diverse vertebrate groups, there is a definite need for future research to include a wider range of species, different pain measures, and different models of pain. However, these studies have provided further proof that fish have a capacity to detect, conceptualize, and subsequently respond to nociceptive stimuli. There is growing scientific evidence to support the case for fish perceiving and experiencing some of the negative affective aspects of pain. It is clear that a painful stimulus does result in adverse changes in behavior and physiology, which may impair the welfare and well-being of fish (Chandroo et al.2004; Correia et al. 2011; Reilly et al. 2008; Roques et al. 2010; Sneddon 2003; Sneddon et al. 2003b; Sneddon 2011; Webber 2011).

The paucity of comprehensive clinical baseline data for the majority of fish species complicates the identification of pain and or distress in fish. Depending on the environment, it may be difficult to observe behavioral changes, especially with secretive species. Most behavioral changes in fish after noxious stimulation occur in the period immediately after the treatment for up to 6 hours, often peaking between 1 and 1.5 hours. Goldfish and trout demonstrate learned avoidance behavior after exposure to a noxious stimulus (Overmier & Hollis 1990; Ehrensing et al. 1982; Sneddon et al. 2003a). Clinical signs ascribed to pain in fish are anomalous behaviors, such as rubbing the affected

area, rocking from side to side with the pectoral fins, decreased activity or swimming behavior, increased gill ventilation (opercular) rates, decreased feeding behavior, color changes, changed postural positions in the water column, increased cortisol levels, and exocytosis of mucous from gill cells. In rainbow trout, the administration of morphine significantly reduced all of the behavioral and physiological changes described above, further demonstrating that they were specifically due to pain (Ashley et al. 2009; Chandroo et al. 2004; Reilly et al. 2008; Sneddon, 2011; Sneddon et al. 2003b; Webber 2011).

Analgesia in Fish Although empirical usage of analgesics in fish has become more widespread in a captive setting, its use in a field setting has been minimal where invasive surgeries such as implantation of intracoelomic electronic transmitters occurs (Harms & Lewbart 2011). The lack of approved analgesics for fish further complicates treatment. There have still been relatively few studies of analgesic use in fish, and varying results highlight the challenge of extrapolating findings between species.

Sladky et al. (2001) demonstrated that red pacu (*Piaractus brachypomus*) anesthetized with eugenol, the active ingredient in clove oil and an effective studied anesthetic in numerous fish species, did not blunt the responses to a noxious stimulus compared with tricaine methanesulfonate (MS-222), and no other published studies have demonstrated an analgesic effect of eugenol in fish. Alpha-2 agonists, such as medetomidine, induce sedation in studied fish but also have failed to demonstrate analgesic activity (Neiffer & Stamper 2009). Local anesthetics, such as lidocaine and benzocaine, have been used for immersion anesthesia, and have been used anecdotally for their local effects, but have not been well studied in a research setting. Mettam et al. (2011) demonstrated that local infiltration of lidocaine (6.25–16 mg/kg) was the most effective analgesic compared with buprenorphine and carprofen in trout being injected with noxious acetic acid.

The elimination half-life of morphine in studied fish species is several fold longer that in mammals, ranging from 12.5 to 37 hours (Nordgreen et al. 2009). Parenteral morphine has been demonstrated to be effective in ameliorating the adverse physiological or behavioral reactions to noxious stimuli in goldfish, winter flounder (*Pseudopleuronectes americanus*), and trout, and to pain from gonadectomy in koi (*Cyprinus carpio*) (Baker et al. 2010; Newby et al. 2007, 2009; Sneddon 2003). However, it also was associated with a marked bradycardia and reduction in cardiac output initially, followed by a significant increase in heart rate for 48 hours afterwards, in treated winter flounder compared with controls. Interestingly morphine was found to be ineffective at studied doses (40 and 50 mg/kg) in goldfish in thermonociception experiments (Nordgreen et al. 2009), indicating the type of noxious stimulus may be important in determining the efficacy of an analgesic in fish. Morphine administered via the water had extremely slow uptake and is not recommended (Newby et al. 2009).

In koi, butorphanol (0.4 mg/kg), but not ketoprofen (2 mg/kg), was effective in reducing postsurgical pain-related behavioral changes, such as decreased activity and feeding behavior (Harms et al. 2005). At higher doses, butorphanol (10 mg/kg) provided antinociceptive activity in koi undergoing gonadectomy, but was associated with respiratory depression and abnormal buoyancy (Baker et al. 2010). However, even at higher doses, neither drug was effective in an elasmobranch, the chain dogfish (*Scyliorhinus rotifer*), for reducing minimum anesthetic concentrations (Davis et al. 2006). Intramuscular buprenorphine (0.01–0.1 mg/kg) did not provide evidence of analgesia in rainbow trout, while the NSAID carprofen did have some analgesic properties at higher doses (2.5 and 5 mg/kg), but decreased activity was noted at the higher dosage (Mettam et al. 2011). Tramadol administered intramuscularly (0.26–2.6 mg/kg) in common carp induced a prolonged dose-dependent analgesic response to a noxious electrical while still maintaining normal swimming and behavior, with analgesic effects lasting greater than 2 hours (Chervova & Lapshin 2000). In the author's experience, meloxicam used empirically at dosages of 0.2–0.3 mg/kg has produced analgesia based on behavioral changes; this remains to be studied scientifically.

Amphibians

Amphibian nociceptive afferents are analogous to the primary afferents of other vertebrates, including mammals, with both lightly and heavily myelinated (Aβ and Aδ, respectively) and unmyelinated (C) afferent fibers found in mixed fiber peripheral sensory nerves (Stevens 2004, 2011). The majority of all impulses induced by noxious stimuli, such as pinching, pinpricks, and heat are conducted by slowly conducting C fibers, while epidermal application of dilute acetic acid evoked Aδ and C fibers to a relatively equal extent (Hamamoto & Simone 2003; Maruhashi et al. 1952). Sensory afferents terminate in the dorsal horn of the spinal cord, and similar to mammals, pain-signaling neurotransmitters, such as substance P, glutamate, and calcitonin, have been identified (Inagaki et al. 1981; Lorez et al. 1981). Amphibian studies have demonstrated responsiveness to α-2 agonists and to local anesthetics. In addition, met-enkepahalin and four types of opioid receptors (μ, κ, δ, and ORL-1) are abundant in the amphibian spinal cord and brain but exhibit less selective binding compared with mammals (Bradford et al. 2005; Newman et al. 2002; Stevens 2004; Walthers et al. 2005). There have only been a few studies that evaluated opioid receptor density in amphibians, with μ receptors being more abundant than κ receptors in leopard frogs (*Lithobates pipiens*), but the reverse found in marine toads (*Bufo marinus*) (Brooks et al. 1994; Newman et al. 2002). Further research is required to elucidate opioid receptor densities in other amphibian species.

Although the spinal ascending nociceptive pathways in amphibians are not clearly defined, a single study in frogs identified that electrical stimulation of the sciatic nerve traveled through the spinal ascending pathways and produced evoked potentials in the thalamus and primordial hippocampus (Munoz et al. 1997; Vesselkin et al. 1971). Thalamocortical projections in anurans are more diffuse and less organized than in mammals, but terminate in the nonolfactory telencephalon as with other vertebrates. Similar to fish, there is minimal cerebral or limbic cortical pallial development but it is likely that other neural pathways have developed for the perception of pain (Stevens 2004, 2011).

Recognition of Pain in Amphibians The acetic acid test has been used for decades to assess amphibian nociception, with application of varying diluted concentrations and monitoring for a wipe response by the hindlimb (Coble et al. 2011; Pezalla 1983; Stevens 2011). Based on this test, dermal exposure to other noxious stimuli is likely to elicit a similar response. More recently, the Hargreaves test has been validated to evaluate thermonociception where heat is applied to the inner thigh of the frog in a specialized apparatus, and the frog is monitored for withdrawal movement of the hindlimb (Coble et al. 2011).

In the author's experience, decreased activity and feeding behavior, color changes, increased reclusive behaviors, and postural changes are associated with pain in amphibians. Painful amphibians also may spend more time in atypical locations (Duncan 2012). Koeller (2009) demonstrated that Eastern red-spotted newts (*Notophthalmus viridescens*) that underwent bilateral forelimb amputation did not eat for 72 hours post surgery when no analgesia was used, while feeding resumed within 24 hours in animals treated with intracoelomic buprenorphine or with butorphanol in their water. In addition, the animals that received no analgesia did not move in response to tapping on the aquarium glass until 72 hours post surgery, while analgesed newts moved at the first post surgical test point at 24 hours. Finally, abnormal postures in nontreated newts were observed for 72 hours post surgery, while 8/10 newts treated with buprenophine or butorphanol had resumed normal postures within 4 hours, and all by 24 hours, post surgery.

Analgesia in Amphibians Numerous analgesics have been studied in a research setting in amphibians for brief noxious stimuli, but very little data exists for analgesic use in a clinical setting for pain. The most effective studied analgesics to date in amphibians are the opioids followed by the α2-agonists, particularly dexmedetomidine. Although the μ-agonist opioids demonstrate more effectiveness compared with κ-agonists, owing to the decreased selective binding of the opioid receptors, both appear suitable for use in amphibians. Amphibians require higher doses of opioids compared with mammals; however, the analgesic effect of the opioid also last longer (Benyhe et al. 1990; Koeller 2009; Stevens 2004, 2011). Tramadol use has not been reported in the literature; however, the author has used it orally in aged marine toads with arthropathies (25 mg/kg PO q 48 hours) with positive clinical results. Further evaluation of tramadol use in amphibians is needed.

Of the few studied NSAIDs in amphibians, flunixin meglumine (25 mg/kg s.c.) has been the most effective for decreasing responsiveness to cutaneous noxious stimulation (Coble et al. 2011; Terril-Robb et al. 1996). Minter et al. (2011) demonstrated that the systemic administration of meloxicam at a dosage of 0.1 mg/kg once daily decreases the circulating serum prostaglandin E2 levels in North American bullfrogs (*Rana catesbeiana*) measured 24 hours after the induction of the inflammatory cascade through surgical muscle biopsies. Meloxicam (0.2 mg/kg s.c.) in African clawed frogs (*Xenopus laevis*) demonstrated a very mild analgesic effect against cutaneous noxious stimuli (Coble et al. 2011). It is quite probable that for analgesic effects, the dose needs to be increased, especially when compared with the flunixin dosage, which is approximately 20- to 25-fold higher than in mammals. The author has seen anti-inflammatory effects of meloxicam when administered parenterally (0.2–0.3 mg/kg) in frogs with cutaneous ulcers. Further research is needed to assess the clinical efficacy and toxicity of NSAID use in amphibians.

Local anesthetics should be used judiciously in amphibians due to potential systemic toxicity associated with dermal absorption; however, they can be very effective when local analgesia is required (e.g., microchip implantation and distal digital amputation). Topical applications of lidocaine, benzocaine, or a prilocaine-lidocaine (EMLA®) have all been used anecdotally for their local effects (Fig. 6.2). However, in one study that evaluated benzocaine and prilocaine-lidocaine as potential topical agents to induce anesthesia in leopard frogs, the latter was associated with 41.7% mortality at a dosage greater than 5 mg/kg (Guenette & Lair 2006).

Reptiles

Similar to mammals and birds, reptiles possess the appropriate neuroanatomical components for nociception with well-developed antinociceptive mechanisms. Aδ nociceptors have been isolated in the oral mucosa

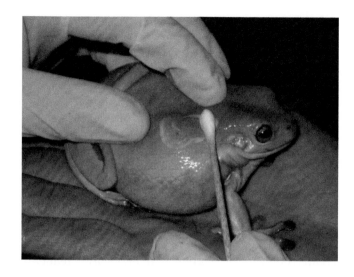

Figure 6.2. Topical application of a local anesthetic cream (lidocaine/prilocaine) in a White's tree frog (*Litoria caerulea*) prior to microchipping.

and facial skin of snakes that are similar to those in primates, and the arrangement of the spinal cord in reptiles is similar to that in mammals. Spinal projections between the brainstem and the superficial layers of the dorsal horn have been identified in Tokay gecko lizards (*Gekko gecko*), and are analogous to those in mammals that promote spinal inhibition. In addition, neurotransmitters responsible for nociceptive modulation in other vertebrates have been identified in reptiles, and nociception can be modulated with analgesics used in other taxa. Opioid receptors are present throughout the central nervous system, although the efficacy of opioid agonists may vary between species. Cyclooxygenase enzymes can be inhibited by the use of nonsteroidal anti-inflammatories in reptiles (Kanui et al. 1990; Kanui & Hole 1992; Liang & Terashima 1993; Mosley 2011; Ng et al. 1986; Reiner 1987; ten Donkelaar & de Boer-van 1987; Schaefffer & Waters 1996; Seebacher & Franklin 2003; Sladky et al. 2007, 2008, 2009; Sladsky 2010).

Recognition of Pain in Reptiles Clinical experience and research demonstrate that reptiles display a number of behaviors that are consistent with pain in mammalian species, including decreased activity levels and appetite, immobility, guarding of painful limbs or regions, changes to ambulation patterns, exaggerated withdrawal, escape or avoidance responses, and attempts to bite. Other clinical signs that may be noted are vocalizations, behavioral changes, closed eyes, color changes, hunched appearance or not resting in a normal posture, excessive scratching, flicking, or biting at painful areas, elevated heart rates, and abnormal respirations (Duncan 2012; Eatwell 2010; Kanui & Hole 1992; Machin 2007; Mosely 2011; Stoskopf 1994). Tortoises can accurately locate a tactile stimulus applied to the shell, and respond by rubbing at the stimulated area with a foot (Rosenberg 1986; Stein & Grossman 1980). However, it is important to realize that some reptiles may suppress some pain-related behaviors when an observer is present (Fleming & Robertson 2006). It is essential to learn the normal repertoire of species-specific behaviors in order to interpret abnormalities that may represent pain.

Analgesia in Reptiles In general, the opioids have been the most studied analgesic in reptile species; however, there are increasing studies with other analgesics being reported. In the anole lizard (*Anolis carolinensis*), intraperitoneally administered morphine at 5 mg/kg slowed the tail-flick response to a noxious stimulus (Mauk et al. 1981). Green iguanas (*Iguana iguana*) demonstrated significantly reduced tail movement after an electrical stimulation when intramuscular morphine (1 mg/kg) was administered (Hawkins 2006), while crocodiles developed significant latencies in response to painful stimuli with maximal effect at 0.3 mg/kg (Kanui & Hole 1992). Morphine also has demonstrated analgesic effects in red-eared sliders (*Trachemys scripta*) and bearded dragons (*Pogona vitticeps*); however, profound long-lasting respiratory depression was noted in the turtles at higher doses. When morphine was administered intrathecally (0.1–0.2 mg/kg) to red-eared slider turtles, it resulted in thermal antinociception of the hindlimbs for up to 48 hours (Mans et al. 2011). Morphine at studied doses was not found to be effective in corn snakes (*Elaphe guttata*). The duration of action may vary considerable between species, and the onset of action of morphine may be delayed for 2–8 hours after administration (Sladky et al. 2007, 2008). Hydromorphone has been used anecdotally by the author in lizards, snakes, and turtles with apparent clinical analgesic effects, although sedation and respiratory depression were noted at dosages higher than 0.5 mg/kg. Transdermal fentanyl patches (2.5 μg/h) applied to prehensile tailed skinks (*Corucia zebrata*) achieved serum concentrations that would equate to effective analgesic levels in human patients (Gamble 2009). Further research with hydromorphone and transdermal fentanyl is needed to evaluate their analgesic effects.

Although butorphanol has been used frequently as an analgesic with variable clinical results, few studies support its analgesic properties in reptiles. In red-eared slider turtles and bearded dragons, it did not yield significant antinociceptive effects (Sladky et al. 2007, 2008). However, in snakes at higher dosages (20 mg/kg), it did result in thermal antinociceptive effects (Sladky et al. 2008). Olesen et al. (2008) demonstrated that butorphanol did not have analgesic properties in ball pythons (*Python regius*). In green iguanas, butorphanol (1 mg/kg) did not have an isoflurane sparing effect on minimum alveolar concentrations (Mosley

et al. 2003); however, analgesia was noted at dosages between 1.5 and 8.0 mg/kg in electrostimulation experiments (Greenacre et al. 2006). Buprenorphine has not demonstrated analgesic activity in red-eared slider turtles or green iguanas, with profound respiratory depression noted in the former species (Greenacre et al. 2006; Sladsky 2010).

Studies with tramadol use in reptiles is limited; however, the drug appears to hold promise as an effective analgesic. In bearded dragons, a significant analgesic effect was noted in electrostimulation experiments at 11 mg/kg (Greenacre et al. 2008). Long-lasting analgesia (up to 96 hours) was noted with oral tramadol administration (10–25 mg/kg) in red-eared sliders; however, a significant decrease in ventilation rates were noted and at the highest dose sedation with flaccid neck and limbs was noted. Dosages of 5 mg/kg did not suppress ventilation and provided analgesia for at least 24 hours. (Baker et al. 2011). The author has noted apparent analgesic effects for 48–72 hours in several species of lizards and snakes with dosages between 10 and 25 mg/kg, with profound sedation and respiratory depression often noted at the higher doses for the first 24 hours.

NSAIDs are the most widely used analgesic in reptiles, with very few clinical studies to evaluate their pharmacokinetics or clinical efficacy (Greenacre et al. 2008; Mosley 2011; Olesen et al. 2008; Read 2004). As such, it is difficult to recommend effective and safe dosing intervals as plasma concentrations of NSAIDs do not always directly correspond with clinical efficacy (Mosley 2011). Meloxicam has been used most frequently by clinicians with no reports of toxicity in reptiles. Daily intramuscular administration of meloxicam (0.2 mg/kg) or carprofen (2 mg/kg) for 10 days in green iguanas did not yield any significant alterations to hematological or serum biochemical parameters (Trnková et al. 2007), and high daily oral doses of meloxicam (1 or 5 mg/kg) for 12 days did not induce any histological changes to renal, hepatic or gastric tissues (Divers et al. 2010). In green iguanas dosed orally or intravenously at 0.2 mg/kg, plasma concentrations associated with analgesia in other species were maintained for 24 hours (Divers et al. 2010). In red-eared sliders, intramuscular administration of meloxicam (0.5 mg/kg) provided for the most consistent clinical pharmacokinetic behavior with a terminal half-life of 7.57 hours, while oral bioavailability was only 37% (Rojo-Solís et al. 2009). Olesen et al. (2008) found no discernable effects on mitigating changes in physiological parameters in ball pythons undergoing surgery when comparing preoperative meloxicam (0.2 mg/kg i.m.) to saline. However meloxicam (0.4 mg/kg i.m.) was effective in significantly decreasing tail movement responses in bearded dragons to electrostimulation, as was carprofen (2 and 4 mg/kg i.m.) and ketoprofen (2 mg/kg i.m.), compared with saline (Greenacre et al.

2008). Ketoprofen bioavailability when administered intramuscularly in green iguanas was 78%, with a longer terminal half-life compared with dogs (Tuttle et al. 2006). The longer half-life of studied NSAIDs necessitates judicious use in compromised reptiles.

Local anesthetics are commonly used for surgical procedures in reptiles, and can be an effective local analgesic (Bennett 1998; Hawkins 2006). Care must be taken to avoid accidental overdose, especially in small patients. Dosages should not exceed 10 mg/kg for lidocaine, 5 mg/kg for bupivicaine, or 25 mg/kg for mepivicaine (Eatwell 2010; Mosley 2011; Wellehan et al. 2006). For smaller patients, less concentrated commercially available solutions (e.g., 1% lidocaine or 0.25% bupivicaine) should be used to minimize the decreased efficacy of local anesthetics when they are diluted (Kanai & Hoka 2006; Kanai et al. 2007). Some clinicians, including the author, prefer to combine these two local anesthetics in a 1:1 ratio to enhance effects and duration, and minimize the potential for toxicity (Eatwell 2010). Clinical evaluation of local anesthetic use in reptiles is rare in the veterinary literature. A technique for a mandibular nerve blockade using 2% mepivicaine was described in crocodilians (Wellehan et al. 2006), and more recently, intrathecal administration of lidocaine (4 mg/kg) or bupivicaine (1 mg/kg) in red-eared sliders resulted in motor block of the hindlimbs for approximately 1 and 2 hours, respectively (Mans et al. 2011). Further research into local anesthetic use in reptiles is needed.

Other drugs such as NMDA antagonists, α-2 agonists, or gabapentin have not been clinically evaluated for their analgesic properties in reptiles, although based on experience in other taxa they may be beneficial (Mosley 2011). Complementary therapies such as acupuncture (Fig. 6.3) and cold laser therapy appear to be

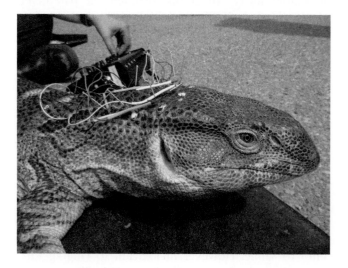

Figure 6.3. Electroacupuncture in a black throated monitor (*Varanus albigularis ionidesi*) for cranial cervical trauma that had resulted in tetraparesis. The monitor had not improved with pharmaceuticals and aqua therapy, but significant clinical improvement was noted within three acupuncture treatments.

valuable based on clinical impressions, and deserve further study as well (Koski 2011).

Birds

The neurological components to respond appropriately to painful stimuli in avian species are analogous to those in mammals, with well-developed antinociceptive mechanisms to diminish pain, and modulation of pain pathways and behavioral responses to painful stimuli with pharmacological agents (Gentle 1992; Hawkins 2006 Machin 2007; Machin & Livingston 2002). Three types of nociceptors have been identified in birds: thermal and mechanical nociceptors, and high threshold nociceptors that are polymodal in nature and respond to mechanical, thermal, and chemical stimulation (Gentle 1992; Gottschaldt et al. 1982; McKeegan 2004; Necker & Reiner 1980). Opioid receptors are detectable as early as 10 days in embryonic chicks (Hendrickson & Lin 1980), and the μ, δ, and κ opioid receptors in birds are similarly distributed in the forebrain and midbrain as seen in mammals, with κ receptors predominating in the few studied species, but with variability existing, even between strains of the same species (Csillag et al. 1990; Mansour et al. 1988; Reiner et al. 1989). Cyclooxygenase enzymes (COX-1 and COX-2) are widely distributed in birds, and can be modulated with NSAIDs (Lu et al. 1995; Mathonnet et al. 2001).

Recognition of Pain in Bird Species In general, similar to many wild species, birds tend not to show overt signs of pain as obvious distress behaviors may attract unwanted attention; rather, they will demonstrate more subtle or cryptic behavioral signs of their discomfort. As there are no universal indicators of pain in birds, the assessment of pain must take into account the species-specific normal behavior and individual behavior, strain, gender, age, concurrent disease states, type of pain, and the environment. In addition, it is important that behavioral observations occur at appropriate times for each species, such as observing nocturnal species at night (Hawkins & Paul-Murphy 2011; Hughes 1990; Machin 2007; Sufka et al. 1992).

Birds that are acclimated to handling may mask physiological changes often associated with pain, such as elevations in body temperature, respiratory rate, or stress hormones. However, birds that are comfortable with their environment also may more readily demonstrate painful behaviors, such as limb guarding or squinting of the eyes (Hawkins 2006; Heatley et al. 2000). In chickens, elevations in blood pressure were consistently associated with painful procedures; however, the measurement of blood pressures is not always feasible (Gentle & Hunter 1991). Immobility is a shared finding across numerous avian species, and in social species, isolative behavior can often be noted (Gentle 1992; Gentle & Hill 1987; Graham 1998; Paul-Murphy & Hawkins 2012). Many bird species that are being handled will respond to acute painful procedures with vocalizations, excessive movement, and escape reactions, but with progression of the painful stimulus will revert to immobility. Normally passive birds may act aggressively when in pain. With prolonged pain, decreased appetite and activity are often noted, especially behaviors such as preening or dust bathing, although in some individuals, particularly with psittacines and mynahs, overgrooming and feather destructive behavior may ensue (Gentle & Hunter 1991; Hawkins & Paul-Murphy 2011).

Analgesia in Birds Based on pharmacodynamic studies and clinical experience, butorphanol is the recommended opioid for use in avian species at a dosages of 1–5 mg/kg intramuscularly every 3–24 hours, as it has poor oral availability (Hawkins 2006; Hawkins & Paul-Murphy 2011; Klaphake et al. 2006; Paul-Murphy et al. 1999; Sanchez-Migallon Guzman et al. 2011; Sladky et al. 2006). In some species, particularly *Buteo sp.* raptors and corvids, it can be associated with profound sedation at the higher dosages. In pharmacokinetic studies, the half-life is only 1–2 hours, so frequent dosing may be necessary depending on clinical need (Paul-Murphy& Hawkins 2012; Riggs et al. 2008; Sanchez-Migallon et al. 2008; Sanchez-Migallon Guzman et al. 2011a). An experimental liposome encapsulated butorphanol holds promise for the future as it provides analgesic effects for 3–5 days after a single subcutaneous injection of 15 mg/kg (Paul-Murphy et al. 2009a; Sladky et al., 2006). Another κ-agonist and partial μ-antagonist that may of future clinical use is nalbuphine hydrochloride. In Hispaniolan Amazon parrots (*Amazona ventralis*), it increased pedal thermal withdrawal thresholds for up to 3 hours after single intramuscular administration of 12.5 mg/kg (Sanchez-Migallon Guzman et al. 2011b).

Other opioids, such as fentanyl and buprenorphine, have demonstrated mixed results in clinical studies. Fentanyl at 0.02 mg/kg intramuscularly in white cockatoos (*Cacatua alba*) was not effective; however, increasing it to 0.2 mg/kg yielded a positive analgesic response but was associated with undesirable hyperactivity (Hoppes et al. 2003). Under constant rate infusion studies in red-tailed hawks (*Buteo jamaicensis*), fentanyl significantly lowered the minimum anesthetic dose of isoflurane by 31–55%, so it may have greater clinical applications as an intraoperative analgesic (Pavez et al. 2011). Buprenorphine administered intra-articularly in domestic fowl, or intramuscularly at 0.1 mg/kg in African gray parrots, failed to demonstrate an analgesic effect (Gentle et al. 1999; Paul-Murphy et al. 1999, 2004a). However, at 0.25 and 0.5 mg/kg in pigeons, it was associated with a positive analgesic response for 2 and 5 hours, respectively, and deserves further study (Gaggermeier et al. 2003).

The pharmacokinetics of tramadol has been studied in bald eagles (*Haliaetus leucocephalus*), red tailed hawks,

peafowl (*Pavo cristatus*), and Hispaniolan Amazon parrots with oral dosages between 5 and 11 mg/kg achieving serum levels equated with analgesia in humans (Black et al. 2010; Souza et al. 2009, 2010, 2011). Preliminary studies on its efficacy against noxious thermal stimuli in Hispaniolan Amazon parrots revealed that a dosage of 30 mg/kg provides analgesia for up to 6 hours, indicating that higher doses may be needed for clinical effect and that significant interspecific variability may exist (Souza et al. 2010).

The most frequently used NSAIDs in avian species are meloxicam, carprofen, and ketoprofen with selective use of celocoxib and piroxicam. Meloxicam is the most commonly used NSAID in zoological medicine, and has shown a wide margin of safety in a large and diverse number of species (Cuthbert et al. 2007; Hawkins & Paul-Murphy 2011; Naidoo & Swan 2008; Naidoo et al. 2008). Significant interspecific variation exists in birds, with elimination half-life in studied species ranging from as short as 30 minutes in ostrich (*Struthio camelus*), to over 3 hours in chickens, and 4 hours in ring-necked parakeets (*Psittacula krameri*) when administered intravenously (Baert & De Backer 2003; Wilson et al. 2005) and 16 hours after oral administration in ring-necked parakeets (Wilson et al. 2005). In Hispaniolan Amazon parrots, intramuscular dosages of 1 mg/kg every 12 hours were needed for effective analgesia for experimentally induced arthritis, but long-term studies have not been carried out to assess for adverse side effects (Cole et al. 2009). Based on the author's clinical experience, an initial dose of 0.2–0.5 mg/kg intramuscularly has proven efficacious in many species, and generally favorable clinical results noted with chronic oral usage at 0.2–0.3 mg/kg up to once daily with no complications. As with the other NSAIDS, further studies are needed to evaluate the pharmacokinetic and pharmacodynamic behavior of meloxicam in various avian taxa, as well as evaluation for adverse effects with chronic administration.

Carprofen has yielded variable results in studied species, with either a very high dose (30 mg/kg) needed to provide analgesia for experimentally induced arthritis in chickens (Hocking et al. 2005; McGeown et al. 1999), or a very short duration of action noted when a lower dose (3 mg/kg) was administered to Hispaniolan Amazon parrots (Paul-Murphy et al. 2009b). Ketoprofen administered orally or parenterally (2 mg/kg) to Japanese quail (*Coturnix japonica*) had a very short half-life of less than 35 minutes despite route of administration (Graham et al. 2005), while in mallard ducks (*Anas platyrhynchos*), an intramuscular dose of 5 mg/kg was associated with decreased levels of the inflammatory mediator thromboxane for up to 12 hours after administration (Machin et al. 2001), and provided analgesia against a noxious stimulus while under isoflurane anesthesia (Machin & Livingston 2002). However, in spectacled (*Somateria fischeri*) and king (*Somateria spectabilis*), eider ducks administration of ketoprofen at 2–5 mg/kg

IM was associated with severe renal tubular necrosis, visceral gout, acute rhabdomyolysis, and death in 40% and 83% of treated males, respectively, although gender-linked behaviors may have increased the susceptibility of these birds to side effects of ketoprofen (Mulcahy et al. 2003). In addition, ketoprofen has proven toxic to studied *Gyps* vulture species at dosages above 1.4 mg/kg (Naidoo et al. 2010).

Piroxicam has not been scientifically studied in avian species, but has been used successfully for the chronic treatment of arthritis in cranes (Paul-Murphy & Hawkins 2012). While other NSAIDS such as flunixin meglumine have been used historically, they have also been associated with a higher degree of undesirable side effects, such renal toxicity and gastrointestinal ulceration (Pereira & Werther 2007). The most severe example of NSAID-induced renal toxicity is the diclofenac-linked severe decline of Asian *Gyps* vulture species (Green et al. 2004; Hussain et al. 2008; Meteyer et al. 2005; Naidoo & Swan 2008; Oaks et al. 2004).

Local anesthetics have been used successfully in a clinical setting, although there are very few scientific studies evaluating efficacy, and none that have evaluated time to effect, or duration of activity. Birds may be more sensitive to the effects of local anesthetics owing to more rapid absorption and delayed absorption compared with mammals, thus lower doses are often indicated to avoid signs of toxicity, such as drowsiness, recumbency, seizures, cardiovascular effects, and death (Hawkins & Paul-Murphy 2011; Hocking et al. 1997). Regional infiltration is generally effective for joints and soft tissue; however, brachial plexus blockade with high dose lidocaine with epinephrine and bupivicaine failed to prevent nerve transmission in chickens and mallard ducks (Brenner et al. 2010; Figueiredo et al. 2008).

Gabapentin has been used at a significantly higher dosage than mammals as an adjunctive treatment for suspected neuropathic pain in a few species, with abatement of self-mutilation (Doneley 2007; Shaver et al. 2009; Siperstein 2007), although based on the author's experience, its efficacy is highly variable, and further studies are indicated. Other drugs, such as NMDA antagonists, have not been evaluated, while complementary therapies, such as acupuncture, physiotherapy, and the use of nutraceuticals, have been anecdotally effective and are in need of further study (Crouch 2009; Koski 2011; Rychel et al. 2011).

Mammals

Despite advances in pain management, compared with the lower vertebrate species, there is still a paucity of scientific studies evaluating species-specific pain responses and analgesia in wild mammals.

Recognition of Pain in Mammals In general, many of the recognized clinical signs associated with pain in domestic mammals may be seen in wild species, although they are often more subtly expressed, especially in prey species that may not display behavioral alterations to a painful event. Often, remote evaluation is needed to truly evaluate the degree of pain. It is important for clinicians to understand the normal behavior of species in order to evaluate for such changes in behavior that may be related to pain (Flecknell 2008; Hawkins 2002).

Objective assessment of pain can be done through evaluation of physiological and biochemical (e.g., alterations in corticosteroid levels) indices and behavior. The former indices are often difficult to assess in the conscious animal. Nonspecific clinical signs, such as tachypnea, trembling, bruxism, salivation, muscle spasms, sweating in species capable of doing so, and dilated pupils, can be associated with pain in mammals, while it is often difficult or impossible to evaluate for more specific changes such as tachycardia or pyrexia in the conscious animal. Changes in facial expressions, such as wrinkling the brow, frowning, or grimacing, are not usually recognized (Williams 2002). Other subjective measures should be evaluated, such as changes in demeanor; altered social interactions; variations in feeding or foraging patterns; changes in posture, mobility, or activity level; alterations of sleep-awake patterns; self-directed behaviors, such as looking, biting, kicking, chewing, or rubbing of painful areas; changes in vocalization; and altered response to touch (Bufalari et al. 2007; Machin 2007; Walker et al. 2010). Any of these measures may be altered with pharmacologic agents. In some social species, pain responses may elicit assistance or directed aggression from conspecifics within the social group (Sanford et al. 1996).

Analgesia in Mammals Much of the analgesic drug selection and doses used in mammals is extrapolated from domestic and laboratory species, although much-needed studies of analgesics in wildlife continue to expand.

Opioids are frequently used for analgesia in a zoological setting, but less frequently with free-ranging wildlife owing to the potential for sedation. Pharmacokinetic (PK) and pharmacodynamic (PD) studies are limited, but include PK of butorphanol in elephants (Tana et al. 2010), PK and PD of butorphanol in llamas (Carroll et al. 2001), PK and PD of morphine in llamas (Uhrig et al. 2007), and PK of fentanyl patches in llamas (Grubb et al. 2005). These studies highlight the need for species-specific studies, as extrapolation from taxonomically related species is not always appropriate.

Even though the duration of activity of butorphanol is relatively short compared with other opioids, it is still frequently used as an analgesic (maned wolf: McNulty et al. 2000; microchiropterans: Wellehan et al. 2001; African lions: Kolata 2002; Egyptian fruit bats: Lafortune et al. 2004; Asian elephants: Abou-Madi et al.

2004; white-tailed deer: MacLean et al. 2006; African hedgehog: Done et al. 2007; otariid seals: Haulena 2007; parma wallabies: Okeson et al. 2009; polar bears: Velguth et al. 2009; prehensile-tailed porcupine: Guthrie & deMaar 2011). Opioid formulations of longer durations such as buprenorphine (lions: Kolata 2002; polar bears: Velguth et al. 2009; hyena: Hahn et al. 2007; pinnipeds: Moore et al. 2010), hydromorphone (squirrel monkey: Wellehan et al. 2004; binturong: Spriggs et al. 2007), fentanyl patches (llama: Grubb et al. 2005; binturong: Spriggs et al. 2007), or epidural morphine are used frequently for analgesia by clinicians in a zoological setting, and are more commonly reported in the literature. Based on clinical experience, tramadol also is an effective analgesic in many species, and its use has been reported in large felids (McCain et al. 2008, 2009), Western lowland gorilla (Rush et al. 2010), binturong (Spriggs et al. 2007), pinnipeds (Moore et al. 2010), and Atlantic bottlenose dolphin (Schmitt & Sur 2012).

Meloxicam is the most widely administered NSAID in zoological species, with increasing applications in free-ranging wildlife. Its pharmacokinetics have been studied in nondomestic species, such as mini-pigs, baboons, and rodents (Busch et al. 1998), and rabbits (Carpenter et al. 2009). It is has been used parenterally or orally in most mammalian families by the author with no observed or reported side effects. Based on the reported literature and the author's experience, oral dosages required for complexed stomached species are higher than those for simple monogastric species. (Chai et al. 2009; Dadone et al. 2011; Okeson et al. 2009; Pye et al. 2008, 2010; Twomey et al. 2010; Whiteside & Black 2004; Whiteside et al. 2006).

Carprofen and ketoprofen also are frequently used NSAIDs for captive and free-ranging mammals. In general, carprofen has been found to be efficacious (Dutton et al. 2002; Mylniczenko et al. 2005; Velguth et al. 2009). However, even in taxonomically similar species, there may be profound difference, as Walker et al. (2011) reported it was not effective in controlling postsurgical pain in Stellar sea lions when administered at dosages suggested by Dold et al. (2004) based on PK and PD studies in California sea lions. The pharmacokinetics of ketoprofen have been studied in elephants (Hunter et al. 2003) and its anecdotal use has been reported in a wide variety of species (golden lion tamarin: Bronson et al. 2005; exotic ruminants: Howard & Richardson 2005; sun bear: Mylniczenko et al. 2005; pinnipeds: Fauquier et al. 2008; Rush et al. 2012; Dennison et al. 2007; koalas: Pye et al. 2008; bongo: Gyimesi et al. 2008; Gyimesi et al. 2011; agoutis: Zimmerman et al. 2009).

NSAIDs, such as phenylbutazone and flunixin meglumine, are still utilized for analgesia, particularly with larger mammalian species (rhinoceros: Wack et al. 2010; Harrison et al. 2011; giraffe: James et al. 2000;

exotic ruminants: Howard & Richardson 2005; Gyimesi et al. 2011; deer: Mansfield et al. 2006; elk: Larsen et al. 2000; Stellar sea lions: Walker et al. 2009; bison: Minter et al. 2011). The PK of phenylbutazone have been carried out in Asian and African elephants (Bechert et al. 2008) and dromedary camel (Kadir et al. 1997), with the PK of flunixin also studied in dromedary camel (Oukessou 1994).

The PK of ibuprofen has been studied in Asian and African elephants (Bechert & Christensen 2007), and its use has been reported in primates (Bronson et al. 2005; Robbins et al. 2009; Wellehan et al. 2004), and Indian rhinoceros (Bertelsen et al. 2004). Its use in carnivore species is not recommended based on side effects noted in domestic canids and felids. Other sporadically used NSAIDs include deracoxib, firocoxib, tepoxalin, etodolcac, tolfenamic acid, and naproxen, which are occasionally reported in the literature (Hohn et al. 2007; Stringer et al. 2012; Williams & Junge 2007). Care should be exercised if using these, as the PK or PD behavior, or the potential negative side effects, are not known.

Corticosteroids are infrequently used for pain management in exotic species owing to the potential negative side effects; however, the use of medium- to long-acting steroids, such as triamcinolone acetate and medroxyprednisolone acetate, have been used successfully for joint infusions in mammals with arthritis refractory to other therapies.

Local anesthetics are frequently used with zoological species, and their use continues to expand in a free range setting. They are effective when used topically, epidurally, intra-articularly, intrapleurally, or intra-abdominally, for specific nerve blocks (such as dental blocks for tooth extractions or endodontic procedures [Fig. 6.4 and Fig. 6.5], or regional nerve blocks), nonspecific infiltration, such as ring blocks or line blocks,

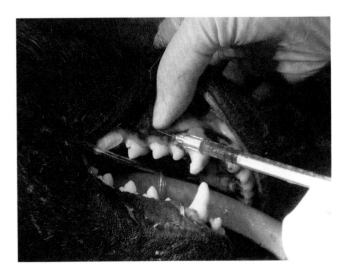

Figure 6.4. Infraorbital nerve block with bupivicaine in a gray wolf (*Canis lupus*) prior to an endodontic procedure.

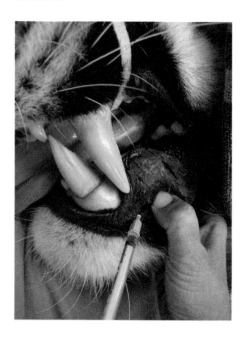

Figure 6.5. Mental nerve block with bupivicaine in an Amur tiger (*Panthera tigris altaica*) for an endodontic procedure. This dental block would be useful for premolar extraction for aging studies as well.

or for intravenous regional blocks (Beasley & Rhodes 2007; Borkowski et al. 2009; Clarke & DeVoe 2011; Dadone et al. 2011; Mansfield et al. 2006; Morges et al. 2009; Mylniczenko et al. 2005; Pye et al. 2010; Schroeder et al. 2010). Care must be taken particularly with smaller species, to avoid approaching toxic dosages (Gyimesi & Burns 2009; Heard 2007).

In a clinical setting, the use of alpha-2 agonists, such as medetomidine, or NMDA antagonists, such as ketamine or amantadine, for analgesia independent from anesthesia are rarely described in the literature for exotic species. Anecdotal evidence suggests that ketamine at 1/10th of the anesthetic dose for a species is efficacious for analgesia or as a constant rate infusion at 0.01–0.02 mg/kg/min, which limits it use in a field setting (Cracknell 2007). The addition of magnesium (Mg^{+2}) with ketamine enhances its analgesic effect (Liu et al. 2001).

Gabapentin use, particularly as part of multimodal therapy for chronic neuropathic pain or chronic disease states such as with osteoarthritis or cancer pain, is apparently effective and warrants further study (Adkesson 2006; Bronson et al. 2008; Vonsy et al. 2009). Other adjunctive therapies, such as oral glucosamine sulfate, chondroitin, omega-3 fatty acid supplementation, or injectable polysulfated glycoaminoglycans, are frequently utilized in a zoological setting for chronic arthritides and are anecdotally effective (Pye et al. 2008; Roush et al. 2010; Stringfield & Wynne 1999; Whiteside et al. 2006); however, there are no supporting scientific studies that clearly demonstrate a benefit

with oral products, and there are legitimate questions of oral biovailability, especially in herbivores. Recent analyses of multiple studies in dogs and humans indicate there is conflicting evidence as to the benefit to glucosamine, chondroitin, green lipped mussels, or methylsulfonylmethane (MSM) supplementation (Aragon et al. 2007; Neil et al. 2005; Teets et al. 2010; Vandeweerd et al. 2012). Further research in their use in zoological species is indicated. Other modalities, such as acupuncture or cold laser therapy, also have produced favorable analgesic responses for osteoarthritis or neuropathic pain, and deserve further study (Cassu et al. 2008; Koski 2011; Maenaka et al. 2006; Rychel et al. 2011; Teets et al. 2010).

Pain in Invertebrates

There is growing scientific evidence that suggests that invertebrate species, especially the more advanced species found in the phyla Arthropoda and Mollusca, have the ability to experience pain, rather than just respond to nociceptive stimuli. This is based on the presence of suitable receptors and central nervous system, responsiveness to analgesics and anesthetics, physiological changes, avoidance learning, protective motor reactions, and cognitive abilities and sentience (Crook and Walters 2011; Barr et al. 2008; Elwood 2011). Many of the advanced invertebrate species have brains that relative to their body weight are larger than those in many vertebrates species, and have complex brain structures for sensory analysis, memory, learning, and decision making, which are analogous to the functions of the cerebral cortex in vertebrate species. (Elwood et al. 2009; Sandeman et al. 1992; Smith 1991).

Behavioral evidence for likely experience of pain has been demonstrated in several invertebrate species through avoidance learning research and protective motor reflexes. Etuarine crabs (*Chasmagnathus granulatus*) associated an electrical shock with a particular location for a minimum of 3 hours after the event, and even 24 hours later in multiple trials (Denti et al. 1988; Fernandez-Duque et al. 1992). Long-term behavioral changes were observed in hermit crabs (*Pagurus bernhardus*) in their shell that were shocked on the abdomen compared with crabs that were not shocked, which included sustained grooming of the abdominal shock location (Elwood 2011; Elwood and Appel 2009). Acetic acid or sodium hydroxide applied to the antenna or eye of glass prawns resulted in an immediate tail flick response followed by increased grooming or rubbing of the affected area. Topical application of the local anesthetic benzocaine markedly decreased these responses but did not interfere with swimming, indicating that analgesia and not anesthesia was achieved (Barr et al. 2008). Finally, some arthropods, such as spiders or crabs, will automize limbs when injected with noxious substances known to be painful in vertebrates, such as the bee or wasp venom or acetic acid, or when exposed to a hot plate or electric shock (Eisner & Camazine 1983; Elwood 2011; Fiorito 1986).

Further research is needed to fully characterize the pain experience and the pharmacokinetics and pharmacodynamics of analgesic drugs in invertebrate species. However, until such research is available, clinicians should consider the administration of analgesics to patients that are being subjected to a procedure that is deemed painful in vertebrates. This includes general anesthesia with a volatile anesthetic, such as isoflurane or sevoflurane, and administration of peri-procedural analgesics, such as local anesthetics (diluted lidocaine, bupivicaine, and benzocaine) (Cooper 2011; Gunkel & Lewbart 2007).

REFERENCES

Abou-Madi N, Kollias GV, Hackett RP, et al. 2004. Umbilical herniorrhaphy in a juvenile Asian elephant (*Elephas maximus*). *Journal of Zoo and Wildlife Medicine* 35(2):221–225.

Adkesson MJ. 2006. The role of gabapentin as an analgesic: potential applications in zoological medicine. Proceedings of the American Association of Zoo Veterinarians, pp. 270–272.

Alvarez FA, Rodriguez-Martin I, Gonzalez-Nunez V, et al. 2006. New kappa opioid receptor from zebrafish *Danio rerio*. *Neuroscience Letters* 405:94–99.

Anand KJS, Hickey PR. 1987. Pain and its effects in the human neonate and fetus. *The New England Journal of Medicine* 317:1321–1329.

Aragon CL, Hofmeister EH, Budsberg SC. 2007. Systematic review of clinical trials of treatments for osteoarthritis in dogs. *Journal of the American Veterinary Medical Association* 230(4):514–521.

Ashley PJ, Sneddon LU, McCrohan CR. 2007. Nociception in fish: stimulus-response properties of receptors on the head of trout *Oncorhynchus mykiss*. *Brain Research* 1166:47–54.

Ashley PJ, Ringrose S, Edwards KL, et al. 2009. Effect of noxious stimulation upon antipredator responses and dominance status in rainbow trout. *Animal Behaviour* 77:403–410.

Baert K, De Backer P. 2003. Comparative pharmacokinetics of three non-steroidal anti-inflammatory drugs in five bird species. *Comparative Biochemistry and Physiology. Toxicology and Pharmacology* 134:25–33.

Baker BB, Sladky KK, Johnson SM. 2011. Evaluation of the analgesic effects of oral and subcutaneous tramadol administration in red-eared slider turtles. *Journal of the American Veterinary Medical Association* 238(2):220–227.

Baker TR, Cummings B, Johnson SM, et al. 2010. Comparative analgesic efficacy of morphine and butorphanol in koi (*Cyprinus carpio*) undergoing gonadectomy. Proceedings of the American Association of Zoo Veterinarians, pp. 203–204.

Barr S, Laming PR, Dick JTA, et al. 2008. Nociception or pain in a decapod crustacean? *Animal Behaviour* 75:745–751.

Beasley JC, Rhodes OE Jr. 2007. Effect of tooth removal on recaptures of raccoons. *The Journal of Wildlife Management* 71(1): 266–270.

Bechert U, Christensen JM. 2007. Pharmacokinetics of orally administered ibuprofen in African and Asian elephants (*Loxodonta africana* and *Elephas maximus*). *Journal of Zoo and Wildlife Medicine* 38(2):258–268.

Bechert U, Christensen JM, Nguyen C, et al. 2008. Pharmacokinetics of orally administered phenylbutazone in African and Asian elephants (*Loxodonta africana* and *Elephas maximus*). *Journal of Zoo and Wildlife Medicine* 39(2):188–200.

Bennett RA. 1998. Reptile anesthesia. *Seminars in Avian and Exotic Pet Medicine* 7(1):30–40.

Benyhe S, Varga E, Hepp J, et al. 1990. Characterization of kappa1 and kappa2 opioid binding sites in frog (*Rana esculenta*) brain membrane. *Neurochemical Research* 15:899–904.

Bertelsen MF, Olberg RA, Mehren KG, et al. 2004. Surgical management of rectal prolapse in an Indian rhinoceros (*Rhinoceros unicornis*). *Journal of Zoo and Wildlife Medicine* 35(2):245–247.

Black PA, Cox S, Macek M, et al. 2010. Pharmacokinetics of tramadol hydrochloride and its metabolite O-desmethyltramadol in peafowl (*Pavo cristatus*). *Journal of Zoo and Wildlife Medicine* 41(4):671–676.

Borkowski R, Citino S, Bush M, et al. 2009. Surgical castration of subadult giraffe (*Giraffa camelopardalis*). *Journal of Zoo and Wildlife Medicine* 40(4):786–790.

Bradford CS, Walthers EA, Searcy BT, et al. 2005. Cloning, heterologous expression and pharmacological characterization of a kappa opioid receptor from the brain of the rough-skinned newt, *Taricha granulosa*. *Journal of Molecular Endocrinology* 34: 809–823.

Brenner DJ, Larsen RS, Dickinson PJ, et al. 2010. Development of an avian brachial plexus nerve block technique for perioperative analgesia in mallard ducks (*Anas platyrhynchos*). *Journal of Avian Medicine and Surgery* 24:24–34.

Brenner GM, Klopp AJ, Deason LL, et al. 1994. Analgesic potency of alpha adrenergic agents after systemic administration in amphibians. *Journal of Pharmacology and Experimental Therapeutics* 270:540–545.

Bronson E, Deem SL, Sanchez C, et al. 2005. Placental retention in a golden lion tamarin (*Leontopithecus rosalia*). *Journal of Zoo and Wildlife Medicine* 36(4):716–718.

Bronson E, Wack A, Johnson B, et al. 2008. Use of oral gabapentin to aid healing of a periparturient pelvic fracture in a common zebra (*Equus burchelli*). Proceedings of the American Association of Zoo Veterinarians, p. 131.

Brooks AI, Standifer KM, Cheng J, et al. 1994. Opioid binding in giant toad and goldfish brain. *Receptor* 4:55–62.

Buatti MC, Pasternak GW. 1981. Multiple opiate receptors: phylogenetic differences. *Brain Research* 218:400–405.

Bufalari A, Adami C, Angeli G, et al. 2007. Pain assessment in animals. *Veterinary Research Communications* 31(Suppl. 1): 55–58.

Busch U, Schmid J, Heinzel G, et al. 1998. Pharmacokinetics of meloxicam in animals and the relevance to humans. *Drug Metabolism and Disposition: The Biological Fate of Chemicals* 26 (6):576–584.

Carli F, Schricker T. 2009. Modification of metabolic responses to surgery by neural blockade. In: *Neural Blockade in Clinical Anesthesia and Pain Medicine*, 4th ed. (MJ Cousins, DB Carr, TT Horlocker, PO Bridenbaugh, eds.), pp. 133–143. Philadelphia: Lippincott Williams & Wilkins.

Carpenter JW, Pollock CG, Koch DE, et al. 2009. Single and multiple-dose pharmacokinetics of meloxicam after oral administration to the rabbit (*Oryctolagus cuniculus*). *Journal of Zoo and Wildlife Medicine* 40(4):601–606.

Carroll GL, Boothe DM, Hartsfield SM, et al. 2001. Pharmacokinetics and pharmacodynamics of butorphanol in llamas after intravenous and intramuscular administration. *Journal of the American Veterinary Medical Association* 219(9):1263–1267.

Cassu RN, Luna SP, Clark RM, et al. 2008. Electroacupuncture analgesia in dogs: is there a difference between uni- and bi-lateral stimulation? *Veterinary Anaesthesia and Analgesia* 35(1):52–61.

Chai N, Hazan T, Wedlarski R, et al. 2009. Treatment of a retroperitoneal abscess by omentalization in an orangutan (*Pongo pygmaeus pygmaeus*). *Journal of Zoo and Wildlife Medicine* 40(2): 350–353.

Chandroo KP, Duncan IJ, Moccia RD. 2004. Can fish suffer?: perspectives on sentience, pain, fear and stress. *Applied Animal Behaviour Science* 86(3):225–250.

Chervova LS, Lapshin DN. 2000. Opioid modulation of pain threshold in fish. *Doklady Biological Sciences: Proceedings of the Academy of Sciences of the USSR, Biological Sciences Sections* 375: 590–591.

Clarke EO, DeVoe RS. 2011. Ovariohysterectomy of three vampire bats (*Desmodus rotundus*). *Journal of Zoo and Wildlife Medicine* 42(4):755–758.

Coble DJ, Taylor DK, Mook DM. 2011. Analgesic effects of meloxicam, morphine sulfate, flunixin meglumine, and xylazine hydrochloride in African-clawed frogs (*Xenopus laevis*). *Journal of the American Association for Laboratory Animal Science* 50(3):355–360.

Coggeshall RE, Leonard RB, Applebaum ML, et al. 1978. Organisation of peripheral nerves of the Atlantic stingray, *Dasyatis sabina*. *Journal of Neurophysiology* 41:97–107.

Cole GA, Paul-Murphy J, Krugner-Higby L, et al. 2009. Analgesic effects of intramuscular administration of meloxicam in Hispaniolan parrots (*Amazona ventralis*) with experimentally induced arthritis. *American Journal of Veterinary Research* 70: 1471–1476.

Cooper JE. 2011. Anesthesia, analgesia, and euthanasia of invertebrates. *ILAR Journal* 52(2):196–204.

Correia AD, Cunha SR, Stevens ED. 2011. A novel behavioural fish model of nociception for testing analgesics. *Pharmaceuticals* 4:665–680.

Cracknell J. 2007. Analgesia in exotics: a review and update. Proceedings of the British Veterinary Zoological Society, pp. 15–24.

Craig AD. 2003. Pain mechanisms: labeled lines versus convergence in central processing. *Annual Review of Neuroscience* 26: 1–30.

Crook RJ, Walters ET. 2011. Nociceptive behavior and physiology of molluscs: animal welfare implications. *ILAR Journal* 52(2):185–195.

Crouch MA. 2009. Egg binding and hind limb paralysis in an African penguin: a case report. *Acupuncture in Medicine* 27(1):36–38.

Csillag A, Bourne RC, Stewart MG. 1990. Distribution of mu, delta, and kappa opioid receptor binding sites in the brain of the one-day-old domestic chick (*Gallus domesticus*): an in vitro quantitative autoradiographic study. *The Journal of Comparative Neurology* 302:543–551.

Cuthbert R, Parry-Jones J, Green RE, et al. 2007. NSAIDs and scavenging birds: potential impacts beyond Asia's critically endangered vultures. *Biology Letters* 3:90–93.

Dadone LI, Whiteside DP, Black SR, et al. 2011. Nasal osteosarcoma and interstitial cell tumor in a Vancouver Island marmot (*Marmota vancouverensis*). *Journal of Zoo and Wildlife Medicine* 42(2):330–334.

Davis MR, Mylniczenko N, Storms T, et al. 2006. Evaluation of intramuscular ketoprofen and butorphanol as analgesics in chain dogfish (*Scyliorhinus retifer*). *Zoo Biology* 25:491–500.

Davis RE, Kassel J. 1983. Behavioral functions of the teleostean telencephalon. In: *Fish Neurobiology, Vol. 2: Higher Brain Areas and Functions* (RE Davis, RG Northcutt, eds.), pp. 238–263. Ann Arbor: University of Michigan Press.

Dennison S, Gulland F, Haulena M, et al. 2007. Urate nephrolithiasis in a northern elephant seal (*Mirounga angustirostris*) and a California sea lion (*Zalophus californianus*). *Journal of Zoo and Wildlife Medicine* 38(1):114–120.

Denti A, Dimant B, Maldonado H. 1988. Passive avoidance learning in the crab *Chasmagnathus granulatus*. *Physiology and Behavior* 43:317–320.

Divers SJ, Papich M, McBride M, et al. 2010. Pharmacokinetics of meloxicam following intravenous and oral administration in green iguanas (*Iguana iguana*). *American Journal of Veterinary Research* 71(11):1277–1283.

Dold C, Haulena M, Gulland FMD. 2004. Pharmacokinetics of oral carprofen in the California sea lion (*Zalophus californianus*).

Proceedings of the American Association of Zoo Veterinarians, pp. 343–345.

Done LB, Deem SL, Fiorello CV. 2007. Surgical and medical management of a uterine spindle cell tumor in an African hedgehog (*Atelerix albiventris*). *Journal of Zoo and Wildlife Medicine* 38(4):601–603.

Doneley B. 2007. The use of gabapentin to treat presumed neuralgia in a little corella (*Cacatua sanguinea*). Proceedings of the Australian Assosiation of Avian Veterinarians Conference, pp. 169–172.

Duncan A. 2012. Reptile and amphibian analgesia. In: *Fowler's Zoo and Wildlife Medicine, Current Therapy*, Vol. 7 (RE Miller, M Fowler, eds.), pp. 247–253. Philadelphia: Elselvier Saunders.

Dunlop R, Laming P. 2005. Mechanoreceptive and nociceptive responses in the central nervous system of goldfish (*Carassius auratus*) and trout (*Oncorhynchus mykiss*). *The Journal of Pain* 6(9):561–568.

Dutton CJ, Duncan M, Price HI. 2002. Hydromyelia in a Reeves' muntjac (*Muntiacus reevesi*). *Journal of Zoo and Wildlife Medicine* 33(3):256–262.

Eatwell K. 2010. Options for analgesia and anaesthesia in reptiles. *In Practice* 32:306–311.

Echteler SM, Saidel WM. 1981. Forebrain connections in the goldfish support telencephalic homologies with land vertebrates. *Science* 212:683–684.

Ehrensing RH, Mitchell GF, Kastin AJ. 1982. Similar antagonism of morphine analgesia by MIF-1 and naxolone in *Carassius auratus*. *Pharmacology, Biochemistry, and Behavior* 17:757–761.

Eisner T, Camazine S. 1983. Spider leg autotomy induced by prey venom injection: an adaptive response to "pain." *Proceedings of the National Academy of Sciences of the United States of America* 80:3382–3385.

Elwood RW. 2011. Pain and suffering in invertebrates? *ILAR Journal* 52:75–184.

Elwood RW, Appel M. 2009. Pain experience in hermit crabs. *Animal Behaviour* 77(5):1243–1246.

Elwood RW, Barr S, Patterson L. 2009. Pain and stress in crustaceans? *Applied Animal Behaviour Science* 118:128–136.

Fauquier DA, Mazet JA, Gulland FM, et al. 2008. Distribution of tissue enzymes in three species of pinnipeds. *Journal of Zoo and Wildlife Medicine* 39(1):1–5.

Fernandez-Duque E, Valeggia C, Maldonado H. 1992. Multi-trial inhibitory avoidance learning in the crab *Chasmagnathus*. *Behavioral and Neural Biology* 57:189–197.

Figueiredo JP, Cruz ML, Mendes GM, et al. 2008. Assessment of brachial plexus blockade in chickens by an axillary approach. *Veterinary Anaesthesia and Analgesia* 35:511–518.

Fiorito G. 1986. Is there "pain" in invertebrates? *Behavioural Processes* 12:383–388.

Fitzgerald M, McIntosh N. 1989. Pain and analgesia in the newborn. *Archives of Disease in Childhood* 64:441–443.

Flecknell P. 2008. Analgesia from a veterinary perspective. *British Journal of Anaesthesia* 101(1):121–124.

Fleming GJ, Robertson S. 2006. Use of thermal threshold test response to evaluate the antinociceptive effects of butorphanol in juvenile green iguanas (*Iguana iguana*). Proceedings of the American Association of Zoo Veterinarians, p. 279.

Gaggermeier B, Henke J, Schatzmann U. 2003. Investigations on analgesia in domestic pigeons (*C. livia*, Gmel., 1789, var. *dom.*) using buprenorphine and butorphanol. Proceedings of the European Association of Avian Veterinarians Conference, pp. 70–73.

Gamble KC. 2009. Plasma fentanyl concentrations achieved after transdermal fentanyl patch application in prehensile tailed skinks, *Corucia zebrata*. *Journal of Herpetological Medicine and Surgery* 18:81–85.

Gentle M. 1992. Pain in birds. *Animal Welfare (South Mimms, England)* 1:235–247.

Gentle MJ, Hill FL. 1987. Oral lesions in the chicken: behavioural responses following nociceptive stimulation. *Physiology and Behavior* 40(7):81–783.

Gentle MJ, Hunter LN. 1991. Physiological and behavioural responses associated with feather removal in *Gallus gallus* var *domesticus*. *Research in Veterinary Science* 50:95–101.

Gentle MJ, Hocking PM, Bernard R, et al. 1999. Evaluation of intra-articular opioid analgesia for the relief of articular pain in the domestic fowl. *Pharmacology, Biochemistry, and Behavior* 63:339–343.

Gottschaldt KM, Fruhstorfer H, Schmidt W. 1982. Thermosensitivity and its possible fine-structural basis in mechanoreceptors in the beak skin of geese. *The Journal of Comparative Neurology* 205:219–245.

Graham DL. 1998. Pet birds: historical and modern perspectives on the keeper and the kept. *Journal of the American Veterinary Medical Association* 212:1216–1219.

Graham JE, Kollias-Baker C, Craigmill AL, et al. 2005. Pharmacokinetics of ketoprofen in Japanese quail (*Coturnix japonica*). *Journal of Veterinary Pharmacology and Therapeutics* 28:399–402.

Green RE, Newton I, Schultz S, et al. 2004. Diclofenac poisoning as a cause of vulture population declines across the Indian subcontinent. *Journal of Applied Ecology* 41:793–800.

Greenacre CB, Takle G, Schumacher JP, Klaphake EK, Harvey RC. 2006. Comparative antinociception of morphine, butorphanol, and buprenorphine versus saline in the green iguana (*Iguana iguana*) using electrostimulation. *Journal of Herpetological Medicine and Surgery* 16(3):88–92.

Greenacre CB, Massi K, Schumacher JP, et al. 2008. Comparative antinociception of various opioids and non-steroidal anti-inflammatory medications versus saline in the bearded dragon (*Pogona vitticeps*) using electrostimulation. Proceedings of the Association of Reptile and Amphibian Veterinarians, pp. 87–88.

Grimm KA, Lamont LA. 2007. Clinical pharmacology. In: *Zoo Animal and Wildlife Immobilization and Anesthesia* (G West, D Heard, N Caulkett, eds.), pp. 3–36. Ames, IA: Blackwell Publishing Ltd.

Grosser T, Yusuff S, Cheskis E, et al. 2002. Developmental expression of functional cyclooxygenases in zebrafish. *Proceedings of the National Academy of Sciences of the United States of America* 99:8418–8423.

Grubb TL, Gold JR, Schlipf JW, et al. 2005. Assessment of serum concentrations and sedative effects of fentanyl after transdermal administration at three dosages in healthy llamas. *American Journal of Veterinary Research* 66(5):907–909.

Guenette SA, Lair S. 2006. Anesthesia of the leopard frog *Rana pipiens*: a comparative study between four different agents. *Journal of Herpetological Medicine and Surgery* 16(2):38–44.

Gunkel C, Lewbart GA. 2007. Invertebrates. In: *Zoo Animal and Wildlife Immobilization and Anesthesia* (G West, D Heard, N Caulkett, eds.), pp. 147–158. Ames. Blackwell Publishing.

Guthrie A, deMaar T. 2011. Metastatic malignant melanoma in a prehensile-tailed porcupine (*Coendou prehensilis*). *Journal of Zoo and Wildlife Medicine* 42(1):121–123.

Gyimesi ZS, Burns RB. 2009. Presumptive benzocaine-induced methemoglobinemia in a slender-tailed meerkat (*Suricata suricatta*). *Journal of Zoo and Wildlife Medicine* 40(2):389–392.

Gyimesi ZS, Linhart RD, Burns RB, et al. 2008. Management of chronic vaginal prolapse in an eastern bongo (*Tragelaphus eurycerus isaaci*). *Journal of Zoo and Wildlife Medicine* 39(4):614–621.

Gyimesi ZS, Burns RB, Campbell M, et al. 2011. Abomasal Impaction in Captive Bongo *Tragelaphus eurycerus*). *Journal of Zoo and Wildlife Medicine* 42:281–290.

Hahn, N, Parker, JM, Timmel, G, et al. 2007. Hyenas. In: *Zoo Animal and Wildlife Immobilization and Anesthesia* (G West, D Heard, N Caulkett, eds.), pp. 437–442. Ames. Blackwell Publishing.

Hamamoto DT, Simone DA. 2003. Characterization of cutaneous primary afferent fibers excited by acetic acid in a model of nociception in frogs. *Journal of Neurophysiology* 90(2):566–57.

Harms CA, Lewbart GA. 2011. The veterinarian's role in surgical implantation of electronic tags in fish. *Reviews in Fish Biology and Fisheries* 21(1):25–33.

Harms CA, Lewbart GA, Swanson CR, et al. 2005. Behavioral and clinical pathology changes in koi carp (*Cyprinus carpio*) subjected to anesthesia and surgery with and without intraoperative analgesics. *Comparative Medicine* 55(3):221–226.

Harrison TM, Stanley BJ, Sikarskie JG, et al. 2011. Surgical amputation of a digit and vacuum-assisted-closure (V.A.C.) management in a case of osteomyelitis and wound care in an Eastern black rhinoceros (*Diceros bicornis michaeli*). *Journal of Zoo and Wildlife Medicine* 42(2):317–321.

Haulena M. 2007. Otariid seals. In: *Zoo Animal and Wildlife Immobilization and Anesthesia* (G West, D Heard, N Caulkett, eds.), pp. 469–478. Ames: Blackwell Publishing Ltd.

Hawkins MG. 2006. The use of analgesics in birds, reptiles, and small exotic mammals. *Journal of Exotic Pet Medicine* 15(3): 177–192.

Hawkins MG, Paul-Murphy J. 2011. Avian analgesia. *The Veterinary Clinics of North America. Exotic Animal Practice* 14(1): 61–80.

Hawkins P. 2002. Recognizing and assessing pain, suffering and distress in laboratory animals: a survey of current practice in the UK with recommendations. *Laboratory Animals*, 36(4): 378–395.

Heard D. 2007a. Lagomorphs. In: *Zoo Animal and Wildlife Immobilization and Anesthesia* (G West, D Heard, N Caulkett, eds.), pp. 647–653. Ames: Blackwell Publishing Ltd.

Heard D. 2007b. Rodents. In: *Zoo Animal and Wildlife Immobilization and Anesthesia* (G West, D Heard, N Caulkett, eds.), pp. 655–663. Ames: Blackwell Publishing Ltd.

Heatley JJ, Oliver JW, Hosgood G, et al. 2000. Serum corticosterone concentrations in response to restraint, anesthesia, and skin testing in Hispaniolan Amazon parrots (*Amazona ventralis*). *Journal of Avian Medicine and Surgery* 14:172–176.

Hendrickson C, Lin S. 1980. Opiate receptors in highly purified neuronal cell populations isolated in bulk from embryonic chick brain. *Neuropharmacology* 13:731–739.

Hess L. 2010. The ethics of exotic animal analgesia. *Journal of Avian Medicine and Surgery* 24(1):72–76.

Hocking PM, Gentle MJ, Bernard R, et al. 1997. Evaluation of a protocol for determining the effectiveness of pretreatment with local analgesics for reducing experimentally induced articular pain in domestic fowl. *Research in Veterinary Science* 63: 263–267.

Hocking PM, Robertson GW, Gentle MJ. 2005. Effects of non-steroidal anti-inflammatory drugs on pain-related behaviour in a model of articular pain in the domestic fowl. *Research in Veterinary Science* 78:69–75.

Hohn N, Parker JM, Timmel G, et al. 2007. Hyenas. In: *Zoo Animal and Wildlife Immobilizaton and Anesthesia* (G West, D Heard, N Caulkett, eds.), pp. 437–442. Ames: Blackwell Publishing.

Hoppes S, Flammer K, Hoersch K, et al. 2003. Disposition and analgesic effects of fentanyl in white cockatoos (*Cacatua alba*). *Journal of Avian Medicine and Surgery* 17:124–130.

Howard LL, Richardson GL. 2005. Transposition of the biceps tendon to reduce lateral scapulohumeral luxation in three species of nondomestic ruminant. *Journal of Zoo and Wildlife Medicine* 36(2):290–294.

Hughes RA. 1990. Strain-dependent morphine-induced analgesic and hyperalgesic effects on thermal nociception in domestic fowl (*Gallus gallus*). *Behavioral Neuroscience* 104:619–624.

Hunter R, Isaza R, Koch DE. 2003. Oral bioavailability and pharmacokinetic characteristics of ketoprofen enantiomers after oral and intravenous administration in Asian elephants (*Elephas maximus*). *American Journal of Veterinary Research* 64(1): 109–114.

Hussain I, Khan MZ, Khan A, et al. 2008. Toxicological effects of diclofenac in four avian species. *Avian Pathology: Journal of the W.V.P.A* 37:315–321.

Ide LM, Hoffmann A. 2002. Stressful and behavioral conditions that affect reversible cardiac arrest in the Nile tilapia, *Oreochromis niloticus* (Teleostei). *Physiology and Behavior* 75:119–126.

Inagaki S, Senba E, Shiosaka S, et al. 1981. Regional distribution of substance P-like immunoreactivity in the frog brain and spinal cord: immunohistochemical analysis. *The Journal of Comparative Neurology* 201:243–254.

James SB, Koss K, Harper J, et al. 2000. Diagnosis and treatment of a fractured third phalanx in a Masai giraffe (*Giraffe camelopardalis tippelskirchi*). *Journal of Zoo and Wildlife Medicine* 31(3):400–403.

Julius D, Basbaum AI. 2001. Molecular mechanisms of nociception. *Nature* 413:203–210.

Kadir A, Ali BH, al Hadrami G, et al. 1997. Phenylbutazone pharmacokinetics and bioavailability in the dromedary camel (*Camelus dromedarius*). *Journal of Veterinary Pharmacology and Therapeutics* 20(1):54–60.

Kanai A, Hoka S. 2006. A comparison of epidural blockade produced by plain 1% lidocaine and 1% lidocaine prepared by dilution of 2% lidocaine with the same volume of saline. *Anesthesia and Analgesia* 102:1851–1855.

Kanai A, Koiso S, Hoka S. 2007. Comparison of analgesia induced by continuous epidural infusion of plain 1% lidocaine and 1% lidocaine prepared by dilution of 2% lidocaine with the same volume of saline. *Journal of Clinical Anesthesia* 19:534–538.

Kanui TI, Hole K. 1992. Morphine and pethidine antinociception in the crocodile. *Journal of Veterinary Pharmacology and Therapeutics* 15:101–103.

Kanui TI, Hole K, Miaron JO. 1990. Nociception in crocodiles: capsaicin instillation, formalin and hot plate tests. *Zoological Science* 7:537–540.

Kehlet H. 1997. Multimodal approach to control postoperative pathophysiology and rehabilitation. *British Journal of Anaesthesia* 78:606–617.

Kehlet H, Wilmore DW. 2002. Multimodal strategies to improve surgical outcome. *American Journal of Surgery* 183:630–641.

Ketz CJ, Radlinsky M, Armbrust L, et al. 2001. Persistent right aortic arch and aberrant left subclavian artery in a white Bengal tiger (*Panthera tigris*). *Journal of Zoo and Wildlife Medicine* 32(2):268–272.

Klaphake E, Schumacher J, Greenacre C, et al. 2006. Comparative anesthetic and cardiopulmonary effects of pre- versus postoperative butorphanol administration in Hispaniolan Amazon parrots (*Amazona ventralis*) anesthetized with sevoflurane. *Journal of Avian Medicine and Surgery* 20:2–7.

Koeller CA. 2009. Comparison of buprenorphine and butorphanol analgesia in the eastern red-spotted newt (*Notophthalmus viridescens*). *Journal of the American Association for Laboratory Animal Science* 48(2):171–175.

Kolata RJ. 2002. Laparoscopic ovariohysterectomy and hysterectomy on African lions (*Panthera leo*) using the ultracision harmonic scalpel. *Journal of Zoo and Wildlife Medicine* 33(3): 280–282.

Koski, AM. 2011. Acupuncture for zoological companion animals. *The Veterinary Clinics of North America. Exotic Animal Practice* 14(1):141–154.

Kuner R. 2010. Central mechanisms of pathological pain. *Nature Medicine* 16(11):1258–1266.

Lafortune M, Canapp SO Jr, Heard D, et al. 2004. A vasectomy technique for Egyptian fruit bats (*Rousettus aegyptiacus*). *Journal of Zoo and Wildlife Medicine* 35(1):104–106.

Larsen RS, Cebra CK, Wild MA. 2000. Diagnosis and treatment of obstructive urolithiasis in a captive Rocky Mountain wapiti

(*Cervus elaphus nelsoni*). *Journal of Zoo and Wildlife Medicine* 31(2):236–239.

Lemke KA, Creighton CM. 2010. Analgesia for anesthetized patients. *Topics in Companion Animal Medicine* 25:70–82.

Lemke KA, Dawson SD. 2000. Local and regional anesthesia. *The Veterinary Clinics of North America. Small Animal Practice* 30: 839–857.

Li X, Keith DE Jr, Evans CJ. 1996. Mu opioid receptor-like sequences are present throughout vertebrate evolution. *Journal of Molecular Evolution* 43:179–184.

Liang YF, Terashima S. 1993. Physiological properties and morphological characteristics of cutaneous and mucosal mechanical nociceptive neurons with A-delta peripheral axons in the trigeminal ganglia of crotaline snakes. *The Journal of Comparative Neurology* 328:88–102.

Liu HT, Hollmann MW, Liu WH, et al. 2001. Modulation of NMDA receptor function by ketamine and magnesium: part I. *Anesthesia and Analgesia* 92(5):1173–1181.

Lorez HP, Kemali M, Substance P. 1981. Met-enkephalin and somatostatin-like immunoreactivity distribution in the frog spinal cord. *Neuroscience Letters* 26:119–124.

Lu X, Xie W, Reed D, et al. 1995. Nonsteroidal antiinflammatory drugs cause apoptosis and induce cyclooxygenases in chicken. *Proceedings of the National Academy of Sciences of the United States of America* 92:7961–7965.

Machin KL. 2007. Wildlife analgesia. In: *Zoo Animal and Wildlife Immobilization and Anesthesia* (G West, D Heard, N Caulkett, eds.), pp. 43–59. Ames: Blackwell Publishing Ltd.

Machin KL, Livingston A. 2002. Assessment of the analgesic effects of ketoprofen in ducks anesthetized with isoflurane. *American Journal of Veterinary Research* 63(6):821–826.

Machin KL, Tellier LA, Lair S, et al. 2001. Pharmacodynamics of flunixin and ketoprofen in mallard ducks (*Anas platyrhynchos*). *Journal of Zoo and Wildlife Medicine* 32:222–229.

MacLean RA, Mathews NE, Grove DM, et al. 2006. Surgical technique for tubal ligation in white-tailed deer (*Odocoileus virginianus*). *Journal of Zoo and Wildlife Medicine* 37(3):354–360.

Maenaka T, Tano K, Nakanishi S. 2006. Positron emission tomography analysis of the analgesic effects of acupuncture in rhesus monkeys. *The American Journal of Chinese Medicine* 34(5): 787–801.

Mans C, Steagall PVM, Lahner LL, et al. 2011. Efficacy of intrathecal lidocaine, bupivicaine, and morphine for spinal anesthesia and analgesia in red-eared sliders (*Trachemys scripta elegans*). Proceedings of the American Association of Zoo Veterinarians, p. 135.

Mansfield KG; Verstraete FJM, Pascoe PJ. 2006. Mitigating pain during tooth extraction from conscious deer. *Wildlife Society Bulletin* 34:201–202.

Mansour A, Khachaturian H, Lewis ME, et al. 1988. Anatomy of CNS opioid receptors. *Trends in Neurosciences* 11:308–314.

Maruhashi J, Mizuguchi K, Tasaki I. 1952. Action currents in single afferent nerve fibres elicited by stimulation of the skin of the toad and the cat. *The Journal of Physiology* 117:129–151.

Mathonnet M, Lalloue F, Danty E, et al. 2001. Cyclo-oxygenase 2 tissue distribution and developmental pattern of expression in the chicken. *Clinical and Experimental Pharmacology and Physiology* 28:425–432.

Matthews G, Wickelgren WO. 1978. Trigeminal sensory neurons of the sea lamprey. *Journal of Comparative Physiology. A, Neuroethology, Sensory, Neural, and Behavioral Physiology* 123: 329–333.

Mauk MD, Olson RD, LaHoste GJ, et al. 1981. Tonic immobility produces hyperalgesia and antagonizes morphine analgesia. *Science* 213:353–354.

McCain S, Souza M, Ramsay E, et al. 2008. Diagnosis and surgical treatment of a Chiari I-like malformation in an African lion (*Panthera leo*). *Journal of Zoo and Wildlife Medicine* 39(3): 421–427.

McCain S, Ramsay E, Allender MC, et al. 2009. Pyometra in captive large felids: a review of eleven cases. *Journal of Zoo and Wildlife Medicine* 40(1):147–151.

McGeown D, Danbury TC, Waterman-Pearson AE, et al. 1999. Effect of carprofen on lameness in broiler chickens. *The Veterinary Record* 144:668–671.

McKeegan DEF. 2004. Mechano-chemical nociceptors in the avian trigeminal mucosa. *Brain Research. Brain Research Reviews* 46: 146–154.

McNulty EE, Gilson SD, Houser BS, et al. 2000. Treatment of fibrosarcoma in a maned wolf (Chrysocyon brachyurus) by rostral maxillectomy. *Journal of Zoo and Wildlife Medicine* 31(3):394–399.

Meteyer CU, Rideout BA, Gilbert M, et al. 2005. Pathology and pathophysiology of diclofenac poisoning in free-living and experimentally exposed oriental white-backed vultures *(Gyps bengalensis)*. *Journal of Wildlife Diseases* 41:707–716.

Mettam JJ, Oulton LJ, McCrohan C, et al. 2011. The efficacy of three types of analgesic drugs in reducing pain in the rainbow trout, *Oncorhynchus myskiss*. *Applied Animal Behaviour Science* 133(3–4):265–274.

Minter LJ, Karlin WM, Hickey MJ, et al. 2010. Surgical repair of a cleft palate in an American bison (Bison bison). *Journal of Zoo and Wildlife Medicine* 41(3):562–566.

Minter LJ, Clarke EO, Gjeltema JL, et al. 2011. Effects of intramuscular meloxicam administration on prostaglandin E2 synthesis in the North American bullfrog (Rana catesbeiana). *Journal of Zoo and Wildlife Medicine* 42(4):680–685.

Mohan S, Stevens CW. 2006. Systemic and spinal administration of the mu opioid, remifentanil, produces antinociception in amphibians. *European Journal of Pharmacology* 534(1):89–94.

Moore RP, Raphael BL, Calle PP. 2010. Use of selective sedatives and analgesics in marine mammals in a large public aquarium. Proceedings of the International Association for Aquatic Animal Medicine Annual Conference, pp. 88–89.

Morges MA, Grant KR, MacPhail CM, et al. 2009. A novel technique for orchiectomy and scrotal ablation in the sugar glider (Petaurus breviceps). *Journal of Zoo and Wildlife Medicine* 40(1): 204–206.

Mosley C. 2011. Pain and nociception in reptiles. *The Veterinary Clinics of North America. Exotic Animal Practice* 14(1):45–60.

Mosley CA, Dyson D, Smith DA. 2003. Minimum alveolar concentration of isoflurane in green iguanas and the effect of butorphanol on minimum alveolar concentration. *Journal of the American Veterinary Medical Association* 222:1559–1564.

Muir WW, Woolf CJ. 2001. Mechanisms of pain and their therapeutic implications. *Journal of the American Veterinary Medical Association* 219(10):1346–1356.

Mulcahy DM, Tuomi P, Larsen RS. 2003. Differential mortality of male spectacled eiders (Somateria fischeri) and king eiders (Somateria spectabilis) subsequent to anesthesia with propofol, bupivacaine and ketoprofen. *Journal of Avian Medicine and Surgery* 17:117–123.

Munoz A, Munoz M, Gonzalez A, et al. 1997. Spinal ascending pathways in amphibians: cells of origin and main targets. *The Journal of Comparative Neurology* 378:205–228.

Mylniczenko ND, Manharth AL, Clayton LA, et al. 2005. Successful treatment of mandibular squamous cell carcinoma in a Malayan sun bear (Helarctos malayanus). *Journal of Zoo and Wildlife Medicine* 36(2):346–348.

Naidoo V, Swan GE. 2008. Diclofenac toxicity in Gyps vulture is associated with decreased uric acid excretion and not renal portal vasoconstriction. *Comparative Biochemistry and Physiology. Toxicology and Pharmacology* 149:269–274.

Naidoo V, Wolter K, Cromarty AD, et al. 2008. The pharmacokinetics of meloxicam in vultures. *Journal of Veterinary Pharmacology and Therapeutics* 31:128–134.

Naidoo V, Wolter K, Cromarty D, et al. 2010. Toxicity of nonsteroidal anti-inflammatory drugs to Gyps vultures: a new threat from ketoprofen. *Biology Letters* 6:339–341.

Necker R, Reiner B. 1980. Temperature-sensitive mechanoreceptors, thermoreceptors, and heat nociceptors in the feathered skin of pigeons. *Journal of Comparative Physiology* 135: 201–207.

Neiffer DL, Stamper MA. 2009. Fish sedation, anesthesia, analgesia, and euthanasia: considerations, methods, and types of drugs. *ILAR Journal* 50:343–360.

Neil KM, Caron JP, Orth MW. 2005. The role of glucosamine and chondroitin sulfate in treatment for and prevention of osteoarthritis in animals. *Journal of the American Veterinary Medical Association* 226(7):1079–1088.

Newby NC, Gamper AK, Stevens ED. 2007. Cardiorespiratory effects and efficacy of morphine sulfate in winter flounder (Pseudopleuronectes americanus). *American Journal of Veterinary Research* 68(6):592–597.

Newby NC, Wilkie MP, Stevens ED. 2009. Morphine uptake, disposition, and analgesic efficacy in the common goldfish (Carassius auratus). *Canadian Journal of Zoology* 87:388–399.

Newman LC, Sands SS, Wallace DR, et al. 2002. Characterization of mu, kappa, and delta opioid binding in amphibian whole brain tissue homogenates. *The Journal of Pharmacology and Experimental Therapeutics* 301:364–370.

Ng TB, Hon WK, Cheng CH, et al. 1986. Evidence for the presence of adrenocorticotropic and opiate-like hormones in the brains of two sea snakes, *Hydrophis cyanocinctus* and *Lapemis hardwickii*. *General and Comparative Endocrinology* 63:31–37.

Nolen RS. 2001. Silent suffering. *Journal of the American Veterinary Medical Association* 219(12):1662.

Nordgreen J, Horsberg TE, Ranheim B, et al. 2007. Somatosensory evoked potentials in the telencephalon of Atlantic salmon (Salmo salar) following galvanic stimulation of the tail. *Journal of Comparative Physiology. A, Sensory, Neural, and Behavioral Physiology* 193:1235–1242.

Nordgreen J, Garner JP, Janczak AM, et al. 2009. Thermonociception in fish: effects of two different doses of morphine on thermal threshold and post-test behaviour in goldfish (Carassius auratus). *Applied Animal Behaviour Science* 119(1–2): 101–107.

Northcutt RG. 1981. Evolution of the telencephalon in nonmammals. *Annual Review of Neuroscience* 4:301–350.

Oaks JL, Meteyer CU. 2012. Non-steroidal anti-inflammatory drugs in raptors. In: *Fowler's Zoo and Wildlife Medicine, Current Therapy, Vol. 7* (RE Miller, M Fowler, eds.), pp. 349–355. Philadelphia: Elsevier Saunders.

Oaks JL, Gilbert M, Virani MZ, et al. 2004. Diclofenac residues as the cause of vulture population decline in Pakistan. *Nature* 427:630–633.

Okeson DM, Esterline ML, Coke RL. 2009. Esophageal diverticula in Parma wallabies (Macropus parma). *Journal of Zoo and Wildlife Medicine* 40(1):168–173.

Okeson DM, Marrow J, Carpenter JW, et al. 2010. Fournier's gangrene syndrome in a chimpanzee (Pan troglodytes). *Journal of Zoo and Wildlife Medicine* 41(1):169–173.

Olesen MG, Bertelsen MF, Perry SF, et al. 2008. Effects of preoperative administration of butorphanol or meloxicam on physiologic responses to surgery in ball pythons. *Journal of the American Veterinary Medical Association* 233:1833–1888.

Ostlund E, Von Euler US. 1956. Occurrence of a substance P-like polypeptide in fish intestine and brain. *British Journal of Pharmacology and Chemotherapy* 11(3):323–325.

Oukessou M. 1994. Kinetic disposition of flunixin meglumine in the camel (Camelus dromedarius). *Veterinary Research* 25(1): 71–75.

Overmier JB, Hollis KL. 1990. Fish in the think tank: learning, memory and integrated behaviour. In: *Neurobiology of Comparative*

Cognition (RP Kesner, DS Olson, eds.), pp. 205–236. Hillsdales: Lawrence Erlbaum.

Paul-Murphy J, Hawkins MG. 2012. Avian Analgesia. In: *Fowler's Zoo and Wildlife Medicine, Current Therapy*, Vol. 7 (RE Miller, M Fowler, eds.), pp. 312–323. Philadelphia: Elsevier Saunders.

Paul-Murphy J, Brunson DB, Miletic V. 1999. Analgesic effects of butorphanol and buprenorphine in conscious African grey parrots (*Psittacus erithacus erithacus* and *Psittacus erithacus timneh*). *American Journal of Veterinary Research* 60:1218–1221.

Paul-Murphy J, Hess J, Fialkowski JP. 2004a. Pharmokinetic properties of a single intramuscular dose of buprenorphine in African grey parrots (*Psittacus erithacus erithacus*). *Journal of Avian Medicine and Surgery* 18:224–228.

Paul-Murphy J, Ludders JW, Robertson SA, et al. 2004b. The need for a cross-species approach to the study of pain in animals. *Journal of the American Veterinary Medical Association* 224(5): 692–697.

Paul-Murphy JR, Krugner-Higby LA, Tourdot RL, et al. 2009a. Evaluation of liposome encapsulated butorphanol tartrate for alleviation of experimentally induced arthritic pain in green-cheeked conures (*Pyrrhura molinae*). *American Journal of Veterinary Research* 70:1211–1219.

Paul-Murphy JR, Sladky KK, Krugner-Higby LA, et al. 2009b. Analgesic effects of carprofen and liposome-encapsulated butorphanol tartrate in Hispaniolan parrots (*Amazona ventralis*) with experimentally induced arthritis. *American Journal of Veterinary Research* 70:1201–1210.

Pavez JC, Hawkins MG, Pascoe PJ, et al. 2011. Effect of fentanyl target-controlled infusions on isoflurane minimum anesthestic concentration and cardiovascular function in red-tailed hawks (*Buteo jamaicensis*). *Veterinary Anaesthesia and Analgesia* 38(4):344–351.

Pereira ME, Werther K. 2007. Evaluation of the renal effects of flunixin meglumine, ketoprofen and meloxicam in budgerigars (*Melopsittacus undulatus*). *The Veterinary Record* 160:844–846.

Pezalla PD. 1983. Morphine-induced analgesia and explosive motor behavior in an amphibian. *Brain Research* 273:297–305.

Pollock PJ, Doyle R, Tobin E, et al. 2008. Repeat laparotomy for the treatment of septic peritonitis in a Bornean orangutan (*Pongo pygmaeus pygmaeus*). *Journal of Zoo and Wildlife Medicine* 39(3):476–479.

Porteros A, García-Isidoro M, Barrallo A, et al. 1999. Expression of ZFOR1, δ-opioid receptor, in the central nervous system of the zebrafish (*Danio rerio*). *The Journal of Comparative Neurology* 412:429–438.

Pye GW, Hamlin-Andrus C, Moll J. 2008. Hip dysplasia in koalas (*Phascolarctos cinereus*) at the San Diego Zoo. *Journal of Zoo and Wildlife Medicine* 39(1):61–68.

Pye GW, White A, Robbins PK, et al. 2010. Preventive medicine success: thymoma removal in an African spot-necked otter (*Lutra maculicollis*). *Journal of Zoo and Wildlife Medicine* 41(4): 732–734.

Read MR. 2004. Evaluation of the use of anesthesia and analgesia in reptiles. *Journal of the American Veterinary Medical Association* 224:547–552.

Reilly SC, Quinn JP, Cossins AR, Sneddon LU. 2008. Novel candidate genes identified in the brain during nociception in common carp. *Neuroscience Letters* 437:135–138.

Reiner A. 1987. The distribution of proenkephalin-derived peptides in the central nervous system of turtles. *The Journal of Comparative Neurology* 259:65–91.

Reiner A, Brauth SE, Kitt CA, et al. 1989. Distribution of mu, delta, and kappa opiate receptor types in the forebrain and midbrain of pigeons. *The Journal of Comparative Neurology* 280:359–382.

Riggs SM, Hawkins MG, Craigmill AL, et al. 2008. Pharmacokinetics of butorphanol tartrate in red-tailed hawks (*Buteo jamaicensis*) and great horned owls (*Bubo virginianus*). *American Journal of Veterinary Research* 69:596–603.

Robbins PK, Pye GW, Sutherland-Smith M, et al. 2009. Successful transabdominal subxiphoid pericardiostomy to relieve chronic pericardial effusion in a Sumatran orangutan (*Pongo abelli*). *Journal of Zoo and Wildlife Medicine* 40(3):564–567.

Rojo-Solís C, Ros-Rodriguez JM, Valls M, et al. 2009. Pharmacokinetics of meloxicam (Metacam) after intravenous, intramuscular and oral administration to red-eared slider turtles (*Trachemys scripta elegans*). Proceedings of the American Association of Zoo Veterinarians, p. 228.

Ronan M, Northcutt RG. 1990. Projections ascending from the spinal cord to the brain in petromyzontid and myxinoid agnathans. *The Journal of Comparative Neurology* 291:491–508.

Roques JAC, Abbink W, Geurds F, et al. 2010. Tailfin clipping, a painful procedure: studies on Nile tilapia and common carp. *Physiology and Behavior* 101:533–540.

Rosenberg M. 1986. Carapace and plastron sensitivity to touch and vibration in the tortoise (*Testudo hermanni* and *T graeca*). *Journal of Zoology (London)* 208:443–455.

Rosenblum PM, Callard IP. 1988. Endogenous opioid peptide system in male brown bullhead catfish, *Ictalurus nebulosus* Lesueur: characterization of naloxone binding and the response to naloxone during the annual reproductive cycle. *The Journal of Experimental Zoology* 245(3):244–255.

Roush JK, Cross AR, Renberg WC, et al. 2010. Evaluation of the effects of dietary supplementation with fish oil omega-3 fatty acids on weight bearing in dogs with osteoarthritis. *Journal of the American Veterinary Medical Association* 236(1):67–73.

Rush EM, Ogburn AL, Hall J, et al. 2010. Surgical implantation of a cardiac resynchronization therapy device in a western lowland gorilla (*Gorilla gorilla gorilla*) with fibrosing cardiomyopathy. *Journal of Zoo and Wildlife Medicine* 41(3):395–403.

Rush EM, Ogburn AL, Garner MM. 2012. Multicentric neurofibromatosis with rectal prolapse in a California sea lion (*Zalophus californianus*). *Journal of Zoo and Wildlife Medicine* 43(1): 110–119.

Rychel JK, Johnston MS, Robinson NG. 2011. Zoologic companion animal rehabilitation and physical medicine. *The Veterinary Clinics of North America. Exotic Animal Practice* 14(1):131–140.

Saidel WM, Marquez-Houston K, Butler AB. 2001. Identification of visual pallial telencephalon in the goldfish, *Carassius auratus*: a combined cytochrome oxidase and electrophysiological study. *Brain Research* 919:82–93.

Sanchez-Migallon GD, Paul-Murphy J, Barker S, et al. 2008. Plasma concentrations of butorphanol in Hispaniolan Amazon parrots (*Amazona ventralis*) after intravenous and oral administration. Proceedings of the Association of Avian Veterinarians Conference, pp. 23–24.

Sanchez-Migallon Guzman D, Flammer K, Paul-Murphy JR, et al. 2011a. Pharmacokinetics of butorphanol after intravenous, intramuscular, and oral administration in Hispaniolan Amazon parrots (*Amazona ventralis*). *Journal of Avian Medicine and Surgery* 25(3):185–191.

Sanchez-Migallon Guzman D, KuKanich B, Keuler NS, et al. 2011b. Antinociceptive effects of nalbuphine hydrochloride in Hispaniolan Amazon parrots (*Amazona ventralis*). *American Journal of Veterinary Research* 72(6):736–740.

Sandeman D, Sandeman R, Derby C, et al. 1992. Morphology of the brain of crayfish, crabs and spiny lobsters: a common nomenclature for homologous structures. *The Biological Bulletin* 183:304–326.

Sanford J, Ewbend R, Molony V, et al. 1996. Guidelines for the recognition and assessment of pain. *The Veterinary Record* 118:334–338.

Schaefffer DO, Waters RM. 1996. Neuroanatomy and neurological diseases of reptiles. *Seminars in Avian and Exotic Pet Medicine* 5(3):165–171.

Schmitt TL, Sur RL. 2012. Treatment of ureteral calculus obstruction with laser lithotripsy in an Atlantic bottlenose dolphin

(*Tursiops truncatus*). *Journal of Zoo and Wildlife Medicine* 43(1): 101–109.

Schroeder CA, Schroeder KM, Johnson RA. 2010. Transversus abdominis plane block for exploratory laparotomy in a Canadian lynx (*Lynx canadensis*). *Journal of Zoo and Wildlife Medicine* 41(2):338–341.

Seebacher F, Franklin CE. 2003. Prostaglandins are important in thermoregulation of a reptile (*Pogona vitticeps*). *Proceedings. Biological Sciences* 270:S50–S53.

Shaver SL, Robinson NG, Wright BD, et al. 2009. A multimodal approach to management of suspected neuropathic pain in a prairie falcon (*Falco mexicanus*). *Journal of Avian Medicine and Surgery* 23:209–213.

Siddall PJ, Cousins MJ. 2009. Introduction to pain mechanisms: implications for neural blockade. In: *Cousin's and Bridenbaugh's Neural Blockade in Clinical Anesthesia and Pain Medicine*, 4th ed. (MJ Cousins, DB Carr, TT Horlocker, et al., eds.), pp. 661–692. Philadelphia: Lippincott Williams and Wilkins.

Siperstein LJ. 2007. Use of neurontin (gabapentin) to treat leg twitching/foot mutilation in a Senegal parrot. Proceedings of the Association of Avian Veterinarians Conference, pp. 81–82.

Sladky KK, Swanson CR, Stoskopf MK, et al. 2001. Comparative efficacy of tricaine methanesulfonate and clove oil for use as anesthetics in red pacu (*Piaractus brachypomus*). *American Journal of Veterinary Research* 62:337–342.

Sladky KK, Krugner-Higby L, Meek-Walker E, et al. 2006. Serum concentrations and analgesic effects of liposome-encapsulated and standard butorphanol tartrate in parrots. *American Journal of Veterinary Research* 67:775–781.

Sladky KK, Miletic V, Paul-Murphy J, et al. 2007. Analgesic efficacy and respiratory effects of butorphanol and morphine in turtles. *Journal of the American Veterinary Medical Association* 230: 1356–1362.

Sladky KK, Kinney ME, Johnson SM. 2008. Analgesic efficacy of butorphanol and morphine in bearded dragons and corn snakes. *Journal of the American Veterinary Medical Association* 233:267–273.

Sladky KK, Kinney ME, Johnson SM. 2009. Effects of opioid receptor activation on thermal antinociception in red-eared slider turtles (*Trachemys scripta*). *American Journal of Veterinary Research* 70:1072–1078.

Sladky K. 2010. Reptile analgesia: is laughter the best medicine for pain. Proceedings of the North American Veterinary Conference, pp. 1708–1710.

Smith JA. 1991. A question of pain in invertebrates. *ILAR Journal* 33:25–31.

Sneddon LU. 2003. The evidence for pain in fish: the use of morphine as an analgesic. *Applied Animal Behaviour Science* 8: 153–162.

Sneddon LU. 2004. Evolution of nociception in vertebrates: comparative analysis of lower vertebrates. *Brain Research. Brain Research Reviews* 46:123–130.

Sneddon LU, Braithwaite VA, Gentle MJ. 2003a. Novel object test: examining nociception and fear in the rainbow trout. *The Journal of Pain* 4:431–440.

Sneddon LU, Braithwaite VA, Gentle MJ. 2003b. Do fishes have nociceptors? Evidence for the evolution of a vertebrate sensory system. *Proceedings. Biological Sciences* B270:1115–1121.

Sneddon LU. 2009. Pain perception in fish: indicators and endpoints. *ILAR Journal* 50(4):338–342.

Striedter GF. 1997. The telencephalon of tetrapods in evolution. *Brain Behavior and Evolution* 49:179–213.

Souza MJ, Martin-Jimenez T, Jones MP, et al. 2009. Pharmacokinetics of oral and intravenous tramadol in bald eagles. *Journal of Avian Medicine and Surgery* 23:247–252.

Souza MJ, Sanchez-Migallon GD, Paul-Murphy J, et al. 2010. Tramadol in Hispaniolan Amazon parrots (*Amazona ventralis*). Proceedings of the Association of Avian Veterinarians Conference, pp. 293–294.

Souza MJ, Martin-Jimenez T, Jones MP, Cox SK. 2011. Pharmacokinetics of oral tramadol in red tailed hawks (*Buteo jamaicensis*). *Journal of Veterinary Pharmacology and Therapeutics* 34(1): 86–88.

Spriggs M, Arble J, Myers G. 2007. Intervertebral disc extrusion and spinal decompression in a binturong (*Arctictis binturong*). *Journal of Zoo and Wildlife Medicine* 38(1):135–138.

Stein P, Grossman M. 1980. Central programme for scratch reflex in turtles. *Journal of Comparative Physiology* 140:287–294.

Stevens CW. 2004. Opioid research in amphibians: an alternative pain model yielding insights on the evolution of opioid receptors. *Brain Research. Brain Research Reviews* 46:204–215.

Stevens CW. 2011. Analgesia in amphibians: preclinical studies and clinical applications. *The Veterinary Clinics of North America. Exotic Animal Practice* 14(1):21–32.

Stoskopf MK. 1994. Pain and analgesia in birds, reptiles, amphibians, and fish. *Investigative Ophthalmology and Visual Science* 35(2):775–780.

Stringer EM, De Voe RS, Linder K, et al. 2012. Vesiculobullous skin reaction temporally related to firocoxib treatment in a white rhinoceros (*Ceratotherium simum*). *Journal of Zoo and Wildlife Medicine* 43(1):186–189.

Stringfield CE, Wynne JE. 1999. Nutraceutical chondroprotectives and their use in osteoarthritis in zoo animals. Proceedings of the American Association of Zoo Veterinarians, pp. 63–68.

Sufka KJ, Hoganson DA, Hughes RA. 1992. Central monoaminergic changes induced by morphine in hypoalgesic and hyperalgesic strains of domestic fowl. *Pharmacology, Biochemistry, and Behavior* 42:781–785.

Tana LM, Isaza R, Koch DE, et al. 2010. Pharmacokinetics and intramuscular bioavailability of a single dose of butorphanol in Asian elephants (*Elephas maximus*). *Journal of Zoo and Wildlife Medicine* 41(3):418–425.

Teets RY, Dahmer S, Scott E. 2010. Integrative medicine approach to chronic pain. *Primary Care: Clinics in Office Practice* 37: 407–421.

ten Donkelaar HJ, de Boer-van HR. 1987. A possible pain control system in a non-mammalian vertebrate (a lizard, *Gekko gecko*). *Neuroscience Letters* 83:65–70.

Teraoka H, Kubota A, Dong W, et al. 2009. Role of the cyclooxygenase 2-thromboxane pathway in 2,3,7,8-tetrachlorodibenzo-p-dioxininduced decrease in mesencephalic vein blood flow in the zebrafish embryo. *Toxicology and Applied Pharmacology* 234:33–40.

Terril-Robb L, Suckow M, Grigdesby C. 1996. Evaluation of the analgesic effects of butorphanol tartrate, xylazine hydrochloride, and flunixin meglumine in leopard frogs (Rana pipiens). *Contemporary Topics in Laboratory Animal Science* 35:54–56.

Trnková S, Knotková Z, Hrdá A, et al. 2007. Effect of non-steroidal anti-inflammatory drugs on the blood profile in the green iguana (*Iguana iguana*). *Veterinarni Medicina Praha (Czech)* 52: 507–511.

Truini A, Cruccu G. 2006. Pathophysiological mechanisms of neuropathic pain. *Neurological Sciences* 27(Suppl. 2): S179–S182.

Tuttle AD, Papich M, Lewbart GA, et al. 2006. Pharmacokinetics of ketoprofen in the green iguana (*Iguana iguana*) following single intravenous and intramuscular injections. *Journal of Zoo and Wildlife Medicine* 37:567–570.

Twomey DF, Boon JD, Sayers G, et al. 2010. Arcanobacterium pyogenes septicemia in a southern pudu (*Pudu puda*) following uterine prolapse. *Journal of Zoo and Wildlife Medicine* 41(1): 158–160.

Uhrig SR, Papich MG, KuKanich B, et al. 2007. Pharmacokinetics and pharmacodynamics of morphine in llamas. *American Journal of Veterinary Research* 68(1):25–34.

Vandeweerd JM, Coisnon C, Clegg P, et al. 2012. Systematic review of efficacy of nutraceuticals to alleviate clinical signs of osteoarthritis. *Journal of Veterinary Internal Medicine* 26(3): 448–456.

Velguth KE, Rochat MC, Langan JN, et al. 2009. Acquired umbilical hernias in four captive polar bears (*Ursus maritimus*). *Journal of Zoo and Wildlife Medicine* 40(4):767–772.

Vesselkin NP, Agayan AL, Nomokonova LM. 1971. A study of thalamo-telencephalic afferent systems in frogs. *Brain, Behavior and Evolution* 4:295–306.

Vonsy JL, Ghandehari J, Dickenson AH. 2009. Differential analgesic effects of morphine and gabapentin on behavioural measures of pain and disability in a model of osteoarthritis pain in rats. *European Journal of Pain* 13(8):786–793.

Wack AN, Miller CL, Wood CE, et al. 2010. Melanocytic neoplasms in a black rhinoceros (*Diceros bicornis*) and an Indian rhinoceros (*Rhinoceros unicornis*). *Journal of Zoo and Wildlife Medicine* 41(1):95–103.

Walker KA, Horning M, Mellish J-AE, et al. 2009. Behavioural responses of juvenile Steller sea lions to abdominal surgery: developing an assessment of post-operative pain. *Applied Animal Behaviour Science* 120(3–4):201–207.

Walker KA, Mellish J-AE, Weary DM. 2010. Behavioural responses of juvenile Steller sea lions to hot-iron branding. *Applied Animal Behaviour Science* 122(1):58–62.

Walker KA, Horning M, Mellish J-AE, et al. 2011. The effects of two analgesic regimes on behavior after abdominal surgery in Steller sea lions. *Veterinary Journal (London, England: 1997)* 190(1):160–164.

Walker SM. 2008. Pain in children: recent advances and ongoing challenges. *British Journal of Anaesthesia* 101(1):101–110.

Walthers EA, Bradford CS, Moore FL. 2005. Cloning, pharmacological characterization and tissue distribution of an ORL1 opioid receptor from an amphibian, the rough-skinned newt *Taricha granulosa*. *Journal of Molecular Endocrinology* 34: 247–256.

Webber ES. 2011. Fish analgesia: pain, stress, fear aversion, or nociception? *The Veterinary Clinics of North America. Exotic Animal Practice* 14(1):21–32.

Weld MM, Maler L. 1992. Substance P-like immunoreactivity in the brain of the gymnotiform fish *Apteronotus leptorhynchus*: presence of sex differences. *Journal of Chemical Neuroanatomy* 5:107–129.

Wellehan JF, Zens MS, Bright AA, et al. 2001. Type I external skeletal fixation of radial fractures in microchiropterans. *Journal of Zoo and Wildlife Medicine* 32(4):487–493.

Wellehan JF, Lafortune M, Heard DJ. 2004. Traumatic elbow luxation repair in a common squirrel monkey (*Saimiri sciureus*) and a bonnet macaque (*Macaca radiata*). *Journal of Zoo and Wildlife Medicine* 35(2):197–202.

Wellehan JF, Gunkel CI, Kledzik D, et al. 2006. Use of a nerve locator to facilitate administration of mandibular nerve blocks in crocodilians. *Journal of Zoo and Wildlife Medicine* 37: 405–408.

Wenger S. 2012. Anesthesia and analgesia in rabbits and rodents. *Journal of Exotic Pet Medicine* 21:7–16.

Whiteside DP, Black SR. 2004. The use of meloxicam in exotic felids at the Calgary Zoo. Proceedings of the American Association of Zoo Veterinarians, pp. 346–349.

Whiteside DP, Remedios AM, Black SR, et al. 2006. Meloxicam and surgical denervation of the coxofemoral joint for the treatment of degenerative osteoarthritis in a Bengal tiger (*Panthera tigris tigris*). *Journal of Zoo and Wildlife Medicine* 37(3): 416–419.

Williams CV, Junge RE. 2007. Prosimians. In: *Zoo Animal and Wildlife Immobilizaton and Anesthesia* (G West, D Heard, N Caulkett, eds.), pp. 367–374. Ames: Blackwell Publishing Ltd.

Williams AC de C. 2002. Facial expression of pain. *The Behavioral and Brain Sciences* 25:439–488.

Wilson GH, Hernandez-Divers S, Budsberg SC, et al. 2005. Pharmacokinetics and use of meloxicam in psittacine birds. Proceedings of the European Association of Avian Veterinarians Conference, pp. 230–232.

Woolf CJ, Chong MS. 1993. Preemptive analgesia: treating postoperative pain by preventing the establishment of central sensitization. *Anesthesia and Analgesia* 77:362–379.

Woolf CJ, Ma Q. 2007. Nociceptors: noxious stimulus detectors. *Neuron* 55:353–364.

Wu CL, Liu SS. 2009. Neural blockade: impact on outcome. In: *Neural Blockade in Clinical Anesthesia and Pain Medicine*, 4th ed. (MJ Cousins, DB Carr, TT Horlocker, PO Bridenbaugh, eds.), pp. 144–158. Philadelphia: Lippincott Williams & Wilkins.

Wullimann MF, Rink E. 2002. The teleostean forebrain: a comparative and developmental view based on early proliferation, *Pax6* activity and catecholaminergic organization. *Brain Research Bulletin* 57:363–370.

Yaksh TL. 2009. Physiologic and pharmacologic substrates of nociception after tissue and nerve injury. In: *Neural Blockade in Clinical Anesthesia and Pain Medicine*, 4th ed. (MJ Cousins, DB Carr, TT Horlocker, PO Bridenbaugh, eds.), pp. 693–751. Philadelphia: Lippincott Williams & Wilkins.

Zimmerman DM, Douglass M, Reavill DR, et al. 2009. Echinococcus oligarthrus cystic hydatidosis in Brazilian agouti (*Dasyprocta leporina*). *Journal of Zoo and Wildlife Medicine* 40(3):551–558.

7 Physical Capture and Restraint

Todd Shury

INTRODUCTION

An important and often overlooked aspect of chemical immobilization of zoo and wild animals is proper physical restraint. How does one get close enough to be able to effectively and safely deliver the appropriate drug combination? Is it better to capture a group of animals or isolate individuals prior to immobilization? Would physical or chemical immobilization be more appropriate? The successful capture and restraint of wild species often requires a combination of physical and chemical restraint using a wide variety of capture and handling devices that are constantly evolving. As a result, there is no single ideal capture or restraint technique that can be successfully utilized for all occasions on a particular species because success depends on many biological, ecological and practical factors including topography, season, climate, age, condition, sex, costs, and logistics (Table 7.1 and Table 7.2).

Many techniques for the capture of free-ranging wildlife have been developed in the latter part of the twentieth century and have been extrapolated from zoos, wildlife parks, and the game ranching industry. This chapter will primarily focus on capture and restraint techniques for free-ranging North American mammalian species, with more limited coverage of reptile, amphibian, and avian species in other parts of the world and in captive situations. Properly applied physical restraint can be the most safe and efficient way to handle even large, dangerous animals if the people involved are knowledgeable about the likely behavior of the target animal(s) under stressful situations and are experienced with the technique being utilized.

Proper physical restraint of wild animals is as much an art as a science, and experience is a critical factor in reducing animal and human injury during physical restraint. Even when people are familiar with the techniques being used, certain people often just have the "knack" for restraining animals without undue injury and suffering. Much has been written and discussed on the topic in the past 30 years, with many old techniques being refined and simplified and completely novel techniques being used for the first time as new technologies become available (Fowler 1995; Fowler & Miller 2003). Many of the physical restraint techniques discussed are applicable to both captive and free-ranging wildlife, while the capture techniques primarily apply to free-ranging situations only. This chapter simply outlines the basic techniques in physical restraint and capture. For a more complete description of species-specific techniques, readers should consult the chapters on specific taxa later in the textbook or consult online references that describe species-specific techniques in detail (refer to Webliography). Several sets of taxon-specific guidelines have also been developed by various societies to help researchers choose capture and restraint techniques that are appropriate for the species being restrained.

MAMMALS

Cervidae, Bovidae, and Antilocapridae (Artiodactylids)

Remote Capture Techniques Many indigenous cultures around the world originally developed physical capture techniques for efficiently harvesting large hoofstock, and some of these techniques have been modified for live capture for wildlife research and intensive game farming over the past 30 years. Some techniques have been developed for mass capture, while others such as helicopter net gunning are designed for individual

Zoo Animal and Wildlife Immobilization and Anesthesia, Second Edition. Edited by Gary West, Darryl Heard, and Nigel Caulkett.
© 2014 John Wiley & Sons, Inc. Published 2014 by John Wiley & Sons, Inc.

Table 7.1. Principles and considerations of humane physical restraint in zoo and wild animals

General Principles	Other Considerations
Must be safe for all people involved	Cost
Must minimize potential for injury and mortality of subject animals	Season
Should be easy to apply with minimal training and experience	Time of day
Should allow rapid return to normal physiological state	Age and sex of animals
Equipment should be quick to set up and take down (portability)	Number of personnel required
Easily implemented regardless of body size or gender of restrainer	Need for adjunct sedative drugs
Should minimize amount of time that animals are restrained	Presence of environmental hazards and predators
	Animal behavior when stressed
	Capture efficiency and selectivity (wild species)

Table 7.2. Comparison of physical capture techniques for free-ranging wildlife

Technique	Cost[a]	Capture Efficiency[b]	Portability[c]	Potential for Injury[d]	Selectivity[e]	Species
Mass capture techniques						
Corral (boma)	Low	High	Low to moderate	Variable	Non-selective	Ungulates, bovids, goats and sheep
Drive nets	Moderate to High	High	Low	Moderate	Non-selective	Ungulates, bovids, goats and sheep
Drop net	Low	Moderate	Moderate	Moderate	Moderately selective	Ungulates, goats and sheep, birds
Rocket net	Low	Moderate	Moderate	High	Moderately selective	Ungulates, birds
Pitfall /coverboard/ funnel traps	Low	Moderate	High	Low	Non-selective	Amphibians, reptiles, small mammals
Individual capture techniques						
Foot snare	Low	Low	High	Low	Moderately selective	Birds, canids, felids, ursids, mustelids
Box traps	Low	Low	Low	Low	Nonselective	Birds, most mammals
Cage traps	Low	Low	Low	Low	Nonselective	Birds, most mammals
Mist nets	Low	High	High	Low	Moderately selective	Birds, bats
Helicopter net gun	High	High	High	Moderate	Highly selective	Ungulates, bovids, goats and sheep, ursids, canids
Foot hold traps	Low	Low	High	Moderate	Moderately selective	Canids, felids, mustelids

[a]Cost per animal captured on a relative basis.
[b]Number of animals that can be quickly captured in a short period of time.
[c]Ease of changing to different capture locations in quickly and efficiently.
[d]Potential for injury to the captured animal.
[e]Ability to avoid capture of nontarget species or individuals.

capture (Table 7.2). Research on the comparative efficacy and level of morbidity and mortality associated with different capture techniques for wild artiodactylids have recently been published (Barrett et al. 1982; Boesch et al. 2011; Conner et al. 1987; DelGiudice et al. 2001; DeYoung 1988; Jacques et al. 2009; Kock et al. 1987a, 1987b; Scotton & Pletscher 1998; Webb et al.

2008). Proper technique selection followed by appropriate training is critical to success when physically restraining zoo and wild animals.

Wild artiodactylids are trapped primarily for research, translocation projects, and population monitoring. Many techniques for physical restraint of domestic, zoo and game farmed cervids and bovids have been developed in North America recently (Fowler 1995; Fowler & Miller 2003; Franzmann 1998; Haigh & Hudson 1993), and boma or corral traps have been extensively used for game capture in Africa for decades (Ebedes et al. 1996; Openshaw 1993).

Box traps are one of the most widely used individual capture techniques, consisting of a wooden or metal structure that is designed to trap a single animal so that it can be physically or chemically restrained. Designs have been developed for the capture of North American ungulates, such as deer (*Odocoileus* spp.), elk (*Cervus elaphus*), moose (*Alces alces*), bighorn sheep (*Ovis canadensis*), and mountain goats (*Oreamnos americanus*) involving baiting animals into the trap followed by a mechanical or remotely operated device to close the trap. Animals are generally baited with hay, grain, fruit, or salt depending on local food preferences. Wooden box traps have been used for several decades in North America to trap white-tailed (*Odocoileus virginanus*) and mule deer (*Odocoileus hemionus*), bighorn sheep, and Rocky Mountain goats. These are essentially a plywood box with a top-hinged door or vertical guillotine slide that is tripped by either a floor plate or cross wire. These traps work best if there are few or no openings to allow light in, as darkness has a calming effect on trapped animals, causing them to struggle less. Once captured, either animals can be chased into a net placed over the opening to the trap and physically restrained, or larger animals can be injected via pole syringe or blow-pipe through a small opening. Care needs to taken to ensure that box traps are placed in relatively flat areas so the trapped animal does not roll down a slope and in areas that are not exposed to the elements. Modifications that make these traps lighter and more portable have been published recently (Anderson & Nielsen 2002).

Clover traps work on the same principle as box traps but are constructed of mesh netting over a steel tubular frame rather than a structure with solid walls. They have been used to successfully capture many ungulates in North America and are considerably lighter and more portable than most box traps because they can be easily collapsed for transport. Animals can either be physically restrained by collapsing the trap or chemically immobilized depending on the extent of restraint required, although recent evidence suggests that chemical immobilization of cervids in Clover traps may be associated with higher morbidity and mortality rates compared with free-range darting (Boesch et al. 2011; Haulton et al. 2001). Disadvantages are that animals may be more exposed to adverse climatic conditions while trapped (e.g., snow, wind, and rain) and may become more stressed as a result of disturbance in urban areas (Anderson & Nielsen 2002). Injuries and mortality can be sustained through capture of more than one animal in a trap or by appendages or legs being caught in netting material that is inappropriately

sized. Clover traps are primarily used for capture of white-tailed deer and mule deer in North America using various baits such as hay, grain, or salt.

Helicopter net gunning was originally developed in New Zealand in the 1970s for capturing red deer (*Cervus elaphus*). It has become a favoured method of capture for North American ungulates over the past twenty years because it can be adapted to a wide variety of animals, allows for selection of different age and sex classes, and large numbers of animals can be handled and captured in a short period of time relative to chemical immobilization (Jacques et al. 2009; Jessup et al. 1988; Webb et al. 2008). It is useful for short, nonpainful procedures such as application of radiotelemetry collars and blood sampling without the need for chemical immobilization.

When painful procedures such as tooth removal or surgery are used with net-gunned animals, adjunct procedures, such as local analgesia, sedation or chemical immobilization must be used to provide adequate analgesia. Intranasal sedation with alpha-2 agonists has been used in elk (Cattet et al. 2004) and reversal can be accomplished with intranasally delivered reversal agents where appropriate (Shury et al. 2010).

Hobbles are generally applied to the ipsilateral front and hind limbs at the level of the metacarphophalangeal joints as a human safety measure following net gun capture. Blindfolds are strongly recommended to reduce stress and calm the animal while being handled. Chase and hazing times (slower, higher altitude flight to push animals out into open areas) need to be kept as short as possible to minimize risk of capture myopathy and hyperthermia. Hazing times are generally less than 10 minutes and chase times are generally less than 2–3 minutes. Temperatures in excess of 42.2°C are potentially life threatening for bighorn sheep (Jessup 1999). Peracute mortality from helicopter net gunning most commonly occurs as a result of cervical fractures and dislocations (Barrett et al. 1982), while subacute mortality also results from capture myopathy and/or hyperthermia (Barrett et al. 1982; Jacques et al. 2009; Kock et al. 1987a). This risk can be minimized by attempting to slow animals prior to net placement by turning them or waiting for deep snow conditions in northern areas and minimizing transport distances and chase times (Jacques et al. 2009).

Bovids and ungulates are generally only safely handled for short periods of 15 minutes or less in lateral recumbency with few complications. If longer periods of restraint are required, reversible sedation with an alpha-2 agonist delivered intranasally or intravenously should be considered as an adjunct procedure.

Net size should be appropriate for the species being captured, with most nets being in the range of 9–17.6m². A lightweight extremely strong material is required for net construction and durability (Barrett et al. 1982). Appropriate mesh size is also important to prevent the animal escaping prematurely and to allow quick entanglement.

Net guns can also be fired from the ground for capture of antelope and other species (Firchow et al. 1986; O'Gara & Yoakum 2004), but care must be taken to ensure that the weights do not hit the animal, causing severe injury. Helicopter net guns have been used to capture bighorn sheep, mountain goats, deer, elk, moose, bison, and antelope in North America. Advantages of net gun capture include selectivity, rapid immobilization so injuries can be avoided, and the ability to release animals quickly without drug residues. Disadvantages include lack of utility in heavily treed environments, and potential for high mortality and morbidity in some species (Barrett et al. 1982; Jacques et al. 2009).

Corral traps or bomas have been used extensively for the mass capture of most artiodactylid species in Europe, North America, and Africa. This is perhaps the oldest and most widely used capture technique for ungulate species for purposes of translocation, research, and testing (Ebedes et al. 2002). Individual animals can then be individually restrained or chemically immobilized once captured. Animals tend to remain quite calm while undisturbed within a boma and large numbers can be captured quickly and effectively in open terrain.

Drive nets are useful to capture ungulate and bovid species where other techniques are not practical, such as heavily treed or steep terrain or in urban environments (López-Olvera et al. 2009; Locke et al. 2004; Mentaberre et al. 2010). Nets are typically strung between poles or trees in an area where animals can be flushed into a narrow opening or other suitable area. It is critical that adequate numbers of people are available to physically restrain animals once they are entangled in the net. One or two people per animal are generally required depending on the size of animals captured. A variation of this technique is drop netting, which works fairly reliably for cervids species and may be useful in mountainous or steep terrain (Conner et al. 1987).

Animals can be driven into nets on foot, by horseback, or by vehicles (snowmobile or truck) or aircraft (helicopter or fixed wing). Care must be taken when using aircraft or vehicles that animals are not chased at excessive speeds or long periods of time as mortality from cervical and leg fractures, capture myopathy, and hyperthermia are often the result (O'Gara & Yoakum 2004). Some researchers have used dense vegetation and water in combination with physical restraint instead of nets for small deer species (Duarte 2008).

Handling and Safety Considerations Most bovids and ungulates that are 60–70 kg weight or less can be physically restrained by a single person of medium build. Larger animals require additional personnel or individuals of large stature for safe physical restraint.

Hobbles that are constructed of leather, canvas or synthetic materials are very useful for safely restraining hooves and legs. Blindfolds are a necessary tool for animals that are to be physically restrained because they reduce stress (Fowler 1995; Mitchell et al. 2003) and protect the eyes from damage. They can be made from a variety of materials but should be able to be removed quickly and should be comfortable for the animal.

Other safety items include foam and rubber balls or hose that can be placed on the sharp tips of horns to prevent injury to handlers for species such as mountain goat, bison (*Bison bison*), and musk oxen (*Ovibos moschatos*). Horns of young bovids and sheep are easily damaged during capture when nets are used due to slippage of horn sheaths that are loosely attached in younger animals. This can lead to moderate to severe blood loss, but long-term damage is usually not severe with the exception of disfigured horns for the remainder of the animal's life. Male cervids and caribou (*Rangifer tarandus*) and reindeer of both sexes should not be captured during the season of antler growth (May–July in northern hemisphere) if possible due to the high vascularity and potential for blood loss and associated pain when rapidly growing antler is damaged. Physical restraint and capture should be avoided on slippery surfaces such as ice and steep slopes due to the potential for injury.

In captive and semi-captive situations, artiodactylids can be easily and efficiently handled in specially designed handling facilities that include chutes, paddocks, and runs specifically designed for each species. The evolution of the game farming industry in North America has led to the development of sophisticated squeezes that utilize drop floors, padded sides, and hydraulics to minimize struggling and injury (Haigh 1999). Individual animal habituation is an important prerequisite, if at all possible for successful physical restraint in these systems regardless of species (Grandin 1993; Meyer et al. 2008). Crash gates are an important component of bison handling systems that allow animals to be more easily restrained in a mechanical or hydraulic neck squeeze (Haigh 1999). Holding pens and runs need to be designed with walls that are high enough to prevent escapes (10 ft or higher for sheep and goats) and designed to minimize injury to animals and humans during use. Points where animals are squeezed into narrow areas need particular attention to detail, and specific flight distances of each species needs to be considered during design.

Captive artiodactylids can be habituated to routine handling procedures, such as venipuncture, vaccination, and/or physical examination with minimal restraint in a chute or box stall depending on individual animal temperament (Citino 2003; Wirtu et al. 2005). The simplest systems use a circular or semicircular tub with movable walls that squeeze the animal between them. It is important to have a large number

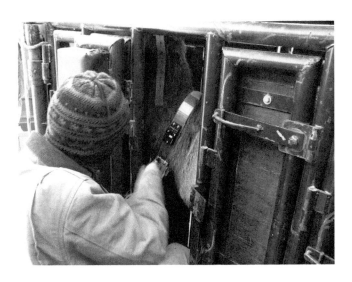

Figure 7.1. Wild elk restrained in a padded manual squeeze near Banff National Park, Canada.

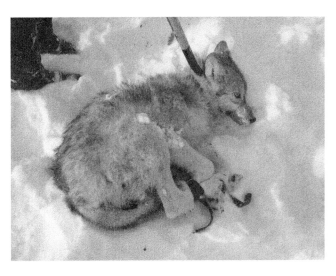

Figure 7.2. Timber wolf physically restrained with hobbles and duct tape on the muzzle for application of a radio collar.

of access panels to be able to gain access to all parts of the animal safely.

Well-designed box chutes have been successfully used for restraint of wild elk in Banff National Park for venipuncture, TB testing, and deworming, and for wild bison and elk in Elk Island National Park in Canada for several decades (Fig. 7.1).

Canidae/Felidae

Remote Capture Techniques Helicopter net gunning has proven to be a very successful method for capturing some large carnivores in North America, including grizzly bears (*Ursus arctos*), black bears (*Ursus americanus*), and wolves (*Canis lupus*). Wolves can be safely restrained after being netted using a forked stick or pole snare to control the muzzle and head of the netted animal. Hobbles are useful to restrain the legs, and nylon dog muzzles or duct tape can be used to restrain the mouth safely without chemical immobilization (Fig. 7.2). Bear species generally require chemical immobilization after netting to safely handle these animals, with the net providing a quick way of immobilizing the animal so it does not injure itself in terrain with natural hazards (water and steep slopes). A common complication of net gunning large carnivores is the ability of the animal to chew its way out of entanglement; therefore, animals need to be either darted or restrained very quickly (within 1 minute) after the net is fired. Medium-sized canids such as coyotes (*Canis latrans*) and wolves have also been captured very successfully with helicopter net gunning. Deep snow conditions are a definite advantage when attempting to capture canids using this method as they are highly maneuverable on bare ground. Snowmobiles and all-terrain vehicles have also been used for capture of coyotes by using a throw net in open, prairie envi-

ronments (Gese & Andersen 1993; Moehrenschlager 2002). African wild dogs have been successfully captured using boma traps following herding by helicopter (English et al. 2008).

Various restraint traps designed to catch animals by a limb are used to capture wolves, coyotes, foxes, procyonids, and some mustelids. The most widely used method of capture utilizes a modified foothold trap designed to minimize injury in captured animals (Earle et al. 2003; Sahr & Knowlton 2000). These traps use padded jaws and laminated jaws to reduce potential for injury on the trapped limb (Kreeger 1999). Swivels and drags are typically used instead of staking traps so that the trap becomes entangled in vegetation reducing the rotational force on trapped limbs.

Other foothold traps such as leg snares are generally constructed of wire cable coated with protective coating and many are activated with a spring. Leg snares have been used for successfully capturing pumas (*Felis concolor*) (Logan & Sweanor 2001; Logan et al. 1999), lions (Panthera leo) (Frank et al. 2003) and Siberian tigers (*Panthera tigris altaica*) (Goodrich et al. 2001) and a modified snare within a oval shaped container called an EGG (EGG Trap Company, Springfield, SD) trap has been widely used for capturing raccoons (*Procyon lotor*) and possums (*Didelphis virginiana*) (Austin et al. 2004; Hubert et al. 1999) with minimal injury. Canada and the United States retain international agreements with the Russian Federation and the European Union to develop humane foothold traps for capture of furbearing animals in the fur trade that came into force in 2007 (refer to Webliography). These traps have been tested to ensure they cause minimal injury to trapped animals (Andelt et al. 1999). Frequent trap checking is critical (minimum every 24 hours) to prevent injury to trapped canids and felids.

When used in winter, limb ischemia, and frostbite can occur as circulation is impaired in the trapped limb, so these types of traps should be used with caution at temperatures below 0°C. Tranquilizer tabs impregnated with propiopromazine or diazepam are a useful adjunct and have been used successfully to tranquilize and reduce injury in trapped wolves (Sahr & Knowlton 2000) and coyotes captured in neck snares (Pruss et al. 2002). Most wild canids up to 60 kg in size can be safely restrained without chemical immobilization for short procedures, such as application of radio collars and venipuncture. Longer or more invasive procedures, such as tooth removal or implant surgery, require chemical immobilization.

Various commercially available and homemade cage or box traps constructed of wire and plastic mesh or completely enclosed wooden or metal boxes are used for capture of procyonids, small- and medium-sized canids, and most felid species (de Wet 1993; Grassman et al. 2004; Harrison et al. 2002; Mudappa & Chellam 2001; Wilson et al. 1996). Animals are baited into the trap which is triggered by a floor plate with a vertical guillotine or hinged door that closes when the animal is inside. Animals can then be hand injected or injected with a pole syringe if chemical immobilization is required. Physical restraint using a snare pole or gloves can be used on smaller species or for restraint of a limb or the muzzle. Extreme care must be exercised with the use of a snare pole when used over the thoracic area. Ensuring that a front limb is ensnared along with the neck or thorax for very short periods of restraint will help prevent asphyxia from thoracic compression. Box traps and cages provide the additional advantage of providing security and safety from predation or attack while the animal is trapped, unlike other restraint devices, such as foothold traps, with the disadvantage that they are not as portable.

Regardless of trap type being used, the frequency of trap checking needs to be 12 to 24 hours or less for most species. The potential for self-injury, hypothermia, hyperthermia, dehydration, frostbite, and other complications is much higher the longer the animal remains restrained or trapped (Cattet et al. 2003). More frequent trap checks are desirable, if possible, in terrain that is easily accessible. A variety of trap-monitoring devices, such as VHF trap transmitters, have been developed to increase the frequency of trap checking in more remote areas (Darrow & Shivik 2008).

Neck snares with stops have been successfully used for capture of coyotes in North America (Pruss et al. 2002), offering an alternative capture technique in areas where foothold traps or box traps are ineffective or prohibited. Tranquilizer tabs are a useful adjunct to help prevent injuries from struggling in a neck snare (Pruss et al. 2002). Circumference of the neck snare is of critical importance to prevent nontarget captures and to decrease the potential for injury and mortality.

Felid species that utilize trees for safety and cover such as puma, jaguar, panthers (*Felis* spp.), bobcat (*Lynx rufus*), and lynx (*Lynx canadensis*) can be captured with the use of trained tracking hounds (Apps 1996, 1999; Deem 2004; Taylor et al. 1998). Treed felids are generally chemically immobilized with a variety of remote drug delivery techniques including blowpipes, pole syringes, dart pistols, and rifles. Injuries occur when dogs attack immobilized animals and when immobilized animals fall from heights greater than 5 m. These are prevented by securely tying up dogs prior to darting and using nets, slings, or inflatable devices to cushion falls. Drug dosage can be a critical factor when chemically immobilizing large felids in trees and needs to be considered when choosing an appropriate drug combination (Beier et al. 2003).

Captive felids in zoo environments are generally captured or restrained with hoop nets, squeeze cages, or chemical immobilization depending on their size. Felid species <14 kg can be safely handled with a net and gloves (Fowler 1995), while larger felids require specialized squeeze crates or snare poles for safe handling. Previous habituation and acclimation to handling facilities is extremely helpful in handling large felids without chemical immobilization for venipuncture and vaccinations. Best practices and trap certification for both live capture and killing traps have been developed for most commercially important furbearer species in the United States and Canada (refer to Webliography).

Handling and Safety Considerations Heavy leather gloves are very useful when handling infant large felids or medium-sized felids as their teeth and claws can inflict serious damage to anyone holding them. Bacterial infections are common sequelae to felid and canid bite wounds, and all bite wounds should be considered contaminated and treated appropriately (Brook 2005). Restraint bags designed for domestic cat restraint are useful for restraint of small- and medium-sized cats for very short procedures, such as venipuncture, injection, or vaccination, while hobbles and blindfolds are often used for larger canids.

Firearm backup is recommended for the larger felids when immobilized in case of spontaneous arousal. Snare poles are useful to restrain the feet of large felids when immobilized as a backup restraint mechanism or strapping them to a table or other flat surface when anesthetized. Small- and medium-sized canids can be easily restrained by hand if the feet and muzzle are adequately restrained (Fig. 7.3).

Ursidae

Remote Capture Techniques Aldrich leg snares have been used as a primary means of capture for various ursid species around the world for both research and management purposes for decades. They have the advantage of being portable, highly efficient, and easy

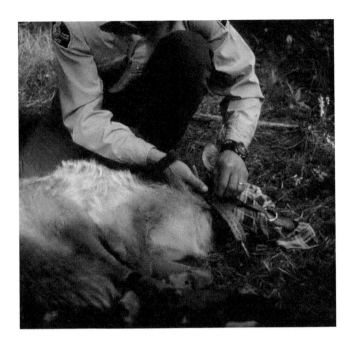

Figure 7.3. Wild coyote physically restrained with hobbles and nylon muzzle after capture in modified foot hold trap.

to set in remote locations (Johnson & Pelton 1980). The basic design involves a braided steel cable that forms a loop and is activated by a spring steel throwing arm (Jonkel 1993) that captures the bear above the carpal joint. These devices are usually anchored to a large tree and set in a hollowed out area in the ground. Injuries are often sustained in leg snares from biting or chewing on digits, fractured limbs, muscle damage, capture myopathy, distal limb edema due to impaired circulation, and cuts and abrasions at the site of contact with the snare cable (Cattet et al. 2003, 2008). Although very uncommon, intraspecific predation has also occurred with the use of these devices for capture of grizzly bears in Canada (Gibeau & Stevens 2002).

Culvert traps are a variation of a box or cage trap on a larger scale and specifically designed for ursids. They were originally made from culverts used for road construction and are manufactured in a wide variety of designs. They have the advantage of protecting the trapped bear from the elements and predators. They have the disadvantage of being quite large and unwieldy and are generally only used in road-accessible areas, although some are designed specifically for use in remote areas and delivered by helicopter. They are used routinely for management of problem black and grizzly bears throughout North America (Jonkel 1993) and for research on Malayan Sun bears (Te Wong et al. 2004). They are also useful for recovering chemically immobilized bears and for transporting them once they are recovered (Caulkett & Cattet 2002). Injuries primarily occur in the oral cavity (lacerations and broken teeth) due to chewing on mesh or openings in

the trap designed for accessing the animal. Mortalities are very rare but can occur when multiple animals are trapped or animals sustain trauma due to falling guillotine doors.

In captive situations, bears are usually isolated individually in separate pens or enclosures prior to chemical immobilization. Sows with dependent cubs may or may not be separated prior to immobilization of the sow depending on the stress level of the individual. Most bears with the exception of cubs <25 kg need to be chemically immobilized to be handled safely. Cubs can be physically restrained or captured with nets or blankets. Climbing gear may be necessary to retrieve cubs of certain species, such as black bears, which routinely climb trees to escape.

Handling and Safety Considerations For safety considerations, it is good practice to have an armed guard equipped with a firearm when capturing and immobilizing adult bears. This is not to protect against the immobilized bear recovering spontaneously, but to protect the immobilization team from other bears that are often attracted to the site (Caulkett & Cattet 2002). Personnel need to be trained in firearm use and must be prepared to use lethal force if necessary.

Hobbles should be applied to the limbs of immobilized bears to restrict mobility if the animal should spontaneously arouse. Equipment and pharmaceuticals to deal with injuries sustained from capture (antibiotics, wound dressings, and antiseptic agents) should be carried in the field when capturing wild bears.

Mustelidae/Procyonidae/Viverridae

Remote Capture Techniques Small- and medium-sized mustelid species—fisher (*Martes pennanti*), marten (*Martes americana*), mink (*Mustela vison*), and weasels (*Mustela* spp.)—can be physically restrained for short procedures using a cone-shaped cotton or mesh bag, which can be used to restrain an animal for examination once it has been captured in a box trap or other device. A method for physical restraint of mink with gloves is described by Fowler (1995) which can be modified for fisher, marten, river otter (*Lontra canadensis*), and small raccoons. Squeeze cages are also useful for mustelids to provide a method of quick restraint for intramuscular injections, such as vaccination or injection of chemical immobilization drugs. Cage traps, box traps and padded foot hold traps are most commonly used for capture of wild mustelids and viverrids (Blundell et al. 1999; Hubert et al. 1996; Serfass et al. 1996). Hancock traps have also been widely used for capture of river otters, although they are not as portable as other trap types and tooth damage is frequent (Blundell et al. 1999). Hoop nets work very well for initial capture of captive mustelids and viverrids in zoos followed by physical restraint with gloves or chemical immobilization.

Homemade box traps made from locally available timber have been used for wolverine (*Gulo gulo*) capture in North America due to the large home ranges and remoteness of habitat (Copeland et al. 1995; Lofroth et al. 2008). Trapped animals are then chemically immobilized with pole syringes or dart pistols. A flashlight is required to visualize the animal as these traps are usually quite dark inside.

Skunks (*Mephitis* spp.) present a formidable challenge if physical restraint is used alone due to their defensive use of spraying musk from their anal sacs when threatened. For this reason, chemical immobilization is always preferred unless extraordinary precautions are taken to prevent contact with the musk (safety glasses and protective clothing).

Handling and Safety Considerations Heavy- or medium weight leather gloves are a necessity for handling most medium and large mustelids and viverrids due to their extremely sharp teeth and propensity for biting when threatened. Most species can be handled by grasping firmly around the base of the head with one hand and the tail with the other hand (Fowler 1995), but a sturdy grip is required due to their extreme flexibility and maneuverability.

Most mustelid species are very susceptible to stress especially when wild animals are held in captivity (Fernández-Morán et al. 2002; Hartup et al. 1999) for a period of time. Skunks, bats, foxes, and raccoons are considered natural reservoirs of rabies virus in North America, so care should be taken to ensure personnel working with these species are vaccinated and trained to avoid exposure. Parasitic zoonoses, such as *Baylascaris* spp., cause severe neurological disease in humans and are also very prevalent in wild mustelids (Kazacos & Boyce 1989) so care should be taken to avoid exposure to feces.

Rodents and Lagomorphs

Remote Capture Techniques Various cage and box traps are widely used for live capture of rodents and lagomorphs. Small wild rodents <1 kg such as mice, voles (Muridae) and ground squirrels (Sciuridae) are typically live trapped in either wire cage traps or metal box traps (Sherman™ or Longworth™ traps) as part of ecological research studies or for pest removal. Specialized protective gear is required for handling certain species of small mammals that carry zoonoses, such as hantavirus and tularemia (see Handling and Safety Considerations). Sherman and Longworth traps are small aluminum box traps that are widely used for capturing small wild rodent species. Insulated bedding in the form of cotton or polyester fiberfill and a food source is required for microtine rodents due to their propensity to develop hypothermia and hypoglycemia (Jones et al. 1996).

Wild lagomorphs are generally trapped in wire cage traps baited with food. Injuries to teeth result from chewing on wire, so wood or plastic boxes with solid sides have been used to prevent this (Sharp et al. 2007). Lagomorphs, especially snowshoe hare, are prone to hypoglycemia (trap sickness) if trapped in box or cage traps, therefore, a source of food should be provided or traps should be checked frequently (Feldhamer et al. 2003).

Aquatic rodents, such as beaver, muskrat, and nutria, can be captured in specialized hinged cage traps called Hancock or Bailey traps or wire cage traps set on land (Rosell & Kvinlaug 1998). Care must be taken to prevent traps from tumbling into water and drowning animals. These species can also be netted from boats or chased from lodges and houses (Rosell & Hovde 2001) into nets.

Pit traps are occasionally used in conjunction with drift fencing for small microtine rodent capture by burying a round metal or PVC container which is 20–40 cm in diameter in the ground 40–50 cm deep (Jones et al. 1996).

Handling and Safety Considerations Mice and rat-sized rodents can be handled with latex exam gloves by grasping the skin over the nape of the neck for short periods of restraint and non-invasive treatments. Larger rodents and lagomorphs require support if picked up or carried in this manner. Rats (*Rattus* spp.) and musk-rats (*Ondatra zibethica*) are usually held by the tail with the feet allowed to grasp a surface such as a wire cage. Heavy leather gloves are required for larger species, such as muskrat, beaver, and nutria, to prevent injury to the handler from biting. Species with haired tails such as squirrels, marmots (*Marmota* spp.), and packrats (*Neotoma* spp.), should not be restrained by the tail only as the hair and skin can easily slip causing severe injury (Fowler 1995). Laboratory techniques that are well developed for mice, rats, guinea pigs, and hamsters often fail to restrain their wild counterparts unless personnel are very experienced in handling these species.

Medium-sized rodent, such as hyrax, agoutis, marmots, and woodchucks, can be netted and restrained manually for injections, quick examinations, venipuncture, and vaccinations. Specially designed squeeze cages that allow the animal to be forced against the side of wire cage or box are very useful for these rodent species.

Most lagomorphs can be manually restrained by grasping them around the base of the head with one hand and supporting the body and restraining the hind legs with the other hand. Severe spinal injuries can result if the hind legs of hares and rabbits are allowed to kick and flail while restrained. Gloves are important to prevent scratches and bites when handling larger hares and rabbits. Nets are useful for initially capturing lagomorphs in small enclosed spaces until they can be manually restrained. Specially designed restraint cages are used for handling domestic lagomorphs in laboratories.

Larger rodent species such as capybara (*Hydrochoerus hydrochaeris*) beaver (*Castor canadensis*), and nutria can be netted and physically restrained for short periods for quick injections or vaccinations only (Fowler 1995). More invasive handling requires chemical immobilization. Beavers should not be hoisted by the tail alone, but can be restrained on the ground using the tail and a hand around the base of the head (Whitelow & Pengelley 1954).

Porcupines (*Erythizon dorsatum*) are specialized rodents with various-sized quills that present a challenge for physical restraint. North American porcupines have barbed quills approximately 1–4 cm long while Old World porcupines such as crested porcupines (*Hystrix* spp.) have extremely long stout quills up to 45 cm long (Fowler 1995) that are capable of severe injury. North American porcupines use their tail as a quill delivery system and contrary to popular belief, are incapable of "shooting" their quills. Sturdy plastic garbage pails or tubs with bottoms cut out can be used to capture porcupines in small enclosures instead of nets where they can be chemically immobilized using a pole syringe or hand injection. Crested porcupines have particularly thin, fragile skin and are prone to injury and laceration from pole syringes (Fowler 1995). Brooms or small plywood boards are useful to safely move porcupines into enclosures or transport containers, although they often tend to go backwards with quills flared rather than forward like most mammals.

Plexiglass or clear plastic induction chambers are very useful for induction of gas anesthesia in rodent species that are not easily handled or prone to injury such as porcupine and voles.

Zoonoses are a major concern with many species of wild and domestic rodents and suitable precautions need to be taken when handling them. Hantaviruses are carried subclinically by several rodent species in North America including the white-footed deer mouse (*Peromyscus maniculatus*), cotton rat (*Sigmodon hispidus*), rice rat (*Oryzomys palustris*), and white-footed mouse (*Peromyscus leucopus*). Prevalence varies dramatically with geographical location and year and so the known carrier species should be considered infected at all times. Virus is shed primarily in saliva, urine and feces so exam gloves and HEPA filters should be worn to prevent transmission while handling. Plague (*Yersinia pestis*) is enzootic in prairie dogs in the American Midwest and great gerbils (Wimsatt & Biggins 2009) in central Asia and is carried by many other wild rodent species. Humans are generally infected through the bite of an infected flea from rodents or from domestic cats that have been exposed to infected rodents and their fleas. Lyme disease caused by the spirochete *Borrelia burgdorferii* is carried primarily by *Ixodes* spp. ticks found on many rodent hosts, but particularly deer mice in eastern and Midwest United States.

Monotremes/Marsupials

Handling and Safety Considerations Medium-sized marsupials with tails such as kangaroos and wallabies can be safely restrained for short procedures by grasping the animal by the tail and grasping the head with the other free hand to control head movement. This is most easily accomplished against a wall or other solid vertical surface. Large male adult kangaroos can be difficult to restrain, and the hind feet are formidable weapons, so blankets or tarps can be used to initially tackle the animal and a minimum of two people are required. Koalas are captured by use of long snare poles or simply grabbed from branches of trees. Other marsupials can generally be restrained by hand and caught with nets.

Primates

Small- and medium-sized non-human primates (monkeys, vervets, and capuchins) are usually captured in box or cage traps or captured manually with long-handled nets (Rocha et al. 2007). Larger ape species, such as oranguatan (*Pongo pygmaeus*) and gorillas (*Gorilla* spp.), require chemical immobilization using remote delivery techniques and are generally not physically restrained with the exception of neonates.

Handling and Safety Considerations Captive primates in the 3–12 kg range can be manually restrained by a person with heavy leather gloves by holding the front limbs and body in one hand and the hind limbs in the other hand. A face mask, shield, or safety glasses are also required for non-human primates due to the risk of zoonotic diseases (see later). Long-sleeved coveralls and leather gloves with sleeve extensions should also be considered to prevent bites and scratches. Most primates possess considerable strength and agility for their size, a fact often underestimated by inexperienced personnel.

Primates and great apes over 12 kg should be chemically immobilized unless extensive training and habituation to procedures has been previously completed. Many zoos and research centres train primates to present limbs through custom-designed restraint cages and boxes for venipuncture, TB testing, vaccinations, and other minor procedures. Great apes such as oranguatans, gibbons, chimpanzees, and gorillas generally require chemical immobilization for safe restraint, unless extensive training has been completed. Commercial squeeze cages are available for most species that facilitate short procedures such as injections and visual exam of TB testing.

When any physical restraint of primate species is going to be necessary, appropriate safety measures should be in place to ensure protection from zoonoses. Herpes

B virus causes a fatal encephalitis in humans and is carried by macaque (*Macaca* spp.) species (Johnson-Delaney 2005). Primate keepers and any staff potentially coming in contact with fecal material or urine need to wear masks, eye protection, and latex gloves as a minimum to prevent exposure when handling animals and when cleaning enclosures. Other potential zoonoses include hepatitis, HIV, Ebola viruses, and many others (Krauss et al. 2003). The potential for reverse zoonoses should also be considered when handling primates, and measures to prevent sick humans from coming in contact with primates should also be considered. Bite wounds can also be quite severe, causing severe pyoderma and fasciitis.

Bats

Remote Capture Techniques Mist nets strung in various configurations, heights, and lengths are a versatile, portable and inexpensive way to capture most bat species. Their use is limited at roost sites where numerous bats could be potentially captured as bats need to be untangled from the net, allowing the capture of single bats usually. Mist nets can be constructed of monofilament nylon, braided nylon, or braided Dacron polyester (Kunz et al. 1996) and set up in numerous configurations wherever bats are found (Kunz et al. 2009). Care must be taken when extracting bats from mist nets, as their delicate wing bones and membranes are easily damaged. Wearing light leather gloves and allowing the bat to bite and hang on is often helpful to allow extraction (Kunz et al. 1996).

Harp traps and Tuttle traps consist of vertical wire strands attached to springs within a rectangular frame that has a cloth or burlap bag attached to the bottom to catch bats that fly into the wires. Larger versions of this trap have been successfully used to capture megachiropteran bat species as well (Tidemann & Loughland 1993). These traps are very useful for capturing bats at roost sites as well.

Handling and Safety Considerations Small bat species (<100 g) can be held in the palm of the hand firmly but gently in a manner as described for passerine birds with the thumb and index finger restraining the head. Larger megachiropterans require two hands to restrain the wings and head effectively. Open weave cloth or mesh bags with drawstring tops are useful for temporary holding or transport of bats (Kunz et al. 2009). Physical restraint should be minimized in most bat species as hyperthermia results from excessive struggling and stress (Heard 1999). Light leather gloves, such as golf gloves, are used for handling microchiropteran species while heavier leather gloves should be used for large pteropid bats.

Injuries to bats can be sustained to patagia, wing bones, and leg bones from improper restraint and attempting to dislodge bats from wire and net surfaces too forcefully (Heard 1999). Personnel working with bats must be vaccinated against rabies, as most species are potential carriers of rabies virus or other lyssaviruses (Heard 2003). Other viruses with zoonotic potential are also carried by bats including Hendra, Nipah, Menangle, and Tioman viruses which are carried by bats in Southeast Asia and Australia (Krauss et al. 2003). An important fungal disease, *Histoplasma capsulatum* has been linked to aerosol inhalation of bat guano in roosting caves, so masks with HEPA filters are recommended when working in caves where bats roost (Huhn et al. 2005).

Suidae/Tapiridae/Tayassuidae

Remote Capture Techniques Tapirs (*Tapirus* spp.) in captive facilities are generally quite docile and many procedures can be accomplished with the animal standing or gently rubbed down and put in an almost hypnotic state. Foot trims, detailed exams, TB testing, radiographs, and venipuncture can often be performed if animals are trained and habituated to these procedures. Tapirs are generally either rubbed along the sides or back with a comb or a gloved hand which will cause them to lie down in ventral or lateral recumbency. If animals cannot be trained to this procedure, chemical immobilization is required. Tapirs can also be gently herded with brooms or boards into squeezes and crates for treatment or injection.

Wild and exotic suid species such as warthogs (*Phacochoerus* spp.), red river hogs, (*Potamochoerus porcus*), babirusa (*Babyrousa babyrussa*), and collared peccaries (*Tayassu tajacu*) can be physically restrained and captured using many of the same techniques used for domestic pigs, including snare poles and ropes, but they are much more difficult to restrain on a kg per kg basis. Most species have extremely sharp teeth and tusks and are capable of causing significant injury or death to people attempting to restrain them. Peccaries and small-sized pig species (<20 kg) can be caught with nets and restrained by stretching them out on a floor or mat by grasping the hind legs and head with gloved hands (Fowler 1995). Adult pigs, warthogs, and babirusa must be either chemically immobilized or run through chutes and trained through operant conditioning to accept procedures such as vaccination and treatment (Morris & Shima 2003).

Camelidae/Giraffidae

Members of this group of wildlife require special handling and restraint procedures, which are well described elsewhere (Bush 2003; Fowler 1995, 1998, 2003; Fowler & Cubas 2001). Typically, large chutes are used to physically restrain giraffes, and a long training and habituation period is generally required to facilitate many routine health procedures such as foot trimming, physical examination, and venipuncture in such facilities. Wild giraffes are often herded into boma corrals to facilitate capture and restraint using vehicles and helicopters. Ropes are often used on chemically immobilized giraffes to enable heavily sedated animals to be properly positioned during the induction and recovery periods. Camelids can generally be restrained in similar fashion to equid species using halters, ropes and specially designed squeezes. Interested readers are referred to the species-specific chapter on camelids and giraffe species later in the textbook for further detail on physical restraint involving these species.

Elephants

Specialized facilities are required to house and allow proper physical restraint of elephants in captivity (refer to Webliography). Capture of adult wild elephants generally involves chemical immobilization using remote drug delivery techniques.

BIRDS

Ratites

Most large ratite species, such as adult ostrich (*Struthio camelus*), can be physically restrained safely and easily for many procedures using custom fitted hoods and appropriate handling facilities, which include triangular stocks, chutes, and boards to herd birds safely. Male ostrich are particularly aggressive during the breeding season and caution should be used when physically restraining an adult male ostrich. Ratites defend themselves with their powerful legs, which can strike out very quickly in a forward direction. Juvenile ratites can be easily restrained by grasping them from behind around the sternum and holding them with the legs dangling. The legs of juvenile ratites are prone to injury and should not be forced into position, but allowed to dangle freely. Once hooded, ostrich are easily restrained or walked short distances into a corner where venipuncture, physical exams, radiographs, ultrasound, and other husbandry procedures can be performed. The head of ostriches can be grasped and pulled toward to the ground to limit the risk of kicking out (Smith 2003). Smaller ratite species, such as emu (Dromaius *novaehollandiae*) and rhea (*Rhea americana*), can also be physically restrained by walking up to the bird and grabbing it from behind with both hands at the base of the wings and restraining the bird either standing or on the ground. Hoods are not applied to emus and rhea as they often become more agitated when hooded. Doing this in a darkened room with solid walls and soft flooring helps avoid injuries. Cassowaries (*Casuarius* spp.) are an exception and chemical immobilization is usually recommended for these birds due to their aggressive nature and ability to seriously injure and kill humans with their sharp and powerful claws. Juvenile cassowaries can be safely physically restrained as described for rheas and emus.

Waterfowl (Anatidae) and Wading Birds (Herons, Cranes, and Storks)

Remote Capture Techniques Remote capture of waterfowl is well described elsewhere (Bookhout 1994; Bub 1991) and consists of using rocket nets, hand nets, nets strung across waterways, and cage traps of various sorts. Capture of wild waterfowl species is often timed to coincide with molting as capture is made easier by the fact that birds cannot fly for a period of several weeks. Appropriate-sized nets can be used to capture birds in enclosures or aviaries where they can be physically restrained for most procedures. Bites can be inflicted on handlers from larger goose and swan species. Injuries to birds are often inflicted on carpi and feet from being crowded into areas with concrete or other hard surfaces, so rubber flooring or mats on walls are often used to decrease injuries in these areas.

Wading birds, such as cranes, storks, and herons, can inflict serious eye damage with their sharp, pointed beaks so safety glasses or face shields are definitely required. These birds are generally herded gently with brooms or boards into corners where they can be grasped by the head and body. The bird is generally held with one arm around the body to restrain the wings and support the body while the other hand restrains the head and neck. The legs are restrained proximal to the hocks only as fractures and capture myopathy result from struggling when attempts are made to restrain the legs more distally (Swenger & Carpenter 1996).

Galliforms (Pheasant, Grouse, and Partridge)

Pheasant, grouse, partridge, and ptarmigan (*Lagopus* spp.) species are fairly easily handled with light gloves to protect from spurs and bites in larger species. Hoop nets are widely used in zoos for capturing these species, which are usually found on the ground. Some male pheasants (*Phasianus* spp.) have sharp spurs that can inflict injury to handlers, and the males can be aggressive during the breeding season. These birds are restrained by holding the bird next to the body, thus restraining the wings between the arm and body, with the other hand restraining the legs. The head does not usually need to be restrained as these species rarely peck once restrained (Fowler 1995).

Wild galliforms are generally trapped in box traps baited with grain or other feedstuff or with mist nets or hoop nets (Mahan et al. 2002; Skinner et al. 1998). Cloth or mesh bags are very useful for holding individual birds for short periods of time or for transport. Birds will settle down considerably if kept in a dark area rather than in bright light. Cardboard boxes are also useful for transport of groups of birds. Capture myopathy and trauma are the main injuries sustained from trapping of wild galliforms (Hofle et al. 2004; Nicholson et al. 2000; Spraker et al. 1987).

Hawks, Owls, and Falcons

Most raptor species can be physically restrained if the talons and wings are restrained adequately to prevent injury to themselves and the handler. Their extremely sharp talons are the main defensive weapon to be avoided when physical restraint is required. Nets are useful to initially capture fully flighted birds in aviaries or pens in appropriately sized nets that will capture the bird without injury.

Hawk species are best restrained with leather gloves by grasping the talons quickly and deftly with one hand with the palm facing toward the chest of the bird. The bird can then be dangled upside down until the wings and head can be grasped. These birds are best held against the chest or side with the wings folded and head facing toward the back of the person holding. Stockinette or mesh bags are useful to restrain birds temporarily for weighing and venipuncture, banding, or radiographs without the need to be holding them. Care needs to be taken to ensure that chest excursions are not restricted when using any physical restraint technique with avian species. The beak also needs to be avoided as painful injuries can be sustained by large hawks, eagles, and owls (Fig. 7.4).

Wild hawks and owls are captured by a variety of methods, including box traps, nets, and leg snares (Bub 1991). Eagles are captured by chasing with vehicles (Ostrowski et al. 2001), on nests or with snares (Hollamby et al. 2004).

Passerines

Remote Capture Techniques Nylon mist nets are the primary method of capture used for free-ranging and captive passerines in large aviaries. Passerine species include the thrushes, sparrows, finches, and others. Many methods of setting these nets have been described depending on the target species and its preferred habitat (arboreal, ground, and wetland). Most species can be

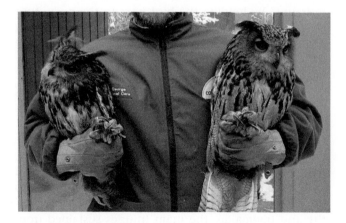

Figure 7.4. Eurasian eagle owls being restrained for examination and weighing following initial capture with a net in a captive enclosure.

held using a banders hold in which the palm of the hand is used to gently cup the body to restrain the wings with the head being restrained between the index and middle fingers (Massey 1999). Many of these species need to be handled as little as possible as they are prone to exertional shock and hypoxia from being overrestrained and not allowing the sternum to lift to allow air exchange in the lungs. The other method of restraint is to hold them in one hand by grasping the legs gently proximal to the hock joints with the index finger between the legs and the thumb and ring finger on either side. This works well if the birds are not flapping and struggling to escape or there is a need to transfer the bird from one person to another. Passerine species should be transported in dark containers or boxes to reduce flapping and struggling and can be removed using a towel or net to initially capture and restrain the bird. Most passerine species have fragile leg bones and rapid metabolic rates, and so injury and mortalities often result from prolonged or rough handling.

Psittacines

Most psittacine species can be physically restrained for most basic procedures, including venipuncture, beak trims, nail trims and physical examinations. Large macaws and parrots often need to be anesthetized for a thorough and less stressful exam. Most captive psittacines can be captured from a perch using a net or towel depending on their level of tameness. Once captured, they are removed from the towel or net by grasping the head and mandible between the fingers of one hand and grasping the feet and wingtips in the other hand. Placing the bird in dorsal recumbency on a table or with a pad or towel underneath will facilitate restraint. Gloves may or may not be used for psittacine restraint based on the temperament and size of the bird being restrained. Care needs to be taken with larger species as they can inflict serious injuries with their powerful beaks. Detailed restraint and exam techniques for psittacines can be found in Romagnano (1999) and Abou-Madi (2001). Smaller species can be restrained as described for passerine birds. Those interested in wild psittacine capture are referred to Bub (1991).

REPTILES

Lizards, Skinks, and Geckos

Lizard species can be safely restrained if the head and tail are adequately restrained to prevent injury to the handler and the animal. Carnivorous lizards (e.g., monitors and tegus) can be particularly difficult to handle while young green iguanas (*Iguana iguana*) and geckos (*Gekkonidae*) are fairly docile to handle. Lizard species should not be restrained solely by the tail as many species can shed their tail (autotomy), so additional support and restraint must be used for the head and

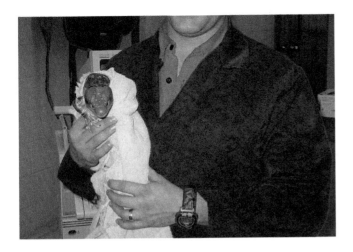

Figure 7.5. Blue-tongued skink restrained in a towel.

body. Small lizard species can be restrained in one hand with the head between thumb and forefinger and the ring and little finder wrapped around the pelvis to restrain the body and tail (Divers 1999). If possible, medium-sized lizards should initially be grabbed over the dorsal pelvic area and pinned against a table or other flat surface and then grabbed behind the head while grabbing the forelegs, to where they can either be wrapped in a towel or held against the body (Fig. 7.5). Towels or hoods placed over the head will facilitate handling of larger lizards, providing a calming effect. Leather gloves are very useful for large iguanas and monitors to prevent bites and scratches. Special precautions need to be taken to avoid the bite of poisonous species such as the Gila monster (*Heloderma suspectum*) and Mexican beaded lizard (*Heloderma horridum*).

REPTILES

Turtles/Tortoises

Most small- and medium-sized chelonians can be grabbed by the shell and supported by the carapace with the other hand. Larger species (e.g., snapping turtle) require more dexterity and skill as well as protective equipment. A variety of aquatic traps have been used for freshwater turtle capture in the wild and detailed references should be consulted prior to wild capture (Dunham et al. 1988; Simmons 2002; Voigt 1980).

AMPHIBIANS

Amphibians can generally just be grabbed by hand and restrained by supporting the body on the opposite hand. Disposable exam gloves should be worn and changed between individual animals to prevent disease transfer and to prevent toxin absorption to restrainers from certain species (e.g., cane toads). Moistened towels or gauze sponges may be useful to gain traction on

slippery amphibian skin but care must be taken not to damage the integument while handling. Wild amphibians are generally captured using pitfall or funnel traps in conjunction with drift fencing or cover boards (Crosswhite et al. 1999; Mitchell et al. 1993).

Regardless of the species or animal being physically restrained, experience and specialized knowledge of anatomy and physiology are mandatory prerequisites to successfully handle most wild and zoo animals without undue distress and suffering. The following chapters outline detailed taxa specific methods for proper physical restraint of the most commonly handled zoo and wild animals. Specialized holding and restraint devices are absolutely necessary in some situations, while smaller or more docile species may only require personal protective equipment.

REFERENCES

Abou-Madi N. 2001. Avian anesthesia. *Veterinary Clinics of North America: Exotic Animal Practice* 4(1):147–167.

Andelt WF, Phillips RL, Schmidt RH, Gill RB. 1999. Trapping furbearers: an overview of the biological and social issues surrounding a public policy controversy. *Wildlife Society Bulletin* 27:53–64.

Anderson RG, Nielsen C. 2002. Modified Stephenson trap for capturing deer. *Wildlife Society Bulletin* 30(2):606–608.

Apps CD. 1996. Bobcat (*Lynx rufus*) habitat selection and suitability assessment in southeast British Columbia. MSc Thesis. Faculty of Environmental Design, University of Calgary, Calgary.

Apps CD. 1999. Space-use, diet, demographics, and topographic associations of lynx in the southern Canadian rocky mountains: a study. In: *Ecology and Conservation of Lynx in the United States* (LF Ruggiero, KB Aubry, SW Buskirk, GM Koehler, CJ Krebs, KS McKelvey, JR Squires, eds.), pp. 351–371. Technical Report RMRS-GTR-30WWW. Fort Collins: U.S. Department of Agriculture, Forest Service, Rocky Mountain Research Station. http://www.fs.fed.us/rm/pubs/rmrs_gtr030 .html (accessed January 20, 2014).

Austin J, Chamberlain MJ, Leopold BD, Burger LW. 2004. An evaluation of EGG and wire cage traps for capturing raccoons. *Wildlife Society Bulletin* 32(2):351–356.

Barrett MW, Nolan JW, Roy LD. 1982. Evaluation of a handheld net-gun to capture large mammals. *Wildlife Society Bulletin* 10:108–114.

Beier P, Vaughan MR, Conroy MJ, Quigley H. 2003. An analysis of scientific literature related to the Florida panther. Final Report. Florida Fish and Wildlife Conservation Commission, Tallahassee, FL.

Blundell GM, Kern JW, Bowyer RT, Duffy LK. 1999. Capturing river otters: a comparison of Hancock and leg-hold traps. *Wildlife Society Bulletin* 27(1):184–192.

Boesch J, Boulanger J, Curtis P, Erb H, Ludders J, Kraus M, Gleed R. 2011. Biochemical variables in free-ranging white-tailed deer (*Odocoileus virginianus*) after chemical immobilization in Clover traps or via ground-darting. *Journal of Zoo and Wildlife Medicine* 42(1):18–28.

Bookhout T. 1994. *Research and Management Techniques for Wildlife and Habitats*, 5th ed. Bethesda: The Wildlife Society.

Brook I. 2005. Management of human and animal bite wounds: an overview. *Advances in Skin and Wound Care* 18(4):197–203.

Bub H. 1991. *Bird Trapping and Bird Banding: A Handbook for Trapping Methods All Over the World*. Ithaca: Cornell University Press.

Bush M. 2003. Giraffidae. In: *Zoo and Wild Animal Medicine*, 5th ed. (ME Fowler, RE Miller, eds.), pp. 625–633. St. Louis: W.B. Saunders.

Cattet M, Stenhouse G, Bollinger T. 2008. Exertional myopathy in a grizzly bear (*Ursus arctos*) captured by leghold snare. *Journal of Wildlife Diseases* 44(4):973–978.

Cattet MR, Caulkett NA, Wilson C, Vandenbrink T, Brook RK. 2004. Intranasal administration of xylazine to reduce stress in elk captured by net gun. *Journal of Wildlife Diseases* 40(3):562–565.

Cattet MRL, Christison K, Caulkett NA, Stenhouse GB. 2003. Physiologic responses of grizzly bears to different methods of capture. *Journal of Wildlife Diseases* 39(3):649–654.

Caulkett N, Cattet MRL. 2002. Anesthesia of bears. In: *Zoological Restraint and Anesthesia* (D Heard, ed.), pp. 1–6. Ithaca: International Veterinary Information Service (IVIS). http://www.ivis.org/special_books/Heard/caulkett/chapter_frm.asp?LA=1 (accessed January 20, 2014).

Citino S. 2003. Bovidae (except sheep and goats) and Antilocapridae. In: *Zoo and Wild Animal Medicine*, 5th ed. (M Fowler, E Miller, eds.), pp. 649–674. St. Louis: W.B. Saunders.

Conner MC, Soutiere EC, Lancia RA. 1987. Drop-netting deer: costs and incidence of capture myopathy. *Wildlife Society Bulletin* 15(3):434–438.

Copeland JP, Cesar E, Peek JM, Harris CE, Long CD, Hunter DLA. 1995. A live trap for wolverine and other forest carnivores. *Wildlife Society Bulletin* 23(3):535–538.

Crosswhite DL, Fox SF, Thill RE. 1999. Comparison of methods for monitoring reptiles and amphibians in upland forests of the Ouachita mountains. *Proceedings of the Oklahoma Academy of Science* 79:45–50.

Darrow PA, Shivik JA. 2008. A pilot evaluation of trap monitors by the USDA Wildlife Services Operational Program. In: *Proceedings of the 23rd Vertebrate Pest Conference* (RM Timm, MB Madon, eds.), pp. 213–217. Davis: University of California Davis.

Deem SL. 2004. Capture and immobilization of free-living jaguars (*Panthera onca*). In: *Zoological Restraint and Anesthesia* (D Heard, ed.). Ithaca: International Veterinary Information Service. http://www.ivis.org/special_books/Heard/deem2/IVIS.pdf (accessed January 20, 2014).

DelGiudice GD, Mangipane BA, Sampson BA, Kochanny CO. 2001. Chemical immobilization, body temperature, and post-release mortality of white-tailed deer captured by Clover trap and net-gun. *Wildlife Society Bulletin* 29(4):1147–1157.

de Wet T. 1993. Physical capture of carnivores. In: *The Capture and Care Manual*. (AA McKenzie, ed.), pp. 255–277. Pretoria: Wildlife Division Support Services and The South African Veterinary Foundation.

DeYoung CA. 1988. Comparison of net-gun and drive-net capture for white-tailed deer. *Wildlife Society Bulletin* 16(3):318–320.

Divers SJ. 1999. Clinical evaluation of reptiles. *Veterinary Clinics of North America: Exotic Animal Practice* 2(2):291–331.

Duarte JMB. 2008. A technique for the capture of free-ranging marsh deer (*Blastocerus dichotomus*). *Journal of Zoo and Wildlife Medicine* 39(4):596–599.

Dunham AE, Morin PJ, Wilbur HM. 1988. Methods for the study of reptile populations. In: *Biology of the Reptilia*, Vol. 16 (C Gans, RB Huey, eds.), pp. 330–386. New York: Alan R. Liss.

Earle RD, Lunning DM, Tuovila VR, Shivik JA. 2003. Evaluating injury mitigation and performance of #3 Victor soft catch traps to restrain bobcats. *Wildlife Society Bulletin* 31(3):617–629.

Ebedes H, Van Rooyen J, du Toit JG. 1996. Game capture. In: *Game Ranch Management* (JduP Bothma, ed.), pp. 271–333. Pretoria: Van Schaik Publishing.

Ebedes H, Van Rooyen J, du Toit JG. 2002. Bomas and holding pens. In: *Game Ranch Management*, 4th ed. (JDP Bothma, ed.), pp. 132–146. Pretoria: Van Schaik Publishing.

English R, Stalmans M, Mills M, Van Wyk A. 2008. Helicopter-assisted boma capture of African wild dogs Lycaonpictus. *Koedoe: African Protected Area Conservation and Science* 36(1):103–106.

Feldhamer GA, Thompson BC, Chapman JA. 2003. *Wild Mammals of North America: Biology, Management and Conservation*, 2nd ed. Baltimore: Johns Hopkins University Press.

Fernández-Morán J J, Saavedra D, Manteca-Vilanova X. 2002. Reintroduction of the Eurasian otter (*Lutra lutra*) in northeastern Spain: trapping, handling, and medical management. *Journal of Zoo and Wildlife Medicine* 33(3):222–227.

Firchow KM, Vaughan MR, Mytton WR. 1986. Evaluation of the hand-held net gun for capturing pronghorns. *The Journal of Wildlife Management* 50(2):320–322.

Fowler ME. 1995. *Restraint and Handling of Wild and Domestic Animals*, 2nd ed. Ames: Iowa State University Press.

Fowler ME. 1998. *Medicine and Surgery of South American Camelids: Llama, Alpaca, Vicuna, Guanaco*. Ames: Iowa State University Press.

Fowler ME. 2003. Camelidae. In: *Zoo and Wild Animal Medicine*, 5th ed. (ME Fowler, RE Miller, eds.), pp. 612–624. St. Louis: W.B. Saunders.

Fowler ME, Cubas ZS. 2001. *Biology, Medicine and Surgery of South American Wild Animals*. Ames: Iowa State University Press.

Fowler ME, Miller RE. 2003. *Zoo and Wild Animal Medicine*, 5th ed. St. Louis: W.B. Saunders.

Frank L, Simpson D, Woodroffe R. 2003. From the field: foot snares, an effective method for capturing African lions. *Wildlife Society Bulletin* 31(1):309–314.

Franzmann AW. 1998. Restraint, translocation and husbandry. In: *Ecology and Management of the North American Moose*. (AW Franzmann, CC Schwartz, eds.), pp. 519–557. Washington, DC: Smithsonian Institution Press.

Gese EM, Andersen DE. 1993. Success and cost of capturing coyotes, *Canis latrans*, from all-terrain vehicles. *Canadian Field Naturalist* 107:112–114.

Gibeau ML, Stevens S. 2002. Grizzly bear monitoring in the Bow River watershed: a progress report for 2002. Eastern Slopes Grizzly Bear Project. http://www.canadianrockies.net/wp-content/uploads/2009/02/report_year9.pdf(accessed January 20, 2014).

Goodrich JM, Kerley LL, Schleyer BO, Miquelle DG, Quigley KS, Smirnov YN, Nikolaev IG, Quigley HB, Hornocker MG. 2001. Capture and chemical anesthesia of Amur (Siberian) tigers. *Wildlife Society Bulletin* 29(2):533–542.

Grandin T. 1993. The effect of previous experiences on livestock behaviour during handling. *Agri-Practice* 14:15–20.

Grassman LI, Austin SC, Tewes ME, Silvy NJ. 2004. Comparative immobilization of wild felids in Thailand. *Journal of Wildlife Diseases* 40(3):575–578.

Haigh JC. 1999. The use of chutes for ungulate restraint. In: *Zoo & Wild Animal Medicine: Current Therapy*, 4th ed. (ME Fowler, RE Miller, eds.), pp. 657–662. St. Louis: W.B. Saunders.

Haigh JC, Hudson RJ. 1993. *Farming Wapiti and Red Deer*. St. Louis: Mosby.

Harrison RL, Barr DJ, Dragoo JWA. 2002. Comparison of population survey techniques for swift foxes (*Vulpes velox*) in New Mexico. *The American Midland Naturalist* 148(2):320–337.

Hartup BK, Kollias GV, Jacobsen MC, Valentine BA, Kimber KR. 1999. Exertional myopathy in translocated river otters from New York. *Journal of Wildlife Diseases* 35(3):542–547.

Haulton S, Porter W, Rudolph B. 2001. Evaluating four methods to capture white-tailed deer. *Wildlife Society Bulletin* 29(1):255–264.

Heard DJ. 1999. Medical management of megachiropterans. In: *Zoo and Wild Animal Medicine, Current Therapy 4*. (RE Miller, ME Fowler, eds.), pp. 344–354. Philadelphia: Saunders.

Heard DJ. 2003. Chiroptera (Bats). In: *Zoo and Wild Animal Medicine*, 5th ed. (E Miller, M Fowler, eds.), pp. 315–333. St. Louis: W.B. Saunders.

Hofle U, Millan J, Gortazar C, Buenes-Tado FJ, Marco I, Villafuerte R. 2004. Self-injury and capture myopathy in net-captured juvenile red-legged partridge with necklace radiotags. *Wildlife Society Bulletin* 32:344–350.

Hollamby S, Afema-Azikuru J, Bowerman WW, Cameron KN, Dranzoa C, Gandolf AR, Hui GN, Kaneene JB, Norris A, Sikarskie JG, Fitzgerald SD, Rumbeiha WK. 2004. Methods for capturing African fish eagles on water. *Wildlife Society Bulletin* 32(3): 680–684.

Hubert GF, Wollenberg GK, Hungerford LL, Bluett RD. 1999. Evaluation of injuries to Virginia opossums captured in the EGG trap. *Wildlife Society Bulletin* 27(2):301–305.

Hubert GF Jr, Hungerford LL, Proulx G, Bluett RD, Bowman L. 1996. Evaluation of two restraining traps to capture raccoons. *Wildlife Society Bulletin* 24(4):699–708.

Huhn GD, Austin C, Carr M, Heyer D, Boudreau P, Gilbert G, Eimen T, Lindsley MD, Cali S, Conover CS, Dworkin MS. 2005. Two outbreaks of occupationally acquired histoplasmosis: More than workers at risk. *Environmental Health Perspectives* 113(5): 585–589.

Jacques C, Jenks J, Deperno C, Sievers J, Grovenburg T, Brinkman T, Swanson C, Stillings B. 2009. Evaluating ungulate mortality associated with helicopter net-gun captures in the northern Great Plains. *The Journal of Wildlife Management* 73(8): 1282–1291.

Jessup DA. 1999. Capture and handling of mountain sheep and goats. In: *Zoo & Wild Animal Medicine: Current Therapy*, 4th ed. (ME Fowler, RE Miller, eds.), pp. 681–687. St. Louis: W.B. Saunders.

Jessup DA, Clark RK, Weaver RA, Kock MD. 1988. Safety and cost-effectiveness net-gun capture of desert bighorn sheep. *Journal of Zoo and Wild Animal Medicine* 19(4):208–213.

Johnson KG, Pelton MR. 1980. Prebaiting and snaring techniques for black bears. *Wildlife Society Bulletin* 8:46–54.

Johnson-Delaney CA. 2005. Safety issues in the exotic pet practice. *Veterinary Clinics of North America: Exotic Animal Practice* 8(3):515–524.

Jones C, McShea WJ, Conroy MJ, Kunz TH. 1996. Capturing mammals. In: *Measuring and Monitoring Biological Diversity: Standard Methods for Mammals*, pp. 115–155. New York: Smithsonian Institution Press.

Jonkel JJ. 1993. *A Manual for Handling Bears for Managers and Researchers* (TJ Thier, ed.), Missoula: U.S. Department of the Interior. Fish and Wildlife Service.

Kazacos KR, Boyce WM. 1989. Baylisascaris larva migrans. *Journal of the American Veterinary Medical Association* 195(7):894–903.

Kock MD, Jessup DA, Clark RK, Franti CE, Weaver RA. 1987a. Capture methods in five subspecies of free-ranging bighorn sheep: an evaluation of drop-net, drive-net, chemical immobilization and the net-gun. *Journal of Wildlife Diseases* 23: 634–640.

Kock MD, Jessup DA, Clark RK, Franti CE. 1987b. Effects of capture on biological parameters in free-ranging bighorn sheep (*Ovis canadensis*): evaluation of drop-net, drive-net, chemical immobilization and the net-gun. *Journal of Wildlife Diseases* 23:641–651.

Krauss H, Weber A, Appel M, Enders B, Isenberg HD, Schiefer HG, Slenczka W, von Graevenitz A, Zahner H. 2003. *Zoonoses: Infectious Diseases Transmissible from Animals to Humans*, 3rd ed. Washington, DC: ASM Press.

Kreeger TJ. 1999. Chemical restraint and immobilization of wild canids. In: *Zoo & Wild Animal Medicine: Current Therapy*, 4th ed. (ME Fowler, RE Miller, eds.), pp. 429–435. St. Louis: W.B. Saunders.

Kunz TH, Tidemann CR, Richards GC. 1996. Small volant mammals in "capturing mammals." In: *Measuring and Monitoring Biological Diversity: Standard Methods for Mammals* (DE Wilson, FR Cole, JD Nichils, R Rudra, MS. Foster, eds.), pp.

122–146. Washington, DC; London: Smithsonian Institution Press.

Kunz TH, Hodgkison R, Weise C. 2009. Methods of capturing and handling bats. In: *Ecological and Behavioral Methods for the Study of Bats*, 2nd ed. (TH Kunz, S Parsons, eds.), pp. 3–35. Baltimore: Johns Hopkins University Press.

Locke SL, Hess MF, Mosley BG, Cook MW, Hernandez S, Parker ID, Harveson LA, Lopez RR, Silvy NJ. 2004. Portable drive-net for capturing urban white-tailed deer. *Wildlife Society Bulletin* 32(4):1093–1098.

Lofroth EC, Klafki R, Krebs JA, Lewis D. 2008. Evaluation of live-capture techniques for free-ranging wolverines. *The Journal of Wildlife Management* 72:1253–1261.

Logan KA, Sweanor LL. 2001. *Desert Puma: Evolutionary Ecology and Conservation of an Enduring Carnivore*, pp. 42–50. Washington, DC: Island Press.

Logan KA, Sweanor LL, Smith JF, Hornocker MG. 1999. Capturing pumas with foot-hold snares. *Wildlife Society Bulletin* 27(1): 201–208.

López-Olvera JR, Marco I, Montané J, Casas-Díaz E, Mentaberre G, Lavín S. 2009. Comparative evaluation of effort, capture and handling effects of drive nets to capture roe deer (*Capreolus capreolus*), Southern chamois (*Rupicapra pyrenaica*) and Spanish ibex (*Capra pyrenaica*). *European Journal of Wildlife Research* 55:193–202.

Mahan BR, Dufford DR, Emerick N, Beissel TJ. 2002. Net and net-box modifications for capturing wild turkeys. *Wildlife Society Bulletin* 30(3):960–962.

Massey GJ. 1999. Physical examination of passerines. *Veterinary Clinics of North America: Exotic Animal Practice* 2(2):357–381.

Mentaberre G, Lopez-Olvera JR, Casas-Diaz E, Bach-Raich E, Marco I, Lavin S. 2010. Use of haloperidol and azaperone for stress control in roe deer (*Capreolus capreolus*) captured by means of drive-nets. *Research in Veterinary Science* 88(3): 531–535.

Meyer LCR, Fick L, Matthee A, Mitchell D, Fuller A. 2008. Hyperthermia in captured impala (*Aepyceros melampus*): a fright not flight response. *Journal of Wildlife Diseases* 44(2):404–416.

Mitchell JC, Erdle SY, Pagels JF. 1993. Evaluation of capture techniques for amphibian, reptile, and small mammal communities in saturated forested wetlands. *Wetlands* 13(2):130–136.

Mitchell KD, Stookey JM, laturnas DK, Watts JM, Haley DB, Huyde T. 2003. The effects of blindfolding on behavior and heart rate in beef cattle during restraint. *Applied Animal Behaviour Science* 85:233–245.

Moehrenschlager A. 2002. Effects of ecological and human factors on the behaviour and population dynamics of reintroduced Canadian swift foxes (*Vulpes velox*). PhD Dissertation. University of Oxford.

Morris PJ, Shima AL. 2003. Suidae and Tayassuidae (wild pigs, peccaries). In: *Zoo and Wild Animal Medicine, Current Therapy 4*. (RE Miller, ME Fowler, eds.), pp. 586–602. St. Louis: W.B. Saunders.

Mudappa D, Chellam R. 2001. Capture and immobilization of wild brown palm civets in western Ghats. *Journal of Wildlife Diseases* 37(2):383–386.

Nicholson DS, Lochmiller L, Stewart MD, Masters RE, Leslie DM. 2000. Risk factors associated with capture-related death in Eastern wild turkey hens. *Journal of Wildlife Diseases* 36: 308–315.

O'Gara BW, Yoakum JD. 2004. *Pronghorn: Ecology and Management*. Boulder: University Press of Colorado.

Openshaw P. 1993. Mass capture techniques. In: *The Capture and Care Manual* (AA Mckenzie, ed.), pp. 138–155. Pretoria: Wildlife Decision Support Services.

Ostrowski S, Fromont E, Meyburg B-U. 2001. A capture technique for wintering and migrating steppe eagles in southwestern Saudi Arabia. *Wildlife Society Bulletin* 29(1):265–268.

Pruss SD, Cool NL, Hudson RJ, Gaboury AR. 2002. Evaluation of a modified neck snare to live-capture coyotes. *Wildlife Society Bulletin* 30(2):508–516.

Rocha VJ, Aguiar LM, Ludwig G, Hilst CLS, Teixeira GM, Svoboda WK, Shiozawa MM, Malanski LS, Navarro IT, Mariño JHF, Passos FC. 2007. Techniques and trap models for capturing wild tufted capuchins. *International Journal of Primatology* 28(1):231–243.

Romagnano A. 1999. Examination and preventative medicine protocols in psittacines. *Veterinary Clinics of North America: Exotic Animal Practice* 2(2):333–356.

Rosell F, Hovde B. 2001. Methods of aquatic an terrestrial netting to capture Eurasian beavers. *Wildlife Society Bulletin* 29(1): 269–274.

Rosell F, Kvinlaug JK. 1998. Methods for live-trapping beaver (*Castor* spp.). *Fauna Norvegica Serie A* 19:1–28.

Sahr DP, Knowlton FF. 2000. Evaluation of tranquilizer trap devices (TTDs) for foothold traps used to capture gray wolves. *Wildlife Society Bulletin* 28(3):597–605.

Scotton BD, Pletscher DH. 1998. Evaluation of a capture technique for neonatal Dall sheep. *Wildlife Society Bulletin* 2(3): 578–583.

Serfass TL, Brooks RP, Swimley TJ, Rymon LM, Hayden AH. 1996. Considerations for capturing, handling, and translocating river otters. *Wildlife Society Bulletin* 24(1):25–31.

Sharp T, Saunders G, Mitchell B. 2007. Live capture of pest animals used in research. Natural Heritage Trust, Government of New South Wales. http://www.environment.gov.au/system/files/resources/dd56dc25-6e77-4700-825b-83fbd12b5371/files/46217-operating-procedure-1.pdf (accessed January 20, 2014).

Shury T, Caulkett N, Woodbury M. 2010. Intranasal naltrexone and atipamezole for reversal of white-tailed deer immobilized with carfentanil and medetomidine. *The Canadian Veterinary Journal* 51(5):501–505.

Simmons JE. 2002. Herpetological Collecting and Collections Management. Revised Edition. Herpetological Circulars #31, Society for the Study of Amphibians and Reptiles.

Skinner WR, Snow DP, Payne NF. 1998. A capture technique for juvenile willow ptarmigan. *Wildlife Society Bulletin* 26(1): 111–112.

Smith D. 2003. Ratites: Tinamiformes (tinamous) and Struthioniformes, Rheiiformes, Cassuariformes (ostriches, emus, cassowaris and kiwis). In: *Zoo and Wild Animal Medicine*, 5th ed. (E Miller, M Fowler, eds.), pp. 94–102. St. Louis: W.B. Saunders.

Spraker TR, Adrian WJ, Lance WR. 1987. Capture myopathy in wild turkeys (*Meleagris gallopavo*) following trapping, handling and transportation in Colorado. *Journal of Wildlife Diseases* 23:447–453.

Swenger SR, Carpenter JW. 1996. General hubsbandry. In: *Cranes: Their Biology, Husbandry and Conservation* (DH Ellis, GF Gee, CW Mirande, eds.), pp. 31–43. Baraboo: National Biological Service and International Crane Foundation.

Taylor SK, Land ED, Lotz M, Roelke-Parker ME, Citino SB, Rotstein D. 1998. Anesthesia of free-ranging Florida panthers (*Felis concolor coryi*), 1981–1998. *Proceedings of American Association of Zoo Veterinarians*, pp. 26–29.

Te Wong S, Servheen CW, Ambu L. 2004. Home range, movement and activity patterns, and bedding sites of Malayan sun bears *Helarctos malayanus* in the rainforest of Borneo. *Biological Conservation* 119(2):169–181.

Tidemann CR, Loughland RA. 1993. A harp trap for large megachiropterans. *Wildlife Research* 20:607–611.

Voigt RC. 1980. New methods for trapping aquatic turtles. *Copeia* 2:368–371.

Webb S, Lewis J, Hewitt D, Hellickson M, Bryant F. 2008. Assessing the helicopter and net gun as a capture technique for white-tailed deer. *The Journal of Wildlife Management* 72:310–314.

Whitelow CJ, Pengelley ET. 1954. A method for handling live beaver. *The Journal of Wildlife Management* 18:533–534.

Wilson DE, Cole FR, Nichols JD, Rudran R, Foster MS. 1996. *Monitoring and Evaluating Biological Diversity: Standard Methods for Mammals.* Biological Diversity Handbook Series. Washington, DC; London: Smithsonian Institution Press.

Wimsatt J, Biggins DE. 2009. A review of plague persistence with special emphasis on fleas. *Journal of Vector Borne Diseases* 46(2): 85–99.

Wirtu G, Cole A, Pope CE, Short CR, Godke RA, Dresser BL. 2005. Behavioural training and hydraulic chute restraint enables handling of eland antelope (*Taurotragus oryx*) without general anesthesia. *Journal of Zoo and Wildlife Medicine* 36(1):1–11.

WEBLIOGRAPHY

http://jjcdev.com/~fishwild/?section=best_management_practices: Association of Fish and Wildlife Agencies Best Management Practices.

http://fisheries.org/docs/policy_useoffishes.pdf: American Society of Ichthyologists and Herpetologists Guidelines for handling fish species.http://www.asih.org/files/hacc-final.pdf: American Society of Ichthyologists and Herpetologists Guidelines for handling herpetiles.

http://www.ccac.ca/Documents/Standards/Guidelines/Wildlife.pdf: Canadian Council on Animal Care (wildlife guidelines).

http://www.aza.org/uploadedFiles/Conservation/Commitments_and_Impacts/Elephant_Conservation/ElephantStandards.pdf: American Association of Zoos and Aquaria Standards for Elephant Management and Care.

http://www.elephantcare.org/Elebase/anesthes.htm: Elephant bibliographic database on anesthesia and restraint.

http://www.environment.gov.au/biodiversity/invasive/publications/humane-control.html: Code of Practice and Standard Operating Procedures for control of feral animals in Australia (Department of Sustainability, Environment, Water, Population and Communities).

http://www.fur.ca/TRS_AIHTS.php?id=points: Fur Institute of Canada, The agreement on international humane trapping standards (AIHTS).

http://www.mammalsociety.org/articles/guidelines-american-society-mammalogists-use-wild-mammals-research-0: The American Society of Mammalogists guidelines for mammal handling and research.

http://www.nmnh.si.edu/BIRDNET/guide/index.html: The Ornithological Council guidelines for bird handling.

http://wildpro.twycrosszoo.org/List_Vols/Wildpro_Gen_Cont.htm: WildPro Multimedia, information on species specific restraint and handling with focus on European species and wildlife rehabilitation.

8 Zoo and Wildlife CPR

Søren Boysen

INTRODUCTION

Cardiopulmonary cerebral resuscitation (CPCR) consists of both basic and advanced life support, as well as postresuscitation care and management. Guidelines have been established in the human profession focusing on evidence-based medicine. Unfortunately, veterinary and wildlife literature is sparse, consisting of a few retrospective studies and no prospective or clinical trials to compare strategies. As such, most veterinary guidelines and recommendations are based on extrapolation from human medicine, experimental animal models, and expert opinion.

In the absence of specific evidence-based veterinary studies, many of the recent human consensus statement guidelines would seem reasonable to apply to veterinary and wildlife patients, at least until such veterinary and wildlife studies can be performed to support or refute these recommendations.

One of the main recurrent themes in recent consensus statements is the increased emphasis on providing minimally interrupted high-quality chest compressions throughout advanced life support interventions. Any interruption in chest compressions decreases survival (Deakin et al. 2010; Neumar et al. 2010). Therefore, chest compressions should only be paused long enough to enable specific interventions and should never exceed 5–10 seconds whenever possible, in order to help minimize no-flow times (Deakin et al. 2010; Neumar et al. 2010).

With the recognized grave prognosis associated with cardiopulmonary arrest (CPA), the other recurrent emphasis in human consensus statements focuses on a "track-and-trigger" system. This system is designed to improve monitoring and to detect the deteriorating patient, which will enable therapeutic interventions, and will hopefully prevent CPA.

Objectives of CPCR

- To apply the knowledge and skills necessary to provide basic and advanced life support in arrested patients
- To be able to systematically organize the personal and equipment necessary to perform basic and advanced life support based on pharmacologic and physiologic principles.

DEFINING BASIC AND ADVANCED LIFE SUPPORT

Basic life support (BLS) is derived from the human profession and generally refers to out-of hospital emergency interventions that are implemented until more advanced procedures can be instituted in a hospital setting. Although classically associated with cardiopulmonary arrest, BLS is used in a number of life-threatening situations (choke, shock, drowning, etc.). It usually focuses on the ABC's (airway, breathing, and circulation) and does not tend to include invasive procedures or pharmacological therapies. In contrast, advanced life support (ALS), which still uses the techniques of BLS, is essentially the application of more advanced procedures designed to further support breathing and circulation. Advanced life support therefore is an extension of BLS. These more advanced procedures often include drugs and invasive procedures (i.e., venous access techniques, open-chest surgery, chest tubes, etc.), which tend to occur in hospital-like environments. Arrests or life-threatening conditions occurring in the field where limited equipment or supplies and fewer highly trained staff are available would be an example of BLS. Arrests occurring in the hospital setting where more advanced procedures can take place

Zoo Animal and Wildlife Immobilization and Anesthesia, Second Edition. Edited by Gary West, Darryl Heard, and Nigel Caulkett.
© 2014 John Wiley & Sons, Inc. Published 2014 by John Wiley & Sons, Inc.

with a greater number of trained staff available will most often include ALS technique.

CARDIOPULMONARY ARREST (CPA) AND CPCR: STRATEGY

In the presence of CPA, it should not take more than 10 seconds to identify that a patient is in a state of arrest and for CPCR measures to be initiated.

Confirm the Presence of an Arrest

Assess Respirations Loss of spontaneous breathing (regard and/or auscultate the thorax): if within 10 seconds there is doubt if the patient is breathing normally act as if it is not normal and intervene. Confusion may exist when animals are in CPA and agonal breaths are present. These agonal breaths must not be confused with respirations and CPA should proceed in their presence.

Assess Heart Beat and Pulses Loss of heart beat (auscultation) and absence of pulses (femoral artery palpation).

Assess Neurologic Responsiveness Loss of consciousness with fixed dilated (unresponsive) pupils.

Pulmonary Arrest without Cardiac Arrest

When respiratory arrest occurs without cardiac arrest (absence of respiratory effort with a palpable pulse) intubate and give 2–4 large breaths. Follow pulse and ECG to be sure the patient does not progress toward complete CPA. If the animal does not start to breathe spontaneously after several seconds, or the partial pressure of carbon dioxide remains greater than 55 mmHg, start positive pressure ventilation using normal resting respiratory rates for the species. If patient progresses to cardiac arrest, begin chest compressions immediately and consider decreasing the respiratory rate to 2/3 the normal resting respiratory rate (see below).

Note: The presence of an ECG waveform does not rule out cardiac arrest (see pulseless electrical activity). A palpable pulse or other means of ensuring spontaneous circulation (i.e., capnography) should be used to rule out cardiac arrest.

The Alphabet of an Arrest: A, B, C

After confirming the presence of CPA, the ABCs of CPCR are the mainstay in applying CPCR. There are six steps of CPCR adapted from the human resuscitation council guidelines: A, B, C and D, E, F.

Airways Verify that the airways are open. Confirm that the respiratory tract is patent (not obstructed by masses or foreign bodies) and intubate the animal as quickly as possible while minimally interrupting chest com-

pressions (If possible, do not stop chest compressions for >5–10 seconds to intubate the patient).

If the animal is intubated at the time of arrest, make sure the tube is patent and in the right location (not esophageal), is not obstructed with mucous, and is not kinked. Also make sure the cuff is inflated in preparation for positive pressure ventilation. It is difficult to provide good lung expansion and tidal volumes when the endotracheal tube cuff is not inflated. High volume low pressure cuffs are preferred over low volume high pressure cuffs due to the risk of pressure necrosis of the tracheal mucosa (Plunkett & McMicheal 2008). In cases where the upper airway is obstructed by something that is not easily removed/corrected (masses or laryngeal collapse for example), a tracheostomy tube may be required to secure the airway. Again, try to minimize the interruption in chest compressions to perform a tracheostomy.

Breathing (Ventilation) Patients that experience CPA should ideally be intubated and ventilated. The optimal tidal volume and respiratory rate (or even inspired oxygen content) to use during CPCR to achieve adequate oxygenation and carbon dioxide removal is unknown, and may vary between individuals, breeds, and species.

Given that blood flow to the lungs is greatly reduced during CPCR, ventilation to perfusion ratios (V/Q) are likely maintained with lower tidal volumes and respiratory rates than is normal for the patient (Neumar et al. 2010). Hyperventilation, which is very common when providing positive pressure ventilation during CPCR, can be harmful because it increases intrathoracic pressures, therefore decreasing venous return to the heart and subsequently cardiac output and cerebral perfusion pressures (Aufderhiede & Lurie 2004; Auferhiede et al. 2004). It is therefore necessary to try and find the balance between hypoventilation (too few breaths or incomplete expansion of the lungs with each breath) and hyperventilation (giving too many breaths at to high a pressure such that cardiac output is impaired). Although this has not been determined in most species, given tidal volume requirements and respiratory rates are generally lower during CPCR than in healthy patients, 2/3 to the lower limit of the normal resting respiratory rate are typically chosen (Neumar et al. 2010; Plunkett & McMicheal 2008).

When providing positive pressure ventilation for the CPCR patient, avoid over inflation of the lungs (if a pressure gauge is available, do not exceed 20 cmH20 pressure), yet make sure the chest rises with each breath delivered (Plunkett & McMicheal 2008). Make sure the endotracheal tube cuff is inflated to ensure adequate tidal volume delivery to the lungs.

Positive pressure ventilation can be delivered by connecting the patient to an anesthetic machine and using the rebreathing bag to deliver a breath, ambu bag, or demand valve depending on the size of the animal and what is more readily available.

Most anesthetic machines contain pressure gauges, which allow pulmonary pressures to be followed during positive pressure ventilation. With anesthetic machines, the pop-off valve can be closed or partially closed during compression of the rebreathing bag to allow filling of the lungs; however, care should be taken not to exceed 20 cmH20 of pressure during compression of the reservoir bag (Deakin et al. 2010; Neumar et al. 2010; Plunkett & McMicheal 2008).

An ambu bag is an inexpensive but very useful piece of equipment to have in the crash cart and can be used with room air until an oxygen source can be located and connected to the ambu bag. Although not common, pressure gauges can also be used with ambu bags. Ideally, the ambu bag should be connected to 100% oxygen using high flow rates. Use of a reservoir bag with the ambu bag (available on some ambu bags) will further increase the inspired oxygen content during positive pressure ventilation (the reservoir bag will fill with oxygen, which the ambu bag draws from during the delivery of a breath, decreasing the chance that the ambu bag will mix room air with the delivered oxygen flow). Avoid overinflating the lungs, but make sure the chest rises with each breath delivered.

Regardless of the positive pressure method used, inspired oxygen content should initially be set at 100% if it is available (Plunkett & McMicheal 2008). Following ROSC and return of spontaneous respirations, the inspired oxygen content should be titrated to a level that provides adequate partial pressure of arterial oxygen or hemoglobin saturation ($PaO_2 \geq 70$ mmHg and $SaO_2 \geq 93\%$) while minimizing the risks of oxygen toxicity.

Circulation In the absence of a palpable pulse or an auscultable heartbeat, and signs consistent with CPA (loss of consciousness and absence of respiratory effort), cardiac massage should be initiated to provide blood flow to the coronary circulation of the heart and cerebral circulation of the brain.

There are two forms of cardiac massage: external cardiac massage and internal cardiac massage.

External Cardiac Massage External cardiac massage (ECM) remains the most commonly used form of cardiac massage in cases of CPA. With a few rare exceptions (open-chest surgery, pleural space diseases, etc.—see later in the chapter), it is the initial starting point for all cases of CPCR.

Although ECM will only generate a small amount of blood flow, if started early and performed properly, it can provide a critical amount of blood flow to the brain and myocardium, which may be sufficient to achieve return of spontaneous circulation (ROSC) or may provide the critical flow needed until more exten-

sive procedures can be instituted (i.e., open-chest cardiac massage).

If ECM is to be successful, given the small flow it can achieve, it is vital that it be performed correctly. In general, compressions should be started immediately upon identification of CPA and interruptions in chest compressions must be kept to an absolute minimum and only for essential interventions (i.e., endotracheal intubation, defibrillation, or catheter placement). When an essential intervention is deemed necessary, interruption in compressions should not exceed 5–10 seconds in duration (Deakin et al. 2010; Neumar et al. 2010).

Technique of External Cardiac Massage: General Upon suspicion of or after confirming an arrest, the identifying individual should start ECM while calling on others for assistance (this may involve an alarm system or air horn in larger hospitals where staff may be spread out). It is best to have a minimum of three people to perform CPCR.

A well-equipped and frequently stocked crash cart (or mobile resuscitation kit for field work) should be readily available and rapidly accessible in areas where an arrest may occur (see appendix on how to stock a crash cart for various situations).

Place the animal in right lateral recumbency if possible (this may not be feasible in patients weighing more than 100 kg). The compressor can stand on the dorsal or ventral aspect of the patient, at the level of the chest, depending on preference (Plunkett & McMicheal 2008).

If at least two people are present, the goal should be to provide respirations as well as cardiac massage.

If only one person is present and the patient is not intubated, then external cardiac massage should be initiated, as the compression and relaxation of the chest during cardiac massage is usually sufficient to provide adequate movement of air within the respiratory system to allow gas exchange to occur (rationale for changing the pneumonic from ABC's of CPCR with at least two individuals present to CAB's if only one person is present) (Deakin et al. 2010; Neumar et al. 2010). Intubate and start positive pressure ventilations as soon as help arrives.

If only one person is present and the patient is already intubated, give 30 chest compressions and two ventilations until help arrives (Deakin et al. 2010; Neumar et al. 2010).

Minimize interruptions and provide high-quality compressions. When interruptions are essential, try to avoid exceeding 5–10 seconds of interrupted compressions.

Providing good quality chest compressions (especially in larger patients) can be exhausting, and it is recommended that the person providing the chest compressions be changed every 2 minutes (Malzer et al. 1996; Orliaguet et al. 1995). The interruption in compressions during the exchange should be minimal.

Maintain the airway, provide oxygen support as soon as possible, and ventilate the lungs with the most appropriate equipment immediately available (see breathing).

Ventilate the patient with PPV at a rate appropriate for the species. Avoid hyperventilating the patient (both rate, pressure, and tidal volume). Slow delivery of breaths, with an inspiratory time of 1 second and enough volume to produce a normal chest rise, should be used (Plunkett & McMicheal 2008).

The importance of uninterrupted chest compressions cannot be over emphasized. In human studies even short interruptions to chest compressions are disastrous for outcome and every effort must be made to ensure that continuous and effective chest compressions are maintained throughout the resuscitation attempt (Deakin et al. 2010; Neumar et al. 2010).

A CPCR leader should monitor the quality of CPR and alternate CPCR providers or technique if the quality of CPCR is poor. Continuous $ETCO_2$, if available, can be used to indicate the quality of CPR: although an optimal target for $ETCO_2$ during CPCR has not been determined, values less than 10 mmHg tend to be associated with failure to achieve ROSC and may indicate that the quality of chest compressions are inadequate.

Provide chest compressions at a rate appropriate for the species; see later.

Avian Patients Avian patients may be placed in dorsal recumbency, and external compressions are performed by compression of the sternum; the method and force applied will depend on the mass of the bird. With very small avian patients compressions can be performed with one or two fingers at a rapid rate (up to 200 minutes), in very large patients, such as ratites, compressions are performed as described later, for mammalian patients >10 kg.

Mammalian Patients ≤1 kg Very small mammalian patients can be placed in lateral recumbency on a solid surface in right lateral recumbency; the person performing CPCR should place two fingers over the chest, immediately caudal to the forelimb. Compressions should be initiated at a rate of 150–200 compressions/ minute. Small mammals can be difficult to intubate, if intubation is possible, intermittent positive pressure ventilation can be initiated at a rate of 20–30 breaths/ minute. If intubation is not possible, mask ventilation may be attempted.

Mammalian Patients 1–10 kg For quadrupeds between 1 and 10 kg in weight, with the animal in right lateral recumbency, place the palm of the hand on the sternum with the fifth to sixth intercostal space between the finger and thumb. This allows direct compression of the heart when the fingers and thumb are squeezed together. The fingers and thumb of the opposite hand can be placed over the first hand if more vigorous compressions are required.

Avoid using only the fingertips to compress the chest as this may result in poorer efficacy and decreased blood flow (Plunkett & McMicheal 2008).

Mammalian Patients 10–100 kg For patients between 10 kg and 100 kg in weight, with the animal in right lateral recumbency, the person performing chest compressions should keep his/her shoulders, elbows, and hands in a straight line so the weight of the upper body is transferred into the compressions via the arms, which will minimize effort and maximize the quality of compressions. With these patients, the widest point of the chest is chosen. For patients exceeding 70 kg, the approach described for patients greater than 250 kg may be more beneficial if the initial response does not appear to be working.

Mammalian Patients 100–250 kg There is no published literature on any technique to perform CPCR in patients between 100 and 250 kg in body weight, and therefore recommendations at this time are based solely on the opinions and experiences of the author. The author tends to use a technique between the techniques described for patients between 10 and 100 kg, and those ≥250 kg. With the patient in right lateral recumbency, the CPR provider can use one foot placed over the widest part of the chest (with the knee and hip in a line over the foot) to perform compressions with the goal to compress the chest by approximately 30% in a 1:1 compression to relaxation rate. Alternatively, the CPR provider, starting in a crouched position, may use one knee to "fall" on the patient at the widest point of the chest just caudal to the left elbow. Again, the idea is to transfer enough force to compress the chest by 30% in a 1:1 compression to relaxation ratio. If this is not achievable, then a change to the technique for patients ≥250 kg should be considered.

Mammalian Patients ≥250 kg There is a paucity of information regarding external cardiac massage in large animal patients, one prospective study has been performed in horses, which demonstrated that the most effective technique of performing thoracic compression in adult horses was to place the animal in right lateral recumbency and induce compressions by having the person performing CPCR fall from a standing or crouched position onto their knee, with the knee striking the chest immediately posterior to the left elbow. Compression rates of 40, 60, and 80 compressions/ minute were compared. A compression rate of 80/ minute resulted in the best improvement in cardiac output. The authors' comment that this technique is

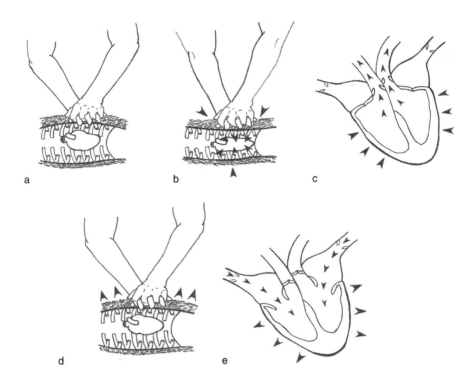

Figure 8.1. (a) The chest in a relaxed state with proper positioning of the hands over the heart. (b) Compression of the heart, between the right and left chest walls. (c) Blood is forced into the aorta and pulmonary artery as the mitral and tricuspid valves are active and act to prevent back flow of blood into the atrii. (d) During relaxation and chest recoil, the heart reexpands. (e) The valves open and blood passively fills the heart.

physically demanding for the operator, and it may be best used intermittently, for short periods, in order to distribute cardiotonic drugs (Hubbel et al. 1993).

Maximizing External Cardiac Massage Experimental studies show that the most effect ECM can provide at best 30–45% of normal cardiac output (Andreka & Fenneaux 2006; Plunkett & McMicheal 2008).

It is well established that the success of establishing coronary and cerebral blood flow during closed CPCR is determined by the quality of the chest compressions. The chest should be compressed approximately 1/3 of the thoracic width at the widest point of the chest (Plunkett & McMicheal 2008).

In addition to the degree of compression, the frequency of compressions is also very important and should follow guidelines for the species and its weight.

Chest compression to chest relaxation time should be approximately 1:1, making sure full chest recoil is attained between each compression relaxation cycle (Plunkett & McMicheal 2008).

Providing compressions greater than recommended for the desired weight and species does not provide any additional advantages and can decrease filling time during the recoil of the relaxation phase. Compressions below the recommended range are associated with a poorer outcome.

In general, there are two theories that have been proposed to help explain the blood flow that is obtained during external cardiac massage: the cardiac pump theory and thoracic pump theory.

The Cardiac Pump Theory With the cardiac pump theory, direct compression of the heart between the two sides of the rib cage results in forward blood flow (Fig. 8.1). Blood flow results because the pressures created on the heart allow the valves (particularly the mitral valve) to function as they would normally (preventing back flow of blood when the heart is compressed, and opening when it is relaxed during decompression/recoil of the chest). This mechanism is probably the most prominent means of blood flow during CPCR in animals less than 15 kg, or during internal cardiac massage (Plunkett & McMicheal 2008).

Blood flow is not influenced as much by the duration of compression as it is by the frequency of compressions.

Although it was initially believed that the cardiac pump theory was responsible for blood flow in animals of any size, subsequent studies in larger animals using ultrasound and angiography have demonstrated that cardiac valves are not functional during external chest compressions (the chest is too wide to compress the heart between the two sides of the chest), and another

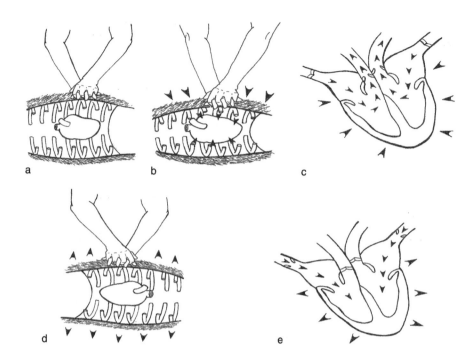

Figure 8.2. (a) The hands are placed over the widest part of the chest. (b) The chest size decreases, but the heart is not directly compressed between the two opposing rib cages. (c) Increases in intrathoracic pressures push blood out of the heart and thorax into the arteries. Note that the tricuspid and mitral valves are open and the heart is acts as a passive conduit. The venous valves play a role in preventing back flow of blood. (d) The chest expands during the relaxation phase. (e) Blood reenters the thoracic vessels and heart passively during the relaxation phase of external CPCR. Note: The heart (and cardiac valves) is passive. There are antireflux valves at the thoracic inlet.

theory has been proposed for blood flow in larger animals (the thoracic pump theory).

The Thoracic Pump Theory With the thoracic pump theory, it is not direct compression of the heart that results in blood flow, but rather the changes in intrathoracic pressure during compressions and relaxation of the chest. With this theory, the heart is a passive conduit and acts similar to a large blood vessel. It is therefore the blood within the thoracic cavity (large vessels and heart) that acts as a blood reservoir. With compression of the chest, the pressures within the thoracic cavity increase, forcing blood to move out of the thorax (Fig. 8.2). Blood is forced cranially through the arterial system due to the presence of valves in the venous system and because the jugular veins are collapsed during the compressive phase of external cardiac massage. This mechanism likely accounts for the majority of blood flow in animals greater than 15 kg in body weight (Plunkett & McMicheal 2008).

Intermittent Abdominal Compression and Continual Abdominal Compression With this technique the abdomen is compressed during the relaxation phase of chest compressions in an effort to move more blood from the abdomen into the thorax. The technique is difficult (but not impossible) to coordinate at frequencies of 80 to 100 compressions per minute. It also

requires an additional person to apply the intermittent abdominal compressions. The risk of regurgitation of stomach contents (due to increased pressures created in the abdomen and sometimes directly on the stomach) is greater with this technique and patients should be intubated. Abdominal trauma with lacerations of the liver and spleen have been reported with these techniques (Plunkett & McMicheal 2008). An alternative to intermittent abdominal compression is continuous abdominal compression where the abdomen is wrapped or pressure is manually applied in a continuous fashion to the abdomen.

Impedance Threshold Device (ITD) The thoracic impedance threshold device is a unidirectional valve that is connected to the end of the endotracheal tube. The valve is sensitive to pressure and will not open until a certain pressure is achieved (it is a spring loaded valve that will typically open around 12 mmHg pressure).

In patients receiving closed chest CPCR without the ITD in place, negative intrathoracic pressures that occur during relaxation help to draw blood back into the chest as air freely enters the mouth, trachea, and lungs. With the ITD in place, the negative pressure in the thoracic cavity during elastic recoil is increased (due to the fact the valve on the ITD remains closed until 12 mmHg pressure is reached), which allows more blood to enter the thorax during the relaxation phase of chest compressions than would normally enter the thorax without the use of this device.

Studies in people have shown improved return of spontaneous circulation and short-term survival when the ITD is used.

Arrests during Anesthesia

If the animal is under anesthesia during the CPA, consider discontinuation of volatile anesthesia or administration of a specific antagonist; if it is safe to do so, this will depend on the species being worked on and the environment.

Confirm the proper connection and function of the anesthetic machine if time permits (tubing free of obstruction, oxygen on and flowing, proper connection to the endotracheal tube, etc.) and begin positive pressure ventilation by using the reservoir bag and pop-off valve. The pop-off valve can be closed or partially closed during compression of the reservoir bag to allow filling of the lungs; however, care should be taken not to exceed 20 cmH20 of pressure during compression of the reservoir bag. At the same time, the chest should visibly rise during delivery of breaths. Ventilate the animal with 100% oxygen if possible.

Frequency of positive pressure ventilations should be based on the lower resting respiratory rate of the species undergoing CPCR (see above).

Begin external chest compressions in the absence of an auscultable heart beat or palpable pulse.

OPEN-CHEST OR INTERNAL CARDIAC MASSAGE

Depending on the situation, species, and quality of life of the patient, open-chest CPR may or may not be a viable option. Given the equipment needed to perform open-chest CPR, the personnel needed, and the intensive postoperative care, including chest tubes, it is generally not a viable option in wildlife under field conditions. However, provided there is a sufficient number of trained staff to perform open-chest CPR and the equipment and facilities necessary to perform the technique and manage the patient postoperatively, it may be possible in some settings.

In the absence of ROSC within 5 minutes of closed chest compressions, or in the face of pleural space disease, rib fractures, pericardial effusions, flail chest, diaphragmatic hernia, severely obese animals (provided the owners are well informed and consent to the procedure), or in cases where the thorax is already open (i.e., sternotomy), or even during open abdominal surgery (where the diaphragm can easily be accessed and incised to allow the hand to be passed into the thorax via the diaphragm to perform direct cardiac massage), open-chest CPCR should be performed (Plunkett & McMicheal 2008).

The advantages of open-chest CPCR are significant: visualization of the heart (visible ventricular fibrillations) and tonicity of flaccidity of the heart, which helps determine venous return and cardiac filling; direct cardiac visualization and cardiac access for administration of CPCR drugs; drainage of the pleural or pericardial spaces if diseased; and finally, manual occlusion of the caudal aorta to divert blood to vital organs and better perfusion of vital organs.

Multiple studies have demonstrated that open-chest CPCR with direct cardiac compressions result in far greater blood flow than closed chest CPCR. As such, through improved cerebral and cardiac flow, the chances of return of spontaneous circulation are much higher. However, if open-chest CPCR is to be attempted it must be done early and should not be delayed until after 10–20 minutes of closed chest CPCR has been attempted. If the chest is going to be opened to improve the chances of CPCR, it must be done early (ideally within 5 minutes of the arrest if closed chest CPCR is not successful in this 5 minute time frame). Always have the materials to perform open-chest CPCR readily available.

Indications for Open-Chest CPCR

- At least 3 people
- CPA during surgery: thoracic or abdominal (can access the chest via an incision through the diaphragm during open abdominal surgery)
- Inability to generate ROSC or good flow during closed chest CPCR
- Intrathoracic disease: pleural or pericardial effusion, diaphragmatic hernia, pneumothorax, and flail chest
- External factors: marked obesity, severe subcutaneous emphysema
- Ineffective external CPCR after 5 minutes (unable to generate good femoral pulses or adequate ETC02).

Technique for Internal Cardiac Massage

1. Place the animal in right lateral recumbency.
2. Rapidly shave and soak the area with alcohol over the left fifth intercostal space (it is better to be dirty and alive than sterile and dead). Shave a 2- to 3-in strip of fur from the sternum ventrally to spine dorsally (the width of the clipper blades in one pass).
3. Make an incision through the skin and subcutaneous tissues over the 5th intercostal space with a scalpel. Start dorsally and cut to the sternum ventrally.
4. With scissors, penetrate the thorax (traverse the muscles to enter the pleural space) at the level of the costocondral junction of the fifth intercostal space. Starting lower than the costocondral junction runs the risk of cutting the internal thoracic

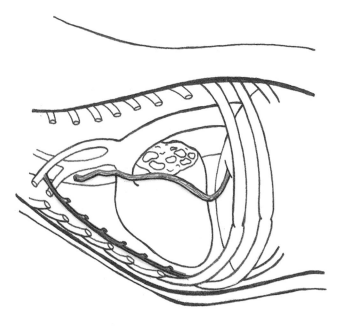

Figure 8.3. Anatomic location of the internal thoracic artery (red) and vagal nerve (yellow) for canid and felid species, which should be avoided when opening the thorax and pericardium respectively.

artery, which runs ventral to the costocondral junction (Fig. 8.3).

5. Retract the ribs (finichetti rib spreaders or manually) to visualize the heart. One can cut or break the ribs to improve visualization and improve exposure if needed; however, do not interrupt compressions of the heart to do this (have an assistant do this).

6. Start cardiac compressions. Take the heart in the palm of the hand and massage from the base to the apex. Wait for the ventricles to refill before the next compression is delivered. If the ventricles do not fill quickly enough to allow 80–100 beats per minute to be delivered, consider increasing venous return by providing abdominal compressions, administering fluids or blood, or having an assistant occlude the caudal vena cava just caudal to the heart. Try to avoid using the fingertips to compress the heart, as this may result in less effective flow rates and increases the risk of traumatic cardiac rupture.

7. The pericardial sac can be opened to improve cardiac massage, to allow visualization of fine ventricular fibrillation, and to help get a feel for cardiac filling between compressions. It is easiest to hook the phrenicopericardiac ligament with the index finger (in a sweeping caudal to cranial direction) and incise the pericardium over the ligament as opposed to cutting the pericardial sac directly over the heart (which runs the risk or accidental laceration of the myocardium).

8. If there is return of spontaneous circulation, the thorax must be copiously lavaged, with warm sterile

saline before closing. A chest tube should be placed prior to chest closure. The chest should then be closed by passing large suture (0) or wire around adjacent ribs. The muscle layers, subcutaneous tissue, and skin are closed routinely.

THE ALPHABET OF AN ARREST: D, E, F

Drugs

Epinephrine Epinephrine remains the gold standard with external cardiac massage through its alpha sympathomimetic effects, particularly its arterial vasoconstricive properties. (Deakin et al. 2010). Despite this, there is no placebo-controlled clinical study to demonstrate that the routine use of any vasopressor at any stage during cardiac arrest increases neurologically intact survival to hospital discharge. Animal models suggest a delay in the delivery of vasopressor drugs following the onset of cardiac arrest may be associated with a worse outcome (Wenzel et al. 1999).

Based on experimental animal models, it has been shown that blood flow during external cardiac massage can be slightly increased with the administration of epinephrine. Principally through its sympathomimetic effects, epinephrine improves the efficacy of ECM through an increase in transdiastolic pressure of the aorta. Note that it is the difference between the aortic pressure and the right atrial pressure during diastole that determines coronary circulation, a primary goal of ECM. Epinephrine may also improve cerebral perfusion through improved carotid flow as a result of redistribution of carotid flow from the external to the internal carotid arteries.

The dosage and frequency of epinephrine varies from 0.01 to 0.1 mg/kg of 1:1000 ratio repeated at 3–5 minute intervals (Neumar et al. 2010). These recommendations are based on "expert opinion" and the optimal dose is unknown. Higher doses have been associated with increased cardiac workload and myocardial injury, although they may be more efficacious in cases of pulseless electrical activity. There are also no data to support repeated doses of epinephrine. However, until further studies can be completed to support or refute epinephrine, or to prove another vasopressor is more efficacious, the standard of care is to administer epinephrine at 3–5 minute intervals during CPCR at a dose of 0.01 mg/kg. Do not discontinue chest compressions to administer epinephrine or any other drug. If 0.01 mg/kg fails to provide ROSC after one to two boluses, a 0.1 mg/kg dose or use of vasopressin can be considered.

Vasopressin The only alternative that has shown promise when compared with epinephrine is vasopressin. Vasopressin is a vasoconstrictor and an antidiuretic. In CPCR models in animals, vasopressin showed greater improvement in cardiac output than epinephrine.

Further studies are needed to confirm any true benefit in morbidity and mortality; however, its use is now accepted and the current recommendation is that an IV dose of vasopressin can be given in place of the first or second dose of epinephrine (Neumar et al. 2010).

Atropine Atropine is a parasympatholytic agent. It inhibits the effects of acetylcholine and increases heart rate. Its primary indication is in situations of increased vagal tone leading to arrest. Atropine is no longer recommended for routine use in the management of PEA/asystole in people (Neumar et al. 2010); however, given there is no evidence to suggest it has detrimental effects during bradycardic or asystolic cardiac arrest, it may still play a role in the veterinary profession for these conditions (see notes on PEA and asystole).

Bicarbonate In humans, the routine administration of sodium bicarbonate during cardiac arrest and CPR or after ROSC is not recommended. It may be beneficial in cases where the arrest was caused by hyperkalemia (i.e., urethral obstruction, uroabdomen, or Addisonian crisis resulting in cardiac arrest due to severe hyperkalemia) or preexisting metabolic acidosis was present. If given, blood gasses should be followed serially to determine response to therapy and the possible need for repeat doses. It is important that ventilation be maintained if bicarbonate is administered to prevent paradoxical CNS acidosis.

Lidocaine and Amiodarone There is no evidence that antiarrhythmics given during cardiac arrest increase survival to discharge. There use may be considered in ventricular fibrillation or pulseless ventricular tachycardia when defibrillation is not available. Amiodarone is recommended over lidocaine in the human literature (Neumar et al. 2010).

Calcium Gluconate, and Glucose All have been used during CPCR; however, they should only be given when indicated (i.e., preexisting conditions).

Routes of CPCR Drug Administration

There are generally five routes of drug administration during CPCR; via a central venous catheter (jugular vein), via a peripheral venous catheter (i.e., cephalic or saphenous), via an intraosseous catheter, via the trachea (through a small 5- to 8-g red rubber tube passed through an endotracheal tube), and intracardiac (only recommended if the chest is open during open-chest CPCR). Do not discontinue cardiac massage during the administration of drugs via any route!

There are many choices to administer drugs during CPCR. Central line administration is the most rapid and preferred route to administer drugs given the proximity of the catheter tip in relation to the heart (Emerman et al. 1998). However, it takes time to place

central lines, they are associated with more risk, and it requires greater skill to place a central line compared to a peripheral line. Unless a central line is already in place, it is recommended that a peripheral catheter be placed and used for CPCR. If there is anticipated difficulty in placing a peripheral line, the newer IO catheters can be placed in under 10 seconds and show equal efficacy to peripheral lines (Neumar et al. 2010).

Drugs delivered via a peripheral venous catheter should be followed by a bolus of fluids (10–20 mL/kg) to push drugs administered peripherally from the venous access site toward the heart to allow drugs to reach the heart (Emerman et al. 1990).

Endotracheal administration is less frequently used in human CPCR due to the unpredictable plasma concentrations achieved when drugs are delivered via this route (Neumar et al. 2010). However, it is still frequently used in the veterinary profession due to the difficulty of placing venous catheters and the cost and availability of alternative routes such as IO catheters. The optimal dose of drug to administer via the tracheal route, for most drugs, is also unknown. If using the endotracheal route the dosage should be two to three times the IV drug dosage. Evidence suggests the dose of epinephrine via the IT route may need to be 3–10 times the IV does (Hornchen et al. 1987). With the exception of bicarbonate all drugs given IV can also be given via the endotracheal route. To ensure the drug reaches the small airways and does not remain in the endotrachdeal tube the author prefers to administer the drugs via a long 5- to 8-g red rubber feeding tube (the tube is passed through the endotracheal tube). A small bolus of 5 mL (the volume of the catheter used) of sterile water (provides more rapid absorption of the drug than 0.9% saline) is then flushed through the red rubber tube following the administration of the drug to ensure the drug does not remain in the catheter. Alternatively the drug can be directly diluted with 5–10 mL of sterile water and injected directly through the endotracheal tube. The patient should also be ventilated with two to three rapid breaths to help distribute the drug within the lungs.

In humans, rapid intraosseous catheters and IO drug administration has all but replaced endotracheal drug administration. All drugs that are administered IV can be given IO at the same dosage. IO drugs should be followed with a bolus of fluids similar to IV drugs in order to push them from the IO space into the circulation and towards the heart. Studies in people have demonstrated that IO injection of drugs achieves adequate plasma concentration in a time comparable to injection through a central venous catheter.

Intracardiac administration of drugs is no longer recommended due to the risk of lacerating coronary vessels, injury leading to arrhythmias and accidental intracardiac muscle injection. Given the evidence to support alternative routes its use should be reserved for cases of open-chest CPCR when the heart can be directly visualized. A drug dose chart is included in Table 8.1.

Electrocardiogram

There are 3 common fatal arrhythmias reported in association with CPA. One may proceed to another.

Ventricular Asystole Ventricular asystole is characterized by an absence of all electrical ventricular activity: The ECG tracing is a flat line (see Fig. 8.4a).

Atropine is no longer recommended for asystole in the human profession given the lack of any demonstrable benefit with its administration. However, in people, most cardiac arrests (including asystole) are

Table 8.1. Cardiopulmonary cerebral resuscitation drug doses

Drug	Dose	2,5 kg	5 kg	10 kg	15 kg	20 kg	25 kg	30 kg	40 kg	50 kg
Epinephrine, 1 : 1000, 1 mg/mL	0.1 mg/kg (0.01 mg/kg)	0.25 0.025	0.5 0.05	1 0.1	1.5 0.15	2 0.2	2.5 0.25	3 0.3	4 0.4	5 0.5
Atropine, 0.5 mg/mL	0.05 mg/kg	0.25	0,5	1	1.5	2	2.5	3	4	5
Lidocaine, 20 mg/mL	2 mg/kg	0.25	0.5	1	1.5	2	2.5	3	4	5
Bicarbonate, 1 mEq/mL	1 mEq/kg	2.5	5	10	15	20	25	30	40	50
External defibrillation	2–5 J/kg	5–12,5	10–25	20–50	30–75	40–100	50–125	60–150	80–200	100–250
Internal defibrillation	0.2–0.5 J/kg	0.5–1.25	1–2.5	2–5	3–7.5	4–10	5–12.5	6–15	8–20	10–25
Vasopressin, 20 u/mL	0.2–0.8 u/kg	0.07	0.13	0.25	0.38	0.5	0.63	0.65	1.0	1.25

Notes: Drugs are in mL per kg, administration IV, double or triple the dose if given endotrachealy.

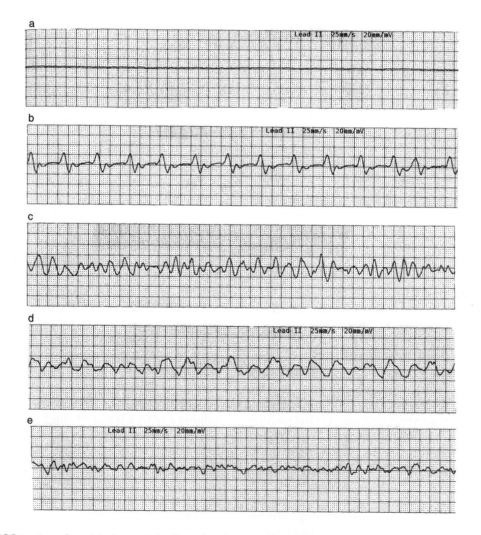

Figure 8.4. (a) ECG tracing of ventricular asystole. Note the absence of any electrical activity (b). An example of pulseless electrical activity (PEA). Note that the ECG tracing can vary from near normal to vary bizarre depending on the electrical activity present. The key to note is that there is synchronous electrical activity from the heart in the absence of a detectable pulse. (c–e) ECG tracing of coarse ventricular fibrillation progressing to fine ventricular fibrillation.

caused by primary myocardial pathology, which is in contrast to many of veterinary patients who experience asystole as a result of increased vagal tone and not primary myocardial pathology. Therefore, given many veterinary patients may arrest without the rhythm being observed, it is still reasonable to administer atropine in conjunction with epinephrine until studies prove otherwise. This is especially true if the arrest may have been the result of increased vagal tone.

Pulseless Electrical Activity This is the most common arrhythmia reported as a cause of arrest in veterinary patients. Electrical mechanical dissociation is characterized by a visible ECG tracing (electrical activity present in cardiac muscle cells), in the absence of myocardial contractility (Fig. 8.4b). There is current passing through the conducting system of the heart resulting in a detectable ECG rhythm, but the muscles fail to contract or fail to contract with sufficient force to generate enough cardiac out put to move blood through the vascular system or produce a palpable pulse. Treatment of this arrhythmia is difficult and often unsuccessful.

Epinephrine is recommended in cases of pulseless electrical activity at a dose of 0.01 to 0.1 mg/kg. When PEA is identified ECM should be started immediately while IV access is secured and epinephrine can be administered. Epinephrine can be continued every 3–5 minutes. Similar to other arrhythmias, ECM should be continued for at least 2 minutes before rapidly checking the rhythm, and interruption in chest compressions should be minimized (less than 5 seconds) while the pulse and rhythm are evaluated. If a pulse is detected, post cardiac care is initiated. If the rhythm does not produce a palpable pulse or asystole is noted, then chest compressions and CPCR should be restarted immediately and continued for 2 minutes before another rhythm check is repeated.

Atropine is no longer recommended for PEA in the human profession given the lack of any demonstrable benefit with its administration. However, as previously discussed asystole, cardiac arrests in veterinary patients often result from increased vagal tone, not myocardial pathology as in humans. Therefore, given many veterinary patients may arrest without the rhythm being observed, it may still be reasonable to administer atropine in conjunction with epinephrine, especially if the arrest may have been the result of increased vagal tone.

Ventricular Fibrillation This is the most common arrhythmia that occurs in people, often as a result of myocardial infarctions. It is characterized by a completely disorganized and anarchic rhythm, which results in complete absence of coordinated or effective ventricular contractions. It may be coarse or fine (Fig. 8.4c–e). By far the best therapy for this arrhythmia is electrical defibrillation, which transiently depolarizes all cardiac cells simultaneously (complete cardiac stand-

still), with the hope they will restart in a synchronized pattern (Deakin et al. 2010; Neumar et al. 2010).

If a defibrillator is available it is still important to emphasize minimizing the duration of the preshock and post-shock pauses and the continuation of compressions during charging of the defibrillator is recommended. It must also be emphasized that compressions should be started immediately following defibrillation and the total time to perform defibrillation should not interrupt chest compressions for more than 5–10 seconds. Deliver a single shock dose and immediately resume chest compressions. Do not interrupt chest compressions to allow rhythm analysis. Instead, continue chest compressions for two minutes, while monitoring response to ECM before checking the rhythm analysis or deciding if a second shock should be delivered.

The earlier defibrillation is delivered following identifications of ventricular fibrillation the greater the chance of success. If an initial single charge fails to convert VF, then three-stacked shocks may be considered. A single shock dose of 2–5 J/kg (preferably biphasic, although monophasic is acceptable) is recommended as a starting current.

Although biphasic defibrillators are phasing out monophasic defibrillators and monophasic defibrillators are no longer being produced, they are likely to play a role in the veterinary profession for many years to come. If given a choice a biphasic defibrillator should be used as they have been shown to be more effective at terminating ventricular arrhythmias at lower energy levels, have demonstrated greater first shock efficacy and have greater first shock efficacy for long duration VF compared to monophasic defibrillators. Wearing rubber gloves has been shown to decrease the risk of an accidental shock being delivered to CPCR givers.

Defibrillation may be transthoracic (external) or transcardiac (internal). If a defibrillator is not available a precordial thump (strong quick thump on the chest wall over the heart, or a direct "flick" of the heart itself if the chest is open) can be attempted. The idea is to traumatically depolarize the heart or stun it. Given the widespread availability of electrical defibrillators in the human profession the precordial thump is no longer recommended; however, in the veterinary profession, where defibrillators or even amiodarone and lidocaine may not be as readily available, the precordial thump may still have some benefit.

Fluids

Resuscitation with fluids is only recommended in cases of confirmed hypovolemia and reflex administration of fluid boluses to arrested patients should be avoided as they can lead to volume overload and pulmonary edema (Deakin et al. 2010). Intravenous fluids are the preferred route of administration. However, in the absence of an intravenous catheter, intraosseous administration is also equally effective. If medications are given during CPCR, a 10-mL/kg fluid bolus should be given through the same catheter as the drug to help ensure it reaches the heart.

MONITORING EFFICACY OF CPCR

Palpation of the femoral pulse is one of the easiest techniques to monitor the efficacy of CPCR without the need for specialized equipment. If CPCR efforts do not produce a palpable femoral pulse then a change in external massage technique or changing to open-chest CPCR should be considered. It should be noted, however, that palpation of a femoral pulse may indicate venous rather than arterial flow (there are no valves in the inferior vena cava), and does not always correlate to effective CPCR. Palpation of a pulse when chest compressions are stopped is a fairly reliable indicator of ROSC (Neumar et al. 2010). Do not discontinue chest compression for more than 10 seconds to assess if a pulse is present or not.

Other methods of assessing efficacy of CPCR include placement of a well-lubricated doppler flow probe on the eye, evaluation of the ECG waveform and measurement of end tidal carbon dioxide.

Measurement of end tidal CO_2 remains one of the most consistent and reliable measures of CPCR and for the detection of ROSC. Unlike ECG analysis, it also does not require an interruption in chest compressions to monitor (Neumar et al. 2010). Although specific parameters have not been established, an end tidal CO_2 of at least 10 mmHg is likely to represent efficacious CPCR (Grmec & Klemen 2001; Kolar et al. 2008; Pokorna et al. 2009). With the return of spontaneous circulation, the end tidal CO_2 will rapidly rise and should reach close to 30 mmHg (Fig. 8.5) (Ahrens et al. 2001; Sehra et al. 2003).

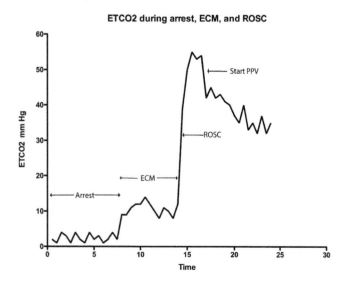

Figure 8.5. End tidal carbon dioxide measurement and its association with cardiac arrest, effective external cardiac message (ECM), return of spontaneous circulation (ROSC) and initiation of positive pressure ventilation (PPV).

In humans, end tidal CO_2 is also used to confirm endotracheal tube placement, which may also be applicable in some animal species, particularly those that are difficult to intubate.

DISCONTINUING CPCR

The risk of permanent severe neurologic injury is significant after 15–20 minutes of CPCR without ROSC. It is therefore reasonable to discontinue CPCR efforts after 20 minutes if ROSC is not reestablished (Plunkett & McMicheal 2008). This time frame may vary depending on the underlying cause, conditions under which CPCR is performed, and ultimately the quality of life of the patient.

PROGNOSIS AND RETURN OF SPONTANEOUS CIRCULATION?

The success of CPCR is dependent on many factors, including the underlying cause, the training of personnel, species, duration of the arrest, and the equipment available. In general, the prognosis is poor with very few patients recovering with normal neurologic function (however, this does vary depending on the underlying cause). The majority of veterinary literature relating to prognosis following CPA is derived from small animals, which demonstrates that 30% of patients will have ROSC, 5–10% will be discharged from the hospital, and 1% will have a return to normal function. Discharge from respiratory arrest alone varies from 25–60% of small animal patients. The chance of rearrest following return of spontaneous circulation is 35–70% in small animal veterinary patients.

CPA caused by anesthesia, drug overdose, increased vagal tone, or electrolyte imbalances tend to have a better prognosis than patients with serious underlying critical illnesses, such as sepsis, SIRS, or neoplasia. Early intervention is also an important factor influencing prognosis, and patients with significant underlying illness (pulmonary or cardiovascular instability, arrhythmias, marked hypothermia, anesthesia) should be monitored closely to help identify patients at increased risk and allow earlier intervention. In addition, well-trained staff (frequent practice of CPCR) with a properly equipped facilities (crash cart (Table 8.2), oxygen, suction, etc.) will further increase the chances of success. Finally, the prognosis also tends to vary with the species affected, with small animal veterinary patients having a better prognosis compared with large animal patients (Fig. 8.6).

There is a very high chance of a second arrest in patients that are successfully resuscitated and have achieved ROSC. Close intensive monitoring is needed, and most patients require vasopressors. Mechanical ventilation may also be necessary for a period of time following ROSC to decrease the chance of a second arrest.

Table 8.2. Sample crash cart setup

Drugs
  Epinephrine 1:1000
  Atropine 1/120 grain
  Lidocaine 2%
  Sodium bicarbonate 8.4%
  Dextrose 50%
  Calcium gluconate 10%
  Dobutamine
  Dopamine
  Dexamethasone SP
  Soludelta cortef
  Naloxone
  Flumazinil
Respiratory
  Endotracheal tubes
  Laryngoscope
  Stylets
  Suction apparatus
  Yankauer suction tip
  Thoracocentesis set (60-cc syringe, three-way IV access stopcock, extension tubing)
  Ambu bag
  Thoracic impedance device
  Chest tubes kits
  Tracheostomy tube kits
  Pulse oximeter

IV fluids and equipment
  Lactated Ringer's
  0.9% Saline
  Hypertonic saline 7.5%
  Hetastarch 6%
  Rapid infuser
  IV catheters, tape, gauze, wrap
  IV sets (pediatric and adult)
  IV extension tubing
  Blood filters (dog and cat)
  Bone marrow needles
  EZIO or other automated IO device
Needles
Syringes
Scalpel blade
Mayo scissors
Sponge forceps
Hemostats

Red rubber tubes (5F and 8F)

Defibrillator/EKG monitor
Doppler monitor/sphygmomanometer/cuffs
Hematocrit tubes, glucometer, lactate meter, azosticks
Serum, EDTA, heparin, and citrate tubes

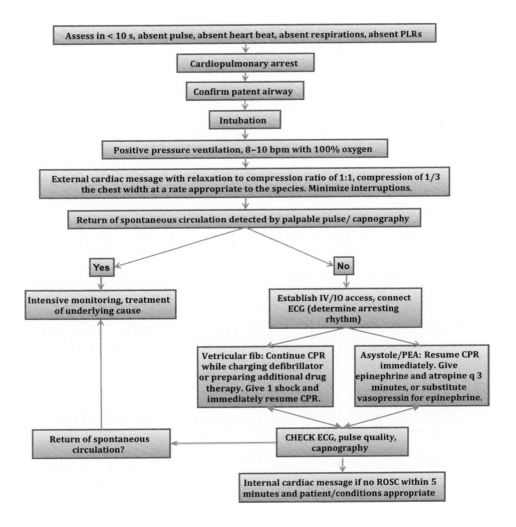

Figure 8.6. Cardiopulmonary resuscitation.

137

REFERENCES

Ahrens T, Schallom L, Bettorf K, et al. 2001. End-tidal carbon dioxide measurement as a prognostic indicator of outcome in cardiac arrest. *American Journal of Critical Care* 10:391–398.

Andreka P, Fenneaux MP. 2006. Haemodynamics of cardiac arrest and resuscitation. *Current Opinion in Critical Care* 12:198–203.

Aufderheide TP, Sigurdsson G, Pirrallo RG, et al. 2004. Hyperventilation-induced hypotension during cardiopulmonary resuscitation. *Circulation* 109:1960–1965.

Aufderhiede TP, Lurie KG. 2004. Death by hyperventilation: A common and life-threatening problem during cardiopulmonary effects of active compression-decompression after prolonged CPR. *Resuscitation* 31:243–253.

Deakin CD, Nolan JP, Sunde K, et al. 2010. European Resuscitation Council Guidelines for Resuscation. *Resuscitation* 81:1293–1304.

Emerman CL, Pinchak AC, Hancock D, et al. 1990. The effect of bolus injection on circulation times during cardiac arrest. *The American Journal of Emergency Medicine* 8:190–193.

Emerman CL, Pinchak AC, Hancock D, et al. 1998. Effect of injection site on circulation times during cardiac arrest. *Critical Care Medicine* 16:1138–1141.

Grmec S, Klemen P. 2001. Does the end-tidal carbon dioxide (EtCO2) concentration have prognostic value during out-of-hospital cardiac arrest? *European Journal of Emergency Medicine* 8:263–269.

Hornchen U, Schuttler J, Stoeckel H, et al. 1987. Endobronchial instillation of epinephrine during cardiopulmonary resuscitation. *Critical Care Medicine* 15:1037–1039.

Hubbel JAE, Muir WW, Gaynor JS. 1993. Cardiovascular effects of thoracic compression in horses subjected to euthanasia. *Equine Veterinary Journal* 25:282–284.

Kolar M, Krizmaric M, Klemen P, et al. 2008. Partial pressure of end-tidal carbon dioxide successfully predicts cardiopulmonary resuscitation in the field: a prospective observational study. *Critical Care (London, England)* 12:R115.

Malzer R, Zeiner A, Binder M, et al. 1996. Hemodynamic effects of active compression-decompression after prolonged CPR. *Resuscitation* 31:243–253.

Neumar RW, Otto CW, Link MS, et al. 2010. American Heart Association Guidelines for Cardiopulmonary Resuscitation and Emergency Cardiovascular Care. *Circulation* 122:S729–S767.

Orliaguet GA, Carli PA, Rozenberg A, et al. 1995. End-tidal carbon dioxide during out-of-hospital cardiac arrest resuscitation: Comparison of active compression-decompression and standard CPR. *Annals of Emergency Medicine* 25:48–51.

Plunkett SJ, McMicheal M. 2008. Cadiopulmonary resuscitation in small animal medicine: an update. *Journal of Veterinary Internal Medicine* 22:9–25.

Pokorna M, Necas E, Kratochvil J, et al. 2009. A sudden increase in partial pressure end-tidal carbon dioxide (P(ET)CO(2))at the moment of return of spontaneous circulation. *The Journal of Emergency Medicine* 38:614–621.

Sehra R, Underwood K, Checchia P. 2003. End tidal CO2 is a quantitative measure of cardiac arrest. *Pacing Clin Electrophsiol* 26:515–517.

Wenzel V, Lindner KH, Krismer AC, et al. 1999. Repeated administration of vasopressin but not epinephrine maintains coronary perfusion pressure after early and late administration during prolonged cardiopulmonary resuscitation in pigs. *Circulation* 99:1379–1384.

9 Field Emergencies and Complications

Jon M. Arnemo, Alina L. Evans, Åsa Fahlman, and Nigel Caulkett

INTRODUCTION

Chemical immobilization of wild animals is a form of veterinary anesthesia conducted under difficult circumstances. The risk of severe side effects, injuries, and death can never be completely eliminated. In addition, all immobilizing drugs are toxic and some are potentially lethal to humans (Haymerle et al. 2010; Kreeger & Arnemo 2012); see Chapter 13 on human safety.

Chemical immobilization of free-ranging wildlife should only be considered when necessary for research or management goals. Captures should be carried out by a team of professionals with proper training, experience, and expertise in wildlife capture, veterinary anesthesia, animal handling, and human and animal first aid and CPR techniques.

All captures must be properly planned, and species-specific capture protocols should be developed. Doses required for immobilization of free-ranging animals are generally higher than those required in captive individuals (Kreeger & Arnemo 2012). In general, overdosing is probably safer than underdosing because extended induction times may cause increased stress and risk of complications.

Chemical immobilization of free-ranging wildlife is a challenging procedure. It is generally not possible to access the patient for a preoperative physical examination or laboratory work. Even if anesthetic risk could be determined, there are generally only a few effective protocols available for each species. Induction of anesthesia in wildlife can be extremely stressful and can result in stress related injuries. Free-ranging wildlife are subject to the elements and are often at risk for hypo- or hyperthermia. Field personnel may be required to work on species for which there is very little background information. Extrapolation between similar species may be required, but can result in unexpected complications. Human and animal safety must also be considered.

Wildlife anesthesia should be a cooperative effort between biologists and veterinarians. A team approach is invaluable and draws on the strengths of the different specialties. It is essential to include experienced personnel on the capture team and to consult with experienced wildlife managers, biologists, and veterinarians to determine anticipated complications, animal behavior when stressed, and the current approaches to dealing with the target species.

PRECAPTURE CONSIDERATIONS

Planning

Before any wildlife capture procedure, an appropriate plan of action must be devised. The species should be researched to determine the most effective and current technique for capture. Communication, evacuation, and first aid protocols for capture personnel must also be established. Field equipment must be carefully selected.

If potentially dangerous animals are targeted, an appropriate firearms backup should be in place. Personnel should be trained in human first aid, firearms safety, and, when applicable, helicopter safety, wilderness survival skills, rock climbing, and avalanche rescue.

Generally the target animal will need to be approached to within 10–40 meters for accurate drug delivery. Animals may be stalked, approached in a vehicle or helicopter or trapped or snared prior to approach. Trapping has the advantage of limiting movement during the capture event, but it can be more stressful than helicopter capture (Cattet et al. 2003b).

Zoo Animal and Wildlife Immobilization and Anesthesia, Second Edition. Edited by Gary West, Darryl Heard, and Nigel Caulkett.
© 2014 John Wiley & Sons, Inc. Published 2014 by John Wiley & Sons, Inc.

Situation

Capture sites should be preplanned and chosen based on their suitability, for example, to avoid roads, communities, and natural hazards, such as rough terrain or open water. The capture should be planned at an appropriate time of the year, for example, ungulates may be captured in winter to decrease the risk of hyperthermia and to allow for tracking in snow or visualization of animals in a deciduous forest. If specific animals are not targeted, the capture team can choose an animal located in a relatively safe capture environment. Current literature and experts in the field should be consulted prior to the capture to ensure the most suitable technique is used. It may be possible to close areas where wildlife are captured to the public.

It is becoming increasingly necessary to immobilize wildlife in urban environments that contain many hazards. In an urban environment, particular attention must be made to traffic. It is often advisable to enlist the help of law enforcement officers for crowd and traffic control. In these situations, attempts at capture usually continue until the animal is under control or euthanized, increasing the risk of injury and adverse effects (e.g., myopathy and hyperthermia). Often, the personnel involved in these captures are wildlife managers, such as wardens or conservation officers. Therefore, it is important to use drug combinations with a rapid onset and a high margin of safety.

Terrain

The ideal capture site should allow good visualization of the animal during the induction period. Particular attention should be paid to open bodies of water, as some species may enter the water after dart placement and be at risk of drowning. Mountainous terrain has obvious risks associated with it. Capture personnel with climbing experience are valuable when working in mountains or canyons. Forest is also hazardous as animals may be difficult to track beneath the canopy. Dogs trained in tracking wildlife species are useful if a darted animal is lost out of sight. Telemetry darts may also be useful in these situations. Some species, such as black bears and mountain lions, may climb trees to escape capture. Equipment should be available to cushion their fall or to facilitate removing the animal from the tree (Fig. 9.1).

Weather

Weather conditions often dictate if wildlife capture is possible. Helicopter work is not possible in high winds or foggy conditions. In remote locations, sudden changes in the weather may be a hazard to personnel. It is important to keep track of current and changing conditions during wildlife capture.

Snow and rain can lead to hypothermia, particularly if wind is also present to enhance convective heat loss. Small mammals are most susceptible to hypothermia.

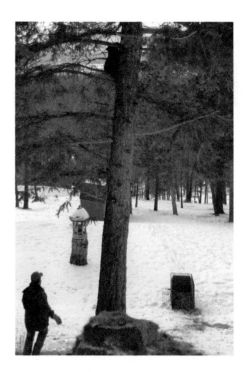

Figure 9.1. Preparation of a cushioned landing area for a bear cub, prior to immobilization in a tree.

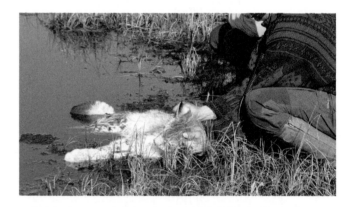

Figure 9.2. Cooling a hyperthermic lynx in a pond.

However, hyperthermia is generally a more serious concern as several of the drug regimens used for wildlife capture impede thermoregulation and lead to hyperthermia (Cattet et al. 2003a; Klein & Klide 1989). Hyperthermia is a serious complication that can be difficult to treat in field situations. When possible, captures in the summer should be planned for the cooler hours of the day. Animals can also become hyperthermic in cold temperatures if they experience physical exertion during the induction period. Also, even in hot tropical climates, small animals can develop hypothermia during anesthesia. Provision should be made to prevent heat loss and to actively cool animals if needed (Fig. 9.2).

Target Species

Prior to embarking on a capture session, it is important to become as familiar as possible with the target species, including a search of current literature and consultation with experts for that species. Nontarget animals may include animals of the right species, but the wrong sex or age class. If traps are used, nontarget species may be caught. Researchers need to anticipate which nontarget species may be trapped, determine if nontarget animals must be anesthetized (e.g., if they are too aggressive to release directly or if they should be marked for other research groups), and be familiar with the best current techniques for anesthesia of these species. Wildlife managers need to be familiar with techniques for all the species they may encounter in the course of their work.

Emergency Equipment

Space limitations dictate what type of equipment can be carried in a field situation. However, capture should not take place unless all necessary equipment can be brought to the animal. A portable oxygen source should be part of the standard field equipment (Fig. 9.3).

Hypoxemia is a common complication of wildlife anesthesia (Caulkett & Arnemo 2007; Read 2003). Oxygen therapy is fundamental for prevention and treatment of hypoxemia during anesthesia. Lightweight aluminum cylinders, combined with a sturdy regulator, are handy for field use. Portable battery-powered oxygen concentrators are also useful, especially in remote locations where logistics with oxygen cylinders can be difficult (Fahlman et al. 2012). Oxygen therapy is further described in Chapter 5.

Equipment for airway support, including appropriately sized endotracheal tubes and a bag valve mask (resuscitator) to enable mechanical ventilation should be included in an emergency kit. As ruminants are

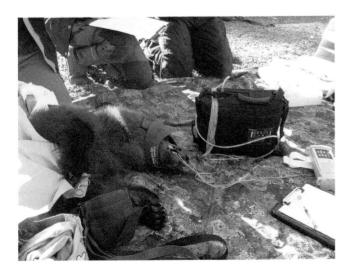

Figure 9.3. Use of a portable oxygen concentrator to provide supplemental inspired oxygen to a brown bear cub.

predisposed to rumenal tympany during anesthesia, it is wise to carry a rumen tube to facilitate decompression of the rumen. A small surgical kit should also be carried to treat lacerations and other injuries (see checklist in Kreeger & Arnemo 2012). Equipment should be carefully chosen to withstand use in a field situation and to be as lightweight and compact as possible.

Immobilizing Drugs

Drug needs must be anticipated; it is wise to budget for at least 50% more drug than is actually needed for the target animals. This will help offset any wasted drug from lost darts or poor dart placement. Resuscitation equipment must be available for use in the target animals. A basic emergency kit containing epinephrine, atropine, local anesthetics, and reversal agents should always be carried. A checklist of emergency drugs can be found in Kreeger and Arnemo (2012).

Capture Techniques

Physical capture, such as net gunning, rocket nets, drive nets, traps, and snares, can induce greater stress than chemical immobilization (Boesch et al. 2011; Cattet et al. 2003b), with higher rates of trauma and mortality (Arnemo et al. 2006; DelGiudice et al. 2001, 2005; Jacques et al. 2009; Webb et al. 2008). Also, injury and even death of humans are not uncommon during physical capture of wildlife (Jessup et al. 1988; López-Olvera et al. 2009). Jessup et al. (1988) reported that over a 12-year period, in New Zealand, there were 127 helicopter crashes and 25 human fatalities during net gun capture of red deer.

Physical restraint should be of short duration, and administration of sedatives or anesthetics are recommended to prevent or reduce distress (Arnemo et al. 2005; Cattet et al. 2004; Mentaberre et al. 2010). In free-ranging wolverines captured with a snare pole, followed by drug injection by hand, the muscular activity related to struggling resulted in similar lactate levels as in wolverines captured by darting from a helicopter (Fahlman et al. 2008). In most cases, chemical immobilization is probably less stressful for a wild animal than handling with physical restraint alone. Contrary to widespread belief, chemical immobilization from a helicopter is perhaps the least stressful capture method for a wide range of mammalian species. In most circumstances, the animal can be rapidly approached, darted, found, handled, and treated, minimizing stress and the risks of capture.

Helicopter Safety

Helicopters can be hazardous, and appropriate training and protective equipment, such as helmets, will help to minimize the risk of injury. Particular attention must be paid to the height of the rotor when entering and exiting the helicopter, especially when landing in

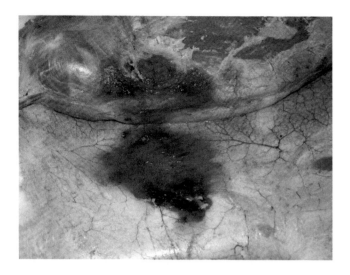

Figure 9.4. Even with lightweight, low velocity darts, impact can cause trauma. This photo shows dart impact trauma in a lynx.

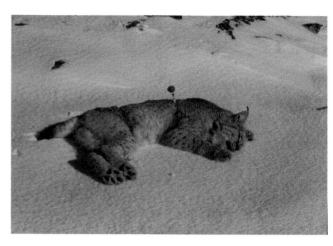

Figure 9.5. Poor dart placement results in a high risk of complications and injury, including pneumothorax.

uneven terrain or on hillsides. A harness that allows only enough room for the darter to attain the proper position is essential. Detailed reviews of helicopter safety are found in Nielsen (1999), Kock and Burroughs (2012) and Chapter 13.

ANIMAL SAFETY CONSIDERATIONS FOR REMOTE DRUG DELIVERY EQUIPMENT

Remote drug delivery systems have the potential to produce serious injury and death, if used inappropriately. The major sources of injury arise from dart impact trauma, high velocity injection of dart contents, and inaccurate dart placement. Dart impact trauma (Fig. 9.4) results from dispersion of energy on dart impact. Impact energy is represented by the following equation: $KE = 1/2M \times V^2$ where M = mass of the dart and V = velocity (Kreeger & Arnemo 2012). High velocity is the major factor resulting in trauma. To minimize trauma, use the lowest velocity that will result in an accurate trajectory at a given distance. Practice with a darting system at a variety of distances is vital to minimize velocity. The other major factor is the mass of the dart. Darts with a lower mass will have less impact energy. This should be a consideration in choice of a darting system, particularly in smaller animals that are more prone to trauma. Inaccurate dart placement can result in injury, most frequently if darts penetrate the abdomen, thorax (Fig. 9.5), or vital structures of the neck. The major factors that can lead to inaccurate dart placement are a lack of practice with the darting system, attempting dart placement over an excessive range, and inherent inaccuracy of the darting system. The final source of injury is related to high velocity injection of dart contents. Systems that expel drug via an explosive charge can produce severe tissue disruption

and trauma (Cattet et al. 2006). These systems should only be used on large, well-muscled animals. Volume of injection should be minimized to decrease the degree of tissue trauma. When possible, darts that deliver their contents via compressed air should be used to minimize trauma. The choice of system depends on the range required, the drug volume used and thus the size of the dart, and individual characteristics of the target animal. A more complete review can be found in Bush (1992), Isaza (2007), Kreeger and Arnemo (2012) and Chapter 11.

COMPLICATIONS

Stress

Fear, chasing, physical restraint, and/or chemical immobilization of wild animals will elicit an acute stress response that may compromise the physiologic homeostasis of an animal and cause distress. The capture event, as well as the immobilizing drugs, influence the physiology and homeostasis of the animal. Muscular activity associated with chasing, excitement and resistance to handling results in lactic acid build-up and an increased body temperature. Increasing lactic acid levels lead to reduced blood pH and subsequent acidosis. Immobilizing drugs interfere with normal respiratory function and thermoregulation, and can lead to respiratory depression, acidosis, hypoxemia and hyperthermia. Blood levels of oxygen and carbon dioxide are closely related to, and affected by, acid–base balance and electrolyte concentrations. Minute changes in body temperature, respiratory patterns, and metabolic demands can alter this balance, resulting in neurological or myocardial dysfunction, multi-organ failure, capture myopathy, or acute mortality (Williams & Thorne 1996). See Chapter 12.

The time of intensive helicopter pursuit and the time of physical restraint should be minimized to decrease the risk of stress-related problems, including capture myopathy, hyperthermia, and trauma. The level of exertion the animal develops can be more important than the duration and distance of helicopter pursuit. In one report, ungulates that were chased rapidly over short distances develop a more severe acidemia compared with if they are run longer distances at slower speed (Harthoorn & van der Walt 1974). The extent of physical exertion may also be influenced by the conditions, including incline, altitude, snow depth, and ambient temperature.

In cases of acute distress, immediate reversal of immobilization and release of the animal should be considered unless effective treatment can be initiated. Emergency drugs including epinephrine, atropine, doxapram, local anesthetics, and reversal agents should always be carried. Fluids for i.v. treatment of shock or hypo- or hyperthermia should be available.

For translocations, administration of short- or long-acting tranquilizers is indicated to prevent distress (Ebedes 1993; Read et al. 2000; Read & McCorkell 2002). Fear is a potent stressor and following capture, a blindfold and earplugs should be used to decrease visual and auditory stimulation.

Induction

Dart placement is the most important determinant of induction time with quickest absorption occurring after injection in large muscle masses, such as the neck, shoulder, or hindquarters. Other factors that may influence induction time include the dose received, the animal's physical condition, age and sex, and its sensitivity to the immobilizing drugs. Animals that are excited or stressed can have induction times that are considerably longer than calm animals. As soon as the dart is placed, the time should be recorded and the animal must be carefully observed to ensure that it is not lost or injured during the induction period.

If a helicopter is used in pursuit, it must retreat so that the animal can be observed with less stress for the animal. The helicopter may need to steer an animal away from potential hazards, such as cliffs or open water.

Initial Assessment

Initial approach to an immobilized animal is a dangerous time. The animal should be observed from a safe distance to determine that there is no purposeful movement. When alpha$_2$–adrenergic agonist-based protocols are used, for example, medetomidine-ketamine and xylazine-tiletamine-zolazepam, there should be no movement of the head or limbs prior to approach. If tiletamine-zolazepam alone or opioids are used, there may be some involuntary movement in adequately immobilized animals. The position of the animal

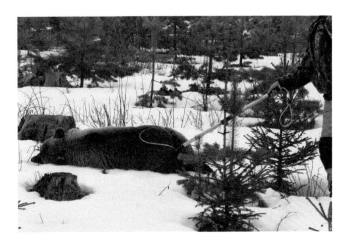

Figure 9.6. Using a pole to check that the bear is safely anesthetized before approaching.

should be observed from a distance to ensure that the position of the head and neck all ensure a patent airway. Respiratory movements can also be observed from a distance. Once it has been determined that the animal is safe to approach, the animal should be cautiously approached accompanied by a firearm backup if necessary. It is important to leave safe exits for the capture team and the animal. Auditory stimulation, such as clapping or shouting, should be employed as the animal is approached to gauge the animal's response. If there is no response to auditory stimulation, the response to tactile stimulation should be gauged. It is advisable to use a stick or pole to extend reach when stimulating the animal (Fig. 9.6). When it is safe, the palpebral reflex can be checked. A set of vital signs, including rectal temperature, respiratory rate, and heart rate, should be obtained. The eyes should be lubricated with an isotonic ophthalmic solution or gel, and a blindfold should be placed to decrease visual stimulation and to protect the cornea from dust and sunlight. Earplugs are useful to minimize auditory stimuli. At this point, hobbles may be considered to limit movement in the event of a sudden recovery.

Anesthetic Depth and Arousal

Depth of anesthesia should be closely monitored throughout the procedure. Factors that increase the risk of sudden arousal include loud noises (especially distress vocalization of young), movement of the animal or changes in the body position, or painful stimuli. Techniques for monitoring depth of anesthesia depend on the anesthetic agent. Tiletamine-zolazepam usually produces reliable anesthesia with predictable signs of recovery. As anesthesia lightens, spontaneous blinking will occur, with carnivores often developing chewing and paw movements. They will start to lift their head and may attempt to raise themselves with their forelimbs. Animals showing signs of recovery, including spontaneous blinking, generally require a "top-up" unless they can be left to recover. The choice of drug depends on the length of the remaining procedures and depth of anesthesia needed. Tiletamine-zolazepam, ketamine, or medetomidine can be used, although top-up doses of tiletamine-zolazepam can significantly prolong recovery, and should only be used if >30 minutes of additional down time is required. Ketamine or medetomidine are drugs of choice if 5–20 minutes of additional time is needed. Top-up drugs can be given intramuscularly or intravenously, with intravenous drugs acting faster with shorter duration than intramuscular drugs.

Respiratory Depression and Hypoxemia

Hypoxemia is a common complication during wildlife anesthesia. Reasons for hypoxemia and respiratory depression, as well as treatment, are discussed in detail in Chapter 5.

Hyperthermia

Rectal temperature should be monitored throughout anesthesia. Most species are prone to hyperthermia. Causative factors include high ambient temperatures, excessive muscular exertion from prolonged pursuit, and interference with normal thermoregulatory mechanisms by anesthetic drugs. Symptoms include rapid, shallow breathing, panting, and weak, rapid, or irregular heart rate, and ultimately, convulsions and death. A rectal temperature of 40°C or 2–3°C greater than normal is cause for concern. Rectal temperatures in excess of 41°C are an emergency and should be treated aggressively. Treatment in the field can include moving the animal into shade, spraying with cold water, cooling in a lake or stream, fanning, packing ice or snow in the inguinal and axillary regions, cool intravenous fluids, and cold water enemas. It is difficult to actively cool large animals, and antagonism of anesthetic agents to allow the animal's normal thermoregulatory mechanisms to recover should be considered. Hyperthermia greatly increases metabolic oxygen demand, and in the face of hypoxemia, is a particularly serious complication. Hyperthermic animals should receive supplemental oxygen.

Intravenous administration of cool fluids can help to decrease body temperature even at low volumes (5–10 mL/kg, repeated if necessary). Hyperthermia may be prevented by avoiding immobilization or capture on very warm days or limiting activities to the coolest part of the day. Avoid prolonged intensive pursuit, keep stress to a minimum, and use the least stressful methods for physical restraint. Protect the animal from direct exposure to the sun.

Hypothermia

Hypothermia is a concern when animals are immobilized during low ambient temperatures, and in young animals, animals with small body masses, and animals in poor body condition. Although body temperature is species specific, hypothermia in most mammals is characterized by a decrease in body temperature to below 35°C. If unchecked, it may result in prolonged recovery, acidosis, and arrhythmias. Causative factors of hypothermia include low ambient temperature, evaporative cooling from windchill, wetness, or precipitation and drugs that impair thermoregulation. Supportive procedures should begin when a declining trend in body temperature is noted and include an immediate attempt to increase body temperature by drying wet animals, covering the animal and providing external heat sources such as hot water bottles. Hypothermia may be prevented by avoiding immobilization or capture on very cold days. Protect the immobilized animal from low ambient temperatures and exposure to wind and precipitation. Keep it warm and dry by covering with blankets or a sleeping bag. Minimize conductive heat loss by maintaining the animal insulated from direct ground contract.

Vomiting and Regurgitation

Vomiting and regurgitation are emergencies in an immobilized animal. If inhalation of stomach contents occurs, aspiration pneumonia can result, requiring prolonged intensive care that usually is not possible for wild animals. In some species, vomiting is a common side effect of opioids and alpha-2 antagonists (Kreeger & Arnemo 2012). Animals should be positioned so that the nose is sloping downwards from the back of the head to decrease the risk of inhaling regurgitated materials. If vomiting occurs in smaller moveable animals, the animal should be placed in sternal recumbency with the head pointed downwards. A long-acting broad-spectrum antibiotic should be considered for animals showing signs of aspiration, such as witnessed aspiration events, rumen contents on the nose, or harsh lung sounds.

Bloat

Bloat during wildlife capture is usually caused by lateral recumbency or by rumenal atony following administration of alpha$_2$–adrenergic agonists. Ruminants should be positioned in sternal recumbeny to reduce the risk of of rumenal tympany. Tympany results from the inability to relieve gases from the rumen or stomach through eructation. Supportive treatment consists of placing the immobilized animal in sternal recumbency with the neck extended and the head forward, permitting saliva to drain. Move the animal from side to side over the brisket and elevate the front quarters of smaller animals. If positioning does not relieve the bloat, insert a lubricated and properly sized tube via the esophagus into the rumen to relieve pressure. Generally, in animals immobilized with alpha$_2$–adrenergic agonists, bloat will resolve following the administration of an alpha-2 antagonist. In the face of severe bloat, procedures should be completed, and the immobilization should be reversed. The last resort is trocharization of the rumen using a large bore (12.5 g or 2.5 mm), long (2.4–3.1″ or 60–80 mm) needle.

Trauma

During the process of immobilization and capture, physical injuries, such as contusions, lacerations, abrasions, punctures, and fractures, may be inflicted on the animal accidentally or as a result of mishandling. Minor lacerations may be flushed, cleaned, and protected with an insect repellant. An appropriate long-acting antibiotic may be given to help prevent infection. Closure may be considered for large lacerations; they should be flushed copiously, cleaned, and debrided. These lacerations are often contaminated, and if they are closed, appropriate drainage must be considered in the closure. Fractures and other serious conditions are difficult to treat effectively and will often require that the animal be euthanized for humane reasons.

Physical trauma may be prevented by taking notice of any hazard in the environment that may cause injury to the animal during capture and by careful handling. If traps, snares, nets, or other forms of manual capture or restraint are used, they should be appropriate for the species, and set by well-trained individuals.

Pneumothorax

An uncommon cause of hypoxemia includes pneumothorax. Dart penetration of the thoracic cavity can result in pneumothorax. It may be possible to treat pneumothorax with thoracocentesis. Equipment should be carried to perform thoracocentesis in the field. See Sigrist (2008) for instructions on thoracocentesis.

Myopathy

Most free–ranging, wild animals exert themselves only infrequently to escape danger. They are not conditioned for running hard over long distances. Chasing wild animals by helicopter or motor vehicle for capture causes a tremendous amount of stress, resulting in intensive muscular activity. The effects of sympathetic exhaustion from sustained stress, combined with intense muscular exertion, are causative factors of various life-threatening syndromes, known as *exertional myopathy* (Paterson 2007; Spraker 1993; Williams & Thorne 1996); see Chapter 15.

Exertional myopathy is difficult to treat and prevention is of utmost importance. Capture myopathy may be prevented by reducing capture stress, fear, and exertion (by limiting chasing time), minimizing visual and auditory stimulation, handling, and restraint of the captured animal and by providing a stress-free recovery environment. More details and treatment options are presented in Chapter 12.

Recovery

Considerations for recovery will vary depending on the choice of drug and the situation. In most situations, reversible drugs are desirable. If reversible drugs are not used, the animal should be observed until it is able to ambulate, to protect itself from other animals, and to avoid environmental hazards. Prior to reversal, equipment should be removed from the capture site. The animal should be placed in a suitable position and the airway should be clear. Typically, one person should remain with the animal to administer the reversal drug and thereafter retreat to a safe distance to observe the animal's recovery. Antagonists should be administered IM unless there is an immediate need for rapid recovery.

Environmental factors during recovery are critical and expected recovery times must be considered. Before reversal agents are given, animals should be placed away from hazards, such as cliffs or open water. They should also be placed out of the wind and sun. In species that move a lot during recovery, such as wolves immobilized with tiletamine-zolazepam, capture personnel should remain at the site to steer the animal away from hazards.

Mortalities

Typically, the highest mortality rates are seen in the early stages of a project; before capture methods are refined, drug doses are adjusted and the immobilization team has gained adequate experience and training. Moreover, an increased risk of mortality may also be seen when captures are carried out for specific purposes, such as health evaluation of animals under environmental or pathogenic stress. Mortalities caused by capture and anesthesia of free-ranging mammals can be grouped into three categories: (1) direct effects of the immobilizing drug, for example, respiratory depression, shock, hyperthermia, and asphyxia due to tympany or vomiting. (2) Indirect effects, for example, drowning during induction or recovery, pneumothorax due to misplacement of darts, and trauma from dart impact. Such mortalities might be a direct consequence of the drug used, for example, etorphine often induces hyperthermia, and this may cause the animal to actively seek water for cooling, with drowning as a possible sequela. (3) Secondary effects caused by the capture process, for example, trauma from traps, long-term effects from chasing or stress (exertional myopathy), separation of dam–offspring, and various problems with radiocollars or implantable transmitters. The secondary effects, however, have nothing to do with the anesthetic risk *per se* and should be treated as a separate entity.

A mortality rate greater than 2% during chemical immobilization is unacceptable for any mammalian species and requires that the anesthetic protocol be reevaluated (Arnemo et al. 2006). By using immobilizing drugs and doses with proven safety, proper remote drug delivery systems, and established capture methods and techniques, a skilled and experienced capture team will minimize the risk of anesthetic mortality.

In the event of mortalities, the situation should be evaluated to assess the cause of the mortality and future preventative measures. A necropsy should be performed either on-site, or the animal should be sent to a diagnostic laboratory. The necropsy can be helpful for determining if the animal was abnormal or if a healthy animal died under anesthesia.

Euthanasia

Equipment or drugs for humane euthanasia should always be carried during animal captures. The method of euthanasia depends on the situation and species. In many countries, the veterinarian is legally responsible for the death of animals, including endangered species, that eat a euthanized carcass. If firearms or bolt guns are used (recommended if the meat will be salvaged), personnel must be trained in the use of the firearms and the appropriate bullet/bolt placement.

CONCLUSION

A thorough understanding of the inherent risks associated with animal capture is indispensible for prevention of capture-related injuries. Careful planning, close monitoring, and early intervention are essential for preventing morbidity and mortality.

REFERENCES

Arnemo JM, Storaas T, Khadka CB, Wegge P. 2005. Use of medetomidine-ketamine and atipamezole for reversible immobilization of free-ranging hog deer (*Axis porcinus*) captured in drive nets. *Journal of Wildlife Diseases* 42:467–470.

Arnemo JM, Ahlqvist P, Andersen R, Berntsen F, Ericsson G, Odden J, Brunberg S, Segerström P, Swenson JE. 2006. Risk of capture-related mortality in large free-ranging mammals: experiences from Scandinavia. *Wildlife Biology* 12:109–113.

Boesch JM, Boulanger JR, Curtis PD, Erb HN, Ludders JW, Kraus MS, Gleed RD. 2011. Biochemical variables in free-ranging white-tailed deer (*Odocoileus virginianus*) after chemical immobilization in clover traps or via ground-darting. *Journal of Zoo and Wildlife Medicine* 42:18–28.

Bush M. 1992. Remote drug delivery systems. *Journal of Zoo and Wildlife Medicine* 23:159–180.

Cattet MRL, Caulkett NA, Stenhouse GB. 2003a. Anesthesia of grizzly bears using xylazine-zolazepam-tiletamine or zolazepam-tiletamine. *Ursus (International Association for Bear Research and Management)* 14:88–93.

Cattet MRL, Christison K, Caulkett NA, Stenhouse GB. 2003b. Physiologic responses of grizzly bears to different methods of capture. *Journal of Wildlife Diseases* 39:649–654.

Cattet MRL, Caulkett NA, Wilson C, Vandenbrink T, Brook RK. 2004. Intranasal administration of xylazine to reduce stress in elk captured by net gun. *Journal of Wildlife Diseases* 40:562–565.

Cattet MRL, Bourque A, Elken BT, Powley KD, Dahlstrom DB, Caulkett NA. 2006. Evaluation of the potential for injury with

remote drug-delivery systems. *Wildlife Society Bulletin* 34:741–749.

Caulkett NA, Arnemo JM. 2007. Chemical immobilization of free-ranging terrestrial mammals. In: *Lumb and Jones' Veterinary Anesthesia and Analgesia*, 4th ed. (WJ Tranquilli, JC Thurmon, KA Grimm, eds.), pp. 807–831. Ames: Blackwell Publishing.

DelGiudice GD, Mangipane BA, Sampson BA, Kochanny CO. 2001. Chemical immobilization, body temperature, and post-release mortality of white-tailed deer captured by Clover trap and net-gun. *Wildlife Society Bulletin* 29:1147–1157.

DelGiudice GD, Sampson BA, Kuehn DW, Powell MC, Fieberg J. 2005. Understanding margins of safe capture, chemical immobilization, and handling of free-ranging white-tailed deer. *Wildlife Society Bulletin* 33:677–687.

Ebedes H. 1993. The use of long-acting tranquilizers in captive wild animals. In: *The Capture and Care Manual. Capture, Care, Accomodation and Transportation of Wild African Animals* (AA Mckenzie, ed.), pp. 71–99. Pretoria: Wildlife Decision Support Services and The South African Veterinary Foundation.

Fahlman Å, Arnemo JM, Persson J, Segerström P, Nyman G. 2008. Capture and medetomidine-ketamine anesthesia in free-ranging wolverines (*Gulo gulo*). *Journal of Wildlife Diseases* 44:133–142.

Fahlman Å, Caulkett N, Arnemo JM, Neuhaus P, Ruckstuhl KE. 2012. Efficacy of a portable oxygen concentrator with pulsed delivery for treatment of hypoxemia during anesthesia of wildlife. *Journal of Zoo and Wildlife Medicine* 43:67–76.

Harthoorn AM, van der Walt K. 1974. Physiological aspects of forced exercise in wild ungulates with special reference to (so-called) over-straining disease. *Journal of the South African Wildlife Management Association* 4:25–28.

Haymerle A, Fahlman Å, Walzer C. 2010. Human exposure to immobilizing agents: results of an online survey. *Veterinary Record* 167:327–332.

Isaza R. 2007. Remote drug delivery. In: *Zoo Animal and Wildlife Immobilization and Anesthesia* (G West, D Heard, N Caulkett, eds.), pp. 61–74. Ames: Blackwell Publishing.

Jacques CN, Jenks JA, Deperno CS, Sievers JD, Grovenburg TW, Brinkman TJ, Swanson CS, Stillings BA. 2009. Evaluating ungulate mortality associated with helicopter net-gun captures in the Northern Great Plains. *Journal of Wildlife Management* 73:1282–1291.

Jessup DA, Clark RK, Weaver RA, Kock MD. 1988. The safety and cost-effectiveness of net-gun capture of desert bighorn sheep (*Ovis canadensis nelsoni*). *Journal of Zoo Animal Medicine* 19:208–213.

Klein LV, Klide AM. 1989. Central alpha 2 adrenergic and benzodiazepine agonists and their antagonists. *Journal of Zoo and Wildlife Medicine* 20:138–153.

Kock MD, Burroughs R. 2012. *Chemical and Physical Restraint of Wild Animals. A Training and Field Manual for African Species*, 2nd ed. Greyton: International Wildlife Veterinary Services (Africa).

Kreeger TJ, Arnemo JM. 2012. *Handbook of Wildlife Chemical Immobilization*, 4th ed. Wheatland: TJ Kreeger.

López-Olvera JR, Marco I, Montané J, Casa-Díaz E, Mentaberre G, Lavín S. 2009. Comparative evaluation of effort, capture and handling effects of drive nets to capture of roe deer (*Capreolus capreolus*), southern chamois (*Rupicapra pyrenaica*) and Spanish ibex (*Capra pyrenaica*). *European Journal of Wildlife Research* 55:193–202.

Mentaberre G, López-Olvera JR, Casa-Díaz E, Fernández-Sirera L, Marco I, Lavín S. 2010. Effects of azaperone and haloperidol on the stress response of drive-net captured Iberian ibexes (*Capra pyrenaica*). *European Journal of Wildlife Research* 56:757–764.

Nielsen L. 1999. *Chemical Immobilization of Wild and Exotic Animals*. Ames: Iowa State University Press.

Paterson J. 2007. Capture myopathy. In: *Zoo Animal and Wildlife Immobilization and Anesthesia* (G West, D Heard, N Caulkett, eds.), pp. 115–121. Ames: Blackwell Publishing.

Read M, Caulkett N, McCallister M. 2000. Evaluation of zuclopenthixol acetate to decrease handling stress in wapiti. *Journal of Wildlife Diseases* 36:450–459.

Read MR. 2003. A review of alpha-2 adrenoceptor agonists and the development of hypoxemia in domestic and wild ruminants. *Journal of Zoo and Wildlife Medicine* 34:134–138.

Read MR, McCorkell RB. 2002. Use of azaperone and zuclopenthixol acetate to facilitate translocation of white-tailed deer (*Odocoileus virginianus*). *Journal of Zoo and Wildlife Medicine* 33:163–165.

Sigrist SE. 2008. Thoracocentesis. In: *Small Animal Critical Care Medicine*. (D Silverstein, K Hopper, eds.), pp. 131–133. St. Louis: W.B. Saunders.

Spraker TR. 1993. Stress and and capture myoptahy in artiodactylids. In: *Zoo and Wildlife Medicine: Current Therapy 3* (ME Fowler, ed.), pp. 481–488. Philadelphia: W.B. Saunders.

Webb SL, Lewis JS, Hewitt DG, Hellickson MW, Bryant FC. 2008. Assessing the helicopter and net gun as a capture technique for white-tailed deer. *Journal of Wildlife Management* 72:310–314.

Williams ES, Thorne ET. 1996. Exertional myopathy (capture myopathy). In: *Noninfectious Diseases of Wildlife* (A Fairbrother, LN Locke, GL Hoff, eds.), pp. 181–193. Ames: Manson Publishing.

10 Euthanasia

Murray Woodbury

INTRODUCTION

Euthanasia is the act of humanely causing the death of an animal. To be considered euthanasia rather than just the termination of a life, the act must minimize any pain, distress, or anxiety experienced by the animal prior to its death. An ideal euthanasia technique would induce a very rapid loss of consciousness in the animal followed by cardiac and respiratory arrest and the loss of brain function (American Veterinary Medical Association [AVMA] 2013). The method would also be reliable, irreversible, and relatively safe for the operator. This ideal method, and indeed many of the recommended techniques for domestic and laboratory animals, are usually not possible in the zoo or under field conditions where many of the factors involved with euthanasia are not well controlled. Under these circumstances, the taking of an animal's life is more often humane killing rather than euthanasia. In zoos and wildlife environments, consideration for factors such as degree of control over the animal, operator and public safety, species peculiarities, and carcass disposal may result in some unavoidable pain and anxiety associated with a rapid and efficient death.

Wildlife and zoo veterinarians and any other person involved with animal research or management are ultimately responsible for the animals under their influence and should be prepared for the possibility of euthanasia in irreversibly diseased or injured animals. They should be familiar with the available techniques for the species and obtain and prepare the required materials and equipment in advance so that correct euthanasia is possible if necessary. Persons actually performing euthanasia should have the appropriate training and experience to ensure that pain and distress are minimized during the procedure.

CONSIDERATIONS FOR WILDLIFE AND ZOO SPECIES

The primary consideration should be providing a quick and painless death whenever possible. In wildlife and zoo situations where the animal is not well confined or restrained, this sometimes means the use of an appropriate caliber firearm to inflict a fatal wound. In free-ranging animals, a fatal headshot may be difficult to accomplish and accidental injury to the animal or an unintended target may be the result. A shot to the heart and lungs is more easily achieved and requires less skill from the operator. Death in this case is not as rapid but it is much more certain under free-ranging conditions (Canadian Council on Animal Care [CCAC] 2003). In other situations, whenever possible the chosen method or combination of methods should involve the use of a chemical or physical technique that first depresses the central nervous system to ensure immediate insensitivity to pain and relief from distress, fear, and apprehension, followed by the irreversible arrest of the animal's respiratory and cardiac function and subsequent brain death.

The practical problems associated with disposal of one large or several individual euthanatized animals and the environmental risks posed to animal scavengers or humans in contact with a carcass euthanatized with toxic chemicals must also be considered. Incineration, burial, or adulteration of the carcass with quick lime are acceptable but not always possible especially with megavertebrates or marine mammals. A chemical-free euthanasia protocol should be used where carcass disposal is not practical or possible.

Consideration should be given to the collection of postmortem samples for diagnostic or research purposes. Where animals are sacrificed for scientific study or disease surveillance the method of euthanasia should

Zoo Animal and Wildlife Immobilization and Anesthesia, Second Edition. Edited by Gary West, Darryl Heard, and Nigel Caulkett.
© 2014 John Wiley & Sons, Inc. Published 2014 by John Wiley & Sons, Inc.

not destroy the tissues or organs of interest. For instance, a gunshot to the brain is not appropriate where animals are to be tested for rabies or other central nervous system diseases.

Methods

The choice of a suitable method of euthanasia depends on the species, size, weight, and behavioral characteristics of the animal. The type of restraint possible, the facilities and equipment available, the number and skill of assisting personnel, and the risks involved should be considered. Economics and the number of animals to euthanatize can also affect the decision.

Literature specific to the species of interest should be consulted when planning euthanasia or activities that could result in euthanasia. Detailed recommendations for euthanasia can be found in the 2013 Guidelines on Euthanasia (formerly the Report of the AVMA Panel on Euthanasia) (AVMA 2013) and the Guidelines on Euthanasia of Nondomestic Animals (American Association of Zoo Veterinarians [AAZV] 2006). Much of the information in this chapter is derived from these sources.

Depending on the chosen method of euthanasia, death results from hypoxia, central nervous system depression, physical damage to the brain, or a combination of these mechanisms. The means of inducing these changes can be chemical, physical, or electrical (Table 10.1). Current guidelines on euthanasia (AVMA 2013) classify methods as acceptable, conditionally acceptable, or generally unacceptable. Conditionally accepted methods are those that may be acceptable for emergen-

cies, or unplanned euthanasia, where rapid killing rather than true euthanasia is achieved. Some unacceptable methods may become acceptable when used in euthanasia protocols where deep anesthesia is provided prior to using the method. Such combined methods are called two-stage protocols, and are especially important when animals cannot be adequately restrained to receive primary methods, such as intravenous euthanasia drugs or a precisely applied physical means of euthanasia. The first stage generally renders the animal unconscious so that it can be approached or humanely restrained for a lethal secondary procedure.

The use of immobilizing drugs followed by a chemical or physical method of euthanasia should be considered to gain control over the movements of free-ranging animals or when close restraint is either too stressful or impossible to achieve in a zoo setting. Immobilizing doses of sedative drugs, usually delivered by a dart gun or blow pipe, can be used to induce a rapid loss of consciousness, permitting the operator direct contact with the animal to subsequently administer suitable chemical or physical euthanasia. An important historical exception to this sequence is when succinylcholine is used as the immobilant drug (Schwartz et al. 1997). Succinylcholine rapidly induces paralysis but offers no analgesia or relief from distress or anxiety and its use as a primary method for euthanasia is not acceptable. In the past, it has been used in free-ranging wildlife because of its rapid onset and the relatively low risk posed from drug residues in the euthanatized animal (AVMA 2013). However, it is imperative to reach the paralyzed animal

Table 10.1.   Euthanasia methods for wildlife and zoo species

Method	Primary Method for These Species	Secondary Method for These Species	Comments
Inhalant agents			
Volatile anesthetic agents		Amphibians, reptiles, small and medium mammals, hoofstock	Requires a follow up method to ensure death. Not generally suitable in the field or for species that breath hold or having low respiratory rates.
Carbon dioxide		Amphibians, reptiles, small and medium mammals, hoofstock	Concentration of CO_2 must be >40% of inspired air. Can be used to render food animals unconscious but not generally recommended for euthanasia.
Carbon monoxide		Reptiles, small and medium mammals, hoofstock	Concentrations >10% in air are explosive. Odorless gas is toxic to humans and generally not used for safety reasons.
Nitrogen, argon		Small and medium mammals	Generally safe for operator. Motor activity continues until death which can be disturbing to viewers.
Chemical agents			
Barbiturates	All species		Ideal for most species but in amphibians and reptiles a secondary physical method is recommended. Creates carcass disposal problems from secondary toxicity. A controlled drug needing accounting.
T-61	All species		Mixture of three drugs. Must be used IV. Not a smooth as barbiturates. Not available in all countries.
Tricaine methanesulfonate (MS-222), Benzocaine HCl	Fish, amphibians		Leave animal in water bath for >10 minutes after resp. ceases. Requires buffering and disposal. Follow-up method needed to ensure death.

Table 10.1. *(Continued)*

Method	Primary Method for These Species	Secondary Method for These Species	Comments
Potassium chloride		Amphibians, small and medium mammals, hoofstock, and megavertebrates	Give by IV or intracardiac injection. Use only on anesthetized animals.
Neuromuscular blockers (succinylcholine, gallamine)		Reptiles, medium mammals, hoofstock, and megavertebrates	Unsuitable method for primary euthanasia but in limited circumstances might be useful for initial immobilization if followed rapidly by acceptable method.
Formalin, alcohols		Amphibians, small reptiles	Prior anesthesia needed. Very small animals only.
Physical methods			
Gunshot to the head or cervical neck	Unrestrained medium sized mammals, hoofstock, and megavertebrates	Large reptiles, small and medium mammals	Appropriate for free ranging animals in secluded areas or as secondary method. Requires operator training and skill. Safety concerns for unintended targets.
Stunning (concussion or electric)		Amphibians, reptiles, small mammals	Generally used in emergency situations when no other means available. Should be followed by a secondary method, for example, exsanguination.
Penetrating captive bolt to the head	Restrained hoofstock	Hoofstock	Adequate restraint or anesthesia needed prior to use. Operator training, skill, and specialized equipment needed.
Cervical dislocation		Small mammals	Small animals only (<200 g). Prior anesthesia recommended
Pithing		Amphibians, reptiles	Prior anesthesia needed. Generally used as a secondary method.
Decapitation		Amphibians, reptiles, small mammals	Prior anesthesia needed. Generally used as a secondary method.
Thoracic compression		Amphibians, reptiles	Not suitable for animals with a diaphragm
Exsanguination		Amphibians, reptiles, small and medium mammals, and megavertebrates	Not a primary method of euthanasia. Useful as a secondary method or confirmation of death.
Hypothermia/rapid freezing		Amphibians, small reptiles, small mammals	Prior anesthesia needed.
Kill traps		Small and medium mammals	Not acceptable in most applications
Maceration	Chicks, very young poultry		Requires special equipment. Birds must be delivered to the macerator without causing injury or distress
Explosives		Megavertebrates	Generally not recommended except when no other means available.

Sources: Guidelines on Euthanasia of Nondomestic Animals, American Association of Zoo Veterinarians (AAZV 2006) and the 2013 AVMA Guidelines on Euthanasia (formerly the 2000 Report of the AVMA Panel on Euthanasia) (AVMA 2013).

as quickly as possible to render it unconscious and insensitive using a secondary method such as a gunshot or penetrating captive bolt to the head. In the case of free-ranging animals, such rapid acquisition of the target animal is usually not possible, and a lethal gunshot should be used as the primary method. In zoo situations, alternate drugs for rendering animals insensible are available, making succinylcholine an obsolete and unacceptable drug for use in euthanasia protocols.

Assessing Death

Verification of death is important for ethical and safety reasons. Animals that recover from attempts at euthanasia can harm nearby personnel through violent physical struggle or defensive acts. Assessing whether death has occurred is especially important when euthanizing potentially dangerous animals and animals that can withstand long periods of anoxia. It is essential that personnel involved with euthanasia be trained to confirm death in the species of concern.

Signs of death include absence of breathing movements, absence of a pulse or a heart beat, discolored mucous membranes with no capillary refill, dilated and fixed pupils, and loss of the corneal reflex. Since none of these signs is universally consistent across species, a physical method of euthanasia such as decapitation or exsanguination should be used as a final step if there is any doubt that death has occurred.

Specific Recommendations

Birds The method most often recommended for birds is the parenteral administration of sodium pentobarbital, preferably intravenously. Exposure to carbon dioxide gas is conditionally acceptable and, which can be used for euthanasia of large numbers of birds. It is also the only chemical method useful for birds intended as food. An overdose of inhalant anesthetics, such as halothane, isoflurane, and sevoflurane, is also conditionally acceptable but should be followed by a method that precludes recovery. Cervical dislocation, stunning, decapitation, or methods causing destruction of the brain, such as gunshot to the head or penetrating captive bolt, are all conditionally acceptable. Methods that are generally unacceptable for birds include potassium chloride injection, thoracic compression, exsanguination, and induction of hypothermia or rapid freezing in liquid nitrogen or dry ice. Where eggs with less than 50% of incubation time are involved, addling (shaking), puncture, freezing, or coating the shell with oil are suitable means.

Amphibians and Reptiles Euthanasia of amphibians is facilitated by their ability to absorb anesthetic drugs through their skin, making immersion in solutions of tricaine methanesulfonate (MS-222) or benzocaine HCl the recommended primary method in these species. Secondary methods such as decapitation, cervical dislocation, or exsanguination should always follow. Electrical or concussive means of stunning followed by decapitation can be conditionally acceptable in circumstances where other methods are not available. Methods that are unacceptable as the sole means of euthanasia include injection of potassium chloride, pithing, exsanguination, and induction of hypothermia or rapid freezing by immersion in liquid nitrogen or dry ice.

Parenteral injection of sodium pentobarbital is recommended as a stand-alone method for both amphibians and reptile species. Conditional chemical methods include inhalation of carbon dioxide gas or fluoridated gas anesthetics, such as halothane. Other conditional means are concussive stunning, decapitation followed by pithing, cervical dislocation, and for species such as crocodilians, captive bolt penetration of the brain. Immersion of smaller reptile species in formalin, formaldehyde, or ethanol is not acceptable without prior deep anesthesia. Potassium chloride injection, carbon monoxide asphyxia, and the use of neuromuscular blockers, such as succinylcholine or gallimine, without prior general anesthesia is unacceptable. Pithing, exsanguination, hypothermia from ice packing and rapid freezing with liquid nitrogen or dry ice are unacceptable except where they are used in a two-stage protocol.

Small- and Medium-Sized Mammals The method most often recommended is sodium pentobarbital injection, preferably intravenously, but also via intracardiac and intraperitoneal routes under some circumstances. Inhalation anesthetics, such as halothane, isoflurane, and sevoflurane, as well as carbon dioxide gas, are conditionally acceptable in small mammals provided another method, usually physical, is used to ensure the termination of life. Physical methods, such as cervical dislocation or decapitation in smaller species, and gunshot or penetrating captive bolt to the head, can be used in medium-sized mammals that are under general anesthesia at the time. Thoracic compression is not suitable in mammals because of the presence of a diaphragm, nor is the induction of hypothermia by refrigerator, refrigerated water, or ice. Rapid freezing with liquid nitrogen is only appropriate for very small mammals already under general anesthesia or newborns and fetuses less than 4 g. Administration of gaseous carbon dioxide, carbon monoxide, argon, or nitrogen is generally unacceptable unless preceded by general anesthesia. Neuromuscular blockade by drugs, such as succinylcholine, is not appropriate as a sole method of euthanasia, but can be used in some circumstances as chemical restraint in a two-stage procedure when followed rapidly by a suitable means of humane killing so that asphyxia and distress are minimized.

Hoofstock In addition to the generally recommended sodium pentobarbital injection, which can be expensive in large animals, administration of a penetrating captive bolt to the brain followed by exsanguination is a recommended method for euthanasia of hoofstock. However, both methods require adequate restraint and close contact with the animal to be effective. Remote delivery of drugs inducing general anesthesia followed by performance of the earlier methods on an immobilized animal is often best. Succinylcholine has been used in some circumstances as a chemical restraint drug in two-stage procedures followed by rapid killing so that asphyxia and animal distress are minimized. However, succinylcholine is not appropriate as a routine immobilizing agent or the sole method of euthanasia. This drug does not render animals unconscious or provide any physical or emotional pain relief. Its use without adjunct drugs or procedures is inhumane and therefore unacceptable (AVMA 2013).

Conditionally acceptable methods applied to hoofstock theoretically include lethal administration of gas anesthetic agents, such as halothane or isoflurane and gunshot to the head or cervical spine region. The latter method, although useful in situations where hands-on methods are not possible, requires operator skill and experience and a suitable firearm and ammunition. Administration of carbon monoxide gas, intravascular or intracardiac potassium chloride solution, or exsanguination are not acceptable without prior general anesthesia.

Megavertebrates and Marine Animals Injection of sodium pentobarbital, although also ideal in these species, requires adequate restraint and large, costly volumes of drug. Prior administration of general anesthesia-inducing drugs such as potent narcotics can facilitate euthanasia with barbiturate. Penetrating captive bolt guns are generally ineffective in such large animals. Gunshot to the head or cervical region of large terrestrial species like elephants and rhinoceros can be appropriate as the sole means of humane killing in some emergency situations and at some locations, but is much less effective with large species such as whales. Explosives have been used to euthanatize beached whales but this method is generally not recommended because of the high level of expertise required and the inherent danger to personnel. Exsanguination is usually acceptable only when used secondary to a procedure that first renders the animal insensible.

SUMMARY

The best method of euthanasia for most captive and free ranging wildlife involves the use of two-stage protocols where the animal is first rendered insensible and then its life is terminated by some efficient and irrevers-

ible means. In those situations, where immediacy and urgency dictate that a more direct method be employed, especially for medium to large species, the use of a firearm is often the quickest and most practical way to humanely end an animal's life under the prevailing circumstances.

REFERENCES

American Association of Zoo Veterinarians (AAZV). 2006. Guidelines on euthanasia of nondomestic animals. American Association of Zoo Veterinarians. http://www.aazv.org/displaycommon.cfm?an=1&subarticlenbr=441 (accessed January 10, 2014).

American Veterinary Medical Association (AVMA). 2013. AVMA Guidelines on euthanasia http://www.avma.org/kb/policies/documents/euthanasia.pdf (accessed May 5, 2014).

Canadian Council on Animal Care (CCAC). 2003. CCAC Guidelines on: the care and use of wildlife. Canadian Council on Animal Care, Ottawa.

Schwartz JA, Warren RJ, Henderson DW, Osborn DA, Kesler DJ. 1997. Captive and field tests of a method for immobilization and euthanasia of urban deer. *Wildlife Society Bulletin* 25(2): 532–541.

11 Remote Drug Delivery

Ramiro Isaza

INTRODUCTION

Practitioners of zoological medicine need to effectively and safely administer anesthetic drugs to nondomestic species. Prior to the development of effective anesthetics and remote delivery systems, veterinary procedures on nondomestic species were either impossible to accomplish or associated with unacceptably high mortality rates. This chapter examines the methods of anesthetic drug delivery with an emphasis on the commercial equipment available to the practitioner in North America.

DIRECT DELIVERY FOR COOPERATIVE ANIMALS

Training for Direct Drug Administration

The technique a clinician selects to administer anesthetic drugs to an animal depends largely on whether or not the animal is cooperative during the preinduction period. Often, the clinician assumes that most nondomestic species are either uncooperative or too dangerous to use traditional routes of drug administration. However, many nondomestic species can be behaviorally restrained following proper training and will often allow the veterinarian to perform a routine physical exam or administer medications on a regular basis. Animals trained for voluntary behavioral restraint are usually well socialized and taught to accept human manipulation. Intramuscular and even intravenous injections can be administered in the same manner as one would treat a domestic animal. For example, a chimpanzee can be trained to place its arm through the cage bars to receive intramuscular injections rather than be subjected to a darting. The more extreme examples are well-trained elephants or whales that permit direct manipulation despite their overwhelming size.

In other nondomestic species, various combinations of mechanical restraints and behavioral training are viable options (see Chapter 8). With proper techniques and safety precautions, manual restraint of smaller nondomestic species for direct-drug administration is often possible. Various mechanical restraint devices, such as horse stanchions or cattle chutes, typically associated with domestic hoofstock, can be adapted for the treatment of nondomestic species (Haigh 1999). An example includes teaching a giraffe or rhinoceros to walk through and stand in a chute for daily physical exams and routine treatments (Fig. 11.1). Once restrained, the animals can be induced with injectable agents or inhalant anesthetics.

In order for any of these methods of direct drug administration to succeed, prior training of the nondomestic animal is critical. Attempting to restrain an animal in an unfamiliar environment for direct drug administration is often unsuccessful, stressful, and dangerous for both the animal and the staff. Consultation with professional trainers and a clearly defined set of target behaviors needed for drug administration is the first step in the process. The trainer's relationship and trust with the animal should not be underestimated. Often an animal will refuse medication offered by a stranger yet will subsequently accept the same medication if presented by the trainer. Effective training prior to the anesthetic procedure can reduce the stress associated with anesthesia and increases the likelihood of compliance.

When feasible, behavioral training and restraint are usually less stressful to the animal, but the veterinarian must be aware of the limitations of this situation. Quiet, well-trained animals may become dangerous if placed in unfamiliar environments such as hospitals, or if given unexpected painful stimulations such as

Zoo Animal and Wildlife Immobilization and Anesthesia, Second Edition. Edited by Gary West, Darryl Heard, and Nigel Caulkett.
© 2014 John Wiley & Sons, Inc. Published 2014 by John Wiley & Sons, Inc.

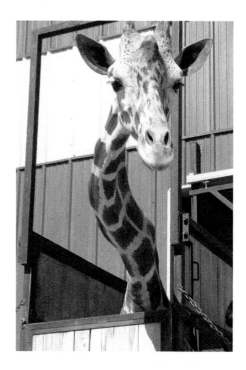

Figure 11.1. Mechanical restraint of a giraffe using a chute.

injections. For example, having the anesthetic procedures begin in the animal's regular enclosure with its usual handler will often facilitate induction.

Manual Drug Delivery Routes for Cooperative Animals

Oral The use of oral anesthetics is occasionally useful in zoological medicine. Some induction agents can be simply sprayed into the oral cavity or placed inside a food item that is then offered to the animal. Oral administration of various anesthetics has been accomplished using pineapple juice, maple syrup, peanut butter, marshmallows, and honey (Thurmon et al. 1996). Oral carfentanil was administered to chimpanzees, tapirs, and bears trans-mucosally by mixing the injectable formulation of the drug into food (Kearns et al. 2000; Mortenson & Bechert 2001; Pollock & Ramsay 2003). The transmucosal formulation of fentanyl was evaluated for use as part of a preanesthetic protocol in great apes (Hunter et al. 2004). Wild animals can be baited with medicated food that is placed in traps or spread out on the ground. One example is the use of oral alpha-chloralose to capture birds (Hayes et al. 2003; Loibl et al. 1988). In situations where animals aggressively open their mouths when provoked, injectable anesthetics can be sprayed into the mouth or the nose for mucosal absorption (Grove & Ramsay 2000). In practice, all of these methods of oral administration are difficult to apply consistently as they require some measure of voluntary cooperation. Also, because the drug needs to be absorbed through the oral or nasal

mucosa, it must remain in contact with the mucosa and not swallowed. Generally, the inductions are prolonged and often unpredictable, but may occasionally work as pre-induction sedation.

Hand-Held Injection Hand injection is the most direct method of administering induction agents to an animal. It usually requires either exceptionally cooperative behavior or restraint for proper placement. For an effective intramuscular injection, even a restrained animal must be approached quietly and given the injection quickly.

The process of administering a hand injection generally involves the following steps:

1. A plastic disposable syringe with Leur-lock hub is selected to avoid needle detachment.
2. A large-gauge needle is selected to prevent breaking the needle during injection and allow fast deposition of the drug.
3. Double check that the needle is firmly attached to the syringe hub.
4. The syringe is loaded with an appropriate dose of the drug.
5. The filled syringe is then grasped between the index and the middle finger with the thumb over the plunger.
6. The injection site is selected.
7. A proper injection technique requires a quick flick of the wrist so that the plunger is pressed as the needle begins to penetrate the skin.

Slower placement of the drug, with aspiration prior to injection, will rarely succeed in unrestrained nondomestic species. The hand injection method of drug administration is considered dangerous for the person injecting the anesthetic. Trauma from bite wounds, kicks, and crushing injuries are common. Of equal concern is the possibility for self-injection subsequent to the animal's sudden movements or exposure to aerosol sprays from a broken syringe. Hand administration of potent narcotics such as carfentanil is therefore not recommended.

Pole Syringes A Pole syringe is essentially a hand injection with the added safety of a long pole. They were primarily developed for use in chute, cage, or trap-restrained animals. This allows the operator to avoid some of the potential trauma associated with direct hand injections. This added safety is, however, at the expense of control of the injection process. Poorly restrained animals invariably react to the needle by moving away or attacking prior to full injection. Similar to the hand injection, the technique requires a quick delivery through a large-gauge needle (14–18g). The needle is inserted in a large muscle, and then the pole is held in position until the drug is deposited.

Three types of pole syringes are available. The manual pressure pole syringe is a typical syringe body with an extended plunger to provide extra length. Once inserted, the plunger is pushed against the resistance of the animal's body. In the second type, the extension pole is attached to the body of the syringe with a second internal extension of the syringe plunger that is manually depressed to deposit the drug. The final type has a mechanism that has a spring or pressurized gas loaded plunger that is triggered when the needle presses on the skin. Although considered safer than hand injection, animals may still react to the needle and cause injury by moving or misdirecting the pole syringe.

REMOTE DELIVERY SYSTEMS FOR UNCOOPERATIVE ANIMALS

Unfortunately, in zoological medicine, many anesthetic procedures are performed on un¬cooperative animals for a variety of reasons. Animals that are not acclimated to human contact generally become agitated and aggressive when approached. This occurs in free-living species or in many captive animals, where routine direct human contact is discouraged. Some species, such as large carnivores or hoofstock, pose significant inherent risks to the veterinarians and keepers that preclude the possibility of using behavioral or physical restraint. Even in cooperative or human-habituated animals, trained behavior can significantly change due to illness or pain so that the training no longer helps facilitate direct anesthetic drug delivery methods (Fig. 11.2).

When injectable anesthetic agents are used in unrestrained nondomestic species, a remote delivery system consisting of a dart and projector is often the most practical option. Darts can be projected via a blowpipe, compressed air projector, or gunpowder cartridge rifle that will be discussed later (Bush 1992). All darts have

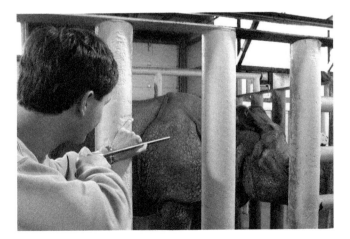

Figure 11.2. Use of a blowpipe for short range injection of a white rhinoceros that would react if hand injected.

four basic components: a drug storage compartment, a method of injecting the drug, a needle to penetrate the skin, and a stabilizer for accurate flight. The commercially available darts differ in their methods of drug expulsion, materials used in their construction, drug payload volumes, and dart attachments, such as the needle or tail. For this chapter, the method of drug delivery will be used to distinguish the darting systems.

Several homemade dart and projector systems have been described in previous literature (Barnard & Dobbs 1980; Haigh & Hopf 1976; Lochmiller & Grant 1983; Warren et al. 1979). This description and discussion of equipment will be limited to those drug delivery systems that are commercially available. The choice of delivery system is subject to the clinician's preferences, needs, or experience, but most commercial systems can be very effective when used by experienced operators. The similarity between available equipment systems allows some interchange of components that can be configured to meet the clinician's specific preferences. However, this interchangeability can also make using these products confusing when mixed together, and may lead to dart failure caused by subtle differences in the darting systems. Generally, it is recommended that one system be purchased, as the manufacturers have developed product lines that are effective and reliable when used as designed.

Historical Development of Remote Delivery Systems

The remote delivery of drugs was first used by indigenous hunters with poison tipped projectiles (Bush 1992; Nielsen 1999). Plant extracts containing curare were used by pre-Columbian South American Indians to produce effective neuromuscular blockage and muscle paralysis in animals. When these poison tipped darts are projected with long blowpipes they could be delivered by experienced hunters with extraordinary precision and with lethal effect. As the purpose of these hunters was to kill, the precision dosage delivery and margin of safety were not important considerations.

Until the second half of the twentieth century, zoological collections relied on manual restraint as the primary means of administering veterinary care. These restraints were dangerous for both the humans and the animals, often resulting in stress, injury, and occasional animal mortalities. In the mid-1950s a remote delivery device was described in the literature (Hall et al. 1953). It consisted of a metal drill bit with a gallamine and glucose paste packed into the groves. The bit was attached to a dart and delivered with a Crossman air gun. Once the animal was paralyzed and the procedure completed, the gallamine was reversed. Although effective, the paste was absorbed slowly, and therefore, a flying syringe was developed to deliver liquid injections (Crockford et al. 1958). This aluminum dart used an acid base reaction to inject the drug. After extensive modifications and improvements to this dart, it became the prototype for many of the modern darts in use today (Bush 1992). Around the same time, Colin Murdoch, a veterinarian and inventor from New Zealand, also developed a series of darts and projectors that became Paxarms. Subsequently, plastic two-chambered gas darts were introduced to zoological

medicine and developed into several commercial darting systems (Bush 1992). For further details, several authors have reviewed the development of darting equipment over the past 40 years (Bush 1992; Fowler 1995; Fritsch 1982; Harthoorn 1976; Nielsen 1999). A listing of currently available darts and delivery systems can be found in Table 11.1.

Table 11.1. Description of currently available darts by manufacturer

Manufacturer and Dart Description	Dart Type	Payload Volume (mL)	Dart Diameter (mm)	Needle Sizes (mm)	Tailpieces	Recommended Projector
Dan-Inject blow dart syringe	2 chamber	1.5, 3	11.8	1.1 × 25 or 1.2 × 38	Orange cloth	12-mm Dan-Inject 1.23 or 1.8-m (2-piece) blowpipe
Telinject blow dart syringe	2 chamber	1, 2	9.5	0.9 × 25 to 1.2 × 38 (3 gauges and 4 lengths)	Yellow cloth	10-mm Telinject 1 or 2-m blowpipe
Telinject blow dart syringe	2 chamber	1, 2, 3	10.8	0.9 × 25 to 1.2 × 38 (3 gauges and 4 lengths)	Orange cloth	11-mm Telinject 1 or 2-m blowpipe
Telinject blow dart syringe	2 chamber	5	14.0	0.9 × 25 to 1.2 × 38 (3 gauges and 4 lengths)	Red with yellow cloth or plastic tailpiece	14.5 Telinject 2.2-m high performance blowpipe
Dist-Inject mini-ject "softy" blow dart syringe	2 chamber	3.8	10.8	1.1 × 25 or 1.2 × 35	Red cloth	11-mm mini-ject 0.9-m blowpipe
Maxi-Ject veterinary syringe dart	2 chamber	1, 2	9.7	1.9 × 25 or 1.2 × 38	Yellow cloth	10mm maxi-ject 2 piece 1-m blowpipe
Maxi-Ject veterinary syringe dart	2 chamber	3	10.7	1.9 × 25 or 1.2 × 38	Red cloth	11-mm maxi-ject 2 piece 1-m blowpipe
Maxi-Ject veterinary syringe dart	2 chamber	5	13.7	1.2 × 38	Red with yellow cloth	14mm maxi-ject 2-piece 1-m blowpipe
TeleDart veterinary syringe dart	2 chamber	1, 2, 3	10.7	0.9 × 25 to 1.2 × 38 (3 gauges and 4 lengths)	Pink Cloth with yellow base	11-mm B11 or B16 blowpipe
Telinject "Vario" molded plastic syringe	2 chamber	1, 3	10.8	1.5 × 20 to 2.0 × 60 (2 gauges and 8 lengths)	Red cloth	11-mm Telinject Vario pistol or rifles
Telinject "Vario" molded plastic syringe	2 chamber	5, 10, 15, 20	12.2	1.5 × 20 to 2.0 × 60 (2 gauges and 8 lengths)	Red with yellow cloth	13-mm Telinject Vario pistol or rifles
Dan-Inject "S" series molded plastic syringe	2 chamber	1.5, 3	10.7	1.5 × 20 or 2.0 × 100	Red cloth	11-mm Dan-Inject model PI pistol or JM/IM injection rifles
Dan-Inject "S" series molded plastic syringe	2 chamber	5, 10	12	1.5 × 20 or 2.0 × 100	Red with white cloth	13-mm Dan-Inject model PI pistol or JM/IM injection rifles
Dist-Inject "mini-ject 2000" molded plastic syringe	2 chamber	3, 5	10.8	1.1 × 25 or 1.2 × 35	Red cloth	11-mm model 45 delta pneumatic 0.35-m blowpipes, or model 70 rifle with 11 barrel insert
Dist-Inject "mini-ject easy" molded plastic syringe	2 chamber	3, 5	10.8	1.1 × 25 or 1.2 × 35	Orange and yellow fins	11-mm model 45 delta pneumatic 0.35-m blowpipes

Table 11.1. (*Continued*)

Manufacturer and Dart Description	Dart Type	Payload Volume (mL)	Dart Diameter (mm)	Needle Sizes (mm)	Tailpieces	Recommended Projector
TeleDart "TD" veterinary syringe dart	2 chamber	1, 2, 3, 5	10.8	1.5 × 20 to 2.0 × 60 (2 gauges and 8 lengths)	Pink with yellow cloth with red base	11-mm model RD206 TeleDart injection pistol or model RD706 TeleDart injection gun
Palmer Cap-Chur aluminum "Air inject" syringe	2 chamber	1, 2, 3, 4, 5	12.5	2.5 × 19 to 2.5 × 38 (11 lengths) (side port with nose plug)	Tetra plastic tail	12.7 Palmer Cap-Chur short, mid, and long range CO_2 projectors
Dist-Inject "mini-ject unic" molded plastic syringe	Chemical	3. 5	10.8	1.1 × 25 or 1.2 × 35	Red cloth	11-mm barrel insert in model 70 or 50 rifles
Pneu-Dart "P" aluminum dart	Explosive	0.5 , 1	12.5	2.0 × 6 to 2.0 × 50 (7 lengths)	Yellow plastic	12.7-mm Blo-Jector blowpipe
Pneu-Dart "P" aluminum dart	Explosive	0.5 , 1, 1.5, 2, 3, 4, 5, 6, 7, 8, 10	12.5	2.0 × 6 to 2.0 × 50 (7 lengths)	Yellow plastic	12.7-mm Oplus-XT gauged CO_2 /pistol, or model 178B air rifle
Pneu-Dart "C" aluminum l dart	Explosive	0.5 , 1, 1.5, 2, 3, 4, 5, 6, 7, 8, 10	12.7	2.0 × 6 to 2.0 × 50 (7 lengths)	Orange plastic	12.7-mm model 193, 194, 196 and 2000 Pneu-Dart cartridge fired rifles
Palmer Cap-Chur aluminum dart	Explosive	0.5, 1, 2, 3, 4, 5, 7, 10, 15, 20	12.6	2.5 × 13 to 2.5 × 76 (11 lengths)	Yarn or plastic "Tetra"	12.7-mm #1300 mid-range pistol, #1200 long-range CO_2 rifle

Dart Types

Two-Chambered Compressed (Pressurized) Gas Darts
These darts are lightweight, two-chambered, and usually made of plastic or occasionally aluminum. The dart body is divided into dual chambers by a movable, rubber syringe plunger in the center (Fig. 11.3).

The anterior drug chamber is bounded by the central plunger and by a syringe hub that accepts a needle at the front of the dart. The posterior gas chamber is bordered anteriorly by the central plunger and a second, smaller movable rubber plunger in the back of the dart. The posterior plunger acts as a one-way valve that allows gas to be inserted through the posterior hub, but then occludes the posterior hub to prevent gas escape. The caudal part of the dart body has a syringe hub that accepts a tailpiece. The dart needles are hollow with a sharp, sealed tip. Several millimeters from the tip, the needles have an opening cut into the side for the medication to come through. A small silicone sleeve is then placed to cover this opening. The needle with the silicone sleeve in place is attached to the anterior hub of the dart (Fig. 11.4).

These darts are charged by placing the drug into the anterior chamber and compressed gas into the back chamber. The pressurized gas may be air introduced manually with an adapter attached to a syringe or butane liquid placed into the posterior chamber of the dart (Fig. 11.5).

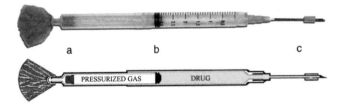

Figure 11.3. Photograph and illustration of a two-chambered compressed gas dart. (a) Posterior plunger that is a one way valve allowing compressed gas to be introduced, but preventing escape. (b) Movable central syringe plunger that divides the two-chambers of the dart. (c) Side-ported needle with a silicone sleeve occluding the port.

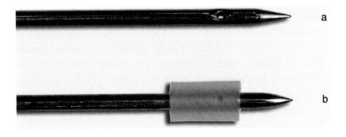

Figure 11.4. Photograph of two side ported needles. (a) This needle has the side port exposed. (b) A similar needle with a silicone sleeve occluding the port.

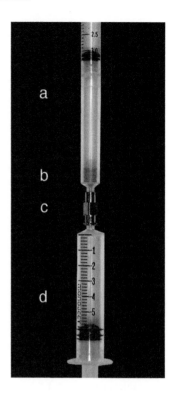

Figure 11.5. Photograph of a two-chambered compressed gas dart being filled. (a) Posterior chamber of the dart. (b) Posterior plunger that is a one way valve allowing compressed gas to be introduced, but preventing escape. (c) Coupler that is needed to allow air to pass from the syringe to the dart. (d) Standard syringe used to force air into the dart.

Leakage of fluid is prevented by the silicone sleeve occluding the needle vent. As the needle enters the skin, the sleeve remains on the skin surface exposing the needle vent. The pressurized gas then pushes the central plunger forward and forces the drug out of the anterior chamber and through the needle. If the darts and needles are cleaned and maintained between usages, they are reusable. The plastic darts can be gas sterilized and the needles can be autoclaved or gas sterilized.

Because this dart type is relatively lightweight with a slow deposition of drug over several seconds, the injection is relatively nontraumatic to the animal. The dart's sharp needles make them ideal for penetration of most skin types. With proper selection of needle lengths and dart sizes, these darts can be used safely on a large variety of species. They are generally used for short ranges and preferably during good weather conditions, as their trajectories are easily affected by wind gusts. The primary disadvantages are that they can be destroyed by hitting unintended solid objects and their complexity makes them prone to dart failures.

Loading a two-chambered plastic dart involves the following steps:

1. An appropriate sized sterilized dart is removed from the package.

2. The dart is inspected for cracks and abnormal shape.
3. The dart is then tested by placing air pressure in both compartments to make sure that the plungers move correctly and that the dart does not leak. A metal connector is needed to couple regular 6 or 12 cc syringes to the hub of the dart and inject air into the posterior chamber.
4. Next, an appropriate-sized, sterile needle is selected. It must be inspected for patency and for the presence of a sharp tip, free of burrs or bends from previous impacts.
5. The needle is then lubricated with sterile ointment and a silicone sleeve is placed over the needle tip and slid down over the needle vent. The sleeve is moved up and down the needle several times to be sure it moves easily before it is placed over the vent opening in the needle.
6. The needle is placed onto a syringe and air is forced into the needle to confirm that the sleeve has occluded the needle vent.
7. The dart is loaded by first displacing the posterior plunger (one-way valve) with a venting pin to make sure the posterior chamber is not pressurized.
8. The central plunger is then positioned to provide the correct volume for the drug in the anterior chamber.
9. The needle of a second syringe containing the drug is inserted through the anterior hub and the anterior chamber is then filled with the drug.
10. The needle with the preplaced silicone sleeve is attached to the dart. This attachment must be secure, with the needle firmly seated on the anterior dart hub.
11. A transparent safety cover is placed over the end of the needle.
12. The dart is held in a vertical position with the needle pointing upwards.
13. The dart is charged with either air or butane placed into the posterior chamber. The air or gas is forced in through the posterior hub, around the one-way valve, and into the posterior chamber of the dart. When properly charged, the rubber plunger at the back of the dart will be firmly pressed against the caudal portion of the posterior chamber.
14. Select the proper tailpiece for the dart. Inspect the tailpiece to ensure that it is clean, dry, and symmetrical.
15. The tailpiece is firmly attached to the posterior hub of the dart making the dart ready for use.

Blow Darts Several types of two-chambered darts use pressurized gas to push the drug into the animal (Fig. 11.6).

The first is the blow dart that is constructed of very lightweight clear medical-grade plastic, similar to the

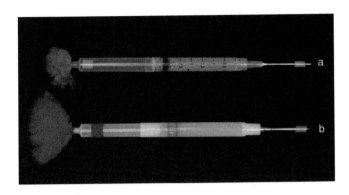

Figure 11.6. Photograph showing the difference between two types of two-chambered compressed gas darts. (a) Blow dart. (b) Molded nylon dart.

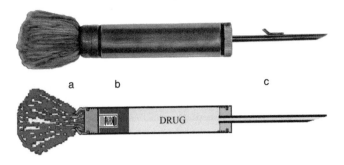

Figure 11.8. Photograph and illustration of a gunpowder explosive-powered dart. (a) Yarn tailpiece that is threaded into the back of the dart body. (b) Movable central syringe plunger, which contains the explosive charge. (c) Forward-ported needle with a wire barb is threaded into the front of the dart body.

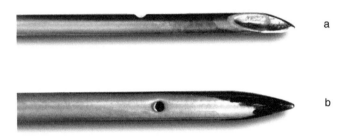

Figure 11.7. Photograph of two needle types used in two types of two-chambered compressed gas darts. (a) A hypodermic needle that has the sharp tip occluded with solder used in blow darts. (b) A thicker, blunter, machined needle used in molded nylon darts.

material used in disposable plastic syringes. The blow dart body usually has a leur-lock syringe tip hub on the anterior drug compartment. The needle of the blow dart is sharp, constructed from a modified hypodermic needle that has a tip that is soldered closed and an opening cut into the side (Fig. 11.7).

Because of the blow dart's lightweight and sharper needles, they are meant to be projected by blowpipes. They are most accurate when used indoors. Blow darts should never be used in CO_2 or gunpowder cartridge propelled projectors as their light construction causes erratic flight at high velocities and they often shatter on impact.

Molded Nylon, Two-Chambered Plastic Darts These darts are heavier than blow darts and constructed of opaque synthetic polyamide polymer plastic (molded nylon). The construction of the dart body is more robust and often reinforced. The anterior hub has a thick collar to better seat the needle and provide additional strength to the needle attachment. These needles are machined from a thicker metal that resists bending or breaking better than the modified hypodermic blow dart needles.

These heavier darts are designed for use in CO_2 or compressed air powered projectors. They have improved

ballistic properties that allow them to fly true at higher velocities. They are also made to withstand greater impact forces. This gives these darts a much greater range and ability to be used outdoors in moderately windy conditions. The blunter needles have no difficulty penetrating most animal skin when powered by these projectors; however, they are ineffective when projected with a blowpipe. When used correctly and at appropriate distances, these darts are safe and cause only minor trauma (Cattet et al. 2006). A variety of needle sizes are available. They can be fitted with barbs to decrease bouncing out of the animal. Impact absorbers can also be placed at the base of the needles to prevent them from penetrating beyond the intended depth and decreasing dart trauma (Wiesner 1998). The potential problems associated with these darts are that they can cause significant trauma when used with gas powered projectors at inappropriate close ranges. Clinical experience has demonstrated that these darts can be imbedded into the soft tissues of animals and can even cause long bone fractures.

Gunpowder Explosive Darts Explosive powered darts use a black gunpowder explosive cap to generate the force needed to discharge the drug. A movable plastic plunger is placed into the center of the dart body to separate the drug from the explosive cap and trigger mechanism (Fig. 11.8).

The anterior chamber holds the drug. The posterior chamber holds a metal explosive unit that contains an explosive cap, a weighted firing pin and a spring that keeps the firing pin away from the cap (Fig. 11.9).

The explosive unit is set behind the caudal aspect of the central plunger, and the back of the dart is sealed with a tailpiece. The needles are hollow, forward, or side ported, and do not need to be capped. The needles come in a large variety of lengths and are usually barbed.

These darts are loaded by placing the drug through the needle lumen and into the anterior chamber. When the dart hits the skin of the animal, the needle

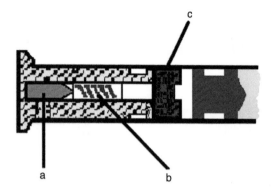

Figure 11.9. Illustration of the tail section and trigger mechanism of a Pneu-Dart gunpowder explosive-powered dart. (a) Movable weight. (b) Spring that holds the weight back. (c) Explosive cap.

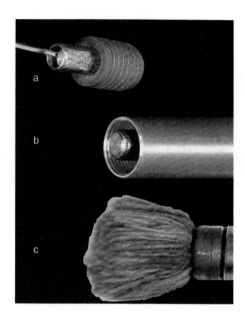

Figure 11.10. Photograph demonstrating the steps in assembling the tail section and trigger mechanism of a Palmer Cap-Chur gunpowder explosive-powered dart. (a) The charge has been placed into the caudal pocket of the central plunger. The needle is pressing the weight and spring to demonstrate the proper orientation of the explosive charge. (b) The plunger and explosive charge have been inserted into the posterior part of the dart body. (c) The yarn tailpiece has been threaded into place.

penetrates and the body of the dart is stopped by the skin surface. The forward momentum of the dart is carried to the metal firing capsule where the small spring is overpowered and the firing pin impacts the cap resulting in an explosion. The resulting expanding gas within the posterior chamber rapidly forces the plunger cranially and the drug out of the needle. The injection occurs within approximately 0.001 seconds and can cause considerable tissue trauma (Cattet et al. 2006; Kreeger 2002). Additionally, the explosive rate of the injection causes a rocket effect that propels the dart out of the animal. For the explosive unit to work, the dart must strike the animal with enough force at a perpendicular angle to the target site to trigger an explosion. This necessary force can result in significant dart trauma in small or delicate species.

Modular Gunpowder Explosive-Powered Darts The Palmer Cap-Chur dart kit comes disassembled in components so the operator can assemble the dart configuration that is needed. The body is an aluminum 12.6 mm (.50 caliber) tube with internally threaded ends. The aluminum syringe barrel comes in various lengths that can hold 0.5–20 mL of drug. The Palmer Cap-Chur charges come in three different power strengths that are selected for the appropriate dart volume; yellow for 0.5–3 mL, orange for 4–10 mL, and red for 15–20 mL. Improper selection of the charge strength can lead to dart failure. The metal explosive charge fits with its closed, rounded, cranial end into a pocket in the caudal aspect of the central plunger (Fig. 11.10).

The explosive unit must be oriented correctly with the open end facing caudally for the dart to discharge. The back of the dart is sealed with a tailpiece that screws into the internally threaded dart body. The needle is threaded into the anterior end of the dart. The needles are hollow, forward ported, and do not need to be capped. The needles come in a large variety of lengths and with several barb styles (Fig. 11.11).

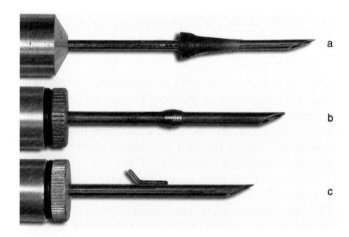

Figure 11.11. Photograph of three needle types used in gunpowder explosive-powered darts. (a) Pneu-Dart needle with a green gel cone collar barb. (b) Palmer Cap-Chur needle with small metal collar. (c) Palmer Cap-Chur needle with wire barb.

This system is one of the oldest commercially available darts and has had many years of proven reliability. The variability in needle length and payload volume (tube size) makes this the most versatile darting system. From one kit, darts can be configured with short needles for carnivores or very large needles and barrels used for elephants and rhinoceroses. The dart components, except the explosive units, are reusable if cleaned and maintained properly. Keeping the dart components sterile is challenging, but using unsterilized equipment may lead to dart induced infections (Bush & Gray 1972). The biggest weakness of the system is that the heavy darts and the explosive discharge of drug lead to tissue damage.

Loading a Palmer Cap-Chur dart involves the following steps:

1. The appropriate-sized sterilized dart components are removed from their packages.
2. The dart parts are inspected for cracks and abnormal shape. The needle, body, and tail are preliminarily assembled to ensure proper threading, and then passed through the syringe barrel of the projector to ensure that the dart passes freely.
3. A sterile, central, rubber plunger is selected and then lubricated. It is placed inside the body of the dart, and the plunger is moved back and forth within the length of the dart body to ensure that it moves easily.
4. The plunger is positioned in the caudal part of the dart body.
5. An appropriate strength metal explosive unit is fitted into the pocket in the caudal aspect of the rubber plunger. It is crucial to make sure that the explosive unit is oriented correctly, with the movable plate exposed caudally.
6. A tailpiece is selected and threaded into the caudal part of the dart body.
7. An appropriate sized needle with an acceptable barb style is selected. It must be inspected for patency and to make sure that it does not have a burr at the tip or is bent from a previous impact.
8. The needle is then threaded onto the cranial part of the dart body.
9. The dart is loaded by passing the needle of a syringe containing the drug through the dart needle lumen and depositing the drug into the anterior chamber of the dart. The syringe needle should be longer than the dart needle and the drug introduced slowly to avoid drug back flow from the dart needle.
10. Sterile water is used to completely fill the remaining volume in the anterior chamber of the dart.

Prefabricated Gunpowder Explosive-Powered Darts Prefabricated versions of the gunpowder explosive-powered darts, such as Pneu-Darts, are commercially available. The explosive system is similar, except that the explosive mechanism is preplaced in the dart by the manufacturers. The dart is made of a combination of aluminum or polycarbonate plastic body, a hollow needle, and a plastic tailpiece. The dart is purchased as a complete unit and cannot be taken apart. The function and limitations are similar to the modular systems.

The simplicity of the prepurchased dart makes this an appealing product. The operator selects the dart volume, needle length, and barb configuration that will be needed for the anesthetic event. Most needles come with a green gelatin collar or barb to prevent the darts from being ejected from the skin when the dart discharges. Loading the dart is a simple matter of placing the drug through the dart needle and into the anterior chamber.

Pneu-Darts come in two types: the first is the "P" dart line, with a yellow tail, that is designed for blowpipes or CO_2 powered projectors. The other dart line is the "C" dart, with orange tailpieces, that are designed for the 22 blank-powered cartridge projectors. The major differences are the diameter of the tailpieces are larger in the "C" dart to help engage the rifled barrel, and the tensile strength of the spring in the explosive unit is weaker in the "P" dart. The Pneu-Dart line has several available configurations that include clear polycarbonate plastic bodies, tri-ported needles, and modified tailpieces to fit other brands of 13-mm projectors.

Loading a Pneu-Dart or similar dart involves the following steps:

1. Select a dart with the appropriate payload size and needle length from the package. Pneu-Dart markets a wide variety of dart sizes and needle combinations that must be preordered prior to the procedure.
2. Note the tailpiece color and package label to make sure that the dart type selected matches the intended projector. A yellow tailpiece indicates the "P" dart line designed for blowpipes or CO_2-powered projectors. An orange tailpiece indicates the "C" dart line designed for the 22 blank-powered cartridge projectors.
3. The dart is inspected for cracks and other manufacturing abnormalities. Make sure that the needle is patent and that the retaining device is correctly installed on the needle.
4. Inspect the dart for dirt or moisture damage that may have compromised sterility or function of the dart during storage and transport.
5. The dart is loaded by passing the needle of a syringe containing the drug through the dart needle lumen and depositing the drug into the anterior chamber of the dart. The syringe needle should be longer than the dart needle, and the drug introduced slowly to avoid drug back flow from the dart needle.
6. Sterile water is used to completely fill the remaining volume in the anterior chamber of the dart.

Miscellaneous Dart Types
Aluminum Two-Chambered Compressed Gas Dart Palmer Cap-Chur produces a two-chambered compressed gas dart that uses a threaded aluminum tube, but the standard explosive charge is replaced with a one-way valve system in the posterior chamber. This dart also has a closed needle with a side port vent and occluding

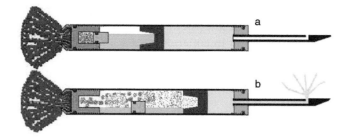

Figure 11.12. Illustration of a chemical reaction-powered dart. (a) Represents the loaded dart prior to impact. The chemical reagents are kept separated by a weight occluding the chemical chambers. (b) Represents the dart after impacting the target and during discharge of the drug. The weight was dislodged and the chemicals have mixed and produced a gas that pushes the central plunger forward.

sleeve over the needle. The function and loading of this dart is similar to the two-chambered gas darts.

Chemical-Powered Darts Chemical darts use an effervescent acid/base reaction to produce gas and thus inject the anesthetic (Fig. 11.12).

The design has a two-chamber configuration with the chemicals placed in the posterior chamber. Prior to discharge the chemicals are kept apart. Upon impact, a variety of mechanisms have been devised to allow the chemicals to mix and produce gas (Bush 1992). No chemical darts are commercially available in the United States, but they are used and available in Africa and Europe (Nielsen 1999). Because the drug compartment is not under pressure, open-ended needles can be used. The advantage is that the darts are easy to load and reliable in most field situations. The injection speed is slower than compressed gas or explosive charged darts, but this slow discharge is usually acceptable. The slow discharge is beneficial in that it causes minimal injection trauma and limited blow back from the dart.

Spring Powered Darts Spring-powered darts are not currently commercially available in the United States. The design is similar to the two-chambered dart, except the posterior chamber is replaced with a spring to provide the injection force. The spring is attached anteriorly to the central plunger and posteriorly to the back of the dart body. Trigger mechanisms usually involve silicone-capped needles that function similarly to the two-chambered darts. The dart body can be constructed of plastic or metal depending on the projector that will be used. The major problem with these darts is that the process of loading the dart is difficult and dangerous due to inadvertent spraying of the drug during the loading process.

Solid Drug Darts Solid drug projectiles can potentially be used to deliver anesthetics or sedatives. The principle of these solid bullets is similar to the original gallamine paste projectiles described from the 1950s.

Several attempts have been made to develop a solid, lightweight, absorbable bullet (Bush 1992). The current versions are made of various materials, such as hydroxypropylcellulose, that dissolve and absorb into the muscle of the animal (Jessup 1993; van de Wijdeven 2002). An example is the BallistiVet system, which was developed for vaccination of domestic livestock, but can be applied to both captive and wild nondomestic species. As in the original descriptions of solid drug injection systems, the limitations of payload size and slow absorption are persistent obstacles in their use for primary induction of anesthesia.

Remote Delivery Projectors
Compressed Gas Projectors
Blowpipes Blowpipes consist of a long lightweight tube with a mouthpiece on one end. A blow dart is placed in the end of the pipe and compressed gas is provided by the operator blowing with a quick, strong breath through the tube. The longer the pipe, the greater the accuracy of the dart. Commercial blowpipes are available from several manufacturers in various pipe lengths, diameters, and shapes of mouthpieces. Selection is based on personal preferences for the mouthpiece and the diameter of the dart type selected.

Usage of a blowpipe requires practice. The pipe is held horizontally and grasped in the hand opposite to the dominant eye. To use a blowpipe correctly, look at the tip of the pipe and aim it at the target. Inhale deeply and then rapidly exhale in a manner that approximates a combination of coughing and spitting through the pipe. Because of the slow dart velocity, the dart will tend to fly in an exaggerated downward arc instead of a straight line. Effective blowpipe range is about 0.5–10 m.

Blowpipes are by far the most versatile, inexpensive, silent, lightweight projectors available. For short ranges, an experienced darter can have exceptional accuracy. The light darts combined with the slow velocity of the dart produce minimal impact and tissue trauma. The operator can adjust the dart speed instantly and therefore deliver the dart as gently as needed. Because darts may occasionally leak and the mouth must be placed on the mouthpiece, it is not recommended to project darts with dangerous drugs such as concentrated narcotics using a blowpipe.

Gauged Blowgun Projectors A modification to the blowpipe is the addition of an external source of compressed gas to eliminate the need for the operator to exhale through the pipe (Fig. 11.13).

These are designed to shoot the heavier machined two-chambered plastic dart or the type "P" Pneu-Darts. The basic components needed are a source of compressed gas, control of the gas pressure with a combination of a pressure gauge and valve system, and a trigger mechanism. These systems can be powered either by

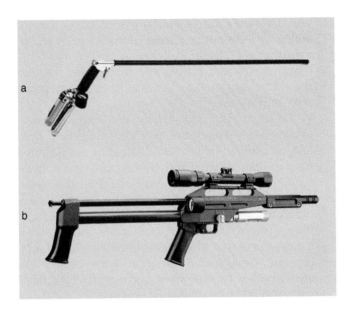

Figure 11.13. Photograph of two Dan-Inject blowgun type projectors. (a) A model CO2 PI pistol with an 11-mm barrel. The pistol is powered with a compressed CO2 cartridge. (b) A JM Special rifle with 11-mm barrel. It is also powered by a compressed CO2 cartridge.

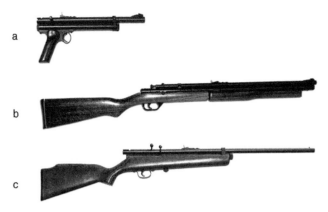

Figure 11.14. Photographs of three compressed gas-powered 12.7 mm (.50 caliber) projectors. (a) Palmer Cap-Chur Model #1300 mid range pistol powered with 2 compressed CO2 cartridges. (b) Pneu-Dart Model 178B air pump rifle. (c) Palmer Cap-Chur Model #1200 long-range rifle powered with two compressed CO2 cartridges.

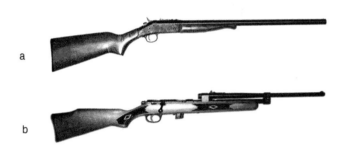

Figure 11.15. Photographs of two cartridge powered 12.7 mm (.50 caliber) projectors. These guns are very powerful and used only outdoors for long range targets. (a) Palmer Cap-Chur Model #1000 extra long-range rifle. (b) Pneu-Dart Model 196 rifle.

air via a foot pump or by compressed carbon dioxide from a pressurized cylinder. Pressure gauges and release valves allow the pressures to be increased or decreased as needed during darting. A detachable, long barrel is then mounted on either a pistol handle or a rifle stock. The projectors can be equipped with a telescopic sight. Often, these projectors have barrels that can be interchanged to accommodate both 11- and 13-mm darts. The pistol is used for short range or indoors where space is limited. The rifles have more accuracy and are used outdoors. Careful selection of the dart type is important, as lightweight plastic blow darts will not fly correctly in these CO_2 powered projectors.

These systems are quiet, reasonably accurate, and a simple means of darting exotics for distances up to 5–30 m. Many veterinarians in zoological collections use this system exclusively.

Air and CO_2 Rifles and Pistols The next group of compressed gas projectors are the pistols and rifles with a barrel permanently mounted onto a triggered compressed gas power source (Fig. 11.14).

The compressed gas power source can be provided by CO_2 cylinders or an attached air pump similar to a pellet gun. These projectors generally lack accurate pressure gauges and valve systems with the ability to change the gas pressure. Instead, they often have two or three preset steps for selecting power levels. They are usually designed for 12.5-mm (.50 caliber) metal darts such as Palmer Cap-Chur and type "P" Pneu-Darts. Due to their short barrels, the pistols are notoriously inac-

curate at long range. In contrast, the rifles can be very accurate at moderate distances. Both systems, when used at short range, can cause significant trauma due to the lack of accurate pressure control.

Gunpowder Cartridge-Powered Rifles These rifles have permanently mounted barrels on a rifle stock. They are powered by .22 caliber blanks that come in several charge strengths with different amounts of gunpowder. In the Palmer Cap-Chur system, brown is the weakest cartridge, followed by green, yellow, and red (Fig. 11.15).

Although they lack pressure gauges, they often have methods of selecting power levels. These rifles are too powerful for short range or indoor use. In contrast to other darting systems, they have the longest effective range and can be used in windy conditions. They have 12.7 mm (.50 caliber) bore and are designed for 12.5-mm metal darts, such as Palmer Cap-Chur or type "C" Pneu-Darts.

Miscellaneous Projector Types

Crossbows and Bows Commercially available darts can be mounted on arrow shafts and delivered with crossbow and conventional bows. In Africa, several Ju/'Hoan bushmen were given arrows with Pneu-Darts attached at the tips. Using these arrows and their archery hunting techniques, they were successfully able to immobilize free-ranging lions and leopards (Stander et al. 1996). Archery based projectors are accurate, but if not controlled, the velocity of the heavy arrows will cause trauma to the animals.

Injection Collars Remote injection collars can be placed on an animal prior to release and used to inject the animal at a later time (Jessup 1993). Commercially available products have been used in white-tailed deer and wolves. The injection is triggered by remote control. Combined with telemetry and a safety collar release if the batteries are low, this can potentially be a valuable tool for wildlife. Application of these collars in zoological collections has been limited, but may be practical in situations that require multiple immobilizations in animals that are difficult to dart.

Darting Accessories

Many manufacturers provide practice darts and targets for their equipment. Usage of these darts is cheaper than using operational darts, and they are consistently weighted to help improve accuracy. Through practice, the operator develops proficiency with the equipment and reliable accuracy. During this practice, it is important to develop an understanding of the proper impact velocity that is needed to prevent excessive trauma.

Laser range finders and binoculars are useful in outdoor darting procedures. Calibrating the projector for selected distances is the best method of consistently producing accurate and atraumatic shots. Once the calibration is completed during practice sessions, using the range finder significantly improves range estimates and allows the operator to make confident and accurate projector settings. The binoculars are useful for selecting the target and then confirming that the dart has hit the animal.

Cleaning and Reusing Darts

Many of the remote drug delivery systems, such as pole syringes, two-chambered compressed gas darts, and the modular gunpowder explosive powered darts, are designed to be reusable. However, for proper function, these darts must be cleaned, maintained, and stored correctly. Specific procedures and maintenance recommendations should be obtained from the dart manufactures and the preferences of the individual practitioner.

General dart cleaning and storage procedures:

1. Every effort should be made to locate and retrieve the dart after the procedure.

2. The retrieved dart should be placed into a labeled and secure container during transport prior to dismantling and cleaning.

3. Using gloves and proper eye protection, the dart should be inspected for residual drug or unreleased internal pressure.

4. While submerged under water, the dart is carefully disassembled. The water provides protection from drug aerosolization and also dilutes any residual drug from the dart. Alternatively, flowing tap water or disassembly in a safety cabinet can be used for this step.

5. After disassembly, each component of the dart is individually cleaned with warm soapy water and then inspected. The dart bodies are inspected for bending or cracks. Needles are inspected for patency, bending, or damaged retention barbs. Needle tips are inspected for sharpness and tip burs. Damaged parts should be discarded or repaired.

6. The dart parts should then be soaked in a disinfectant solution, carefully rinsed, and individually dried.

7. The dart components should be lubricated according to manufactures recommendations.

8. The darts components are then sorted and packaged in sealable containers or surgical instrument wrappers.

9. Finally, the dart components should be sterilized according to manufacturer's recommendations.

Drug delivery Problems

Dart Failure Although darts and their projectors have become indispensable tools in zoological medicine, dart failures are common. The most important factor causing a dart to miss the target is operator error from inexperience with the darting system. Each darting system has individual characteristics that must be learned by the operator. Accuracy and consistency are only developed with persistent practice.

Unfortunately, all darting systems are prone to high failure rates, and even when the darts hit their intended target, many fail to discharge. As the complexity of the darts increase, this becomes the most important factor leading to dart failure. Careful preparation and testing of the darts is an essential step prior to each darting. The various darting systems each have their critical or failure prone components that must be carefully checked by the operator. Maintaining the equipment in portable organized kits helps ensure that the proper components are available and facilitates the darting procedures (Fig. 11.16).

Examples of common problems are explosive charges that fail to fire, blocked dart needles, and central plungers that stick. Ambient temperatures can affect dart function and the performance of compressed gas darts. In very cold temperatures, darts may fracture on impact, drugs can freeze or become thick, and compressed gas exerts less pressure, causing incomplete discharges.

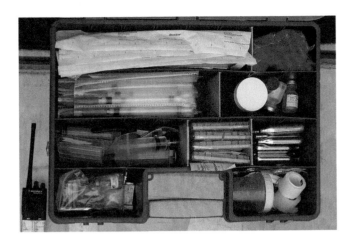

Figure 11.16. Photograph of a darting kit with essential components separated into compartments. Note that a radio is included to provide emergency communications.

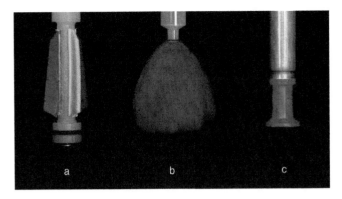

Figure 11.17. Photograph of three types of dart tails. (a)Four fin tail from a Dist-Inject mini-ject easy dart. (b) Cloth tail from a Dan-Inject molded S series dart. (c) Plastic tail from a Pneu-Dart C dart.

Drug Failure The selection of anesthetic drugs is beyond the scope of this chapter, but can definitely cause immobilization failures. Improper deposition of the darted drugs can also produce unexpected results. Darts that deposit drugs into vascular structures or medullary cavities of bones can have rapid onset similar to intravenous administration. Conversely, deposition into skin, subcutaneous space, tendons, or other poorly vascularized tissues can have slow absorption. Some clinicians recommend the usage of hyluronidase to improve absorption of drugs injected with darts (Kock 1992).

Drug interactions when mixed into a syringe must be considered, but have been poorly studied. Environmental conditions, such as freezing or heating, may also alter drug potency. Long-term storage of drugs in preloaded darts is questionable, as the drugs potency and purity may change with time (Kreeger et al. 2002).

Aerodynamics of Darts Darts have poor ballistic properties when compared with bullets or arrows. With variable shapes and shifting liquids, they are often very erratic in flight. As an example, bent darts or needles damaged by previous impacts can radically alter the flight trajectory. Aside from the shape, the velocity of the dart as it exits the projector is an important variable in prediction of the dart's trajectory. Fast muzzle velocities produce flat flight trajectories similar to a bullet. Although accurate, these faster velocities are associated with severe impact trauma and dart malfunctions. Further, all darts, even when properly loaded and balanced, will destabilize at very high velocities. This forces all darting systems to use relatively slow muzzle velocities. At these slower velocities, the darts tend to form a downward arced trajectory that is increased as the darting distance increases. This arc must be anticipated, and an experienced darter will compensate appropriately.

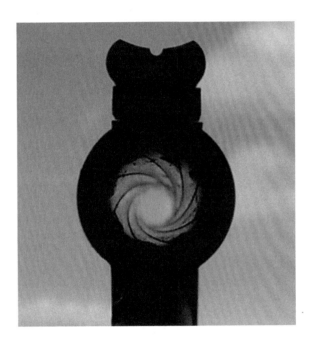

Figure 11.18. Photograph through the barrel of a rifle barrel showing the spiral riffling needed to cause a dart to spin on its horizontal axis during flight.

The tailpiece is designed to provide the dart with aerodynamic stability (Fig. 11.17).

Available tails range from finned tails similar to archery arrows, which are considered the best, to cloth tail stabilizers that can cause problems if they are asymmetrical. Rifling of the projector barrel is a method of increasing flight stability by forcing the projectile to spin on its horizontal axis (Fig. 11.18).

Unfortunately, few darts are capable of engaging the rifled barrel surface and therefore do not spin in flight. Additionally, some dart tails, such as cloth and finned configurations, actually resist the horizontal spin that the rifled barrel is intended to provide.

In addition to the aerodynamic considerations of unobstructed flight, environmental conditions associated with outdoor darting can have significant effects on dart trajectories. Objects such as plants may deflect the dart. Winds and wind gusts can cause darts to fly in unexpected directions. Helicopter down drafts can also affect darts. Due to their light weight, plastic darts are particularly prone to this problem.

Animal Injury Severe tissue injury, including hemorrhage, necrosis, and bone fractures, can occur whenever darts are used. Any projectile with a needle can cause injury when it hits an animal in an unexpected location. Sudden movements from the targeted animal can lead to inadvertent injury to either the target or other animals in the group. Examples of dart injuries to the eye, thorax, abdomen, and testicles are common. It is ultimately the operator's responsibility to only take shots that are likely to hit the expected target.

The site selection for darting is important. In most animals, the muscles of the upper hind legs are the safest selection. Occasionally, the base of the neck or the triceps can be targeted. When selecting the site, the animal must have sufficient muscle mass to allow for injection of the drug and safe impact of the dart. Most darting systems have a variety of needle selections that must be chosen to limit tissue trauma while effectively providing penetration and injection of the drug into the muscle. Needle length is selected on the thickness of the animal's skin and the expected depth of the muscle mass. Inappropriately long needles have the potential to fracture bones on impact. Thickness of the needle is dependent on the potential for the needle to break on impact, and broken dart needles retained in muscle tissue have been reported (Cohn 1998).

Darts primarily cause trauma on impacting the animal in direct relationship to the kinetic energy of the dart (Karlsson & Stahling 2000; Kreeger 2002). This energy can be estimated by knowing the mass and speed of the dart at impact in the following relationship: $KE = 1/2 (Mass)*(Velocity)^2$. It is important to note that the velocity is squared and therefore has the greatest influence on the injuries caused on impact. Thus, heavy darts are not always more harmful for the animal (Kreeger 2002). All darts require enough kinetic energy for the needle to enter the skin and trigger discharge, but excessive amounts are associated with trauma and dart failure. In extreme situations, the whole dart can be imbedded into the muscle or fracture a bone.

Darts can also injure tissues by forceful injection of drug (Cattet et al. 2006). This is particularly true of large-bore, open-ended needles that are discharged with explosive force. Evidence of tissue injury and necrosis has been documented with these types of darts (Cattet et al. 2006; Wiesner 1998).

Needle trauma caused by movement of the needle after discharge can be significant. Often, the first reaction of a darted animal is to jump, run, or remove the dart. Barbs and collars on many dart needles are designed to keep the darts in the animals, but if they are retained for long periods or forcefully removed, they can lead to injury.

Infection of the dart site is generally rare, but can cause serious complications to routine darting procedures. The needle of the dart enters unprepared and often grossly contaminated skin. Some darts have been shown to directly introduce hair and other foreign material deep into the dart injection sites (Cattet et al. 2006). Unsterile darts and contaminated drugs can further inoculate the injection site. Once bacteria are introduced into the dart wound, they grow well in the traumatized tissues associated with the dart site. This combination of trauma, large needles, and unprepared injection site can produce significant and deep wounds that are likely to develop into clinical infections. Inspection of the dart site and local wound care during the anesthetic procedure is always recommended. Many practitioners also recommend the use of prophylactic antibiotics; however, the effectiveness of a single antibiotic injection is questionable and has not been prospectively evaluated. To minimize dart site infection, most darting systems can be sterilized prior to use and aseptic techniques can be used during the dart preparation (Bush & Gray 1972).

Human Safety Concerns during Darting Procedures

Dart projectors should be considered firearms and treated with the same precautions and basic gun safety to prevent accidental discharges. As in animals, the ballistic properties of all darts are able to inflict serious injuries to people. Darts are subject to radical changes in trajectory when they are deflected by wind, obstacles, and bouncing off animals. It is therefore imperative that the operator considers the position of all the personnel around, and particularly behind, the target before the trigger is pulled.

All the dart systems described earlier are designed to automatically discharge drugs, making them even more dangerous when they hit a human. In rare occasions, darts may expel the drug prior to full needle penetration or after bouncing out of the skin. In these cases, the drug can be aerosolized or sprayed onto the surface of the animal and can be a source of drug exposure. Emergency plans to deal with accidental drug exposure need to be in place prior to the immobilization procedures. It is important to have effective emergency communication equipment, such as a cellular telephone or two-way radios.

The most important safety considerations are proper planning and familiarization with the drug delivery method selected. Having each procedure well planned is essential so that everyone is cognizant of their roles and safety considerations. Prior practice and familiarization with the equipment make the operator more confident and effective in delivery of the anesthetics. Ultimately, the responsibility for the safety of an anesthetic delivery is on the anesthetists and the operator of the equipment.

CONCLUSIONS

The methods of drug delivery to nondomestic species are essential to the practice of zoo animal and wildlife anesthesia. However, these methods are often complicated and must be learned and practiced before application. Each remote delivery system has both advantages and significant limitations. Practitioners interested in obtaining equipment should familiarize themselves with all the available systems. Commercial websites often provide detailed information and information on specific product lines. Classes and conference lectures can provide valuable comparative information and often provide the opportunity to use several products. Additional information is also available in other publications that describe the usage of this equipment for specific applications (Kock & Burroughs 2012; Kreeger et al. 2002).

REFERENCES

Barnard S, Dobbs JS. 1980. A handmade blowgun dart: its preparation and application in a zoological park. *Journal of the American Veterinary Medical Association* 177:951–954.

Bush M. 1992. Remote drug delivery systems. *Journal of Zoo and Wildlife Medicine* 23:159–180.

Bush M, Gray CW. 1972. Sterilization of projectile syringe. *Journal of the American Veterinary Medical Association* 161:672–673.

Cattet MR, Bourque A, Elkin BT, Powley KD, Dahlstrom DB, Caulkett NA. 2006. Evaluation of the potential injury with remote drug-delivery systems. *Wildlife Society Bulletin* 34:741–749.

Cohn DL. 1998. Foreign body in a chimpanzee (*Pan troglodytes*). *Revue de medecine veterinaire* 149:1021–1022.

Crockford JA, Hayes FA, Jenkins JH, Feurt SD. 1958. An automatic projectile type syringe. *Veterinary Medicine* 53:115–119.

Fowler ME. 1995. *Restraint and Handling of Wild and Domestic Animals*, 2nd ed. pp. 36–56. Ames: Iowa State University Press.

Fritsch R. 1982. Injection systems. In: *Handbook of Zoo Medicine* (HG Klos, EM Lang, eds.), pp. 15–23. New York: Van Nostrand Reinhold Co.

Grove DM, Ramsay EC. 2000. Sedative and physiologic effects of orally administered α_2-adrenoceptor agonists and ketamine in cats. *Journal of the American Veterinary Medical Association* 216:1929–1932.

Haigh JC. 1999. The use of chutes for ungulate restraint. In: *Zoo and Wild Animal Medicine, Current Therapy 4* (ME Fowler, RE Miller, eds.), pp. 657–662. Philadelphia: W.B. Saunders.

Haigh JC, Hopf HC. 1976. The blowgun in veterinary Practice: its uses and preparation. *Journal of the American Veterinary Medical Association* 169:881–883.

Hall TC, Taft EB, Baker WH, Aub JC. 1953. A preliminary report on the use of Flaxedil to produce paralysis in white-tailed deer (*Odocoileus virginianus borealis*). *The Journal of Wildlife Management* 17:516–520.

Harthoorn AM. 1976. Syringes and projectors. In: *The Chemical Capture of Animals* (AM Harthoorn, ed.), pp. 159–191. London: Cox and Wyman.

Hayes MA, Hartup BK, Pittman JM, Barzen JA. 2003. Capture of sandhill cranes using alpha-chloralose. *Journal of Wildlife Diseases* 39:859–868.

Hunter RP, Isaza R, Carpenter JW, Koch DE. 2004. Clinical effects and plasma concentrations of fentanyl after transmucosal administration in three species of great ape. *Journal of Zoo and Wildlife Medicine* 35:162–166.

Jessup DA. 1993. Remote treatment and monitoring of wildlife. In: *Zoo and Wild Animal Medicine, Current Therapy 3* (ME Fowler, ed.), pp. 499–504. Philadelphia: W.B. Saunders.

Karlsson T, Stahling S. 2000. Experimental blowgun injuries, ballistic aspects of modern blowguns. *Forensic Science International* 112:59–64.

Kearns KS, Swenson B, Ramsey EC. 2000. Oral induction of anesthesia with droperidol and transmucosal carfentanil citrate in chimpanzees (*Pan troglodytes*). *Journal of Zoo and Wildlife Medicine* 31:185–189.

Kock MD. 1992. Use of hyaluronidase and increased etorphine (M99) doses to improve induction times and reduce capture-related stress in the chemical immobilization of the free-ranging black rhinoceros (*Diceros bicornis*) in Zimbabwe. *Journal of Zoo and Wildlife Medicine* 23:181–188.

Kock MD, Burroughs RB. 2012. Chemical and physical restraint of wild animals; A training and field manual for African species. International Wildlife Veterinary Services (Africa). Greyton, South Africa.

Kreeger TJ. 2002. Analyses of immobilizing dart characteristics. *Wildlife Society Bulletin* 30:968–970.

Kreeger TJ, Arnemo JM, Raath JP. 2002. *Handbook of Wildlife Chemical Immobilization, International Edition*. Fort Collins: Wildlife Pharmaceuticals.

Lochmiller RL, Grant WE. 1983. A sodium bicarbonate-acid powered blow-gun syringe for remote injection of wildlife. *Journal of Wildlife Diseases* 19:48–51.

Loibl MF, Clutton RE, Marx BD, McGrath CJ. 1988. Alpha-chloralose as a capture and restraint agent of birds: therapeutic index determination in the chicken. *Journal of Wildlife Diseases* 24:684–687.

Mortenson J, Bechert U. 2001. Carfentanil citrate used as an oral anesthetic agent for brown bears (*Ursus arctos*). *Journal of Zoo and Wildlife Medicine* 32:217–221.

Nielsen L. 1999. *Chemical Immobilization of Wild and Exotic Animals*. Ames: Iowa State University Press.

Pollock CG, Ramsay EC. 2003. Serial immobilization of a brazilian tapir (*Tapirua terrestrus*) with oral detomidine and oral carfentanil. *Journal of Zoo and Wildlife Medicine* 34:408–410.

Stander P, Ghau X, Tsisaba D, Txoma X. 1996. A new method of darting: stepping back in time. *African Journal of Ecology* 34:48–53.

Thurmon JC, Tranquilli WJ, Benson GJ. 1996. Anesthesia of wild, exotic, and laboratory animals. In: *Lumb and Jones' Veterinary Anesthesia*, 3rd ed. (JC Thurmon, WJ Tranquilli, GJ Benson, eds.), pp. 686–735. Baltimore: Williams & Wilkins.

van de Wijdeven GGP. 2002. Development and assessment of mini projectiles as drug carriers. *Journal of Controlled Release* 85:145–162.

Warren RJ, Schauer NL, Jones JT, Scanlon PF, Kirkpatrick RL. 1979. A modified blow-gun syringe for remote injection of captive wildlife. *Journal of Wildlife Diseases* 15:537–541.

Wiesner H. 1998. Tierschutzrelevante neuentwicklungen zur optimierung der distanzimmobilisation. *Tierarztliche Praxis* 26:225–233.

12 Capture Myopathy

Jessica Paterson

INTRODUCTION

Capture myopathy (CM) is a noninfectious, metabolic disease of wild and domestic animals that can lead to significant morbidity and mortality. The condition is most commonly associated with pursuit, capture, restraint, and transportation of animals. CM may also manifest secondary to other diseases, or as a result of natural hazards encountered in the environment. It is characterized by metabolic acidosis, muscle necrosis, and myoglobinuria. Clinical signs include muscle stiffness, severe muscle pain, ataxia, paresis, torticollis, prostration, and paralysis. Animals typically become obtunded, anorexic, and unresponsive. Death can occur from within minutes or hours of capture to days or weeks after the inciting event.

CM has been described in a remarkably wide range of vertebrate species, primarily within the mammalian and avian taxa. A very similar condition has been reported in poikilotherms, including fish (Holloway & Smith 1982) (Hassanein 2010) and amphibians (Williams & Thorne 1996). A syndrome resembling CM has also been documented in lobsters (Ridgway et al. 2007). The disease has never been described in reptiles.

CM shares many similarities with the myodegenerative disorders of domestic cattle, sheep, horses, and swine, as well as exertional rhabdomyolysis (ER) in humans. The factors that contribute to the onset of CM can be highly unpredictable, and the manifestations of the disease often vary between species and individuals. Treatment generally has a low success rate, although recoveries have been recently documented and will be discussed later in the chapter. There continues to be a much greater emphasis on prevention in the literature.

HISTORY

CM has been termed muscular dystrophy, white muscle disease, overstraining disease, capture disease, cramp, leg paralysis, spastic paresis, stress myopathy, transport myopathy, incipient myopathy, degenerative polymyopathy, muscle necrosis, and idiopathic muscle necrosis throughout the literature. The condition is now most commonly referred to as CM, exertional myopathy, or exertional rhabdomyolysis. One of the earliest reports of lesions consistent with CM was reported in a white-tailed deer (*Odocoileus virginianus*) in 1955 (Hadlow 1955). The first description of the pathology of CM was in a Hunter's hartebeest (*Damalisicus hunteri*) (Jarrett et al. 1964). Throughout the late 1960s and early 1970s, CM was described in many free-ranging African ungulates (Basson et al. 1971; Harthoorn & Van Der Walt 1974; Hofmeyr et al. 1973; Mugera & Wandera 1967). CM in other African mammalian species, including baboons (McConnell et al. 1974) and flamingoes (Young 1967), were also documented during the same time period.

The first documentation of CM in North America was most likely in mountain goats (*Oreamnos americanus*) in British Columbia (Hebert & Cowan 1971). The condition in these mountain goats was described as white muscle disease, but the findings more accurately fit CM. CM was reported throughout the late 1970s in several species of North American ungulates including white-tailed deer (Wobeser et al. 1976), elk (Lewis et al. 1977), moose (Haigh et al. 1977), pronghorn (Chalmers & Barrett 1977), and bighorn sheep (Demartini & Davies 1977).

THE HUMAN COMPARATIVE

CM is very similar to exertional rhabdomyolysis syndrome described in people (Warren et al. 2002). There

Zoo Animal and Wildlife Immobilization and Anesthesia, Second Edition. Edited by Gary West, Darryl Heard, and Nigel Caulkett.
© 2014 John Wiley & Sons, Inc. Published 2014 by John Wiley & Sons, Inc.

are hundreds of causes of rhabdomyolysis identified in people that are classified as either being acquired or inherited (Warren et al. 2002). Exertional rhabdomyolysis is one of eight forms of human-acquired rhabdomyolyis (Warren et al. 2002) and has traditionally been associated with military training (Smith 1968) and exhaustive endurance sports (Lin et al. 2006). Current research has recognized new exercise-related hyperthermic syndromes such as "white-collar rhabdomyolysis" (Knochel 1990) and raver's hematuria (Sultana & Byrne 1996). Rhabdomyolysis has also been associated with people sustaining a TASER® shock, although the incidence rate is low and the evidence is controversial (Sanford et al. 2011).

Rhabdomyolysis is one of the leading causes of acute renal failure (ARF) in human patients (Vanholder et al. 2000). Progression of rhabdomyolysis to myoglobinuria and ARF was first described in humans during the London Blitz (Bywaters & Beall 1941). Civilians suffering from crush injuries died from ARF within 8 days of hospital presentation despite treatable, localized limb injury (Bywaters & Beall 1941).

ETIOLOGY

Exertional rhabdomyolyis, or CM, in animals is distinguishable from other types of rhabdomyolysis by its pathophysiology, as it affects both skeletal and cardiac muscles in response to extreme stress and muscular exertion (Williams & Thorne 1996). It is a complex and multifactorial disease. Spraker (1993) theorized that CM is an inherent mechanism that facilitates a symbiotic relationship between predator and prey. The prey animal experiences a relatively quick and painless death after capture by its predator, thus allowing the predator to conserve energy.

Other authors argue that CM develops in wild animals after an unnatural degree of stress and physical exertion (such as experienced during hunting or live capture) for which they are maladapted (Bateson & Bradshaw 1997; Harthoorn 1980). These authors believe CM is an iatrogenic disease and does not develop under the conditions of stress and predation naturally encountered in the wild. Chalmers and Barrett (1982) suggested that the stresses of fear and anxiety are the triggering mechanisms for CM that may be modified by genetic or acquired predispositions to the disease. These factors in turn may be exacerbated by iatrogenically induced circumstances, such as overexertion, disturbance, excessive handling, transportation, and shock (Chalmers & Barrett 1982).

PREDISPOSING FACTORS

There are many predisposing or contributing factors for CM. These factors can be placed into seven categories and remembered with the mnemonic SECONDS (Table 12.1).

Table 12.1. Predisposing or contributing factors for capture myopathy

S	Species
E	Environment
C	Capture related
O	Other diseases
N	Nutrition
D	Drugs
S	Signalment

Species

Prey species are considered the most susceptible to CM in the mammalian taxa, particularly ungulates. Highly susceptible African species include zebra, giraffe, nyala, tsessebe, duiker, roan antelope, red hartebeest, eland, springbok, kudu, giraffe, and female impala (Ebedes et al. 2002). North American species with apparent increased susceptibility to CM include white-tailed deer (Beringer et al. 1996) and pronghorn (Chalmers & Barrett 1977). Fallow and hog deer in Australia appear to be more excitable, and thus more susceptible to CM, compared with species such as rusa and samba deer (Presidente 1978).

The long-legged wading birds are particularly predisposed to CM within the avian taxa. The combination of struggle during capture and restraint in bags or cages where the birds cannot stand increases their susceptibility to CM (Green 2003).

Reports of CM in carnivores are rare but the disease can occur under certain conditions. A grizzly bear succumbed to CM approximately 10 days after capture by a leghold snare (Cattet et al. 2008). A retrospective analysis reported serum biochemistry results consistent with CM in 6% of grizzly bears (7/119) and 18% of black bears (29/165) trapped with leghold snares (Cattet et al. 2008). Captive-raised and free-ranging red foxes caught in foothold traps developed exertional rhabdomyolysis (Kreeger et al. 1990). A captive mountain lion was successfully treated after being diagnosed with myopathy due to secondary thiafentanil intoxication (Wolfe & Miller 2005).

Environment

Environmental factors that can increase the incidence of CM include extremes in ambient temperature, rain, and high humidity. The need for animals to negotiate steep terrain, difficult footing, or water hazards can also hasten the onset of CM.

Capture Related

Capture-related factors that contribute to CM comprise the largest category. Capture techniques that involve high chase speeds, prolonged exertion without rest, excessive handling, prolonged restraint, restraint that promotes struggling from unnatural positioning, crating, transport, subjection to fear stimuli over periods of time, and renewed stresses, such as repeated moving and transport predispose animals to CM. Injuries induced by capture techniques, or by other animals, can also increase the incidence of CM. Eccentric exercises (when muscles are lengthening while trying to contract) have been positively correlated with a higher incidence of ER in humans (Lin et al. 2006).

Other Diseases

Underlying diseases and infections can make an animal more susceptible to CM. Severe worm and tick infections cause anemia and weaken the animal. Heartworm infection may compromise cardiopulmonary circulation. Animals that have utilized water sources that have a high salt content may have preexisting renal damage (Ebedes et al. 2002).

Nutrition

Nutrition is one area commonly overlooked as a contributing factor to CM. Animals with a preexisting vitamin E or selenium deficiency may be predisposed to developing CM (Hebert & Cowan 1971). Individuals on a high nutritional plane and carrying excess body fat, such as premigratory birds, may also be at higher risk. Providing food, water, and nutritional supplements to captured animals, particularly during prolonged transport or upon reaching the new destination, may reduce the incidence of CM (Ebedes et al. 2002).

Drugs

Rhabdomyolysis is a frequent complication of illicit drug consumption in humans and a frequent finding in drug-related deaths (Welte et al. 2004). It is estimated that toxins and drugs play a role in up to 80% of adult human cases of rhabdomyolysis (Gabow et al. 1982). Opiates are one of the most frequently implicated in primary drug-induced rhabdomyolysis (Warren et al. 2002). Controversial human literature suggests that abuse of mu opioids may lead to rhabdomyolysis through a directly myotoxic effect (Warren et al. 2002).

Potent mu opioids, such as fentanyl, etorphine, carfentanil, and thiafentanil, are often used in combination with alpha-2 agonists, butyrophenones, benzodiazepines, and cyclohexamines for wildlife capture. Wildlife species immobilized with opioid-based combinations frequently demonstrate side effects, such as excitement (Haigh 1990), spontaneous movement (Haigh 1990; Paterson et al. 2009), muscle rigidity (Haigh 1990; Paterson et al. 2009), hypoventilation, catecholamine release (Schumacher et al. 1997), and hyperthermia (Jessup 1984). These effects, combined with hypoxemia and elevated fluid loss, may significantly increase the risk of CM. It is important to recognize that nonopioid drug combinations can also cause similar side effects and predispose anesthetized animals to CM (Caulkett et al. 2000).

Signalment

In addition to species susceptibility described previously, the age and sex of an animal may also contribute to CM susceptibility. Extremely old and extremely young animals may be the most susceptible to CM in certain circumstances (Ebedes et al. 2002). Postrelease mortality was higher in yearling pronghorn compared with adults captured by helicopter-released net guns (Jacques et al. 2009). Human literature suggests males have a higher risk of developing severe ER (Lin et al. 2006). Some authors theorize that estrogens have a protective effect therefore reducing the risk for women (Lin et al. 2006). Male red knots were more likely to develop CM compared to females after cannon-net capture and banding (Rogers et al. 2004). Heavily pregnant African ungulates are considered more susceptible to CM than nonpregnant females (Ebedes et al. 2002).

Recent retrospective studies in bears and roe deer have shown differences in postcapture behavior between males and females of different ages (Morellet et al. 2009) and reproductive status (Cattet et al. 2008; Morellet et al. 2009). These variations in response to the capture process may indicate which individuals are more susceptible to morbidity and mortality from CM.

PATHOPHYSIOLOGY

Spraker (1993) described the pathogenesis of CM as involving three primary components: perception of fear, sympathetic nervous and adrenal systems, and muscular activity. The normal physiology related to these components has been described in detail by Spraker (1993). The pathophysiology of CM has also been extensively reviewed by Chalmers (1982), Spraker (1993), and Williams and Thorne (1996), and therefore is not discussed in detail in this chapter. Briefly, CM results from altered blood flow to the tissues and exhaustion of normal aerobic energy, particularly in skeletal muscle. Exhaustion of ATP in muscle cells leads to decreased delivery of oxygen and nutrients, increased production of lactic acid, and inadequate removal of cellular waste products (Spraker 1993). Damaged muscle cells undergo necrosis to a varying degree. Myoglobin released from these cells cause tubular necrosis in the kidneys and acute renal failure (Vanholder et al. 2000). Similar necrosis of cardiac tissue can occur as well (Williams & Thorne 1996).

CLINICAL AND PATHOLOGICAL SYNDROMES

Rhabdomyolysis literally means "dissolution of striped (skeletal) muscle" (Warren et al. 2002). Exertion-induced rhabdomyolysis leads to the breakdown of skeletal muscle fibers with leakage of intracellular contents, including creatinine kinase (CK) and myoglobin into the blood. Current diagnosis of rhabdomyolysis in humans requires the presence of tetraparesis, CK elevation more than 10 times the upper reference limit, myoglobin-uria, hyperkalemia, and coagulopathy (Melli et al. 2005). A CK concentration greater than 10,000 U/L in horses is indicative of myopathy (reference range 60–330 U/L) (Volfinger et al. 1994). Significant muscle injury in captured grizzly and black bears was diagnosed at CK levels greater than 387 U/L (reference range 0–387 U/L) and 421 U/L (reference range 0–421 U/L), respectively (Cattet et al. 2008; Teare 2002).

Despite the common mechanism of muscle breakdown, CM can manifest differently and have varying sequelae depending on the species, the individual, and the circumstances. One classification system defined four temporal syndromes of CM: hyperacute, acute, subacute, and chronic (Harthoorn 1973). Spraker (1993) also described four primary CM syndromes: capture shock, ataxic myoglobinuric, ruptured muscle and delayed peracute. The latter classification scheme will be discussed in detail in this chapter. When classifying specific clinical signs and gross and histologic findings into different syndromes of CM, it is important to recognize that the pathogenesis of CM is a continuum; some animals may show clinical signs and pathology that overlap one or more syndromes.

Capture Shock Syndrome
Acute death syndrome can occur during immobilization or within a short time after capture. Death usually occurs within 1–6 hours postcapture. Clinical signs include depression, hyperpnea/tachypnea, tachycardia, elevated body temperature, weak thready pulses, and death. Serum biochemical findings include elevations in serum aspartate aminotransferase (AST), creatinine phosphokinase (CK), and lactate dehydrogenase (LDH) enzymes. The most common postmortem lesions include severe small intestinal and hepatic congestion along with pulmonary congestion and edema. Frank blood and blood-tinged contents may be found within the lumen of the small intestine.

Histologic findings may include small areas of necrosis in skeletal muscle, brain, liver, heart, adrenal glands, lymph nodes, spleen, pancreas, and renal tubules. These lesions are most pronounced if the animal was hyperthermic. Small thrombi may occasionally be found in the capillaries in various organs (Spraker 1993).

Ataxic Myoglobinuric Syndrome
Literature suggests that this is the most commonly observed among the four syndromes. It may become evident several hours to several days postcapture. Clinical signs may include mild to severe ataxia, torticollis, and myoglobinuria. Serum enzymes (AST, CK, and LDH) and blood urea nitrogen (BUN) levels are elevated. Animals demonstrating mild signs are the most likely to survive. Animals with moderate to severe symptoms have a higher mortality.

Gross lesions can be seen in the kidneys and skeletal muscle. The kidneys are swollen and dark. The urinary

bladder is empty or contains a small amount of brownish urine (Fig. 12.1).

The cervical and lumbar muscles, as well as the flexor and extensor muscles of the limbs (appendicular skeleton) contain multifocal, pale, soft, dry areas, accentuated by small white foci in a linear pattern. The lesions are bilateral but not symmetrical. They are subtle in animals that die within 1–2 days after capture, but they are more pronounced in chronic cases. Animals with prolonged survival may have small ruptures within the necrotic muscles. Well-demarcated, gross changes to the hindlimb musculature of a nilgai and a Grant's zebra can be seen in Figure 12.2 and Figure 12.3, respectively.

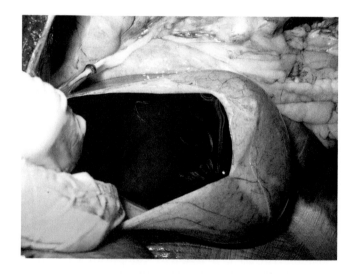

Figure 12.1. Incised urinary bladder of the same white-tailed deer as pictured in Figure 12.4 demonstrating marked myoglobinuria (photo courtesy of Dr. Douglas Whiteside).

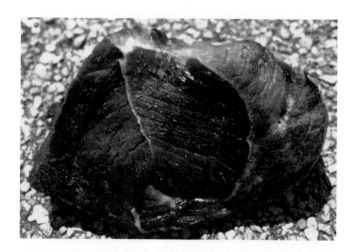

Figure 12.2. Hindlimb adductor muscle of a nilgai diagnosed with capture myopathy after escaping from a zoo exhibit. The animal survived for 1 week postescape. Note the sharp demarcation between normal muscle on the left-hand side and the affected adductor muscle on the far right that has a pale, dry appearance (photo courtesy of Dr. Scott Citino).

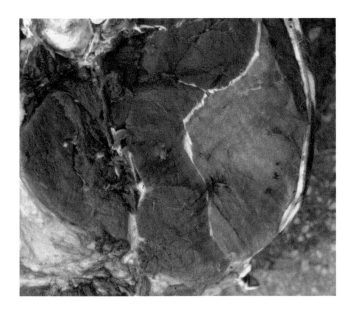

Figure 12.3. Gluteal musculature of a Grant's zebra diagnosed with capture myopathy. The affected muscle is on the far right. It is pale in color, appears to have a dry surface and it is isolated from normal muscle by a septum of deep fascia (photo courtesy of Dr. Scott Citino).

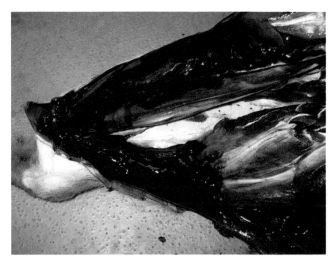

Figure 12.4. Left hindlimb of a captive white-tailed deer diagnosed with capture myopathy and exhibiting ruptured muscle syndrome. The left lateral musculature is exposed with the tarsus on the left. Note the marked subcutaneous hemorrhage surrounding the hindlimb muscles proximal to the tarsus (photo courtesy of Dr. Douglas Whiteside).

Histologic lesions are primarily localized to the renal cortex and skeletal muscle. Renal lesions are characterized by dilatation of tubules, moderate to severe tubular necrosis, and protein (myoglobin) casts. Muscular lesions are characterized by acute rhabdomyolysis. Myocytes are markedly swollen, with loss of striations and fragmentation and cleavage of myofibrils. Sarcolemmal nuclei are pyknotic in multiple areas. Sarcolemmal proliferation usually begins within 3 days of capture (Spraker 1993).

Ruptured Muscle Syndrome

Clinical signs of this syndrome do not usually manifest until 24–48 hours postcapture and animals initially appear normal. Physical exam findings include a marked drop in the hindquarters and hyperreflexion of the hock due to unilateral or bilateral rupture of the gastrocnemius muscle. Extreme elevations in AST, CK, and LDH are present. Blood urea nitrogen may be within normal limits or slightly elevated. Although most animals with ruptured muscle syndrome die within a few days, some may survive for several weeks.

Gross examination reveals massive subcutaneous hemorrhage of the rear limbs (as seen in Fig. 12.4), and multifocal small to large, pale, soft lesions in the forelimb, hindlimb, diaphragm, cervical, and lumbar muscles. Muscular lesions are similar to those described for the ataxic myoglobinuric syndrome but they are more severe and widespread. Lesions are bilateral but not symmetrical. Multiple, small to large ruptures may be found in necrotic muscle bodies. The gastrocnemius, subscapularis, middle and deep gluteal, semitendinosus, and semimembranosus muscles are often ruptured.

Histologic lesions are primarily located within the skeletal muscles and they are characterized by severe, diffuse necrosis. More extensive sarcolemmal proliferation, fibrosis, and muscular regeneration are evident in ruptured muscle syndrome compared to the ataxic myoglobinuric syndrome (Spraker 1993).

Delayed Peracute Syndrome

This syndrome is rare but can be seen in animals that have been in captivity for at least 24 hours. The animals appear normal if they are left undisturbed. When disturbed, captured, or acutely stressed, they will try to escape or run but stop abruptly and stand or lie still for a few moments. During this period, their eyes begin to dilate and death ensues within several minutes. These animals die in ventricular fibrillation and have elevated AST, CK, and LDH. There are usually no lesions, or a few small pale foci within the skeletal muscle at necropsy. When present, histologic lesions are characterized by mild to moderate rhabdomyolyis throughout the skeletal muscle, especially in the hindlimbs (Spraker 1993).

A syndrome called delayed acute CM was identified in three roe deer (Montané et al. 2002). These deer died 48 hours, 72 hours, and 8 days post-capture while being housed in a large enclosure. The authors reported no clinical signs of CM in the deer after capture or while housed in the enclosure until an unobserved, human-initiated pursuit took place. The animals most likely died 14, 41, and 21 hours, respectively, after the disturbance. Although the etiology is similar to delayed peracute syndrome, confirming a common pathogenesis based on available evidence is not possible.

DIFFERENTIAL DIAGNOSES

Differential diagnoses for CM in wildlife may include white-muscle disease, plant toxicities such as *Cassia occidentalis*, *Cassia obtusifolia*, and *Karwinskia humboldtiana* (Chalmers & Barrett 1982), malignant hyperthermia, early tetanus, hypocalcemia, and myositis. This is not an exhaustive list. Conclusive diagnosis of CM depends on history, clinical signs, clinical pathology, and gross and microscopic pathology (Chalmers & Barrett 1982).

TREATMENT

Treatment of CM generally has a low success rate, although animals have been rehabilitated with intensive efforts (Businga et al. 2007; Clark & Clark 2002; Rogers et al. 2004; Smith et al. 2005; Wolfe & Miller 2005). Costs and logistics associated with treating wild animals, particularly in field situations, pose significant challenges. Potential treatment options are discussed below.

Analgesia

Animals suffering from CM can experience severe muscle pain. Analgesia should be considered from an ethical and prognostic point of view. The distress and anxiety resulting from pain will make this disease more difficult to treat. Analgesics used will vary depending on the affected species. Judicious use of nonsteroidal anti-inflammatories is an option provided there is no concurrent steroid administration or indication of renal dysfunction. Opioid administration with or without a sedative should also be considered. Corticosteroids may alleviate pain and help preserve lysosomal membrane and capillary integrity (Muir et al. 2000b).

Dantrolene

Dantrolene sodium is a lipid soluble hydantoin analog used to treat and prevent malignant hyperthermia in humans and exertional rhabdomyolysis in horses (McKenzie et al. 2004). Dantrolene suppresses the release of calcium from the sarcoplasmic reticulum (Krause et al. 2004). Side effects associated with dantrolene include neurologic deficits, muscular weakness, and hepatoxicity (McKenzie et al. 2004). Dantrolene was used in the successful treatment of severe rhabdomyolysis in a dog (Wells et al. 2009). There are no reports of dantrolene administration for the treatment of CM in wildlife or zoo animals. The drug would be impractical for field use due to its light sensitivity, insolubility, and expense (McKenzie et al. 2004).

Muscle Relaxants

Benzodiazepines, including diazepam, midazolam, and zolazepam, are centrally acting muscle relaxants that reduce muscle spasms and spasticity (Muir et al. 2000a).

Benzodiazepines are also anticonvulsants and may aid in calming obtunded and/or debilitated animals (Muir et al. 2000a; Wolfe & Miller 2005). Methocarbamol is another centrally acting muscle relaxant that has been used to successfully treat CM in a rhea (Smith et al. 2005). Limited pharmacokinetic data is available for this medication in veterinary species.

Dietary Supplements

Vitamin E and selenium are biological antioxidants administered as a prophylaxis or treatment for CM (Abbott et al. 2005; Businga et al. 2007). The efficacy of these supplements is contentious. Abbott et al. (2005) suggested increased survival rates in northern bobwhites injected with vitamin E and selenium after capture and relocation, although the study lacked adequate sample size. Rio Grande wild turkeys showed no improvement in survival when individuals were treated with vitamin E and selenium during trapping and relocation (Schutz 2009). Successful treatment of CM in birds has been achieved with (Businga et al. 2007) and without (Rogers et al. 2004; Smith et al. 2005) vitamin E and selenium supplementation.

Parentrovite was a balanced formulation of B vitamins with vitamin C in parenteral form. The drug was withdrawn from the human market in 1989. Parentrovite was administered to tsessebe to treat locomotory and capture stress but no conclusions could be made as to its effectiveness (Harthoorn & Harthoorn 1976). Reported use of multivitamin formulations for the treatment of CM could not be found in any recent literature.

Coenzyme Q_{10} and L-carnitine were administered to a dog with rhabdomyolysis with the intention of supporting oxidative metabolism (Wells et al. 2009). These two nutrients are critical cofactors in cellular reactions required for energy production (Freeman & Rush 2005). Coenzyme Q_{10} is also an antioxidant (Freeman & Rush 2005).

Hyperbaric Oxygen

Hyperbaric oxygen has been used as an adjunctive therapy in humans for severe rhabdomyolysis and acute renal failure (Abdullah et al. 2006). Hyberbaric oxygen (HBO_2) induces high oxygen partial pressure in all tissues, inhibits toxin formation, and promotes wound healing (Abdullah et al. 2006). The popularity of this therapy in veterinary medicine is increasing and may become more accessible in the future, particularly for highly valued captive animals.

Sodium Bicarbonate

Sodium bicarbonate is used to treat acidemia and alkalinize the urine. Approximately 4 mEq/kg of sodium bicarbonate administered intravenously was successful in resolving metabolic acidosis and reducing mortality in captured zebra (Harthoorn & Young 1974). Alkalinizing the urine can reduce the risk of tubular obstruction by myoglobin casts; however, myoglobin is also intrinsically nephrotoxic (Lane & Phillips 2003). Blood gas analysis should ideally be used to titrate sodium bicarbonate therapy. Excessive administration may produce metabolic alkalosis or paradoxic cerebrospinal fluid acidosis (Muir et al. 2000b). The practicality of using this therapy in the field is limited.

Fluid Therapy

Intravascular volume expansion with balanced electrolyte solutions is effective in treating metabolic acidosis, hyperkalemia, dehydration, and myoglobinuria. Intravenous fluid therapy may also help to offset hypotension that occurs in some cases of CM. Parenteral fluid therapy was part of the successful management protocol for greater sandhill cranes (Businga et al. 2007), a rhea (Smith et al. 2005), and a mountain lion (Wolfe & Miller 2005).

Nutritional Support

Animals suffering from CM will usually not meet their nutritional requirements voluntarily. Decreased body condition, nutritional deficiencies, and weight loss may significantly impact prognosis. Nutritional supplementation was a vital component in the successful treatment of avians, including Australian shorebirds (Rogers et al. 2004), greater sandhill cranes (Businga et al. 2007), and a rhea (Smith et al. 2005).

Physical Therapy

Authors reporting successful treatment of CM in avians have stressed the importance of physical therapy for restoring muscle coordination, strength, and function (Businga et al. 2007; Rogers et al. 2004; Smith et al. 2005). Recumbent or severely debilitated birds have been supported in slings and gradually reintroduced to weight-bearing exercise (Rogers et al. 2004; Smith et al. 2005). Wading birds may recover from early symptoms of CM if their legs are bathed in water (Clark & Clark 2002). Physical therapy is relatively easy to perform on a small bird (or sedated ratite in the case of the rhea). Providing effective muscle support and exercise in other species may be challenging especially as it can take days to weeks for muscle function to return.

PREVENTION

Possible modes of preventing CM will depend largely on the species being captured, the goal of capture, the resources available, and the environment in which the capture is taking place. Operators must recognize environmental limitations, such as extremes in temperature or terrain. Handling should be minimal and performed by experienced personnel. Transportation must be as brief as possible and appropriate for the species and individual. Wild animals will also adapt better to

capture and confinement with prior training and desensitization.

Drugs chosen for immobilization should be tailored for rapid induction, rapid recovery, efficient delivery, and physiologic stability. Duration of anesthesia should be as short as possible and oxygen supplementation is generally recommended. Administration of tranquilizers, such as acepromazine (López-Olvera et al. 2007; Montané et al. 2007), azaperone (Mentaberre et al. 2010), haloperidol (Mentaberre et al. 2010), or long-acting alpha-2 agonists, such as zuclopenthixol acetate (Read et al. 2000), can aid in reducing stress during handling, transport, and confinement.

Researchers are continuously refining capture techniques and identifying methods of trapping that are more or less likely to cause CM. Culvert trapping and aerial darting resulted in less morbidity and mortality in black bears and grizzly bears compared with leghold snares (Cattet et al. 2008). Dugongs were more efficiently and safely caught manually at the surface of the water versus hoop-netting (Lanyon et al. 2006). Radio-controlled up-net enclosures were found superior to other traps for capturing chamois and may prove successful for a variety of ungulate species (Dematteis et al. 2010). Similar netting innovations have also been described for birds (Bush 2008). Jacques et al. (2009) found the probability of capture-related, postrelease mortality in pronghorn decreased by 58% when transport distance was reduced from 14.5 to 0 km (initial mortality was 25/281 or 8.9%). Similarly, capture-related, postrelease mortality decreased by 69% in pronghorn and white-tailed deer (initial mortality: 3/208 or 1.4%) when helicopter pursuit time decreased from 9 minutes to less than 1 minute (Jacques et al. 2009).

A recent retrospective analysis suggested a capture-related mortality rate of greater than 2% be considered unacceptable in any large mammalian species (Arnemo et al. 2006). The following study provides a case-specific, yet universally applicable example of how CM can be minimized (Harthoorn 1980). From 1973 to 1978, the mortality rate in captured and relocated animals in Traansval provincial reserves in South Africa dropped from 15% to 1.1% (Harthoorn 1980). The high mortality rate was attributed to net capture with prolonged restraint, the capture of individuals rather than family groups, individual crating and transport, prolonged holding in slatted pens, further handling and transport after a rest period, and a sudden change in food. Survival rates were improved by reducing chase speeds, allowing periodic rests during drives over long distances, an almost a total absence of handling, capturing family or herd groups, transporting to the destination immediately after capture with no holding or quarantine, using plastic sheeting or Hessian funnels and corrals, reducing fear and stress by eliminating shouting and other noise, and ensuring minimal contact between the animals and the capture personnel.

CONCLUSIONS

CM remains a frustrating and poorly understood condition despite being frequently reported in veterinary literature. Its unpredictable and multifactorial nature poses a distinct challenge to those who study the disease. Developing a consistently effective treatment for CM will require a better understanding of how to stop the physiologic cascade once it has been triggered. The key to preventing CM lies in understanding the behavior and physiology of individual species. Wildlife capture must be carried out sparingly and with great planning and precision. Ultimately, the welfare of the animal must always be the first priority.

REFERENCES

Abbott CW, Dabbert CB, Lucia DR, et al. 2005. Does muscular damage during capture and handling handicap radiomarked northern bobwhites? *The Journal of Wildlife Management* 69: 664–670.

Abdullah MS, Al-Waili NS, Butler G, et al. 2006. Hyperbaric oxygen as an adjunctive therapy for bilateral compartment syndrome, rhabdomyolysis and acute renal failure after heroin intake. *Archives of Medical Research* 37:559–562.

Arnemo JM, Ahlqvist P, Andersen R, et al. 2006. Risk of capture-related mortality in large free-ranging mammals: experiences from Scandinavia. *Wildlife Biology* 12:109–113.

Basson PA, McCully RM, Kruger SP, et al. 1971. Disease conditions of game in southern Africa; recent miscellaneous findings. *Veterinary Medical Review* 2/3:313–340.

Bateson P, Bradshaw EL. 1997. Physiological effects of hunting red deer (*Cervus elaphus*). *Proceedings. Biological Sciences* 264: 1707–1714.

Beringer J, Hansen LP, Wilding W, et al. 1996. Factors affecting capture myopathy in white-tailed deer. *The Journal of Wildlife Management* 60:373–380.

Bush KL. 2008. A pressure-operated drop net for capturing greater sage-grouse. *Journal of Field Ornithology* 79:64–70.

Businga NK, Langenberg J, Carlson L. 2007. Successful treatment of capture myopathy in three wild greater sandhill cranes (*Grus canadensis tabida*). *Journal of Avian Medicine and Surgery* 21:294–298.

Bywaters EG, Beall D. 1941. Crush injuries with impairment of renal function. *British Medical Journal* 1:427–432.

Cattet M, Stenhouse G, Bollinger T. 2008. Exertional myopathy in a grizzly bear (*Ursus arctos*) captured by leghold snare. *Journal of Wildlife Diseases* 44:973–978.

Cattet MR, Boulanger J, Stenhouse G, et al. 2008. An evaluation of long-term capture effects in ursids: implications for wildlife welfare and research. *Journal of Mammalogy* 89:973–990.

Caulkett NA, Cattet MR, Cantwell S, et al. 2000. Anesthesia of wood bison with medetomidine-zolazepam/tiletamine and xylazine-zolazepam/tiletamine combinations. *The Canadian Veterinary Journal. la Revue Veterinaire Canadienne* 41:49–53.

Chalmers GA, Barrett MW. 1977. Capture myopathy in pronghorns in Alberta, Canada. *Journal of the American Veterinary Medical Association* 171:918–923.

Chalmers GA, Barrett MW. 1982. Capture myopathy. In: *Noninfectious Diseases of Wildlife* (GL Hoff, JW Davis, eds.), pp. 84–94. Ames: Iowa State University Press.

Clark J, Clark N. 2002. Cramp in captured waders: suggestions for new operating procedures in hot conditions and a possible field treatment. *Wader Study Group Bulletin* 98:49.

Demartini JC, Davies RB. 1977. An epizootic of pneumonia in captive bighorn sheep infected with *Muellerius* sp. *Journal of Wildlife Diseases* 13:117–124.

Dematteis A, Giovo M, Rostagno F, et al. 2010. Radio-controlled up-net enclosure to capture free-ranging Alpine chamois *Rupicapra rupicapra*. *European Journal of Wildlife Research* 56:535–539.

Ebedes H, Van Rooyen J, Du Toit JG. 2002. Capturing wild animals. In: *Game Ranch Management*, 4th ed. (JDP Bothma, ed.), pp. 382–430. Pretoria: Van Schaik Uitgewers.

Freeman LM, Rush JE. 2005. Nutritional modulation of heart disease. In: *Textbook of Veterinary Internal Medicine*, 6th ed. (SJ Ettinger, EC Feldman, eds.), pp. 579–583. St. Louis: Elsevier Saunders.

Gabow PA, Kaehny WD, Kelleher SP. 1982. The spectrum of rhabdomyolysis. *Medicine (Baltimore)* 61:141–152.

Green GH. 2003. Capture myopathy ("cramp") in waders. *Bulletin Wader Study Group* 68:29.

Hadlow WJ. 1955. Degenerative myopathy in a white-tailed deer, *Odocoileus virginianus*. *The Cornell Veterinarian* 45:538–547.

Haigh JC. 1990. Opioids in zoological medicine. *Journal of Zoo and Wildlife Medicine* 21:391–413.

Haigh JC, Stewart RR, Wobeser G, et al. 1977. Capture myopathy in a moose. *Journal of the American Veterinary Medical Association* 171:924–926.

Harthoorn AM. 1973. Physiology and therapy of capture myopathy, 2nd annual report. Pretoria, South Africa: Transvaal Nature Conservation Division, Pretoria.

Harthoorn AM. 1980. Exertional myoglobinaemia in black wildebeest, and the influence of graduated exercise. *Journal of the South African Veterinary Association* 51:265–270.

Harthoorn AM, Harthoorn LM. 1976. Parentrovite as a supportive therapy for locomotory stress in tsessebe. *Journal of the South African Veterinary Association* 47:219–222.

Harthoorn AM, Van Der Walt K. 1974. Physiological aspects of forced exercise in wild ungulates with special reference to (so-called) overstraining disease. 1. Acid-base imbalance and PO2 levels in blesbok, *Damaliscus dorcas phillipsi*. *Journal of South African Wildlife Management Association* 4:25–28.

Harthoorn AM, Young E. 1974. A relationship between acid-base balance and capture myopathy in zebra, *Equus burchelli*, and an apparent therapy. *The Veterinary Record* 95:337–342.

Hassanein LH. 2010. The physiological and physical response to capture stress in sharks. *The Plymouth Student Scientist* 4:413–422.

Hebert DM, Cowan IM. 1971. White muscle disease in the mountain goat. *The Journal of Wildlife Management* 35:752–756.

Hofmeyr JM, Louw GM, du Preez JS. 1973. Incipient capture myopathy as revealed by blood chemistry of chased zebras. *Madoqua* 1:45–50.

Holloway HLJ, Smith CE. 1982. A myopathy in North Dakota walleye, *Stizostedion vitreum* (Mitchill). *Journal of Fish Diseases* 5:527–530.

Jacques CN, Jenks JA, Deperno CS, et al. 2009. Evaluating ungulate mortality associated with helicopter net-gun captures in the Northern Great Plains. *The Journal of Wildlife Management* 73:1282–1291.

Jarrett WFH, Jennings FW, Murray M, et al. 1964. Muscular dystrophy in a wild Hunter's antelope. *East African Wildlife Journal* 2:158–159.

Jessup DA. 1984. Immobilization of captive mule deer with carfentanil. *Journal of Zoo Animal Medicine* 15:8–10.

Knochel JP. 1990. Catastrophic medical events with exhaustive exercise: "white collar rhabdomyolysis." *Kidney International* 38:709–719.

Krause T, Gerbershagen MU, Fiege M, et al. 2004. Dantrolene: a review of its pharmacology, therapeutic use and new developments. *Anaesthesia* 59:364–373.

Kreeger TJ, White PJ, Seal US, et al. 1990. Pathological responses of red foxes to foothold traps. *The Journal of Wildlife Management* 54:147–160.

Lane R, Phillips M. 2003. Rhabdomyolysis. Has many causes, including statins, and may be fatal. *BMJ (Clinical Research Ed.)* 327:115–116.

Lanyon JM, Slade RW, Sneath HL, et al. 2006. A method for capturing dugongs (*Dugong dugon*) in open water. *Aquatic Mammals* 32:196–201.

Lewis RJ, Chalmers GA, Barrett MW, et al. 1977. Capture myopathy in Elk in Alberta, Canada: a report of three cases. *Journal of the American Veterinary Medical Association* 171:927–932.

Lin H, Chie W, Lien H. 2006. Epidemiological analysis of factors influencing an episode of exertional rhabdomyolysis in high school students. *The American Journal of Sports Medicine* 34:481–486.

López-Olvera JR, Marco I, Montané J, et al. 2007. Effects of acepromazine on the stress response in Southern chamois (*Rupicapra pyrenaica*) captured by means of drive-nets. *Canadian Journal of Veterinary Research* 71:41–51.

McConnell EE, Basson PA, de Vos V, et al. 1974. A survey of diseases among 100 free-ranging baboons (*Papio ursinus*) from the Kruger National Park. *The Onderstepoort Journal of Veterinary Research* 41:97–167.

McKenzie EC, Valberg SJ, Godden SM, et al. 2004. Effect of oral administration of dantrolene sodium on serum creatine kinase activity after exercise in horses with recurrent exertional rhabdomyolysis. *American Journal of Veterinary Research* 65:74–79.

Melli G, Chaudhry V, Cornblath DR. 2005. Rhabdomyolysis: an evaluation of 475 hospitalized patients. *Medicine* 84:377–385.

Mentaberre G, López-Olvera JR, Casas-Díaz E, et al. 2010. Use of haloperidol and azaperone for stress control in roe deer (*Capreolus capreolus*) captured by means of drive-nets. *Research in Veterinary Science* 88:531–535.

Montané J, Marco I, Manteca X, et al. 2002. Delayed acute capture myopathy in three roe deer. *Journal of Veterinary Medicine. A, Physiology, Pathology, Clinical Medicine* 49:93–98.

Montané J, Marco I, López-Olvera JR, et al. 2007. Effect of acepromazine on the signs of capture stress in captive and free-ranging roe deer (*Capreolus capreolus*). *The Veterinary Record* 160:730–738.

Morellet N, Verheyden H, Angibault J-M, et al. 2009. The effect of capture on ranging behaviour and activity of the European roe deer *Capreolus capreolus*. *Wildlife Biology* 15:278–287.

Mugera GM, Wandera JG. 1967. Degenerative polymyopathies in east African domestic and wild animals. *The Veterinary Record* 80:410–413.

Muir WW, Hubbell JE, Skarda RT, et al. 2000a. Drugs used for preanesthetic medication. In: *Handbook of Veterinary Anesthesia*, 3rd ed. (JA Schrefer, ed.), pp. 19–40. St. Louis: Mosby, Inc.

Muir WW, Hubbell JE, Skarda RT, et al. 2000b. Cardiac emergencies. In: *Handbook of Veterinary Anesthesia*, 3rd ed. (JA Schrefer, ed.), pp. 475–495. St. Louis: Mosby.

Paterson JM, Caulkett NA, Woodbury MR. 2009. Physiologic effects of nasal oxygen or medical air administered prior to and during carfentanil-xylazine anesthesia in North American elk (*Cervus canadensis manitobensis*). *Journal of Zoo and Wildlife Medicine* 40:39–50.

Presidente PJA. 1978. Diseases and parasites of captive rusa and fallow deer in Victoria. *Australian Deer* 3:23–38.

Read M, Caulkett N, McCallister M. 2000. Evaluation of zuclopenthixol acetate to decrease handling stress in wapiti. *Journal of Wildlife Diseases* 36:450–459.

Ridgway ID, Stentiford GD, Taylor AC, et al. 2007. Idiopathic muscle necrosis in the Norway lobster, *Nephrops norvegicus* (L.): aetiology, pathology and progression to bacteraemia. *Journal of Fish Diseases* 30:279–292.

Rogers DI, Battley PF, Sparrow J, et al. 2004. Treatment of capture myopathy in shorebirds: a successful trial in northwestern Australia. *Journal of Field Ornithology* 75:157–164.

Sanford JM, Jacobs GJ, Roe EJ, et al. 2011. Two patients subdued with a TASER(R) device: cases and review of complications. *The Journal of Emergency Medicine* 40:28–32.

Schumacher J, Citino SB, Dawson R Jr. 1997. Effects of a carfentanil-xylazine combination on cardiopulmonary function and plasma catecholamine concentrations in female bongo antelopes. *American Journal of Veterinary Research* 58:157–161.

Schutz TPJ. 2009. An evaluation of vitamin E and selenium as a treatment for capture myopathy in Rio Grande wild turkeys (*Meleagris gallopavo intermedia*) [Dissertation]. Tarleton State University.

Smith KM, Murray S, Sanchez C. 2005. Successful treatment of suspected exertional myopathy in a rhea (*Rhea americana*). *Journal of Zoo and Wildlife Medicine* 36:316–320.

Smith RF. 1968. Exertional rhabdomyolysis in naval officer candidates. *Archives of Internal Medicine* 121:313–319.

Spraker TR. 1993. Stress and capture myopathy in artiodactyls. In: *Zoo and Wild Animal Medicine, Current Therapy*, 3rd ed. (ME Fowler, ed.), pp. 481–488. Philadelphia: W.B. Saunders.

Sultana SR, Byrne DJ. 1996. "Raver's" haematuria. *Journal of the Royal College of Surgeons of Edinburgh* 41:419–420.

Teare JA. 2002. Reference ranges for physiological values in captive wildlife. Apply Valley, MN.

Vanholder R, Sever MS, Erek E, et al. 2000. Rhabdomyolysis. *Journal of the American Society of Nephrology* 11:1553–1561.

Volfinger L, Lassourd V, Michaux JM, et al. 1994. Kinetic evaluation of muscle damage during exercise by calculation of amount of creatine kinase released. *The American Journal of Physiology* 266:R434–R441.

Warren JD, Blumbergs PC, Thompson PD. 2002. Rhabdomyolysis: a review. *Muscle and Nerve* 25:332–347.

Wells RJ, Sedacca CD, Aman AM, et al. 2009. Successful management of a dog that had severe rhabdomyolysis with myocardial and respiratory failure. *Journal of the American Veterinary Medical Association* 234:1049–1054.

Welte T, Bohnert M, Pollak S. 2004. Prevalence of rhabdomyolysis in drug deaths. *Forensic Science International* 139:21–25.

Williams ES, Thorne ET. 1996. Exertional myopathy. In: *Noninfectious Diseases of Wildlife*, 2nd ed. (A Fairbrother, LL Locke, GL Hoff, eds.), pp. 181–193. Ames: Iowa State University Press.

Wobeser G, Bellamy JE, Boysen BG, et al. 1976. Myopathy and myoglobinuria in a wild white-tailed deer. *Journal of the American Veterinary Medical Association* 169:971–974.

Wolfe LL, Miller MW. 2005. Suspected secondary thiafentanil intoxication in a captive mountain lion (*Puma concolor*). *Journal of Wildlife Diseases* 41:829–833.

Young E. 1967. Leg paralysis in the greater flamingo and lesser flamingo (*Phoenicopterus ruber roseus* and *Phoeniconaias minor*) following capture and transportation. *International Zoo Yearbook Zoological Society of London* 7:226–227.

13 Human Safety during Wildlife Capture

Nigel Caulkett and Todd Shury

INTRODUCTION

Capture and anesthesia of zoo and wild animals is inherently dangerous for the people who carry it out. These risks can be elevated in free-ranging situations where the capture team may be subject to environmental threats. Prior to any capture, procedure steps must be taken to recognize potential risks to personal safety, and every attempt should be made to reduce the risk of injury. In the event of injury, there must be a well-thought-out treatment and evacuation plan to deal any and all situations.

This chapter will discuss some of the major risks to human safety that may be encountered during the capture and handling of wildlife. It will discuss methods to reduce risk, and finally it will discuss how to prepare for and deal with emergency situations.

RISKS TO HUMAN SAFETY DURING WILDLIFE CAPTURE AND HANDLING

Hazard Assessment

It is important to perform a hazard assessment of any novel job site prior to commencing work. The hazard assessment should identify any potential hazards and identify what steps can be taken to reduce the risks from these potential hazards. Ideally, a written document should be created that outlines these steps. Everyone on the capture team should be made aware of the risks and any precautionary measures that will be taken. Once personnel have been briefed of the risks and mitigation strategies, they should sign off that they have been briefed.

Environmental Risks

Before working in any environment it is important to be aware of potential hazards. Weather conditions can pose a risk, particularly in areas where personnel may be exposed to extremes of temperature. In some environments, the weather may change very quickly; heavy fog or snow can disable helicopter flight and leave a crew stranded. Personnel should be well prepared for the weather conditions and terrain that may be encountered in their environment. In areas that have rapidly changing weather conditions, clothing should be carried to protect from adverse weather conditions. Work on animals in mountainous terrain requires a knowledge of mountaineering and the use of ropes and harnesses in potentially dangerous locations (Fig. 13.1).

Adequate water supplies are vital in any environmental condition. In remote areas, personnel should be prepared to spend the night outdoors if it is not possible to return to base. Altitude can be a problem if personnel are not properly acclimated. Personnel should be aware of potentially dangerous mammals, reptiles, or insects in a given environment. Communication is vital in emergency situations and a reliable method of communication should be established. In areas where cellular phones do not function, VHF radios may be an option. Satellite telephones function in most parts of the world.

Disease risks should be evaluated for a given environment, and steps should be taken to prevent exposure to infectious disease. Public health professionals should be consulted to determine disease threats and vaccine requirements or malaria prophylaxis in a given region. In some environments, the political situation can be hazardous. Capture personnel should be aware of human-related risk factors in a given environment.

Equipment Related Risks
Remote Delivery Equipment
Dart rifles and pistols have the potential to induce severe trauma if they are used inappropriately (Bush 1992; Cattet et al. 2006). They should be treated with

Zoo Animal and Wildlife Immobilization and Anesthesia, Second Edition. Edited by Gary West, Darryl Heard, and Nigel Caulkett.
© 2014 John Wiley & Sons, Inc. Published 2014 by John Wiley & Sons, Inc.

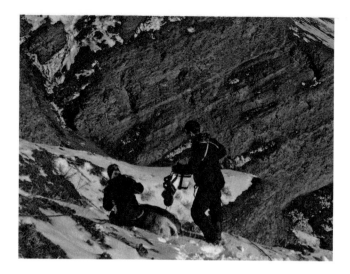

Figure 13.1. The use of ropes to approach a bighorn sheep on a cliff edge.

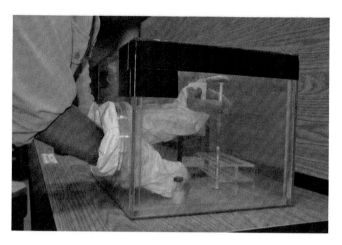

Figure 13.2. Loading a dart in a "splash box" (image courtesy of Dr. Keith Amass).

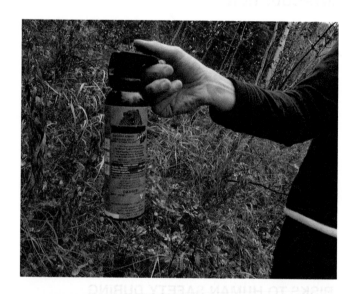

Figure 13.3. Bear deterrent spray.

the same respect as firearms. Personnel using dart rifles and pistols should have appropriate firearms training and practice firearms safety rules.

Dart loading is a potentially hazardous procedure. The risk of drug exposure is increased during dart loading and during charging of darts that utilize compressed gas for their discharge. Darts should never be loaded alone, and should always be loaded on a steady surface, that is, never in a moving vehicle. There should be sufficient water available to dilute spills, and protective clothing (i.e., safety glasses, gloves, and coveralls) should be worn to prevent exposure to drugs. Darts should always be covered, to contain leaks, when they are charged. Loaded darts should always be stored in a sealed, impenetrable, leak proof container. An alternative solution is to load and pressurize darts inside a sealed container that can contain leaks or spills. The original concept, developed by Dr. Jerry Haigh, has been further refined and advocated to prevent exposure to hazardous drugs (K. Amos, personal communication). An example of a "splash box" can be found in Figure 13.2.

Firearms and Pepper Spray

A firearm backup is essential when working with potentially dangerous animals. Everyone working around firearms should receive firearms safety training, and only very experienced personnel should be in charge of providing the firearm backup.

It is important to choose a firearm that has sufficient impact energy to rapidly incapacitate the target species.

In some situations, animals other than the immobilized animal may be the major threat. In these situations, it is advisable to assign a dedicated person to the task of guarding the capture crew. Bear deterrent spray has proven to be an effective deterrent to bear attacks and should be considered as a nonlethal option of repelling wildlife attacks. It has been well studied as an alternative to firearms during bear attacks. A study of 72 adverse bear encounters in Alaska, between 1985 and 2006, revealed that pepper spray stopped undesirable behavior in 92% of brown bear incidents, 90% of black bear incidents, and 100% of polar bear incidents. When pepper spray was used, 98% of individuals deploying the spray were uninjured, and when injuries did occur, they were minor (Smith et al. 2008). This is very convincing evidence of the utility of pepper spray, given the nonlethal nature of this deterrent, it should be considered as a first line of defense. It is important to note that 14% of individuals using the spray experienced effects of the spray themselves (Smith et al. 2008), and that as this study documents use in bears, this may not be applicable to other wildlife species (Fig. 13.3).

Compressed Gas

Care must always be taken when transporting or delivering oxygen. Aluminum D or E cylinders can be easily transported in the field. It is important to secure the tanks as impact damage to the neck of the cylinder can result in a rapid escape of gas and create a missile. Oxygen should never be used around open flames or grease. People using compressed gasses should have appropriate safety training. In situations where it is undesirable to transport compressed gas, portable oxygen concentrators are proving to be a useful alternative to compressed gas cylinders.

Traps and Snares

Traps, snares, and nets are frequently used to facilitate physical capture. Net guns have the potential to induce severe injury if the victim is struck by a weight. Net guns are frequently used from a helicopter. Nets have the potential to induce a crash if they are deployed into the main or tail rotor.

Leg hold traps and snare springs can produce significant bruising or crush injuries. Culvert traps that have heavy guillotine-type doors can induce significant injury.

Helicopters

Wildlife capture work often involves low level highly technical flying. Capture may occur at altitude and sometimes in inclement weather. Helicopter crashes have been a significant cause of injury and death during wildlife capture work (Jessup et al. 1988). A highly skilled, experienced pilot and a well maintained aircraft is vital in these situations. It is also very important to make safe decisions about the weather conditions before embarking on a capture expedition.

Personnel working around helicopters should receive safety training. Helmets and fireproof clothing may decrease the risk of mortality during a helicopter crash.

Animal-Related Risks
Trauma

Animal-induced trauma is very frequent in personnel working with zoo and wild animals. In 1998, a special report in the *Journal of Zoo and Wildlife Medicine* reported a 61.5% incidence of major animal-related injuries in zoo veterinarians (Hill et al. 1998). The most frequently reported injuries were animal bites and kicks. Scratches, crush injuries, and horn wounds were also reported. This report recommended the use of long-sleeved shirts, lab coats, leather gloves, and face shields to protect from injury (Hill et al. 1998). A report on large carnivore attacks on people details some of the risk factors involved and number of attacks by species. This study discusses attacks in general, not attacks in zoo or wildlife capture situations (Löe & Röskaft 2004)

Zoonotic Infections

Zoonotic infections are relatively common in zoo and wildlife workers (Adejinmi & Ayinmode 2008; Stetter et al. 1995). These infections range from simple irritations to life threatening conditions. The study quoted a 30.2% incidence of zoonotic disease in zoo veterinarians. The most common infection was ringworm (reported by 28 veterinarians), followed by psittacosis (24 veterinarians) (Hill et al. 1998). Allergies are also a fairly common occupational hazard among zoo workers (Herzinger et al. 2005; Krakowiak et al. 2002). Simian retroviruses and herpesviruses can present a risk to animal workers and nonhuman primates in primate colonies; an excellent review of these risks and steps to decrease the risk of exposure is available (Weston Murphy et al., 2006.

Careful handling, protective clothing, and up-to-date vaccination status are important to prevent the transmission of zoonotic disease.

Drug-Related Risks
Anesthetic Gasses

Anesthetic gasses are commonly utilized by zoo veterinarians. Ninety-one percent of zoo veterinarians have reported using inhalant anesthetics and 10.9% reported an adverse exposure (Hill et al. 1998). The most commonly reported effects with halothane and isoflurane were headaches, dizziness, sleepiness, and light headedness (Hill et al. 1998). Nitrous oxide exposure was associated with dizziness and sleepiness. Chronic occupational exposure to nitrous oxide has been associated with decreased fertility and increased rate of abortion in dental assistants (Rowland et al. 1992).

Occupational exposure to all gas anesthetics should be minimized. The best method to minimize exposure is the use of an active scavenging system. In addition to active scavenging, delivery equipment should be well maintained to minimize leaks. It is further recommended that anesthetic gas exposure should be periodically monitored by an industrial hygienist (Hill et al. 1998).

Drugs Used for Remote Delivery

Drugs designed for remote delivery are often very potent. While this allows for the delivery of small volumes, it also increases the risk of intoxication from exposure to the drug. Capture drugs must always be handled with respect, and the level of vigilance must always be high. It is a good practice to always wear disposable gloves when drugs are handled. A face shield is also recommended when working with potent narcotics or concentrated medetomidine. Coveralls can be quickly removed if a drug is spilled on them. If a human antagonist is available, it should be drawn up and ready to administer. One should never work alone, and everyone on the capture team should be trained in first aid and CPR. It is important to maintain an increased level of vigilance during the handling of drug vials, the loading and unloading of darts, and during pressurization of darts that utilize compressed air or butane for injection.

Potent Narcotics

Potent narcotics are commonly used for the capture and handling of ungulates. They are a group of drugs that demand respect and care in handling. The three drugs in common usage are etorphine, carfentanil, and thiafentanil. Carfentanil has been quoted to be 10,000 times as potent as morphine (Van Bever et al. 1976). Thiafentanil has been quoted to be 6000 times the potency of morphine (Stanley et al. 1988). Not only are these drugs potent, but they are also formulated in a relatively concentrated solution to increase their utility for remote delivery. Carfentanil is commercially available as a 3 mg/mL solution. Thiafentanil is typically used as a 10 mg/mL solution. These factors, taken together, will increase the risk of a significant human intoxication with exposure to a very small volume of drug.

There are several reports of human intoxication in the literature. Most of these reports detail human intoxication with etorphine (Anonymous 1976; Sheridan 1981; Summerhays 1976). One human fatality was reported from accidental injection of etorphine (Anonymous 1976). There is very little information concerning human intoxication from carfentanil or thiafentanil (Haymerle et al. 2010). It is likely that minor intoxications are not reported due to embarrassment (Haigh 1989).

The ultra potent narcotics have a high therapeutic index in comparison with older drugs, such as morphine (Wax et al. 2003). The therapeutic index of carfentanil in rats is 10,600 (Van Bever et al. 1976). It has been argued that the high therapeutic index may confer a higher level of safety in the event of human exposure. In October 2002, the Russian military used an "incapacitating gas" to end a hostage crisis at the Moscow Dubrovka Theater. The gas was most likely a mixture of carfentanil and halothane (Wax et al. 2003). Unfortunately, 127 of the 800 hostages died and 650 of the survivors required hospitalization. Given the high therapeutic index, this number of deaths was not anticipated by Russian officials (Wax et al. 2003). Obviously, it was not appropriate to directly extrapolate animal data to human beings (Wax et al. 2003). This incident stresses the need for a high level of vigilance when these agents are used.

A study published in 2010 (Haymerle et al. 2010) surveyed European zoo and wildlife practitioners and reviewed the literature regarding exposure to drugs used in wildlife capture and anesthesia. In 18 cases of exposure, the vast majority of individuals did not suffer severe symptoms; 2 of 18 individuals required administration of a narcotic antagonist. This study stressed the importance of proper personal protective gear and

the availability of a pharmacological antagonist (Haymerle et al. 2010)

Given the potential risks of these agents and their widespread use, it is surprising that there are very few published reports of accidental human intoxication. It is possible that this is the result of education and safe practice by zoo and wildlife veterinarians. A survey found that 65.1% of zoo veterinarians reported using ultrapotent narcotics and immobilizing agents (Hill et al. 1998). Of those who used these drugs, 86.7% had a written emergency protocol, 92.3% wore gloves, and 76.2% wore eye protection (Hill et al. 1998). This good standard of practice probably limits the incidence of adverse drug exposure in zoo veterinarians.

Prevention of exposure to potent narcotics is the best way to avoid intoxication. Protective clothing, gloves, and an eye shield should always be worn when these drugs are handled. Full face protection can be advantageous to prevent oral, ocular, or nasal exposure.

Symptoms of narcotic overdose in humans include nausea, dizziness, respiratory depression, and miosis. This can progress to coma and cardiovascular collapse with severe intoxication (Haigh & Haigh 1980). Rapid administration of a specific narcotic antagonist is vital in the face of severe intoxication. Naloxone has been advocated for this purpose, but it must be administered at a high dose, and due to its short half-life, repeated dosing will probably be required. A dose of 0.53–2 mg/kg of naloxone may be required to antagonize the effects of carfentanil in humans (Petrini et al. 1993). This may require up to 14 10 mL vials of 1 mg/mL naloxone (Petrini et al. 1993). In emergent situations, it would be ideal to administer naloxone via intravenous administration; this may be difficult due to lack of training in human IV access, or due to the challenges of functioning well in an emergent situation. Intranasal administration of naloxone has proven to be a viable alternative to intravenous administration in a prehospital setting (Barton et al. 2005). This may well be a good option to treat intoxication with potent narcotics in field situations. Naltrexone is commonly used to antagonize potent opioids in wildlife (Allen 1989). It has the advantage of a long half-life, which reduces the risk of renarcotization following antagonism of carfentanil (Allen 1989). Naltrexone is available as a 50 mg tablet for human use. It is advocated for the treatment of narcotic addiction and alcoholism. An oral formulation is less useful than an injectable form in emergent situations, particularly when intoxication may include nausea, vomiting, or coma. The oral formulation of naltrexone could prove useful after initial antagonism with naloxone, particularly in remote locations where medical help is difficult to access.

Intoxication from a large dose of an opioid can occur very rapidly. Personnel should always work in teams and everyone should be trained in first aid with a current CPR certificate. The major threat to life from opioid overdose is from respiratory depression. A means of assisting respiration, such as rescue breathing with a pocket mask or ambu bag can provide the respiratory support that is required until the intoxication is treated. If oxygen is available it should also be utilized during rescue breathing.

Alpha-2 Agonists

There are several published reports that detail human deaths or intoxication from xylazine (Capraro et al. 2001; Carruthers et al. 1979; Fyffe 1994). In most of these reports, xylazine was self-administered, either in a suicide attempt or for recreational use. Intoxication is commonly characterized by bradycardia, hypotension, and respiratory depression. Treatment of xylazine intoxication is typically supportive care and the use of assisted, or controlled ventilation (Capraro et al. 2001; Carruthers et al. 1979; Fyffe 1994). Alpha-2 antagonists, such as yohimbine and tolazoline, are not typically used to treat xylazine intoxication in humans.

The use of xylazine has been widespread in veterinary medicine. It has proved to be an extremely useful drug for wildlife capture and handling. In recent years, there has been a drive to develop alpha-2 agonists with increased potency and specificity for the alpha-2 receptor. Medetomidine has proven to be a very effective drug for wildlife capture and handling. It can be formulated in a concentrated solution of 10–40 mg/kg. This concentration, combined with its high potency, makes medetomidine very attractive for wildlife handling. This same factor will increase the risk of human intoxication with a very small volume exposure. Dexmedetomidine is the pharmacologically active d-isomer of medetomidine. Dexmedetomidine is marketed in the United States as Precedex® (Hospira Inc., Lake Forest IL). Precedex is typically administered as an IV loading dose of 1 μg/kg, followed by an infusion of 0.2–0.7 μg/kg/h. Side effects at this dose include transient hypertension (during the loading dose), bradyarrhythmias, and hypotension. This dose is used to induce sedation and facilitate ventilation of ICU patients. An IV dose of 75 μg (total) induced significant bradycardia and an 18% reduction in blood pressure (compared with baseline) in human volunteers (Kallio et al. 1989). This dose would be equivalent to approximately 150 μg of medetomidine. If medetomidine is formulated to a concentration of 10 mg/mL, this dose will be contained in 0.015 mL of solution. A dose of 120 μg of medetomidine has been reported to induce sleep in 50% of human males (Scheinin et al. 1998). This dose is equivalent to 0.003 mL of 40 mg/mL medetomidine (Haymerle et al. 2010). It is obvious from these examples that the formulation of medetomidine routinely used in wildlife anesthesia is extremely potent and deserves the same degree of respect that is given to potent opioids.

Treatment of exposure to a toxic dose of an alpha-2 agonist will be supportive, as no alpha-2 antagonist is currently approved for human use. In a field situation, the victim may benefit from administration of supplemental inspired oxygen and ventilatory support as needed. Airway protection will also be important if the victim becomes comatose. Heart rate and blood pressure should be monitored. Rapid evacuation to a medical facility is vital for the victim to receive appropriate treatment for hypotension and respiratory depression.

Phencyclidine Derivatives

There are two phencyclidine derivatives that are commonly used for wildlife anesthesia. Ketamine is typically used in combination with an alpha-2 agonist or a benzodiazepine tranquilizer. Telazol® and Zoletil® are 1 : 1 combinations of tiletamine, an arylcyclohexamine structurally related to phencyclidine and zolazepam, a benzodiazepine tranquilizer. There are case reports that detail human fatalities with self-administration of Telazol (Chung et al. 2000; Cording et al. 1999). These drugs are typically used to produce a state of dissociative anesthesia. One of the major side effects of ketamine is bizarre hallucinations; this has limited its utility in human anesthesia. Ketamine is a common drug of abuse. Its effects appear rapidly and include visual hallucinations and a dream-like state (Gahlinger 2004). Undesired side effects include confusion, delirium, tachycardia, palpitations, hypertension, and respiratory depression (Gahlinger 2004). A severe intoxication will result in loss of consciousness and the accompanying risks of respiratory depression or airway loss.

Ketamine is often snorted, with a typical abuse dose of 20 mg into each nostril (Stodder Cuddy 2004). It can be seen from the earlier discussion that a relatively low dose exposure of ketamine or tiletamine could produce intoxication. A low dose intoxication, which resulted in confusion or disorientation, could prove hazardous in a wildlife capture environment. In the event of a low dose intoxication, the victim should be removed from the capture team, reassured, closely monitored, and evacuated to a medical facility for observation. In the event of a high dose intoxication, the unconscious victim should receive supplemental oxygen, airway support, and rescue breathing if required. The victim should be rapidly evacuated to a medical facility for treatment.

EMERGENCY PREPAREDNESS

Every effort should be made to identify the risks associated with a planned capture procedure. It is always best to take steps to minimize the risk of human or animal injury. A preimmobilization plan will identify risks and allow the capture team to anticipate complications and take steps to mitigate risk. Unfortunately, risk reduction is not always 100% successful; therefore, it is vital to develop an emergency response protocol that can be initiated if an accident occurs.

Preimmobilization Plan

A preimmobilization plan should identify potential risks associated with a capture event or research project. Many of these risks are outlined earlier. All members of the capture team should be briefed on these risks prior to the capture. The plan should outline everyone's role on the capture team. A team leader is typically identified. The plan should ensure that everyone on the capture team is appropriately trained in wildlife handling techniques. Anyone working directly with the animal should receive appropriate training in chemical immobilization. Ideally, everyone on the team should receive training in first aid and hold a current CPR certificate. If this is not possible, at least two team members should have this training. Personnel should be trained in the proper use of darting equipment. Helicopter safety and firearms training may be indicated. Additional training may be required. This may include training in communications, survival, or terrain-specific training, such as cold water survival or avalanche rescue. Field equipment should be checked prior to a capture event. First aid kits and human antidotes should be carried, and team members must know how to access and use them. Appropriate clothing should be carried for the terrain and weather conditions.

A system of communications should be established between capture team members and with any personnel that will be required for evacuation or medical treatment of an accident victim. An emergency response plan will need to be developed. This plan must clearly outline the steps that will be taken in the event of an emergency. The plan should be well thought out and flexible enough to deal with any foreseeable emergency.

Emergency Response Protocol

An emergency response protocol should be developed prior to commencing work on a project and should be in place at any facility where there is a significant risk to human safety from wildlife or zoo animal capture and handling. These protocols are often quite specific for a facility or location, and will need to be revised if wildlife capture is initiated in a new location. Good examples of a specific emergency response protocols can be found in the following references (Petrini et al. 1993; Tolo & Keyler 1998). The emergency response protocol should be developed in consultation with physicians who may be required to treat the victim and with emergency medical services (EMS) personnel who may be required to treat and transport the victim. The main components to the protocol are consultation with medical professionals, communication, treatment, and evacuation.

Consultation with Medical Professionals

In any true emergency, time to treatment is probably the most important factor that will determine outcome. Emergency room physicians may not be familiar with drugs that are commonly used for wildlife capture. Development of an emergency response protocol should include a visit to the hospital that a victim will be evacuated to in the event of an emergency. Drug package inserts and information regarding the capture drugs should be given to the medical staff that may be required to treat the victim. The effects of most of these drugs can be extrapolated from similar drugs used in human medicine. The visit should also include a means to set up a communication link, from the field, to assist with initial stabilization of the victim. In some locations, the victim may require evacuation by the capture crew. It is preferable to have the victim evacuated by EMS whenever it is available. The development of the emergency response protocol should include a visit to the ambulance service that would transport the victim. Ideally, a paramedic should be dispatched to stabilize the victim. Stabilization in the field may include venous access and possibly intubation and ventilation, this treatment can be lifesaving. Again, the effects of the drugs and antagonists should be discussed.

Communication

A reliable method of communication should be established with EMS and with the hospital. This may be as simple as a cellular telephone. In remote locations, VHF radios may be used, either directly to EMS or via a dispatcher. Satellite telephones are very useful for this purpose as they can be used from very remote locations. A communications link is vital in an emergency situation.

Treatment and Evacuation

In the event of an emergency, timely treatment in the field will have a major influence on outcome. In remote locations, where access to EMS is difficult, capture team members should receive advanced first aid training. A first aid kit must be carried with appropriate equipment to treat a major traumatic incident. The accident victim should never be left alone, and help should be summoned as soon as possible. In the event of a drug intoxication, the key to a successful outcome will be the rapid administration of antagonists and supportive care. The unconscious victim should receive airway support and oxygenation. Rescue breathing can be lifesaving in the face of respiratory arrest. Rescue breathing can be learned through a CPR course. Ideally, advanced training should be taken to become certified in the use of pocket masks, oral airways, oxygen therapy, and ambu bags. This will facilitate ventilation with a high inspired concentration of oxygen.

An evacuation plan must be developed for every situation. Ideally, EMS should be used for the evacuation. Paramedics and EMT's are experts in this field and can ensure that the victim is cared for appropriately during transport. In remote locations, the capture team may need to evacuate the victim. The evacuation should be to the closest location for ambulance access, or directly to the hospital. If helicopters are used, it will be important to determine the best location for landing if there is not an established landing pad. The victim must never be left alone and should always be closely attended by someone who is trained in advanced first aid.

Capture and handling of wild animals is not without risk. It is vital to carefully plan for emergencies, as time spent planning and preparing for an emergency will generally dictate the outcome.

REFERENCES

Adejinmi JO, Ayinmode AB. 2008. Preliminary investigation of zooanthroponosis in a Nigerian zoological garden. *Veterinary Research* 2:38–41.

Allen JL. 1989. Renarcotization following carfentanil immobilization of nondomestic ungulates. *Journal of Zoo and Wildlife Medicine* 20:423–426.

Anonymous. 1976. Inquest-veterinary surgeon's immobilon death "accidental." *The Veterinary Record* 98:414.

Barton ED, Colwell CB, Wolfe T, et al. 2005. Efficacy of intranasal naloxone as a needless alternative for treatment of opioid overdose in the prehospital setting. *The Journal of Emergency Medicine* 29:265–271.

Bush M. 1992. Remote drug delivery systems. *Journal of Zoo and Wildlife Medicine* 23:159–180.

Capraro AJ, Wiley JF, Tucker JR. 2001. Severe intoxication from xylazine inhalation. *Pediatric Emergency Care* 17:447–448.

Carruthers SG, Wexler HR, Stiller CR. 1979. Xylazine Hydrochloride (Rompun) overdose in man. *Clinical Toxicology* 15:281–285.

Cattet M, Bourque A, Elkin B, et al. 2006. Evaluation of the potential for injury with remote drug delivery systems. *Wildlife Society Bulletin* 34:741–749.

Chung H, Choi H, Kim E, et al. 2000. A fatality due to injection of tiletamine and zolazepam. *Journal of Analytical Toxicology* 24:305–308.

Cording CJ, DeLuca R, Camporese T, et al. 1999. A fatality related to the veterinary anesthetic Telazol. *Journal of Analytical Toxicology* 23:552–555.

Fyffe JJ. 1994. Effects of xylazine on humans: a review. *Australian Veterinary Journal* 71:294–295.

Gahlinger PM. 2004. Club drugs: MDMA, gamma-hydroxybutyrate (GHB), Rohypnol, and ketamine. *American Family Physician* 69:2619–2626.

Haigh JC. 1989. Hazardous drugs in zoo and wildlife medicine: an update. Proceedings of the American Association of Zoo Veterinarians, p. 69–71.

Haigh JC, Haigh JM. 1980. Immobilizing drug emergencies in humans. *Veterinary and Human Toxicology* 22(2):94–98.

Haymerle A, Fahlman A, Walzer C. 2010. Human exposures to immobilizing agents: results of an online survey. *The Veterinary Record* 167:327–332.

Herzinger T, Scharrer E, Placzek M, et al. 2005. Contact urticaria to giraffe hair. *International Archives of Allergy and Immunology* 138:324–327.

Hill DJ, Langley RL, Morrow WM. 1998. Occupational injuries and illnesses reported by zoo veterinarians in the United States. *Journal of Zoo and Wildlife Medicine* 29:371–385.

Jessup DA, Clark RK, Weaver RA, et al. 1988. The safety and cost-effectiveness of net-gun capture of desert bighorn sheep (*Ovis canadensis nelsoni*). *Journal of Zoo Animal Medicine* 19:208–213.

Kallio A, Scheinin M, Koulu M, et al. 1989. Effects of dexmedetomidine, a selective á₂-adrenoceptor agonist on hemodynamic control mechanisms. *Clinical Pharmacology and Therapeutics* 46:33–42.

Krakowiak A, Palczyński C, Walusiak J, et al. 2002. Allergy to animal fur and feathers among zoo workers. *International Archives of Occupational and Environmental Health* 75(Suppl.):S113–S116.

Löe J, Röskaft E. 2004. Large carnivores and human safety: a review. *Ambio* 33:283–288.

Petrini KR, Keyler DE, Ling L, et al. 1993. Immobilizing agents: developing an urgent response protocol for human exposure. Proceedings of the AAZV, pp. 147–155.

Rowland AS, Baird AA, Weinberg CR, et al. 1992. Reduced fertility among women employed as dental assistants exposed to high levels of nitrous oxide. *The New England Journal of Medicine* 372:993–997.

Scheinin H, Aantaa R, Antilla M, et al. 1998. Reversal of the sedative and sympatholytic effects of dexmedetomidine with a specific alpha2-adrenoceptor agonist atipamezole: a pharmacokinetic and dynamic study in healthy volunteers. *Anesthesiology* 89:574–584.

Sheridan V. 1981. Immobilon incident. *The Veterinary Record* 108:503.

Smith T, Herrero S, Debruyn T, et al. 2008. Efficacy of bear deterrent spray in Alaska. *The Journal of Wildlife Management* 72:640–645.

Stanley TH, McJames S, Kimball J, et al. 1988. Immobilization of elk with A 3080. *The Journal of Wildlife Management* 52:577–581.

Stetter MD, Mikota SK, Gutter AF, et al. 1995. Epizootic of *Mycobacterium bovis* in a zoologic park. *Journal of the American Veterinary Medical Association* 207:1618–1621.

Stodder Cuddy ML. 2004. Common drugs of abuse: part II. *The Journal of Practical Nursing* 54:5–31.

Summerhays G. 1976. Overdosage with nalorphine hydrobromide following self-inflicted injury with Immobilon. *The Veterinary Record* 99:236.

Tolo D, Keyler D. 1998. Field management of inadvertent carfentanil (Wildnil™)/etorphine (M99™) human exposure. Proceedings of the American Association of Zoo Veterinarians and American Association of Wildlife Veterinarians, Omaha, NB, pp. 501–502.

Van Bever WF, Niemegeers CJ, Schellekens KH, et al. 1976. N-4-Substituted 1-(2-arylethyl)-4-piperindyl-N-phenylpropanamides, a novel series of extremely potent analgesics with unusually high safety margin. *Arzneimittel-Forschung* 26:1548–1551.

Wax PM, Becker CE, Curry SC. 2003. Unexpected "gas" casualties in Moscow: a medical toxicology perspective. *Annals of Emergency Medicine* 41:700–705.

Weston Murphy H, Miller M, Ramer J, et al. 2006. Implications of simian retroviruses for captive primate population management and the occupational safety of primate handlers. *Journal of Zoo and Wildlife Medicine* 37:219–233.

Section II

Invertebrates, Fish, Reptiles, and Amphibians

14 Invertebrates

Cornelia I. Mosley and Gregory A. Lewbart

INTRODUCTION

What sort of topic is invertebrate anesthesia and analgesia? A better first question might be "what exactly are invertebrates?" The invertebrates are a collection of animals, comprising more than 95% of the earth's species, unified by the lack of a vertebral column. Barnes and Ruppert (1994) stated invertebrates are a group of unrelated taxa that share no universal "positive" traits.

Depending on the text or specialist(s), there are currently over 30 recognized phyla of invertebrates (not including the protozoans). Many of these phyla be considered "obscure," but for no better reason than they may contain few species, microscopic representatives, or have no *obvious* economic value. In reality, each phylum and its members are important to the diversity and survival of the planet, even if the group is only studied by a small number of scientists. Unfortunately, relatively little is known about the veterinary, and more specifically, anesthesia/analgesia aspects, of many of these taxa. Writing a comprehensive book chapter for all invertebrate phyla would be an inefficient task. Consequently, we have elected to include, at least in this chapter, the most economically important and "visible" metazoan taxonomic groups.

The science of taxonomy is a dynamic and at times controversial branch of biology. We have elected to use the taxonomic terminology currently described in Ruppert et al. (2004), with the knowledge that some invertebrate zoologists may utilize a slightly different nomenclature for some groups.

Invertebrate anesthesia is still in its infancy and little research has been done to improve the understanding of the various anesthetic agents in this group of animals (Table 14.1). The goal of this chapter is to provide an overview of anesthetic concerns and techniques in more commonly anesthetized invertebrates. It should be emphasized that more research is necessary to better understand and improve anesthesia in the different, and frequently unrelated, invertebrate species.

TAXONOMIC GROUPS

Mollusks

Anatomy, Physiology, and Natural History The mollusks are a diverse and large group of animals that occupy terrestrial, freshwater, and marine environments. There are probably about 100,000 described extant species in this huge phylum. Some are extremely important to the environment because of their ability to filter water and consume debris and detritus. Economically, they are one of the most important taxa on earth, and provide billions of dollars annually as a source of food, animals for pets, display, and research, and as jewelry, artwork, and the lucrative shell-collecting hobby.

Details of molluscan natural history, anatomy, and physiology can be found in a number of references, including Ruppert et al. (2004); Lewbart (2012), and any general invertebrate zoology text. Malacology is the term used to describe the study of mollusks.

Despite their wide variety of function and form, nearly all mollusks have the following traits in common at some point in their life history: a muscular foot for locomotion, gills for respiration, a calcareous shell for protection and a mantle to secrete it, ciliated planktonic larvae for dispersal, and a chitinous radula for feeding.

We have elected to divide up the mollusks into three separate groups. It should be noted that only the most economically important classes are discussed, as these are the groups that have received some attention with

Zoo Animal and Wildlife Immobilization and Anesthesia, Second Edition. Edited by Gary West, Darryl Heard, and Nigel Caulkett.
© 2014 John Wiley & Sons, Inc. Published 2014 by John Wiley & Sons, Inc.

Table 14.1. Immobilization and anesthetic drugs used in invertebrates

Invertebrate	Anesthetic Agent	Dosage	Induction Time	Recovery	Comments	Source
Gastropods						
Snails	Ethanol (5%)					Flores et al. (1983)
	Ethanol (21.9%) + menthol (0.042%)				10% Listerine solution	Woodall et al. (2003)
Great pond snail	Sodium pentobarbital	0.4 mg/mL H_2O	8 hours		Low mortality rate	Martins-Sousa et al. (2001)
	Isoflurane	MAC: 1.09%	<10 minutes	<10 minutes	Induction excitement	Girdlestone et al. (1989)
	1-Phenoxy-2-propanol	8–16 mmol/L	1.5 hours		Stir solution well to avoid tissue damage	Wyeth et al. (2009)
Sea snails	Magnesium sulfate or Mg Cl_2	Intracoelomic	2–5 minutes		Good muscle relaxation	Clark et al. (1996)
Abalone	2-Phenoxyethanol	0.5–3 mL/L	1–3 minutes	5–20 minutes		White et al. (1996)
	Benzocaine	100 mg/L	13–28 minutes			Edwards et al. (2000)
	Magnesium sulfate	4–22 g/100 mL water	5–8 minutes	3–35 minutes	Larger size = higher dosage	White et al. (1996)
	Sodium pentobarbital	1 mL/L	15 minutes 34–78 minutes	<80 minutes	Decrease in HR Size dependent induction/recovery timing	Aquilina and Roberts (2000) Sharma et al. (2003)
Cephalopods						
Cuttlefish	Ethanol	15–30 mL/L >10–15 mL/L	1 minutes	20 minutes	Transient excitement	Harms et al. (2006)
Octopus	Mg Cl_2	6.8 g/L	6–12 minutes			Gore et al. (2005)
	Ethanol	20 mL/L (2%)	4 minutes	2.5 minutes	Excitement, not effective in cold water species	Andrews and Tansey (1981)
	Mg Cl_2 (7.5%)/H_2O	50/50	1.5–13 minutes	1–10 minutes	Smooth induction and recovery	Messenger et al. (1985); Culloty and Mulcahy (1992)

	Agent	Dosage	Induction	Recovery	Notes	References
Bivalves						
Oysters	Propylene phenoxetol (1% solution)	1–3 mL/L	6–15 minutes	<30 minutes	Dosage is species dependent	Norton et al. (1996); Mills et al. (1997)
	Mg Cl$_2$ (3.5%)		1–2 hours	90 minutes	Variable effects, long induction and recovery, species + temperature dependent, see text for details	Norton et al. (1996); Mills et al. (1997), Culloty et al. (1992); and others
Scallops	Mg Cl$_2$	30–50 g/L	2–6 minutes	10 minutes	Drug of choice	Heasman et al. (1995)
	Chloral hydrate	4 g/L	10–25 minutes	20–30 minutes	Variable effects, temperature dependent	Heasman et al. (1995)
Arachnida						
Spiders and scorpions	Isoflurane/sevoflurane	3–5%/4–6%	5–15 minutes	3–20 minutes	Induction chamber system	Pizzi (2012); Melidone and Mayer (2005); Cooper (2001)
Crustaceans						
Crayfish	Lidocaine	0.4–1 mg/g IM	1.5 minutes	5–30 minutes		Brown et al. (1996)
	Ketamine	40–90 μg/g IM	1 minutes	1–2 hours, Dose dependent.	Variable response	Brown et al. (1996)
Giant crab	Ketamine	25–100 μg/kg IV	15–45 seconds	8–40 minutes	Brief induction excitement	Gardner (1997)
	Xylazine	16–22 mg/kg IV	3–5 minutes	25–45 minutes	Bradycardia high dosages (70 mg/kg IV)	Gardner (1997); Oswald (1977)
Crabs	Procaine	25 mg/kg IV	20–30 seconds	2–3 hours	Excitatory phase, very long duration	Oswald (1977)
Blue crab	Lidoaine	70 mg/kg IV	12.5 seconds	2–3 minutes	Very short duration	Quesada et al. (2011)
	Ketamine	20 mg/kgIV	1 minutes	5 minutes	Reliable and deep anesthesia	Quesada et al. (2011)
Small crabs	Clove oil	0.125 mL/L	16 minutes	2.5 hours	Add xylazine (20 mg/kg) for greater effects	Gardner (1997)
Lobster	Eugenol	75–100 ppm	10 minutes	8 minutes	Euthanasia at long durations	Waterstrat et al. (2005)
Echinoderms						
Seastar	MgCl$_2$	7.5–8%				Harms (2012); McCurley and Kier (1995)
Sea urchin	MS222	1–10 g/L				Hendler et al. (1995); O'Neill (1994)
	Menthol	2.5–5%				Costello and Henley (1971)
	MgCl$_2$	5–20 mmol/L				Arafa et al. (2007)

193

regards to anesthesia and analgesia. Classes not covered include the Aplacophora, Monoplacophora, Polyplacophora (chitons), and Scaphopoda (tusk or tooth shells).

Gastropods

Anatomy, Physiology, and Natural History The gastropods are a large, important, and easily recognized group that includes the abalone, snails, nudibranchs, and sea hares, among others. Most are aquatic and have a well-developed head with eyes and other sensory organs, an external shell, muscular foot, and gills within a chamber for respiration. There are many exceptions, however, and one need only examine a common garden slug (no shell or gills and terrestrial) to appreciate the exceptions and diversity within the taxon.

Physical Restraint Gastropods are generally slow-moving and easy to restrain manually or with a protective container. While most gastropods are harmless to humans, members of the tropical genus *Conus* can inflict serious injury or even death with small toxic "harpoons," which are modified teeth from the radula.

Anesthetic Agents Used and Techniques Garden and pond snails can be anesthetized with menthol or 5% ethanol (Flores et al. 1983) or inhalant agents such as isoflurane (Girdlestone et al. 1989). A commercial 10% Listerine® solution (ethanol 21.9%, menthol 0.042%) in normal *Lymnaea* saline is commonly used to anesthetize pond snails (*Lymnaea*) in research settings (Woodall et al. 2003). Sodium pentobarbital at 0.4 mg/mL in water has been reported in freshwater snails (*Biomphalarias)* with a very slow onset (8 hours), but good effects and a low mortality rate (Martins-Sousa et al. 2001).

The drug of choice in queen conch (*Strombus gigas*) is magnesium chloride (30 g/L) (Acosta-Salmon & Davis 2007). Other agents (2-phenoxethanol, menthol, benzocaine, and MS-222) failed to produce muscle relaxation.

Anesthesia via isoflurane for terrestrial snails requires an anesthetic chamber with the ability for fresh gas inflow and waste gas scavenging (Girdlestone et al. 1989). The minimum anesthetic concentration (MAC) of isoflurane in the pond snail is reported as 1.09 (Girdlestone et al. 1989). Induction is fast (<10 minutes), but an excitatory period is common. One disadvantage of using inhalant anesthesia is the need to take the animal out of the chamber for the procedure, which results in fluctuation of anesthetic depth and increased pollution. Furthermore, the depth of anesthesia may not be adequate for surgical procedures.

An anesthesia level reached in snails is defined when body and tentacle withdrawal response to gentle stimulation is absent. Tentacle withdrawal reflex remaining under inhalant anesthesia may suggest an insufficient depth for surgery (Girdlestone et al. 1989).

Ketamine and propofol do not induce anesthesia and might even show an excitatory, not a depressant, effect (Woodall & McCrohan 2000). Ketamine in combination with xylazine may have toxic effects (Martins-Sousa et al. 2001).

Some nudibranchs (marine gastropods), such as the opalescent sea slug (*Hermissede crassicornis*) and *Tritonia diomedea*, have been successfully anesthetized with 1-phenoxy-2-propanol (PP) via bath application (Wyeth et al. 2009). An initial concentration of 8 mmol/L in appropriate water volume is recommended and can be increased to 16 mmol/L. Induction time can be 1.5 hours to achieve adequate muscle relaxing effects. It is important to stir the solution thoroughly to avoid tissue damage from undissolved PP (Wyeth et al. 2009).

Bigger sea snails, such as the California sea hare (*Aplysia californica*), can be anesthetized with intracoelomic administration of magnesium sulfate or magnesium chloride (Clark et al. 1996). Induction is fast (2–5 minutes) and smooth, leading to good muscle relaxation. Halothane and MS-222 seem to be ineffective (administered as immersion or intracoelomic) in this species (Clark et al. 1996).

Abalone Abalones (*Haliotis* sp.) are commercially farmed and frequently require physical examination and sizing, pearl seeding, and removal from holding tanks for maintenance and harvesting (White et al. 1996). Removal of abalones from the substratum is often only possible with mechanical assistance due to their ability to tightly adhering to the substratum. This forced removal may result in injury with slow recovery or even death. Therefore, a muscle relaxing or anesthetic agent may be necessary to avoid stress and mechanical injuries related to dislodging. Protocols used in abalones for removal include ethanol (3%), 2-phenoxyethanol (1–2 mL/L), benzocaine (100 mg/L), magnesium sulfate (2–24 g/100 mL), and sodium pentobarbital (1 mL/L) (Aquilina & Roberts 2000; Edwards et al. 2000, Sharma et al. 2003). Magnesium sulfate is administered in water (4–22 g/100 mL), with dose ranges depending on size of the abalone (higher doses for larger animals) (White et al. 1996). Induction time is fast (5–8 minutes) and recovery is uneventful (3–35 minutes, depending on dose and anesthesia time). Phenoxyethanol is administered at 0.05–0.3 mL/100 mL and also shows a fast induction period (1–3 minutes) and a recovery time of 5–20 minutes (White et al. 1996). Nembutal (sodium pentobarbital, 1 mL/L = 60 mg/L) produces good muscle relaxation with an induction time of 15 minutes and complete recovery (Aquilina & Roberts 2000; Sharma et al. 2003). In Sharma's study, induction time was size dependent, with larger animals needing longer time for complete relaxation (78 minutes) than smaller animals (34 minutes) (Sharma at al., 2003). A 50% decrease in heart rate occurred during anesthesia and further decline continued when anesthesia was prolonged. Recovery was completed in all abalones by 80 minutes (Sharma et al. 2003). The water should be held at a temperature between 16 and 23°C for reliable effects (Aquilina & Roberts 2000; Sharma et al. 2003).

Clove oil (0.5–1.5 mL/L) and propylene phenoxytol (2.5 mL/L) are not recommended since both agents can cause unacceptable high mortalities (Aquilina & Roberts 2000; Edwards et al. 2000). Tricaine methanesulfonate (MS-222) at 1 g/L and benzocaine (0.1 g/L) are ineffective as muscle relaxants in these abalone species (Aquilina & Roberts 2000). During induction, both MS-222 and propylene phenoxytol cause major excitation, resulting in copious mucus production and loss of pigment (Aquilina & Roberts 2000).

Recovery from any anesthetic includes thorough washing of the abalone and exposure to fresh flowing seawater at their optimal temperature (18°C) until muscle strength returns.

Cephalopods

Anatomy, Physiology, and Natural History This group of predatory and specialized mollusks includes such familiar forms as the squids, cuttlefish, octopuses, and the chambered nautilus. Most of these animals are pelagic and have the ability for fast locomotion. They have closed circulatory systems, high metabolic rates, and advanced nervous systems that include excellent vision and tactile senses. Most have an internal skeleton (shell), with the exceptions being the octopuses (no shell) and the nautilus (external shell). Other interesting features of most members include the ability to "ink" when disturbed or threatened, suction-cup discs on the arms, and internal fertilization. All of the approximately 700 extant species are marine.

Physical Restraint Generally, these animals are difficult to handle, other than for a quick move or relocation, without sedation. Buckets, plastic nets, or other objects may be used to capture or restrain cephalopods.

Anesthetic Agents Used and Techniques Cephalopods should ideally be anesthetized in their own seawater to maintain the mineral balance. The two most commonly used anesthetic agents in these marine invertebrate species are magnesium chloride ($MgCl_2$) and ethanol.

Cuttlefish (*Sepia officinalis*) have been successfully anesthetized with 1.5–3% ethanol (15–30 mL/L) diluted in seawater (Harms et al. 2006). Inductions are rapid (1 minute), especially at higher doses, and dilution to a lower concentration (10–15 mL/L) to decrease the risk of overdosing should be considered. During inductions with lower concentrations of ethanol, occasional transient excitement has been noticed (Harms et al. 2006). If the procedure cannot be performed in the water,

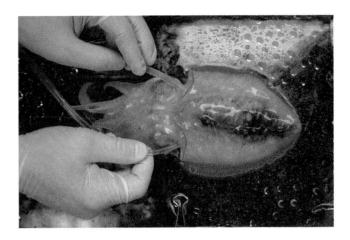

Figure 14.1. A recirculating anesthesia system containing dilute ethanol with an anesthetized cuttlefish (*Sepia officinalis*). Note that two irrigating tubes are being used, one for each set of gills (photo courtesy of J. Bolynn).

anesthesia is maintained with a recirculating anesthesia system (Lewbart & Harms 1999) (Fig. 14.1). The anesthetic concentration of the water is adjusted over time to the depth of anesthesia desired.

If magnesium chloride ($MgCl_2$) is used as an anesthetic agent in cuttlefish, a 7.5% MgCl stock solution can be prepared with distilled water (Gore et al. 2005; Scimeca & Forsythe 1999). This stock solution is mixed with a known amount of seawater to prepare an anesthetic concentration suitable for induction. A final concentration of 6.8 g/L (100 mL of the stock solution mixed with 1 L of seawater) has been reported to have an induction time of 6–12 minutes without side effects (Gore et al. 2005). Due to the size of the cuttlefish, a total water volume of 6–8 L is commonly needed. Induction is usually smooth and without a period of excitation. Decreasing the concentration via dilution may be necessary over time to adjust the depth of anesthesia.

Octopuses (*Octopus vulgaris*) are anesthetized in a similar manner. Two commonly employed anesthetic agents are ethanol and $MgCl_2$. Ethanol (2% v/v in seawater) can produce excitement during the short induction time (increased respiratory rate, attempts to climb out of the solution and ink ejection) (Andrews & Tansey 1981). Induction time has been reported to be 4 minutes and time to full recovery as 2.5 minutes (Andrews & Tansey 1981). Ethanol (2%) does not seem to be effective in coldwater species (below 15°C) (I.G. Gleadall, pers. comm., 2006).

Long-term anesthesia (5 hours) in longfin squids (*Doryteuthis pealii*) with magnesium chloride (0.15 mol $MgCl_2$ seawater solution) has been successfully achieved (Mooney et al. 2010). The animals were placed into the $MgCl_2$ solution until relaxed and nonresponsive with decreasing respiratory rate, then recovered in a $MgCl_2$ free tank and reimmersed when lightened. Increasing

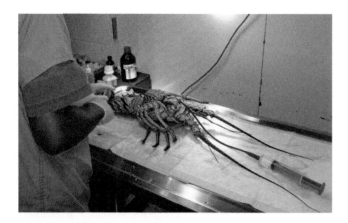

Figure 14.2. Spiny lobster (*Panularis* spp.) anesthesia: This adult spiny lobster has been anesthetized with a eugenol immersion, followed by eugenol gill perfusion, for some diagnostic procedures (photo courtesy of M. Mehalick).

duration of anesthesia was noted with subsequent immersions (20–111 minutes) (Mooney et al. 2010).

Overall, $MgCl_2$ is the preferred anesthetic agent in cephalopods. It is used by preparing an isotonic solution of 7.5% $MgCl_2.6H_2O$ (in distilled water) mixed with an equal volume of seawater (Messenger et al. 1985; Scimeca & Forsythe 1999). Induction time lies between 1.5 and 13 minutes with a short period of hyperventilation, then a gradual increase in arm flaccidity and righting reflexes; it is considered to be very smooth (Culloty & Mulcahy 1992; Messenger et al. 1985). Respiration will decrease and even cease if the anesthetic concentration is not decreased. The gills should be intermittently or constantly perfused with anesthetic seawater (Fig. 14.2). Time of recovery from $MgCl_2$ is fairly quick (1–10 minutes), but dependent on length and type of procedure (up to 20–60 minutes after prolonged procedures).

There is a controversy whether $MgCl_2$ produces adequate sedation and analgesia by blocking nerve transmission and neurotransmitter release, or acts only as a neuromuscular blocking agent (Clark et al. 1996). Differences in vertebrate versus invertebrate anatomy/physiology, as well as routes of administration seem to play a role in the effects, but the issue remains unresolved (Clark et al. 1996). An analgesic should be added to the protocol for any painful procedure to assure adequate patient care.

The use of urethane has been reported (Andrews & Tansey 1981; Gleadall 1991; Messenger et al. 1985) and was routinely used in the 1970s and 1980s, but despite good anesthetic effects, the traumatic effects on the animals were severe (excitement during the induction phase). Chloroform, chloral hydrate, gallamine, and CO_2 are unsuitable anesthetic agents in cephalopods as they can cause high mortality (Garcia-Franco 1992; Gleadall 1991; Mooney et al. 2010).

It should be emphasized that hypothermia, despite its popularity in the literature, is not an adequate anesthetic and should not be used in this group of animals due to its lack of analgesic and muscle relaxing properties. Mortalities and distress have been reported (Bower et al. 1999; Mooney et al. 2010). The underestimation of cardiovascular and respiratory system compromise during hypothermia, as well as in the phase of warming, may be one of the leading causes.

For recovery, the cephalopod is placed into a container with anesthesia-free seawater. Ideally, the water in this container is circulated and aerated. If spontaneous respiration is not present, gentle and slow mantle massage can be used until normal respiration is restored. The tentacles remain extended and flaccid in the first phase of the recovery and will retract in response to light pinching with progressive awakening (Harms et al. 2006).

Resuscitation of cephalopods includes squeezing and relaxation of the whole mantle/body for water circulation over the gills and hemolymph through the body (Harms et al. 2006). Anesthesia-free water should be directed over the gills for a washout effect.

Cephalopods are commonly monitored by visualization of their respiratory rate and pattern. Normal awake values for *O. vulgaris* in a weight range from 100 to 800 g are 26–30 breath/min (Andrews & Tansey 1981). The cardiovascular system is assessed by placing a Doppler probe on the dorsal area (above the aorta) or behind the gills (above either branchial heart) to monitor heart rate and blood flow. A pulse oximeter will likely give false readings due to the presence of hemocyanin instead of hemoglobin, but may be used for heart rate. In transparent species (espesially with $MgCl_2$), the pallial organs can be observed. Depth of anesthesia is difficult to assess in cephalopods. One guideline is that the level of anesthesia seems adequate when no response to tactile and surgical stimuli is present (withdrawal of appendices or movement, contraction of the skin around the eye in response to pressure on the eyeball, withdrawal of the animal in response to a pinch of the skin over the eye [Andrews & Tansey 1981]). Further indicators of anesthetic depth are the flaccidity of the arms, loss of normal posture, and inability to regain normal posture after disturbance (Andrews & Tansey 1981). Respiration usually remains spontaneous and varies in depth and rate with the level of anesthesia (Mooney et al. 2010); a depression or cessation is a sign of critical deep levels of anesthesia.

Bivalves

Anatomy, Physiology, and Natural History This large and economically important group of highly evolved mollusks includes the clams, mussels, oysters, and scallops. They lack a well-developed head, are generally nonvisual (the scallops are an exception), feed by filtration utilizing the gills for food transport, and utilize a muscular and sometimes large foot for locomotion. All of the approximately 8000 described extant species are aquatic, and nearly 80% of these are marine.

Physical Restraint Most bivalves are easy to handle and restrain safely. Nearly all will tightly close their calcareous valves when handled or disturbed and may require sedation or physical manipulation (prying) to open the valves, which are held fast by strong adductor muscles.

Anesthetic Agents Used and Techniques

Oysters Oysters are commonly anesthetized for pearl harvesting and seeding. There are four major pearl oyster species used in the cultured pearl industry (Mamangkey et al. 2009). Unfortunately every oyster species seems to be responding differently to the various anesthetic agents (Mamangkey et al. 2009).

Propylene phenoxetol can be used as a 1% solution to anesthetize oysters (*Pinctada albino, Pinctada margaritifera,* and *Pinctada maxima* and *Pteria penguin*) in a dose range from 1 to 3 mL/L. Higher doses induce a rapid and relative deep level of anesthesia (Mills et al. 1997) and may need decreasing throughout the procedure to decrease recovery time (Norton et al. 1996). Generally, concentrations are dependent on species and study design, and recommendations vary: 1–2 mL/L are safe and effective for most oyster species (Mills et al. 1997; Norton et al. 1996), but Mamangkey et al. (2009) recommend 2.5 mL/L for *P. maxima*, Kishore (2011) suggests 3.0 mL/L for *P. penguin*, and O'Connor and Lawler (2002) recommend 2.2 mL/L for *Pinctada imbricate* and *P. albina.*

The oyster should be placed hinge down in the solution, leaning against the walls of the aerated container to facilitate monitoring. Induction time is reported to be between 6 and 15 minutes. Adequate anesthesia is reached when the oyster gapes wide enough to part the gill curtain inside the shell and shows no responsiveness to handling (Mills et al. 1997) or contraction of the tissue to a stimulus (Norton et al. 1996). A decrease in stress from handling before placing oysters into the anesthesia container will improve the anesthetic effects and opening. Recovery time with propylene phenoxetol is short (10–30 minutes), although it depends on length of procedure, concentration of anesthetic, and temperature (Kishore 2011; Norton et al. 1996). Recovery tanks should be aerated.

The muscle contractility in invertebrates is dependent on the interaction between Ca^{2+} and Mg^{2+}. Magnesium chloride works via the Mg^{2+} effect of inhibiting the facilitating effect of Ca^{2+} at the synaptic transmission (Altura et al. 1987; Namba et al. 1995), and it is suspected that it works mainly as a muscle relaxant rather than an anesthetic.

Magnesium chloride has variable effects on oysters. Some studies describe little effect in pearl oysters

(*P. maxima*) (Mills et al. 1997; Norton et al. 1996), mainly due to long induction times (1–2 hours). Culloty and Mulcahy (1992) reported good anesthetic effects in flat oysters (*Ostrea edulis*), but also long induction and recovery times (90 minutes) at 3.5%. Suquet et al. (2009, 2010) found flat oysters (*O. edulis*) and Pacific oysters (*Crassostrea gigs*) can be successfully anesthetized for gonad sampling by maintaining them for 2–3 hours in a 50 g/L $MgCl_2$ bath at 19°C (1/3 seawater; 2/3 freshwater). A study in Sydney rock oysters (*Saccostrea glomerata*) found $MgCl_2$ to be the only effective agent as a muscle relaxant at a concentration of 50 g/L with an onset time of 30 minutes to 6 hours (Butt et al. 2008). The effect of $MgCl_2$ seems dependent on species, concentration, duration, and water temperature with significant variable times to effect (Namba et al. 1995; Suquet et al. 2009, 2010).

Tricaine methanesulfonate and chloral hydrate are not effective in oysters (slow induction and recovery) and are associated with complications (death; some of it may be related to the low pH of unbuffered MS-222) (Norton et al. 1996).

Eugenol often produces a high mortality in oysters (Mamangkey et al. 2009; Suquet et al. 2009). Benzocaine also has a high mortality in a dose-dependent manner in the Pacific oyster (Suquet et al. 2009), but worked well in *P. maxima, Pinctada fucata, P. margaritifera,* and *P. penguin* at 1200 mg/L with a fast induction time of about 10–16 minutes (Acosta-Salmon et al. 2005; Kishore 2011; Mamangkey et al. 2009). Cases of body and/or mantle collapse have been reported with the use of benzocaine (Acosta-Salmon et al. 2005; Kishore 2011). Another disadvantage of using benzocaine is its inability to dissolve in seawater, which leads to an extensive preparation process (Acosta-Salmon et al. 2005; Kishore 2011; Mamangkey et al. 2009).

A drug that dissolves well and provides effective anesthesia with short induction time (13 minutes) and over 95% survival rate in *P. maxima* is 2-phenoxyethanol (3 mL/L) and can be recommended for this oyster species (Mamangkey et al. 2009).

Scallops Anesthesia in scallops may be required, but mainly for muscle relaxation. In general, the depth of anesthesia/relaxation is adequate when handling and stimulating of the mantle tissue fails to stimulate shell closure. Recovery is often defined as the regained ability for shell closure in response to handling (Heasman et al. 1995).

Magnesium chloride is the drug of choice in scallops due to its rapid and consistent induction and recovery. The agent is predissolved in seawater and then added to the aerated induction container to reach a concentration of 30–50 g/L. Induction times at these concentrations are quick and in the range of 2–6 minutes. Recovery time in scallops anesthetized with $MgCl_2$ seems to be consistently short (10 minutes) regardless of concentration used or temperature (Heasman et al. 1995).

Chloral hydrate has variable effects in scallops, with significant changes in induction and recovery at different concentrations and temperatures (Heasman et al. 1995). A concentration of 4 g/L produces anesthesia in about 10–25 minutes, if temperature is held at 24°C. Lower temperatures will significantly slow the induction period. Higher concentrations will shorten the induction time, but can result in high mortality. Recovery time at 4 g/L is between 20 and 30 minutes, but varies widely depending on temperature (and concentration). Aerated seawater recovery tanks and continuously flushing with seawater will facilitate recovery.

Other drugs have been examined for scallop anesthesia with little success. MS-222 causes hyperactivity and hyperextension, benzocaine causes an initial hyperactivity, metomidate results in shell closure, ethanol does not seem to have any effect, and magnesium sulfate leads to high mortality (Heasman et al. 1995).

Giant Clams   Giant clams (*Tridacna* sp.) have been anesthetized with propylene phenoxetol (Mills et al. 1997).

Arachnida

Introduction   The arachnids are a large class of approximately 70,000 described species of terrestrial carnivorous chelicerates (Ruppert et al. 2004). All Chelicerata, a group that also includes the horseshoe crabs, scorpions, and sea spiders (Pycnogonida), belong to the phylum Arthropoda. Spiders, mites, and ticks make up the bulk of the arachnid species. Less conspicuous arachnids include the whip spiders, microwhip spiders, harvestmen, pseudoscorpions, tick spiders, and sun spiders. Tarantulas (Mygalomorphae) represent an important group of commonly kept arachnids that frequently require medical care.

Spiders (Araneae)

Anatomy, Physiology, and Natural History The spiders comprise one of the largest orders in the class Arachnida (which belongs in the subphylum Chelicerata). There are approximately 40,000 described species of spiders (Araneae) belonging to 3000 genera, with thousands more species as yet undescribed (Ruppert et al. 2004).

Spiders range in size from a body of less than a millimeter to over 9 cm for large tropical tarantulas (Ruppert et al. 2004). The basic spider body plan includes two large segments, the cephalothorax and the abdomen, connected to each other by the pedicel. All spiders have four pairs of walking legs, paired chelicerae, and paired pedipalps. The fangs are located at the tip of the chelicerae and are used to immobilize prey, frequently by injecting venom. The male pedipalps are usually modified to aid in sperm delivery. The spinneret is located at the distal end of the abdomen and is used to spin silk, an ability that virtually all spiders possess and use for a variety of functions.

Spiders are carnivorous and perform most of their digestion outside of the gastrointestinal (GI) tract (food is digested in a cavity adjacent to the mouth and the liquefied food is then ingested). The GI tract is divided into the foregut (mouth, pharynx, and esophagus), midgut (many branching cecae), and a short hindgut (Ruppert et al. 2004).

Spiders breathe through book lungs, trachea, or both. Tarantulas have two pairs of book lungs that are found on the ventral aspect of the abdomen. Most spiders have just one pair of abdominal book lungs and a pair of tracheae. Other combinations and modifications on these two plans are found within the order (Ruppert et al. 2004).

Spiders possess an open circulatory system with the hemolymph functioning in oxygen transport, immune defense, waste removal, and limb mobility through hydrostatic pressure. The heart is large and located in the dorsal abdominal segment. Most spiders excrete uric acid as well as adenine and guanine as their nitrogenous waste products. Malphigian tubules absorb these compounds from the hemolymph and direct them into the cloacal chamber, where they are excreted with the feces (Ruppert et al. 2004).

Spiders have two main nerve centers located in the cephalothorax: the subesophageal and supraesophageal ganglia. Spiders sense their environment in a number of ways, including vision, tactile reception, chemoreception, and vibration detection. These are accomplished with four pairs of eyes, tactile hairs, chemosensory hairs, and slit sense organs, respectively (Ruppert et al. 2004).

Sexes are separate in spiders and fertilization is generally internal. Female spiders produce egg sacs that may contain thousands of young, and there are varying degrees of parental care among spiders. While most spiders probably do not live longer than 2 years, some female tarantulas may live for several decades (Pizzi 2012).

Physical Restraint Physical restraint is commonly used to handle and transport spiders (Fig. 14.3). However, some tarantula species are capable of shedding urticating hairs, which can be quite irritating, especially to individuals allergic to these structures. Other drawbacks to manual restrain are injury to the animal and potential envenomation of the handler. It is advisable to wear latex gloves when handling spiders and to be cautious of dropping the spider or having it leap or fall to the ground.

Anesthetic Agents Used and Techniques Spiders are most commonly and successfully anesthetized with inhalant anesthetic agents. Many agents (halothane, isoflurane,

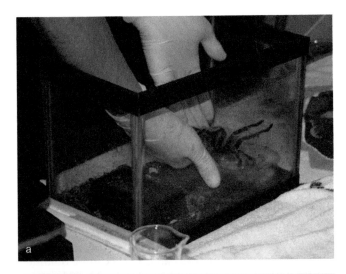

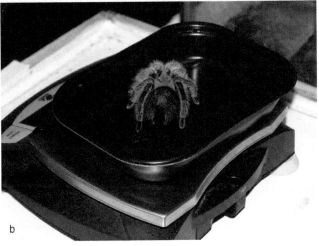

Figure 14.3. (a) Wearing latex gloves, or other protective measures, should be taken when handling many invertebrates, like this rose hair tarantula (*Grammostola rosea*). (b) Sensible physical capture and restraint are used to obtain a weight from this rose hair tarantula (photos courtesy of M. Mehalick).

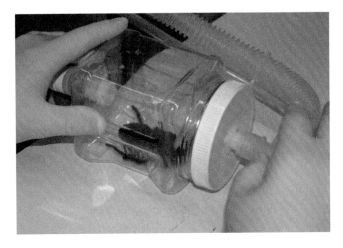

Figure 14.4. Inhalant anesthetic chamber for terrestrial invertebrates. Pictured here is an anesthetized rose hair tarantula (5% isoflurane) (photo courtesy of M. Mehalick).

sevoflurane, and desflurane) have been used, although halothane will not be available in the near future in North America. Of the potent inhalant anesthetics, halothane is least desirable for invertebrate anesthesia, because of the high likelihood of potential toxicity for personnel during gas delivery.

Several different induction chambers have been described (Cooper 2001; Melidone & Mayer 2005; Pizzi 2012) and used successfully for delivering inhalant anesthesia to spiders. These chambers are either commercially available induction chambers (invertebrate-specific or regular small mammal induction chambers) with appropriate fresh gas inflow and scavenging outflow, or simple self-made clear plastic containers (Fig. 14.4). Plastic containers without the use of an inflow and outflow system may be used by placing a cotton wool swab soaked with a small amount of inhalant agent into the box. The spider itself should be placed in a separate smaller container with small pores. The smaller container holding the spider is placed into the larger box, allowing the inhalant to diffuse into the box with the spider while ensuring that the spider cannot come into direct contact with the inhalant-soaked cotton swab. This method is not ideal because of the higher exposure risk to the personnel of the anesthetic agent, less control of the amount of anesthetic given to the spider, and higher risk of overdose. An induction chamber using anesthetic gas given via a precision vaporizer is much preferred. The advantages of the chamber technique are convenience of use, low cost, and safety to the patient associated with the set up. The disadvantage associated with this type of system is that the animal can only be temporarily sedated or anesthetized. For any physical examination or surgery, the animal is removed from the chamber, which limits the time for any procedure before the animal recovers. This may require repeated inductions, but also increases the exposure of the clinician and staff to the anesthetic gases. A surgery chamber has been developed (Melidone & Mayer 2005) that allows the clinician to perform the surgery or other manipulations on the animal without taking the animal out of the chamber.

Another interesting technique is to induce the spider in an anesthetic chamber and then place its abdomen (with the associated book lungs/tracheae) into a smaller chamber "sealed" with a latex glove (Fig. 14.5). This technique appears to have some merit when a procedure must be performed on the cephalothorax or limbs (Dombrowski 2006).

The most commonly used anesthetic agents for spiders are isoflurane and sevoflurane (Cooper 2001; Melidone & Mayer 2005; Pizzi 2012). The animal is placed into the chamber and the chamber is filled with

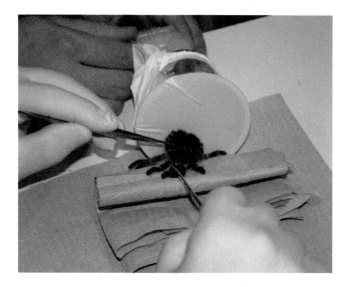

Figure 14.5. Since the spider's respiratory intake is located in the abdominal segment it appears that at least some species can be maintained on inhalant anesthesia, as shown here, while the limbs and cranial body parts are examined or manipulated. This is a rose hair tarantula (*Grammostola rosea*) (photo courtesy of M. Mehalick).

the anesthetic gas (about 3–5% for isoflurane; 4–6% for sevoflurane). To increase the filling time in larger chambers, the oxygen flow rate is high at the beginning (1–3 L/min), but can be decreased to a minimum if there are no major leaks in the system (300–1000 mL/min). Oxygen flow lower than 200 mL/min decreases the accuracy of the vaporizer and may decrease the amount of anesthetic agent in the chamber due to the uptake of the animal; the amount of CO_2 in the chamber may also be increased using low fresh gas flows. An appropriate scavenging system is necessary to decrease pollution and exposure of the staff to anesthetic gases. With increasing depth of anesthesia, the vaporizer can be adjusted (decreased over time). The MAC of the different anesthetic agents in spiders has not been determined.

Other agents, such as carbon dioxide (CO_2) and nitrogen (N_2), as well as hypothermia, have been used to immobilize spiders (Madsen & Vollrath 2000; Pizzi 2012). No reports about the amount of nitrogen used or the quality of nitrogen anesthesia could be found. Carbon dioxide is administered as a gas in a chamber, often producing 98% saturation. Dilution with air or oxygen is hard to achieve, resulting in an increased risk for mortalities (Pizzi 2012). Hypothermia is not an anesthetic and does not provide analgesia; hypothermia itself is considered to be painful, and should therefore not be used as an anesthetic.

Observing the spider for righting reflexes and leg movements assists monitoring depth of anesthesia. During induction it may take 10–15 minutes with several attempts of the spider to move and reposition

itself, until full immobilization has occurred. During the procedure leg movements in response to stimuli is an obvious sign of insufficient depth of anesthesia. An increase in heart rate and respiratory rate may be seen, but is often unrecognized. A deep level of anesthesia is more difficult to evaluate, and slow respiratory rate and low heart rates are often the only way to assess a patient for an excessive depth of anesthesia. An analgesic administered for painful stimulations may make it easier for the clinician to maintain a consistent level of anesthesia.

Respiratory rate is observed at the cranial lateral side of the animal. The heart rate can often only be monitored in larger spiders. The heart lies under the dorsal surface of the body. With a Doppler (pinpoint-crystal head) placed over the heart area a rate can be obtained. Normal heart rates are considered to be 30–70 beats per minute in large spiders and up to 200 beats per min in smaller species.

After turning off the inhalant and maintaining the animal on fresh oxygen flow or room air, the recovery from anesthesia is gradual and can take between 3 and 20 minutes, depending on the ambient room temperature and the depth of anesthesia during the procedure. Slow leg movements and righting attempts occur and increase over time. When fully awake, the animal should be returned to its enclosure and maintained at its preferred ambient temperature. Feeding after anesthesia should be withheld for 48 hours (Pizzi 2012).

Scorpions

Anatomy, Physiology, and Natural History   There are about 1200 species of scorpions. Most are nocturnal and found in warm climates, such as the tropics and subtropics (Ruppert et al. 2004). They belong to the order Scorpiones and share many traits with their arachnid cousins, the spiders.

The basic anatomical plan consists of a cephalothorax, segmented abdomen, and telson, sometimes referred to as the sting (Ruppert et al. 2004). Although scorpions are infamous for their stinger and venom, a scorpion envenomation is rarely fatal to humans and normally induces only pain and discomfort. Scorpions can range in size from less than 10 mm to just over 20 cm.

Scorpions differ from spiders and most other arachnids in that they have a well-developed ventral nerve cord and exhibit viviparity with extended maternal care of the young in most species (Ruppert et al. 2004). For a more detailed account of scorpion anatomy, physiology, and natural history, please refer to Frye (2012) or Ruppert et al. (2004).

Physical Restraint   Direct handling should be kept to a minimum for both the safety of the handler and the animal. Clear plastic containers, and in some cases, utensils, such as long forceps, can be employed for moving an animal from one place to another (Frye 2012).

Anesthetic Agents Used and Techniques Scorpions are anesthetized similarly to spiders (see earlier section). An induction chamber using anesthetic gas in oxygen given via a precision vaporizer is preferred. Isoflurane or sevoflurane can be used.

Crustaceans

Anatomy, Physiology, and Natural History The crustaceans are a large and diverse group of arthropods that are all aquatic at some stage of their life history. Some authors consider this group, with over 40,000 described species, a subphylum of the phylum Mandibulata (Ruppert et al. 2004). Other workers still consider it a class of mandibulate arthropods that have two pairs of antennae, biramous appendages, compound eyes, segmented excretory organs, a well-developed protective carapace, and an aquatic nauplius larva (Noga et al. 2012). The majority of the most conspicuous and economically important crustaceans belong to the order Decapoda, which includes the crabs, crawfish, hermit crabs, lobsters, and shrimp.

Physical Restraint Some species can be manually restrained with gloved hands, or in some cases, with the help of utensils such as nets or tongs (Fig. 14.6). Since some crustaceans, such as lobsters and large crabs, can cause serious injury to handlers, care should be taken when manipulating or restraining these animals.

Anesthetic Agents Used and Techniques Crustaceans can be anesthetized with various agents. Depending on the animal's size and procedure, MS-222, isobutyl alcohol, eugenol, and intramuscular or intravenous

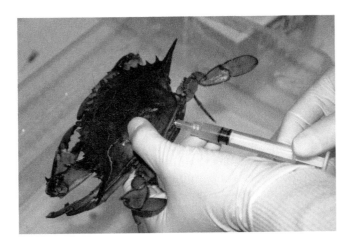

Figure 14.6. This blue crab (*Callinectes sapidus*) is being manually restrained while hemolymph is collected (photo courtesy of M. Mehalick).

injections of various anesthetics have been reported (Brown et al. 1996; Coyle et al. 2005; Ferraro & Pressacco 1996; Gardner 1997; Oswald 1977; Quesada et al. 2011). Tricaine methanesulphonate is generally accepted as a noneffective agent to produce anesthesia in decapods (Gardner 1997; Oswald 1977) and only very high doses show some effect (>1 g/L) with very slow induction time (Brown et al. 1996; Gardner 1997).

Lidocaine (0.4–1 mg/g) can be injected intramuscularly into the tail and lasts for about 5–30 minutes in crayfish, depending on the dose administered, with an average induction time of 1.5 minutes (Brown et al. 1996). Lidocaine (70 mg/kg) administered intravenously to the blue crab (*Callinectes sapidus*) resulted in a light anesthesia with short induction time (12.5 seconds) and short duration of two to three minutes (Quesada et al. 2011).

Ketamine has been used in crawfish (40–90 mcg/g), (Brown et al. 1996), in Australian giant crabs (*Pseudocarcinus gigas*) (0.025–0.1 mg/kg IV) (Gardner 1997), and in blue crabs (20 mg/kg, IV) (Quesada et al. 2011) with variable response. Ketamine given intramuscularly to crawfish will provide consistent anesthesia (induction time: 1 minutes) for over 10 minutes (40 mcg/g) to almost 2 hours (>90 mcg/g) without excitatory side effects during induction or recovery (Brown et al. 1996). When ketamine alone was given to the giant crab intravascularly, a short period of excitement occurred, but induction time was fast (15–45 seconds) (Gardner 1997). Duration of anesthesia was dose dependent and lasted between 8 and 40 minutes. The blue crab showed reliable and deep anesthesia with ketamine administered IV for a short period of time (5 minutes) after a fast induction within a minute (Quesada et al. 2011). When ketamine (20 mg/kg) is administered with xylazine (20 mg/kg), greater depth with good muscle relaxation can be achieved (Quesada et al. 2011).

Tiletamine-zolazepam at 30 mg/kg IV also provides a smooth and relaxed anesthesia (induction time 37.5 seconds, duration 5 minutes) (Quesada et al. 2011).

Xylazine has shown good anesthetic effects in adult giant crabs, when used at doses between 16 and 22 mg/kg IV (Gardner 1997) or in common shore crabs at 70 mg/kg IV (Oswald 1977). Induction seems to be smooth and fairly fast (3–5 minutes), and immobilization lasts 25–45 minutes (depending on the dose administered). Side effects, such as bradycardia, extrasystoles, and dysrhythmias, have been reported with high doses (70 mg/kg) (Oswald 1977). Xylazine alone (20 mg/kg, IV) administered to the blue crab only resulted in light anesthesia of short duration (Quesada et al. 2011).

An intravascular injection can be performed in adult giant and blue crabs through the arthropodial membrane, either midline between the cephalothorax and first abdominal segment, or dorsally at a 45° angle between carapace and the coxa of the swimming period (Gardner 1997; Oswald 1977; Quesada et al. 2011) using a small needle (25 or 27 gauge). The needle is gradually advanced until hemolymph is obtained and the drug is then administered (Quesada et al. 2011).

Intracardiac administration of drugs such as ketamine has been reported in the blue crab, but resulted in high mortality rate (Quesada et al. 2011) and therefore should be reserved for euthanasia. Intracardiac injections are performed by advancing a 25-gauge needle through the midline of the arthrodial membrane of the hinge of the carapace by aiming the needle toward the cervical groove, in which the pericardial sinus is situated (Quesada et al. 2011).

Etomidate (16 mg/kg) has been used in the blue crab, but showed no anesthetic effects (Quesada et al. 2011). Propofol seems to be contraindicated in the blue crab as it only produces light anesthesia with severe distress at 20 mg/kg IV. Distress was expressed by twitching, tremors, and limb autotomy (Quesada et al. 2011). Similarly, pentobarbital (60 mg/kg IV) resulted in unreliable anesthesia with violent dysphoria (Quesada et al. 2011).

Procaine (25 mg/kg IV) has also been used in crabs and provides good anesthesia with a very short induction time (20–30 seconds). This included a 10-second long excitatory phenomena that lead to tonic contraction before paralysis. Duration was very long (2–3 hours) with slow recoveries (Oswald 1977) and may be reserved for long-term experimental anesthesia.

For smaller crabs, in which an IV or IM injection is impractical, clove oil can be used as a bath treatment and has shown a 16-minute onset of anesthesia at a dose of >0.125 mL/L and a long recovery phase (2.5 hours). Once the animal is anesthetized, a reduction of concentration is necessary, because clove oil at 0.125 mL/L over a longer period of time is also used for euthanasia (Gardner 1997).

In shrimp, clove oil (eugenol) has become increasingly popular to anesthetize or sedate shrimp to reduce stress during transport. Benefits of eugenol are the apparent safety for shrimp and the lack of withdrawl time for consumption in some countries (Akbari et al. 2010; Coyle et al. 2005; Parodi et al. 2012). Some studies have looked at the effect of eugenol in different type of shrimp species. The Indian shrimp (*Fenneropenaeus indicus*) has been successfully sedated with eugenol (1.3–3.7 mg/L) (Akbari et al. 2010). Eugenol and Aqui-S™ (active ingredient is isoeugenol) have also been used to sedate and anesthetize freshwater prawn *Fenneropenaeus indicus*) (Coyle et al. 2005). The effect on induction and recovery time is dose dependent (100–300 mg/L) with a higher safety margin for eugenol over Aqui-S (Coyle et al. 2005). The optimal dose of eugenol in white shrimp was 175 μL/L, producing rapid induction and recovery (Parodi et al. 2012). The essential oils *Lippia alba* (1000 μ/L) and *Aloysia triphylla*

(300 μL/L) also produce sedation and anesthesia in white shrimp (Parodi et al. 2012).

Tricaine methanesulphonate and 2-phenoxyethanol were found to be ineffective to sedate freshwater prawns (Coyle et al. 2005).

Eugenol is also commonly used for sedation and immobilization in lobsters to facilitate handling and diagnostic procedures. When eugenol is added to the water at 75–100 ppm, the American lobster (*Homarus americanus*) becomes reliably immobilized within 10 minutes (Waterstrat & Pinkham 2005). After transferring the animal to an aerated flow-through aquarium, recovery was achieved in 8 minutes (Waterstrat & Pinkham 2005).

Lobsters (*Homarus americanus*) can be euthanized with injectable potassium chloride (KCl) causing cardiac arrest (Battison et al. 2000). A 330-mg/mL solution of KCl is prepared and 1 g/kg is injected into the hemolymph sinus containing the ventral nerve cord (Battison et al. 2000). This sinus can be accessed by a 20-gauge needle placed at the base of the second pereiopod (walking leg). The leg can be rotated internally and extended caudally. The needle is advanced until hemolymph is reached and the KCl solution is injected (Battison et al. 2000). Following a 15-second period of rigid extension of the claws and legs, cardiac arrest will be achieved in 1–2 minutes and can be confirmed by a Doppler (Battison et al. 2000).

Monitoring Crustaceans Crustacean heart rates can be assessed by applying ECG pads with ample gel on the shell above the heart. Alternatively a Doppler probe placed on the carapace over the heart can be used (Noga et al. 2012; Quesada et al. 2011). The normal heart rate for lobsters is between 5 and 20 beats per minute with a circadian influence (higher at night) (Aguzzi et al. 2004) and 30–70 beats per minute for the shore crab (Styrishave et al. 2003), depending on pH and temperature. Battison et al. (2000) reported heart rates of 19–60 with a mean around 40, depending on temperature. The blue crab showed a heart rate around 180 beats per minute under water, but when taken out of water, precipitously dropped to a few beats/min (Quesada et al. 2011).

Depth is evaluated in crustaceans by the relaxation of the body and the ability to withdraw extremities and very slow withdrawal of their antennae (Gardner 1997). A deep anesthesia is considered when complete limb immobility is achieved and abdominal flap and chelae are relaxed. A loss of righting response and loss of defense behavior marks induction, and its return will characterize recovery (Gardner 1997; Quesada et al. 2011).

Insects

Anatomy, Physiology, and Natural History The insects are an incredibly diverse and numerous group that some taxonomist term the Hexapoda. With nearly a million described species, they are the true taxonomic champion of sheer species numbers and diversity. Most species are terrestrial, some are aquatic, and the only habitat they have not exploited is the ocean (some are found in the intertidal zone). Insects are arthropods with three major body segments (head, thorax, and abdomen) and three pairs of legs. Most have keen eyesight, well-developed mouthparts, sensory antennae, and wings. They have an open circulatory system that contains hemolymph and gases are exchanged through spiracles that open into a system of tracheae. Most species lay eggs following internal fertilization.

Physical Restraint In most cases, insects can be handled and restrained manually without risk to the animal or handler. In some cases, gloves are recommended as a protective measure and various utensils can be employed to immobilize or restrain insects. Much depends on the size and species of insect being worked with (Fig. 14.7).

Anesthetic Agents Used and Techniques Carbon dioxide (CO_2) gas remains popular for immobilization of insects in entomological research, although multiple side effects, including convulsion and excitation at induction, are well recognized and mortality is high (Champion de Crespigny & Wedell 2008; Nicolas & Sillans 1989; Valles & Koehler 1994). Its use remains controversial, and a more progressive approach would be the use of a volatile anesthetic agent, such as isoflurane or sevoflurane. This requires a chamber apparatus to allow for appropriate delivery and scavenging of the inhalant agent (Walcourt & Ide 1998).

The use of ether (diethyl ether) is limited due to its high flammability, but ethyl acetate has been used in

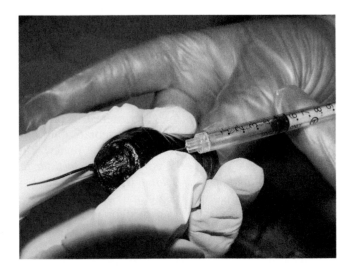

Figure 14.7. Hemolymph collection from a Madagascar hissing cockroach (*Gromphadorhina portentosa*): This mature male hissing cockroach has been sedated with inhalant isoflurane for hemolymph collection.

the green lacewing (*Chrysoperla rufilabris*) (Loru et al. 2010). A few drops of ethyl acetate are placed on a cotton ball in an induction chamber, and the insect is observed until movement ceases, at which point the treatment is removed (Loru et al. 2010). Ethyl acetate seems to have a small margin of safety and therefore overdosing and mortality are a concern.

Echinoderms

Anatomy, Physiology, and Natural History The echinoderms are a diverse phylum of about 6000 extant marine species in six classes that all share, at least at some point in their life history, pentamerous radial symmetry. Familiar members of this phylum include the sea lilies, feather stars, sea stars, brittle stars, sea urchins, sea biscuits, sand dollars, and sea cucumbers. Echinoderms have a water vascular system that is used for feeding, locomotion, and transport of coelomocytes used in the immune response. Nearly all species have a skeleton composed of calcareous ossicles, and in some cases, these ossicles are fused to form an external structure called the test (e.g., sea urchins). The nervous system is composed of a nerve ring with associated radial nerves (there are no ganglia). Fertilization is external, and most species have planktonic larval forms.

Physical Restraint Many species can be readily handled safely and effectively without anesthesia or sedation. Most tend to be slow moving and quite hardy (one exception being the brittle stars). Certain species of sea urchins can inflict a painful "sting" with movable, sharp spines. Nets, tongs, and gloves can aid in the safe handling of many species.

Anesthetic Agents Used and Techniques Echinoderms can be anesthetized/immobilized with $MgCl_2$, MS-222 or menthol (Harms 2012). Ideally, the sea star (starfish) is anesthetized in its own seawater (i.e., the water they are adapted to in their aquarium), to keep temperature and water content (including pH and salinity) consistent. To a known amount of that water, an $MgCl_2$ solution (7.5–8% in tap or seawater) is administered. A 1:1 mixture has been reported (McCurley & Kier 1995), and may be necessary for induction, but adjustments over time during maintenance of anesthesia may have to be made (gradually administer more seawater). Tricaine methanesulphonate can be used in a concentrated form (1–10 g/L in seawater) (Hendler et al. 1995; O'Neill 1994). Other reported anesthetic agents are menthol (2.5–5% in sterile seawater) (Costello & Henley 1971) and propylene phenoxetol (2 mL/L in seawater) (Hendler et al. 1995; Van den Spiegel & Jangoux 1987).

Recommendations for anesthetizing adult sea urchins (*Paracentrotus lividus*) are made by Arafa et al. (2007). A range of $MgCl_2$ can be used (5–20 mmol/L), but least mortality rate for longer anesthesia times (transports etc.) is achieved with 5 mmol/L. Sea urchins are not good at regulating changes in osmotic and ionic levels, therefore, it is important that the magnesium concentration has the same tonicity as the animal/seawater (Arafa et al. 2007; Namba et al. 1995). Magnesium chloride at 5 mmol/L has similar osmotic pressure, which makes it the ideal concentration for anesthetizing adult sea urchins for longer periods of time (Arafa et al. 2007). Juvenile green sea urchins (*Strongylocentrotus droebachiensis*) can be paralyzed for detachment with potassium chloride (KCl) (0.25–5%) (Hagen 2003). Duration of paralysis is dose dependent (10 minutes for 0.25%, 24 hours at 5%). No mortality was seen under 5%, but will increase to 100% at a 10% concentration of KCl (Hagen 2003). Magnesium chloride at 10% will also reach a state of paralysis and detachment, lower doses being ineffective. 2-phenoxyethanol is effective at 3%, but the narrow safety margin (lethal dose is 4%) makes it a less recommended anesthetic agent for juvenile green sea urchins (Hagen 2003).

PAIN MANAGEMENT

Whether invertebrates feel pain is still an unanswered topic of debate. The crux of the argument may lie in the differentiation between nociception and pain per se. Nociception describes the neurophysiologic components leading to the sensation of pain, but excludes the central perception of nociceptive input that ultimately leads to the sensation of pain. In other words, nociception is an involuntary rapid reflex response and lacks the negative emotional response or feeling associated with pain (Bateson 1991; Broom 2001). In respect to animals, "pain" has been defined as an "aversive sensation and feeling associated with actual or potential tissue damage" (Broom 2001). In humans and mammals, this pain experience resulting from nociception is created in the cerebral cortex, leading to learned avoidance and modified species-specific behaviors (Nieuwenhuys 2012). Although invertebrates do not possess a central nervous system with a well-described cortex or similar structure it has been shown that a nociceptive response is present in invertebrates (Kavaliers et al. 1983; Mather 2011; Smith & Lewin 2009). Various parts of the nociceptive system have been described and seem to be similar across the wide range of invertebrate taxa (Elwood 2011; Tobin & Bargmann 2004). Multidendritic polymodal nociceptive neurons with naked endings attached to epidermal cells (Goodman 2003; Hwang et al. 2007; Nicholls & Baylor 1968), and unmyelinated nociceptive fibers (Smith & Lewin 2009) similar to the C-fibers of vertebrates, are present. An upregulation of the nociceptive system after noxious stimulation resulting in long-term hypersensitization has been explained (Walters 1987).

Invertebrates do not possess a brain-like structure that is homologous to the human cortex, and wide differences exist across the invertebrate phyla (Crook & Walters 2011; Elwood 2011). Nevertheless, many invertebrates have an incredible complex brain configuration that certainly is different from the mammalian brain, but is suspected to have structures that are analogous to a cortex with the ability to experience pain, sensory analysis, memory, and learning (Broom 2007; Elwood 2011; Smith 1991). Invertebrates that lack appropriate processing centers may only be capable of a rapid reflexive unconscious response to a noxious stimulus (Crook & Walters 2011). Further research is needed to give us a better understanding in this matter. Opioid receptor systems may have a functional role in invertebrate nociception (Fiorito 1986; Kavaliers 1988; Kavaliers & Hirst 1983; Kavaliers et al. 1983; Smith 1991), although there are controversial opinions (Crook & Walters 2011; Dores et al. 2002). The animals' response to mechanical, chemical, and electrical stimulation is seen by withdrawal and escape behaviors (Elwood et al 2009). This response is decreased or slowed when an analgesic is used (Kavaliers & Hirst 1983; Lozada et al. 1988; Maldonado & Miralto 1982). It is not yet clear if this decreased response is due to a sedative or an analgesic effect of the drug. Two interesting studies in fruit flies and glass prawns have addressed this problem by showing a change in behavior without the decrease in activity when an analgesic agent was administered (Barr et al. 2008; Maney & Dimitrijevic 2005).

Certain species (*Drosophila* sp., *Chasmagnathus granulatus, Pagurus clarkia*, and *Pagurus bernhardus*) expressed a learning of avoidance of noxious stimuli over various periods of time, which indicates ability for memory to decrease risk for potential future damage (Denti et al. 1988; Elwood & Appel 2009; Kawai et al. 2004; Yarali et al. 2008).

However, due to limited conclusive data, no definitive answer exists for the debate of whether invertebrates perceive pain and would suffer emotional stress from it. Evidence from behavioral studies that crustaceans and mollusks experience pain, or a "painlike state", seem to be consistent (Crook & Walters 2011; Elwood 2011), but further research is necessary to confirm and clarify this.

Presently, there is an emerging interest in bringing more evidence to the debate of invertebrate pain and in particular animal welfare. For further review, the reader is referred to a special edition of the *Institute for Laboratory Animal Research Journal* (ILAR) (Smith 2011). In the United Kingdom, the octopus is covered under the same animal welfare act as vertebrates, due to the increasing evidence for pain perception found in cephalopods (Crook & Walters 2011).

Until the question of pain in invertebrates is clearly answered, it should be taken into account that some invertebrate species seem to have the capacity of a painlike experience, and an analgesic should be considered for any animal that is subjected to a painful procedure. On the other hand, the use of analgesics in invertebrate species is not common, and little research has been done examining methods of administration of analgesics, dosing, and the effects and impact of the different analgesics on the patient, the anesthesia, and the recovery.

Until more research is published, drugs with analgesic properties are recommended to anesthetize invertebrates when invasive procedures are performed to avoid potential nociceptor activation and painlike sensation. Hypothermia and CO_2 do not possess analgesic properties and inhalant agents or $MgCl_2$ may be preferred. Although inhalant agents do not possess true analgesic properties, they do render mammalian patient insensible to painful stimuli when administered at sufficient anesthetizing doses. Unfortunately, the insensibility to painful stimuli only lasts as long as the animal is anesthetized, so if the procedure is expected to be associated with significant postoperative pain, the administration of an analgesic is advisable. Different general options may include: the use of a local anesthetic, such as 2% benzocaine applied topically to a specific site (Barr et al. 2008) or diluted lidocaine (0.5–1 mg/mL) also for topical administration, and the use of an opioid and/or an nonsteroidal anti-inflammatory drug (NSAID).

EUTHANASIA

Invertebrates play an important role in laboratory research. Historically, no thorough guidelines or rules were available for euthanizing invertebrates, despite ongoing improvements in regulations for euthanasia in different vertebrate species (American Veterinary Medical Association [AVMA] Panel on Euthanasia 2000). Main reasons were primarily the fact that invertebrates are not covered by the U.S. laboratory animal guidelines and do not need an IACUP. Animal welfare has recently been an emerging topic in North America, following Europe's lead, and over the last few years, suggestions for euthanasia of invertebrates have been made throughout the literature (Battison et al. 2000; Hackendahl &Mashima 2002; Reilly 2001; Cooper 2012; Bennie et al. 2012; Pizzi 2012). Very recently, great progress has been made by including invertebrates into the "2013 Edition of the AVMA Guidelines for the Euthanasia" from the "Panel on Euthanasia" (AVMA 2013), with specific suggestions on euthanasia techniques.

Due to the wide variety of invertebrate species, anatomical differences and major difficulties to confirm death in these species, it is in general suggested to perform a two-step euthanasia protocol (AVMA 2013). This involves a chemical induction of anesthesia, commonly an overdose, that causes presumed death (step 1), followed by an additional physical or chemical method that causes destruction of the nervous system (brain or major ganglia) (step 2) (AVMA 2013). Acceptable step 1 methods for invertebrates are dependent on the species and the effectiveness of a specific anesthetic agent. For aquatic invertebrates immersions into magnesium salts, eugenol, or ethanol are listed in the guidelines as acceptable step 1 methods (AVMA 2013). The adjunctive methods (step 2) in aquatic species can be physical (pithing, freezing, or boiling) or chemical (70% alcohol or 10% formalin) (AVMA 2013). It is explicitly stated that any method that is listed under acceptable step 2 techniques is not accepted as a sole method or as a first step method (AVMA 2013). The guidelines also state that any method, that does not cause rapid death, in particular hypoxia, anoxia, or death by caustic chemicals or traumatic injury without the loss of consciousness prior to it, is unacceptable (AVMA 2013).

For terrestrial invertebrates, an overdosing injection of pentobarbital into the circulating hemolymph or intracoelemic is recommended by the AVMA, when possible, and can be used as a single method.

Also acceptable is an overdose of inhalant anesthetics or CO_2 with adjunct methods, such as a physical or chemical destruction of the nervous system (AVMA 2013). It is important to keep in mind that the nervous system is different in every species, and that decapitation alone may be an unsuitable technique.

Battison et al. (2000) described the intracardiac injection of KCl in lobsters, which causes rapid immobilization and death. This method has been further developed by Bennie et al. (2012) in various anesthetized terrestrial invertebrate species. Bennie et al. injected KCl (100 µL/g) directly into the thoracic ganglion ("targeted hyperkalosis"), and achieved immediate paralysis and death. Centipedes seem to need a higher KCl concentration (20% v/w) than other terrestrial invertebrates (Bennie et al. 2012).

The new guidelines are a step further into the right direction, but there still is an enormous need for improvement and research to assure ethically acceptable ways to euthanize members of this diverse group of animals. More species-specific research is needed on this topic. As mentioned earlier, the ability of invertebrates to respond to noxious stimuli and show different types of stress responses is well recognized.

It should be our goal as veterinarians to treat every living creature with respect and promote the well-being of these animals and trying to provide a stress-free environment, even when the perception of pain is not fully understood. Animal welfare should have priority over the success of a research study, and euthanasia should be performed by a method that is effective, painless, and fast.

REFERENCES

Acosta-Salmon H, Davis M. 2007. Inducing relaxation in the queen conch *Strombus gigas* (L.) for pearl production. *Aquaculture (Amsterdam, Netherlands)* 262:73–77.

Acosta-Salmon H, Martinez-Fernandez E, Southgate CP. 2005. Use of relaxants to obtain saibo tissue from the blacklip pearl oyster (*Pinctada margaritifera*) and the Akoya pearl oyster (*Pinctada fucata*). *Aquaculture (Amsterdam, Netherlands)* 246 (1–4):160–170.

Aguzzi J, Abello P, Depledge MH. 2004. Endogenous cardiac activity rhythms of continental slope *Nephrops norvegicus* (Decapoda: Nephropidea). *Marine and Freshwater Behaviour and Physiology* 37(1):55–64.

Akbari S, Khoshnod MJ, Rajaian H, et al. 2010. The use of Eugenol as an anesthetic in transportation of With Indian shrimp (*Fenneropenaeus indicus*) post larvae. *Turkish Journal of Fisheries and Aquatic Sciences* 10(3):423–429.

Altura BM, Altura BT, Carella A, et al. 1987. Mg^{2+}–Ca^{2+} interaction in contractility of vascular smooth muscle: Mg^{2+} versus organic calcium channel blockers on myogenic tone and agonist-induced responsiveness on blood vessels. *Canadian Journal of Physiology and Pharmacology* 65:729–745.

Andrews PLR, Tansey EM. 1981. The effects of some anesthetic agents in *Octopus vulgaris*. *Comparative Biochemistry and Physiology* 70C:241–247.

Aquilina B, Roberts R. 2000. A method for inducing muscle relaxation in the abalone, *Haliotis iris*. *Aquaculture (Amsterdam, Netherlands)* 190:403–408.

Arafa S, Sadok S, Abed AE. 2007. Assessment of magnesium chloride as an anesthetic for adult sea urchins (*Paracentrotus lividus*): incidence on mortality and spawning. *Aquaculture Research* 38:1673–1678.

AVMA. 2013. AVMA guidelines for the euthanasia of animals: 2013 edition. https://www.avma.org/KB/Policies/Documents/euthanasia.pdf (accessed January 17, 2014).

AVMA Panel on Euthanasia. 2000. Report of the AVMA panel on euthanasia. *Journal of the American Veterinary Medical Association* 218(5):669–696.

Barnes RD, Ruppert EE. 1994. *Invertebrate Zoology*, 6th ed. Philadelphia: Saunders College Publishing.

Barr S, Laming PR, Dick JTA, et al. 2008. Nocicpetion or pain in a decapod crustacean? *Animal Behaviour* 75:745–751.

Bateson P. 1991. Assessment of pain in animals. *Animal Behaviour* 42:827–839.

Battison A, MacMillan R, MacKenzie A, et al. 2000. Use of injectable potassium chloride for euthanasia of American lobsters (*Homarus americanus*). *Comparative Medicine* 50:545–550.

Bennie NAC, Loaring CD, Bennie MMG, et al. 2012. An effective method for terrestrial arthropod euthanasia. *The Journal of Experimental Biology* 215(24):4237–4241.

Bower JR, Sakurai Y, Yamamoto J, et al. 1999. Transport of the ommastrephid squid *Todarodes pacificus* under cold-water anesthesia. *Aquaculture (Amsterdam, Netherlands)* 170:127–130.

Broom DM. 2001. Evaluation of pain. In: *Pain: It's Nature and Management in Man and Animals*, Royal Society of Medicine International Congress Symposium Series, Vol. 246 (EJL Soulsby, D Morton, eds.), pp. 17–25. London: Royal Society of Medicine.

Broom DM. 2007. Cognitive ability and sentience: which aquatic animals should be protected? *Diseases of Aquatic Organisms* 75:99–108.

Brown PB, White MR, Chaille J, et al. 1996. Evaluation of three anesthetic agents for crayfish (*Orconectes virilis*). *Journal of Shellfish Research* 15(2):433–435.

Butt D, O'Connor SJ, Kuchel R, et al. 2008. Effects of the muscle relaxant, magnesium chloride, on the Sydney rock oyster (*Saccostrea glomerata*). *Aquaculture (Amsterdam, Netherlands)* 275:342–346.

Champion de Crespigny F, Wedell N. 2008. The impact of anesthetic techniques on survival and fertility in *Drosophila*. *Physiological Entomology* 33:310–315.

Clark TR, Nossov PC, Apland JP, et al. 1996. Anesthetic agents for use in the invertebrate sea snail, *Aplysia californica*. *Contemp Top Lab Anim Sci* 35 (5): 75–79.

Cooper JE. 2001. Invertebrate anesthesia. In: exotic anesthesia and analgesia (D Heard ed.). *The Veterinary Clinics of North America. Exotic Animal Practice* 4(1):57–67.

Cooper JE. 2012. Insects. In: *Invertebrate Medicine* (GA Lewbart, ed.), pp. 267–283. Ames: Wiley-Blackwell.

Costello DP, Henley C. 1971. *Methods of Obtaining and Handling Marine Eggs and Embryos*, 2nd ed. Woods Hole: Marine Biological Laboratory.

Coyle SD, Dasgupta S, Tidwell TH, et al. 2005. Comparative efficacy of anesthetics for the freshwater prawn *Macrobrachium rosenbergii*. *Journal of the World Aquaculture Society* 36:282–290.

Crook RJ, Walters ET. 2011. Nociceptive behavior and physiology of molluscs: animal welfare implications. *ILAR Journal* 52(2):185–195.

Culloty SC, Mulcahy MF. 1992. An evaluation of anesthetics for *Ostrea edulis* (L.). *Aquaculture (Amsterdam, Netherlands)* 107(2–3):249–252.

Denti A, Dimant B, Maldonado H. 1988. Passive avoidance learning in the crab *Chasmagnathus granulatus*. *Physiology and Behavior* 43:317–320.

Dombrowski D 2006. Personal communication/unpublished data.

Dores RM, Lecaude S, Bauer D, et al. 2002. Analyzing the evolution of the opioid/orphanin gene family. *Mass Spectrometry Reviews* 21:220–243.

Edwards S, Burke C, Hindrum S, et al. 2000. Recovery and growth effects of anaesthetic and mechanical removal on greenlips (*Haliotis laevigata*) and blacklip (*Haliotis rubra*) abalone. *Journal of Shellfish Research* 19(1):510.

Elwood RW. 2011. Pain and suffering in invertebrates? *ILAR Journal* 52(2):175–184.

Elwood RW, Appel M. 2009. Pain in hermit crabs? *Animal Behaviour* 77:1243–1246.

Elwood RW, Barr S, Patterson L. 2009. Pain and stress in crustaceans? *Applied Animal Behaviour Science* 118:128–136.

Ferraro EA, Pressacco L. 1996. Anesthetic procedures for crustaceans. An assessment of isobutanol and xylazine as general anaesthetics for *Squilla mantis* (Stomapoda). *Memorie di Biologia Marina e di Oceanografia* 12:471–475.

Fiorito G. 1986. Is there "pain" in invertebrates? *Behavioural Processes* 12:383–388.

Flores DV, Salas PJI, Vedra JPS. 1983. Electroretinography and ultrastructural study of the regenerated eye of the snail *Cryptomphallus aspera*. *Journal of Neurobiology* 14(3):167–176.

Frye F. 2012. Scorpions. In: *Invertebrate Medicine*. (GA Lewbart, ed.), pp. 223–234. Ames: Wiley-Blackwell.

Garcia-Franco M. 1992. Anaesthetics for the squid *Sepioteuthis sepioidea* (Mollusca: Cephalopoda). *Comparative Biochemistry and Physiology* 103C(1):121–123.

Gardner C. 1997. Options for humanely immobilizing and killing crabs. *J Shellfish Res* 16(1):219–224.

Girdlestone D, Cruickshank SGH, Winlow W. 1989. The actions of 3 volatile anaesthetics on the withdrawal response of the pond snail *Lymnaea stagnalis*. *Comparative Biochemistry and Physiology* 92C(1):39–43.

Gleadall IG. 1991. Comparison of anaesthetics for octopuses. *Bulletin of Marine Science* 49(1–2):663.

Goodman MB. 2003. Sensation is *painless*. *Trends in Neurosciences* 26:643–645.

Gore SR, Harms CA, Kukanich B, et al. 2005. Enrofloxacin pharmacokinetics in the European cuttlefish, *Sepia officinalis*, after a single i.v. injection and bath administration. *Journal of Veterinary Pharmacology and Therapeutics* 28:433–439.

Hackendahl N, Mashima TY 2002. Considerations in aquatic invertebrate euthanasia. Proceedings of the American Association of Zoo Veterinarians, pp.324–329.

Hagen N. 2003. KCl induced paralysis facilities detachment of hatchey reared juvenile green sea urchins, *Strongylocentrotus droebachiensis*. *Aquaculture (Amsterdam, Netherlands)* 216:155–164.

Harms CA. 2012. Echinoderms. In: *Invertebrate Medicine*. (GA Lewbart, ed.), pp. 365–379. Ames: Wiley-Blackwell.

Harms CA, Lewbart GA, Woolard KD, et al. 2006. Surgical excision of mycotic (*Cladosporium* sp.) granulomas from the mantle of a cuttlefish (*Sepia officinalis*). *Journal of Zoo and Wildlife Medicine* 37:524–530.

Heasman MP, O'Connor WA, Frazer AWJ. 1995. Induction of anesthesia in the commercial scallop, *Pecten fumatus* Reeve. *Aquaculture (Amsterdam, Netherlands)* 131:231–238.

Hendler G, Miller JE, Pawson DL, et al. 1995. *Sea stars, sea urchins and allies: Echinoderms of Florida and the Caribbean.* pp. 21–27. Washington, DC: Smithsonian Institution Press.

Hwang RY, Zhong L, Xu L, et al. 2007. Nociceptive neurons protect *Drosophila* larvae from parasitoid wasps. *Current Biology* 17:2105–2116.

Kavaliers M. 1988. Evolutionary and comparative aspects in nociception. *Brain Research Bulletin* 21:923–931.

Kavaliers M, Hirst M. 1983. Tolerance to morphine-induced thermal response in terrestrial snail, *Cepaea nemoralis*. *Neuropharmaology* 22:1321–1326.

Kavaliers M, Hirst M, Teskey GC. 1983. A functional role for an opiate system in snail thermal behavior. *Science* 220(4592): 99–101.

Kawai N, Kono R, Sugimoto S. 2004. Avoidance learning in crayfish (*Procambarus clarkia*) depends on the predatory imminence of the unconditioned stimulus: a behavior approach to learning in invertebrates. *Behavioural Brain Research* 150: 229–237.

Kishore P. 2011. Use of 1-prpylene phenoxetol and benzocaine to anesthetise *Pteria penguin* (Roeding, 1798) for mabe production. SPC Pearl Oyster Information Bulletin No. 19:29–33.

Loru L, Sassu A, Fois X, et al. 2010. Ethyl acetate: a possible alternative for anaesthetizing insects. *Annales de la Societe Entomologique de France. Societe Entomologique de France* 46(3–4):422–424.

Lewbart GA, ed. 2012. *Invertebrate Medicine*. Ames: Wiley-Blackwell.

Lewbart GA, Harms CA. 1999. Building a fish anesthesia delivery system. *Exotic DVM* 1(2):25–28.

Lozada M, Romano A, Maldonado H. 1988. Effects of morphine and naloxone on a defensive response of the crab *Chasmagnathus granulatus*. *Pharmacology Biochemistry and Behavior* 30: 635–640.

Madsen B, Vollrath F. 2000. Mechanism and morphology of silk dawn from anesthetized spiders. *Die Naturwissenschaften* 87: 149–153.

Maldonado H, Miralto A. 1982. Effects of morphine and naloxone on a defensive response oft eh mantis shrimp (*Squilla mantis*). *Journal of Comparative Physiology. A* 147:455–459.

Mamangkey NGF, Acosta-Salmon H, Southgate PC. 2009. Use of anaesthetics with the silver-lip pearl oyster, *Pinctada maxima* (Jameson). *Aquaculture (Amsterdam, Netherlands)* 288:280–284.

McCurley RS, Kier WM. 1995. The functional morphology of starfish tube feet: the role of a crossed-fiber helical array in movement. *The Biological Bulletin* 188:197–209.

Maney H, Dimitrijevic N. 2005. Fruit flies for anti pain drug discovery. *Life Sciences* 76:2403–2407.

Martins-Sousa RL, Negrao-Correa D, Bezerra FSM, et al. 2001. Anesthesia of *Biomphalaria* spp. (Mollusca, Gastropoda): sodium pentobarbital is the drug of choice. *Memorias Do Instituto Oswaldo Cruz* 96(3):391–392.

Mather JA. 2011. Philosophical background of attitudes toward and treatment of invertebrates. *ILAR Journal* 52:205–212.

Melidone R, Mayer J. 2005. How to build an invertebrate surgery chamber. *Exotic DVM* 7(5):8–10.

Messenger JB, Nixon M, Ryan KP. 1985. Magnesium chloride as an anesthetic for cephaolpods. *Comparative Biochemistry and Physiology* 82C(1):203–205.

Mills D, Tlili A, Norton J. 1997. Large-scale anesthesia of the silver-lip pearl oyster, *Pinctada maxima* Jemeson. *J Shellfish Res* 16(2):573–574.

Mooney TA, Lee W-J, Hanlon RT. 2010. Long-duration anesthetization of squid (*Doryteuthis pealeii*). *Marine and Freshwater Behaviour and Physiology* 43(4):297–303.

Namba K, Kobayashi M, Aida S, et al. 1995. Persistent relaxation of the adductor muscle of Oyster *Crassostrea gigas* induced by magnesium ion. *Fisheries Science* 61(2):241–244.

Nicholls JG, Baylor DA. 1968. Specific modalities and receptive fields of sensory neurons in the C leech. *Journal of Neurophysiology* 31:740–756.

Nicolas G, Sillans D. 1989. Immediate and latent effects of carbon dioxide on insects. *Annual Review of Entomology* 34:97–116.

Nieuwenhuys R. 2012. The insular cortex: a review. *Progress in Brain Research* 195:123–163.

Noga EJ, Hancock AL, Bullis RA. 2012. Crustaceans. In: *Invertebrate Medicine*. (GA Lewbart, ed.), pp. 235–254. Ames: Wiley-Blackwell.

Norton JH, Dashorst M, Lansky TM, et al. 1996. An evaluation of some relaxants for use with pearl oysters. *Aquaculture (Amsterdam, Netherlands)* 144:39–52.

O'Connor AW, Lawler FN 2002. Propylene phenoxetol as a relaxant for the pearl oysters *Pinctada imbricate* and *Pinctada albino*. *Asian Fisheries Science* 15:53–59.

O'Neill PL. 1994. The effect of anesthesia on spontaneous contraction of the body wall musculature in the astereroid *Coscinasterias calamaria*. *Marine Behaviour and Physiology* 24: 137–150.

Oswald RL. 1977. Immobilization of decapod crustaceans for experimental purposes. *Journal of the Marine Biological Association of the United Kingdom* 57:715–721.

Parodi TV, Cunha MA, Heldwein CG, et al. 2012. The anesthetic efficacy of eugenol and the essential oils of *Lippia alba* and *Aloysia triphylla* in post-larvae and sub-adults of *Litopenaeus vannamei* (Crustacea, Penaeidae). *Comparative Biochemistry and Physiology. C* 155:462–468.

Pizzi R. 2012. Spiders. In: *Invertebrate Medicine*. (GA Lewbart, ed.), pp. 187–221. Ames: Wiley-Blackwell.

Quesada RJ, Smith CD, Heard DJ. 2011. Evaluation of parenteral drugs for anesthesia in the blue crab (*Callinectes sapidus*). *Journal of Zoo and Wildlife Medicine* 42(2):295–299.

Reilly RS. 2001. *Euthanasia of Animals Used for Scientific Purposes*, 2nd ed., pp. 98–99. ANZCCART.

Ruppert EE, Fox RS, Barnes RD. 2004. *Invertebrate Zoology: A Functional Evolutionary Approach*, 7th ed. Belmont: Thompson-Brooks/Cole.

Scimeca JM, Forsythe JW. 1999. The use of anesthetic agents in cephalopods. Proceedings of the International Association for Aquatic Animal Medicine 27, p. 88.

Sharma PD, Nollens HH, Keogh JA, et al. 2003. Sodium pentobarbitone-induced relaxation in the abalone *Haliotis iris* (Gastropoda): effects of animal size and exposure time. *Aquaculture (Amsterdam, Netherlands)* 218:589–599.

Smith ES, Lewin GR. 2009. Nocicptors: a phylogenetic view. *Journal of Comparative Physiology. A* 195:1089–1106.

Smith J. 1991. A question of pain in invertebrates. *ILAR Journal* 33(1–2):25–31.

Smith S., ed. 2011. Spineless wonders: welfare and use of invertebrates in the laboratory and classroom. Special edition of the *Institute for Laboratory Animal Research Journal* 52(2).

Styrishave B, Andersen O, Depledge MH. 2003. In situ monitoring of heart rates in shore crabs *Carcinus maenas* in two tidal estuaries: effects of physico-chemical parameters on tidal and diel rhythms. *Marine and Freshwater Behaviour and Physiology* 36(3): 161–175.

Suquet M, De Kermoysa G, Gonzalez Araya R, et al. 2009. Anaesthesia in Pacific oyster, *Crassostrea gigas*. *Aquatic Living Resources* 22:29–34.

Suquet M, Gonzales Araya R, Lebrun L, et al. 2010. Anaesthesia and gonad sampling in the European flat oyster (*Ostrea edulis*). *Aquaculture (Amsterdam, Netherlands)* 308:196–198.

Tobin DM, Bargmann CI. 2004. Invertebrate nociception: behaviors, neurons and molecules. *Journal of Neurobiology* 61: 161–174.

Valles SM, Koehler PG. 1994. Influence of carbon dioxide anesthesia on chlopyrifos toxicity in the German cockroach (*Dictyptera: Blattellidae*). *Journal of Economic Entomology* 87(3): 709–713.

Van den Spiegel D, Jangoux M. 1987. Cuverian tubules of the holothuroid *Holothuria forskali* (Echinodermata): a morphofunctional study. *Marine Biology* 96:263–275.

Walcourt A, Ide D. 1998. A system for the delivery of general anesthetics and other volatile agents to the fruit-fly *Drosophila melanogaster*. *Journal of Neuroscience Methods* 84:115–119.

Walters ET. 1987. Site specific sensitization of defensive reflexes in Aplysia: a simple model of long-term hyperalgesia. *Journal of Neuroscience* 7:400–407.

Waterstrat PR, Pinkham L. 2005. Evaluation of eugenol as an anesthetic for the American lobster *Homarus americanus*. *Journal of the World Aquaculture Society* 36(3):420–424.

White HI, Hecht T, Potgieter B. 1996. The effect of four anaesthetics on *Haliotis midae* and their suitability for applicationj in commercial abalanone culture. *Aquaculture (Amsterdam, Netherlands)* 140:145–151.

Woodall AJ, McCrohan CR. 2000. Excitatory actions of propofol and ketamine in the snail *Lymnaea stagnalis*. *Comparative Biochemistry and Physiology* 127C:297–305.

Woodall AJ, Naruo H, Prince DJ, et al. 2003. Anesthetic treatment blocks synaptogenesis but not neuronal regeneration of cultured *Lymnaea* neurons. *Journal of Neurophysiology* 90: 2232–2239.

Wyeth RC, Croll RP, Willows AOD. 2009. 1-Phenoxy-2-propanol is a useful anaesthetic for gastropods used in neurophysiology. *Journal of Neuroscience Methods* 176:121–128.

Yarali A, Niewalda T, Chen YC, et al. 2008. "Pain relief" learning in fruit flies. *Animal Behaviour* 76:1173–1185.

15 Bony Fish (Lungfish, Sturgeon, and Teleosts)

Natalie D. Mylniczenko, Donald L. Neiffer, and Tonya M. Clauss

INTRODUCTION

Do fish need to be anesthetized? Do fish feel pain? Fish welfare has become a hot topic for the last several years, in particular, the ability of fish to feel pain has come under considerable scrutiny. We need to consider this notion as it questions the need for anesthesia or analgesia altogether in this taxon. The previous version of this chapter as well as many recent publications (Braithwaite & Boulcott 2007; Posner 2009; Sneddon 2009) have thorough reviews on the subject. In brief, fish display robust, neuroendocrine and physiologic stress responses to noxious stimuli. Acute and chronic stress negatively affects fish health. Consequently, there is a need to identify and then reduce these stressors in individuals and groups.

Although examination and sample collection can be performed using manual restraint, for many minor procedures, chemical immobilization is safer for both fish and handler. In addition, many procedures are preferably performed out of water. In most fish, this stimulates struggling that requires restraint (Harms & Bakal 1995). That said, we will attempt to describe some methods in which fish can be restrained without anesthesia but with minimal restraint and stress.

Chemical immobilization is routinely utilized to reduce excitement and trauma related to hyperactivity that can occur during routine handling for vaccinations, hormonal implants or injections, roe or milt collection, sorting, tagging, and transportation of fish (Cooke et al. 2004; Harms 1999; Kumlu & Yanar 1999; Myszkowski et al. 2003; Ross 2001). In addition to acute trauma causing mortality and morbidity, integument damage results in acute to chronic osmoregulatory disturbances and increased susceptibility to pathogens (Kumlu & Yanar 1999; Ross 2001). Chemical immobilization during transport reduces metabolism, leading to decreased oxygen demand and waste (i.e., CO_2 and ammonia) production (Cooke et al. 2004; Crosby et al. 2006; Guo et al. 1995; Ross 2001).

Major or surgical procedures require anesthesia to prevent movement and remove any doubt in the debate over pain (Harms & Bakal 1995; Myszkowski et al. 2003; Ross 2001). At the very least, movement and physiologic changes in response to nociception are minimized.

STRESS AND ANESTHESIA

Fish restraint activates the hypothalamo–pituitary–interrenal (HPI) axis, resulting in cortisol release causing various secondary stress responses (Bressler & Ron 2004; Myszkowski et al. 2003; Ross and Ross 2008; Small 2003; Small & Chatakondi 2005). Cortisol release suppresses feeding and immune function, and alters reproductive productivity (Bressler & Ron 2004; Iversen et al. 2003; Myzkowski, 2003; Small 2003; Small & Chatakondi 2005).

Although anesthesia minimizes handling stress, it is inherently stressful (Bressler & Ron 2004) and a strong potentiator of catecholamine release, especially in salmonids (Rothwell et al. 2005; Zahl et al. 2010). Anesthesia-associated catecholamine release is likely due to hypoxemia rather than acidemia or direct drug effects (Ross & Ross 2008; Rothwell et al. 2005). However, unbuffered inhalants (immersives) (e.g., MS-222) do induce a stress response. Hypoxemia is usually due to drug-induced hypoventilation (decreased buccal movement). In air-breathing fish, hypoxemia can be exacerbated by preventing anesthetized fish access to the water's surface (Rantin et al. 1993, 1998).

Zoo Animal and Wildlife Immobilization and Anesthesia, Second Edition. Edited by Gary West, Darryl Heard, and Nigel Caulkett.

Hypoventilation with decreased water flow in the buccal cavity usually leads to reflex bradycardia and dorsal aortic hypotension producing a progressive hypoxemia (Ross 2001).

Despite the earlier-mentioned effects, chemical sedation or anesthesia produce a lower stress response when compared with drug-free handling and transport. This conclusion is based on comparison of circulating cortisol levels, as well as secondary indicators such as blood glucose, hematocrit (HCT), hemoglobin (Hgb), lactate, and osmolarity (Bressler & Ron 2004; Crosby et al. 2006; Hseu et al. 1996; Small & Chatakondi 2005).

Of the commonly used drugs, only metomidate consistently and significantly blocks HPI activation (Davis & Griffin 2004; Iversen et al. 2003; Zahl et al. 2010) in a broad range of species (e.g., red drum, *Sciaenops ocellatus*, Thomas & Robertson 1991; Atlantic salmon, *Salmo salar*, Iversen et al. 2003, Olsen et al. 1995; hybrid striped bass, *Morone chrysops* × *Morone saxatilis*, Davis & Griffin 2004; channel catfish, *Ictalurus punctatus*, Small 2003; and Atlantic cod and Atlantic halibut, Zahl et al. 2010).

The effect of clove oil (eugenol and isoeugenol) on cortisol secretion in fish is inconclusive. In channel catfish, no significant increase in cortisol concentrations were observed following 30 minutes of undisturbed clove oil anesthesia or when subjected to confinement and reduced oxygen levels while exposed to isoeugenol (AQUI-S™) (Small 2003, 2004; Small & Chatakondi 2005). However, in the same species anesthetized with AQUI-S and exposed to high unionized ammonia concentrations, cortisol was not suppressed (Small 2004). In Atlantic salmon smolts, clove oil and AQUI-S suppressed cortisol secretion while in adults only high dosages had the same effect (Iversen et al. 2003). In a different study, isoeugenol was found to have the same effect as MS-222 on stress but did not reach levels of cortisol as high as with MS-222 (Zahl et al. 2010). In seabream (*Sparus* sp.) exposed to clove oil (Bressler & Ron 2004) and rainbow trout (Small & Chatakondi 2005) exposed to both clove oil and AQUI-S, cortisol concentrations increased in response to handling. In gilthead seabream (*Sparus aurata*) exposed to clove oil (Bressler & Ron 2004) and hybrid striped bass exposed to both compounds (Davis & Griffin 2004), similar increases in circulating cortisol and glucose occurred. In red pacu (*Piaractus brachypomus*), exposure to eugenol increased glucose, HCT, and Hgb (Sladky et al. 2001) while in a related tropical freshwater species, tambaqui (*Colossoma macropomum*), no increase in glucose was noted (Roubach et al. 2005).

Except for low MS-222 dosages that depress (not block) the stress response in some fish (e.g., Chinook salmon, *Oncorhynchus tshawytscha*, and hybrid striped bass), immersive anesthetic drugs minimally inhibit the HPI response (Davis & Griffin 2004). Elevated cortisol and/or hyperglycemia occur in MS-222 exposed channel catfish (Small 2003; Small & Chatakondi 2005), Atlantic salmon (Olsen et al. 1995), hybrid striped bass (Davis & Griffin 2004), and red drum (Thomas & Robertson 1991). Similar elevations occur in gilthead bream exposed to benzocaine (Bressler & Ron 2004). Increased cortisol, with or without hyperglycemia, has also been associated with quinaldine exposure in red drum (Thomas & Robertson 1991), channel catfish (Small 2003), and hybrid striped bass (Davis & Griffin 2004). In four marine teleost species, the physiologic effects of 2-phenoxyethanol varied between species with significant elevations of HCT in red snapper (*Lutijanus argentimaculatus*), Hgb in gray mullet (*Mugil cephalus*), and osmolarity of black porgy (*Acanthopagrus schlegeli*), but no changes in milkfish (*Chanos chanos*) (Hseu et al. 1996).

Limited information on the effects of injectable drugs on the HPI response exists. In bonito (*Sarda chiliensis*), ketamine/medetomidine did not significantly alter HCT, Hgb, or glucose, although baseline values were not provided (Williams et al. 2004).

It has been argued that the stress-induced corticosteroid response is not harmful and is essential for recovery from severe acute or prolonged stressors. A transient, relatively small elevation of cortisol does not necessarily reduce immunocompetency, but may instead bolster it (Bressler & Ron 2004; Davis & Griffin 2004; Small 2003; Thomas & Robertson 1991). Based on this argument, drugs that suppress the HPI (e.g., metomidate) are contraindicated in fish. However, the contrary argument is that typical husbandry and handling procedures do not result in high stress levels associated with chronic immunosuppression (Bressler & Ron 2004; Davis & Griffin 2004; Small 2003; Thomas & Robertson 1991). For anesthetics that do not block the HPI, the intensity and duration of the stress response either depends on the duration of exposure or is drug, dosage, and species dependent (Bressler & Ron 2004; Gomes et al. 2001; Thomas & Robertson 1991).

In addition to affecting the stress response, some anesthetics are immunosuppressive. This effect may be caused by direct interaction with immune components or indirectly through the nervous system. For example, in gilthead seabream, both humoral and cellular immune responses were significantly depressed by benzocaine (Bressler & Ron 2004). However, clove oil does not cause significant immunosuppression in the same species demonstrating the variability between species and drug effects (Bressler & Ron 2004). Metomidate associated blockade of the HPI is thought to prevent immunosuppression (Davis & Griffin 2004).

TAXONOMY, ANATOMY, PHYSIOLOGY, AND BEHAVIOR

Fish number upwards of 30,000 species and comprise more than 40% of all extant chordates. Of these, teleosts (Teleostei: class Acinopterygii) comprise about 96% of living fish species. Other groups include other members of class Acinopterygii or ray-fined fishes (sturgeon, gar, bichir, paddlefish, and bowfin), class Sarcopterygii or lobe-finned fishes (lungfishes and coelacanths), class Agnatha or jawless fish (hagfishes and lampreys), and class Chondrichthyes (elasmobranchs and chimeras) (Bond 1996; Harms 2003).

The majority of immobilization studies involve only a handful of teleosts. Extrapolation to all species is potentially harmful and negligent without consideration of the wide range of anatomic, physiologic, and behavioral differences. For example, benzocaine kills cod (*Gadus morhua*) at the same dosage that is safe and effective in Atlantic salmon (Hansen et al. 2003; Mattson & Riple 1989). Even within families, there can be marked variation in preferred environmental parameters. Consequently, knowledge of taxonomy and natural history is essential for developing anesthetic regimens in fish.

Respiration

All fish have gills though the degree of reliance on these structures for respiration varies across class, order, and family. Most fish force water over the gills through rhythmic movements of their lower jaw and opercula (buccopharyngeal respiration). However, some species utilize ram ventilation (forcing water over the fish gill by swimming through the water column) with minimal opercular movement. Some teleosts (e.g., tuna, family Scombridae, tribe Thunnini) are obligate ram ventilators, with gilling alone not providing sufficient ventilation to meet metabolic demands. These species swim forward continuously with mouth slightly agape to develop the pressure head necessary for sufficient water flow over the gills. Failure to perfuse the gills during anesthesia results in suffocation (Brill & Bushnell 2001; Bushnell & Jones 1994). Tuna also rely on constant forward speed to produce lift from their pectoral fins for hydrostatic equilibrium (Brill & Bushnell 2001). Consequently, during recovery of ram ventilating species, it is necessary to hold the fish with sufficient water flow over the gills via a pump mechanism until adequate voluntary forward motion of the sedated animal returns. Walking the animal or pulling the animal manually through the water to ventilate is a favored option among fish enthusiasts; however, this does not always provide adequate ventilation, and a pump is strongly encouraged to move water over the gills, particularly with pelagic fish species.

In responses to hypoxic environments or other selective pressures, many species have evolved anatomical, physiologic, and behavioral adaptations to meet their ventilatory needs (Graham 1997). In addition to elaboration of the basic gill design for improved oxygen extraction, a diverse array of accessory respiratory organs has evolved, with a number of species capable of utilizing atmospheric air. For many, increased aerial gas exchange surface exists in portions of the alimentary canal (i.e., buccal and pharyngeal cavities) either as a direct proliferation of the respiratory surface in the lumen or as a single or a pair of pouches extending from it (Ishimatsu & Itazawa 1993). Alternatively, branchial diverticulae may develop as in anabantoids (gouramis, bettas, and climbing gouramis) (Graham 1997).

Many species take in atmospheric air with a behavior termed aquatic surface respiration (ASR). The fish position their mouths to skim the air/water interface that is richer in oxygen. Some species (e.g., pacu, *Piaractus mesopotamicus*) respond to hypoxic conditions by developing temporary dermal swellings of the lower jaw to facilitate ASR (Rantin et al. 1993, 1998). Others (e.g., channids [snakeheads] and anabantoids) employ alternate filling of an air-breathing chamber (laryrinth organ in anabantoids) with air and water during aerial ventilation (Ishimatsu & Itazawa 1993).

Lungfish (the sister group to tetrapods) and polypterids (bichirs and reedfish) possess true lungs with ventrally situated pneumatic duct openings in the alimentary canal instead of a traditional gas or "swim" bladder (Graham 1997). Of these, the African (*Propterus* sp.) and South American (*Lepidosiren* sp.) lungfish are obligatory air-breathers (Bassi et al. 2005; Graham 1997). The Australian lungfish possesses gills as well as a lung (Lenfant et al. 1966). Interestingly, unlike water-breathing fishes, the air-breathing lungfish will alter ventilation to compensate for metabolic acid–base changes, but there is likely an extrarenal component involved as with water breathing fish (Gilmour et. al. 2007). Although anatomically challenging, it is theoretically possible to cannulate the pneumatic duct of lungfish for administration of inhalant anesthesia; this has been done experimentally with animals under controlled experiments (Pack, et al, 1992). Conceivably, chamber induction (while somewhat submerged) may be possible but has not been reported. Alternatively, sterile percutaneous trocharization of the lung could be attempted. The Australian lungfish is the only facultative breather in the group, but when placed in immersive anesthetics, will attempt to breathe air and not respirate with its gills. However, immersion anesthesia with MS-222 has been accomplished in lungfishes and is a viable option if the animals are managed appropriately under anesthesia either by ensuring oxygenation once sedated via oxygen gas (or oxygenated water in animals with gills) and prevent drowning (DeLaney et al. 1976; Lenfant et al. 1966; N. Mylniczenko, pers. exp., 2004).

Understanding the range of fish respiration is important for anesthesia for two reasons. First, immersion uptake and induction rate is linked to oxygen demand. For fish that depend primarily or entirely on dissolved oxygen in water, induction rates are shorter compared with those of air-breathing species. Responding to confinement or hypoxic anesthetic baths, the latter pull air from the water surface and reduce opercular movement. Some may temporarily stop opercular activity (Hseu et al. 1997). Decreased branchial contact with the water results in a slower rate of anesthetic uptake. For example, 2-phenoxyethanol induction in hypoxia tolerant tilapia (*Oreochromis mosambicus*) and molly (*Poecilia velifera*) is significantly longer than in black porgy (*Acanthopagrus schlegeli*) and Japanese sea perch (*Lateolabrax japonicus*) (Hseu et al. 1997). To circumvent this issue, injectable anesthetics can be used for induction of species capable of aerial respiration (e.g., anabantoids) (Bruecker & Graham 1993). Second, although many fish that utilize an accessory respiratory organ retain gills for aquatic gas exchange, effective gill tissue is so reduced in some species (e.g., channids, lepidosirenid lungfish, and clariids or walking catfish), they will succumb or "drown" if denied access to atmospheric air (Ishimatsu & Itazawa 1993; Peters et al. 2001). These species are maintained in very shallow water, or on a moist substrate, until capable of reaching the water: air interface regardless of anesthetic route used.

Arapaima and other osteoglossids are also obligate air breathing fishes that use a modified swim bladder for respiration (Brauner et al. 2004). Focused spraying of immersion drugs, such as benzocaine and eugenol, on the gills is an effective method of induction (Honczaryk & Inoue 2009, 2010). Researchers have used MS-222 at 25, 50, 75, and 100 mg/L in juveniles, finding that 100 mg/L concentration was ideal for their project (Hinostroza & Serrano-Martínez 2013). In a different study, chloroform was used via gas mask with rapid induction times, but longer than expected recoveries; regardless, the anesthesia was considered successful (Carreiro, et. al, 2011). One of the authors (Mylniczenko) has experiences using high dose MS-222 (1 g/L) over the gills to sedate larger species, as well as low dose immersion MS-222 (25 ppm) in combination with valium (1 mg/kg PO) for transport. Ketamine has shown to be successful orally in this species for transport (Raines & Clancy 2009). There is also concern that these fish are at high risk for not recovering their air-breathing reflexes once anesthetized (Chu-Koo et al. 2008), though the authors have not experienced this (Carreiro et al. 2011). Still, caution must be exercised as the arapaima are very sensitive species and can drown without air access. As described with the lungfish, intubation can be attempted in their swim bladders (Farrell 1978).

Although notable exceptions exist (e.g., tarpon, *Megalops atlanticus*), few marine species have evolved adaptations for hypoxic environments other than surface piping or migrating from the area. Consequently, marine species may be less tolerant of hypoxic conditions during anesthesia in comparison with the freshwater species discussed earlier (Rothwell et al. 2005).

Metabolism

Most fish are ectothermic with metabolism dependent on ambient temperature. Though exceptions exist for some cold-adapted species, lower temperatures are usually associated with prolonged induction and recovery times during either inhalant/immersion or parenteral anesthesia (Gelwicks & Zafft 1998). This effect is reversed at higher temperatures (Detar & Mattingly 2004; Gomes et al. 2001; Peters et al. 2001; Stehly & Gingerich 1999). During immersion anesthesia, this relationship is primarily related to altered respiratory rate. Blood acid–base status is temperature dependent. Increased temperature leads to acidemia and hypercapnia, which stimulate hyperventilation. This decreases induction and recovery times for drugs taken up or eliminated from the gills (Aguiar et al. 2002; Stehly & Gingerich 1999).

Some fish have evolved various degrees of endothermy. They have the capacity to conserve metabolic heat in slow-twitch muscle, viscera, brain, and eyes, and to elevate body tissue temperature above ambient (Bushnell & Jones 1994). The most studied are tuna (family Scombridae), which have many anatomical and physiologic adaptations that promote endothermy. Tuna gills have large surface areas and thin epithelia compared with other fish (Brill & Bushnell 2001; Bushnell & Jones 1994). For example, gill surface areas are approximately 7–9× larger and gill blood–water barrier thickness an order of magnitude less than those of rainbow trout (Brill & Bushnell 2001). The net result is enhanced oxygen uptake. Red cells with elevated hemoglobin are circulated by proportionally large hearts with high cardiac outputs (Blank et al. 2004; Bushnell & Jones 1994) to well vascularized tissues. High myoglobin levels and aerobic enzymes enhance tissue oxygen extraction. Enzyme activity is particularly high in muscle; aerobic oxidation rates are 3–5× greater than other teleosts (Bushnell & Jones 1994). Elevated enzymatic activity and counter-current heat exchangers raise muscle temperatures (Cooper et al. 1994). Endothermy leads to increased rate of anesthetic uptake and metabolism compared with similarly sized ectothermic species. More primitive Scombrids (e.g., bonitos, seerfishes, and mackerels) are not endothermic and lack physiologic characteristics of tuna, such as the vascular countercurrent heat exchange mechanism. However, aerobic enzyme activity is similar, and these scombrids represent a transition between ectothermy and tuna endothermy (Brill & Bushnell 2001; Williams et al. 2004).

All teleost fish have an anatomic separation between aerobic, slow-oxidative muscles (red muscle), and anaerobic, fast-twitch, glycolytic muscles (white muscle). In many species, a distinct pattern of highly oxygenated slow oxidative muscle runs along the midline of the body. Given the increased capillarization, injection of anesthetic agents into this region may result in more rapid induction times compared with injections administered elsewhere (Williams et al. 2004), but in reality, this layer is very thin and has large variation in thickness and location, making consistent injections difficult.

Integument

Although most fish possess scales, marked variation in distribution and structure exist. This has implications for administration of parenteral drugs by hand and remote injection. Species (e.g., tarpon and arapaima) that have large, hard scales are difficult to dart or pole-syringe, while even large cobia (*Rachycentron canadum*) are relatively easy to inject.

For many fish, the skin is a respiratory organ, responsible in some species for up to 30% of oxygen uptake (Bruecker & Graham 1993). Most marine species have well vascularized skin capable of significant cutaneous gas exchange (Ishimatsu & Itazawa 1993). Though scaleless species (e.g., catfish, Siluriformes) are better designed for cutaneous respiration, capacity often varies with age class. Younger fish, regardless of size, tend to have thinner skin and less developed scalation favoring greater oxygen uptake (Myszkowski et al. 2003). Fish species that produce larvae lacking gills require skin respiration the first 9–15 days until full differentiation of secondary gill lamellae (Oikawa et al. 1994). Like other respiratory organs, skin is a route for immersion drug uptake and presumably excretion (Ferreira et al. 1984). The efficiency of uptake is dependent on scalation and, similar to gill tissue, lipid content of the skin. For example, some scaleless types of common carp (*Cyprinus carpio*) with high skin lipid content are much more efficient at cutaneous anesthetic uptake than rainbow trout with their small, densely packed scales and comparatively lower lipid content (Ferreira et al. 1984). In some instances, skin may actually be more efficient than other respiratory organs. For example, in the electric eel (*Electrophorus electricus*), quinaldine uptake across the skin was higher than the gills (Walsh & Pease 2002).

Size

Minimum effective anesthetic concentration is directly correlated with increasing body mass (Oikawa et al. 1994). This relationship is also true for toxic concentration. For example, MS-222 LC_{50} increases with growth in rainbow trout (*Oncorhynchus mykiss*), brown trout (*Salmo trutta*), lake trout (*Salvelinus namaycush*), large-mouth bass (*Micropterus salmoides*), and channel catfish (Oikawa et al. 1994).

ENVIRONMENTAL AND OTHER FACTORS

Temperature

In addition to metabolism, dissolved oxygen (DO) concentrations are influenced by temperature. At higher temperatures, DO decreases exacerbating any anesthetic-induced hypoxia. Warmer temperatures also promote solubilization of immersion anesthetics while cooler temperatures promote precipitation.

pH

The pH of immersion solutions will influence efficacy, possibly by affecting the ratio of charged to uncharged molecules. In general, decreased efficacy is seen as the pH drops due to increased ionization that interferes with absorption. Unfortunately, most immersion anesthetics (e.g., MS-222 and quinaldine) in solutions are acidic, requiring buffering agents (e.g., sodium bicarbonate) to neutralize the pH. In addition to promoting immersion anesthetic efficacy (Ferreira et al. 1984), buffers prevent metabolic acidemia, a condition precipitated by anesthetic-induced hypoxemia and anerobic metabolism. Saltwater, with its higher pH and greater natural buffering capacity compared with freshwater, may not require addition of buffering agents (Harms & Bakal 1995; Harms 1999; Oikawa et al. 1994; Ross 2001; Ross & Ross 2008). The greater efficacy and safety of immersion anesthetics in sea water was demonstrated in mullet (*Mugil cephalus*) (Sylvester 1975). For a given concentration of MS-222, decreased efficacy and increased toxicity was noted in freshwater acclimated compared with saltwater housed mullet. At some institutions, it is common practice to err on the side of caution and buffer marine water with sodium bicarbonate at a 2 : 1 ratio (2 parts bicarb, 1 part MS-222 based on weight). Alternatively, the pH of the anesthetic water can be measured and the pH adjusted accordingly. Regardless of the method used, one should keep in mind that pH shifts may potentially have metabolic effects on the fish not solely related to anesthetic efficacy especially if exposure is prolonged. That said, in an unpublished study (T. Clauss, pers. exp., 2011) with crevalle jacks, there was no significant short-term difference in blood gas values from fish anesthetized in buffered or unbuffered MS-222. Regardless, species differences exist and without a controlled study as this one, it is advised to buffer or measure water pH.

Nitrogenous Compounds

Build up of nitrogenous compounds, particularly ammonia and nitrite, can damage or induce changes in gill morphology that affect uptake and clearance of immersion anesthetics. In addition, compromised oxygen uptake affects metabolism, including that of parenteral and immersion anesthetic agents, and can lead to acidemia. Water that has an animal in it for a long period of time, or when immersion water is reused, has the risk of nitrogenous compound elevations; water changes during the procedure will ameliorate these effects; additionally, measuring the water's ammonia content during the procedure will remove all concerns.

Drug Concentration or Dosage

At a given temperature, higher concentration immersions or drug dosages generally decrease induction and increase recovery times. However, recovery time from some immersions is independent of concentration (Hseu et al. 1997, 1998).

Drug Exposure Time

Increased immersion anesthetic exposure time usually results in increased recovery time. This effect is often associated with progressive hypoxemia and metabolic acidemia due to prolonged hypoventilation. Some immersion drugs (e.g., MS-222) continue to increase in brain and muscle despite blood equilibration. Therefore, an initially satisfactory drug dosage can produce progressively deeper anesthesia and respiratory arrest, even during recovery when the fish is in anesthetic-free water (Ross 2001). Thus, using graded anesthesia, higher dose rapid induction and lower dose maintenance levels is a sound practice. This practice has shown to reduce overall levels of physiologic stress in some species (Matsche 2011).

VASCULAR ACCESS

Most fish fall under a similar body plan and accessing their blood vessels is fairly straightforward. In large fish, spinal needles might be required due to the depth of the vessels. The ventral tail vein is accessible on the ventral midline or laterally under the lateral line (Fig. 15.1a,b). Cardiac puncture is sometimes the only viable options in species, where the tail is either covered by large, thick scales (parrot fish, arowana, and arapaima) that prevent access without removal of scale or where removal would result in significant skin exposure (Fig. 15.2). Cardiac puncture can be achieved by moving the operculum and inserting the needle through the skin that is cranial to the bulbus arteriosis/ventricle or ventrally through the body wall. Access to the dorsal aorta is also available through the oral cavity, midline and immediately posterior to the hard palate (Fig. 15.3). In some fishes (e.g., Australian lungfish), there is a periorbital sinus that can also be reached through the oral cavity.

Catheterization of fishes is not a minimally invasive process and is not routinely utilized, but possible (Ostrander 2000). In certain settings, typically research, dorsal aorta cannulization can be performed, but requires anchoring specialized tubing through the roof of mouth and through the rostrum and affixation to the dorsal fin or muscle of the fish (Smith & Bell 1964; Sovio et al. 1972). The ventral aorta is cannulated in a similar fashion but using the lower jaw. The caudal vein has also been catheterized and uses similar tubing as with the earlier cannulas (Ostrander 2000). With either method, the tubing of the setup must be affixed to the animal in order to prevent slippage of the catheter. In

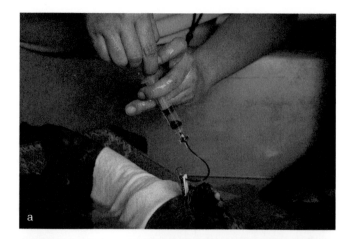

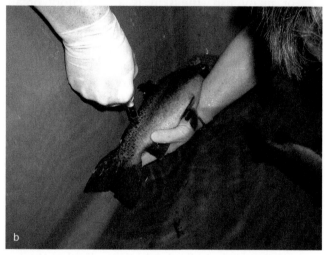

Figure 15.1. (a) Midline caudal tail venipuncture in a grouper (*Epinephelus itajara*) using an 18-gauge spinal needle and extension set. A chamois is placed on the tail to hold the animal in place within a sling during the venipuncture. (b) Lateral approach to caudal vein in a rainbow trout (*Onchorynchus mykiss*).

fast-moving fishes, maintaining such catheters is nearly impossible, therefore confinement may be necessary which carries its own obvious stressors (Sumpter et al. 1986). Additionally, anatomical features of some fishes make some of these approaches impossible.

IMMOBILIZATION METHODS AND TECHNIQUES

Manual Restraint

Manual restraint when used appropriately can be used for managing simple, short procedures or when preparing the animal for induction of anesthesia. For procedures lasting longer than several minutes, it is better to use chemical immobilization. Animals that are habituated or domesticated tolerate handling restraint better than nonacclimatized fish. See also the operant conditioning section in this chapter.

Considerations for human safety with manual restraint should include bites, stings, abrasions, and

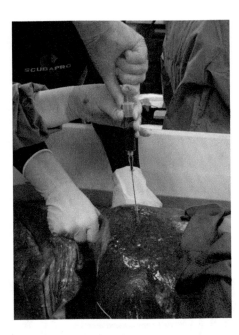

Figure 15.2. Cardiac venipuncture in a grouper (*Epinephelus lanceolatus*) using a 16-gauge spinal needle.

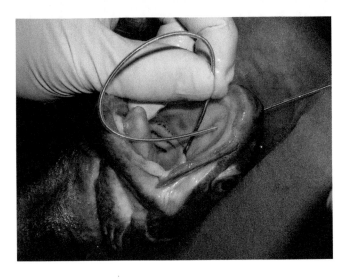

Figure 15.3. Cannulation of the dorsal aorta in a rainbow trout (*Onchorynchus mykiss*).

physical trauma due to thrashing. Even with chemical immobilization, the following should be considered so that appropriate safety precautions are utilized. Venom can occur in the dorsal or pectoral spines of scorpionfish, toadfish, rabbitfish, and a number of other fishes (Williamson et al. 1996). Sharp spines or other protuberances, such as with the acanthuridae (tangs and surgeonfish) or some tetraodontidae (porcupine pufferfishes), can cause significant damage without protective wear. Teeth have vast anatomic variety and can be crushing, puncturing, and macerating. In some species, pharyngeal teeth deep in the oral cavity can

cause trauma, particularly if the handler is unaware of their presence. Finally, there is the unique group of electric animals (electric eels, Mormyridiformes, and Gymnotiformes) that pose varying risks. An electric eel can produce 550 V (~1 amp) (Harms 2003), while the elephant nose mormyrids produce 500 Hz (Von der Emde 1998). Wearing gloves that do not transmit electric current is beneficial.

In regard to animal safety, the tubular, soft bodied fishes are particularly challenging to hold without crushing them. Further, the mucus on the skin of fishes is very slippery and in some species, copious. This not only poses a risk for not being able to securely restrain but it can be a source of long-term negative consequences should the mucus be removed. Wearing latex gloves that have been rinsed free of powder (an irritant to fish) helps with minimizing damage to fish skin and mucus, but can make secure handling more challenging. Wet material, such as cloth diapers and chamois used for automobiles, are both soft and smooth and can be useful in restraining some fish without damaging or altering the skin and mucous layer. Some fishes are scaleless and require more delicate handling in order to avoid abrading the skin. Additionally, keeping the basic facts in mind, such as that fish lack eyelids, will help in avoiding simple mistakes.

Nets of varying sizes and configurations (dip, seine, and box) are the most obvious tool for catching and restraining many fishes. For delicate skinned fish, nets made of plastic or very soft fine mesh are needed, but alternately, clear plastic bags can be used. In some circumstances, as in large exhibits, even the hook and line approach has been successfully used; note, however, that as with wild fishes, hook traumas can be fatal, as can exhaustive exercise.

Animals that struggle should be sedated. The concept of "learned helplessness" as with mammals is not an appropriate parallel to draw. The fish that "gives up" is stressed and depleted of energy. Anticipation of how a fish will manage manual restraint is crucial.

Larger fish can also be netted and then slung, but need care when lifting; the integrity of the net must be solid. These animals should only be moved for purposes of sedation and no further manipulation due to human and animal safety concerns. One method of recent use in elasmobranch restraint (see Chapter 16) is also an effective method for larger teleosts, such as grouper. This entails the use of a large vinyl bag with a narrow end that is open to allow water flow and a larger opening to catch the animal; this technique is best used on partially sedated or sedated animal. At the Seas, Walt Disney World, Orlando, FL, a large grouper in a 6-million-gallon aquarium was presedated with oral valium, moved into the bag, and then further sedated with high doses of tricaine methanesulfonate and safely brought to the surface. The bag was borrowed from uShaka Marine World Durban, South Africa

(G. Drysdale, pers. comm., 2013), where it is used predominantly in elasmobranchs.

An additional important consideration for manual restraint is time out of the water. In several studies, exposure to air increased mortality rates of angler caught fishes (Ferguson & Tufts 1992; Gingerich et al. 2007). In another study, while there were no mortality rates, there was significant morbidity (Schreer et al. 2005). Severity is species variable, as fishes that require oxygen-rich environments (e.g., trout) are more profoundly affected by air exposure and become acidotic with even short exposure times to air.

Operant Conditioning

Operant conditioning in fish is not a new concept (Couvillon 1984; Sison & Garlai 2010; Wright & Eastcott 1982), but the general trend of utilizing it for husbandry practices in aquaria has only gained popularity in the last few years. Many fish can be trained to move into certain areas of their enclosure, to swim into nets, crates or pools. The size of the animal is not a restriction, as schools of small fish can be as efficiently trained as large fishes. In larger animals, operant conditioning can be an invaluable tool to isolate animals for brief exams, treatments or for facilitating chemical administration for inducing anesthesia (Fig. 15.4a,b).

Methods for induction of anesthesia usually reduce the area where an animal can swim so that immersion anesthetics can be used in smaller volumes, injections are more achievable, or so that high dose inhalation agents (discussed later) can be administered with ease. Corralling animals into smaller areas with baffles, bringing them over slings (Fig. 15.5) and allowing the sling to come up around the animal's body, moving them into small inflatable pools, and finally, moving them into "squeeze" areas (Fig. 15.6) are all methods that facilitate examination, minor procedures (e.g., praziquantel immersion treatments), as well as anesthetic induction. Training animals to shift into containers like a PVC box or a trash bin are also good options to get closer contact.

Fish cognitive abilities allow individuals or groups to respond to visual, auditory or olfactory cues, and as such they can be trained much like you would train any higher vertebrate (Couvillon 1984; Sison & Garlai 2010; Wright & Eastcott 1982).

General Suggestions for Anesthesia

Before anesthetizing an unfamiliar species the anesthesiologist should perform a review of the available literature. Despite limited fish anesthesia publications, a literature search using the scientific name, along with words or phrases such as "physiology," "anatomy," "site fidelity," "fecundity," and "population assessment," will identify studies that required sedation or anesthesia. Table 15.1, while listing anesthetic regimens for representatives of many families, is far from exhaustive and was accomplished, in part, as suggested

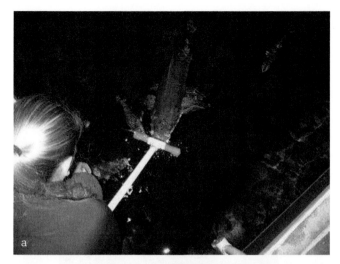

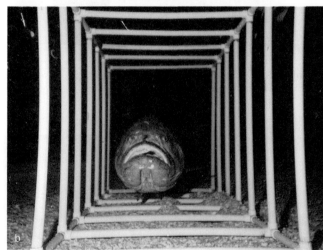

Figure 15.4. (a) Operant conditioning of a cobia (*Rachycentron canadum*). Note the animal is targeting on a T-shaped piece of PVC. (b) Operant conditioning of a grouper (*Epinephelus itajara*). The animal swims into a PVC box, which can then be closed/secured to reduce the functional swimming space of the animal.

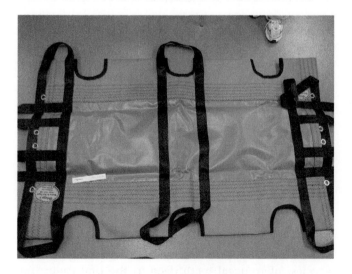

Figure 15.5. Sling designed to lift large aquatic animals.

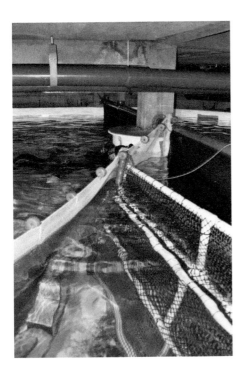

Figure 15.6. Squeeze device designed from PVC and plastic mesh. To the left of the squeeze is a net that reduced the spaced of the tank. The animal was corralled into the right side of the PVC/mesh (the animal is in the far right bottom corner).

earlier. Careful review of age class and body size in the literature should be taken into account when using these dosages and regimens because many studies utilize young or small fish. For example, drug dosages used in salmon smolts may not be effective in ocean ranging adults.

Regardless of available information, the anesthetic regimen for an untested species should be tried through to recovery using one or a small group of fish. Start at the low end of the recommended dosage range and work up to the desired effect (Harms & Bakal 1995; Ross 2001; Stetter 2001). However, in a species whose anesthetic tolerance is known, use a high dosage for a smoother and more rapid induction. Once induced, a lower immersion maintenance dosage is usually appropriate (Harms 1999). Rapid capture or in-enclosure anesthesia will reduce stress and facilitate smoother inductions. As mentioned, utilizing graded anesthesia (high induction, low maintenance dose) is a stress reducing method of anesthesia (Matsche 2011).

Preanesthetic Preparations

Where possible, the following should be performed prior to induction:

1. Baseline behavioral parameters (i.e., ventilation, caudal fin stroke rate, and overall activity level) should be recorded for comparison during anesthesia.
2. Although aspiration pneumonia is not a concern, it is not uncommon for fish to regurgitate material

that clogs gill rakers and contributes to water quality degradation. Additionally, if the regurgitant is fine and covers the gill lamellae, then suffocation can theoretically occur (sestonosis). Fasting for 12–24 hours (one feeding cycle) limits regurgitation and decreases nitrogenous waste production (Harms & Bakal 1995; Stetter 2001).
3. Containers with adequate water for transportation, induction, maintenance, and recovery should be available (Harms 1999; Stetter 2001). This is particularly important when water is used for immersion anesthesia. If the procedure occurs next to the animal's tank, it can be used for recovery. This assumes monitoring is possible and other specimens will not traumatize or predate the fish during recovery.
4. The physical (e.g., temperature) and chemical (e.g., pH and salinity) variables of all water used must be matched to those of the fish's source water. It is important to remember that the typically smaller water volumes used for anesthetic procedures will warm or chill to the temperature of the room air, thus water temperature should be monitored during the procedure and maintained as consistently as possible. Dissolved oxygen is maintained >5 ppm (mg/L) with 6–10 ppm ideal (Harms 1999; Stetter 2001).
5. For out of water procedures, a plan is made to prevent drying of the skin, fins, and eyes. This can include coverage with clear plastic drapes, bubble wrap, soft cloth (chamois or microfiber), and regular rinsing of tissues with water from a syringe or a small portable atomizer (Harms 1999; Ross 2001).
6. Capture techniques should be considered and the procedure discussed with all staff involved especially with large fishes.

Immersion (Inhalant) Anesthesia

Inhalant anesthesia via immersion in the water is analogous to gaseous anesthesia in terrestrial animals. The anesthetic in solution is ventilated by the fish, enters the bloodstream through the gills ± accessory respiratory organs ± the skin and passes rapidly to the central nervous system. When returned to drug-free water, drugs or their metabolites are excreted mostly via the gills and presumably accessory respiratory organs. Some elimination also occurs through the kidneys, liver, and presumably the skin (Ross 2001; Walsh & Pease 2002). Unlike in terrestrial vertebrates, any water soluble drugs or metabolites excreted from fish will be continuously absorbed through the body surface and gills, while being simultaneously metabolized and eliminated (Oikawa et al. 1994). This is problematic for assessing dosage effects and performing pharmokinetic studies, unless flowthrough systems or closed systems with inline carbon filters are utilized. This is significant when considering reusing the same water for multiple fishes; while it is unknown how much metabolism of drug occurs per volume of anesthetic water, it is in the

Table 15.1. Selected anesthetic agents used in selected bony fish (lungfish, sturgeon, and teleosts)

Class Osteichthyes Taxa	Drug	Dose	Route	Wt/Age	Temp (°C)	Comments	Reference
Subclass Sarcopterygii (coelacanths/lungfish) Order Ceratodontiformes Family Ceratodontidae							
Neoceratodus forsteri (Australian lungfish)	MS-222	100 mg/L	IM	Adult		Possess gills but may cease ventilation, may need to ventilate for the animal. Drowning is a potential hazard as this species has a single lung. Anesthetic induction is often long and may require some manual restraint until fully sedate.	N. Mylnczenko, unpubl.
Order Lepidosireniformes Family Lepidosirenidae							
Lepidosiren paradoxa (South American lungfish)	Benzocaine	Induction: 1 g/L Maintenance: 0.25 g/L	IN	577 ± 12 g	25	Obligate air breathers—prevent drowning. Induction: within 10 minutes. Maintained by flushing 0.25 g/L solution over gills. Recovery within 1 hour.	Bassi et al. (2005)
Family Protopteridae							
Protopterus annectens (West African lungfish)	Medetomidine plus Ketamine	0.053 mg/kg 5.26 mg/kg	IM	1.33 kg		Obligate air breathers—prevent drowning. Provided mild sedation, but not adequate for diagnostics without physical restraint. No reversal given. Recommend higher dose.	D. Neiffer, unpubl.
Protopterus aethiopocus (African lungfish)	MS-222	0.5%	IM	2–14 kg		Used for catheter placement into the branchial arch	DeLaney et al. (1976)
Subclass Actinopterygii Subdivision Chondrostei (sturgeons, paddlefish) Order Acipenseriformes Family Acipenseridae							
Acipenser oxyrhynchus desotoi (Gulf of Mexico sturgeon)	Medetomidine plus ketamine Atipamezole	0.06 mg/kg 6 mg/kg 0.30 mg/kg	IM IM	4-year-old 3.6 ± 1.2 kg	21.6 ± 3.1	Light plane of anesthesia for minor diagnostic procedures within 10 minutes. Mild bradycardia and respiratory depression noted. Atipamezole administered 30 minutes after immobilizing agents. Full recovery by 30 minutes. No mortality.	Fleming et al. (2003)
	Propofol	6.5 mg/kg	IV	4-year-old 3.6 ± 1.2 kg	21.6 ± 3.1	Light plane of anesthesia for minor diagnostic procedures within 5 minutes. Mild bradycardia and respiratory depression noted, with the latter persisting for 60 minutes. Fish remained quiet and unresponsive for 40 minutes. At 60 minutes, 70% were struggling at preinjection levels. All fish fully recovered within 120 minutes. No mortality.	Fleming et al. (2003)

Species	Agent	Dose	Route	Life stage	Weight	Temp (°C)	Comments	Reference
Acipenser transmontanus (white sturgeon)	Clove oil	50–100 mg/L	IN		206–363 g		Induction: 3–6 minutes. Recovery: 4.5–8.5 minutes. No mortality.	Taylor and Roberts (1999)
	Ketamine	77–88 mg/kg	IM		5–7.7 kg		Induction: 4–7 minutes. Effect lasted 6 hours.	Williams et al. (1988)
Acipenser ruthenus × *Huso huso* (hybrid Sterlet and Beluga sturgeon)	MS-222	100–125 mg/L	IN		1.36–2.34 kg		Variable effect from mild sedation to light anesthesia. $N = 10$.	D. Neiffer, unpubl.
Subdivision Teleostei								
Order Anguilliformes (eels)								
Family Anguillidae								
Anguilla reinhardtii (long-finned eel)	Benzocaine dissolved in ethanol (1:10)	60–80 mg/L	IN	Adults		17–25	Induction within 6 minutes.	Walsh and Pease (2002)
	Clove oil	100 mg/L	IN	Adults		17–25	Induction within 6 minutes. Recovery within 4 minutes.	Walsh and Pease (2002)
Moray eels								
Anguilla rostrata (American eel)	MS-222	90–100 ppm	IN				Sedation rated excellent. Examination performed.	D. Neiffer, unpubl.
	MS-222	75 mg/L	IN					
Family Muraenidae								
Gymnothorax funebris (green moray)	MS-222	50–100 mg/L	IN	Adults			Suitable for examination. Animals that gulp air at surface may take longer to induce. Make sure animal is enclosed in a confined area since prone to leaping.	E. Chittick, unpubl.
Gymnothorax vicinus (purplemouth moray)	MS-222	50–100 mg/L	IN	Adults			Suitable for examination. Animals that gulp air at surface may take longer to induce. Make sure animal is enclosed in a confined area since prone to leaping.	E. Chittick, unpubl.
Order Batrachoidiformes								
Family Batrachoididae								
Opsanus beta (Gulf toadfish)	MS-222	670 mg/L buffered with NaOH	IN	Sexually mature fish		24–26	Once fish was induced they were wrapped in anesthetic solution soaked paper towels for 30 minute surgical placement of venous cannula. Species considered tolerant of air exposure, and it was not necessary to irrigate gills. pH = 8	Gilmour et al. (1998)
Opsanus tau (oyster toadfish)	MS-222	50–250 mg/L	IN	Adults	675 ± 46 g	20	Slight sedation at 50 mg/L. Decreasing respiratory rate and ability to maintain equilibrium from 100–250 mg/L. Cessation of voluntary respiratory activity at 300 mg/L. These later fish resumed gilling 14 minutes after anesthetic withdrawal and all fish regained equilibrium within 23 minutes of anesthetic withdrawal.	Palmer and Mensinger (2004).

(Continued)

Table 15.1. (*Continued*)

Class Osteichthyes Taxa	Drug	Dose	Route	Wt/Age	Temp (°C)	Comments	Reference
Order Beryciformes **Family Holocentridae**							
Holocentrus ascensionis (longjawed squirrelfish)	MS-222	70–85 mg/L	IN	160–500 g		Variable sedation (mild to heavy) for examination.	D. Neiffer, unpubl.
Bloodspot squirrelfish	MS-222	100 mg/L	IN				T. Clauss, unpubl.
Myripristis jacobus (blackbar soldierfish)	MS-222	50–100 mg/L	IN	140–390 g		Variable sedation (mild to heavy) for examination.	D. Neiffer, unpubl.
Order Characiformes **Family characidae**							
Brycon cephalus (matrinxã)	MS-222 buffered with CaCO₃	150 mg/L	IN	Juveniles 31.56 ± 8.08 g	25	Time to anesthesia: 5.62 ± 0.53 minutes. Anesthesia duration: 10 minutes. Recovery: 5.19 + 3.07 minutes. Mortality: 0% at 150 mg/L, 16.7% at 200 mg/L, and 33.3% at 300 mg/L. Pronounced stress response at 200 and 300 mg/L. pH = 6.3	Roubach et al. (2001)
Colossoma macropomum (tambagui [aka large or black pacu]	Benzocaine dissolved in acetone (10 g/100 mL)	100–150 mg/L	IN	Juvenile 9.32 ± 3.7 g	24	Induction: 0.11–1.01 minutes. Recovery following exposure for 10 minutes: 2.32–9.04 minutes. Recovery following exposure for 30 minutes: 30 ± 20 minutes. Fish exposed to ≥220 mg/L exhibited stress response. Mortality 30% at 350 mg/L. pH = 6.5	Gomes et al. (2001)
	Eugenol dissolved in alcohol to make 1:2 stock solution	65 mg/L 65 mg/L	IN IN	Juveniles 56.6 ± 7.7 g Sub-adults 1100 ± 90.7 g	26–27	Stage necessary for handling reached in 1.45 minutes and a surgical stage in 2.54 minutes. Recovery: 6.82 ± 3.73 minutes. Exposure for 30 minutes was not associated with mortality. Dose up to 100 mg/L considered safe. Stage necessary for handling in 1.48 minutes and surgical stage in 3.77 minutes. Exposure for 30 minutes. Recovery: 3.79 ± 0.89 minutes. No mortality. Dose up to 100 mg/L considered safe.	Roubach et al. (2005)
	MS-222	30 mg/L	IN	Adult		In-tank sedation then transport	N. Mylniczenko, unpubl.
	Medetomidine, Butorphanol, Midazolam	100 μg/mkg 1 mg/kg 1 mg/kg	IM	Adult		Used in combination prior to euthanasia with MS-222. Very light sedation.	N. Mylniczenko, unpubl.

Species	Agent	Dose	Route	Size/Age	Temp (°C)	Comments	Reference
Piaractus brachypomus (red pacu)	MS-222 buffered 1:1 with NaHCO₃	100, 200 mg/L	IN	4 years old adults 500–727 g	20–23	Induction: 100 mg/L average 550 seconds; 200 mg/L average 350 seconds. Recovery: 300–500 seconds. pH = 5.5 = 7.0	Sladky et al. (2001)
	Eugenol dissolved in 95% ethanol (1:9)	50, 100, 200 mg/L	IN	4 years old adults 500–727 g	20–23	Induction: 50 mg/L average 300 seconds; 100 and 200 mg/L average 200 seconds. Recovery: 550–600 seconds. Resuscitation required in >50% fish exposed to 100–200 mg/L. pH = 5.5–7.0	Sladky et al. (2001)
Piaractus mesopotamicus (pacu caranha)	Benzocaine (1 g dissolved in 0.L liter ethanol.	99 mg/L	IN	Adults 315.2–745.2 g	15–35	Used for surgical implantation of ECG electrodes, buccal and opercular catheters. Sufficient level of anesthesia without interruption of spontaneous breathing.	Aguiar et al. (2002) Rantin et al. (1998)
Pygocentrus cariba (cariba piranha)	MS-222	70–90 mg/L	IN	Adult		Good anesthesia for mass removal, ocular aspirations and assist feeding	T. Clauss, unpubl.
Pygocentrus nattereri (red-bellied piranha)	MS-222	70–100 mg/L	IN	Adult		Good anesthesia for minor and surgical procedures	N, Mylniczenko and T. Clauss, unpubl.

Family Erythrinidae

Species	Agent	Dose	Route	Size/Age	Temp (°C)	Comments	Reference
Hoplias lacerdae (giant trahira)	Benzocaine (1 g in 0.1-L ethanol)	50 mg/L	IN	Adults 375 ± 47 g	25 ± 1	Provided light anesthesia for brief procedures including ECG electrode and buccal catheter placement. Spontaneous breathing present.	Rantin et al. (1993)
Hoplias malabaricus (tiger characin)	Benzocaine (1 gram in 0.1-L ethanol)	50 mg/L	IN	Adults 312 ± 47 g	25 ± 1	Provided light anesthesia for brief procedures including ECG electrode and buccal catheter placement. Spontaneous breathing present.	Rantin et al. (1993)

Order Cypriniformes
Family Cyprinidae

Species	Agent	Dose	Route	Size/Age	Temp (°C)	Comments	Reference
Carassius auratus (goldfish)	2-PE	0.25–0.35 mL/L 0.45 mL/L	IN	3.93 ± 1.99 g	24	Provided light sedation. Provided anesthesia with loss of equilibrium.	Kaiser and Vine (1998)
Ctenopharyngodon idella (grass carp)	MS-222	100 mg/L for induction; 75 mg/L for maintenance	IN	1.0–2.5 kg	22	Induction within 5 minutes. Allowed for surgical implantation of radio transmitters. Recovery took 5–25 minutes. Mortality occurred with 100 mg/L at temperatures >31°C.	Schramm and Black (1984)
	2-PE mixed with 500 mL tank water and added to chamber.	0.2 mL/L 0.4 mL/L	IN	Brood stock 3–12 kg	25	Induction to light sedation in 2–3 minutes. Females stripped of ova with this dose. Induction to anesthesia in 5–10 minutes. Males stripped of milt with this dose.	McCarter (1992)

(Continued)

Table 15.1. (*Continued*)

Class Osteichthyes Taxa	Drug	Dose	Route	Wt/Age	Temp (°C)	Comments	Reference
Cyprinus carpio (koi/common carp)	MS-222	100–200 mg/L	IN	123 ± 53 g	22–27	Utilized for exploratory celiotomy. pH = 6.9–7.5	Harms et al. (2005)
	MS-222 buffered with NaHCO$_3$	200 mg/L	IN	144 ± 44 g	23–25	Induction within 2 minutes. Level sufficient for deep IM injection and phlebotomy. Recovery within 2 minutes. pH = 7.4–7.6	Yanong et al. (2005)
	Alphaxalone-alphadolone (Saffan®)	0.3 mL/kg	IM	2 kg.		Sedation with partial loss of equilibrium. Able to be netted, but responsive	Harvey et al., (1988)
Epalzeorhynchos bicolor (red-tail black shark)	MS-222	100 mg/L	IN	Juveniles 1.4 ± 0.4 g	25.5	Anesthesia sufficient for handling and vaccination. pH = 7.5	Russo et al. (2006)
Hypophthalmichthys molitrix (silver carp)	2-PE mixed with 500-mL tank water and added to chamber.	0.2 mL/L 0.4 mL/L	IN	Brood stock 3–12 kg	25	Induction to light sedation in 2–3 minutes. Induction to anesthesia in 5–10 minutes.	McCarter (1992)
Phoxinus erythrogaster (Southern redbelly dace)	MS-222 buffered with NaHCO$_3$	60 mg/L	IN	Adults and juveniles 0.35–4.46 g	11–21	Induction to total loss of equilibrium in 5–13 minutes. Recovery: <2 minutes with faster recovery at higher temperatures. Mortality: 0%. pH = 7.0–7.9	Detar and Mattingly (2004)
	Clove oil dissolved in ethanol (1:10)	40–60 mg/L	IN	Adults and juveniles 0.35–4.46 g	11–21	Induction to total loss of equilibrium within 3 minutes. Recovery: <5 minutes with faster recovery at higher temperatures. No mortality. pH = 7.0–7.9	Detar and Mattingly (2004)
Phoxinus cumberlandensis (blackside dace)	Clove oil	40 mg/L	IN	Adults and juveniles	4–19	Used for anesthesia in the field during elastomer tag placement and fin clipping.	Detar and Mattingly (2004)
Rhinichthys atratulus (blacknose dace)	MS-222 unbuffered with significant pH drop.	300–500 mg/L	IN	Adults		Light anesthesia within 3 minutes. Allowed for handling. Recovery following 9 minutes exposure: 4–7 minutes. Exposure to this dose range beyond 15 minutes associated with mortality.	MacAvoy and Zaepfel (1997)
Rutilus rutilus (roach)	Clove oil dissolved in 95% ethanol at 1:10 ratio.	4 mg/L	IN	71 grams	15	Provided sedation for 6 hours without loss of equilibrium at which time fish is removed from anesthetic. Considered useful for transport. No mortality.	Hoskonen and Pirhonen (2004)
Tinca tinca (tench)	2-PE	0.5 g dm^{-3}	IN	Juveniles 0.08–1.82 g	25	Induction time: 2.2–12.6 minutes. Recovery after 15 minutes exposure: 1.1–3.3 minutes. Recommended for short term anesthesia. pH = 7.5–8.0	Myszkowski et al. (2003)

Order / Family / Species	Agent	Dose	Route	Weight / Age		Notes	Reference
Order Cyprinodontiformes							
Family Poeciliidae							
Poecilia velifera (sailfin molly)	2-PE	600 mg/L	IN	Adults 1.56 + 0.27 g	23	Induction: 7.50 ± 11.97 minutes. Recovery (fish placed in fresh water immediately after induction): 1.28 ± 2.53 minutes.	Hseu et al. (1997)
Xiphophorus maculatus (southern platyfish)	MS-222	30 mg/L	IN	Adults 1.71 ± 0.36 g		Provides light sedation.	Guo et al. (1995)
	Metomidate	1 mg/L	IN	Adults 1.71 ± 0.36 g		Provides light sedation.	Guo et al. (1995)
	Quinaldine sulfate	10 mg/L	IN	Adults 1.71 ± 0.36 g		Provides light sedation.	Guo et al. (1995)
	2-PE	220 mg/L	IN	Adults 1.71 ± 0.36 g		Provides light sedation.	Guo et al. (1995)
Order Gadiformes							
Family Gadidae							
Gadus morhua (Atlantic cod)	MS-222	75 mg/L	IN	84 ± 5 g	8.4	Anesthesia within 4 minutes. Exposure time 2.8–3.4 minutes. Recovery time 3.7–7.1 minutes.	Mattson and Riple (1989)
	Benzocaine dissolved in ethanol.	40 mg/L	IN	101 ± 6 g	9.5	Anesthesia reached within 3 minutes. Exposure time 2.1–3.2 minutes. Recovery time 3.9–10.8 minutes. Mortality 50% at 75–100 mg/L.	Mattson and Riple (1989)
	Metomidate	5 mg/L	IN	101 ± 6 g	9.6	Anesthesia reached within 4 minutes. Exposure time 4.8–10.8 minutes. Recovery time 8.2–19.2 minutes. Used for sorting and handling broodstock.	Mattson and Riple (1989)
Order Gasterosteiformes							
Family Syngnathidae							
Hippocampus erectus (lined seahorse)	MS-222	60–100 mg/L	IN	Adult		Low-end dose adequate for radiographs and minimally invasive procedures	N. Mylniczenko and T. Clauss, unpubl.
Hippocampus reidi (longsnout seahorse)	MS-222	25 mg/L	IN			Provided mild sedation.	D. Neiffer, unpubl.
	MS-222	75–100 mg/L	IN	Adult		Good sedation for blood draw, assist feed and injectable treatments	N. Mylniczenko, unpubl.
Phycodurus eques (leafy seadragon)	MS-222	50–100 mg/L	IN	Adult		Under 60 mg/L very light sedation and not sufficient for assist feeding or oral examination. Above 80 mg/L occasionally noted longer recoveries.	N. Mylniczenko and T. Clauss, unpubl.
Phyllopteryx taeniolatus (weedy seadragon)	MS-222	50–100 mg/L	IN			Same as above	
Syngnathus scovelli (pipefish)	MS-222	75 mg/L	IN			Sedation rated as good. Topical treatments performed.	D. Neiffer, unpubl.

(Continued)

223

Table 15.1. (*Continued*)

Class Osteichthyes Taxa	Drug	Dose	Route	Wt/Age	Temp (°C)	Comments	Reference
Order Gonorynchiformes Family Chanidae							
Chanos chanos (milk fish)	2-PE	400 mg/L	IN	23.99 ± 1.07 g	28	Provided total loss of equilibrium allowing phlebotomy.	Hseu et al. (1996)
Order Lophiiformes Family Antennariidae							
Antennarius maculattus (warty frogfish)		50–60 mg/L	IN			Heavy sedation for radiographs and swim bladder aspiration	T. Clauss, unpubl.
Antennarius ocellattus (ocellated frogfish)	MS-222	30–80 mg/L	IN	350–450 g		Sedation rated fair to excellent (higher doses better). Examination and topical treatments performed.	D. Neiffer, unpubl.
Antennarius striatus (striated frogfish)	MS-222 buffered with NaHCO₃	100 mg/L	IN	Adults		Diagnostics performed.	Yanong et al. (2003)
Histrio histrio (sargassumfish)	MS-222	30 mg/L	IN			Sedation adequate for examination and injections.	D. Neiffer, unpubl.
Order Osteoglossiformes Family Mormyridae							
Gnathonemus petersii (elephantnose fish)	Alfaxalone-alfadolone	2 mg/L for induction 1.5 mg/L for maintenance	IN	Average 15 grams and 15 cm	23	Loss of equilibrium and cessation of opercular movement at 20 minutes. Recovery took average of 17 minutes following 2.5 hours exposure.	Peters et al. (2001)
Order Perciformes Family Acanthuridae							
Acanthurus bahianus (ocean surgeonfish)	MS-222	50–75 mg/L	IN			Sedation rated fair to good. Examinations performed.	D. Neiffer, unpubl.
Acanthurus chirurgus (doctorfish)	MS-222	50–75 mg/L	IN			Provided surgical anesthesia for enucleation.	D. Neiffer, unpubl.
Acanthurus coeruleus (blue tang)	MS-222	85 mg/L	IN			Sedation rated excellent. Examination and topical treatment performed.	D. Neiffer, unpubl.
Acanthurus leucosternon (powder blue surgeonfish)	MS-222	50–78 mg/L	IN			Sedation rated excellent. Diagnostic examination performed.	D. Neiffer, unpubl.
Acanthurus sohal (Sohal tang)	MS-222	50 mg/L	IN			Sedation rated good. Diagnostic examination performed.	D. Neiffer, unpubl.
Family Anarhichadidae							
Anarhichas lupus (Atlantic wolffish)	MS-222	50–75 mg/L	IN			Physical exam, blood draw	N. Mylniczenko, unpubl.
Anarrhichthys ocellatus (wolf eel)	MS-222	90–100 mg/L				Lower than 90 not adequate for blood draw	T. Clauss, unpubl.

	Drug	Dose	Route	Weight	Comments	Reference
Family Carangidae						
Carangoides ruber (bar jack)	MS-222	75 mg/L	IN	70 g	Sedation rated as good. Adequate for examination and enucleation.	D. Neiffer, unpubl.
Caranx crysos (blue runner)	MS-222	80 mg/L	IN		Sedation rated as good. Diagnostic examinations performed.	D. Neiffer, unpubl.
	Alphaxalone-alphadolone (Saffan)	1.5 mL/kg	IM	1.5 kg	Anesthesia with marked depression of ventilation.	Harvey et al., (1988)
Caranx latus (horse-eye jack)	MS-222	70–80 mg/L	IN		Sedation rated as good to excellent. Examinations performed.	D. Neiffer, unpubl.
Caranx melampygus (Ulua)	Metomidate	80–100 mg/kg	IM	20–35 kg	Sedation with partial loss of equilibrium within 2–5 minutes. More than one dart used to deliver total dose. Able to be netted, but responsive. Recovered within 30 minutes.	Harvey et al., (1988)
	Alphaxalone-alphadolone (Saffan)	0.4 mL/kg	IM	18 kg	Light sedation with partial loss of equilibrium. Directed net avoidance.	Harvey et al., (1988)
Selene vomer (lookdown)	MS-222	75–125 mg/L	IN		Varied effect from mild sedation to light anesthesia (125 mg/L) for examinations.	D. Neiffer, unpubl.
Seriola lalandi (yellowtail amberjack)	Tiletamine-zolazepam (35-mg active powder in gel capsules)	8–9 mg/kg	PO	6–9 kg	Sedation first noted at 6–8 hours. At this point, fish trapped in hand-held net for examination, phlebotomy, and translocation. Animal remained responsive to the touch. Maximum sedation at approximately 12 hours. Recovery ranged from 12 to 48 hours. Mortality: 4/14 died due to unplanned consumption of additional oral doses (Total averaging 15–20 mg/kg).	Steers and Sherrill (2001)
Seriola dumerili (greater amberjack)	Metomidate	80 mg/kg	IM	9 kg	Sedation with partial loss of equilibrium within 2–5 minutes. Able to be netted, but responsive. Recovered within 30 minutes.	Harvey et al., (1988)
	Alphaxalone-alphadolone (Saffan)	0.3 mL/kg	IM	8 kg	Sedation with partial loss of equilibrium. Able to be netted, but responsive.	Harvey et al., (1988)
Trachinotus carolinus (Florida pompano)	MS-222	75–100 mg/L	IN		Provided sedation to light anesthesia for examinations, tagging, and ocular surgery.	D. Neiffer, unpubl.
Family Centrarchidae						
Lepomis macrochirus (bluegill sunfish)	Isoeugenol (AQUI-S™)	20 mg/L	IN	Juveniles-young adults 213 ± 118g 12 ± 2	Induction within 3 minutes. Total exposure time ≤15 minutes. Recovery within 8 minutes. Useful for basic handling procedures. pH = 8.1	Stehly and Gingerich (1999)
	Isoeugenol	20 mg/L	IN	Fry-fingerlings 0.54 ± 0.2g	Induction within 4.1 minutes. Total exposure time ≤15 minutes. Recovery within 5 minutes. Useful for basic handling procedures. pH = 8.1	

(Continued)

225

Table 15.1. (*Continued*)

Class Osteichthyes Taxa	Drug	Dose	Route	Wt/Age	Temp (°C)	Comments	Reference
Micropterus salmoides (largemouth bass)	MS-222	50 mg/L for induction 25 mg/L for maintenance				Provided sufficient sedation for transport.	Cooke et al. (2004)
	Clove oil dissolved in ethanol (1:9)	5–9 mg/L 15–20 mg/L		fingerlings and subadults	21	Time to deep sedation: 368 seconds. Sufficient for transport (reduced activity while maintaining equilibrium). Recovery: 417 seconds Time to moderate anesthesia 651 seconds. Recovery: 1699 seconds	D. Neiffer, unpubl.
Family Centropomidae							
Centropomus undecimalis (common snook)	MS-222	50–60 mg/L	IN			Provided mild sedation for diagnostic examinations.	
Lates calcarifer (Asian sea bass)	Clove oil dissolved in boiled water	6–9 mg/L		42 ± 9.74 g	29–30	Induction: 1.8–4.5 minutes. Exposed to clove oil for 4 minutes. Recovery: 0.5–5.0 minutes. No mortality, though some distal gill filament necrosis noted with repeated exposure to 9 mg/L.	Afifi et al. (2001)
Family Cichlidae							
Amphilophus citrinellus (*Cichlasoma citrinellum*) (Midas cichlid, red devil)	MS-222	150 mg/L for induction; 60 mg/L for maintenance.	IN	800 g		Induction in 8 minutes. Flow rate of maintenance solution = 3 L/min. Procedure duration (partial swim bladder resection) = 71 minutes	Lewbart et al. (1994)
	Ketamine	30 mg/kg	IV	206 ± 36 g	22 ± 2	Fish sedated first in buffered MS-222 (100–125 mg/L) for 8–10 minutes at which point fish became unresponsive. Fish removed to from bath and ketamine was injected. Induction: <10 seconds. In some fish, complete cessation of ventilation occurred while in other intermittent coughing or rapid ventilation was noted. Anesthesia lasted 1–41 minutes, with balance regained at 57–263 minutes.	Bruecker and Graham (1993)
Oreochromis mossambicus (Mozambique tilapia)	2-PE	600 mg/L	IN	Juveniles 3.83 ± 0.55 g	30	Induction: 7.43 + 13.25 minutes. Recovery (fish placed in fresh water immediately after induction): 1.38 + 1.77 minutes.	Hseu et al. (1997)
	MS-222	100 mg/L	IN	Juveniles and adults			N. Mylniczenko, unpubl.
(African cichlid)	MS-222	110–150 mg/L	IN			Light sedation at low range	T. Clauss, unpubl.

Species	Agent	Dose	Route	Size	N	Notes	Reference
Family Chaetodontidae							
Chaetodon pelewensis (Pelewensis butterfly)	MS-222	50–75 mg/L	IN	100 g		Sedation rated as good. Examination performed.	D. Neiffer, unpubl.
Chaetodon semilarvatus (red-lined butterflyfish)	MS-222	75–80 mg/L	IN			Provided mild to heavy sedation. Examination and topical treatments performed.	D. Neiffer, unpubl.
Heniochus acuminatus (black and white heniochus)	MS-222	90 mg/L	IN			Sedation rated as good. Diagnostic examination performed.	D. Neiffer, unpubl.
Heniochus sp. (bannerfish)	MS-222	90 mg/L	IN			Provided heavy sedation for diagnostic examinations.	D. Neiffer, unpubl.
Family Ephippidae							
Chaetodipterus faber (Atlantic spadefish)	MS-222	50–100 mg/L	IN	0.22–2.32 kg		Effect varied from mild sedation at lower doses to surgical anesthesia at 100 mg/L. N = 11.	D. Neiffer, unpubl.
Family Gobiidae							
Afurcagobius tamarensis (Tammar River goby)	Clove oil in ethanol at ratio 1:5	40 mg/L	IN		18	Induction within 3 minutes. Recovery within 5 minutes. Sufficient for handling and measurement.	Griffiths (2000)
Bathygobius cocosensis (Cocos frill-goby)	Clove oil in ethanol at ratio 1:5	40 mg/L	IN		18	Induction within 3 minutes. Recovery within 5 minutes. Sufficient for handling and measurement.	Griffiths (2000)
Favonigobius lateralis (goby)	Clove oil in ethanol at ratio 1:5	40 mg/L	IN		18	Induction within 3 minutes. Recovery within 5 minutes. Sufficient for handling and measurement.	Griffiths (2000)
Family Grammatidae							
Pseudoanthias sp. (*Anthias* sp.)	MS-222	77 mg/L	IN	Adult		Sedation rated excellent. Diagnostic examination performed.	D. Neiffer, unpubl.
Gramma loreto (royal gramma)	MS-222	65–90 mg/L	IN			Sedation rate as good. Diagnostic examinations performed.	D. Neiffer, unpubl.
Family Haemulidae							
Haemulon chrysargyreum (smallmouth grunt)	MS-222	100 mg/L	IN			Provided surgical anesthesia for kidney culture.	D. Neiffer, unpubl.
Haemulon flavolineatum (French grunt)	MS-222	100 mg/L	IN			Provided surgical anesthesia for enucleation and kidney culture.	D. Neiffer, unpubl.
Haemulon plumieri (white grunt)	MS-222	85–100 mg/L	IN			Sedation rated good. Examinations performed.	D. Neiffer, unpubl.
Haemulon sciurus (bluestripe grunt)	MS-222	30–90 mg/L	IN			Most sedations rated as good. Diagnostic examinations, injections, and enucleation (1 case) performed.	D. Neiffer, unpubl.
Haemulon melanurum (Cottonwick)	MS-222	80 mg/L	IN			Sedation rated as good. Examination performed.	D. Neiffer, unpubl.

(Continued)

Table 15.1. (*Continued*)

Class Osteichthyes Taxa	Drug	Dose	Route	Wt/Age	Temp (°C)	Comments	Reference
Haemulon aurolineatum (tomtate)	MS-222	100 mg/L	IN			Sedation rated good. Examination performed.	D. Neiffer, unpubl.
Anisotremus virginicus (porkfish)	MS-222	100 mg/L	IN			Provided surgical anesthesia for enucleation and kidney culture.	D. Neiffer, unpubl.
Family Kyphosidae							
Girella elevata (black drummer)	Clove oil in ethanol at ratio 1:5	40 mg/L	IN		18	Induction within 3 minutes. Recovery within 5 minutes. Sufficient for handling and measurement.	Griffiths (2000)
Microcanthus strigatus (convict tang)	MS-222	75 mg/L	IN			Provide heavy sedation.	D. Neiffer, unpubl.
Scorpis lineolatus (silver sweep)	Clove oil in ethanol at ratio 1:5	40 mg/L	IN		18	Induction within 3 minutes. Recovery within 5 minutes. Sufficient for handling and measurement.	Griffiths (2000)
Family Labridae							
Halichoeres radiatus (puddingwife)	MS-222	50–100 mg/L	IN			Sedation rated as good. Diagnostic examinations performed.	D. Neiffer, unpubl.
Thalassoma duperreyi (saddle wrasse)	MS-222	90 mg/L	IN			Sedation rated as good. Diagnostic examinations performed.	D. Neiffer, unpubl.
Cheilinus undulates (Napolean Wrasse)	MS-222	100 mg/L	IN			Induction at 100 mg/L, maintenance at 50 mg/L. Excellent for transport and physical exam.	N. Mylniczenko, unpubl.
Family Lateolabracidae							
Lateolabrax japonicus (Japanese seaperch)	2-PE	400 mg/L	IN	48.98 ± 3.47 g	29	Provided total loss of equilibrium allowing phlebotomy.	Hseu et al. (1996)
	2-PE	400 mg/L	IN	Juveniles, 4.4 + 0.86 g	28	Induction: 2.13 + 0.45 minutes. Recovery (fish placed in fresh water immediately after induction): 0.69 + 0.15 minutes.	Hseu et al. (1997)
	2-PE	400 mg/L	IN	Juveniles, 4.8 ± 1.46 g	24	Induction: 1.75 ± 0.16 minutes. Recovery (fish placed in non-medicated water immediately after induction): 0.49 ± 0.08 minutes.	Hseu et al. (1997)
Family Lobotidae							
Lobotes surinamensis (tripletail)	MS-222	80–90 mg/L	IN			Sedation sufficient for examinations and jaw debridement (one individual).	D. Neiffer, unpubl.
Family Lutjanidae							
Lutjanus apodus (schoolmaster)	MS-222	125 mg/L	IN			Provided surgical anesthesia for kidney culture.	D. Neiffer, unpubl.
Lutjanus sp. (Snapper)	Metomidate	50 mg/kg	IM	14 kg		Anesthesia with marked depression of ventilation. Two or more darts used to deliver total.	Harvey et al., (1988)

Species	Drug	Dose	Route	Size/Weight	Temp (°C)	Comments	Reference
Ocyurus chrysurus (yellowtail snapper)	MS-222	75–85 mg/L	IN	50–120 g		Effect varied from mild to heavy sedation. Examinations performed. N = 17.	D. Neiffer, unpubl.
	Medetomidine plus ketamine	1.1–1.7 27–42 mg/kg (ratio M:K averages 24:1)	IM	2.35–3.65 kg (N = 6)		All fish injected by dives using jab stick. Initial effect seen in 4–12 minutes. For complete injections, mild to moderate sedation achieved. Fish netted and transferred to MS-222 bath for phlebotomy. Fish culled as part of disease surveillance and thus no reversal agent given.	D. Neiffer, unpubl.
Lutjanus argentimaculatus (mangrove red snapper)	2-PE	400 mg/L	IN	39.21 ± 2.08 g	29	Provided total loss of equilibrium allowing phlebotomy.	Hseu et al. (1996)
Family Moronidae							
Dicentrarchus labrax (sea bass)	Quinaldine sulfate with diazepam	7.5 mg/L 2 mg/L	IN	Juveniles 8–9 g	24–25	Induction time 1–2 minutes. Recovery time 4–6 minutes. Provides deep anesthesia suitable for marking, surgery, and handling. "Note: quinaldine sulfate alone at 15 mg/L associated with 10% mortality and at 20–25 mg/L, associated with 30–100% mortality. pH = 7.9–8.2	Yanar and Kumlu (2001)
	Quinaldine sulfate with diazepam	5 mg/L 2 mg/L	IN	Juveniles 8–9 g	24–25	Induction time 1–2 minutes. Recovery time 3–5 minutes. Provides light anesthesia suitable for transportation. pH = 7.9–8.2	Yanar and Kumlu (2001)
Morone saxatilis (striped bass)	MS-222	20 mg/L	IN	Adult, 48–81 cm	21	Prior to placement in bath, gills were sprayed twice with MS-222 solution (3200 mg/L). Procedure: Mock intracoelomic transmitter placement. Induction: 38–58 seconds. Recovery after 5 minutes exposure to drug: 156–272 seconds. No mortalities. "Note from author (DN): species appears to be sensitive to MS-222.	Jennings and Looney (1998)
Morone saxatilis (striped bass)	Benzocaine dissolved in 100% ethanol at 1 g/30 mL	55–80 mg/L	IN	Juvenile and Adults 0.118–3.5 kg	11–22	Induction in 3 minutes. Recovery in 1.5–14.25 minutes.	Gilderhus et al. (1991)
Morone saxatilis × *chrysops* (hybrid striped bass)	MS-222	25 mg/L	IN	87 ± 24.4 g	23	Light sedation.	Davis and Griffin (2004)
	Clove oil	8 μl/L	IN	87 ± 24.4 g	23	Light sedation.	Davis and Griffin (2004)
	Isoeugenol (AQUI-S)	3.6 mg/L	IN	87 ± 24.4 g	23	Light sedation.	Davis and Griffin (2004)
	Quinaldine sulfate	8.3 mg/L	IN	87 ± 24.4 g	23	Light sedation.	Davis and Griffin (2004)
	Metomidate	1.5 mg/L	IN	87 ± 24.4 g	23	Light sedation.	Davis and Griffin (2004)

(Continued)

Table 15.1. (Continued)

Class Osteichthyes Taxa	Drug	Route	Dose	Wt/Age	Temp (°C)	Comments	Reference
Family Mugilidae							
Mugil cephalus (gray mullet)	2-PE	IN	400 mg/L	38.49 ± 3.85 g	31	Provided total loss of equilibrium allowing phlebotomy.	Hseu et al. (1996)
Myxus elongates (sand gray mullet)	Clove oil in ethanol at ratio 1:5	IN	40 mg/L		18	Induction within 3 minutes. Recovery within 5 minutes. Sufficient for handling and measurement.	Griffiths (2000)
Family Mullidae							
Pseudupeneus maculatus (spotted goatfish)	MS-222	IN	30–50 mg/L			Heavy sedation.	D. Neiffer, unpubl.
Family Tripterygiidae							
Enneapterygius rufopileus (redcap triplefin)	Clove oil in ethanol at ratio 1:5	IN	40 mg/L		18	Induction within 3 minutes. Recovery within 10 minutes. Sufficient for handling and measurement.	Griffiths (2000)
Family Osphronemidae							
Colisa labiosus (thick-lipped gourami)	MS-222 buffered with sodium bicarbonate	IN	200 mg/L for induction. 80 mg/L for maintenance.	8 g		Induction: 90 seconds. Total anesthesia time = 47 minutes. Flow rate of maintenance fluid = 12.1 mL/min. Gill motion throughout procedure. Full recovery by 23 minutes. Surgical mass removal.	Harms and Bakal (1995)
Trichogaster trichopterus (threespot gourami)	MS-222 buffered with NaHCO$_3$	IN	400 mg/L 60 mg/L	19 ± 3 g	23–25 28–29	Induction within 2 minutes. Level sufficient for deep IM injection and phlebotomy. Recovery within 2 minutes. pH = 7.4–7.6 Level sufficient to induce light sedation within 4 minutes.	Yanong et al. (2005) Crosby et al. (2006)
	Metomidate	IN	0.8 mg/L		28–29	Level sufficient to induce light sedation within 4 minutes.	Crosby et al. (2006)
	Quinaldine	IN	5 mg/L		28–29	Level sufficient to induce light sedation within 4 minutes.	Crosby et al. (2006)
Family Percidae							
Perca fluviatilis (European perch)	Clove oil dissolved in 95% ethanol at 1:10 ratio.	IN	6 mg/L	17 g	15	Provided sedation for 6 hours without loss of equilibrium at which time fish removed from anesthetic. Considered useful for transport. No mortality.	Hoskonen and Pirhonen (2004)
Perca flavescens (yellow perch)	Isoeugenol (AQUI-S)	IN	20 mg/L	Juveniles–young adults 126 ± 50.1 g	12 ± 2	Induction within 3 minutes. Total exposure time ≤15 minutes. Recovery within 8 minutes. Useful for basic handling procedures. pH = 8.1	Stehly and Gingerich (1999)
	Isoeugenol (AQUI-S)	IN	20 mg/L	Fry–fingerlings 1.1 ± 0.22 g	12 ± 2	Induction within 4.1 minutes or less. Total exposure time ≤15 minutes. Recovery within 5 minutes. Useful for basic handling procedures. pH = 8.1	Stehly and Gingerich (1999)

Species	Agent	Dose	Route	Weight/Size	Temp (°C)	Comments	Reference
Stizostedion vitreum (walleye)	Isoeugenol (AQUI-S)	50 mg/L	IN	Juveniles-young adults 58.3 ± 12.2g	12 ± 2	Induction averaged 4.3 minutes. Total exposure time <15 minutes. Recovery within 8 minutes. Useful for basic handling procedures. pH = 8.1	Stehly and Gingerich (1999)
	Isoeugenol (AQUI-S)	50 mg/L	IN	Fry-fingerlings 0.8 ± 0.16g	12 ± 2	Induction averaged 3.9 minutes. Total exposure time <15 minutes. Recovery within 5 minutes. Useful for basic handling procedures. pH = 8.1	Stehly and Gingerich (1999)
Family Pomacanthidae							
Centropyge bicolor (bicolor angelfish)	MS-222	75 mg/L	IN			Sedation rated excellent. Diagnostic examination performed.	D. Neiffer, unpubl.
Pomacanthus arcuatus (gray angelfish)	MS-222	50–100 mg/L	IN	0.2–1.7 kg		Provided mild to heavy sedation with a few animals considered lightly anesthetized at 100 mg/L. Diagnostic exams and topical treatments performed. N = 16	D. Neiffer, unpubl.
Pomacanthus paru (French angelfish)	MS-222	50–80 mg/L	IN	0.40–1.95 kg		Provided mild to heavy sedation with a few animals considered excessively deep at 70–80 mg/L range. Diagnostic examinations performed. N = 8	D. Neiffer, unpubl.
Pomacanthus semicirculatus (Koran angelfish)	MS-222	60–85 mg/L	IN			Variable sedative effect (fair to excellent). Diagnostic exams and topical treatments performed. N = 2	D. Neiffer, unpubl.
Family Pomacentridae							
Abudefduf saxatilis (sergeant major)	MS-222	100 mg/L	IN			Provided surgical anesthesia for kidney culture.	D. Neiffer, unpubl.
Amphiprion percula (Percula clownfish)	MS-222	50–75 mg/L	IN			Provided mild to heavy sedation for examinations.	D. Neiffer, unpubl.
Chromis cyanea (blue chromis)	MS-222	75 mg/L	IN			Sedation rated as good. Examination performed.	D. Neiffer, unpubl.
Chromis multilineata (brown chromis)	MS-222	75 mg/L	IN			Sedation rated as good. Examination and transport.	D. Neiffer, unpubl.
Dascyllus melanurus (four-stripe damselfish)	MS-222	90 mg/L	IN			Sedation rated as good. Diagnostic examination performed.	D. Neiffer, unpubl.
Dascyllus trimaculatus (domino damselfish)	MS-222	50–75 mg/L	IN			Provided heavy sedation for examinations.	D. Neiffer, unpubl.
Family Rachycentridae							
Rachycentron canadum (cobia)	Medetomidine with Ketamine	0.122–0.240 mg/kg 6–13.5 mg/kg	IM	24–40 kg		Injected using spring-loaded pole syringe. Dose resulted in mild sedation. Supplemental dose of 0.100-mg/kg medetomidine and 2.8-mg/kg ketamine necessary for final capture. MS-222 at 50mg/L has been used for maintenance during examinations, skin biopsies, and one enucleation. Reversal with atipamezole at 5× total mg dose of medetomidine given IM.	D. Neiffer, unpubl.

(Continued)

Table 15.1. *(Continued)*

Class Osteichthyes Taxa	Drug	Dose	Route	Wt/Age	Temp (°C)	Comments	Reference
Family Scaridae							
Scarus coelestinus (midnight parrotfish)	MS-222	75 mg/L	IN			Provided light anesthesia for diagnostic examination.	D. Neiffer, unpubl.
Scarus guacamaia (rainbow parrotfish)	MS-222	50–75 mg/L	IN	2.03–7.45 kg		Effect varied from moderate sedation to light anesthesia. Diagnostic examinations performed. $N = 4$.	D. Neiffer, unpubl.
Scarus vetula (queen parrotfish)	MS-222	50–75 mg/L	IN			Provided mild to heavy sedation. Diagnostic examinations performed.	D. Neiffer, unpubl.
Sparisoma aurofrenatum (redband parrotfish)	MS-222	75 mg/L	IN			Provided surgical anesthesia for enucleation.	D. Neiffer, unpubl.
Family Sciaenidae							
Sciaenops ocellatus (red drum)	MS-222	80 mg/L	IN		26–27	Anesthesia induced in 2.5–6 minutes. Sufficient for handling and phlebotomy. pH = 7.7–7.8	Thomas and Robertson (1991)
	Metomidate	7 mg/L	IN		26–27	Anesthesia induced in 3–7 minutes. Sufficient for handling and phlebotomy. pH = 7.7–7.8	Thomas and Robertson (1991)
	Quinaldine sulfate	20 mg/L	IN		26–27	Anesthesia induced in 2–4 minutes. Sufficient for handling and phlebotomy. pH = 7.7–7.8	Thomas and Robertson (1991)
Family Scombridae							
Sarda chiliensis (bonito)	Ketamine plus Medetomidine Atipamezole	4 mg/kg 0.4 mg/kg 2 mg/kg	IM IM	2.7 ± 0.6 kg	19.5–20.5	Injections placed in red lateral muscle, immediately ventral to the lateral ridge below the lateral line, posterior and dorsal to the end of the pectoral fin. Induction: 8.9 ± 2.1 minutes. Anesthesia time: 19.0 ± 3.8 minutes. Recovery following injection of atipamezole: 7.7 ± 8.5 minutes. Mortality in fish receiving atipamezole dose <5× medetomidine dose. pH = 7.8–7.9	Williams et al. (2004)
Scomber japonica (Pacific mackerel)	Ketamine plus Medetomidine Atipamezole	53–228 mg/kg 0.6–4.2 mg/kg 5× Medetomidine dose.	IM IM	0.33–0.40 kg	19.5–20.5	Injected placed in red lateral muscle, immediately ventral to the lateral ridge below the lateral line, posterior and dorsal to the end of the pectoral fin. Induction: 4–21 minutes (mean = 9 minutes) for 37 fish; 45–56 minutes for 8 fish. Anesthesia time: 1–52 minutes (mean = 16 minutes). Recovery following atipamezole: 2–12 minutes (mean = 5 minutes). pH = 7.8–7.9	Williams et al. (2004)

232

Species	Agent	Dose	Route	Weight	Temp	Comments	Reference
Thunnus thynnus (bluefin tuna)	MS-222	90 mg/L	IN			Oxygenated water over gills at 12–20L/min following induction until recovery. Minor surgical procedures, ultrasonographic examinations, and serial blood sampling.	Sylvia et al. (1994)
	MS-222	75 mg/L	IN			Induction rapid and deep. For short procedures, fish captured and dosed in vinyl bag with supplemental oxygen provided. For longer procedures, fish captured in stretcher and transferred to large pool containing MS-222. Once induced, fish transferred to exam table with oxygenated anesthetic water directed over gills. In either case, recovery involved directing anesthetic free water over gills until fish capable of forward swimming motion.	Cooper et al. (1994)
Family Serranidae							
Epinephelus itajara (goliath grouper)	MS-222	75–95 mg/L	IN	7.7–106.2 kg		Provided mild to heavy sedation. Diagnostic examinations, injections, and topical treatments performed. N = 5.	D. Neiffer, unpubl.
Epinephelus lanceolatus (Queensland grouper)	MS-222	95–125 mg/L	IN	3.4–10 kg		Effect varied from heavy sedation to anesthesia (swim bladder surgeries and sampling). N = 6.	D. Neiffer, unpubl.
Epinephelus ongus (white-streaked grouper)	MS-222	1 g/L, 75 mg/L	IN	Adult		Induction with high dose power sprayer over gills, following by maintenance in lower dose	N. Mylniczenko, unpubl.
Epinephelus polyphekadion (camouflage grouper)	MS-222	80 mg/L	IN	610 g		Good for diagnostics (clips and scrapes)	T. Clauss, unpubl.
	Clove oil	10 mg/L	IN			Suitable for sampling and for transportation.	Afifi et al. (2001)
Epinephelus morio (red grouper)	MS-222	80 mg/L	IN	0.51–8.64 kg		Effect ranged from mild sedation to light anesthesia. Examinations performed. N = 7.	D. Neiffer, unpubl.
Mycteroperca bonaci (black grouper)	MS-222	80–100 mg/L	IN	183–800 g		Provided adequate sedation for examination. N = 5	D. Neiffer, unpubl.
Mycteroperca venenosa (yellowfin grouper)	MS-222	50 mg/L	IN			Provided adequate sedation for examination.	D. Neiffer, unpubl.
Family Siganidae							
Siganus lineatus (rabbitfish)	Clove oil	100 mg/L	IN	Juveniles 7–39 g	27–29	Time to anesthesia <3 minutes. Time to recovery <5 minutes. Suitable for examination. No mortality observed.	Soto and Burhanuddin (1995)

(Continued)

Table 15.1. (Continued)

Class Osteichthyes Taxa	Drug	Dose	Route	Wt/Age	Temp (°C)	Comments	Reference
Family Sparidae							
Acanthopagrus schlegelii (black porgy)	2-PE	400 mg/L	IN	11.55 ± 3.47 g	29	Provided total loss of equilibrium allowing phlebotomy.	Hseu et al. (1996)
Calamus pennatula (pluma porgy)	MS-222	50–100	IN			Suitable for evaluation of exophthalmia though 100 mg/L excessive in one case.	D. Neiffer, unpubl.
Chrysophrys auratus (New Zealand snapper, squirefish)	Isoeugenol (AQUI-S)	120 mg/L for induction; 60 mg/L for maintenance.	IN	861.3 ± 64.6 g	11 ± 0.2	Time to surgical anesthesia was 20–25 minutes. During surgery (cannula placement) 60 mg/L oxygenated solution flushed continuously over gills. Poor survival with possible relation to prolonged surgery and/or hypoxemia.	Rothwell et al. (2005)
Pagrus major (red seabream, porgy)	MS-222	100 mg/L with no buffering 50 mg/L with no buffering	IN IN	595 days old, 320 g post-hatch larvae, 0.00022 g	20	Induction: 3–5 minutes. 100% recovery after 30 minutes exposure. Observations: maintained Stage III anesthesia; pH = 7.2. Induction: 3–5 minutes. 100% recovery after 30 minutes exposure. Note: no gills in this species at this age—all skin absorption. Maintained Stage III anesthesia; pH = 7.7	Oikawa et al. (1994)
Rhabdosargus sarba (*Sparus sarba*) (goldlined seabream)	MS-222	100 mg/L	IN	Juvenile 3.2 + 0.15 g	27–29	Induction: 1.31 ± 0.06 minutes. Recovery: 0.63 ± 0.03 minutes. No mortality. pH = 8.1	Hseu et al. (1998)
	Benzocaine dissolved in 95% ethanol	50 mg/L	IN	Juvenile 3.2 + 0.15 g	27–29	Induction: 1.94 ± 0.03 minutes. Recovery: 0.52 ± 0.04 minutes. No mortality. pH = 8.1	Hseu et al. (1998)
	Quinaldine dissolved in 95% ethanol	9 μL/L	IN	Juvenile 3.2 + 0.15 g	27–29	Induction: 1.19 ± 0.11 minutes. Recovery: 0.40 ± 0.03 minutes. No mortality. pH = 8.1	Hseu et al. (1998)
	Quinaldine sulfate	20 mg/L	IN	Juvenile 3.2 + 0.15 g	27–29	Induction: 2.40 ± 0.11 minutes. Recovery: 0.51 ± 0.02 minutes. No mortality. pH = 8.1	Hseu et al. (1998)
	2-PE	400 μL/L	IN	Juvenile 3.2 + 0.15 g	27–29	Induction: 1.25 ± 0.08 minutes. Recovery: 0.51 ± 0.04 minutes. No mortality. pH = 8.1	Hseu et al. (1998)
Sparus aurata (gilthead seabream)	Benzocaine dissolved in 100% ethanol (1:20)	22.5 μL/L	IN	220 ± 15 g	24 ± 0.5	Used for diagnostic sampling. Loss of sensation and equilibrium within 8 minutes. Recovery within 90 seconds of transfer to anesthetic free water. No mortality.	Bressler and Ron (2004)
	Clove oil dissolved in 100% ethanol (1:5)	44.5 μL/L	IN	220 ± 15 g	24 ± 0.5	Used for diagnostic sampling. Loss of sensation and equilibrium within 8 minutes. Recovery within 90 seconds of transfer to anesthetic free water. No mortality.	Bressler and Ron (2004)

Agent	Dose	Route	Size/Age	Temp (°C)	Comments	Reference
Quinaldine sulfate (plus diazepam)	5 mg/L, 1 mg/L	IN	Juveniles 6–7 g	25–26	Use for light anesthesia and transportation. Induction: 1–2 minutes. Recovery: 2–4 minutes. Observations: opercular rate 150/min, which is less than opercular rate when quinaldine sulfate is used alone to reach the same level of anesthesia. Mortality 0%. pH = 7.9–8.2	Kumlu and Yanar (1999)
Quinaldine sulfate (plus diazepam)	7.5 mg/L, 1 mg/L	IN	Juveniles 6–7 g		Use for deep anesthesia, marking, handling and surgery. Induction: 0–1 minute. Recovery: 3–5 minutes. Observations: opercular rate 170/min, which is less than operuclar rate observed when quinaldine sulfate is used alone to reach the same level of anesthesia. Mortality: 0%. pH = 7.9–8.2	
Quinaldine sulfate	10 mg/L	IN	Juveniles 6–7 g		Light anesthesia achieved. Induction: 0–1 minute. Recovery: 3–5 minutes. Observations: opercular rate 190/min. All fish remained sensitive to external stimuli. Mortality: 0% at light sedation dose, but 30–100% at deep sedation dose of 15–20mg/L. In these cases, opecular rate increased to 190/min and then ceased. pH = 7.9–8.2	
Family Sphyraenidae *Sphyraena barracuda* (great barracuda)						
MS-222	30 mg/L, 50 mg/L	IN	Adult		Lower dose for whole tank sedation, higher dose for transport. Once transported, blood was drawn from the animal.	N. Mylniczenko, unpubl.
	100 mg/L	IN	Juvenile		Excellent sedation for physical exam and treatments	N. Mylniczenko, unpubl.
Family Terapontidae *Bidyanus bidyanus* (silver perch)						
Benzocaine	20 mg/L	IN	682 ± 99 g		Used for sedation during transport	Kildea et al. (2004)
Clove oil	15 and 50 mg/L	IN	682 + 99 g		15 mg/L sufficient for light handling, tagging, and harvesting (exposure time 60 minutes). 50 mg/L produced anesthesia suitable for surgical procedures (exposure time 30 minutes).	Kildea et al. (2004)
AQUI-S	15 mg/L	IN	682 + 99 g		Sufficient for light handling, tagging, and harvesting (exposure time 60 minutes).	Kildea et al. (2004)
Family Toxotidae *Toxotes jaculatrix* (Archerfish)						
MS-222	90–100 mg/L	IN				N, Mylniczenko and T. Clauss, unpubl.

(Continued)

Table 15.1. (*Continued*)

Class Osteichthyes Taxa	Drug	Dose	Route	Wt/Age	Temp (°C)	Comments	Reference
Family Zanclidae							
Zanclus cornutus (Moorish idol)	MS-222	75 mg/L	IN			Sedation rated as excellent. Examination performed.	D. Neiffer, unpubl.
Order Pleuronectiformes							
Family Paralichthyidae							
Paralichthys lethostigma (southern flounder)	MS-222	75 mg/L	IN			Provided adequate sedation for examination.	D. Neiffer, unpubl.
Family Pleuronectidae							
Hippoglossus hippoglossus (halibut)	MS-222	250 mg/L	IN	2915 + 592 g	9–10	Induction to anesthesia = 250–282 seconds. Dose allowed for handling and phlebotomy. Recovery time 495–649 seconds.	Malmstrøm et al. (1993)
	Metomidate	20–30 mg/L	IN	2915 ± 592 g	9–10	Induction to anesthesia = 189–310 seconds. Dose allowed for handling and phlebotomy. Recovery time 220–320 seconds.	Malmstrøm et al. (1993)
		9 mg/L	IN	Age 12 months	10.3 ± 0.5	Though times not given, induction considered rapid and recovery prolonged. Respiration was depressed. See information on same study results in turbot (*Scophthalmus maximus*) in this table.	Hansen et al. (2003)
		3 mg/kg (50-mg/mL soln. diluted with 0.9% NaCl to 3 mg/mL)	IV			No information on use, induction, or recovery, but good tissue distribution measured. No mortalities.	
Family Scopthalmidae							
Scophthalmus maximus (turbot)	Metomidate	9 mg/L	IN	Age 8 months	18 ± 0.5	Induction: 0.28–1.83 minutes. Recovery following 10 minutes exposure: 19–38 minutes. Observations: opercular movement ceased 2.16–4.50 minutes into bath and resumed 0.63–2.98 minutes after placing in nonmedicated water. Heart rate was depressed. No mortality.	Hansen et al. (2003)
		7 mg/kg (concentration in a minced fish feed: cod liver oil emulsion delivered by gavage.	PO	Age 8 months, 228 g		Induction: 2.5–5 minutes. Recovery time 11–35 minutes. Observations: Induction based on loss of balance/motor control and inability to right self. Recovery considered complete when fish righted self. No mortalities.	
		3 mg/kg (50 mg/mL solution diluted with 0.9% NaCl to 3 mg/mL)	IV	Age 8 months, 228 g		No information on use, induction, or recovery, but good tissue distribution measured. No mortalities	

Order Salmoniformes
Family Salmonidae

Species	Agent	Dose	Route	Weight	Temp (°C)	Comments	Reference
Oncorhynchus kisutch (coho salmon)	Clove oil	25 mg/L	IN	5.47–12.72 kg		Induction: 2.5–3.5 minutes. Exposed for 10 minutes. Recovery: 7.5–13 minutes. No mortality.	Taylor and Roberts (1999)
	Ketamine	30 mg/kg	IV	1.857 ± 0.102 kg	15	Injected into dorsal aorta via cannula. Caused immediate cessation of ventilation for 10–300 seconds with loss of equilibrium. Ventilation rate recovered within 1–2 hours.	Graham and Iwama (1990)
	Alphaxalone-alphadolone (Saffon)	0.5–1.0 mL/kg	IM	2–3 kg		Sedation with partial loss of equilibrium. Able to be netted, but responsive.	Harvey et al. (1988)
Oncorhynchus nerka (sockeye salmon)	Clove oil	50 mg/L	IN	Adults	9–10	Fish could be handled within 3 minutes for measurement, esophageal implants, and fin clips. Recovery within 10 minutes following 15 minutes exposure.	Woody et al. (2002)
Oncorhynchus tshawytscha (Chinook salmon)	MS-222	100 mg/L with 300-mg/L NaHCO₃	IN	844–1562 g	12.5 ± 2.5	Resulted in light anesthesia. Recovery following 5 minutes exposure occurred within 5 minutes.	Rothwell et al. (2005)
	MS-222 buffered 1:1 with NaHCO₃	50 mg/L	IN	Juveniles 40.2 + 0.6 g		Provided deep anesthesia within 2 minutes.	Cho and Heath (2000)
	Benzocaine dissolved in ethanol at 1 g/30 mL	25–35 mg/L	IN	Juveniles 80 g	7–17	Induction: 1–3.25 minutes. Recovery following 15 minutes exposure: 2.25–18.5 minutes. Provided light to heavy sedation.	Gilderhus (1989)
	Clove oil in 1:10 ratio with 95% ethanol.	20 mg/L	IN	Juveniles 40.2 + 0.6 g		Provided deep anesthesia within 2 minutes.	Cho and Heath (2000)
	Isoeugenol (AQUI-S)	60 mg/L	IN	844–1562 g	12.5 ± 2.5	Sedation with partial loss of equilibrium. Suitable for handling.	Rothwell et al. (2005)
	Isoeugenol (AQUI-S)	120 mg/L	IN	844–1562 g	12.5 ± 2.5	Resulted in surgical anesthesia within 10 minutes for placement of vascular cannula. Recovery within 5–8 minutes.	Rothwell et al. (2005)
	Metomidate	42 mg/kg	IM	9 kg		Light sedation with partial loss of equilibrium. Directed net avoidance.	Harvey et al., (1988)
Oncorhynchus mykiss (rainbow trout)	Benzocaine	20 mg/L	IN	100–500 g	10	Provided adequate sedation within 30 seconds to permit weighing and injections.	Oswald (1978)
	Benzocaine dissolved in ethanol at 1 g/30 mL to make stock solution	25–40 mg/L; 30–45 mg/L	IN	Juveniles 2–500 g; Adults 0.68–2.04 kg	7–17	Induction: 1.25–5.5 minutes. Recovery following 15 minutes exposure: 4–16 minutes. Provided light to heavy sedation. Induction: 2.25–4.5 minutes. Recovery following 15 minutes exposure: 5.5–13.5 minutes. Provided light to heavy sedation.	Gilderhus (1989)

(Continued)

238

Table 15.1. (Continued)

Class Osteichthyes Taxa	Drug	Dose	Route	Wt/Age	Temp (°C)	Comments	Reference
	Clove oil dissolved in ethanol at a ratio of 1:10	2–5 mg/L 40–60 mg/L	IN IN	Age 6 months 20.46 ± 0.73 g	9.1 ± 0.2	Recommended for sedation suitable for 6–8 hours transport. Provided deep anesthesia following 3–6 minutes exposure.	Keene et al. (1998)
	Isoeugenol (AQUI-S)	20 mg/L 20 mg/L	IN IN	Juveniles–young adults 754 ± 145 g Fry fingerlings 4.1 ± 1.4 g	12 ± 2	Induction within 3 minutes. Total exposure time ≤15 minutes. Recovery within 8 minutes. Useful for basic handling procedures. pH = 8.1 Induction within 4.1 minutes or less. Total exposure time ≤15 minutes. Recovery within 5 minutes. Useful for basic handling procedures. pH = 8.1	Stehly and Gingerich (1999)
	Ketamine	50 mg/L	IM	100–500 g	10	Anesthesia generally within 5–10 minutes. Anesthesia persisted for 20 minutes at 130 mg/ and 50–80 minutes at 150 mg/kg. Apnea requiring assisted ventilation occurred in 30% fish. Recovery took up to 90 minutes and was characterized by excitement and ataxia.	Oswald (1978)
	Ketamine	30 mg/kg	IV	365 ± 26 g		Injected into dorsal aorta via cannula. Caused immediate cessation of ventilation for 10–300 seconds with loss of equilibrium. Ventilation rate recovered to preanesthesia values within 1–2 hours.	Graham and Iwama (1990)
	Medetomidine Atipamezole	5–20 mg/L 30–80 mg/L (6× medetomidine dose)	IN IN	300–400 g	10 ± 0.2	Exposure for 10 minutes. Considered to be a good sedative, but not anesthetic. Exposed to atipamezole for 7–10 minutes. Exposure to 80 mg/L atipamezole resulted in panic-like reactions.	Horsberg et al. (1999)
	Alphaxalone-alphadolone (Saffan)	130 and 150 mg/kg	ICe or ⅔ ICe + ⅓ IM	100–500 g	10	Induction within 5–10 minutes. Doses of 18 mg/kg produced anesthesia. Lower doses only produced sedation. Recovery generally complete within 2 hours. Doses >18 mg/kg associated with apnea and prolonged recoveries (3–6 hours).	Oswald (1978)
	MS-222 buffered 1:1 with NaHCO₃	50–100 mg/L	IN	Adult 0.6–2 kg		70–75 ppm provides excellent anesthesia for invasive procedures.	N. Mylniczenko, unpubl.
Salvelinus namaycush (lake trout)	Isoeugenol (AQUI-S)	50 mg/L 20–50 mg/L	IN IN	Adult Juveniles–young adult 167–1399 g	12 ± 2	Induction in 2.5–3.9 minutes. Total exposure time ≤15 minutes. Recovery within 8 minutes. Useful for basic handling procedures. pH = 8.1	Stehly and Gingerich (1999)
Salmo salar (Atlantic salmon)	Benzoak (20% benzocaine)	30–100 mg/L	IN	31–44 g	15	Provided sedation for 6 hours without loss of equilibrium at which time fish removed from anesthetic. Considered useful for transport. No mortality.	Hoskonen and Pirhonen (2004)

Species	Anesthetic agent	Route	Dose	Size/age	Temperature (°C)	Comments	Reference
	Clove oil dissolved in 95% ethanol at 1:10 ratio.	IN	5 mg/L	31–44 g	15	Provided sedation for 6 hours without loss of equilibrium at which time fish removed from anesthetic. No mortality. Considered useful for transport.	Hoskonen and Pirhonen (2004)
	Clove oil dissolved in 95% ethanol at 1:10 ratio.	IN	8 mg/L	1-year-old smolts 44.7 ± 12.8 g	5.4 ± 0.2	Anesthesia attained in 2.2–8.1 minutes. Exposure to 100 mg/L for >6 minutes may result in cessation of voluntary respiration.	Iversen et al. (2003)
	Clove oil dissolved in ethanol at 1:10 ratio.	IN	30–100 mg/L	1-year-old smolts 44.7 + 12.8 g	5.4 ± 0.2	Anesthesia attained in 2.2–8.1 minutes. Exposure to 100 mg/L for >6 minutes may result in cessation of voluntary respiration.	Iversen et al. (2003)
	Isoeugenol (AQUI-S)	IN	30–100 mg/L	1-year-old smolts 44.7 + 12.8 g	5.4 ± 0.2	Anesthesia attained in 2.2–6.2 minutes.	Iversen et al. (2003)
	Metomidate	IN	2–10 mg/L	1-year-old smolts 44.7 + 12.8 g	5.4 ± 0.2	Anesthesia attained in 3.0–17.4 minutes. Exposure to 100 mg/L for >6 minutes may result in cessation of voluntary respiration.	Iversen et al. (2003)
Salmo trutta (brown trout)	Clove oil dissolved in 95% ethanol at 1:10 ratio.	IN	8 mg/L	100–500 g	10	Provided adequate sedation within 30 seconds to permit weighing and injections.	Oswald (1978)
	Benzocaine	IN	50 mg/L	100–500 g	10	Induction generally in 5–10 minutes.	Oswald (1978)
	Ketamine	IM	130 and 150 mg/kg	100–500 g	10	Anesthesia persisted for 20 minutes at 130 mg/kg and 50–80 minutes at 150 mg/kg. Apnea requiring assisted ventilation occurred in 30% of fish. Recovery took up to 90 minutes and was characterized by excitement and ataxia.	Oswald (1978)
	Alphaxalone-alphadolone (Saffan)	ICe or 2/3 ICe + 1/3 IM	12–18 mg/kg	100–500 g	10	Induction within 5–10 minutes. Doses of 18 mg/kg produced anesthesia. Lower doses only produced sedation. Recovery generally complete within 2 hours. Doses >18 mg/kg associated with apnea and prolonged recoveries (3–6 hours).	Oswald (1978)
	Alphaxalone-alphadolone (Saffan)					Induction within 5–10 minutes. Doses of 18 mg/kg produced anesthesia. Lower doses only produced sedation. Recovery generally complete within 2 hours. Doses >18 mg/kg associated with apnea and prolonged recoveries (3–6 hours).	Oswald (1978)
Coregonus lavaretus (whitefish)	Clove oil dissolved in 95% ethanol at 1:10 ratio.	IN	3 mg/L	31–44 g	15	Provided sedation for 6 hours without loss of equilibrium at which time fish removed from anesthetic. Considered useful for transport. No mortality.	Hoskonen and Pirhonen (2004)

Order Scorpaeniformes
Family Anoplopomatidae

(Continued)

Table 15.1. (Continued)

Class Osteichthyes Taxa	Drug	Dose	Route	Wt/Age	Temp (°C)	Comments	Reference
Anoplopoma fimbria (sablefish)	Metomidate	62 mg/kg	IM	3 kg		Light sedation with partial loss of equilibrium. Directed net avoidance.	Harvey et al., (1988)
	Alphaxalone-alphadolone (Saffan)	0.3–0.4 mL/kg (need mg)	IM	3–5 kg		Light to heavy sedation with some fish exhibiting directed net avoidance. Recovery within 90 minutes.	Harvey et al., (1988)
Family Sebastidae							
Sebastes caurinus (copper rockfish)	Metomidate	100 mg/kg	IM	2 kg		Anesthesia with marked depression of ventilation. Recovery taking several hours.	Harvey et al., (1988)
	Gallamine triethiodide	1–4 mg/kg	IM	1–3 kg		Up to 2 hours until effect noted. Effect ranged from sedation (fish could be netted but were responsive) to anesthesia with marked depression of ventilation.	Harvey et al., (1988)
Sebastes sp.	MS-222	80–110 mg/L	IN			Good sedation for invasive procedures (ocular surgery)	N, Mylniczenko and T. Clauss, unpubl.
Family Scorpaenidae							
Pterois sp. (dwarf lionfish)	MS-222	75 mg/L	IN			Sedation rated as good. Diagnostic examinations performed.	D. Neiffer, unpubl.
Taenianotus triacanthus (leaf scorpionfish)	MS-222	50–90 mg/L	IN			Provided mild to good sedation. Diagnostic examination performed. $N = 3$.	D. Neiffer, unpubl.
Order Siluriformes							
Family Clariidae							
Clarias gariepinus North African catfish	Alphaxalone-alphadolone	24 mg/kg	IM	Average 1150 g	24	Preanesthetized by squirting a few mL of 2-PE on gills, which induced almost immediate immobility. Once alphaxalone-alphadolone is injected, the gills were rinsed with fresh water. Surgical anesthesia at 26 ± 8 minutes. Artificial respiration required by pumping gills. If the investigators assured that either the fish could reach the water surface from time to time during recovery or the fish were placed in shallow water (≤15 cm), the fish survived. If these precautions were not taken, mortality occurred.	Peters et al. (2001)
Family Ictaluridae							
Ictalurus furcatus (blue catfish)	MS-222	60–120 mg/L	IN			Low range good for minimally invasive procedures	T. Clauss, unpubl.
(*Ameiurus nebulosus*) (*Ictalurus nebulosus*) (brown bullhead catfish)	Alphaxalone-alphadolone	24 mg/kg	IM	56–255 g	18	Injection given just behind first dorsal fin. Induction: within minutes. Gradually lost balance and eventually ventilation ceased. Artificial respiration required by pumping water over gills at ~100 mL/min. Surgical anesthesia required on average 20 minutes. Time until recovery of opercular movements averaged 207 minutes.	Peters et al. (2001)

Species	Anesthetic	Dose	Route	Life stage/weight	Temperature (°C)	Comments	Reference
Ameiurus melas (*Ictualurus melas*) (black bullhead catfish)	Alphaxalone-alphadolone	24 mg/kg	IM		18	Injection given just behind first dorsal fin. Event very similar to brown bullhead above	Peters et al. (2001)
Ictalurus punctatus (Channel catfish)	MS-222	100 mg/L	IN	Adult 1.1 + 0.04 kg	14.5	Anesthesia: 4.5 ± 0.8 minutes. Fish immediately transferred to anesthetic free water with recovery time of 1.7 ± 0.2 minutes. Survival 100% at 24 hours. Dose considered useful for basic handling procedures.	Small and Chatakondi (2005)
	Clove oil	100–150 mg/L (no ethanol added directly to water and aerated strongly prior to addition of fish).	Inhalant	Fingerlings 19.12 ± 4.32 g	23	Induction: Within 1 minute. Recovery: Following 10 minutes exposure to 100mg/L, recovery occurred within 4 minutes. Recovery prolonged (>10 minutes) after exposure to 150mg/L. Exposure to 100mg/L for ≥20 minutes associated with increasing mortality. Exposure to 300mg/L for 10 minutes resulted in 50% mortality. pH = 7.6	Waterstrat (1999)
	Isoeugenol (AQUI-S)	2.5 mg/L	IN	Juveniles 62 ± 11.3 g	26	Sedation achieved in all fish. No mortality with exposure from 30 minutes to 24 hours. pH = 8.6	Small (2004)
	Isoeugenol (AQUI-S)	40–60 mg/L	IN	Adult 1.1 ± 0.04 kg	14.5	Time to anesthesia: 3.7–3.9 minutes. Fish immediately transferred to anesthetic free water with recovery time of 2.8–5.3 minutes. Survival 100% at 24 hours. Dose considered useful for basic handling procedures.	Small and Chatakondi (2005)
	Metomidate hydrochloride	6 mg/L	IN	Juvenile to adult 3–810 g	26	Induction: 0.46–2.31 minutes. Rapid recovery after 60 minutes exposure (2.01–2.52 minutes). Note: 65% mortality at 16mg/L. pH = 8.6.	Small (2003)
	Metomidate hydrochloride	1.5 mg/L	IN	Juveniles 62 ± 11.3 g	26	Sedation achieved in all fish. No mortality with exposure from 30 minutes to 24 hours. pH = 8.6.	Small (2004)
Family Pangasiidae *Pangasius* sp. (Pangasius catfish)	Isoeugenol (AQUI-S)	20 mg/L	IN	Juvenile-young adults 335 ± 92.0 g	12 ± 2	Induction in 5.3 minutes. Total exposure time ≤15 minutes. Recovery within 8 minutes. Useful for basic handling procedures. pH = 8.1.	Stehly and Gingerich (1999)
	Isoeugenol (AQUI-S)	20 mg/L	IN	Fry-fingerlings 1.3 + 0.16 g		Induction within 4.1 minutes or less. Total exposure time ≤15 minutes. Recovery within 5 minutes. Useful for basic handling procedures. pH = 8.1.	

(Continued)

Table 15.1. (Continued)

Class Osteichthyes Taxa	Drug	Dose	Route	Wt/Age	Temp (°C)	Comments	Reference
Family Siluridae							
Kryptopterus bicirrhis (Glass catfish)	Alphaxalone-alphadolone	4.8 mg/L for induction 2.4 mg/L for maintenance	IN	Check on age, but likely adults 2–7 g	23–27	Opercular movements disappeared after 5 minutes exposure at which time fish transferred to maintenance. Artificial respiration given by pumping water through mouth and across gills at 7–10 mL/min. Recovery in ~ 30 minutes after being placed in clean water.	Peters et al. (2001)
Order Tetraodontiformes							
Family Balistidae							
Canthidermis maculata (rough triggerfish)	MS-222	45–75 mg/L	IN			Provided mild to heavy sedation. Diagnostic examinations performed.	D. Neiffer, unpubl.
Family Diodontidae							
Diodon holocanthus (balloonfish)	MS-222	75–80 mg/L	IN	0.38–1.16 kg		Sedative effect rated fair to good. Diagnostic exams and topical treatments performed. $N = 5$.	D. Neiffer, unpubl.
	MS-222	100–125 mg/L	IN	0.38–0.42 kg		Provided surgical anesthesia for removal of fungal granulomas from integument and resection of coelomic musculature.	D. Neiffer unpubl.
Diodon hystrix (porcupinefish)	MS-222	75–80 mg/L	IN			Mild to moderate sedation. Diagnostic examinations performed. $N = 2$.	D. Neiffer, unpubl.
Family Monocanthidae							
Aluterus scriptus (scrawled filefish)	MS-222	50–60 mg/L, 75–100 mg/L	IN	0.44–2.35 kg		Sedation rated as good to excellent. Diagnostic examinations performed. Heavy sedation with cessation of gilling	D. Neiffer, unpubl.
Meuschenia trachylepis (filefish)	Clove oil in ethanol at ratio 1:5	40 mg/L	IN		18	Induction within 3 minutes. Recovery within 5 minutes. Sufficient for handling and measurement.	Griffiths (2000)
Monacanthus tuckeri (slender filefish)	MS-222	50 mg/L	IN			Provided mild sedation. Diagnostic examination performed	D. Neiffer, unpubl.
Family Tetraodontidae							
Arothron nigropunctatus (dogface puffer)	MS-222	70–75 mg/L	IN			Provided mild to heavy sedation. Diagnostic examinations performed. $N = 3$.	D. Neiffer, unpubl.
	MS-222	100 mg/L	IN	360 g		Provided surgical anesthesia for removal of skin lesion.	D. Neiffer, unpubl.
Sphoeroides testudineus (checkered puffer)	MS-222	70–100 mg/L	IN	280–330 g		Variable effect from mild sedation to light anesthesia. Examinations and topical laser surgeries performed. $N = 6$.	D. Neiffer, unpubl.

Notes: Where possible, the most recently accepted scientific name is used. Anesthesia was not the focus of some articles, with only limited information provided.
[a]IM, intramuscular; IN, inhalant/immersion; PO, orally; IV, intravenous; ICe, intracoelomic; 2-PE, 2-phenoxyethanol; MS-222, tricaine methanesulfonate.

authors' experience that with multiple animals, there is degradation of water quality and inductions are longer, but this is highly variable based on the number of fish and the volume of water used.

Immersion drugs must be water soluble or utilize a water-soluble solvent as a vehicle. For simple, short procedures, the required drug concentration is made up in an aerated container to which fish are transferred or drugs are added directly to the water containing the fish. In the latter situation, a buffer (e.g., sodium bicarbonate) is added. It is always preferable to use water from the fish's tank or pond to make the anesthetic solution prior to drug administration to minimize acute drops in pH (Harms 1999; Ross 2001). Ideally, spontaneous ventilation is maintained during short procedures.

For large fish, where immersion is impractical or dangerous to handlers, drugs may be applied directly to the gills. Inexpensive plastic pump spray bottles (e.g., unused bug sprayers) are ideal for this application (Fig. 15.7). When used by divers, the addition of a harmless dye (e.g., food coloring) helps identify distribution of the anesthetic.

Regardless of application, anesthetic solutions are most accurately made using a measured volume of a standard stock solution. However, preparing stock solutions of expensive powdered anesthetic drugs (e.g., MS-222) is uneconomical if used infrequently because potency decreases over time (Ross 2001). Alternatively, preweighed drug packets are recommended. Waterproof quick reference charts and known volume containers are useful for procedure set up. More importantly, they enable quick modification of drug dosage level.

Ventilation, even in animals that are apparently ventilating on their own, is an important tool to perform. It is akin to providing oxygen to mammals sedated with injectables. Simply, a syringe and plastic tubing can be utilized with care to ventilate each side of the animal's gills. With longer procedures (>10 minutes), debilitated fish, species that are slow to recover, and all but the shortest out-of-water proce-

dures, an artificial ventilation system can be used (Fig. 15.8). The animal is held in shallow water or placed on a fenestrated surface in lateral recumbency or in dorsal recumbency in a soft holder (foam, soft cloth, and sponge).

Aerated anesthetic solution is delivered across the gills from a bifurcated pipe or mouthpiece placed in the buccal cavity (Fig. 15.9). Nonrecirculating or recirculating systems can be used. In its simplest form, a nonrecirculating system uses an IV fluid bag and drip set. Resealable bags are easier for preparation, but used sealed bags with an opening cut in the end suffice. Flow rate is controlled by the drip set valve. Aeration of the anesthetic water with an air stone in the IV bag ensures

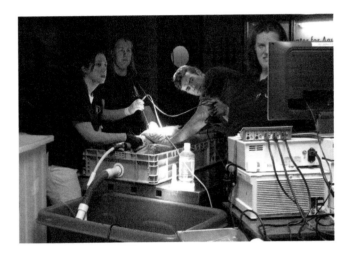

Figure 15.8. A simple recirculating system that enables delivery of anesthetic water from a reservoir to the gills and recycling of the effluent back to the fish by use of submersible pump.

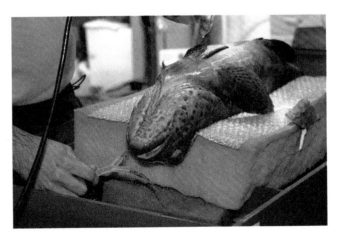

Figure 15.9. A goliath grouper (*Epinephelus itajara*) positioned in dorsal recumbency in a foam holder during anesthesia with MS-222. Note the bifurcated mouthpiece being placed in the buccal cavity for delivery of oxygenated anesthetic water to both sets of gill arches, normograde.

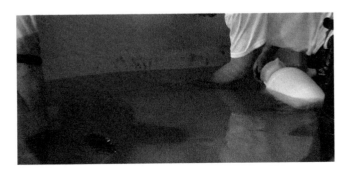

Figure 15.7. A large grouper (*Epinephalus* sp.) being anesthetized using a pump sprayer to deliver concentrated MS-222 into the oral cavity of the animal.

near-saturation of oxygen and removal of dissolved CO_2. Used water is collected, but not recycled (Harms 1999; Ross 2001; Stetter 2001). This system is suitable for small- to medium-sized fish depending on reservoir volume, drip set tube diameter, and the rate at which fluid can be delivered.

Recirculating systems enable delivery of anesthetic water from a reservoir to the gills and recycling of the effluent back to the fish. This recycling is either done manually (refill elevated reservoir with collected effluent) or with a submersible pump. When using pumps electrical safety for the operator must be considered. Flow rate can be controlled by a valve on the tube leading to the mouth. Minimum effective flow rate during fish anesthesia has not been determined; 1–3 L/min/kg are recommended. Low delivery rates fail to keep the gills on both sides wet, reducing gas exchange. High flow rates can result in alimentary anesthetic delivery and gastric dilatation, which may also occur due to depth of anesthesia and low sphincter tone. Both scenarios can be alleviated with the use of a "Y" or "T" plastic piece that equally distributes water over both gill arches. Oxygenation of the water should be provided. Recirculating systems are used in large fish where cost and waste water concerns make conservation of anesthetics and water paramount (Harms 1999; Ross 2001; Stetter 2001).

Regardless of method used, adjusting the delivered drug concentration in response to anesthetic depth is difficult. One option is to prepare measured volumes of anesthetic-free water and concentrations of anesthetic solution. These solutions are placed in separate bags or reservoirs and used in either recirculating or nonrecirculating systems. Alternatively, a syringe or turkey baster is used to rapidly deliver small amounts of fluid directly to the gills without disconnecting the fish from the system (Harms 1999).

The flow is usually normograde to achieve optimal gas and anesthetic exchange. During oral surgery, flow is reversed, if necessary, for surgical access. However, retrograde flow nullifies the normal countercurrent exchange mechanism and may damage the gills. The size or anatomy of some fish (e.g., filefish [Monocanthidae], triggers [Balistidae], or eels [Muraenidae]) (Fig. 15.10) make placement of a bifurcated buccal tube difficult. In these species, some retrograde flow is used to ensure all gill tissue is adequately perfused.

In some circumstances, whole tank anesthesia is required to move fishes out of their systems. When this occurs, sufficient supportive staff for induction, transport, and recovery will be necessary. Using lower doses that tranquilize the animals enough for safely moving into transports would be sensible versus full sedation, but this will be species specific as well as animal specific (individual temperament, disease state, and size). This method has shown to result in the least amount of stress when compared with capturing animals out of

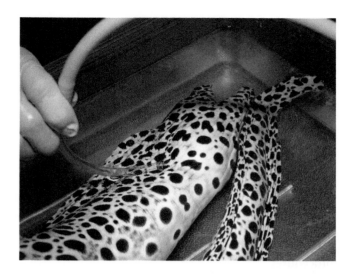

Figure 15.10.   Laced moray eel (*Gymnothorax favagineus*) receiving retrograde ventilation in preparation for an oral surgery.

the tank and transferring to an induction tank (Caamano Tubio et al. 2010).

Parenteral Anesthesia

In addition to inhalation, anesthetics are delivered orally, intravenously (IV), intramuscularly (IM), and intracoelomically (ICe). Oral administration is rarely used because precise dosing is difficult and the rate and degree of absorption is uncertain (Harms 2003). However, a few examples of successful oral drug use exist (Hansen et al. 2003; Harms & Bakal 1995; Harvey et al. 1988; Raines & Clancy 2009; Steers & Sherrill 2001). Intravenous injection is the fastest delivery method, with rapid induction and usually short duration of effect. However, this route has limited clinical use because it requires either manual restraint or prior administration of drugs by another route to allow IV access (Fleming et al. 2003; Hansen et al. 2003).

Intramuscular is the most common parenteral route. The major challenge with this route is that muscle is comprised of both red and white muscle with the white muscle taking up a majority of the muscle mass. In comparison with white muscle, the red muscle is aerobic and most likely the ideal set of muscles for appropriate metabolism and pharmacokinetics. However, because of location and low percentage of muscle mass, it is unlikely that an injection will be in the correct location, particularly if it needs to be administered quickly. Additionally, not all fish have both types of muscle, instead being composed of completely white muscle. ICe has an increased risk of visceral damage, and drugs must pass through the serosal surface, making induction time erratic. Both IM and

ICe routes are used in larger fish because many are kept in large volume aquariums or pens where adding waterborne anesthetics is impractical and because injection site trauma is less problematic in larger specimens (Harms 1999; Harvey et al. 1988; Williams et al. 1988). Injected fish will stop swimming and begin to drop through the water column with or without obvious gilling. However, when approached by divers with a net, they will often arouse and swim with directed movement. The diver retreats and allows the drugs more time to act and/or supplemental drug injections are made. Regardless of ease of capture, parenteral anesthetics are unpredictable and often do not provide adequate sedation or anesthesia, thus requiring supplemental inhalation anesthesia. Hypoxemia during the induction is a concern as ventilatory ability is compromised. Additionally, ventilatory support is necessary during maintenance of parenteral immobilization drugs, and particularly during recovery if prolonged (Harms 1999).

Injections are made by hand syringe, pole syringe (or modified pole syringe [Fig. 15.11]), or a darting system.

Examples of darting systems include a modified Hawaiian sling (Fig. 15.12), pneumatic spear guns, and a laser-aimed underwater gun (Harms 1999; Harvey et al. 1988; Williams et al. 1988).

The latter propels darts from a distance of 1- to 2-m (4–7 ft) that inject pneumatically upon impact and remain attached after jettisoning the lightweight spear shaft. The Hawaiian sling and pneumatic spear guns should be used with caution and are usually used for euthanasia as they are very powerful and it is hard to control the force of the impact on the animal. Both barbless and barbed needles are used for large active and heavily scaled or sluggish fish, respectively (Harvey et al. 1988). A complication of dart use is injection site trauma and scale loss, with some fish requiring local or systemic wound treatment. Intramuscular injections will often result in leakage of some injected drug as the needle falls out or is withdrawn and the surrounding muscles contract (Harms & Bakal 1995; Peters et al. 2001). Consideration to injection volume is important as fish cannot retain much fluid due to muscle inelasticity. A final thought is that when divers are underwater, there is refraction between the divers mask and the water, thus affecting the aim.

If the fish is in hand for injection, the needle is placed directly on dorsal midline between epaxial muscles, and then laterally inserted into a muscle bundle to reduce drug loss (Harms & Bakal 1995). Filtered food dye can be added to the contents of the syringe, so injection success can be judged. Alternatively, fluoroscein stain or methylene blue dye is used (Harvey et al. 1988).

A first consideration when using parenteral anesthetics is human safety. The large dosages and drug volumes required make accidental injection a possibility for handlers (Harvey et al. 1988). The authors recommend reference to drug exposure protocols for hoofstock when using large enough doses that may adversely affect the handler.

MONITORING

Anesthetic Depth

Various schemes are used to describe anesthetic depth in fish with no consensus (Detar & Mattingly 2004; Myszkowski et al. 2003; Oikawa et al. 1994). This makes comparison of regimens between and within species difficult when reviewing the literature. Common criteria used in defining anesthetic depth or level include

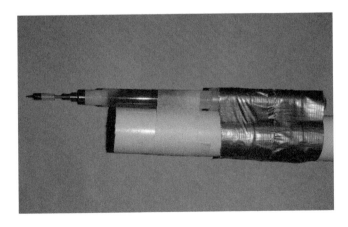

Figure 15.11. Modified pole syringe system: a commercially available spring-loaded syringe capable of injecting 5 cc of solution is loaded and charge. The dart setup is backed into a syringe case taped to a PVC pipe, and the dart is taped with paper tape that can easily fall off when the animal is injected. Filtered food dye has been added to the contents of the syringe so injection success can be judged.

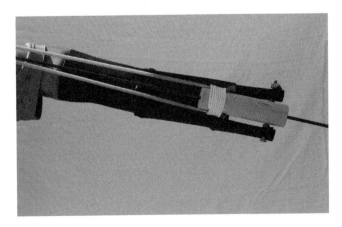

Figure 15.12. An example of a Hawaiian sling. It is recommended that this only be used for long distances with skilled users or for euthanasia purposes due the power of the propulsion of the tip.

activity, reactivity to stimuli, equilibrium (righting reflex), muscle tone, and respiratory and heart rates. Broad stages include sedation, narcosis or loss or equilibrium, and anesthesia; each stage is further subdivided further into light and deep planes (Harms 2003; Stetter 2001). Depending on the species, drug, and dosage used, some stage components are unrecognized (Harms 1999; Stetter 2001). Conversely, some signs attributed to drug effect are instead responses to stress. For example, Gulf of Mexico sturgeon (*Acipenser oxyrinchus de soti*) often turns into a ventral/dorsal position when stressed (Fleming et al. 2003). Therefore, loss of the righting reflex is not used to determine anesthetic stage in this species.

For most fish, induction occurs in 5–10 minutes with immersion drugs, but can be prolonged using other routes. During induction swimming, respiratory rate and reaction to stimuli decreases. As the fish becomes anesthetized, there is loss of equilibrium and response to stimuli. At a surgical anesthetic plane, there is total loss of muscle tone and a further decrease, but not cessation, in respiratory rate. A firm squeeze at the base of the tail or insertion of a needle into the peduncle is used to determine response to stimuli; if the animal does not respond, general anesthesia has been achieved (Harms 2003; Stetter 2001; Storms & Mylniczenko 2004). Some species go through excitement during immersion induction and may traumatize themselves (Harms 1999; Stetter 2001).

Cardiopulmonary

Respiratory and cardiac rate changes are useful in assessing anesthetic depth. Both usually decrease with increased anesthetic dosage and anesthetic time. Respiratory rates are determined in the perianesthetic period by observing opercular movement (Harms 1999, 2003; Stetter 2001). However, in some species (e.g., scombrids), opecular movement is minimal to nonexistent, and potentially nondetectable in some species due to anatomy (frogfish, cowfish, etc). Additionally, passage of oxygenated water over the gills of any anesthetized fish with ceased opercular movement will maintain adequate ventilation, at least in the short term. This is accomplished because of the large differential between respiratory and cardiac arrest. The heart will still supply fresh arterial blood to the gills, allowing for adequate gas exchange.

In species with thin pliable body walls and proportionally large hearts, heart beats are observed directly, but for most, it is neither visible nor palpable (Harms 1999; Harms & Bakal 1995). In these species, heart rate is monitored using cardiac ultrasonography, Doppler flow probes, or electrocardiography (Harms 1999; Harms & Bakal 1995; Ross 2001). During cardiac ultrasonography, the probe is placed into the opercular slit of medium to large fish, or directly over the heart in smaller or small scaled/scaleless species (Fig. 15.13).

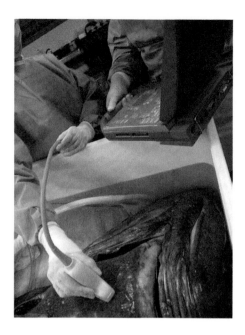

Figure 15.13. Ultrasonography is a useful tool for monitoring heart rate in fish. In specimens of sufficient size, the probe can be placed into the opercular slit as in this goliath grouper (*Epinephelus itajara*). Alternatively, the probe is placed directly over the heart in smaller specimens or small-scaled/scaleless species.

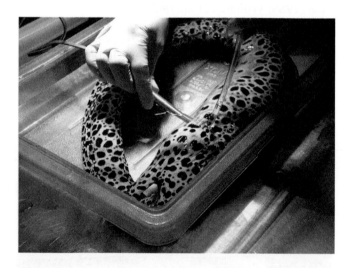

Figure 15.14. Doppler flow is also used for monitoring heart rate in fish with probes placed as described for ultrasonography. This figure demonstrates placement of the probe onto the area of the heart in a laced moray eel (*Gymnothorax favagineus*).

Doppler probes are placed in the same locations (Fig. 15.14). Regarding electrocardiogram, electrodes can be clamped lightly to the surface of the fins, with the pectoral and anal fins being a good combination (Ross 2001). Subcutaneous placement of needle electrodes minimizes skin trauma, reduces the chance of grounding out the ECG signal by contact with a wet external surface, and improves signal quality (Harms 1999). In

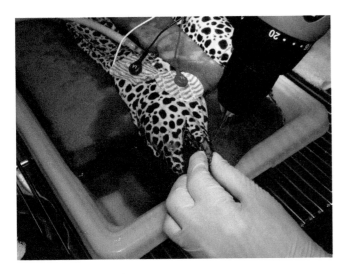

Figure 15.15. While not always practical, is it possible to monitor the ECG of fish, as with this laced moray eel (*Gymnothorax favagineus*). Note the retrograde placement of a ventilation tube in the opercular slit.

some species, use of human electrodes may work as well (Fig. 15.15). Pulse oximetry is not effective for measuring hemoglobin saturation in fish (Harms 1999; Ross 2001).

If the animal is stable, respiratory and heart rates are measured and recorded every 2–5 minutes. It is important to focus on trends because normal rates are not known for most species. Additionally assessing quality of the rhythm and if using ultrasound, contractility can be helpful, particularly if a baseline has been observed. Anesthetized fish generally have slower heart rates than terrestrial animals of similar size (Stetter 2001).

Other variables that are visually or palpably monitored include equilibrium, jaw tone, color of fin margin (pallor = hypoxemia, hypotension, or peripheral vasoconstriction), response to touch or surgical stimuli, and gill color (pallor = hypoxemia, hypotension, hypovolemia, or asystole) (Harms & Bakal 1995; Stetter 2001). Because of the relative low blood pressure of fishes, blood pooling can occur normally and occur in the dependent portions of the body, particularly when animals are not in the water where hydrostatic forces keep this pooling from occurring (Sandblom & Axelsson 2007).

An effective way to monitor respiratory efficiency is periodic blood gas sampling to determine oxygenation, carbon dioxide, and pH. Venous samples are easier to collect, and useful information about physiological trends is obtained. Other blood variables used to assess metabolic status include HCT, glucose, and lactate. Lactate is a critical metabolite that has been instrumental in evaluating fish responses to hypoxia and exertion (Heming 1989; McDonald & Milligan 1992). There is species variation in tolerance of both hypoxia and exertion that must be taken in account; regardless, changes in blood gas values indicate an unstable anesthetic event. Small size or debilitation may preclude collection of even a single sample from some individuals.

Water Quality

After cardiorespiratory function, water quality monitoring is critical to reducing anesthetic morbidity and mortality. Assuming aeration, DO, and temperature are appropriate and constant, ammonia concentration is of greatest concern. Ammonia concentrations will rise, and buffering capacity will decrease during prolonged procedures and when multiple fish are sequentially anesthetized in the same system. More alkaline water, as in marine systems, enhances ammonia toxicity. Ammonia concentrations are easy to measure with tank side kits. Alternatively, the handler uses other indicators of deteriorating water quality (e.g., surface foam formation due to increased protein from fish slime) (Harms 1999). Some species (e.g., Gulf toadfish, *Opsanus beta*) are facultatively ureotelic and ureogenic. In contrast to most teleosts that are obligate ammonioteles, the toadfish switches to ureotelism in response to moderate stressors (e.g., anesthesia), excreting the majority of its nitrogenous waste as urea (Gilmour et al. 1998). Consequently, ammonia level measurement as a guide to water quality is inaccurate for this and similar species.

Declining water quality during anesthesia is corrected with a partial water change. The handler either adds water containing a known anesthetic concentration or, when reducing anesthetic depth, a known volume of clean water to the system.

RECOVERY

Recovery from immersion anesthesia begins when the fish is placed in drug-free water (Ross 2001). Even when using oral or parenteral drugs, moving to clean water is important, as some of these drugs and their metabolites may be excreted into the water and be reabsorbed across the gills and/or skin. The recovery water is aerated, with the fish's mouth oriented toward water flow. In an artificial ventilaton system, clean drug-free water is passed over the gills until spontaneous ventilation returns. Alternatively, if the fish is not spontaneously ventilating, it is pulled forward through the water with its mouth open; however, assisted ventilation is preferred. Dragging the animal backwards through water may cause gill damage and should be avoided. Most fish fully recover within 5–15 minutes from immersion anesthetics, but this number can be highly variable. Recoveries extending >10 minutes indicate either excessive anesthetic dosage or a medically compromised animal (Ross 2001; Stetter 2001). In comparison, recovery from oral and parenteral agents is often greater. The time is dependent on route, rate of drug metabolism, and if a reversal agent is used. As the fish recovers, respirations increase, muscle tone returns, fin movements start, and the fish swims with progressively less ataxia until full equilibrium is regained. Some fish go through an erratic porpoising phase and are prevented from escaping from tank (Harms 1999). Certain individuals may need to be manually restrained during this period to prevent damage to eyes and body.

RESUSCITATION

Marked hypoventilation or apnea is usually not alarming. If cardiac output is maintained and oxygenated water is flowing appropriately over the gills, tissue gas exchange is probably adequate. Decreasing the anesthetic concentration or moving the fish to anesthetic-free water until respirations resume (Stetter 2001) are recommended. If involved in a major procedure (e.g., exploratory coeliotomy), the latter is not advisable. In either scenario, the anesthetist takes advantage of the "buccal flow/heart rate" reflex; increasing water flow through the buccal cavity accelerates heart rate. The subsequent increase in gill blood flow more rapidly eliminates immersion drugs and hastens recovery. However, too rapid a flow may not allow adequate exchange, thus a balance much be achieved. Unresponsive fish are given standard mammalian emergency drugs, such as doxapram, corticosteroids, and fluids. The authors' have observed positive response to doxapram administration (5 mg/kg IV, IM [or both at the same time], ICe or even over the gills) in several cases of erratic respirations or respiratory arrest. Controversy over the use of epinephrine versus norepinephrine in fish exists and is an area in need of further investigation. At this time, epinephrine appears to be an effective drug for critical situations.

ANESTHETIC DRUGS

General Comments

Of the definitions of "anesthesia," the following is perhaps more acceptable given the controversy regarding pain perception in fish: "Anesthesia is a biological state induced by an external agent which results in the partial or complete loss of sensation or loss of voluntary neuromotor control through chemical or non-chemical means" (Bressler & Ron 2004).

Rather than listing a few cross taxa dosage recommendations for several commonly used drugs, the authors have taxonomically arranged cited and anecdotal dosages for representative species from most orders (Table 15.1). Some extrapolation is always necessary, but the more species-based data one can refer to, the more accurate the educated guess.

Inhalant (Waterborne or Immersion) Drugs

Tricaine Methanesulfonate (MS-222) Tricaine methansulfonate (MS-222) is a benzocaine derivative with a sulfonate radical, which accounts for its water solubility and increased acidity over the parent compound (Harms 1999; Oikawa et al. 1994). It is absorbed across the gill epithelium (±skin) and biotransformed in liver and probably kidney. It is cleared primarily through the gills as free and acetylated forms, with additional metabolites eliminated in urine and bile (Harms 1999). Tricaine powder is directly mixed into the anesthetic chamber or administered as a stock solution of 10 g/L (10,000 mg/L). The latter is unstable in light and is kept in a dark container. Oily residues in buffered stock solutions indicate the presence of a desulfonation product and decreased potency.

MS-222 is acidic and is more effective and safe in its neutralized form. Solutions are buffered to the pH of the holding water before immersing the fish. Although sodium bicarbonate is primarily used, other buffers include imidazole, sodium hydrogen phosphate, sodium hydroxide, and calcium carbonate. Exact amounts are measured out or the powdered buffer is incrementally mixed into the anesthesia chamber until the solid no longer dissolves and saturation is reached (Harms 1999; Oikawa et al. 1994; Roubach et al. 2001; Stetter 2001).

There has been some dispute in the literature regarding the susceptibility of some sturgeon subspecies to MS-222, suggesting they are refractory to standard doses of MS-222 (Fleming et al. 2003); however, other groups have used MS-222 with no resistance at typical inductive doses (Hernandez-Divers et al. 2004; Feng et al. 2011; Matsche 2011). The reasons for this discrepancy can include subspecies variations and environmental parameters (e.g., temperature), which may affect metabolism. In one study of sturgeon anesthesia, it was found that when compared with medetomidine/ketamine and even clove oil, MS-222 resulted in much higher negative physiologic effects (Di Marco et al. 2011).

The margin of safety is narrower with young fish in warm, soft water, and there is species variation (Harms 1999; Roubach et al. 2001). In all age groups, MS-222 can be associated with hypoxemia resulting from drug-induced hypoventilation (Davis & Griffin 2004; Harms & Bakal 1995; Oikawa et al. 1994). MS-222 is a suspected carcinogen (Detar & Mattingly 2004) and in humans may cause reversible retinal deficits (Bernstein et al. 1997). A chronically exposed ichthyologist developed decreased vision, photophobia, and photopsia that resolved after terminating MS-222 contact for 7 months (Bernstein et al. 1997). While this article suggests that fish can have similar effects, a recent paper showed that koi carp exposed for 13 days to clinically relevant concentrations of MS-222 showed no changes in retinal structure or function (Bailey et al. 2013). Personnel with regular occupational exposure should wear gloves to prevent systemic absorption of this retinotoxic drug.

MS-222 is the only FDA-approved anesthetic for fish and, consequently, is widely used in United States aquaculture. However, there is a 21-day withdrawal period prior to human consumption or release to the wild. This makes its use impractical or incompatible with some farming operations and field work (Detar & Mattingly 2004; Sladky et al. 2001; Waterstrat 1999).

Benzocaine Benzocaine, the parent compound to MS-222, is similar in pharmacology, but is much less water soluble. Consequently, a stock solution in ethanol or acetone (100 g in 1 L) or propylene glycol is prepared prior to its use. The stock solution is kept in a dark bottle and held at room temperature (Harms & Bakal 1995; Iversen et al. 2003) Its relative insolubility may account for its usefulness in species sensitive to MS-222. For example, striped bass (*Morone saxatilis*) are very sensitive to MS-222, but are effectively anesthetized in benzocaine solutions (55–80 mg/L) (Hseu et al. 1998).

Other advantages include low toxicity to humans at the concentrations used, and it can be removed from aquaculture facility effluents using activated carbon filtration. Even if not filtered, breakdown in water is approximately 4 hours, making it less likely to cause environmental contamination. Exposure also does not impair fish growth or reproductive capacity (Gomes et al. 2001; Hseu et al. 1998).

Efficacy and sensitivity to benzocaine is species and dosage related (Gomes et al. 2001; Heo & Shin 2010) and it can stimulate the stress response as discussed previously. The only other major concern is its fat solubility, which may result in prolonged recovery in older and gravid fish (Iversen et al. 2003). It is one of the few drugs shown to be effective for safe anesthesia of arapaima (Honczaryk & Inoue 2010). A recent paper in Crucian carp noted it to be a safe rapid agent with low increases in stress biomarkers (glucose and cortisol) (Heo & Shin 2010). In Atlantic cod, induction and recovery times were found to increase with increasing body weight. Additionally, it was found that recovery times were longer with benzocaine versus MS-222, even at half the dose of MS-222. In combination with metomidate though, induction times did decrease (but not as much as medetomidiate and MS-222) (Zahl et al. 2009).

Clove Oil, Eugenol, Isoeugenol, and AQUI-S Clove oil is a mixture of compounds, of which the phenolic eugenol comprises 85–95%. Isoeugenol and methyleugenol make up the remaining 5–15% of active ingredients. Commercially available clove oil has approximately 84% eugenol, but it is possible to purchase 100%, even at local natural product stores. Clove oil and isoeugenol are "generally recognized as safe" (GRAS) by the FDA as a food additive for humans. Eugenol is similarly approved for use in animal feeds and is used in dental cement for temporary fillings. (Harper 2003). AQUI-S contains primarily isoeugenol (Iversen et al. 2003; Kildea et al. 2004). Clove oil and/or AQUI-S are approved as legal anesthetics with no withdrawal period in Australia, Chile, Finland, New Zealand, and the Faroe Islands(Hoskonen & Pirhonen 2004), but neither clove oil, any component of clove oil, nor AQUI-S is approved for use as a fish anesthetic in the United States (Bressler & Ron 2004; Davis & Griffin 2004; Harper 2003; Stetter 2001). AQUI-S was under review as a possible approved drug for zero withholding days (Young 2009), but due to carcinogenic effects in mice, has been now strictly prohibited (http://www.fws.gov/fisheries/aadap/aquis.htm, accessed 5/7/2014). However, AQUI-S 20E is available in the United States under the Investigational New Animal Drug (INAD) program (Aquatactics Fish Health, Kirkland, WA).

Clove oil and eugenol are incompletely water soluble, particularly at cold temperatures. A 1 : 10 mixture of either in 95% ethanol yields a 100-mg/mL stock solution. Final concentrations of 40–120 mg/L are used for most species (the contribution of ethanol to the anesthetic effect is nil at these concentrations) (Harms 2003).

In addition to use in aquaculture, research, and aquaria, clove oil is regularly employed in marine field studies for sampling tide pool and tropical reef fish assemblages (Ackerman & Bellwood 2002; Griffiths 2000; Marnane 2000). For tide pools, the volume is estimated, and the drug is administered as in an anesthetic chamber. For reef surveys, a section is covered with mesh net covered in turn by a nylon cloak. A solution of clove oil mixed with ethanol is then pumped into the netted area to temporarily immobilize all fish (as a reminder, clove is not a U.S. approved drug). Rotenone, an effective and nonselective ichthyocide, has historically been utilized for this purpose, but is more controversial given increasing conservation and environmental concerns (Ackerman & Bellwood 2002). This application of clove oil may be of use in captive exhibits that often have elaborate rock or coral work, making removal of fish for medical or maintenance reasons difficult.

Compared with other immersion anesthetics, clove oil results in more rapid induction times and consistent anesthesia (Bressler & Ron 2004; Detar & Mattingly 2004; Sladky et al. 2001). However, isoeugenol (AQUI-S) is considered more effective (Ross 2001). Although clove oil recoveries are also consistent, they are longer compared with other drugs (e.g., MS-222) (Detar & Mattingly 2004; Sladky et al. 2001). Other claimed advantages include efficacy at a range of water temperatures, availability, lower expense, and handler safety (Bressler & Ron 2004; Detar & Mattingly 2004; Gladden et al. 2010). As mentioned previously, the effect of clove oil and its components on the stress response is variable with suppression in some cases and activation in others. Unlike metomidate, the mechanism of action remains unknown (Small & Chatakondi 2005).

Although increased safety compared with other immersion drugs has been claimed (Detar & Mattingly 2004), a narrow safety margin compared with MS-222 has been reported. In red pacu, most fish exposed to eugenol (100 mg/L) required resuscitation, and the risk of ventilatory failure increased with increasing dosages (Sladky et al. 2001). An explanation for ventilatory failure and medullary collapse in some fish is a neuro-toxic or hepatotoxic effect similar to those described in mammals (Sladky et al. 2001). On the note of low safety margin, in a study on *Astyanax altiparanae*, concentrations of 50–150 mg/L were assessed, with the 50 mg/L concentration deemed as the most efficacious and safe for deep anesthesia with rapid inductions (1.5 minutes) but with mortalities of >80% at 75 mg/L (Pereira da Silva et al. 2009). Alternatively, it may be a function of the physical properties of eugenol oil or increased duration of exposure. As an oil, eugenol coats anatomic structures and its persistence on gill epithelia may block gaseous diffusion (Sladky et al. 2001). In addition, mild gill necrosis due to repeated exposure to low dose eugenol (9 mg/L) has been reported (Afifi et al. 2001). Along with safety concerns, some fish are very sensitive to small increases in concentration, acutely losing equilibrium. This is a problem when controlling concentrations in large tanks, and clove oil and its components may not be suitable as transport drugs in sensitive species (Hoskonen & Pirhonen 2004).

Clove oil at 18–20 uL/L has also been used for long-term transports (up to 48 hours) in *Haplochromis obliquidens*, with some mortalities at the higher end range (reiterating the narrow safety margin); additionally, ammonia levels were higher in those containers with anesthetized fish (Kaiser et al. 2006). In beluga, *Huso huso*, that were exposed to clove oil at doses of 500–3000 mg/L, it was noted that cortisol, glucose, and lactate levels were lower, at the higher dosages with faster inductions (Hoseini et al. 2010). In the authors' experience, this tends to be true with many anesthetics.

A more novel approach has been to utilize clove powder mixed in water rather than oil. In sturgeon, the powder has been used in juvenile great sturgeon from 175 to 350 mg/L, with negative side effects being limited to increases in hematocrit, hemoglobin, and total erythrocyte count, but with a return to normal within 24 hours (Mohammadizarejabad et al. 2010).

Although the analgesic effects of eugenol in humans result from the inhibition of prostaglandin H synthase (Keene et al. 1998), proof of analgesia in fish does not exist (Sladky et al. 2001). In red pacu, fish anesthetized with eugenol were more likely to react to a hypodermic needle puncture than fish anesthetized with tricaine methanesulfonate, raising the question of appropriateness of clove oil or related compounds for invasive or markedly noxious procedures.

In a recent examination of AQUI-S in small freshwater *Melanoteania australis*, 80 mg/L was most efficacious with rapid induction times (lower doses resulted in long inductions and recoveries), but mortality rates increased after exposure times of >15 minutes. This concentration is higher than those used for other freshwater fish, which usually use 20–60 mg/L, but these fish were all coldwater animals (Young 2009). In koi carp, isoeugenol was used at 20, 40, 80, and at 500 mg/L, noting that mortalities occurred only at the high range, and even in those animals, no pathology was observed (Gladden et al. 2010).

Metomidate   Metomidate is a nonbarbiturate imidazole. Available in Canada under the trade name Marinil, it is not licensed in the United States, but is available for investigational use (Harms 1999). It is readily water soluble and is stored in tight light protected containers. In addition to inhalation, the drug can be given orally (Hansen et al. 2003; Harvey et al. 1988).

Metomidate suppresses cortisol response to anesthesia. It blocks adrenocorticotropic hormone stimulation of steroidogenesis, even when exogenous ACTH is injected intracoelomically. This occurs by a direct effect on the interrenal gland and the mitochondrial cytochrome P_{450}-dependent enzymes that catalyze the synthesis of cortisol (Davis and Griffin 2004; Iversen et al. 2003; Small & Chatakondi 2005). Cortisol synthesis blockade may cause the anesthetized fish to transiently turn very dark. This may be due to reduced cortisol production terminating the negative feedback loop on ACTH synthesis. As ACTH synthesis is linked to melanocyte stimulating hormone production, both compounds increase with the associated color change occurring (Harms 1999; Harms & Bakal 1995).

In addition to sedation and anesthesia for minor procedures, metomidate is useful for limiting transport trauma. Fish transported while immobilized are damaged by contact with the container sides and bottom. Metomidate dosages that suppress the cortisol stress response still allow maintenance of equilibrium (Davis & Griffin 2004; Harms 1999; Kilgore et al. 2009).

Metomidate is a hypnotic, inducing sleep rather than general anesthesia. This is reflected in maintenance of opercular respiration for twice as long at the effective concentration as other immersions (Mattson & Riple 1989). Additionally, muscle fasciculations occur at low dosages, indicating incomplete relaxation (Harms 1999). Metomidate is probably a poor analgesic and should not be used alone for major surgical or noxious procedures (Hansen et al. 2003; Harms 1999).

In some marine species, metomidate has a wider therapeutic range compared with benzocaine (Hansen et al. 2003). Among freshwater tropical fish, gouramis are very sensitive to metomidate, and its use in cichlids (Cichlidae) in water of pH < 5 is contraindicated (Harms 1999). In Atlantic cod, recovery times were found to increase with increasing body weight, but not induction times. When metomidate was used in combination with MS-222 or benzocaine, overall reduction of dose of both MS-222 and benzocaine were possible, with marked reduction of both induction and recovery time (Zahl et al. 2009).

Quinaldine and Quinaldine Sulfate Quinaldine sulfate (QS) is a strongly acidic, highly water-soluble powder that must be buffered. Rather than adding powder directly to the water, QS is administered as a stock solution (10 g/L). Its parent compound, Quinaldine, is a yellowish oily liquid and must be dissolved in acetone or alcohol prior to mixing in water. Due to high lipid solubility, quinaldine tends to accumulate in the brain more than QS (Harms 1999; Hseu et al. 1998; Ross 2001). Like MS-222 and most immersions, quinaldine and QS depress the CNS sensory centers. Unlike MS-222, neither drug is metabolized by fish and is excreted entirely unchanged (Harms 1999; Hseu et al. 1998).

Though not approved for use in the United States (Harms 1999), QS is common in aquaculture elsewhere because of its relatively low cost. This has also made quinaldine a popular tool for collection of fishes from tidal pools and small lagoons (Ross & Ross 2008). Other reported advantages include effectiveness at very low concentrations, purported low toxicity and wide safety margin, and short fish recovery time (Kumlu & Yanar 1999).

Despite claims of safety, mortality occurs in some species. For example, in gilthead seabream, low dosage QS (15–20 mg/L) resulted in 30–100% mortality (Kumlu & Yanar 1999). In addition, quinaldine can be an irritant and has caused corneal damage in salmonids (Harms & Bakal 1995; Ross and Ross 2008). Also of importance are studies that demonstrate that fish exposed to quinaldine or QS alone retain a strong reflex response to being touched, even when they have totally lost equilibrium and are deeply anesthetized. This, along with the potential lack of analgesia, makes them inappropriate for transportation, handling, and surgical or similarly noxious procedures (Cullen 1996; Harms 1999; Kumlu & Yanar 1999).

To reduce toxicity, and increase efficacy and analgesia, some researchers have combined diazepam with QS. As demonstrated in gilthead seabream, sea bass (*Dicentrarchus labrax*), and cichlids (*Cichlasoma nigrofasciatum*), addition of diazepam to the QS bath results in fish entering a deeper anesthetic plane at lower QS dosages. This occurs with lower to no mortality, improved muscle relaxation, and reduced excitement in confined spaces (e.g., transport boxes) (Bircan-Yildrim et al. 2010; Kumlu & Yanar 1999; Yanar & Kumlu 2001). Nondepolarizing neuromuscular blocking agents (gallamine triethiodide, tubocurarine chloride, and pancuronium bromide) IM eliminate the reflex responses in fish anesthetized by quinaldine alone (Kumlu & Yanar 1999). However, these combinations do not provide analgesia.

2-Phenoxyethanol 2-phenoxyethanol (2-PE) is a clear or straw-colored oily liquid. It has a faintly aromatic odor and is moderately water soluble. 2-PE was used initially in aquaculture to treat ichthyophoniasis and other fungal, bacterial and parasitic diseases. Less expensive than many anesthetics, 2-PE has been widely used for sedation, particularly in fish transportation, as well as general anesthesia (Hseu et al. 1996, 1997; Ross 2001). Another advantage is that it causes no pH change when added to sea water (Hseu et al. 1998).

2-PE produces hypoventilation and has poor analgesia (Oswald 1978). Also, sustained and regular exposure to 2-PE solution causes a neuropsychological syndrome in some handlers (Hseu et al. 1998). Additionally, 2-PE may not completely cease involuntary movements, so muscle twitching is possible. Other negative aspects to the drug include no block of the stress response and cardiovascular activity is significantly reduced (Fredricks et al. 1993; Molinero & Gonzalez 1995).

In a recent article, over 102 species (30 families) of a variety of sizes and ages were moved from one aquarium to another using 2-PE exclusively at an average dosage of 0.15 mL/L with maintenance in the immersion for up to 330 minutes. In general, the procedure was smooth, with very little (mostly none) excitation noted in most of the species (Vaughan et al. 2008). Due to the numbers of animals, they are not all included in the table in this chapter and the reader is referred to the original paper. Similarly, at Ocean Park, Hong Kong (K. Larson, pers. comm., 2011) 2-PE has become the anesthetic product of choice for their anesthetic events, and as earlier, they also use it to catch fish out of large aquaria with divers in the water.

Isoflurane There are limited published studies evaluating chlorofluorocarbon-based anesthetics in fish, and care is exercised in their use. Isoflurane is considered safe and effective in freshwater and marine fish at concentrations ranging from 0.4 cc to 0.75 cc isoflurane/L H_2O for induction and 0.25 cc isoflurane/L H_2O for maintenance (Stetter 2001). Isoflurane liquid is vaporized and bubbled through the water or is directly added to the anesthetic chamber. The latter involves spraying the drug through a 25-gauge needle beneath the surface of the anesthetic chamber. This allows small drug droplets to be distributed in the water (Stetter 2001). Anesthetic depth is difficult to control and, due to insolubility in water, localized areas of higher concentrations may occur, resulting in overdosage. In addition, volatilization and difficulty in scavenging waste gas is a hazard to personnel (Harms 1999; Ross 2001). This is addressed, to some extent, by attaching a funnel system to a standard scavenging system and placing it immediately above the anesthetic chamber (Stetter 2001). Given the disadvantages associated with its use, a number of researchers and clinicians recommend the use of isoflurane or similar drugs only as a last-resort anesthetic, for euthanasia, or not at all (Harms 1999; Ross 2001). A recent paper rejuvenated interest in this drug for fish anesthesia, utilizing it in combination with MS-222 which resulted in safer anesthetics for zebrafish, which have high mortalities with long MS-222 sedations (Huang et al. 2010).

Ketamine and Xylazine Traditionally used intramuscularly or intravenously, the drugs ketamine and xylazine can also be used as an immersion. In a study utilizing these drugs in various combinations as a bath for carp (*Cyprinus carpio*) resulted in smooth inductions with sufficient anesthetic time to perform minor procedures (Al-Hamdani et al. 2010).

Medetomidine One novel use of this drug is as an antifouling agent used for barnacle control. The drug is incorporated into marine paints and prevents the settling of barnacle and tubeworm larvae on surfaces coated with the paint. To assess the potential for effects on nontarget species in the vicinity of such paints, studies have been performed with low dose long-term immersion baths. In one of these studies 0.5- to 50-nM medetomidine baths were used; mostly fry were affected, and side effects noted were body paleness, decreased oxygen consumption, and decreased respiratory (Lennquist et al. 2010). Sedative effects were not noted, as it was not the scope of the study, but all the side effects were reversible when animals were removed to clean water. In rainbow trout it produced sedation but not analgesia. Bradypnea was observed during immobilization with an increase in respiration occurring after addition of atipamezole to the recovery water at 6× the medetomidine concentration (Horsberg et al. 1999).

Carbon Dioxide Carbon dioxide for immobilization is obtained from three sources: CO_2 gas, sodium bicarbonate ($NaHCO_3$), or carbonic acid (H_2CO_3) (Gelwicks & Zafft 1998; Prince et al. 1995). Use of carbon dioxide gas involves diffusing compressed CO_2 gas through air stones into water. The $NaHCO_3$ (baking soda) method involves mixing a specific amount of the drug with water to release CO_2. Carbonic acid immobilization involves mixing equal volumes of sulfuric acid (H_2SO_4) and $NaHCO_3$ solutions in water to form carbonic acid and liberate CO_2 (Gelwicks & Zafft 1998; Prince et al. 1995).

Carbon dioxide gas and $NaHCO_3$ methods are popular, but cumbersome for many field applications (Gelwicks & Zafft 1998; Prince et al. 1995). In comparison, the materials needed for carbonic acid immobilization are compact, and concentrations are easily controlled, making it more applicable to field work (Gelwicks & Zafft 1998). The carbonic acid method has its own disadvantage in that $NaHCO3$ and H_2SO_4 solutions are designed to react completely, and accuracy is essential. If one solution is mixed incorrectly, water chemistry (i.e., pH) will be significantly affected. Safe handling of concentrated H_2SO_4 requires protective gloves, clothing, and glasses and work under a fume hood (Gelwicks & Zafft 1998). The acid is added to the water, not the reverse.

Regardless of method, CO_2 use has many disadvantages. Concentrations in water are difficult to control and oxygen must be maintained at high levels. Blood gases and acid–base balance are markedly altered (Harms 1999; Prince et al. 1995). To address the latter concern, some handlers use $NaHCO_3$ with CO_2 gas for its buffering effect (Prince et al. 1995). Alternatively, some handlers mix $NaHCO_3$ with glacial acetic acid to yield carbon dioxide concentrations sufficient for immobilization while limiting acid-base shifts (Prince et al. 1995).

Following immersion in water with a high CO_2 concentration, there is a rapid decrease in blood pH and increase in blood CO_2 concentration. Low blood pH results in less efficient oxygen transport to tissues, including the brain. The resulting cerebral hypoxia causes an overall inhibition of spontaneous activity of the CNS and the observed "anesthetic" effect (Gelwicks & Zafft 1998; Harms & Bakal 1995). When fish are returned to freshwater, CO_2 diffuses out of the gills, blood pH rapidly returns to normal levels, and fish recover. One may expect these changes in blood pH and subsequent cerebral hypoxia to produce morbidity. However, rainbow trout appear tolerant of these changes in blood pH. Recent studies provide conflicting evidence regarding effectiveness and safety of carbonic acid (Gelwicks & Zafft 1998).

Although touted to decrease the stress response, CO_2 has questionable analgesia (Prince et al. 1995; Ross 2001) and is not appropriate for invasive procedures.

In the United States, the primary advantage of using CO_2 is that it is "generally regarded as safe, and there are not restrictions on its use which is appealing to both aquaculture and field work" (Gelwicks & Zafft 1998; Harms 1999). However, many handlers feel it should be used for immobilization or euthanasia as a last resort (Harms 1999).

Other Immersion Agents There are more esoteric drugs that have been tried in fishes, usually in an effort to find an inexpensive and easy-to-use drug with no tissue residues. They include tobacco (nicotine) (Agokei 2010), menthol (Simoes & Gomes 2009), avocado pear (Adebayo et al. 2010), and crotalaria, among others (Ramanayaka & Atapattu 2006). To obtain details on the use of these drugs, the reader is referred to the original papers.

Of additional interest is also the use of diazepam as an immersion, and while not overtly sedative, it does show evidence of an anxiolytic effect, which may prove useful in other combinations. Zebrafish, in particular, are used as a model for behavioral pharmacology research, as anxiety behaviors have been described in this species with amelioration after exposure to anxiolytic drugs. Clonazepam, bromazepam, diazepam, and ethanol significantly reduced shoal cohesion and tank exploration. These benzodiazepines and buspirone, as well as ethanol also increased time spent in light versus dark areas (and thus less "hiding"). Whereas propranolol and chlordiazepoxide had no effects (Bencan et. al. 2009; Gebauer et. al. 2011). Nicotine, which has anxiolytic effects in rodents and humans, showed similar responses in the zebrafish. Different dosages of these drugs provided little to no sedation, with the exception of 20 mg/L of chlordiazepoxide (Bencan et al. 2009; Gebauer et al. 2011).

Some historical drugs include chloral hydrate, urethane, chlorobutanol, and diethyl ether, none of which are recommended for use in fish any longer (McFarland & Klontz 1969).

Oral Anesthetics

Metomidate In addition to being used as an immersion, metomidate has been administered orally by high pressure syringe as a supplement in fish partially immobilized by remote injection (Harvey et al. 1988) and to turbot (*Scophthalmus maximus*) via stomach tube for rapid and complete immobilization (Hansen et al. 2003).

Diazepam In addition to being combined with QS for immersion anesthesia (Yanar & Kumlu 2001), diazepam impregnated pellets have been fed to American shad (*Alosa sapidissima*), resulting in a slow anesthetic induction (Harms & Bakal 1995). The authors regularly use oral diazepam as an oral presedative in larger fishes at dosages of 0.5–1.5 mg/kg, with higher dosages likely being necessary. This is an area requiring much more investigation on efficacy and safety in its use in fishes.

Ketamine Ketamine, when gavaged orally to goldfish (*Carassius auratus*) and hybrid striped bass (*Morone saxatilis*), showed notable sedative effects and animals allowed themselves to be netted; further, an arapaima sedated by this method tolerated slinging (Raines & Clancy 2009).

Tiletamine-Zolazepam Though designed to be used as an injectable drug combination, successful sedation and translocation of >70% of a population of captive yellowtail jacks (*Seriola lalandi*) was performed using tiletamine-zolazepam (TZ) powder packed in gelatin capsules placed in food items. Mortalities were attributed to anesthetic overdosage from fish consuming greater than one medicated food item (Steers & Sherrill 2001).

Injectable Anesthetics

Ketamine Hydrochloride Ketamine is used alone or in combination with alpha$_2$-agonists (Harms 1999). Intramuscular injection is the most common route and requires high dosages in teleosts and sturgeons when used alone (Bruecker & Graham 1993; Fleming et al. 2003; Williams et al. 1988). When available in the lyophilized form, a concentrated solution permitting a

smaller volume IM injection can be prepared (Oswald 1978). IV administration, though rarely reported, uses dosages 1/3 to 1/2 of those used IM. Ketamine has been used for capture and manipulation of a number of marine and freshwater species (Williams et al. 1988) and for short-duration procedures and transport (Bruecker & Graham 1993; Oswald 1978). Ketamine IV in coho salmon (*Oncorhynchus kisutch*), rainbow trout, and Midas cichlids (*Heros citrinellum*) reduces the oxygen demand during handling (Bruecker & Graham 1993; Oswald 1978).

Regardless of administration route, ketamine alone has a species-specific effect in fish often characterized by incomplete anesthesia, periods of apnea, and prolonged recovery with excitement when used (Bruecker & Graham 1993; Graham & Iwama 1990; Oswald 1978). To reduce dosage and apnea, and improve anesthesia, ketamine is often combined with the reversible alpha-2-adrenergic agonist, medetomidine. This combination provides safe and effective anesthesia in some species (Williams et al. 2004), but respiratory depression, bradycardia (Fleming et al. 2003), and incomplete immobilization is noted in others. For the latter reason, either ketamine or a ketamine/medetomidine (K/M) combination is more appropriate as an aid to restraint rather than a substitute for immersion anesthesia during major procedures. One of the authors (Neiffer) has found K/M particularly useful in capture of fish from large-volume aquaria. Following sedation or slowing down with K/M, staff is able to net the fish and transfer them to an MS-222 bath for maintenance and evaluation. In sturgeon (*Acipenser* hybrids), IV medetomidine 0.04 mg/kg and ketamine 4 mg/kg had slower inductions and longer recoveries than MS-222 or clove oil, but interestingly had fewer physiologic effects than the MS-222 or clove oil (DiMarco 2011).

Medetomidine Medetomidine is usually combined with ketamine and reversed with atipamezole. One of the authors (Mylniczenko) found that in black pacu, medetomidine (100 μg/kg IM) in combination with midazolam (1 mg/kg IM) and butorphanol (1 mg/kg IM), did not produce adequate anesthesia to result in ataxia or allow any invasive testing or significant animal manipulation, but did allow sedation for removal into a small transport and then for euthanasia with MS-222.

Xylazine In rainbow and brown trout, the lowest effective dose of xylazine (100 mg/kg) consistently produced apnea. Convulsant activity occurred during induction and recovery, making it difficult to ensure artificial ventilation because the convulsions frequently dislodged the water supply. In addition, gross ECG disturbances were detected. Consequently, xylazine is not recommended in salmonids (Oswald 1978). Given the proven usefulness of medetomidine in other teleost species, xylazine is not the preferred alpha₂-agonist for any fish.

Tiletamine-Zolazepam IM administration of TZ was used in one study at dosages of 5–20 mg/kg in multiple saltwater species (not noted in the abstract). Even at dosages of 60 mg/kg, this group did not experience any mortalities. At higher dosages, animal did have prolonged recoveries, some up to 72 hours (Garcia-Parrage et al. 2007). The greatest advantage of using TZ was lower volumes of drug required as the drug is purchased as a powder and can be reconstituted to high concentrations with good effect and no supersaturation.

Propofol Propofol IV has been used successfully for rapid induction in Gulf of Mexico sturgeon, but caused significant respiratory depression. This complication was addressed by passing oxygenated water across gills. In addition to respiratory depression, uncomplicated bradycardia was noted (Fleming et al. 2003). At one facility (Neiffer), propofol in an African lungfish (*Protopterus annectens*) was associated with mortality. It is not certain if this was directly drug related or due to an obligate air-breathing fish being recovered in water that was too deep to allow surface access.

Alfaxalone-Alfadolone A combination steroid anesthetic, alfaxalone/alfadolone (A/A), mainly depresses CNS activity while leaving the integumentary sensory system operational. This makes it very valuable for research in sensory physiology including mechanoreceptors (Peters et al. 2001). However, it is no longer marketed in the United States. An advantage of A/A is its cardiac chronotropic and inotropic stimulatory effect with vasodilation of the gill capillaries. This seems to ensure adequate oxygenation of the blood compared with many other anesthetics (Oswald 1978). As with all drugs, species differences are seen. In a collection of marine and freshwater species A/A was effective, but not consistent for capture of free swimming individuals (Harvey et al. 1988). In several catfish species, A/A provided surgical anesthesia lasting several hours (Peters et al. 2001). In rainbow and brown trout, A/A produces similar long sleep times, but it is difficult to give a dose that simultaneously abolishes locomotion yet preserves ventilation (Oswald 1978).

Lidocaine Lidocaine yields variable results as an immersion anesthetic. However, it is effective as an injectable local anesthetic in fish, alone or in combination with other drugs (Harms & Bakal 1995; Park et al. 2011).

Miscellaneous Drugs Galamine triethiodide IM has been used for capture and handling of large tank fish, providing a smooth induction of paralysis following injection (Harvey et al. 1988). It is worth considering for noninvasive procedures or as an adjunct to anesthetic

agents. A combination of etorphine-acetylpromazine (Large Animal Immobilon™) has been used in trout for anesthesia, but given the human accidental exposure risks (Oswald 1978) and availability of other agents, its use is not recommended. Ethanol is an anesthetic of last resort. Anesthetic depth is variable and difficult to control. However, in nonclinical situations or for euthanasia, ethanol is sometimes available when other drugs are not (Harms & Bakal 1995).

NONCHEMICAL ANESTHESIA

Electroshock is a common fisheries tool for group immobilization to tag, survey, or remove animals from an area. It is often coined "electroanesthesia"; however, this is a misnomer, as animals are not truly anesthetized. The process results in electronarcosis or stunning, but when the intensity of the current is too high, it can result in severe muscle tetany and spinal injuries (Schreck et al. 1976). While this method can be used appropriately and there are reports that when done properly there are few deleterious effects, one author (Mylniczenko) has experienced long-term immunocompromise and resulting secondary infections in animals collected by this manner. Additionally, the acute effects can be very dramatic and mimic exhaustive exercise. Finally, this method does not have much practical application for the aquarium but may be a tool used to collect specimens coming into quarantine or utilized during field work. There should be caution for human safety when using electricity in water and for collateral damage of nontarget animals in the vicinity of the shock.

Hypothermia is not an appropriate method of anesthesia but had been used historically to induce light anesthesia and for transport; the physiologic effects are too great for its consideration as an anesthetic.

ANALGESIA

Most sources define analgesia as the absence of pain in the presence of stimuli that would normally be painful without the loss of consciousness. The less used definition seems more universally acceptable, as it includes absence of noxious stimulation as well as pain in the definition (Blood & Studdert 1988; Thurmon et al. 1996). Numerous contemporary articles exist on the topic of analgesia in fishes (Neiffer & Stamper 2009; Sneddon 2009; Weber 2011). Putting aside the question of pain perception, fish have μ and κ opiate receptors throughout the brain, making it reasonable to expect some effect of opioid treatments in fish experiencing noxious stimuli (Harms et al. 2005).

Despite increased interest, limited information on the use of analgesics in fish exists. In one of the earliest studies, the lips of juvenile rainbow trout were injected with 0.1-mL acetic acid. This resulted in a marked increase in opercular rate compared to controls, and anomalous behaviors including rocking from side to side and lip rubbing against the gravel and tank sides. Administration of high morphine dosages significantly reduced the opercular rate and the noxious stimulus-related behaviors. These fish also returned to normal eating behavior faster. Thus, morphine appears to act as an analgesic or at least antinociceptive in this and presumably other teleost fish (Sneddon 2003; Sneddon et al. 2003). In a later study, koi carp (*Cyprinus carpio*) underwent exploratory celiotomy and were treated with butorphanol, ketoprofen, or saline. Only koi injected with butorphanol exhibited no significant differences between pre- and postsurgery caudal fin beat frequency and vertical position in the water column. This suggests a mild behavioral sparing effect compared with the ketoprofen-treated and saline control groups (Harms et al. 2005). Fish can become tolerant of morphine, and naloxone reduces its effects (and presumably butorphanol) (Rose 2002). Regardless of the pain perception controversy, it appears that analgesic drugs have application in reducing stress associated with noxious stimuli in teleosts and presumably other bony fish. Additionally, some drugs that attain immobility are devoid of analgesic effects and should not be used alone for surgical or similarly noxious procedures.

In trout treated with ketoprofen or butorphanol, the amount of MS-222 needed for antinociception was lower using the drugs than without; this technique was modeled after the MAC (minimal alveolar concentration) sparing studies performed in mammals (Davis et al. 2006; Mylniczenko 2012). Not only was there an anesthetic sparing effect occurring, but there were dose-dependent responses as well.

EUTHANASIA

When necessary, overdosage of immobilization drugs is an acceptable means of euthanasia (Harms & Bakal 1995). Inhalant (immersion) drugs at 5–10× the anesthetic concentration for a particular species are usually chosen, although injectable agents can also be used (Ross and Ross 2008). MS-222 is most often used. However, many fish in large exhibits require induction first with parenteral drugs (e.g., medetomidine/ketamine), then euthanasia in an MS-222 bath. Alternatively, in fish too large for a bath, inhalant (immersion) is poured directly over the gills (Harms & Bakal 1995). Cessation of opercular movements sometimes indicates a fish has expired, but is not definitive and should not be used as the sole parameter for confirmation of death. Cardiac asystole usually lags behind brain death since fish myocardial cells utilize local glycogen stores for energy and do not need blood glucose (Stetter 2001). Use of Doppler flow probes, ultrasonography, or electrocardiography is recommended to confirm asystole. To be certain, additional anesthetic

drug or pentobarbital are administered IV into the heart or caudal vein (Ross 2001). Alternatively, cranial concussion, decapitation, spinal transection, or exsanguination is performed once the fish is deeply anesthetized (Harms & Bakal 1995). While euthanasia with baking powder or Alka-Seltzer™ tablets has been utilized and is considered an acceptable euthanasia method, MS-222 is the quicker and has less physiologically altering technique. The reader is directed to review euthanasia principles for fish as outlined by the American Veterinary Medical Association (AVMA) and by Yanong et al. (2009). Unacceptable methods of euthanasia include asphyxiation and hypothermia.

FIELD IMMOBILIZATION

Immobilization of fishes in the field is a fairly commonplace event. Considerations for immobilizing fish in remote areas include having portable equipment that can connect to car batteries or portable generators/batteries. It is important to consider guidelines for approved drugs (U.S. Fish and Wildlife Service, The Aquatic Animal Drug Approval Partnership 2010) and to observe withdrawal periods. Alternately, there are tags available that state "do not consume" that are affixed to the fish.

Typically for field procedures, unless invasive, animals are not anesthetized with chemicals. Hook and line, net, trawl, and electroanesthesia fishing are methods used to capture free-range fish, each technique carrying its own risk to the animal from hypoxia, trauma, exhaustion, and major physiologic disturbances. These must be considered for long-term management or survival of the animals.

When using source water, clarity must be considered as some water bodies may have turbid water, algal blooms, or high tannins. This can complicate visualization of induction or recovery in these animals. Temperature shifts throughout the course of the day will greatly modify temperatures in holding vats.

POSTANESTHETIC CHALLENGES

Once animals are placed into recovery water, ensuring adequate ventilation is critical. The authors prefer using an electronic pump to facilitate oxygenated water flow, but many aquarists prefer moving the animal through the water column (see previous section on this topic). Determining when to release the animal requires skilled staff that is aware of normal swimming behavior. Staff should be prepared to retrieve the animal if rather than swimming away it falls to the bottom of the water column (or if aggressed upon). Observation of the animal for the next 24–48 hours is recommended for observing any morbidity or mortality associated with the procedure. As with all anesthetic procedures in animals, restraining a compromised animal with either manual or chemical methods carries a risk for increased morbidity or mortality.

ACKNOWLEDGMENTS

Special thanks to Charlene Burns, Dr. M. Andrew Stamper, Jane Capobianco, DeAnne Fanta, and Dr. Beth Nolan from Walt Disney World, Orlando, FL, and Lynda Leppert from the Georgia Aquarium, Atlanta, GA for their assistance with chapter preparation.

REFERENCES

Ackerman JL, Bellwood DR. 2002. Comparative efficiency of clove oil and rotenone for sampling tropical reef fish assemblages. *Journal of Fish Biology* 60:893–901.

Adebayo OT, Fasakin EA, Popoola OM. 2010. Use of aqueous extracts of avocado pear, *Pyrus communis*, leaf as anaesthetic in gonadectomy of African catfish, *Clarias gariepinus*. *Journal of Applied Aquaculture* 22:117–122.

Afifi SH, Al-Thobaiti S, Rasem BM. 2001. Multiple exposure of Asian sea bass (*Lates calcarifer*, Centropomidae) to clove oil: a histological study. *Journal of Aquaculture in the Tropics* 16:131–138.

Aguiar LH, Kalinin AL, Rantin FT. 2002. The effects of temperature on the cardio-respiratory function of the neotropical fish, *Piaractus mesopotamicus*. *Journal of Thermal Biology* 27:299–308.

Al-Hamdani AH, Ebrahim SK, Mohammad FK. 2010. Experimental xylazine-ketamine anesthesia in the common carp (*Cyprinus carpio*). *Journal of Wildlife Diseases* 46:596–598.

Bailey KM, Hempstead JE, Tobias JR, Borst LB, Clode AB, Posner LP. (2013). Evaluation of the effects of tricaine methanesulfonate on retinal structure and function in koi carp (*Cyprinus carpio*). *Journal of the American Veterinary Medical Association* 242(11):1578–1582.

Bassi M, Klein W, Fernandes MN, Perry SF, Glass ML. 2005. Pulmonary oxygen diffusing capacity of the South American lungfish, *Lepidosiren paradoxa*: physiological values by the Bohr method. *Physiological and Biochemical Zoology* 78:560–569.

Bencan Z, Sledge D, Levin ED. 2009. Buspirone, chlordiazepoxide, and diazepam effects in a zebrafish model of anxiety. *Pharmacology, Biochemistry, and Behavior* 94:75–80.

Bernstein PS, Digre KB, Creel DJ. 1997. Retinal toxicity associated with occupational exposure to the fish anesthetic MS-222. *American Journal of Ophthalmology* 124:843–844.

Bircan-Yildrim Y, Genc E, Turan F, Cek S, Yanar M. 2010. The anaesthetic effects of quinaldine sulphate, muscle relaxant diazepam and their combination on convict cichlid, *Cichlasoma nigrofasciatum* (Gunther, 1867) juveniles. *Journal of Animal and Veterinary Advances* 9:547–550.

Blank JM, Morrissette JM, Landeira-Fernandez AM, Blackwell SB, Williams TD, Block BA. 2004. In situ cardiac performance of Pacific bluefin tuna hearts in response to acute temperature change. *The Journal of Experimental Biology* 207:881–890.

Blood DC, Studdert VP. 1988. *Bailliere's Comprehensive Veterinary Dictionary*. Philadelphia: W.B. Saunders.

Bond CE. 1996. *Biology of Fishes*, 2nd ed. Philadelphia: Saunders College Publishing.

Braithwaite VA, Boulcott P. 2007. Pain perception, aversion, and fear in fish. *Diseases of Aquatic Organisms* 75:131–138.

Brauner CJ, Matey V, Wilson JM, Bernier NJ, Val AL. 2004. Transition in organ function during the evolution of air-breathing: insights from *Arapaima gigas*, an obligate air-breathing teleost from the Amazon. *The Journal of Experimental Biology* 207:1433–1438.

Bressler K, Ron B. 2004. Effect of anesthetics on stress and the innate immune system of gilthead bream (*Sparus aurata*). *Israeli Journal of Aquaculture* 56:5–13.

Brill RW, Bushnell PG. 2001. The cardiovascular system of tunas. In: *Tuna: Physiology, Ecology, and Evolution* (BA Block, ED Stevens, eds.), pp. 79–119. San Diego: Academic Press.

Bruecker P, Graham M. 1993. The effects of the anesthetic ketamine hydrochloride on oxygen consumption rates and behavior in the fish *Heros (Cichlasoma) citrinellum* (Gunther, 1864). *Comparative Biochemistry and Physiology. C: Comparative Pharmacology* 104:57–59.

Bushnell PG, Jones DR. 1994. Cardiovascular and respiratory physiology of tuna: adaptations for support of exceptionally high metabolic rates. *Environmental Biology of Fishes* 40:303–318.

Caamano Tubio RI, Weber RA, Aldegunde M. 2010. Home tank anesthesia: a very efficient method of attenuating handling stress in rainbow trout (*Oncorhynchus mykiss*, Walbaum). *Journal of Applied Ichthyology* 26:116–117.

Carreiro CRP, Furtado-Neto MAA, Mesquita PEC, Bezerra TA. 2011. Sex determination in the giant fish of Amazon Basin, *Arapaima gigas* (Osteoglossiformes, Arapaimatidae), using laparoscopy. *Acta Amazonica* 41(3):415–420.

Cho GK, Heath DD. 2000. Comparison of tricaine methansulphonate (MS-222) and clove oil anaethesia effects on the physiology of juvenile Chinook salmon, *Oncorhynchus tshawytscha* (Walbaum). *Aquaculture Research* 31:537–546.

Chu-Koo F, Dugué R, Aguilar MA, Daza AC, Bocanegra FA, Veintemilla, CC, Duponchelle F, Renno JF, Tello S, Nuñez J. 2008. Gender determination in the Paiche or *pirarucu* (*Arapaima gigas*) using plasma vitellogenin, 17b-estradiol, and 11-ketotestosterone levels. *Fish Physiology and Biochemistry* 35:125–136.

Cooke SJ, Suski CD, Ostrand KG, Tufts BL, Wahl DH. 2004. Behavioral and physiological assessment of low concentrations of clove oil anaesthetic for handling and transporting largemouth bass (*Micropterus salmoides*). *Aquaculture (Amsterdam, Netherlands)* 239:509–529.

Cooper R, Krum H, Tzinas G, Sylvia P, Belle S, Kaufman L. 1994. A preliminary study of clinical techniques utilized with bluefin tuna (*Thunnus thynnus* Linnaeus): a comparison of some captive and wild caught blood parameters. *Proceedings of the International Association for Aquatic Animal Medicine* 25:26–36.

Couvillon PA. 1984. Performance of goldfish (*Carassius auratus*) in patterned sequences of rewarded and nonrewarded trials. *Journal of Comparative Psychology* 98:333–344.

Crosby TC, Hill JE, Watson CA, Yanong RPE. 2006. Effects of tricaine methanosulfonate, hypno, metomidate, quinaldine, and salt of plasma cortisol levels following acute stress in three-spot gourami, *Trichogaster trichopterus*. *Journal of Aquatic Animal Health* 18:58–63.

Cullen LK. 1996. Muscle relaxants and neuromuscular block. In: *Lumb and Jones' Veterinary Anesthesia*, 3rd ed. (JC Thurmon, WJ Tranquilli, GJ Benson, WV Lumb, eds.), pp. 337–364. Baltimore: Williams and Wilkins.

Davis KB, Griffin BR. 2004. Physiological responses of hybrid striped bass under sedation by several anesthetics. *Aquaculture (Amsterdam, Netherlands)* 233:531–548.

Davis MR, Mylniczenko N, Storms T, Raymond F, Dunn JL. 2006. Evaluation of intramuscular ketoprofen and butorphanol as analgesics in chain dogfish (*Scyliorhinus retifer*). *Zoo Biology* 25(6):491–500.

DeLaney RG, Shub C, Fishman AP. 1976. Hematologic observations on the aquatic and estivating African lungfish, *Protopterus aethiopicus*. *Copeia* 1976(3):423–434.

Detar JE, Mattingly HT. 2004. Response of southern redbelly dace to clove oil and MS-222: effects of anesthetic concentration and water temperature. *Proceedings of the Annual Conference of the Southeastern Association of Fish and Wildlife Agencies* 58: 219–227.

Di Marco P, Petochi T, Longobardi A, Priori A, Finoia MG, Donadelli V, Corsalini I, Marino G. 2011. Efficacy of tricaine methanesulfonate, clove oil, and medetomidine-ketamine and their side effects on the physiology of sturgeon hybrid *Acipenser naccarii* × *Acipenser baerii*. *Journal of Applied Ichthyology* 27:611–617.

Farrell AP. 1978. Cardiovascular events associated with air breathing in two teleosts, *Hoplerythrinus unitaeniatus* and *Arapaima gigas*. *Canadian Journal of Zoology* 56(4):953–958.

Feng G, Zhuang P, Zhang L, Kynard B, Shi X, Duan M, Liu J, Huang X. 2011. Effect of anaesthetics, MS-222 and clove oil, on blood biochemical parameters of juvenile Siberian sturgeon (*Acipenser baerii*). *Journal of Applied Ichthyology* 27:595–599.

Ferguson RA, Tufts L. 1992. Physiologic effects of brief air exposure in exhaustively exercised rainbow trout (*Oncorhynchus mykiss*): indications for catch and release fisheries. *Canadian Journal of Fisheries and Aquatic Sciences* 49:1157–1162.

Ferreira JT, Schoonbee HJ, Smit GL. 1984. The uptake of the anesthetic benzocaine hydrochloride by the gills and the skin of three freshwater fish species. *Journal of Fish Biology* 25:35–41.

Fleming GJ, Heard DJ, Floyd RF, Riggs A. 2003. Evaluation of propofol and medetomidine-ketamine for short-term immobilization of Gulf of Mexico sturgeon (*Acipenser oxyrinchus desoti*). *Journal of Zoo and Wildlife Medicine* 34:153–158.

Fredricks KT, Gingerich WH, Fater DC. 1993. Comparative cardiovascular effects of four fishery anesthetics in spinally transected rainbow trout, *Oncorhynchus mykiss*. *Comparative Biochemistry & Physiology* 104C(3):477–483.

Garcia-Parrage D, Alvaro T, Valls M, Malabia A. 2007. Tiletamine-Zolazepam injectable anesthesia: an easy technique to handle fish in large volume aquaria. Proceedings of the International Association for Aquatic Animal Medicine, pp. 25–27.

Gebauer DL, Pagnussat N, Piato AL, Schaefer IC, Bonan CD, Lara DR. 2011. Effects of anxiolytics in zebrafish: similarities and differences between benzodiazepines, buspirone, and ethanol. *Pharmacology, Biochemistry, and Behavior* 99:480–486.

Gelwicks KR, Zafft DJ. 1998. Efficacy of carbonic acid as an anesthetic for rainbow trout. *North American Journal of Fisheries Management* 18:432–438.

Gilderhus PA. 1989. Efficacy of benzocaine as an anesthetic for salmonid fishes. *North American Journal of Fisheries Management* 9:150–153.

Gilderhus PA, Lemm CA, Woods LC. 1991. Benzocaine as an anesthetic for striped bass. *Progressive Fish Culturist* 53:105–107.

Gilmour KM, Perry SF, Wood CM, Henry RP, Laurent P, Part P, Walsh PJ. 1998. Nitrogen excretion and the cardiorespiratory physiology of the gulf toadfish, *Opsanus beta*. *Physiological Zoology* 71:492–505.

Gilmour KM, Euverman RM, Esbaugh AJ, Kenney L, Chew SF, Ip YK, Perry SF. 2007. Mechanisms of acid–base regulation in the African lungfish *Protopterus annectens*. *The Journal of Experimental Biology* 210(11):1944–1959.

Gingerich AJ, Cooke SJ, Hanson KC, Donaldson MR, Hasler CT, Suski CD, Arlinghaus R. 2007. Evaluation of the interactive effects of air exposure duration and water temperature on the condition and survival of angled and released fish. *Fisheries Research* 86:169–178.

Gladden JN, Brainard BM, Shelton JL, Camus AC, Divers SJ. 2010. Evaluation of isoeugenol for anesthesia in koi carp (*Cyprinus carpio*). *American Journal of Veterinary Research* 71:859–866.

Gomes LC, Chippari-Gomes AR, Lopes NP, Roubach R, Araujo-Lima CARM. 2001. Efficacy of benzocaine as an anesthetic in juvenile tambaqui, *Colossoma macropomum*. *Journal of the World Aquaculture Society* 32:426–431.

Graham JB. 1997. *Air-Breathing Fishes: Evolution, Diversity, and Adaptation*. San Diego: Academic Press.

Graham MS, Iwama GK. 1990. The physiological effects of the anesthetic ketamine hydrochloride on two salmonid species. *Aquaculture (Amsterdam, Netherlands)* 90:323–332.

Griffiths SP. 2000. The use of clove oil as an anaesthetic and method for sampling intertidal rockpool fishes. *Journal of Fish Biology* 57:1453–1464.

Guo FC, Teo LH, Chen TW. 1995. Effects of anaesthetics on the water parameters in a simulated transport experiment of platyfish, *Xiphophorus maculatus*. *Aquaculture Research* 26:265–271.

Hansen MK, Nymoen U, Horsberg TE. 2003. Pharmokinetic and pharmacodynamic properties of metomidate in turbot (*Scophthalmus maximus*) and halibut (*Hippoglossus hippoglossus*). *Journal of Veterinary Pharmacology and Therapeutics* 26:95–103.

Harms CA. 1999. Anesthesia in fish. In: *Zoo and Wild Animal Medicine, Current Therapy 4* (ME Fowler, RE Miller, eds.), pp. 158–163. Philadelphia: W.B. Saunders.

Harms CA. 2003. Fish. In: *Zoo and Wild Animal Medicine, Current Therapy 5*. (ME Fowler, RE Miller, eds.), pp. 2–20. St. Louis: W.B. Saunders.

Harms CA, Bakal RS. 1995. Techniques in fish anesthesia. *Journal of Small Exotic Animal Medicine* 3:19–25.

Harms CA, Lewbart GA, Swanson CR, Kishimori JM, Boylan SM. 2005. Behavioral and clinical pathology changes in koi carp (*Cyprinus carpio*) subjected to anesthesia and surgery with and without intra-operative analgesics. *Comparative Medicine* 55:221–226.

Harper C. 2003. Status of clove oil and eugenol for anesthesia of fish. *Aquaculture Magazine* 29:41–42.

Harvey B, Denny C, Kaiser S, Young J. 1988. Remote intramuscular injection of immobilizing drugs into fish using a laser-aimed underwater dart gun. *Veterinary Record* 20:174–177.

Heming TA. 1989. Clinical studies of fish blood: importance of sample collection and measurement techniques. *American Journal of Veterinary Research* 50:93–97.

Heo GJ, Shin G. 2010. Efficacy of benzocaine as an anaesthetic for Crucian carp (*Carassius carassius*). *Veterinary Anaesthesia and Analgesia* 37:132–135.

Hernandez-Divers SJ, Bakal RS, Hickson BH, Rawlings CA, Wilson HG, Radlinsky M, Hernandez-Divers SM, Dover SR. 2004. Endoscopic sex determination and gonadal manipulation in Gulf of Mexico sturgeon (*Acipenser oxyrinchus desotoi*). *Journal of Zoo and Wildlife Medicine* 35:459–470.

Hinostroza ME, Serrano-Martínez E. 2013. Efecto anestésico del metasulfonato de tricaína en paiches (*Arapaima gigas*) juveniles. *Revista de Investigaciones Veterinarias del Perú* 24(4):451–458.

Honczaryk A, Inoue LAKA. 2009. Anestesia do pirarucu po aspersão direta nas brânquias do eugenol em solucão aquosa. *Ciência Rural* 39:577–579.

Honczaryk A, Inoue LAKA. 2010. Anestesia do pirarucu por aspersão da benzocaina diretamente nas brânquias. *Ciência Rural* 40:204–207.

Horsberg TE, Burka JF, Tasker RAR. 1999. Actions and pharmacokinetic properties of the (alpha$_2$)-adrenergic agents, medetomidine and atipamezole, in rainbow trout (*Oncorhynchus mykiss*). *Veterinary Anaesthesia and Analgesia* 26:18–22.

Hoseini SM, Hosseini SA, Nodeh AJ. 2010. Serum biochemical characteristics of beluga, *Huso huso* (L.), in response to blood sampling after clove powder solution exposure. *Fish Physiology and Biochemistry* 37:567–572.

Hoskonen P, Pirhonen J. 2004. The effect of clove oil sedation on oxygen consumption of six temperate-zone fish species. *Aquaculture Research* 35:1002–1005.

Hseu J-R, Yeh S-L, Chu Y-T, Ting Y-Y. 1996. Effects of anesthesia with 2-phenoxyethanol on the hematological parameters of four species of marine teleosts. *Journal of the Fisheries Society of Taiwan* 23:43–48.

Hseu J-R, Yeh S-L, Chu Y-T, Ting Y-Y. 1997. Different anesthetic effects of 2-phenoxyethanol on four species of teleosts. *Journal of the Fisheries Society of Taiwan* 24:185–191.

Hseu J-R, Yeh S-L, Chu Y-T, Ting Y-Y. 1998. Comparison of efficacy of five anesthetics in goldlined sea bream, *Sparus sarba*. *Acta Zoologica Taiwanica* 9:11–18.

Huang W-C, Hsieh Y-S, Chen I-H, Wang C-H, Chang H-W, Yang C-C, Ku T-H, Yeh S-R, Chuang Y-J. 2010. Combined use of MS-222 (tricaine) and isoflurane extends anesthesia time and minimizes cardiac rhythm side effects in adult zebrafish. *Zebrafish* 7:297–304.

Ishimatsu A, Itazawa Y. 1993. Anatomy and physiology of the cardiorespiratory system in air-breathing fish, *Channa argus*. In: *Advances in Fish Research* (BR Singh, ed.), pp. 55–70. Delhi: Narendra Publishing House.

Iversen M, Finstad B, McKinley RS, Eliassen RA. 2003. The efficacy of metomidate, clove oil, Aqui-S™, and Benzoak® as anaesthetics in Atlantic salmon (*Salmo salar* L.) smolts and their potential stress-reducing capacity. *Aquaculture (Amsterdam, Netherlands)* 221:549–566.

Jennings CA, Looney GL. 1998. Evaluation of two types of anesthesia for performing surgery on striped bass. *North American Journal of Fisheries Management* 18:187–190.

Kaiser H, Vine N. 1998. The effect of 2-phenoxyethanol and transport packing density on the post-transport survival rate and metabolic activity in the goldfish, *Carassius auratus*. *Aquarium Sciences and Conservation* 2:1–7.

Kaiser H, Brill G, Cahill J, Collett P, Czypionka K, Green A, Orr K, Pattrick P, Scheepers R, Stonier T, Whitehead MA, Yearsley R. 2006. Testing clove oil as an anaesthetic for long-distance transport of live fish: the case of the Lake Victoria cichlid, *Haplochromis obliquidens*. *Journal of Applied Ichthyology* 22:510–514.

Keene JL, Noakes DLG, Moccia RD, Soto CG. 1998. The efficacy of clove oil as an anaesthetic for rainbow trout, *Oncorhynchus mykiss* (Walbaum). *Aquaculture Research* 29:89–101.

Kildea MA, Allan GL, Kearney RE. 2004. Accumulation and clearance of the anaesthetics clove oil and Aqui-S™ from the edible tissue of silver perch (*Bidyanus bidyanus*). *Aquaculture (Amsterdam, Netherlands)* 232:265–277.

Kilgore KH, Hill JE, Powell JF, Watson CA, Yanong RP. 2009. Investigational use of metomidate hydrochloride as a shipping additive for two ornamental fishes. *Journal of Aquatic Animal Health* 21:133–139.

Kumlu M, Yanar M. 1999. Effects of the anesthetic quinaldine sulphate and muscle relaxant diazepam on sea bream juveniles (*Sparus aurata*). *Israeli Journal of Aquaculture* 51:143–147.

Lenfant C, Johansen K, Grigg GC. 1966. Respiratory properties of blood and pattern of gas exchange in the lungfish *Neoceratodus forsteri* (Krefft). *Respiratory Physiology* 2:1–21.

Lennquist A, Hilvarsson A, Förlin L. 2010. Responses in fish exposed to medetomidine, a new antifouling agent. *Marine Environmental Research* 69(Suppl.):S43–S45.

Lewbart GA, Stone DA, Love NE. 1994, Surgical management of a swim bladder disorder in a red devil cichlid (*Cichlasoma citrinellum*). Proceedings of the International Association for Aquatic Animal Medicine, pp. 141–143.

MacAvoy SE, Zaepfel RC. 1997. Effects of tricaine methanesulfonate (MS-222) on hematocrit: first field measurements on blacknose dace. *Transactions of the American Fisheries Society* 126:500–503.

Malmstrøm T, Salte R, Gjøen HM, Linseth A. 1993. A practical evaluation of metomidate and MS-222 as anaesthetics for Atlantic halibut (*Hippoglossus hippoglossus* L.). *Aquaculture (Amsterdam, Netherlands)* 113:331–338.

Marnane MJ. 2000. Site fidelity and homing behaviour in coral reef cardinalfishes. *Journal of Fish Biology* 57:1590–1600.

Matsche MA. 2011. Evaluation of tricaine methanesulfonate (MS-222) as a surgical anesthetic for Atlantic Sturgeon *Acipenser oxyrinchus oxyrinchus*. Special Issue: Proceedings of the 6th International Symposium on Sturgeon Wuhan,

China, October 25–31, 2009. *Journal of Applied Ichthyology* 27 (2):600–610.

Mattson NS, Riple TH. 1989. Metomidate, a better anesthetic for cod (*Gadus morhua*) in comparison with benzocaine, MS-222, chlorobutanol, and phenoxyethanol. *Aquaculture (Amsterdam, Netherlands)* 83:89–94.

McCarter N. 1992. Sedation of grass carp and silver carp with 2-phenoxyethanol during spawning. *Progressive Fish Culturist* 54:263–265.

McDonald DG, Milligan CL. 1992. The cardiovascular system. In: *Fish Physiology*, Vol. 12A (WS Hoar, DJ Randall, AP Farrell, eds.), p. 78. San Diego: Academic Press.

McFarland WN, Klontz GW. 1969. Anesthesia in fishes. *Federal Proceedings* 28:1535–1540.

Mohammadizarejabad A, Bastami KD, Sudagar M, Motlagh SP. 2010. Haematology of great sturgeon (*Huso huso* Linnaeus, 1758) juvenile exposed to clove powder as an anaesthetic. *Comparative Clinical Pathology* 19:465–468.

Molinero A, Gonzalez J. 1995. Comparative effects of MS 222 and 2-phenoxyethanol on gilthead sea bream (*Sparus aurata* L.) during confinement. *Comparative Biochemistry and Physiology. A, Comparative Physiology* 111A(3):405–414.

Mylniczenko ND. 2012. Chapter 22: Medical management of rays. In: *Fowler's Zoo and Wild Animal Medicine Current Therapy*, Vol. 7 (RE Miller, ME Fowler, eds.), pp. 170–176. St. Louis: Elsevier Saunders.

Myszkowski L, Kaminski R, Wolnicki J. 2003. Response of juvenile tench *Tinca tinca* (L.) to the anaesthetic 2-phenoxyethanol. *Journal of Applied Ichthyology* 19:142–145.

Neiffer DL, Stamper MA. 2009. Fish sedation: anesthesia, analgesia, and euthanasia: considerations, methods, and types of drugs. *ILAR Journal* 50:343–346.

Oikawa S, Takeda T, Itazawa Y. 1994. Scale effects of MS-222 on a marine teleost, porgy *Pagrus major*. *Aquaculture (Amsterdam, Netherlands)* 121:369–379.

Olsen YA, Einarsdottir IE, Nilssen KJ. 1995. Metomidate anaesthesia in Atlantic salmon, *Salmo salar*, prevents plasma cortisol increase during stress. *Aquaculture (Amsterdam, Netherlands)* 134:155–168.

Ostrander G, ed. 2000. *The Laboratory Fish*. San Diego: Academic Press.

Oswald RL. 1978. Injection anesthesia for experimental studies in fish. *Comparative Biochemistry and Physiology. C: Comparative Pharmacology* 60:19–26.

Pack AI, Galante RJ, Fishman AP. 1992. Role of lung inflation in control of air breath duration in African lungfish (*Protopterus annectens*). *American Journal of Physiology* 262:R879–R884.

Palmer LM, Mensinger AF. 2004. Effect of the anesthetic tricaine (MS-222) on nerve activity in the anterior lateral line of the oyster toadfish, *Opsanus tau*. *Neurophysiology* 92:1034–1041.

Park IS, Park SJ, Gil HW, Nam YK, Kim DS. 2011. Anesthetic effects of clove oil and lidocaine-HCl on marine medaka (*Oryzias dancena*). *Lab Animal* 40:45–51.

Pereira da Silva EM, Franco de Oliveira RH, Rosa Ribeiro MA, Pereira Coppola M. 2009. Anesthetic effect of clove oil on lambari. *Ciência Rural* 39:1851–1856.

Peters RC, Van den Hoek B, Bretschneider F, Struik ML. 2001. Saffan®: a review and some examples of its use in fishes (Pisces: Teleostei). *Netherlands Journal of Zoology* 51:421–437.

Posner LP. 2009. Pain and distress in fish: a review of the evidence. *ILAR Journal* 50:327–328.

Prince AMJ, Low SE, Lissimore TJ. 1995. Sodium bicarbonate and acetic acid: an effective anesthetic for field use. *North American Journal of Fisheries Management* 15:170–172.

Raines JA, Clancy MM. 2009. Sedation by orally administered ketamine in goldfish, *Carassius auratus*; hybrid striped bass, *Morone saxatilis* x *M. chrysops*; and ocellated river stingray, *Pota-*

motrygon motoro. Journal of the World Aquaculture Society 40: 788–794.

Ramanayaka JC, Atapattu NSBM. 2006. Fish anaesthetic properties of some local plant material. *Tropical Agricultural Research and Extension* 9:1–6.

Rantin FT, Glass ML, Kalinin AL, Verzola RMM, Fernandes MN. 1993. Cardio-respiratory responses in two ecologically distinct erythrinids (*Hoplias malabaricus* and *Hoplias lacerdae*) exposed to graded environmental hypoxia. *Environmental Biology of Fishes* 36:93–97.

Rantin FT, Guerra CDR, Kalinin AL, Glass ML. 1998. The influence of aquatic surface respiration (ASR) on cardio-respiratory function of the serrasalmid fish *Piaractus mesopotamicus*. *Comparative Biochemistry and Physiology* 119:991–997.

Rose JD. 2002. The neurobehavioral nature of fishes and the question of awareness and pain. *Reviews in Fisheries Science* 10: 1–38.

Ross LG. 2001. Restraint, anaesthesia, and euthanasia. In: *Manual of Ornamental Fish*, 2nd ed. (WH Wildgoose, ed.), pp. 75–83. Gloucester: BSAVA.

Ross LG, Ross B. 2008. *Anaesthetic and Sedative Techniques for Aquatic Animals.* Oxford: Blackwell Science, Ltd.

Rothwell SE, Black SE, Jerrett AR, Forster ME. 2005. Cardiovascular changes and catecholamine release following anaesthesia in Chinook salmon (*Oncorhynchus tshawytscha*) and snapper (*Pagrus auratus*). *Comparative Biochemistry and Physiology. A, Comparative Physiology* 140:289–298.

Roubach R, Gomes LC, Val AL. 2001. Safest level of tricaine methanesulfonate (MS-222) to induce anesthesia in juveniles of matrinxã, *Brycon cephalus. Acta Amazonica* 31:159–163.

Roubach R, Gomes LC, Fonesca FAL, Val AL. 2005. Eugenol as an efficacious anaesthetic for tambaqui, *Colossoma macropomum* (Cuvier). *Aquaculture Research* 36:1056–1061.

Russo R, Yanong RPE, Mitchell H. 2006. Dietary beta-glucans and nucleotides enhance resistance of red-tail black shark (*Epalzeorhynchos bicolor*, Family Cyprinidae) to *Streptococcus iniae* infection. *Journal of the World Aquaculture Society* 37:298–306.

Sandblom E, Axelsson M. 2007. The venous circulation: a piscine perspective. *Comparative Biochemistry and Physiology. A, Comparative Physiology* 148:785–801.

Schramm HL, Black DJ. 1984. Anesthesia and surgical procedures for implanting radio transmitters into grass carp. *Progressive Fish Culturist* 46:185–190.

Schreck CB, Whaley RA, Maughan OE, Solazzi M. 1976. Physiological responses of rainbow trout (*Salmo gairdneri*) to electroshock. *Journal of the Fisheries Research Board of Canada* 33:76–84.

Schreer JF, Resch DM, Gately ML, Cooke SJ. 2005. Swimming performance of brook trout after simulated catch and release angling: looking for air exposure thresholds. *North American Journal of Fisheries Management* 25:1513–1517.

Simoes LN, Gomes LC. 2009. Menthol efficiency as anesthetic for juveniles Nile tilapia Oreochromis niloticus. *Arquivo Brasileiro de Medicina Veterinária e Zootecnia* 61(3):613–620.

Sison M, Garlai R. 2010. Associative learning in zebrafish (*Danio rerio*) in the plus maze. *Behavioural Brain Research* 207:99–104.

Sladky KK, Swanson CR, Stoskopf MK, Loomis MR, Lewbart GA. 2001. Comparative efficacy of tricaine methanesulfonate and clove oil for use as anesthetics in red pacu (*Piaractus brachypomus*). *American Journal of Veterinary Research* 62:337–342.

Small BC. 2003. Anesthetic efficacy of metomidate and comparison of plasma cortisol responses to tricaine methanesulfonate, quinaldine, and clove oil anesthetized channel catfish, *Ictalurus punctatus. Aquaculture (Amsterdam, Netherlands)* 218:177–185.

Small BC. 2004. Effect of isoeugenol sedation on plasma cortisol, glucose, and lactate dynamics in channel catfish, *Ictalurus punctatus*, exposed to three stressors. *Aquaculture (Amsterdam, Netherlands)* 238:469–481.

Small BC, Chatakondi N. 2005. Routine measures of stress are reduced in mature channel catfish during and after Aqui-S anesthesia and recovery. *North American Journal of Aquaculture* 67:72–78.

Smith LS, Bell GR. 1964. A technique for prolonged blood sampling in free-swimming salmon. *Journal of the Fisheries Research Board of Canada* 21:711–717.

Sneddon LU. 2003. The evidence for pain in fish: the use of morphine as an analgesic. *Applied Animal Behaviour Science* 83: 153–162.

Sneddon LU. 2009. Pain perception in fish: indicators and endpoints. *ILAR Journal* 50:338–342.

Sneddon LU, Braithwaite VA, Gentle MJ. 2003. Do fishes have nociceptors:evidence for the evolution of the vertebrate sensory system. *Proceedings. Biological Sciences* 270:1115–1121.

Soto CG, Burhanuddin CG. 1995. Clove oil as a fish anaesthetic for measuring length and weight of rabbitfish (*Siganus lineatus*). *Aquaculture (Amsterdam, Netherlands)* 136:149–152.

Sovio A, Westman K, Nyholm K. 1972. Improved method of dorsal aorta catheterization: haematological effects followed for three weeks in rainbow trout (*Salmo gairdneri*). *Finnish Fisheries Research* 1:11–21.

Steers JE, Sherrill J. 2001. Use of oral tiletamine-zolazepam for sedation and translocation of captive yellowtail jacks (*Seriola lalandi*). Proceedings of the International Association for Aquatic Animal Medicine, pp. 168–170.

Stehly GR, Gingerich WH. 1999. Evaluation of Aqui-S™ (efficacy and minimum toxic concentration) as a fish anaesthetic/sedative for public aquaculture in the United States. *Aquaculture Research* 30:365–372.

Stetter MD. 2001. Fish and amphibian anesthesia. *Veterinary Clinics of North America Exotic Animal Practice* 4:69–82.

Storms TN, Mylniczenko ND. 2004. Pain and analgesia in fish: unanswered questions. Proceedings of the American Association of Zoo Veterinarians.

Sumpter JP, Dye HM, Benfey TJ. 1986. The effects of stress on plasma ACTH, alpha-MSH, and cortisol levels in salmonid fishes. *General and Comparative Endocrinology* 62:377–385.

Sylvester JR. 1975. Factors influencing the efficacy of MS-222 to striped mullet (*Mugil cephalus*). *Aquaculture (Amsterdam, Netherlands)* 6:163–169.

Sylvia P, Belle S, Cooper R, Krum H. 1994. Handling, restraint, anesthesia and surgery in the bluefin tuna (*Thunnus thynnus*). Proceedings of the American Association of Zoo Veterinarians, p. 189.

Taylor PW, Roberts SD. 1999. Clove oil: an alternative anaesthetic for aquaculture. *North American Journal of Aquaculture* 61: 150–155.

Thomas P, Robertson L. 1991. Plasma cortisol and glucose stress responses of red drum (*Sciaenops ocellatus*) to handling and shallow water stressors and anesthesia with MS-222, quinaldine sulfate, and metomidate. *Aquaculture (Amsterdam, Netherlands)* 96:69–86.

Thurmon JC, Tranquilli WJ, Benson GJ. 1996. History and outline if animal anesthesia. In: *Lumb and Jones' Veterinary Anesthesia*, 3rd ed. (JC Thurmon, WJ Tranquilli, GJ Benson, WV Lumb, eds.), pp. 3–4. Baltimore: William and Wilkins.

U.S. Fish and Wildlife Service, The Aquatic Animal Drug Approval Partnership. 2010. A quick reference guide to: approved drugs for use in aquaculture. http://www.fws.gov/fisheries/aadap/PDF/Quick%20Reference%20Guide%20to%20Approved%20Drugs_FINAL2%20POSTER%2026jan2010.pdf (accessed on February 16, 2014).

Vaughan DB, Penning MR, Christison KW. 2008. 2-phenoxyethanol as anaesthetic in removing and relocating 102 species of fishes representing from Sea World to uShaka Marine World South Africa. *Onderstepoort Journal of Veterinary Research* 75:189–198.

Von der Emde G. 1998. Electroreception. In: *The Physiology of Fishes* (DH Evans, ed.), pp. 313–343. Boca Raton: CRC Press.

Walsh CT, Pease BC. 2002. The use of clove oil as an anaesthetic for the longfinned eel, *Anquilla reinhardtii* (Steindachner). *Aquaculture Research* 33:627–635.

Waterstrat PR. 1999. Induction and recovery from anesthesia in channel catfish, *Ictalurus punctatus*, fingerlings exposed to clove oil. *Journal of the World Aquaculture Society* 30:250–255.

Weber ES III. 2011. Fish analgesia: pain, stress, fear aversion, or nociception? *Veterinary Clinics of North America Exotic Animal Practice* 14:21–32.

Williams TD, Christiansen J, Nygren S. 1988. Intramuscular anesthesia of teleosts and elasmobranchs using ketamine hydrochloride. Proceedings of the American Association of Zoological Parks and Aquariums, pp. 132–135.

Williams TD, Rollins M, Block BA. 2004. Intramuscular anesthesia of bonito and Pacific mackerel with ketamine and medetomidine and reversal of anesthesia with atipamezole. *Journal of the American Veterinary Medical Association* 225:417–421.

Williamson JA, Fenner PJ, Burnett JW, Rifkin JF. 1996. *Venomous and Poisonous Marine Animals: A Medical and Biological Handbook*, 4th ed. Sydney: University of New South Wales Press.

Woody CA, Nelson J, Ramstad K. 2002. Clove oil as an anaesthetic for adult sockeye salmon: field trials. *Journal of Fish Biology* 60:340–347.

Wright DE, Eastcott A. 1982. Operant conditioning of feeding behaviour and patterns of feeding in thick-lipped mullet, *Crenimugil labrosus* (Risso) and common carp, *Cyprinus carpio* (L.). *Journal of Fish Biology* 20:625–634.

Yanar M, Kumlu M. 2001. The anaesthetic effects of quinaldine sulphate and/or diazepam on sea bass (*Dicentrarchus labrax*) juveniles. *Turkish Journal of Veterinary and Animal Sciences* 25: 185–189.

Yanong RP, Curtis EW, Terrell SP, Case G. 2003. Atypical presentation of mycobacteriosis in a collection of frogfish (*Antennarius striatus*). *Journal of Zoo and Wildlife Medicine* 34:400–407.

Yanong RPE, Curtis EW, Simmons R. 2005. Pharmacokinetic studies of florfenicol in koi carp and threespot gourami *Trichogaster trichopterus* after oral and intramuscular treatment. *Journal of Aquatic Animal Health* 17:129–137.

Yanong RPE, Hartman KH, Watson CA, Hill JE, Petty BD, Francis-Floyd R. 2009. Fish slaughter, killing, and euthanasia: a review of major published US guidance documents and general considerations of methods. http://www.esf.edu/animalcare/documents/Yanong-FishEuth_FA15000_b.pdf (accessed on February 16, 2014).

Young MJ. 2009. The efficacy of the aquatic anaesthetic Aqui-S™ for anaesthesia of a small freshwater fish, *Melanotaenia australis*. *Journal of Fish Biology* 75:1888–1894.

Zahl IH, Kiessling A, Samuelsen OB, Hansen MK. 2009. Anaesthesia of Atlantic cod (*Gadus morhua*): effect of preanaesthetic sedation and importance of body weight, temperature, and stress. *Aquaculture (Amsterdam, Netherlands)* 295:52–59.

Zahl IH, Kiessling A, Samuelsen OB, Olsen RE. 2010. Anesthesia induces stress in Atlantic salmon (*Salmo salar*), Atlantic cod (*Gadus morhua*), and Atlantic halibut (*Hippoglossus hippoglossus*). *Fish Physiology and Biochemistry* 36:719–730.

16 Elasmobranchs and Holocephalans

Natalie D. Mylniczenko, Tonya M. Clauss, and M. Andrew Stamper

INTRODUCTION

The class Chondrichthyes is comprised of nearly 1200 extant species worldwide (Compagno 1999) belonging to two subclasses, Elasmobranchii and Holocephalii. They are probably the most successful of all fishes based on historical endurance in the fossil records (Grogan & Lund 2004). Elasmobranchs (sharks and batoids) represent 96% of the cartilaginous fishes, while the Holocephalans (chimeras and elephant fish) represent only 4% (Compagno 1999), and as such, elasmobranchs are the primary focus in this chapter. With so many different species and such variety of anatomical and physiological characteristics among them, immobilization and anesthesia can be challenging. Additionally, much of the information relied upon for anesthesia in cartilaginous fishes has been anecdotal.

Due to the variable and often inconsistent reactions to drugs intra- and interspecies, extrapolation of drug doses between species is often difficult and unpredictable. Growth of the aquatic animal medicine field has resulted in a greater breadth of clinical experience with teleost and elasmobranch fishes. This has led to some generalities that can be applied to facilitate safe and effective immobilization and anesthesia.

Various situations arise that require fish to be immobilized, including research and clinical procedures, as well as field activities. As mentioned in Chapter 15, however, the debate over the necessity for chemical immobilization and anesthesia in fish continues. Elasmobranchs do possess opioid receptors and receptor-like DNA sequences and cyclooxygenase. There is, however, histological evidence some axonal layers are missing from the spinal cords of some species. This suggests transmission of pain to the central nervous system is either limited, not possible or at the very least different from pain transmission in "higher" animals (Davis et al. 2006; Rose 2002; Snow et al. 1993). Regardless of this neuroanatomical evidence, these animals (unless behaviorally conditioned) often respond negatively to even mildly invasive stimuli, such as injections. Decisions on whether to manually or chemically immobilize an animal should be based on the invasiveness of the procedures planned, the duration of time the animal will need to be immobilized, experience and capabilities of staff involved, and human and animal safety. When chemical immobilization is deemed necessary, determination of what drug or drug combination should be used depends on the level and duration of sedation or anesthesia desired, method and feasibility of delivery of the drug, and ability to safely support and monitor the animal through recovery.

ANATOMY AND PHYSIOLOGY

A full discussion of the anatomy and physiology of the cartilaginous fishes is outside the scope of this chapter, and has been well described in detail in other texts (Carrier et al. 2004, 2011; Hamlett 1999; Oetinger & Zorzi 1995; Smith et al. 2004). Some of their unique characteristics, however, should be taken into account when considering immobilization and anesthesia as they may have a direct impact on the outcome of a procedure. The stress response is one such factor.

As with teleost fish, elasmobranchs possess a functional hypothalamic-pituitary-interrenal (HPI) axis based on the presence of adrenocorticotropic hormone (ACTH), which regulates interrenal production of 1α-hydroxycorticosterone (1α-OHB), a primary corticosteroid, which is produced only in elasmobranchs and which is currently difficult to study since there are no

Zoo Animal and Wildlife Immobilization and Anesthesia, Second Edition. Edited by Gary West, Darryl Heard, and Nigel Caulkett.

available assays for its measurement (Anderson 2012; Idler & Truscott 1966, 1967, 1968, 1969; Truscott & Idler 1968, 1972). Comparatively, cortisol is not present in elasmobranchs, while it is the primary corticosteroid in teleost fish (Skomal & Bernal 2011). Corticosterone (CS) is also found in measurable concentrations in some elasmobranch species (Rasmussen & Crow 1993; Rasmussen & Gruber 1990, 1993; Snelson et al. 1997), but 1α-OHB has been shown to be the dominant hormone. It is likely that early reports of cortisol and CS levels were due to interference with the 1α-hydroxycorticosterone under certain assays (fluorimetric). CS assays are currently being used as an indirect measure of 1α-OHB. However, CS also shows elevations with the reproductive cycle. Interpretation of the results of CS assays must, therefore, take these effects into account (Anderson 2012; Skomal & Bernal 2011).

There are few studies of the role of the HPI axis in regulating the elasmobranch primary stress response. Catecholamines increase immediately after a stressor and peak after the cessation of the event (Randall & Perry 1992). Manire et al. (2007) found both a short and long-term CS response to capture and handling stress in bonnethead sharks (*Sphyrna tiburo*). These reports suggest a relationship between stress and the activity of the interrenal gland. The secondary stress response has been studied more than the primary response; receiving a lot of attention in the last several years (Adrian Van Rijn & Reina 2010; Frick & Reina 2009; Karsten & Rice 2004; Mandelman & Farrington 2007; Mandelmann & Skomal 2009; Marshall et al. 2012; Naples et al. 2012; Renshaw et al. 2012). This information can be very useful in assessing elasmobranchs, and clinical applications will be discussed later in this chapter.

Chemical immobilization and anesthesia can decrease the stress response associated with handling, as well as decrease the chance of injury to the people, animals, and equipment involved. An adequately anesthetized fish is easier to handle and manipulate, providing more diagnostic opportunities.

The response to a drug is dependent on many factors including drug receptor type and tissue distribution, method of administration, body temperature, hepatic biotransformation, blood distribution, renal function, and respiratory mechanism and function. These, among other factors, explain the frequent variation of drug effect seen in elasmobranchs both within and between species. Drug-binding sites are molecular locations on target tissues. The use of mammalian anesthetic drugs in elasmobranchs may result in several possible outcomes: (1) they may bind to the same active binding site and produce the desired effect; (2) there may be a chemically similar binding site, but one that triggers a different physiological function resulting in a completely different response; (3) there may be a

lower number of binding sites resulting in a weakened response or conversely, there may be more binding sites thus requiring more drug to fill these sites; (4) the binding site may be slightly different in anatomy resulting in the inability to bind; or (5) there may be no binding sites at all resulting in no effect. Drugs can also bind with blood proteins or other nontarget tissue, thus altering the amount of drug available and the effect on target tissue.

Drug administration in elasmobranchs may be via inhalation/immersion, injection (intravenous, intramuscular, and intracoelomic) or orally. Some drugs that produce a notable response when administered intravenously may produce little to no response when delivered intramuscularly or orally (Clauss et al. 2011; Mylniczenko, pers. exp.). Drugs delivered intramuscularly may produce variable responses dependent upon the injection site on the animal's body. As with some teleosts, sharks have red and white muscles (Fig. 16.1a). In most sharks, the red (myotomal) muscles are located more laterally along the body of the fish and are aerobic versus the more predominant anaerobic, white muscle. Injection into white muscle is most likely since it is the predominant anaerobic muscle type. Anesthetic injections in the red muscle may result in more rapid induction times as has been noted in some teleosts (Williams et al. 2004). Due to the variable density of vasculature associated with myotomal muscle bodies (Bernal et al. 2001; Bernal & Graham 2001; Totland et al. 1981), however, drug uptake can still be relatively unpredictable.

Active sharks (e.g., hammerhead [*Sphyrna mokkaran*] and blacktip [*Carcharhinus limbatus*]) have a higher percentage of myotomal muscles (up to 22%) than less active sharks (e.g., nurse shark [*Ginglymostoma cirratum*] and epaulette [*Hemiscyllium ocellatum*]) (Bone 1999). The even more active sharks from the Lamnidae (e.g., porbeagle [*Lamna nasus*], mako [*Isurus oxyrinchus*], white [*Carcharodon carcharias*]) family, and the common thresher shark from the Alopiidae family have a similar muscular plan, except that the myotomal framework is unique and similar to that of scombrid teleosts (e.g., tuna and mackerel). In these species, the red muscle is condensed into a solid piston-like muscle mass that is found closer to the vertebrae (Bernal et al. 2001; Carey et al. 1985; Graham & Dickson 2000, 2001; Graham et al. 1983; Sepulveda et al. 2005). In these highly active elasmobranchs, the vascular supply to this red muscle is through a set of lateral vessels that give rise to a counter-current heat exchange system (retia mirabilia). This allows conservation of metabolically derived heat, giving these sharks some endothermic abilities. The red muscle temperature may be elevated significantly above ambient (Bernal et al. 2003; Bone & Chubb 1983; Carey et al. 1971) and produce regional endothermy. Environmental temperature may have little to no impact on the metabolic rates of these endothermic sharks. Ambient

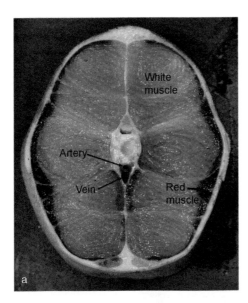 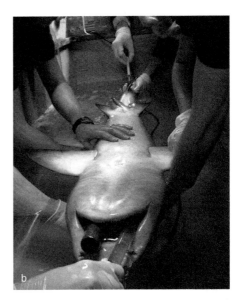

Figure 16.1. (a) Cross section of the tail of a blacktip reef shark (*Carcharhinus melanopterus*) demonstrating the more vascular or "red" muscle in comparison with the "white" muscle. Note the location of the artery and vein in comparison to the vertebral column. (b) Assisted ventilation in a sandbar shark (*Carcharhinus plumbeus*). There is a PVC tube in place to keep the mouth open. A continuous flow pump is used to direct oxygenated water over the gills. Water flow out of the gill slits determines appropriate positioning.

temperature, however, plays a major role in controlling the metabolic rates of the majority of elasmobranchs, which are ectothermic. Body temperature, therefore, must be considered as it impacts metabolic rates, determines enzyme activity, and may influence drug elimination and duration of effect.

In most studied animals, the liver metabolizes certain drugs to either active or inactive forms. Elasmobranch liver size and composition is species dependent, but is overall larger than other animals and more lipid rich. In the normal animal, it can account for up to 23% of body weight and as much as 80% may be lipid (Holmgren & Nilsson 1999). The pharmacodynamics of drugs are dependent, in part, on their lipophilic or lipophobic solubility, as well as the amount of hepatic cellular exposure. This adds an additional layer of complexity to drug metabolism in elasmobranchs. Unfortunately, there is very little pharmacokinetic data in elasmobranchs, especially with regard to anesthetics.

The kidney is very different to that of mammals, having a higher filtration rate and different selectivity (Lacy & Reale 1999). These differences may influence drug elimination rates. Like reptiles and other nonmammals, elasmobranchs have a renal-portal system that allows blood from the caudal half of the animal to drain directly into the kidneys. Historically, injections in the caudal half of the body were avoided in reptiles and fish as theory suggested the renal portal system may enhance the nephrotoxicity or influence renal excretion of drugs. Studies in reptiles, however, found no significant difference in drug metabolism when injections were given in the fore or hind limbs suggesting the renal portal system

has little, if any, negative influence on drug metabolism (Beck et al. 1995; Holz, 1999; Holz et al. 2002). Based on the studies in reptiles, it is unlikely the renal portal system poses a threat to drug action or metabolism in elasmobranchs.

The basic function of the respiratory system is the exchange of gases (oxygen, pH, and carbon dioxide). While simplistic in theory, elasmobranchs manage their metabolic exchange of these gases differently. The elasmobranchs can be classified into categories based on their methods of respiration: pelagic (open water), intermediary, and benthic. Examples of these include: (1) pelagic: black tip (*C. limbatus*) and blue shark (*Prionace glauca*); (2) intermediate: sand tiger shark (*Carcharhinus taurus*) and brown shark (*Carcharhinus plumbeus*); (3) benthic: Japanese wobbegong (*Orectolobus japonicas*) and the nurse shark (*G. cirratum*). Many pelagic elasmobranchs rely on ram ventilation, forcing water over their gills by swimming constantly. The nonpelagic animals are able to pump water over their gills and can rest on the bottom for extended periods of time. These animals tend to have a higher tolerance for lower oxygen environmental conditions (Mylniczenko et al. 2007). The nonpelagic animals can further be divided into intermediate or benthic respirators. Benthic animals are those that spend much of their active time on the sea bottom, while the intermediates swim more than they rest. The classifications are not strict. In general, benthic animals are able to buffer acidemia and/or manage hypoxemia more efficiently. This is critical because activity (such as capture) will significantly affect elasmobranch blood gases and physiologic status. In general, there are few obligate ram ventilators in aquaria, but these animals need additional care during anesthesia and recovery to ensure adequate ventilation.

Most benthic sharks and batoids have an additional respiratory feature, the spiracle, located dorsally behind the eyes. This opening may serve as an alternate route for channeling water over the gills when the mouth of these elasmobranchs is in contact with the sediment or substrate. It is suggested that the spiracle function is voluntary to prevent sand entry into the gills (Butler 1999). During anesthesia, ventilation may occur either via the mouth or through the spiracles. The advantage to ventilation via the mouth is flow may easily be directed over both gill sets simultaneously (Fig. 16.1b). Specific modifications are necessary to achieve simultaneous flow over both gill sets when water is directed through the spiracles.

Other physiological or anatomical factors that may influence drug response include gill surface area to body weight ratio, lipid content, stress, health status, and body condition changes associated with age, season, sexual maturity, and nutrition. There are, therefore, many variables that need to be considered when anesthetizing elasmobranchs.

CAPTURE

Many elasmobranchs housed in public aquaria share large systems with mixed species. Catching these animals can be challenging and even dangerous to both the people and animals involved. Retrieving these animals may be done either by using behavioral conditioning, manually using a variety of techniques or with chemical immobilization. Regardless of the method used, minimizing distress and maintaining safety should be primary goals. Elasmobranchs are very responsive to behavioral conditioning and training techniques. The benefits of animal training programs include enrichment, better animal control and monitoring, reduced stress during handling, implementation of advanced husbandry techniques, enhanced education programs, and positive associations between animals and caretakers (Baker 1991). Operant conditioning is a process by which a subject produces a behavior in the presence of a cue on the condition of achieving desirable outcomes or avoiding undesirable consequences. A number of facilities have achieved impressive results through operant conditioning and behavioral modification (Fig. 16.2a,b).

Behaviors as seemingly simple as target training or station feeding can be invaluable. Staff from the International Zoological Applications at Parque Nizuc, Cancun, Mexico successfully trained a group of nurse sharks (*G. cirratum*), southern stingrays (*Dasyatis americana*) and chupare stingrays (*Himantura schmardae*) to do a number of advanced husbandry and veterinary

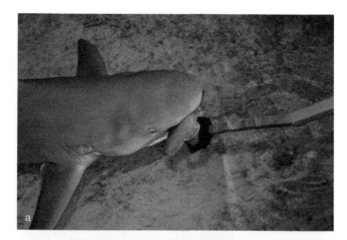

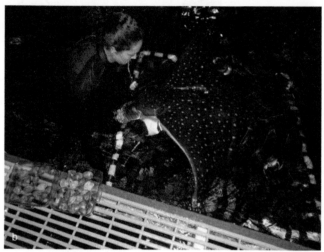

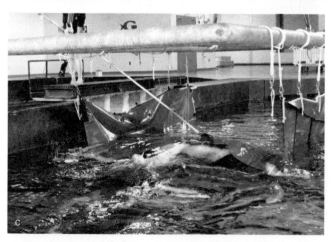

Figure 16.2. (a) A sandbar shark (*Carcharhinus plumbeus*) target feeding during a training session. (b) An eagle ray (*Aetobatus narinari*) targeting over a stretcher in a training session. (c) Behaviorally conditioning a manta ray (*Manta alfredi*) to swim into and through a stretcher (photo credit: Georgia Aquarium).

procedures, including shifting areas of the exhibit, stretcher training, and layouts for ultrasound examination (Sabalones et al. 2004). Animal care staff at the Georgia Aquarium, Atlanta, GA, conditioned four manta rays (*Manta birostris*) to swim into and through

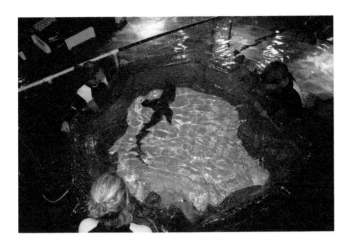

Figure 16.3. A partially deflated swimming pool in a larger medical pool used to corral a sandbar shark (*Carcharhinus plumbeus*) into a smaller area for anesthesia. The pool was measured for volume when fully inflated and in the water in order to provide accurate dosing with immersion anesthesia.

a stretcher to enable physical examinations and collection of morphometric data (Fig. 16.2c). Similarly, at the John G. Shedd Aquarium, Chicago, IL, sharks and sawfish were trained to swim into a deflated swimming pool (which is then inflated once the animal is captured) or into a chute/restraint device for induction of anesthesia (Fig. 16.3). Behavioral management in some of the larger elasmobranchs is arguably a necessity as manually catching and restraining can be difficult, if not impossible, and has the potential to cause significant stress and possible injury to the staff and animal(s).

When animals are not conditioned to present behaviorally for exams or other procedures, more invasive capture techniques must be used and may or may not involve administration of drugs. Staff at the Melbourne Aquarium in Melbourne, Australia routinely caught four adult broadnose sevengill (*Notorynchus cepedianus*) sharks out of the "Oceanarium" for ultrasound examination using a 300-cm, clear vinyl bag with Velcro® closures. The narrow end of the bag was covered with a nylon mesh to enable water flow to be directed at the head of the shark. Three divers operated the bag, one at the closed end and two at the entrance. A fourth diver guided the nonanesthetized shark into the bag. The bag and shark were then brought into a holding area for the procedures (Daly et al. 2007). A similar set-up is used at uShaka Marine World Durbin, South Africa for the capture of their animals. They utilize the device, however, only for sedated animals due to the species they regularly work with (Fig. 16.4a). At the Georgia Aquarium in Atlanta, Georgia, staff periodically catch unanesthetized large batoids (e.g., bowmouth (*Rhina ancylostoma*) (Fig. 16.4b) and giant guitar fish (*Rhynchobatus djiddensis*), sawfish (Fig. 16.4c–e),

and pink whiprays (*Himantura fai*) from a 6.4 million gallon exhibit using a large box net. The square PVC frame and attached knotless net is sunk to the exhibit floor. Divers in SCUBA corral the target animal over the net and people at the surface then haul the net up rapidly. The animal may then be restrained manually or chemically. Smaller sharks, such as bonnetheads and blacktips, may be caught via a hoop net when they approach a feeding station. Though this technique has proven successful much of the time, care should be taken not to over use this technique as the behavior of showing up to station for feeding may be broken if a negative event occurs frequently.

In some cases, a net draped across the width of a tank and pushed across the length of the enclosure can be used to both encourage animals into a medical pool and to limit the overall size of the area animals need to be captured in. This technique also allows the possibility to significantly reduce the depth of the area by bringing the bottom of the net to a more comfortable depth (Fig. 16.4f,g). Disadvantages include the amount of staff/divers required to execute a "catch up" as well as catching multiple animals and nontarget animals. Animals such as sawfish in these situations are difficult to manage and need to be excluded.

Drugs may also be used to assist in retrieving elasmobranchs from an exhibit or holding system. Immersion anesthetics are often impractical (but possible) due to tank size and presence of other animals. However, divers may spray very concentrated immersion agents such as tricaine methanesulfonate (MS-222) or eugenol directly over the gills of an animal to sedate it long enough to gain physical control. Injectable drugs may be delivered while the animal is swimming. This is usually done intramuscularly, but intravenous anesthetics have been delivered to a variety of rays and whale sharks by staff at the Okinawa Churaumi Aquarium in Okinawa, Japan (Yanagisawa, pers. comm., 2011) and to whale sharks at the Osaka Aquarium KAIYUKAN in Osaka, Japan (Ito, pers. comm., 2011). When dealing with the more active or aggressive animals, diligent care must be taken when administering drugs via pole syringe, nearby darting apparatus, and especially when hand injecting. Animals, when surprised, even if partially sedated, may turn around on a diver and inflict harm in their effort to ward off a threat. The speed of the animal and the trauma from their teeth or skin cannot be underestimated. Oral medications may also be delivered if the animal in question is target or station trained. Oral doses required to sedate elasmobranchs are often quite high and the amount of drug required may be volume limiting or cause the animal to regurgitate the food item it is delivered in. As with injectable agents, the response to oral anesthetics is often unpredictable. Anesthetics and sedation will be discussed in greater detail later in this chapter.

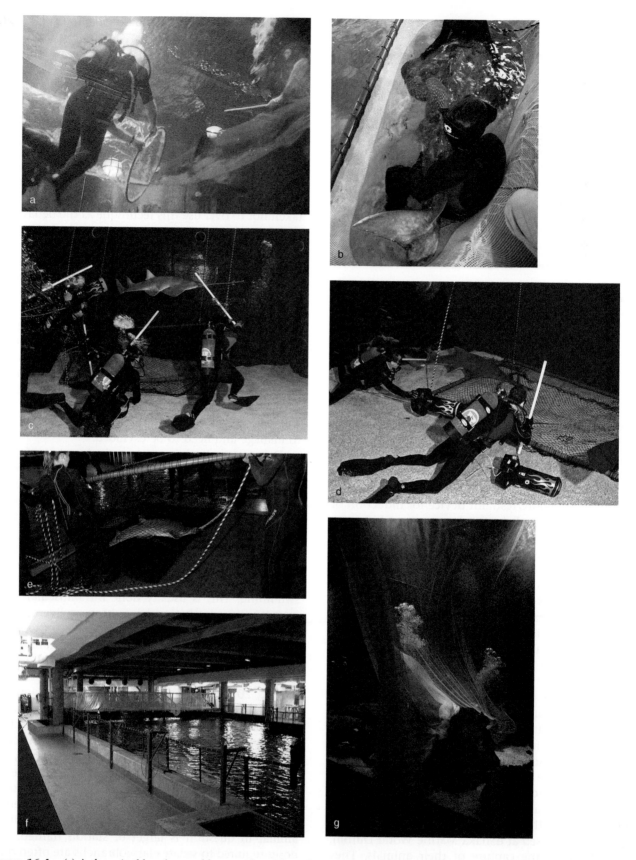

Figure 16.4. (a) A clear vinyl bag (a round hoop at the wide end and a narrower hole, to allow for water flow, at the distal portion of the bag) used to guide a shark into the bag for transport to the surface of the water and further restraint into a sling (photo credit: Gavin Drysdale, uShaka Marine World Durbin, South Africa). (b) Restraint of a bowmouth guitarfish (*Rhina ancylostoma*) in a partially submerged boxnet (photo credit: Georgia Aquarium). (c, d, and e) Retrieval of a largetooth sawfish (*Pristis microdon*) from an exhibit utilizing a boxnet. SCUBA divers corral the animal over the submerged net which is then quickly hoisted to the surface (photo credit: Marj Awai, Georgia Aquarium). (f) A metal bridge across an enclosure with a net (wall-to-wall) that extends to the depth of the tank. The bridge and net can move across the entire tank to isolate animals or push them from one end to the other. (g) The same net as in Figure 16.4b with an underwater view of divers maneuvering the net over coral heads in the enclosure's bottom.

PHYSICAL RESTRAINT

Tonic immobility (TI) or hypnosis is one form of physical restraint used in a variety of elasmobranchs. Tonic immobility is induced by placing an animal in dorsal recumbency. Though these animals, especially batoids, may go through a period of marked excitability during the initial catch and handling, once in this hypnotic state, they are subdued. The level of restraint and duration of effect is highly variable between species. This technique has been reported in a variety of elasmobranchs, including the clearnose skate (*Raja eglanteria*), cownose ray (*Rhinoptera bonasus*), southern stingray (*D. americana*), blacktip reef shark (*Carcharhinus melanopterus*), Caribbean reef shark (*Carcharhinus perezii*), leopard shark (*Triakis semifasciata*), swellshark (*Cephaloscyllium ventriosum*), whitetip reef shark (*Triaenodon obesus*), and shovelnose guitarfish (*Rhinobatos lentiginosus*). When immobilized with TI, the blood pressure and heart rate of *C. melanopterus* decreased significantly. Branchial irrigation improved blood pressure in these animals, but heart rate was unchanged (Davie et al. 1993; Henningsen 1994). This indicates a vagal nerve response with the ability to have physiologic shifts based on ventilator support. Some aquaria report that pinching the dorsal fin will have a calming effect on some species, akin to reptile ocular–vagal responses; however this is anecdotal and not recommended as a standalone method of restraint.

Manual restraint in species that do not experience TI or when it is unsuccessful can be challenging and induce stress responses in the animal. Even when not utilizing manual restraint for an entire procedure, it is often necessary at the onset of a chemical immobilization. In those cases, rapid restraint either by netting or by hand is recommended if it can be done safely. Pursuing animals for prolonged periods frequently results in rapid elevations of lactate and acidemia. Only experienced staff should be involved with manual restraint of elasmobranchs. Even some of the smallest species are extremely strong, thus increasing the chances of injury to people and animals. Some additional human safety factors to consider include (1) abrasions from the placoid scales in sharks, (2) sharp teeth, spines, or crushing plates in the oral cavity, (3) barbs on stingrays, and in some of the freshwater ray species, the surrounding epidermal bumps are venomous (Mylniczenko 2010). To mitigate these issues, under dangerous situations, it is advisable to utilize baffles made of mesh and PVC or some other shielding device (Fig. 16.5), to wear appropriate gloves that prevent bite and crush injuries (e.g., Kevlar gloves), and in some circumstances, to wear suits that prevent bodily injury (e.g., chain mail suits specifically designed to work with dangerous aquatic animals). Ideally, in case of traumatic injury, there should also be an emergency diver evacuation plan in place and access

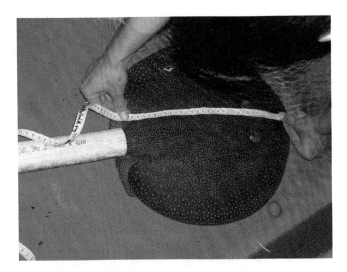

Figure 16.5. A PVC safety tube placed over the tail of a freshwater stingray (family Potamotrygonidae).

to first aid either by trained personnel or a nearby emergency response unit.

Chimaerids offer unique handling challenges in that they are soft-skinned and have ambient light restrictions (because they have an all-rod retina they must minimize the amount of light that enters the retina). These animals should be handled with soft mesh or plastic nets and corralled under water as they are very sensitive to net trauma. Ideally, procedures should be conducted in low light. They have a spine that precedes the first dorsal fin that contains weak venom, therefore staff should handle cautiously.

VASCULAR ACCESS

Access to elasmobranchs vasculature is often determined by the size and position of the animal rather than which vessel is most ideal. The largest blood vessel accessible with the animal in dorsal recumbency, in both sharks and rays, is the artery or vein that lies along the midline just ventral to the vertebral column (Fig. 16.1 and Fig. 16.6a). These vessels are located by placing the needle just posterior to the base of the trailing edge of the first or second anal fins in sharks or just caudal to the vent in rays. The needle is directed anteriorly at an angle of 30–90°, relative to the body, and inserted until the needle tip meets cartilage (approximately 4 cm for a 10 kg shark) to penetrate the vessel (Stoskopf et al. 1984). In large-bodied species and mature animals, needles may become plugged during penetration of the cartilage wall protecting the vessel. A spinal needle (with a removable stylet protecting the needle aperture) is used in these larger animals. However, longer needles may be difficult to place accurately on midline, therefore careful threading is necessary.

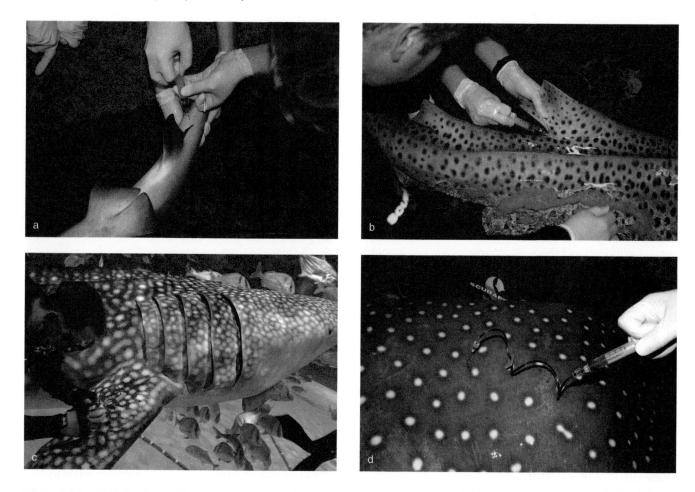

Figure 16.6.   (a) Collection of blood from a ventral tail vessel in a whitetip reef shark (*Triaenodon obesus*). (b) Collection of blood from the dorsal sinus in a vessel in a zebra shark (*Stegostoma fasciatum*). (c) Underwater collection of blood from the pectoral fin vasculature of a whale shark (*Rhincodon typus*) under behavioral control using a specialized feeding technique (photo credit: Georgia Aquarium). (d) Collection of blood from the wing vessel in an eagle ray (*Aetobatus narinari*).

There is a vascular plexus associated with the dorsal fins that is commonly referred to as the "dorsal sinus" (Fig. 16.6b). The first and second dorsal fins have this plexus and it can be found in most shark species as well as numerous batoids. It is a viable access port for blood collection as well as drug administration and is considered an access point to the secondary circulatory system. The reader is cautioned with interpretation of blood work from this site as it does have variations compared to the central vasculature system (Mylniczenko et al. 2006). Regardless, various species have been successfully anesthetized using this route.

The pectoral fin vasculature in large sharks, such as whale sharks, as well as wing vessels in rays, can be used for either blood collection or administration of intravenous drugs (Fig. 16.6c). The wing vessel in rays can be found by palpating the cartilaginous rays and then placing the needle in front of the cartilage, advancing the needle slowly with slight negative pressure in the syringe until a flash is obtained (Fig. 16.6d).

Catheterization of the ventral coccygeal vein or dorsal sinus is possible, but difficult to maintain. When successful, it permits medications to be given in a direct, consistent manner over a long period of time.

PREANESTHETIC CONSIDERATIONS

Ideally, preanesthetic assessment will include a thorough history of the fish, information on water quality conditions and husbandry practices, remote observation (preferably in the original habitat) and familiarization with any unique characteristics of the species or individual. Fish often present to the clinician when they are already systemically ill. This represents an anesthetic risk, particularly since the etiology will likely be unknown until an examination is conducted.

Determining if water quality conditions may be a contributing factor in a disease process is important, and evaluation prior to sedation can be helpful. If the fish has been transported to the clinician, the water quality variables of the transport vessel should be tested as well. Observation of fish in their primary habitat or even in a transport or holding vessel is useful for assessing swim patterns, posture, general appearance and demeanor, as well as obtaining respiratory rates.

Even minimal handling can be stressful to healthy fish. A full clinical examination or blood work prior to anesthesia may, therefore, not be feasible or reasonable. The stress and potential trauma associated with manual restraint for diagnostics and morphometrics may be more risky than anesthetizing a fish without that information. When the body weight cannot be safely obtained prior to anesthesia, other methods exist for estimation, such as the length-to-weight ratio data exist for some species. When this information is not available, blind estimates may have to be made if oral or injectable anesthetics are used. However, this may greatly affect the quality and depth of the anesthesia. If this is the case, a weight and fork length should be taken and documented for future work.

As with most other animals, it is preferable fish be fasted prior to anesthesia so the anesthetic water and/ or the procedure container are not fouled if regurgitation or elimination occurs. Caretakers should be instructed to bring additional water with them that may be used if the transport water is fouled and/or for recovery from anesthesia.

Once an animal is removed from its primary habitat, all actions associated with transport, handling, and anesthesia should be swift and precise to minimize the stress response. Ideally, a preanesthetic meeting is conducted to ensure animal and human safety by outlining the goals of the capture, procedure, and recovery process, as well as identifying the responsibilities for each person that is partaking in the event. Thorough preparation prior to an anesthetic procedure is essential in providing fish with the best opportunity for a full recovery.

CHEMICAL IMMOBILIZATION

The use of chemical restraint can provide a safer, less stressful procedure for the fish and staff involved. Minimization of movement and the ability to perform procedures with a fish out of the water often reduces handling time. Some diagnostic techniques and procedures cannot be adequately performed when animal movement occurs (e.g., magnetic resonance imaging, computed tomography, and standard radiography), and thus chemical immobilization is essential. The authors have compiled cited and anecdotal dosages of anesthetics used in various species of elasmobranchs (Table 16.1). Anesthetics may be delivered via inhalation, injection or per os.

Immersion (Inhalation) Anesthesia

Waterborne or immersion anesthesia is still the most widely used method for sedating or anesthetizing elasmobranchs and holocephalans. The chemical in aqueous solution is ventilated by the fish, passes into the blood via the gills, and is delivered to the central nervous system. An extensive discussion of immersion anesthetics, including delivery techniques, mechanisms of action, metabolism and clearance, as well as advantages and disadvantages, can be found in Chapter 15. The same principles used in boney fish also apply to elasmobranchs and holocephalans. Immersion anesthetics are most commonly administered with the fish submerged in a specified concentration of the drug. Depending on clinician preference, a higher concentration of a drug may be used to induce anesthesia, with a lower concentration being used to maintain the preferred plane of anesthesia. These chemicals have the advantage of being relatively safe to deliver, and the concentration can be modified by addition or dilution of the solution. One disadvantage of immersion medications is the large amount of drug needed when immobilizing animals in large bodies of water, such as those many captive elasmobranchs inhabit. As previously mentioned, some waterborne anesthetics may be delivered in high concentration via direct administration to the gills. Gilbert and Kritzler (1960) anesthetized large sharks and rays with MS-222 (1 g/L) delivered through a hand pump sprayer while animals were free swimming. Care must be taken with this approach, as some of these larger specimens are predatory and delivery requires the anesthetist to be in very close proximity to the mouth of the animal. An alternative that facilitates the use of immersion anesthetics is training or conditioning fish to shift into smaller bodies of water, such as secondary systems or smaller containers. An example of the latter is an inflatable pool submerged partially deflated in the main tank (Fig. 16.3). Air is then added to fully inflate the pool once the water is in the body of the pool. In large elasmobranchs, even after an animal is moved to a smaller container, the volume of drug needed for adequate immobilization can still be great. The technique of applying high concentrations of the anesthetic over the gills via the gill slits or through the spiracles, if present, can further reduce the volume of drug needed (Fig. 16.7a–c).

Tricaine Methanesulfonate (MS-222) This water-soluble, benzocaine derivative is used at a range of 50–150 mg/L to anesthetize both sharks and batoids (Larid & Oswald 1975). The concentration is varied with species and procedures performed. If delivering via a hand pump, even higher concentrations will likely be necessary for induction (1–2 g/L). One author (Stamper) has used up to 25 g/L. The drug is acidic and requires buffering. Sodium bicarbonate is the most commonly used buffering agent and is usually mixed at a ratio of two parts buffer to one part drug based on weight. Cavin and Innis (pers. comm.) have modified their protocols to an effective concentration of 5–6 g/L

Table 16.1. Anesthetic and immobilization drugs used in elasmobranchs

Species	Common Name	Drug	Dose or Dosage	Route of Administration	Body Wt (kg)	Population	Age Class	Water Temp (C°)	Comments	Reference
Squalus acanthias	Spiny dogfish	Hexobarbital	20mg/kg	IV					Recovery of righting reflex—3 hours.	Adamson and Guarino (1972)
Squalus acanthias	Spiny dogfish	Sodium pentobarbital	20mg/kg	IV					Recovery of righting reflex—6–8 hours.	Adamson and Guarino (1972)
Squalus acanthias	Spiny dogfish	Thiopental	20mg/kg	IV					Recovery of righting reflex—3 hours.	Adamson and Guarino (1972)
Carcharhinus plumbeus	Sandbar shark (brown shark)	Dexmedetomidine + ketamine	0.03mg/kg + 2mg/kg	IM		0.1.0	3 years		Added saline to make a 1mL injection. Purpose of exam: mass removal.	Boylan, pers. comm.
Carcharhinus plumbeus	Sandbar shark (brown shark)	Dexmedetomidine + ketamine + midazolam	0.036mg/kg + 7mg/kg + 0.5mg/kg	IM	21				Able to swim animal into a net	Boylan, pers. comm.
Carcharhinus taurus	Sand tiger shark	Medetomidine + diazepam + ketamine	0.5mg + 7.5mg + 50mg	IM		1.0.0				Boylan, pers. comm.
Carcharhinus taurus	Sand tiger shark	Medetomidine + midazolam hydrochloride + ketamine	0.5mg + 7.5mg + 50mg	IM		1.0.0				Boylan, pers. comm.
Ginglymostoma cirratum	Nurse shark	Quinoline salts	0.075–0.1mM	Immersion	4.0/21.0/4.5	1.2.0			Blood levels reached fairly constant value within 15 minutes	Brown et al. (1972)
Negaprion brevirostris	Lemon shark	Quinoline salts	0.075–0.1mM	Immersion	5.7 / 7.0	1.1.0			Blood levels reached fairly constant value withinn 15 minutes	Brown et al. (1972)
Negaprion brevirostris	Lemon shark	Quinoline salts	0.15mM	Immersion	5.7/7.0/4.1	3.0.0	young	26.5	Quickly produced anesthesia; drug enters brain rapidly	Brown et al. (1972)
Squalus acanthias	Spiny dogfish	Medetomidine + ketamine	200µg/kg + 4mg/kg	IM		0.0.15			Adequate for sedation, not for surgical anesthesia	Cavin et al. (2007)
Squalus acanthias	Spiny dogfish	Propofol	5mg/kg	IV		0.0.15			Good for surgical anesthesia	Cavin et al. (2007)
Carcharhinus taurus 1	Sand tiger shark	Dexmedetomidine + ketamine	0.05mg/kg + 10mg/kg	IM		1.0			Induction. Used repeatedly (some dosage variation) with varied results, some recoveries rapid, some prolonged (days).	Cavin and Innis, pers. comm.
Carcharhinus taurus 1	Sand tiger shark	MS-222	90mg/L	Immersion		1.0			Maintenance; plan to reduce to 70mg/L MS-222	Cavin and Innis, pers. comm.
Carcharhinus taurus 1	Sand tiger shark	MS-222	12.5g/L	Spray to gills		1.0			35 minutes after injection	Cavin and Innis, pers. comm.

Species	Common name	Drug	Dose	Route		Comments	Reference
Carcharhinus taurus 2	Sand tiger shark	Dexmedetomidine + ketamine	0.03 mg/kg + 3 mg/kg	IM	1.0	Induction for transport. Slightly reactive and ventilating well. Intermittent and prolonged periods of resting on the bottom.	Cavin and Innis, pers. comm.
Carcharhinus taurus 2	Sand tiger shark	MS-222	12.5 g/L	Spray to gills	1.0	Technique performed underwater by divers, not sprayed directly onto the gills. This concentration is highly acidic; currently used at 5–6 g/L buffered 4:1 with bicarb (20–24 g/L).	Cavin and Innis, pers. comm.
Carcharhinus taurus 3	Sand tiger shark	Dexmedetomidine + ketamine	0.03 mg/kg + 3.3 mg/kg	IM	0.0.1	Rapid induction within 11 minutes with minimal respiration	Cavin and Innis, pers. comm.
Carcharhinus taurus 3	Sand tiger shark	MS-222	70 mg/L	Immersion	0.0.1	Maintenance (very short period of time)	Cavin and Innis, pers. comm.
Carcharhinus taurus 4	Sand tiger shark	Dexmedetomidine	0.03 mg/kg	IM	0.0.1	Good sedation—removed from tank after 20 minutes	Cavin and Innis, pers. comm.
Carcharhinus taurus 5	Sand tiger shark	Dexmedetomidine + Ketamine	0.03 mg/kg + 3.3 mg/kg	IM	0.1	Rapid induction within 11 minutes with minimal respiration	Cavin and Innis, pers. comm.
Carcharhinus taurus 5	Sand tiger shark	MS-222	70 mg/L	Immersion	0.1	Maintenance; increased to 90 mg/L due to mild arousal	Cavin and Innis, pers. comm.
Carcharhinus taurus 6	Sand tiger shark	Dexmedetomidine	0.03 mg/kg	IM	0.1	Good sedation—removed from tank after 20 minutes	Cavin and Innis, pers. comm.
Carcharhinus taurus 6	Sand tiger shark	MS-222	50 mg/L	Immersion	0.1	Transport bin	Cavin and Innis, pers. comm.
Ginglymostma cirratum 2	Nurse shark	Dexmedetomidine	~0.03 mg/kg	IM	0.1	Induction; minimal sedation after 30 minutes	Cavin and Innis, pers. comm.
Ginglymostma cirratum 2	Nurse shark	MS-222	25 g/L	Spray to gills	0.1	20 minutes of spraying (in tank) before sedated enough	Cavin and Innis, pers. comm.
Ginglymostoma cirratum	Nurse shark	MS-222	20 g/L	Spray to gills	0.1	5 minutes of spraying in stretcher	Cavin and Innis, pers. comm.
Ginglymostoma cirratum 1	Nurse shark	Dexmedetomidine + ketamine	0.05 mg/kg + ~9 mg/kg	IM	0.1	Induction	Cavin and Innis, pers. comm.
Ginglymostoma cirratum 1	Nurse shark	MS-222	90 mg/L	Immersion	0.1	Maintenance	Cavin and Innis, pers. comm.
Trygonorrhina fasciata	Fiddler ray	MS-222	90 mg/L	Immersion		Blood and morphometrics	Clauss and Hatcher, pers. comm.

(Continued)

Table 16.1. (Continued)

Species	Common Name	Drug	Dose or Dosage	Route of Administration	Body Wt (kg)	Population	Age Class	Water Temp (C°)	Comments	Reference
Pristis microdon	Largetooth sawfish	Propofol	2.0–3.0 mg/kg	IV dorsal sinus	64.7–112.5	4.1	adult		2–8 min initial effect; 45–63 min full recovery; good for animal moves, exam, debridement of wounds	Clauss and Hatcher, pers. comm.
Taeniuria meyeni	Blotched fantail ray	Propofol	3 mg/kg	IV	57	0.1	adult		Hook removal from esophagus; 2 min initial effects; top up with 1.5 mg/kg at 36 min due to increased GVR & resistance to manipulation; 88 min recovery	Clauss and Hatcher, pers. comm.
Carcharhinus melanopterus	Blacktip reef shark	Propofol	3 mg/kg	IV dorsal sinus	17.5	0.1	adult		<1 min initial effect; 40–60 min swimming; endoscopy of uterus	Clauss and Hatcher, pers. comm.
Carcharhinus melanopterus	Blacktip reef shark	Propofol	2.5 mg/kg	IV	22.6	0.1	adult		Pregnant; good plane at 4 min; 50 min swimming	Clauss and Hatcher, pers. comm.
Sphyrna tiburo	Bonnethead shark	Propofol	4 mg/kg	IV dorsal sinus	1.4–4.65	1.3	adult		1–3 min initial effect; 48–64 min swimming	Clauss and Hatcher, pers. comm.
Carcharhinus taurus	Sand tiger shark	Propofol	2.56–3.77 mg/kg	IV dorsal sinus	85–116.5	3.3	adult		4–6 min adequate plane; 2–4 hour swimming	Clauss and Hatcher, pers. comm.
Urogymnus asperrimus	Porcupine ray	MS-222	80 mg/L	Immersion	89	0.1	adult		Ultrasound, blood, endoscopy	Clauss and Hatcher, pers. comm.
Notorynchus cepedianus	Broadnose sevengill shark	None—dorsal recumbancy		Tonic immobilization		0.4.0	adult	17–22.5	10-minute ultrasonography exams	Daly et al. (2007)
Dasyatis violacea	Pelagic Stingray	MS-222	80–100 mg/L	Immersion	50		2–6 years	20		Ezcurra, pers. comm.
Squatina californica	Angel shark	MS-222	80–100 mg/L	Immersion				10–14		Ezcurra, pers. comm.
Torpedo californica	Pacific electric ray	MS-222	80–100 mg/L	Immersion	0.5 kg			10–14		Ezcurra, pers. comm.
Rhinoptera bonasus	Cownose stingray	Eugenol	25–75 mg/L in 50% ethanol	Immersion			Adult		Deep sedation not achieved at 25 mg/L. Recovery times longer than with MS-222	Grusha (2005)
Aetobatus narinari	Spotted eagle ray	Alphaxalone-alphadolone (Saffan)	0.35 mL/kg	IM	54	0.0.1			Achieved the deepest state within 1 hour with disorientation, slowed swimming, bumping into tank walls, net avoidance	Harvey et al. (1988)

Species	Common name	Drug	Dose	Route			Age	Effect	Reference
Carcharhinus limbatus	Blacktip shark	Alphaxalone-alphadolone (Saffan)	0.4 mL/kg	IM	21	0.0.1		Achieved deepest state within 1 hour, partial loss of equilibrium, settling or rising to surface, allowed netting but still responsive to touch	Harvey et al. (1988)
Dasyatis alta	Brown stingray	Alphaxalone-alphadolone (Saffan)	0.2–0.3 mL/kg	IM	15	0.0.2		Deepest state within 1 hour: partial loss of equilibrium, settling or rising to surface, allowed netting but still responsive to touch	Harvey et al. (1988)
Dasyatis alta	Brown stingray	Alphaxalone-alphadolone (Saffan)	0.85 mL/kg	IM	18	0.0.1		Deepest state within 1 hour: disorientation, slowing of swimming, bumping into tank walls, net avoidance	Harvey et al. (1988)
Raja binoculata	Skate	Alphaxalone-alphadolone (Saffan)	0.25 mL/kg	IM	50	0.0.1		Deepest state within 1 hour: partial loss of equilibrium, settling or rising to surface, allowed netting but still responsive to touch	Harvey et al. (1988)
Squalus acanthias	Spiny dogfish	Alphaxalone-alphadolone (Saffan)	0.3–0.5 mL/kg	IM	3/2	0.0.2		Deepest state within 1 hour: disorientation, slowing of swimming, bumping into tank walls, net avoidance	Harvey et al. (1988)
Squalus acanthias	Spiny dogfish	Alphaxalone-alphadolone (Saffan)	1.5 mL/kg	IM	4	0.0.2		Deepest state within 1 hour: complete loss of equilibrium and cessation of swimming, no response to touch, marked depression of ventillation	Harvey et al. (1988)
Squalus acanthias	Spiny dogfish	Metomidate hydrochloride	30 mg/kg	IM	3	0.0.1		Deepest state within 1 hour: disorientation, slowing of swimming, bumping into tank walls, net avoidance	Harvey et al. (1988)
Ginglymostoma cirratum	Nurse shark	Medetomidine + ketamine	70–100 μg/kg + 8–10 mg/kg	IM			Adult	Poor to mild sedation; often ketamine was repeated at 5 mg/kg doses and medetomidine at 30 mcg/kg	Kilbourn, pers. comm.
Hemiscyllium ocellatum	Epaulette shark	Tiletamine + zolazepam	20 mg/kg	IM			Adult	Allowed some manipulation (rolling over) but could not perform invasive procedures	Kilbourn, pers comm.

(Continued)

Table 16.1. (Continued)

Species	Common Name	Drug	Dose or Dosage	Route of Administration	Body Wt (kg)	Population	Age Class	Water Temp (C°)	Comments	Reference
Carcharhinus taurus	Sand tiger shark	Medetomidine + butorphanol	0.1mg/kg + 0.3mg/kg	IM	160	1.0	Adult		Swimming more deeply in 4 minutes after injection. Able to guide shark for transport after 12 minutes. Sternal recumbancy and ideal for transport in 20 minutes.	Larson, pers. comm.
Chiloscyllium spp.	Bamboo shark	2-Phenoxyethanol	0.02ml/L	Immersion		0.0.1			Sedated for radiographs	Larson, pers. comm.
Orectolobus japonicus	Japanese wobbegong	Propofol	2.2mg/kg	IV		0.0.1			Spontaneous gill movement ceased at 3 minutes, returned at 55 minutes. Spontaneous movement at 148 minutes, full recovery at 153 minutes.	Larson, pers. comm.
Pristis microdon	Largetooth sawfish	2-Phenoxyethanol	0.1–0.17mL	Immersion		0.0.6			0.1ml/L not adequate for transport; 0.0145ml/L markedly sedate, full recovery 90 minutes later.	Larson, pers. comm.
Raja erinacea	Little skate	2-Phenoxyethanol	0.11mL/L	Immersion		0.0.1			Deep sedation for minor surgical procedure. Excellent sedation, fast recovery.	Larson, pers. comm.
Rhina ancylostoma	Bowmouth guitarfish	Propofol	2.22mg/kg	IV		0.0.1				Larson, pers. comm.
Rhinoptera bonasus	Cownose stingray	2-Phenoxyethanol	0.2mL/L	Immersion		0.0.2			Sedated for ultrasound	Larson, pers. comm.
Squalus acanthias	Spiny dogfish	Azaperone	4mg/kg	Spray on gills	1–5	10.11.0			Ideal for capture & confinement; still exhibit normal swimming	Latas (1987)
Carcharhinus plumbeus	Sandbar shark (brown shark)	Etomidate	40mg + 40mg 15 minutes later	IM	~45	1.0.0	20 years	23–27	Procedure for diagnostics; induced TI at 29 minutes	Lécu et al. (2011)
Carcharhinus plumbeus	Sandbar shark (brown shark)	Eugenol 99%/ethanol (1:8)	30mg/L	Immersion	40	1.0.0	20 years	23–27	Hook removal; stage II at 5 minutes, stage III at 10 minutes	Lécu et al. (2011)
Aetobatus narinari	Spotted eagle ray	MS-222	75mg/L	Immersion	14.5–82	0.0.6			Average to good sedation	Mylniczenko, pers. comm.

Species	Common name	Drug	Dose	Route			Notes	Reference
Aetobatus narinari	Spotted eagle ray	MS-222	40 mg/L	Immersion			Slightly light sedation	Mylniczenko, pers comm.
Aetobatus narinari	Spotted eagle ray	MS-222	50 mg/L	Immersion	avg 2.2; 1@40	0.0.8	Good	Mylniczenko, pers comm.
Aetobatus narinari	Spotted eagle ray	MS-222	60 mg/L	Immersion	2–2.5		Good to deep sedation	Mylniczenko, pers comm.
Carcharhinus acronotus	Blacknose shark	Medetomidine + Ketamine	0.07–0.1 mg/kg + 5.5–8.8 mg/kg	IM	15-Oct		Variable effects but did not achieve more than light sedation without supplementation of the same drugs. One animal death.	Mylniczenko, pers comm.
Carcharhinus acronotus	Blacknose shark	MS-222	150 mg/L	Immersion	6.9		Good	Mylniczenko, pers comm.
Carcharhinus falciformis	Silky shark	MS-222	100 mg/L	Immersion	9.5		Fair	Mylniczenko, pers comm.
Carcharhinus plumbeus	Sandbar shark (brown shark)	Medetomidine + Ketamine	0.1 to 0.12 mg/kg + 5–7 mg/kg	IM	26–65			Mylniczenko, pers comm.
Carcharhinus plumbeus	Sandbar shark (brown shark)	MS-222	100 mg/L	Immersion	9.5		Good	Mylniczenko, pers comm.
Carcharhinus taurus	Sand tiger shark	Medetomidine + Ketamine	0.1 mg/kg + 5–8 mg/kg	IM	110		Variable effects from very light sedation to heavy sedation.	Mylniczenko, pers comm.
Carcharhinus taurus	Sand tiger shark	MS-222	85 mg/L	Immersion	avg 92		Good	Mylniczenko, pers comm.
Chiloscyllium spp.	Bamboo shark	MS-222	60 mg/L	Immersion	0.17–2	0.0.4	Good	Mylniczenko, pers comm.
Chiloscyllium spp.	Bamboo shark	MS-222	60 mg/L	Immersion	2.344		Good	Mylniczenko, pers comm.
Dasyatis americana	Southern stingray	MS-222	50 mg/L	Immersion	11.7–28.48	0.0.7	Good	Mylniczenko, pers comm.
Dasyatis americana	Southern stingray	MS-222	55 mg/L	Immersion		0.0.4	Average to good sedation	Mylniczenko, pers comm.
Dasyatis americana	Southern stingray	MS-222	60 mg/L	Immersion	4.66–43.31	0.0.28	Good	Mylniczenko, pers comm.
Dasyatis americana	Southern stingray	MS-222	70 mg/L	Immersion	13.1	0.0.3	Good	Mylniczenko, pers comm.
Dasyatis americana	Southern stingray	MS-222	75 mg/L	Immersion	9.98–45.83		Good	Mylniczenko, pers comm.
Dasyatis americana	Southern stingray	MS-222	80 mg/L	Immersion	5.29–25.8	0.0.3	Good	Mylniczenko, pers comm.

(*Continued*)

Table 16.1. (Continued)

Species	Common Name	Drug	Dose or Dosage	Route of Administration	Body Wt (kg)	Population	Age Class	Water Temp (C°)	Comments	Reference
Hemiscyllium ocellatum	Epaulette shark	MS-222	75 mg/L	Immersion					Good	Mylniczenko, pers. comm.
Rhinobatos spp.	Guitarfish	MS-222	75 mg/L	Immersion	0.5–1.1	0.0.6			Good	Mylniczenko, pers. comm.
Rhinoptera bonasus	Cownose stingray	MS-222	50 mg/L	Immersion	2.39–21.9	0.0.12			Light to good	Mylniczenko, pers. comm.
Rhinoptera bonasus	Cownose stingray	MS-222	55 mg/L	Immersion	17.95	0.0.2			Slightly light	Mylniczenko, pers. comm.
Rhinoptera bonasus	Cownose stingray	MS-222	60 mg/L	Immersion	2.39–24.36	0.0.8			Consider higher dose for longer/invasive exam	Mylniczenko, pers. comm.
Rhinoptera bonasus	Cownose stingray	MS-222	65 mg/L	Immersion	10.11	0.0.2			Slightly light	Mylniczenko, pers. comm.
Rhinoptera bonasus	Cownose stingray	MS-222	70 mg/L	Immersion	2.39–24.36	0.0.13			Deep	Mylniczenko, pers. comm.
Rhinoptera bonasus	Cownose stingray	MS-222	75 mg/L	Immersion	2.2–10.05	0.0.10			Average to good	Mylniczenko, pers comm.
Rhinoptera bonasus	Cownose stingray	MS-222	80 mg/L	Immersion	2.28 to 13.5	0.0.15			Recovery tends to be a bit slow, but otherwise normal	Mylniczenko, pers. comm.
Rhinoptera bonasus	Cownose stingray	MS-222	83 mg/L	Immersion					Good	Mylniczenko, pers. comm.
Rhinoptera bonasus	Cownose stingray	MS-222	85 mg/L	Immersion	4.3–20.9	0.0.10			Average to good	Mylniczenko, pers. comm.
Rhinoptera bonasus	Cownose stingray	MS-222	88 mg/L	Immersion					Good	Mylniczenko, pers. comm.
Rhinoptera bonasus	Cownose stingray	MS-222	90 mg/L	Immersion	4.3				Slightly light	Mylniczenko, pers. comm.
Rhinoptera bonasus	Cownose stingray	MS-222	93 mg/L	Immersion	4.3				Prolonged recovery; average good	Mylniczenko, pers. comm.
Rhinoptera bonasus	Cownose stingray	MS-222	95 mg/L	Immersion	avg 20				In recovery, breathing was slightly shallow and rapid	Mylniczenko, pers. comm.
Rhinoptera bonasus	Cownose stingray	MS-222	100 mg/L	Immersion	avg 8				Good to deep	Mylniczenko, pers. comm.

Sphyrna tiburo	Bonnethead shark	MS-222	50 mg/L	Immersion	0.9–3.4	0.0.16	Good; maintenance	Mylniczenko, pers. comm.
Sphyrna tiburo	Bonnethead shark	MS-222	100 mg/L	Immersion	0.9–3.4	0.0.16	Good; induction	Mylniczenko, pers. comm.
Stegostoma fasciatum	Zebra shark	MS-222	60 mg/L	Immersion	34.47		Good	Mylniczenko, pers. comm.
Taeniuria lymma	Blue spotted or ribbontail stingray	MS-222	50 mg/L	Immersion	2.05	0.0.3	Slightly light	Mylniczenko, pers. comm.
Taeniuria lymma	Blue spotted or ribbontail stingray	MS-222	60 mg/L	Immersion	avg 2.2		Slightly light	Mylniczenko, pers. comm.
Taeniuria lymma	Blue spotted or ribbontail stingray	MS-222	65 mg/L	Immersion	2.178		Good	Mylniczenko, pers. comm.
Taeniuria lymma	Blue spotted or ribbontail stingray	MS-222	70 mg/L	Immersion	1.2–2	0.0.2	Good to deep	Mylniczenko, pers. comm.
Taeniuria lymma	Blue spotted or ribbontail stingray	MS-222	50 mg/L	Immersion			Good	Mylniczenko, pers. comm.
Taeniuria lymma	Blue spotted or ribbontail stingray	MS-222	70 mg/L	Immersion			Good	Mylniczenko, pers. comm.
Taeniuria lymma	Blue spotted or ribbontail stingray	MS-222	60 mg/L	Immersion	0.129		Good	Mylniczenko, pers. comm.
Triakis semifasciata	Leopard shark	MS-222	60–65 mg/L	Immersion	5–8.86	0.0.4	Good	Mylniczenko, pers. comm.
Urobatis halleri	Haller's round ray	MS-222	60–70 mg/L	Immersion	0.3–1.2	0.0.2	Good	Mylniczenko, pers. comm.
Urobatis halleri	Haller's round ray	MS-222	60 mg/L	Immersion	0.875		Slightly light	Mylniczenko, pers. comm.

(Continued)

Table 16.1. (Continued)

Species	Common Name	Drug	Dose or Dosage	Route of Administration	Body Wt (kg)	Population	Age Class	Water Temp (C°)	Comments	Reference
Urobatis jaimacensis	Yellow stingray	MS-222	50 mg/L	Immersion	0.914				Dose should be increased for more invasive procedures; average good	Mylniczenko, pers. comm.
Urobatis jaimacensis	Yellow stingray	MS-222	60 mg/L	Immersion	0.87				Good	Mylniczenko, pers. comm.
Urobatis jaimacensis	Yellow stingray	MS-222	65 mg/L	Immersion	1				Good to deep	Mylniczenko, pers. comm.
Urobatis jaimacensis	Yellow stingray	MS-222	70 mg/L	Immersion	0.5–1	0.0.8			Good to deep	Mylniczenko, pers. comm.
Carcharhinus taurus	Sand tiger shark	Diazepam	0.1 mg/kg	IM			Adult		High individual variability. 20 minutes for induction, assessment by pulling the tail or dorsal fin. If not too active, place into a stretcher and into a transport container. If after about 30 minutes the animal is still too active, then inject about 20% more. We found the drug lasts for at least 5 hours.	McEwan, pers. comm.
Ginglymostoma cirratum	Nurse shark	Medetomidine + ketamine	75 µg/kg + 7.5 mg/kg	IM	20 kg		Juvenile			Mulican, pers. comm.
Carcharhinus melanopterus	Blacktip reef shark	Midazolam hydrochloride	0.05–0.1 mg/kg	IM					Used as a premedication administered immediately after netting appeared to decrease stress or hyperexcitability during induction	Mylniczenko, pers. exp.
Carcharhinus plumbeus	Sandbar shark (brown shark)	Diazepam	1.2–1.6 mg/kg	PO					Followed by MS222 staged anesthesia.	Mylniczenko, pers. exp.

Species	Common name	Drug	Dose	Route	Weight		Age	Comments	Reference
Carcharhinus plumbeus	Sandbar shark (brown shark)	Midazolam hydrochloride	0.05–0.1 mg/kg	IM				Premedication administered immediately after netting as animals became larger and more difficult to handle to decrease stress during induction	Mylniczenko, pers. exp.
Carcharhinus plumbeus	Sandbar shark (brown shark)	MS-222	50–125 mg/L	Immersion		24–25.5		High dose induction around transport, then switched to a manageable transport for exam to the low dose. Usually 100 mg/L to 50 mg/L.	Mylniczenko, pers. exp.
Chiloscyllium punctatum	Brownbanded bamboo shark	Medetomidine + Midazolam hydrochloride + Butorphanol	0.1 mg/kg + 1 mg/kg + 1 mg/kg	IM + IV			Adult	No response from IM doses, IV dosages produced light sedation that allowed handling and minor procedures (transponder, blood draws, pin prick to evaluate).	Mylniczenko, pers. exp.
Dasyatis americana	Southern stingray	Guaifenisin	10–40 mg/kg	IV	20–25 kg	0.1	Adult	Initial induction with MS-222, then increased sedation with increasing dosage of guaifenisin to stage 2; notable period of asystole at onset of injection with rapid return to normal rhythm.	Mylniczenko, pers. exp.
Dasyatis americana	Southern stingray	Isoeugenol	15–30 mg/L	Immersion			Adult	Habituated rays that are often handled needed the lower doses for good effect. These animals at 30 mg/L showed dramatic decreased ventilations, improved at lower doses.	Mylniczenko, pers. exp.
Himantura granulata	Mangrove whipray	MS-222	125 mg/L	Immersion		2.2		These animals at 30 mg/L showed dramatic decreased ventilations, improved at lower doses.	Mylniczenko, pers. exp.

(*Continued*)

Table 16.1. *(Continued)*

Species	Common Name	Drug	Dose or Dosage	Route of Administration	Body Wt (kg)	Population	Age Class	Water Temp (C°)	Comments	Reference
Hydrolagus collia	Spotted ratfish	MS-222	125 mg/L	Immersion		1.1			Induction	Mylniczenko, pers. exp.
Hydrolagus collia	Spotted ratfish	MS-222	100 mg/L	Immersion		1.1			Maintenance	Mylniczenko, pers. exp.
Potamotrygon castexi	Vermiculate river stingray	MS-222	125 mg/L	Immersion		0.1				Mylniczenko, pers. exp.
Potamotrygon menchacai	Tiger ray	MS-222	125 mg/L	Immersion		4.1				Mylniczenko, pers. exp.
Pristis zijsron	Green sawfish	Diazepam	0.4 mg/kg	PO					Premedication 1 hour prior to any attempted handling because the animal was considered dangerous to handlers	Mylniczenko, pers. exp.
Pristis zijsron	Green sawfish	MS-222	125 mg/L	Immersion		0.1			Induction	Mylniczenko, pers. exp.
Pristis zijsron	Green sawfish	MS-222	100 mg/L	Immersion		0.1			Maintenance	Mylniczenko, pers. exp.
Taeniuria lymma	Blue spotted or ribbontail stingray	Butorphanol	0.2 mg/kg	IM						Mylniczenko, pers. exp.
Aetobatus narinari	Spotted eagle ray	MS-222	125 mg/L	Immersion		2.2			Induction	Naples et al. (2012)
Aetobatus narinari	Spotted eagle ray	MS-222	100 mg/L	Immersion		2.2			Maintenance	Naples et al. (2012)
Carcharhinus melanopterus	Blacktip reef shark	MS-222	50–125 mg/L	Immersion				24–25.7	High dose induction around transport, then switched to a manageable transport for exam to the low dose. Usually 100 mg/L to 50 mg/L.	Naples et al. (2012)
Carcharhinus melanopterus	Blacktip reef shark	MS-222	125 mg/L	Immersion		15.3			Induction dose	Naples et al. (2012)
Carcharhinus melanopterus	Blacktip reef shark	MS-222	100 mg/L	Immersion		15.3			Maintenance dose	Naples et al. (2012)

Species	Common name	Agent	Concentration	Route		Purpose	Reference
Carcharhinus plumbeus	Sandbar shark (brown shark)	MS-222	100 mg/L	Immersion	3.3	Maintenance	Naples et al. (2012)
Cephaloscyllium ventriosum	Swell shark	MS-222	50–125 mg/L	Immersion	14	High dose induction around transport, then switched to a manageable transport for exam to the low dose. Usually 100 mg/L to 50 mg/L.	Naples et al. (2012)
Cephaloscyllium ventriosum	Swell shark	MS-222	125 mg/L	Immersion	1.1	Induction	Naples et al. (2012)
Cephaloscyllium ventriosum	Swell shark	MS-222	100 mg/L	Immersion	1.1	Maintenance	Naples et al. (2012)
Chiloscyllium plagiosum	White spotted bamboo shark	MS-222	125 mg/L	Immersion	6.7	Induction	Naples et al. (2012)
Chiloscyllium plagiosum	White spotted bamboo shark	MS-222	100 mg/L	Immersion	6.7	Maintenance	Naples et al. (2012)
Heterodontus francicsci	Hornshark	MS-222	50–125 mg/L	Immersion	14	High dose induction around transport, then switched to a manageable transport for exam to the low dose. Usually 100 mg/L to 50 mg/L.	Naples et al. (2012)
Heterodontus francicsci	Hornshark	MS-222	125 mg/L	Immersion	1.1.1	Induction	Naples et al. (2012)
Heterodontus francicsci	Hornshark	MS-222	100 mg/L	Immersion	1.1.1	Maintenance	Naples et al. (2012)
Orectolobus japonicus	Japanese wobbegong	MS-222	125 mg/L	Immersion		Induction	Naples et al. (2012)
Orectolobus japonicus	Japanese wobbegong	MS-222	100 mg/L	Immersion		Maintenance	Naples et al. (2012)
Stegastoma fasciatum	Zebra shark	MS-222	50–125 mg/L	Immersion	24-25.8	High dose induction around transport, then switched to a manageable transport for exam to the low dose. Usually 100 mg/L to 50 mg/L.	Naples et al. (2012)

(Continued)

Table 16.1. *(Continued)*

Species	Common Name	Drug	Dose or Dosage	Route of Administration	Body Wt (kg)	Population	Age Class	Water Temp (C°)	Comments	Reference
Stegastoma fasciatum	Zebra shark	MS-222	125 mg/L	Immersion		3.4			Induction	Naples et al. (2012)
Stegastoma fasciatum	Zebra shark	MS-222	100 mg/L	Immersion		3.4			Maintenance	Naples et al. (2012)
Triaenodon obesus	Whitetip reef shark	MS-222	50–125 mg/L	Immersion				24–25.6	High dose induction round transport, then switched to a manageable transport for exam to the low dose. Usually 100 mg/L to 50 mg/L.	Naples et al. (2012)
Triaenodon obesus	Whitetip reef shark	MS-222	125 mg/L	Immersion		6.10			Induction	Naples et al. (2012)
Triaenodon obesus	Whitetip reef shark	MS-222	100 mg/L	Immersion		6.10			Maintenance	Naples et al. (2012)
Triakis semifasciata	Leopard shark	MS-222	50–125 mg/L	Immersion				14	High dose induction around transport, then switched to a manageable transport for exam to the low dose. Usually 100 mg/L to 50 mg/L.	Naples et al. (2012)
Triakis semifasciata	Leopard shark	MS-222	125 mg/L	Immersion		1.2			Induction	Naples et al. (2012)
Triakis semifasciata	Leopard shark	MS-222	100 mg/L	Immersion		1.2			Maintenance	Naples et al. (2012)
Carcharhinus plumbeus	Sandbar shark (brown shark)	MS-222	125 mg/L	Immersion		3.3			Induction	Naples et al. (2012)
Dasyatis americana	Southern stingray	Isoeugenol	15.7 mg/L	Immersion			Adult		Smooth induction, good light sedation.	Neiffer et al. (2009)
Dasyatis americana	Southern stingray	Medetomidine + Midazolam hydrochloride + Butorphanol	0.05 mg/kg + 0.4 mg/kg + 0.4 mg/kg	IV			Adult		20 minute induction, highly variable responses.	Neiffer et al. (2009)
Carcharhinus leucas	Bull shark	Medetomidine	0.1 mg/kg	IM			Adult		15–20 minutes for induction; able to guide into PVC sock in 1 hour.	Penning (2012)

Species	Common name	Drug	Dose	Route		Stage	Comments	Reference
Aetobatus narinari	Spotted eagle ray	Medetomidine	0.1 mg/kg	IM			15–20 minutes for induction; able to guide into PVC sock in 1 hour.	Penning (2012)
Carcharhinus brevipinna	Spinner shark	Medetomidine + Butorphanol	0.1 mg/kg + 0.065 mg/kg	IM			15–20 minutes for induction; able to guide into PVC sock in 1 hour.	Penning (2012)
Carcharhinus obscurus	Dusky shark	Medetomidine	0.1 mg/kg	IM			One death, suspected due to other disease process	Penning (2012)
Carcharhinus taurus	Sand tiger shark	Medetomidine	0.1 mg/kg	IM	275	Adult		Penning (2012)
Carcharhinus taurus	Sand tiger shark	Medetomidine + Butorphanol	0.1 mg/kg + 0.065 mg/kg	IM			One death, suspected due to other disease process	Penning (2012)
Galeocerdo cuvier	Tiger shark	Medetomidine	0.1 mg/kg	IM	250	Adult	15–20 minutes for induction; able to guide into PVC sock in 1 hour.	Penning (2012)
Galeocerdo cuvier	Tiger shark	Medetomidine + Ketamine	0.1 mg/kg + 5 mg/kg	IM	250	Adult	15–20 minutes for induction; able to guide into PVC sock in 1 hour.	Penning (2012)
Rhynchobatus djiddensis	Giant guitarfish	Medetomidine + Butorphanol	0.1 mg/kg + 1 mg/kg	IM				Penning (2012)
Potamotrygon motoro	Ocellated river stingray	Ketamine	50 mg/kg	PO	0.093–0.1 0.0.4 (75–78F)		Stage 2 at 10 minutes: loss of equilibrium, very slow swimming, decreased opercular movement, loss of muscle tone	Raines and Clancy (2009)
Carcharhinus taurus	Sand tiger shark	Medetomidine + Ketamine	60.0–80.0 μg/kg + 5–10 mg/kg	IM	21–22	Adult	Animals had scoliosis and lordosis; one animal was euthanized for medical reasons; not recovered	Snyder et al. (1998)
Carcharhinus taurus	Sand tiger shark	Medetomidine + Ketamine	70.0–80.0 μg/kg + 4 mg/kg	IM	24	Adult		Stamper, pers. exp.
Carcharhinus acronotus	Blacknose shark	Medetomidine + Ketamine	59.2–70.4 μg/kg + 2.8 mg/kg	IM	25.5	Juvenile		Stamper, pers. exp.
Carcharhinus plumbeus	Sandbar shark (brown shark)	Medetomidine + Ketamine	87 μg/kg + 5.4 mg/kg	IM	24.5	Adult		Stamper, pers. exp.

(Continued)

Table 16.1. (Continued)

Species	Common Name	Drug	Dose or Dosage	Route of Administration	Body Wt (kg)	Population	Age Class	Water Temp (C°)	Comments	Reference
Chiloscyllium plagiosum	White spotted bamboo shark	Medetomidine + Ketamine	60 µg/kg + 3.0 mg/kg	IM			Adult	23.4		Stamper, pers. exp.
Carcharhinus taurus	Sand tiger shark	Ketamine	10 mg/kg	IM	158	0.1.0	adult			Tuttle and Dunn (2003)
Carcharhinus leucas	Bull shark	2-Phenoxyethanol	0.15 ml/L	Immersion					70-minute induction time	Vaughan et al. (2008)
Carcharhinus taurus	Sand tiger shark	2-Phenoxyethanol	0.15 ml/L	Immersion		0.0.8			70-minute induction time	Vaughan et al. (2008)
Notorynchus cepedianus	Broadnose sevengill shark	Ketamine	80 mg/kg	IM	29				5 minutes to first effect, then 45 minutes to slow swimming, 60 minutes easily caught in net and then moved to net	Vogelnest et al. (1994)
Ginglymostoma cirratum	Nurse shark	Sodium pentobarbital	20 mg/L	IM	2–10				5 minutes slowed activity; 20 minutes weak gilling and swimming	Walker (1972)
Ginglymostoma cirratum	Nurse shark	Sodium pentobarbital	40 mg/L	IM	2–10				2 minutes to anesthesia, weak gilling; 2 hours, return of gilling; 24 hours, rights and swims	Walker (1972)
Ginglymostoma cirratum	Nurse shark	Sodium pentobarbital	10 mg/L	ICe	2–10				1 hour: slowed activity, gilling, rights and swims	Walker (1972)
Ginglymostoma cirratum	Nurse shark	Sodium pentobarbital	40 mg/L	ICe	2–10				25 minutes to anesthesia, gilling; 50 minutes, loss of gilling; 7 hours, return of gilling; 30 hours, rights; 42 hours, slowed activity	Walker (1972)
Ginglymostoma cirratum	Nurse shark	Sodium pentobarbital	60 mg/L	ICe	2–10				3 minutes to anesthesia, gilling lost; 42 hours, weak gilling; 54 hours, rights and swims slowly	Walker (1972)
Ginglymostoma cirratum	Nurse shark	Sodium pentobarbital	10 mg/L	IV	2–10				1 minute to anesthesia, loss of gilling; 20 minutes, return. of gilling; 3 hours, weakly rights	Walker (1972)
Ginglymostoma cirratum	Nurse shark	Sodium pentobarbital	20 mg/L	IV	2–10				1 minute to anesthesia, loss of gilling; 3 hours, return of gilling; 5 hours, weakly rights	Walker (1972)

								Died	Walker (1972)
Ginglymostoma cirratum	Nurse shark	Sodium pentobarbital	60 mg/L	IV	2–10				
Carcharhinus leucas	Bull shark	Detomidine + ketamine	128 μg/kg	IM	85.7	Adult	23	No effect, injection thought to be complete	Walsh, pers. comm.
Carcharhinus leucas	Bull shark	Medetomidine + ketamine	90 μg/kg WHERE IS THE KET DOSE	IM	85.7	Adult	23	Abnormal animal; became recumbent after handling; redosed with half supplemental.	Walsh, pers. comm.
Ginglymostoma cirratum	Nurse shark	Medetomidine + ketamine	90 μg/kg + 9.0 mg/kg	IM	68 kg	Adult	26		Walsh, pers. comm.
Negaprion brevirostris	Lemon shark	Medetomidine + ketamine	90 μg/kg + 4.5 mg/kg	IM		Adult	26	Both animals blanched after drug adminstration; Noted leakage from injection sites-undetermined amount, became recombant after handling	Walsh, pers. comm.
Triaenodon obesus	Whitetip reef shark	Medetomidine + ketamine	90 μg/kg + 4.5 mg/kg	IM		Juvenile	27	Animal was abnormal; infection and scoliosis; Stopped gilling unless touched	Walsh, pers. comm.
Chiloscyllium punctatum	Brownbanded bamboo shark	2-Phenoxyethanol	200 mg/L	Immersion	2.3–3.9		26.1–26.9	Light sedation	Yanagisawa, pers. comm.
Chiloscyllium punctatum	Brownbanded bamboo shark	2-Phenoxyethanol	300–350 mg/L	Immersion	2.3–3.9		26.1–26.9	Deep narcosis—surgical anesthesia	Yanagisawa, pers. comm.
Chiloscyllium punctatum	Brownbanded bamboo shark	2-Phenoxyethanol	400 mg/L	Immersion	2.3–3.9		26.1–26.9	Deep	Yanagisawa, pers. comm.
Chiloscyllium punctatum	Brownbanded bamboo shark	Medetomidine + ketamine	400 μg/kg + 20 mg/kg	IM	5.0		20.0–21.0	Stage 3	Yanagisawa, pers. comm.
Chiloscyllium punctatum	Brownbanded bamboo shark	Medetomidine + ketamine	800 μg/kg + 40 mg/kg	IM	3.7		20.0–21.0	Stage 3	Yanagisawa, pers. comm.
Chiloscyllium punctatum	Brownbanded bamboo shark	Medetomidine + ketamine	100 μg/kg + 5 mg/kg	IM	3.8–3.9		26.1–26.7	Stage 2 Plane 1–Plane 2	Yanagisawa, pers. comm.
Chiloscyllium punctatum	Brownbanded bamboo shark	Medetomidine + ketamine	200 μg/kg + 10 mg/kg	IM	2.3–3.5		26.1–26.7	Stage 2 Plane 2	Yanagisawa, pers. comm.
Chiloscyllium punctatum	Brownbanded bamboo shark	Propofol	2.5 mg/kg	IV	5.1		22.0–25.0	Stage 2–Stage 3 Plane1	Yanagisawa, pers. comm.
Chiloscyllium punctatum	Brownbanded bamboo shark	Propofol	4.0 mg/kg	IV	4.55		22.2–22.5	Stage 3: Stop swimming	Yanagisawa, pers. comm.

(*Continued*)

Table 16.1. (Continued)

Species	Common Name	Drug	Dose or Dosage	Route of Administration	Body Wt (kg)	Population	Age Class	Water Temp (C°)	Comments	Reference
Chiloscyllium punctatum	Brownbanded bamboo shark	Propofol	5.0 mg/kg	IV	4.86			21.7–21.9	Apnea	Yanagisawa, pers. comm.
Chiloscyllium punctatum	Brownbanded bamboo shark	Propofol + fentanyl citrate	2.5 mg/kg + 1.5 µg/kg	IV	3.6			21	Stage 2–Stage 3 Plane 1	Yanagisawa, pers. comm.
Chiloscyllium punctatum	Brownbanded bamboo shark	Propofol + fentanyl citrate	2.0 mg/kg + 5 µg/kg	IV	4.0			29	Stage 3	Yanagisawa, pers. comm.
Carcharhinus leucas	Bull shark	Medetomidine	200 µg/kg	IM	3.85		1 year	25	Stopped swimming, apnea, did not recover.	Yanagisawa, pers. comm.
Carcharhinus leucas	Bull shark	Medetomidine + ketamine	100 µg/kg + 5 mg/kg	IM	4		1 year	25	Slow swimming, recovered but died the subsequent day.	Yanagisawa, pers. comm.
Carcharhinus leucas	Bull shark	Medetomidine + ketamine	150 µg/kg + 7.5 mg/kg	IM	3.9		1 year	25	Slow swimming, recovered but died the subsequent day.	Yanagisawa, pers. comm.
Carcharhinus leucas	Bull shark	Medetomidine + ketamine	200 µg/kg + 10 mg/kg	IM	—		1 year	25	Stopped swimming, apnea, did not recover.	Yanagisawa, pers. comm.
Nebrius ferrugineus	Tawny nurse shark	Midazolam hydrochloride + propofol	0.75 mg/kg + 1.0 mg/kg	IM + IV					Stage 2 Plane 2	Yanagisawa, pers. comm.
Nebrius ferrugineus	Tawny nurse shark	Propofol	1.5 mg/kg	IV	7.25				Stage 2 Plane 2–Stage 3 Plane 1	Yanagisawa, pers. comm.
Nebrius ferrugineus	Tawny nurse shark	Propofol	1.0 mg/kg	IV	10.8			28.6	Stage 2 Plane 2–Stage 3 Plane 1	Yanagisawa, pers. comm.
Nebrius ferrugineus	Tawny nurse shark	Propofol	1.5 mg/kg	IV	10.7			28.6	Stage 2 Plane 2–Stage 3 Plane 1	Yanagisawa, pers. comm.
Rhincodon typus	Whale shark	Midazolam hydrochloride	3.0 mg/kg	IM	1,500			29.9	Stage 2 Plane 2 (animal in poor condition)	Yanagisawa, pers. comm.
Rhincodon typus	Whale shark	Midazolam hydrochloride + propofol	6.0 mg/kg + 1.5 mg/kg	IM + IV	1,300			28.9	Midazolam = slow swimming; propofol = stopped swimming. Stage 3 Planes 2–4	Yanagisawa, pers. comm.
Stegostoma fasciatum	Zebra shark	Midazolam hydrochloride + propofol	1.5 mg/kg + 1.0 mg/kg	IM + IV					Stage 2 Plane 2	Yanagisawa, pers. comm.
Chiloscyllium plagiosum	White spotted bamboo shark	MS-222	50 mg/L	Immersion				25.0–26.68	Light anesthesia	Zimmerman et al. (2006)

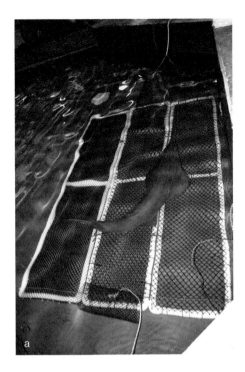
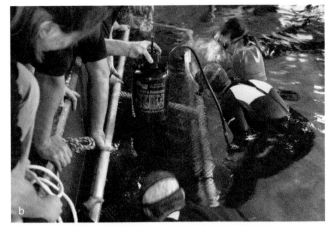
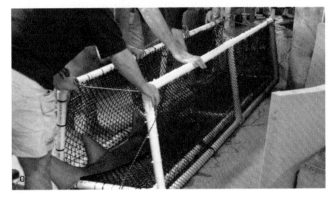

Figure 16.7. (a) Target training a green sawfish (*Pristis zijsron*) to swim over a foldable restraint device. (b) The same animal, within the folded restraint device, now in the shape of a prism with the animal's head at the far end of the photo. Divers are administering high dose MS-222 over the gills of the animal through the device. (c) The same animal, fully anesthetized and pulled from the water, ready for examination.

MS-222 buffered 4:1 with sodium bicarbonate (20–24 g/L). When the same anesthetic water is used to anesthetize multiple animals, it is necessary to monitor the pH as shifts may occur. The authors recommend monitoring water quality or changing water after every third animal.

A direct linear relationship exists between MS-222 concentration and time to muscular relaxation (Dunn & Koester 1990). A wide variety of elasmobranch species will achieve a surgical plane of anesthesia (i.e., stage 3) using MS-222 (75–95 mg/L), but species-specific responses are common (Dunn & Koester 1990). Many sharks have been anesthetized using a low concentration (50 mg/L) as a "preanesthetic" dose followed by higher concentrations (≤85 mg/L) for maintenance (Davis, pers. comm. 2006). This "preanesthetic" concentration is reported to reduce the excitement phase and lower overall maintenance level of MS-222. Conversely, the authors prefer high dose induction (150 mg/L), especially in pelagic animals, with removal to a lower maintenance dose (50–75 mg/L). This regimen has resulted in rapid anesthesia, decreased excitement phase, better blood gas measurements, and better planes of anesthesia.

Gilbert and Wood (1957) describe a field technique of bringing large lemon sharks (*Negaprion brevirostris*) up to the water surface with a hook and line and then applying a high concentration of MS-222 (1 g/L) with a pump hand sprayer. Effects were noted within 15 seconds, and the animals were anesthetized within 1 minute. It is recommended the patient's head remain out of water, and only buffered MS-222 be applied to the gills if utilizing this technique.

MS-222 excretion in the piked dogfish (*Squalus acanthias*) is primarily through the gills and is a function of cardiac output (Maren et al. 1968). Elimination of MS-222 into the water can result in a positive feedback of increasing anesthetic concentration if the heart slows, resulting in a possible overdose if the animals are not closely monitored. Utilizing a system, such as the drip system described in Chapter 15, whereby the drug is administered, and then discarded, can prevent an overdose problem. MS-222 anesthesia is the preferred anesthetic for holocephalans. In the authors' experience, 80–110 mg/L buffered MS-222 provides excellent anesthesia and good recovery.

Clove Oil (Eugenol), Aqui-S™/Aqui-S 20E™ (Isoeugenol) The active ingredient in clove oil is a phenolic compound, eugenol. It is commercially available and inexpensive. The active ingredient in Aqui-S™/Aqui-S

20E™ is isoeugenol. This anesthetic is commercially produced by Aqui-S New Zealand LTD and Aqui-S 20E is available in the United States under the INAD (Investigation New Animal Drug) program (Aquatactics Fish Health, Kirkland, WA).

The use of eugenol and isoeugenol is well established in teleosts (see Chapter 15), but controlled studies in elasmobranchs are limited. Clove oil (25–50 mg/L) was used to anesthetize epaulette sharks (*H. ocellatum*) and shovel nose rays (*Rhinobatus typus*) without complication (Grusha 2005). Grusha (2005) performed controlled studies with cownose rays (*R. bonasus*) using eugenol (25, 50, and 75 mg/L) dissolved in 50% ethanol, as well as MS-222 (100 mg/L). Effects were similar for all four treatment groups. The animals anesthetized with 25 mg/L eugenol, however, did not reach a plane of deep sedation. Recovery times were generally longer for the animals anesthetized with 50 and 75 mg/L eugenol compared with the rays anesthetized with MS-222. In a recent study with southern stingrays (*D. americana*) eugenol (20 mg/L), isoeugenol (15.7 mg/L), and MS-222 (55–65 mg/L) were compared. Induction-associated excitation was observed in all three groups, with a lower percentage observed with eugenol. Animals anesthetized with isoeugenol had a greater number of animals that didn't respond to stimuli. Cardiac rates were stable and similar for all regimens. Median time from placement in recovery water to release was 9 minutes for the MS-222 group and 12 minutes for both the eugenol and isoeugenol groups. Minor variations were noted, but overall, all the agents provided adequate anesthesia for short-term immobilizations and minor procedures (Neiffer et al. 2009). Similarly, one author (Mylniczenko, pers. exp.) has used this drug at doses from 15 to 30 mg/L. Higher doses produced hypoventilation and apnea in some animals, especially habituated or frequently anesthetized animals. Recoveries at higher dosages were also prolonged. Excitation seemed to be less or absent compared with MS-222 induction. Aqui-S foams the water, causing decreased patient visibility. There is a commercially available product designed to mitigate this issue (AQUI-S antifoam, Aquatactics Fish Health, Kirkland, WA). Lécu et al. (2011) anesthetized a male sandbar shark (*C. plumbeus*) with eugenol 99% and ethanol (1 : 8 respectively) at 30 mg/L for a laparotomy procedure to remove a hook from the coelom. Stage 2 anesthesia was reached in 5 minutes, and stage 3 anesthesia was reached within 10 minutes. The shark was maintained at 30 mg/L for 40 minutes and was then reduced to 15 mg/L for the remaining 46 minutes of anesthesia. The recovery period was prolonged, potentially due to the combination of tonic immobility and chemical immobilization, but consistent autonomous swimming resumed just over 3 hours after the procedure was concluded and the shark was returned to the main exhibit.

2-Phenoxyethanol (2-PE) 2-Phenoxyethanol, a glycol ether, is a clear or straw-colored oily liquid. It has a faintly aromatic odor and is moderately water soluble. 2-PE was used initially in aquaculture to treat ichthyophoniasis and other fungal, bacterial, and parasitic diseases. Less expensive than many anesthetics, 2-PE has been widely used for sedation, particularly in fish transportation, as well as general anesthesia (Hseu et al. 1996, 1997; Ross 2001). Another advantage is it causes no pH change when added to sea water (Hseu et al. 1995).

At uShaka Marine World in Durban, South Africa, 2-PE was mixed with tap water in plastic containers and poured directly into the water of two aquatic systems in an effort to translocate all of the teleost and elasmobranch fishes to new exhibits. Concentration increments of 0.05 mL/L were added every 30 minutes to the exhibit to a final concentration of 0.150 mL/L. Excitation events were recorded, and the fishes were removed according to their effective induction to anesthesia based on loss of equilibrium. No excitation was noted in the eight sand tiger sharks (*C. taurus*), but excitation was noted at 0.100 mL/L in the two Zambezi sharks (*C. leucas*). Members of both species were guided into stretchers at the first signs of anesthesia to prevent physical injury due to collision with walls or viewing windows. Anesthesia at 0.150 mL/L lasted 70 minutes in both species. All sharks recovered well (Vaughan et al. 2008).

According to Oswald (1978), 2-PE may cause hypoventilation, and it has poor analgesic properties. Sustained regular exposure can cause a neurophysiological syndrome in some individuals, thus staff handling 2-PE are advised to wear personal protective gear, such as gloves and masks (Hseu et al. 1995).

Metomidate and Etomidate Etomidate and metomidate are GABA agonists and provide a more rapid induction and recovery than MS-222. Etomidate is more effective in alkaline water and higher water temperature, but is not affected by total hardness. In adult sandbar sharks (*C. plumbeus*), 10 mg/L of either drug induced stage II anesthesia in approximately 2–4 minutes. This stage was characterized by an absence of response to positional changes, decreased respiratory rate to approximately normal, total loss of equilibrium, no righting response, decreased muscle tone, some response to strong tactile and vibrational stimuli, and adequate restraint for external sampling (e.g., gill biopsy). Increasing the dose to 20 mg/L reduced induction time to ≤1 minute, but anesthetic depth was more difficult to control. Although etomidate is considerably more potent than metomidate in freshwater teleosts, this difference was not observed in sandbar sharks. Recovery from stage II plane 2 took approximately 3–5 minutes for metomidate. Recovery from deeper planes was considerably prolonged (>1 hour), possibly due to decreased cardiac output (Stoskopf 1986).

Halothane/Oxygen/Nitrous Oxide Halothane (2-bromo-2-chloro-1,1,1-trifluoroethane) is an inhalation anesthetic typically used in air breathing animals, including previous use in humans. Dunn and Koester (1990) used halothane (1.5% for induction, then 0.5–0.8% for maintenance) in nitrous oxide (100–200 mL/min) and oxygen (200–300 mL/min) for anesthesia of guitarfish (*Rhinobatas* sp.) and skates (*Raja* sp.). A precision vaporizer was used to add halothane to a mixture of nitrous oxide and oxygen which was then introduced into the water through an aerator. This combination provides easy control of anesthetic depth, shorter recovery and a very high survival rate. A major disadvantage is contamination of the working environment room with halothane and nitrous oxide. Isoflurane (1-chloro-2,2,2-trifluoroethyl difluoromethyl ether) and sevoflurane (fluoromethyl 2,2,2-trifluoro-1-(trifluoromethyl) ethyl ether) can be used in the same manner. The advantages and disadvantages of isoflurane and sevoflurane are similar to those noted for halothane and, hence, use of anesthetics requiring gas vaporizers is not common practice in fish medicine.

Oxygen The use of oxygen for sedation (hyperoxia or hyperoxygenation) is common practice in aquaria, but its use is largely anecdotal with scant available references. This oxygen narcosis is used for transport or minor procedures. Hyperoxygenated (>100%, usually 120–180%) water is flushed across the gills via a power head or ventilation system. Reported signs of oxygen sedation include depressed respiratory effort, behavioral changes, and in some cases, loss of equilibrium (Stamper, pers. exp.). Since the oxygen is not provided under pressure, "gas bubble disease" does not occur.

Prolonged exposure to elevated oxygen will depress ventilation and produce hypercapnia (likely the cause of narcosis) and potentially life-threatening acidemia (Spotte 1992). The use of oxygen narcosis for immobilization, therefore, should be limited in duration, and monitoring of blood gas variables is recommended. Hyperoxygenation, even in short bursts, can also result in elevated plasma cortisol levels (Sundh et al. 2009). Chronic exposure in fish also increased permeability of cell membranes and pathogen susceptibility (Sundh et al. 2009). Oxygen toxicity, when administration of oxygen levels exceeds biotransformation and clearance, can occur (Manning 2002). Consequently, the positive and negative aspects of hyperoxygenation must be considered in balance.

Injectable Anesthesia
Injectable anesthetics are an alternative when waterborne anesthesia is impractical due to large water volume, or as mentioned previously, when sedation is

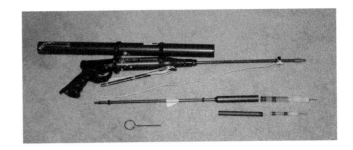

Figure 16.8. An underwater dart system with laser apparatus (AQUADART, Harvey et al. 1988).

necessary to safely capture animals from primary exhibits. The popularity of injectable anesthesia has grown as more controlled studies offer clinicians a better understanding of the effects the drugs may have on various species. Intramuscular (IM) delivery is the most common, however, intravenous (IV) and intracoelomic (ICe) administration are used in some situations.

Delivery IM is typically achieved by hand injection, pole syringe, Hawaiian sling (Chapter 15), or remotely through either an underwater laser aimed dart gun (Fig. 16.8), (AQUADART, Harvey et al. 1988) or other similar remote injection devices.

A newer "homemade setup" is described for immobilizing large fishes and may prove useful for large elasmobranchs as well (Garcia-Parrage et al. 2007). When setting up a dart on a pole or extension, an air-charged dart as used in zoo practice (Chapter 11) is placed against a barrier at the caudal end. This is then attached to a sturdy pole (Chapter 15). Whether an animal is free swimming or manually restrained, IM injections should be delivered quickly, ensuring reduced contact or handling time. This in turn reduces the chance of injury to the animal and people involved. The safety precautions taken when injecting free swimming animals are described earlier. Challenges of underwater darting include judgment of distance, refraction from the facemask (making targeting less accurate), and getting a full discharge of darts under water (reduces gas pressure in the dart) is less reliable than on land. Increased water depth markedly changes these parameters. With the earlier-mentioned laser aimed dart gun these issues are reduced. The cost and availability of this unit, however, make it impractical for use (Harvey, pers. comm., 2012).

As mentioned previously, many sharks have both red and white muscle (Fig. 16.1). The red, oxidative myotomal muscles usually comprise less than 10% of the body mass and consist of relatively small, well-vascularized, myoglobin-rich fibers. White myotomal muscles comprise approximately 50% of body mass and consist of less vascularized, myoglobin poor fibers. In fishes, other than the scombrids, lamnid sharks, and the common thresher shark, the red muscle usually occurs as a relatively thin layer directly beneath the

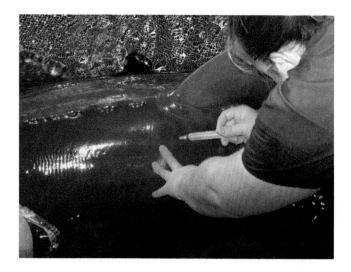

Figure 16.9. Intramuscular injection into the dorsal saddle just ventrolateral to the first dorsal fin in a giant guitarfish (*Rhynchobatus djiddensis*) (photo credit: Georgia Aquarium.)

skin, gradually becoming more abundant in the posterior regions of the body (Greer-Walker & Pull 1975). Injection into different muscles will theoretically affect drug absorption. Some of the variability in response to IM drugs within a species may be due to this anatomical variation in blood supply.

The recommended site for IM injection is the dorsal saddle (Fig. 16.9). This area surrounds the first dorsal fin and extends laterally to just above the lateral line, from the posterior gill slit caudal to a point halfway between the first and second dorsal fins (Stoskopf et al. 1984). The protective denticles and epidermis make needle penetration of the integument difficult and often require the use of a heavy needle (20–22 gauge in small species, 16–18 gauge in larger species) for IM injections. Unfortunately, shark skin does not have a great degree of contractibility and muscle is at a positive resting potential. Injection site leakage is, therefore, a problem in many injections (Stamper, pers. exp.). To minimize leakage, it is recommended the needle be angled either anteriorly or posteriorly, depositing the drug away from the injection site. If remotely injected darts are used to administer a drug, the dart should be left in the animal until it has become sedated, thus preventing drug leakage. Barbed or collared needles can be used, but they result in more skin/muscle trauma. Additionally, if the animal is not sedated sufficiently it may remain in the skin/muscle for a long period of time. In some situations, bone wax (mix of beeswax and isopropyl palmitate), Ilex® skin protectant paste, or other water-insoluble substances may be used to cover or plug the injection site when the needle is removed. In rays, the volume of drug to be administered must be considered as the musculature and cartilaginous rays prevent retention of high volumes. In one of the authors experience (Stamper), higher

volumes resulted in slow absorption or increased leakage of drug. This can be mitigated by using dyes to detect leakage.

Skeletomuscular movement helps blood and lymph circulate (Gruber & Keyes 1981) and has a direct impact on IM drugs, which may not be adequately absorbed in sedentary animals. Anesthetic induction time may be erratic or delayed in these animals, and injection of large volumes of drugs may form a sterile abscess (Tyler & Hawkins 1981).

Intravenous injection is the most reliable anesthetic delivery route, providing more rapid induction and often a shorter duration of effect. Locations for vascular access are described above. Walker (1972) calculated a circulation time of 1–2 minutes for indigo cyanine green injected in the caudal tail vein of nurse sharks (*G. cirratum*). Slow circulation in elasmobranchs may delay the onset of effect of an IV drug when compared with onset times of other classes of animals. The main disadvantage with IV administration is most animals must be appropriately restrained for drug delivery. Some exceptions were previously described in which a diver swims next to an animal while administering a drug via the vasculature associated with the dorsal or pectoral fins.

ICe (into the body cavity) injection is an additional option. It requires drugs to pass through the serosal membranes of the coelomic cavity organs, making anesthetic induction time erratic. Needle insertion at an acute angle directed anteriorly to the pelvic girdle on the right side of the abdominal wall minimizes the possibility of puncturing any internal organs, particularly the liver, which is easily damaged. In addition to unpredictable induction times and the possibility of organ puncture, other disadvantages of ICe administration include risk of peritonitis, as well as the need to place an animal in dorsal recumbency to administer the injection.

Injectable Anesthetics

No published reports were found on batoid injectable anesthesia; however, recent procedures using a combination of midazolam, medetomidine, and butorphanol were successful in producing sedation adequate for minimally invasive procedures (Neiffer, pers. comm. 2011). The protocol included initial immersion in isoeugenol (15.7 ppm), followed by midazolam (0.2–0.3 mg/kg IV), medetomidine (0.035–0.05 mg/kg IV), and butorphanol (0.2–0.3 mg/kg IV), and immediate transfer to isoeugenol-free saltwater for the remainder of the anesthetic event. Recovery was complete after administration of reversal with flumazenil (0.01 mg/kg IV), atipamezole (0.228 mg/kg IV), and naltrexone (0.280 mg/kg IV).

Acepromazine   Intrasinus administration of acepromazine (0.5 and 4 mg/kg), a phenothiazine derivative, in *S. tiburo* resulted in no clinical responses (Clauss, pers. exp.).

Alfaxalone-Alfadolone Alfaxalone-alfadolone (Alfathesin®) is a steroid anesthetic (no longer marketed in the United States) that had been used in the piked dogfish (1.5 mL/kg), the brown ray (*Raja miraletus*) (0.2–0.3 mL/kg), the skate (*Dipturus batis*) (0.2 mL/kg), the blacktip shark (*C. limbatus*) (0.4 mL/kg), and the spotted eagle ray (*Aetobatus narinari*) (0.3 mL/kg) (Harvey et al. 1988). The anesthetic response was highly variable from minimal effect in the eagle ray to immobilization in the dogfish.

Azaperone Azaperone, a butyrophenone, reduces response to environmental stimuli without motor impairment or sedation. Preliminary studies in piked dogfish (*Squalus acanthias*) showed the most efficacious application of azaperone is directly over the gills rather than by injection. No effect was noted when animals were injected with the drug IM. However, an effect was observed when the drug (4 mg/kg) was deposited on the gill filaments and the animal held out of water for several seconds (Latas 1987). At 4 hours, drugged animals, compared with control animals, showed no flight response. Blood glucose levels were unaffected. Tranquilized animals were more likely to feed compared with control animals that exhibited several days of anorexia after blood collection. They were capable of negotiating tank walls and returned to normal behavior within 24 hours. The advantages of using azaperone include uninterrupted swimming patterns, normal gill ventilation, and normal cardiovascular function (Latas 1987).

When administered intrasinus to *S. tiburo*, a range of responses were seen. These include variable induction times (10–40 minutes), ability to handle animals, and highly varied recovery times. At the higher dosages, bottom settling was noted as well as a slow, coordinated swim pattern with obstacle avoidance. If given IM, there were no responses at 12 mg/kg, but higher dosages were not tried (volume limiting) (Clauss, pers. exp.).

Carfentanil Citrate Carfentanil citrate, an ultrapotent opioid, failed to achieve any effect in a nurse (*G. cirratum*) and a lemon shark (*Negaprion brevirostris*) at a dosage of 0.25 mg/kg (normal hoofstock dosages are 1–6 ug/kg) (Stoskopf 1986, 1993). This seems unusual as sharks do possess μ opioid-like receptors and peptides (Li et al. 1986; Lorenz et al. 1986). It is conceivable that as with amphibians (Wright & Whitaker 2001), the amount of receptors binding requires much higher amounts than those published in other animals.

Chloral Hydrate Chloral hydrate is a hypnotic sedative whose mechanism of action is not well understood. When given intrasinus to bonnethead sharks (*Sphyrna tiburo*) at 60–80 mg/kg, reactions were variable from intermittent uncoordination with little obstacle avoidance to settling on the bottom and tolerance of handling. Additionally, the drug caused minor skin reaction at the injection site (Clauss, pers. exp).

Detomidine Hydrochloride Dormosedan® (detomidine hydrochloride) is an α2 agonist. Two trials using relatively high amounts of detomidine (115 μg/kg IM)/ketamine (4.5 mg/kg IM) in a single bull shark (*Carcharhinus leucas*) showed little effect (Clauss, pers. exp.). Atipamezole was given in equal volumes to the detomidine (5× times the microgram dose) for reversal.

Dexmedetomidine This α2 agonist is gaining more popularity since medetomidine can now only be purchased at compounding pharmacies in concentrated form. It has been used in *C. plumbeus*, *C. taurus*, and *G. cirratum* at dosages of 0.03 mg/kg alone and in combination with ketamine. See also the comments on medetomidine and ketamine combinations and their side effects.

Diazepam Diazepam in sand tiger sharks, *C. taurus* (0.1 mg/kg IM) provided satisfactory sedation in one institution, but more research is indicated to define dosages (McEwan, pers. comm., 2011). The authors feel diazepam does not provide sufficient sedation despite use at multiple dosages.

Etomidate Etomidate (0.4–1.3 mg/kg IM) has been used as an induction agent for *C. taurus* and *C. plumbeus* by either darting or by pole syringe. The higher dosages resulted in more rapid induction. The drug formulation is very thick and can result in leakage from the injection site. Anesthetic effects were noted as variable, but resulted in animals that would allow manual restraint and tonic immobility. Ultrasound assessment of these animals noted no cardiac effects (Lecu, pers. comm., 2012).

Guaifenesin The mechanism of guaifenisin is unknown but is believed to depress or block nerve impulse transmission and has sedative qualities. It is commonly used for continuous rate infusions in hoofstock species to maintain muscle relaxation and offer rapid recoveries. Guaifenisin IV was used in *D. americana* after 5–10 minute induction in buffered MS222 (50 ppm), which was enough to allow turning the animal over for IV administration of the drug (Mylniczenko, pers. exp.). The drug was given as a bolus at dosages of 10–40 mg/kg to observe effects in hopes of identifying a continuous rate infusion dose for longer procedures. At the low dosages, this drug provided very little sedative effect and only showed sedation (stage 2) at the higher dosages, with rapid recoveries at all dosages. The only negative effect was a brief cessation of cardiac rhythm, asystole (identified by continual observance via ultrasound), which rapidly returned to a normal rhythm. One other institution has used the drug (20 mg/kg) in a bowmouth guitarfish (*Rhina ancylostoma*) for treatment of a suspected muscular condition and showed minor sedative effects as well (Naples, pers. comm., 2011).

Haloperidol Haloperidol lactate is a neuroleptic butyrophenone used as a tranquilizer in mammals. It is used to facilitate transports of flighty animals and to decrease stress. Its calming effects make it a possible desirable drug for elasmobranchs. During trials in bonnethead sharks (*Sphyrna tiburo*), using the lactate form (2–10 mg/kg) intrasinus, only one animal out of five showed a response (incoordination and hyperexcitability) at the higher dosage. There was also considerable skin reaction to the drug. In general, haloperidol was not considered successful for sedation or adequate tranquilization at the dosages tested (Clauss, pers. exp.). The use of haloperidol decanoate has not been documented in elasmobranchs.

Ketamine Hydrochloride Ketamine hydrochloride is an analgesic and cataleptic cyclohexamine. Ketamine provides good peripheral analgesia (pain relief) in mammals through suppression of dorsal horn cell activity in the spinal cord, but provides little visceral analgesia. Seizure-like muscle spasms due to spinal reflex firing are occasionally noted in elasmobranchs (Stoskopf 1993). For these reasons, it is preferably used in combinations with other anesthetics, but has been used alone at very high dosages (50–80 mg/kg). Recovery is often prolonged and animals are disoriented for long periods of time (another reason to use in combination with reversible anesthetics).

Medetomidine Medetomidine has been used in combination with ketamine in several shark species, including sand tiger shark (*C. taurus*), blacknose shark (*Carcharhinus acronotus*), sandbar shark (*C. plumbeus*), and nurse shark (*G. cirratum*) to ameliorate muscle spasms that can occur with ketamine alone (Snyder et al. 1998; Tuttle & Dunn 2003). See medetomidine/ketamine combinations for effects. Atipamezole is used as the reversal agent at standard mammalian dosages.

Midazolam As a benzodiazepine receptor agonist, midazolam can result in sedation and anxiolytic activity. When used at dosages of 1–5 mg/kg IM as a sole agent in *S. tiburo*, *C. melanopterus*, and *C. plagiosum* the authors have not found the drug to be useful. However, when used in combination with other drugs, induction times do seem to decrease as does the physical excitement phase (Mylniczenko, pers. exp.). When administered intrasinus in *S. tiburo*, there was notable hyperexcitability and ataxia at 4–5 mg/kg in two animals, while at 8 mg/kg death occurred in one animal (Clauss, pers. exp.).

Propofol Propofol is a sedative-hypnotic (Miller 2001; Mitchell et al. 2001) and has been administered at 2.5 mg/kg IV over 30 seconds to spotted bamboo sharks

(*Chiloscyllium plagiosum*), achieving a surgical anesthetic level by 5 minutes. Righting response returned within 60 and 75 minutes in four and two of the sharks, respectively. Respiration and heart rates remained stable throughout the anesthetic period. Using the drug at 1–2 mg/kg IV in *C. plagiosium*, *D. americana*, and *O. japonicas*, inductions were very smooth and provided long sedations, but recoveries were prolonged (>30 minutes) (Mylniczenko, pers. exp.). When used intrasinus in *S. tiburo*, at 2.5 mg/kg, slight incoordination was noted but no anesthesia. At 5 mg/kg, however, induction was rapid, a surgical plane of anesthesia was achieved, and marked respiratory suppression occurred with return to gilling >35 minutes post induction. The animals returned to swimming >65 minutes after induction, which is not practical for ram ventilators (Clauss, pers. exp.). In the spiny dogfish (*S. acanthias*), a minimum of 5 mg/kg IV was necessary to achieve a surgical stage of anesthesia (Cavin et al. 2007). With *C. limbatus*, 2.5–3.0 mg/kg delivered intrasinus resulted in rapid induction (<1 minute) and a surgical plane of anesthesia with persistent shallow, irregular spontaneous ventilation. Sharks returned to normal gilling 35–45 minutes post induction and normal swimming in 55–75 minutes (Clauss, pers. exp.).

Sodium Pentobarbital Sodium pentobarbital (10 mg/kg) produced satisfactory general surgical anesthesia in nurse sharks (*Ginglymosoma cirratum*) when administered rapidly IV (Walker 1972). Slow injection resulted in an erratic response. Intraperitoneal absorption was slow and response was variable, while IM injection resulted in only slightly improved response. Serum half-life was approximately 15 seconds with a second half-life of several days, due to an inability of the animals to excrete the drug through their gills or kidneys. An anesthetic IV dose (10 mg/kg) resulted in loss of ventilatory movements (gilling) within 1 minute. Gilling returned after 10 minutes and a weak righting response was observed at 3 hours. A higher IV dose (20 mg/kg) resulted in a rapid loss of gilling that did not return by 3 hours. A weak righting response was only observed after 5 hours. A high IV dose (60 mg/kg) resulted in death. Larger, more active sharks require smaller doses per kilogram than smaller, sedentary specimens. For example, sandbar and bull sharks (6 mg/kg IV) responded similarly to the nurse shark (10 mg/kg IV) (Walker 1972).

Tiletamine/Zolazepam Tiletamine/zolazepam (12 mg/kg) administered to a lemon (*Negaprion brevirostris*) and a sand tiger (*C. taurus*) shark produced irritability, rapid swimming, and unrestrained biting (Stoskopf 1986, 1993). Dosages of 5–20 mg/kg IM in *C. plagiosum* showed very little response even at the high dosage (some animals allowed being turned over for a few seconds) (Kilborne, unpubl. data, 1999).

Xylazine Xylazine in bony fish (teleosts) is a convulsant and causes major changes in the electrocardiogram (Oswald 1978). Used in combination with ketamine (12 mg/kg), xylazine (6 mg/kg) in sand tiger shark (*C. taurus*), lemon shark (*Negaprion brevirostris*), sandbar shark(*C. plumbeus*), and nurse shark (*Ginglymosoma cirratum*) variably ameliorated the muscle spasms that can occur with ketamine alone (Stoskopf 1993). Yohimbine hydrochloride administered IV to a nurse shark immobilized with xylazine/ketamine caused arousal (Stoskopf 1986).

Injectable Anesthetic Combinations

Several drug combinations have been or are currently being investigated for immobilization or anesthesia of elasmobranchs. Stoskopf (1986) showed xylazine (6 mg/kg) and ketamine (12 mg/kg) satisfactorily immobilized (between stage I and III) sand tiger (*C. taurus*) ($n = 4$), lemon (*N. brevirostris*) ($n = 4$), sandbar (*C. plumbeus*) ($n = 9$), and nurse sharks (*G. cirratum*)($n = 5$). Andrews and Jones (1990) also found xylazine (7.5 mg/kg) and ketamine (16.5 mg/kg) produced light anesthesia adequate for the safe transport of adult sandbar sharks (*C. plumbeus*).

One popular combination is IM medetomidine and ketamine at varying dosages (see Table 16.1). General dosages range from 90–100 ug/kg medetomidine and 4–5 mg/kg ketamine. Usually initial effects take 20–40 minutes, but results can be erratic. These effects vary from complete anesthesia with recumbency (some within 5 min), animals showing partial signs with no recumbency (despite additional dosing), and animals showing almost no sedative effects. There also appears to be a great variation between species in their responses to similar dosages under the same conditions. Additionally, recoveries are highly variable, with reports of immediate recoveries to some deaths several days later. Anorexia is a common complaint post procedure. Cavin and Innis (pers. comm.) sedated three adult sand tigers with variable inductions and recoveries. Recoveries of 6–10 hrs with one not swimming until 24 hrs; all swam abnormally slowly and did not eat for 2–3 weeks after the exam.

Penning and his team (2012) have successfully used medetomidine and butorphanol for multiple procedures in several elasmobranchs. Medetomidine (0.1 mg/kg IM) and butorphanol at (0.65 mg/kg IM) proved very successful with several *Carcharinus* species. Moderate success was achieved with giant guitarfish *(R. djiddensis)* by increasing the butorphanol dosage to 1 mg/kg. Inductions started at approximately 20 minutes, but animals were not handled until 45 minutes, considered a minimum time to avoid stimulation for successful sedation. The animals were then guided into a plastic sock (described above) and transported. In some instances, the sharks lay on the bottom of the tank, while others continued to glide very slowly. Reversals were given for rapid and full recoveries. The team noted

the addition of ketamine seemed to increase the frequency of phantom biting or biting at the stimulating activities. In these situations, they offered a bite stick for the animal to hold onto (Penning, pers. comm.).

In bamboo sharks (*C. plagiosum*), midazolam (1–5 mg/kg), medetomidine (80–90 μk/kg), and butorphanol (0.5–1 mg/kg) had little to no effect IM, but minor sedative effects IV. With the latter route, the animals tolerated being turned over and stayed dorsally recumbent for several seconds to several minutes (Mylniczenko, pers. exp.).

Oral (PO)

Oral sedation of elasmobranchs is not widely practiced and rarely reported (Clauss et al. 2011; Raines & Clancy 2009). It holds potential for management of animals in large aquaria and for improving capture of animals for further immobilization. In one study, four ocellated river stingrays (*Potamotrygon motoro*) were offered ketamine-injected earthworms at a dosage of 20 mg/kg; within 15 minutes, the animals were easily netted and placed into dorsal recumbency, but did not reach anesthetic depths (Raines and Clancy 2009). In a different study, multiple sedatives were used with bonnethead sharks (*S. tiburo*), comparing oral (via capsule in food) and IV injectable drugs (Clauss, pers. exp.). The oral drugs produced little effect, even at doses considered high for other species. These drugs included chloral hydrate (no sedative response at 300 mg/kg), ketamine (no sedative response at 30 mg/kg), and haloperidol lactate (no sedative response at dosages up to 50 mg/kg). Haloperidol showed no sedative effects at 10 mg/kg in *Triakis semifasciata*, but did show behavioral modifying effects (decreased stereotypy) (Mylniczenko, pers. exp.). The authors have also used diazepam at dosages from 1 to 40 mg/kg (most at the 1–10 mg/kg range) with variable anxiolytic effects or appetite stimulation effects. There were no overt sedative effects in a variety of species: sawfish (*Pristis zijsron*), brown sharks (*C. plumbeus*), blacktip reef shark (*C. melanopterus*), leopard (*Triakis semifasciata*), blotched fantail ray (*Taeniura meyeni*), bowmouth (*Rhina ancylostoma*), and whale sharks (*Rhincodon typus*). More research is indicated to evaluate the usefulness of oral sedation in elasmobranchs.

Nonspecific "Reversal" Drugs

Doxapram Hydrochloride Doxapram hydrochloride has been noted to produce dramatic arousal and stimulation in anesthetized elasmobranchs and should be used with caution because animals can become extremely excited and dangerous (Stoskopf 1986).

MONITORING

In captive animals, a quiet environment without predatory tank mates should be used for anesthetic induction and maintenance. Several baseline physiological variables should be monitored. Ventilation rates are recorded if the animal is actively pumping water through the gills and not ram ventilating (i.e., using forward motion to force water through the gills). Caudal fin strokes are measured to determine the onset of drug effect; this activity is usually the first to be reduced.

After an animal becomes ventrally recumbent, the righting reflex, respiration, and heart rate should be closely monitored. Although animals may appear to be ventilating well, bradycardia and an increased resistance to gill capillary flow (as erythrocytes accumulate within the capillary bed and become swollen) has been noted to possibly cause hypoxemia (Tyler & Hawkins 1981). Therefore, the authors strongly advise assisted ventilated even with voluntary gill movement. Gill ventilation rate and rhythm can be monitored visually. If respiration becomes erratic, slows significantly, or ceases, the animal must be manually ventilated by directing water flow over the gills. Respiratory effectiveness is best assessed with periodic blood gas analysis to determine oxygenation, carbon dioxide, pH, and lactate levels. Large changes in blood chemistry can occur during the stress of capture and handling elasmobranch fishes (Frick & Reina 2009; Mandelmann & Skomal 2009; Naples et al. 2012). Respiratory, metabolic, and lactic acidosis are common. In elasmobranchs, lactic acid is produced in large quantities during hyperactivity and the resultant acidemia is usually corrected by hydrogen ions buffering or through gill excretion (a much slower process). This is why lactate levels will continue to rise in elasmobranchs for up to 12 hours after the inciting event (Piiper & Baumgarten 1969). Experiments with larger spotted dogfish (*Scyliorhinus stellaris*) indicated PaCO$_2$ was increased immediately after exercise, but returned to baseline within 1 hour. The pH gradually decreased, reaching a minimum in the second hour and returned to baseline within 8 hours. Lactate concentrations increased slowly to very high levels reaching a maximum of 220 mg% within 6–8 hours after exercise (Piiper & Baumgarten 1969). The pH may, therefore, correct itself in an animal that has sufficient buffering capacity, but this is largely determined by the animal's respiratory mode and method of oxygen metabolism (Chapman & Renshaw 2009; Cliff & Thurman 1984; Frick & Reina 2009; Manire et al. 2001; Piiper & Baumgarten 1969). Benthic animals tolerate and correct acidemia more readily than pelagic.

Handheld analyzers offer rapid analysis at poolside or on a boat and some automatically adjust calculations for lower body temperature. If they do not, then correction for ambient water temperature is necessary, or alternately, evaluation or trends should be followed rather than actual values. The pH appears to be a critical variable to monitor. For the authors, animals with corrected values under 7.0 are unlikely to recover, even

when chemical restraint is not utilized. A temperature corrected pH of 7.2 is usually associated with imminent recovery from anesthesia. Lactate levels are useful for anticipating problems that may occur later or for evaluating handling/anesthetic events. Further investigation is needed to determine lactate values that would indicate that an animal is at increased risk. These values vary by species. Under circumstances of continued pH decline and/or lactate elevation, the authors have treated animals with fluids solely or in combination with sodium bicarbonate and/or sodium acetate therapy.

Another factor to consider when evaluating blood gas variables is the location used for blood collection. In larger specimens, the dorsal sinus is often used for blood collection due to ease of access. Several variables, however, have been shown to be inaccurate for the animal's baseline state. Not only is hematocrit lower at this site compared with the tail (Mylniczenko et al. 2006), blood gas values are also different. In particular, pH and lactate are not accurate or "real-time" when measured in blood samples collected from the dorsal sinus (Naples et al. 2012). The collected sample from the tail is likely to be arterial if the needle tip is moved just off the cartilage as the vessel abuts the vertebrae.

Heart rate is monitored using either an ultrasound or Doppler flow detection probe placed over the heart. It is located along the ventral midline just caudal to the gill openings (Fig. 16.10). The heart rate will vary between species and in response to stress and temperature. Most unanesthetized fish will have a heart rate between 30 and 70 beats per minute, depending on animal size, species, and condition (Lewbart 2001). In addition to heart rate, the contraction quality and rhythm are critical to examine. Changes, such as weak

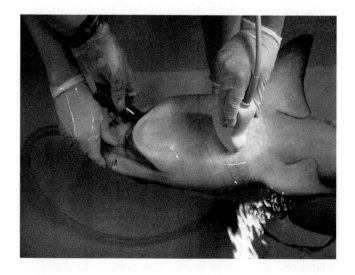

Figure 16.10. Cardiac ultrasound of a whitetip reef shark (*Triaenodon obesus*).

contractions and dysrhythmias, may indicate the animal is doing poorly under anesthesia and must be recovered. If contractions appear to be weak, then evaluation of the animal's calcium is warranted, particularly ionized calcium, which can be monitored with a handheld analyzer. Normally, this value is greater than the readable limit of some portable units (>2.5 mmol/L). If it is reading below this value, and the animal has weak contractions, then the animal should be recovered and/or calcium administered to manage the relatively lower calcium levels (Mylniczenko, pers. exp.).

Anesthetic stages in elasmobranchs are similar to mammals and teleost fish (Chapter 15). Stages are gauged by activity, reactivity to stimuli, equilibrium, muscle tone, respiratory rate and heart rate (Ross & Ross 2008). The period between respiratory and cardiac arrest, however, is greater because the respiratory capillaries are able to exchange oxygen and carbon dioxide when water flow over the gills is maintained via assisted ventilation. Stages of anesthesia are highly variable between animals (both intra and interspecies) and between drugs.

During an immobilization procedure, it is also important to monitor and control the water quality of the anesthesia or restraint system as poor or altered water variables may negatively impact the animal(s). Temperature fluctuations may also occur if the water volume is small and should be controlled. Hyper or hypothermia can impact metabolism and recovery. Dissolved oxygen should be maintained close to 100% and may require the addition of supplemental air stones with or without supplemental oxygen. If animals have not been adequately fasted, buildup of nitrogenous waste due to elimination may result, requiring water changes or chemical additions. Waterborne anesthetics, in particular MS-222, can lower the pH of the water and will require buffering.

RECOVERY CONSIDERATIONS AND POSTANESTHETIC CHALLENGES

All safety precautions exercised for induction and maintenance should continue to be a priority during recovery from anesthesia. An isolated environment is preferable. Ideally, the recovery container or tank will be easily accessible for the staff but will also be large enough to allow the animal space to swim as it progresses through stages of recovery. Water in recovery containers should be well aerated. The water flow should be aimed toward the fish's mouth if the animal is respiring spontaneously. Assisted ventilation directly over the gills may be necessary if the fish is not respiring, if the respiration rate is slow or irregular, or if the animal is still sedate from anesthesia. An alternative to using the ventilation system is pulling the fish forward

through the water with its mouth open. However, in the authors' experience, this method is inferior to the use of a ventilation system.

Animals should continue to be monitored carefully during recovery. Care should be taken when monitoring requires any touching or handling as some fish may exhibit erratic behavior to this stimulus. If a fish is respiring spontaneously and attempting to regain normal posture in the water column, it is often best left untouched to avoid erratic movements and added stress. However, if an animal is in danger of injuring itself due to erratic movements, restraint may be necessary (Harms 1999). Additionally, if animals are released prior to being able to maneuver in the water column, they may swim briefly and then fall to the bottom of the recovery pool. This is not an issue with buccopharyngeal breathers, but can be problematic with pelagic animals; the animal must be retrieved and continue to be supported through recovery. It is important to have experienced personnel involved when making judgment calls of this nature. As a fish recovers from anesthesia, the respiratory rate should increase and the rhythm should stabilize. Muscle tone and fin movements should return followed by progressively less ataxia. Careful observation is important, and staff should be readily available to intervene if the fish becomes distressed or the recovery process halts.

Recovery from immersion anesthesia begins when the fish is placed in anesthesia-free water. With most immersion anesthetics, the authors find that time to full recovery is seldom greater than 10 minutes. During the recovery process, the water in the tank may need to be changed as anesthetics and their metabolites may be excreted from the fish into the water and potentially reabsorbed. The same process is theoretically possible with oral or parenteral drugs as they, too, may be excreted into the water and reabsorbed. Recovery from oral or parenteral anesthetics technically begins after the drug is administered and fully metabolized. Faster recovery in some cases is facilitated by administering reversal agents. However, there is no reversal for some drugs, and in those situations, it is up to the fish to fully metabolize and clear the drug(s) for full recovery to occur. Recovery time from oral and parenteral agents is dependent on the route of administration, rate of metabolism, use of reversal agents, health status of the patient, and the species. As has been mentioned previously, the response to anesthetics and associated recoveries varies considerably both within a species and between species of elasmobranchs.

Extended recovery periods may occur with excessive anesthetic dosage, in a medically compromised animal or for unknown pharmacokinetic reasons. Due to the tremendous variation in response to anesthesia, extrapolation of doses is challenging and can potentially result in prolonged recoveries or other unpredictable scenarios. At the New England Aquarium, two sand tiger sharks (*C. taurus*) anesthetized with dexmedetomidine (0.03 mg/kg) and ketamine (3.0 mg/kg), followed by MS-222 (70–90 mg/L) immersion, had markedly different recovery times. Even after reversal with atipamezole, one shark did not begin to swim until 6 hours after reversal and return to the exhibit tank. The other shark did not begin to swim until 24 hours after reversal (Cavin and Innis, pers. comm., 2011). At the Living Seas with Nemo and Friends® (Walt Disney World, Orlando, FL), highly variable responses to a similar drug combination were noted and ranged from no response to rapid induction; recoveries were also highly varied, such as a quick return to normal versus different degrees of abnormal behavior, including swim gait abnormalities, anorexia, and prolonged lethargy for up to 7 days in the same species.

Care should be taken not to abandon recovery or resuscitation attempts prematurely in apneic fish as respiratory arrest may precede cardiac arrest by extended periods of time. In the authors' experience, anesthetics such as propofol may produce respiratory arrest for periods in excess of 30 minutes followed by full recovery when the sharks are artificially ventilated. Four bonnethead sharks (*S. tiburo*) at the Georgia Aquarium were anesthetized with propofol (5.0 mg/kg) administered into the first dorsal sinus. Spontaneous respirations ceased within three minutes. The sharks were artificially ventilated with a submersible pump and monitored closely. Gilling resumed in all four animals within 36–52 minutes after propofol administration. Fish with persistent apnea or bradypnea that also experience bradycardia, abnormal blood gases, or other physiological challenges may be given doxapram. The authors have observed positive response to doxapram (5 mg/kg IV, IM, ICo, or over the gills) in several cases of respiratory arrest. Caution should be used when administering doxapram as it may cause hyperexcitability, especially in sharks.

In some situations, it may be necessary to provide supportive care and/or emergency drugs, such as atropine, corticosteroids, fluids, or other therapeutics. In cases of shock or physiological collapse, corticosteroids, such as methylprednisolone, prednisolone, or dexamethasone, may be given with the caveat that it is unknown if steroid therapy is effective in elasmobranchs. In the authors' experience, corticosteroid administration has been subjectively helpful in some cases and no adverse effects have been noted.

Emergency fluid therapy should take into account the animal's osmotic balance as well as any imbalances or deficiencies that may be present. Elasmobranchs are hyperosmotic to their environment with urea, NaCl, and trimethylamine oxide being the major osmoregulatory plasma components (Olson 1999). Elasmobranch Ringers, a balanced salt solution, is made by adding NaCl (8 g/L) and urea (21 g/L) to phenol red-free Hank's balanced salt solution (Andrews & Jones 1990). Alternatively, if Hank's balanced salt solution is not available, 0.9% NaCl or Normosol R with of additional NaCl (8 g/L) and urea (21 g/L) may be used. Thorough summaries on the osmoregulation of elasmobranchs as it is currently understood can be found in the literature (Anderson et al. 2007; Hammerschlag 2006). Greenwell et al. (2003) provides an overview of the clinical implications involved with elasmobranch osmoregulation including additional guidelines on the principles of fluid administration. The fluids are ideally administered through a needle or catheter placed in the caudal vein or the dorsal sinus, but may also be administered intracoelomically or orally. No rates of fluid administration have been published based on scientific studies, but the authors use maintenance doses of 7–10 mL/kg. Fluid volumes reportedly as high as 66 mL/kg/d have been given following surgical procedures and routine handling (Greenwell et al. 2003). Some elasmobranchs appear to respond to oral freshwater administration at 1–3% body weight in less severe situations. When metabolic acidemia occurs, if the fish is unable to compensate and does not respond to increased oxygen supplementation and fluid therapy, it may be beneficial to administer an alkalinizing agent such as sodium bicarbonate or sodium acetate. Care should be taken not to over correct causing an alkalosis or electrolyte imbalance.

As with other classes of animals, administration of emergency medications varies by case and should be governed by individual animal needs. Table 16.2 lists emergency and supportive care therapeutics the authors have used that has been valuable when working with elasmobranchs and holocephalans.

FIELD IMMOBILIZATION

Immobilization of elasmobranchs in the field has been in practice for many years. Live release biological assessments and subsequent tagging and tracking provide valuable information on factors such as population dynamics, spatial patterns, foraging behavior, and health status of free ranging animals. These activities have become increasingly common practice as scientists try to understand the causes and significance of changing or declining populations and relationships to ocean health.

Generally, animals are manually restrained after hook and line, long line, or trawl net capture, but other techniques may be employed as warranted. In these situations, naïve animals are being placed under the rigors of extreme exercise and are particularly vulnerable to exertional rhabdomyolosis (Chapter 12), hypoxemia and lactic acidemia, hook and handling trauma, and stomach eversion. Pelagic (ram ventilating) species are especially susceptible to stress and exhaustion and

Table 16.2. Drugs used for emergency and supportive care in anesthetized elasmobranchs

	Elasmobranch and Holocephalan Emergency Medications		
Drug	Dosage	Route	Indication
Atropine	0.02–0.2 mg/kg	IV, IM, IP	Bradycardia, arrythmia, organophosphate poisoning
Glycopyrrolate	0.01 mg/kg	IV, IM	Bradycardia, arrythmia
Epinephrine	0.2 mL/kg	IV, IM, IP	Bradycardia, cardiac arrest
Doxapram	2–10 mg/kg	IV, IM, over gills; may cause hyperexcitability	Apnea, respiratory arrest
Furosemide	2–3 mg/kg	IV, IM, IP	Excessive coelomic fluid, generalized edema
Dexamethasone	1–2 mg/kg	IV, IM, IP	Stress, shock, trauma
Methyl-prednisolone acetate	30 mg/kg initial, 15 mg/kg follow-up		
Prednisolone sodium succinate	5–30 mg/kg		
Midazolam	0.5 mg/kg	IV, IM	Seizures
Diazepam	1–2 mg/kg		
Calcium gluconate	0.2–1.5 mL/kg	IV, IP	Muscle fasiculations, tetany, dysrhythmias, decreased myocardial contractility
Calcium lactate/calcium glycerophosphate	10 mg/kg	IV, IM, IP	
Sodium bicarbonate	0.5–1 mEq/kg	IV, IM, IP	Acidosis
Sodium acetate	1 mEq/kg diluted ~ 1:10 with fluids	IV, IP	
Hank's balanced salt solution + 8 g/L NaCland 21 g/L urea	7–10 mL/kg	IV, IP, PO	Dehydration, shock, fluid loss, hypovolemia, hypotension
0.9% NaCl + 8 g/L NaCl and 21 g/L urea	7–10 mL/kg		

can have a poor chance of survival; however, this is highly species dependent (Mandelman & Skomal 2009). Location of release may also have an impact on survivability. Predatory fish, including other elasmobranchs, may take the opportunity to predate a tired, recently released animal, particularly if the area has been chummed to attract additional specimens for capture. Often, however, there is no control in the matter as the animals are mainly caught and released in open water. Capture–release scenarios that result in the least impact to the animal are imperative.

Experienced handlers are required as the space on a boat or dock is limited, areas on deck are potentially unstable, or wet and animals are strong and often very agitated (see previous comments in this chapter about manual restraint and safety). If the animals will be out of the water for any length of time, it is advised to safely ventilate them with the water they were just pulled from. If animals are to be maintained in live wells, consider the time in the well, volume of water, oxygen delivery to the water, swim-glide pattern (usually nonexistent under these circumstances), and number of animals in the well (more animals means more consumption of oxygen, crowding, and excretion of biological end products).

In some scenarios with animals too large to be hauled onto the deck, they must be restrained in the water along the side of the boat or dock (Fig. 16.11). Under these circumstances, even more expertise and potentially specialized equipment is important for

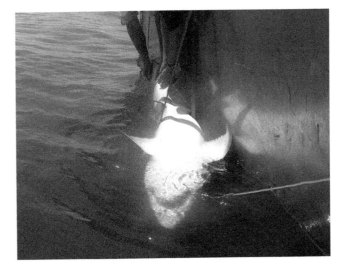

Figure 16.11. Collection of blood from a free-ranging sand tiger shark (*Carcharias taurus*) during a population health assessment project in Delaware Bay (photo credit: Georgia Aquarium).

human and animal safety. Though rare, when capture and immobilization involves extremely large specimens, such as white sharks, whale sharks, or manta rays, specialized water craft is also necessary.

It is rare to use anesthesia for field immobilization procedures for a number of reasons: speed, efficiency, space, and most importantly regulations governing using drugs in potential food fish (U.S. Fish and Wildlife Service, The Aquatic Animal Drug Approval Partnership 2010). It is important to note that if elasmobranchs are to be retained in captivity for extended periods of time, there may be restrictions against release or there may be special permitting required, but this is highly variable by state in the United States.

When health assessments occur during field immobilization projects, additional considerations include having portable equipment that can connect and operate on generators, batteries, or plugged into the vessel's electrical, as well as having adequate, safe storage and preservation capacity for biological specimens. Weather and water conditions may change rapidly and in turn may complicate sample collection, processing, and safe handling. Having seaworthy staff, experienced in biological sample processing is beneficial.

With any field immobilization technique, speed and precision is essential to reduce the stress on the animal and improve viability on release. Ultimately, limited handling or limited time in a live well is best. Some researchers have developed techniques for collecting samples and attaching tracking or identification devices without physically restraining the animals. These methods usually involve less stress or physical exertion for the animal, but may present a different set of safety hazards for the people involved.

Some studies have assessed the impacts of catching elasmobranchs for science, sport or accidentally as by-catch. Blood acid-base status can be utilized to gauge the magnitude of the stress response, which is dependent on the nature of the capture and the metabolic capacity of the animal in question (Mandelmann & Skomal 2009). Changes in blood glucose, electrolytes, osmolality, and hematocrit have also been documented in various species of elasmobranchs after capture (Wells et al. 1986; Wendelaar Bonga 1997; Hoffmayer & Parsons 2001; Manire et al. 2001; Moyes et al. 2006). Regardless of collection technique, captured fish experience distress caused by the cumulative impacts of physical trauma and physiological stress (Skomal 2007). The importance of swift and meticulous capture, handling, and release cannot be underestimated and can greatly improve survivability in field immobilization activities.

EUTHANASIA

The goal of euthanasia should be the rapid loss of consciousness. This can be accomplished by an overdosage of immobilization drugs. Inhalant (immersion) drugs at 5–10× the anesthetic concentration for a particular species can be chosen (Ross & Ross 2008). Elasmobranchs, however, may require sedation first with parenteral drugs then euthanasia with a drug such as pentobarbital, following all of the previously stated techniques. Use of Doppler flow probes, ultrasonography, or electrocardiography is recommended to confirm asystole. Severing the spinal cord at the brain stem (decapitation) or exsanguination are alternatives to chemotherapeutic euthanasia and can be performed once the fish is anesthetized. The reader is directed to review euthanasia principles for fish as outlined by the American Veterinary Medical Association (AVMA). Unacceptable methods of euthanasia include asphyxiation and hypothermia.

ACKNOWLEDGMENTS

Portions of this chapter have previously been published in Smith M, Warmolts D, Thoney D, Hueter R. (eds.) 2004, The elasmobranch husbandry manual: captive care of sharks, rays and their relatives (a special publication of the Ohio Biological Survey). The authors would like to thank Mike Walsh, Ilze Berzins, Lisa Naples, Don Neiffer, Lynda Leppert, Nicholas Parnell, and Nicole Hatcher for their assistance in preparing the manuscript.

REFERENCES

Adamson RH, Guarino AM. 1972. The effect of foreign compounds on elasmobranchs and the effect of elasmobranchs on foreign compounds. *Comparative Biochemistry and Physiology. A, Comparative Physiology* 42(1):171–182.

Adrian Van Rijn J, Reina RD. 2010. Distribution of leukocytes as indicators of stress in the Australian swellshark, *Cephaloscyllium laticeps*. *Fish and Shellfish Immunology* 29:534–538.

Anderson WG. 2012. The endocrinology of 1α-hydroxycorticosterone in elasmobranch fish: a review. *Comparative Biochemistry and Physiology. A, Comparative Physiology* 162:73–80.

Anderson WG, Taylor JR, Good JP, Hazon N, Grosell M. 2007. Body fluid volume regulation in elasmobranch fish. *Comparative Biochemistry and Physiology. A, Comparative Physiology* 148: 3–13.

Andrews JC, Jones RT. 1990. A method for the transport of sharks for captivity. *Journal of Aquaculture and Aquatic Sciences* 5: 70–72.

Aquatic Animal Drug Approval Partnership. 2010. *Quick Reference Guide to Approved Drugs for Use in Aquaculture*. Washington, DC: U.S. Fish and Wildlife Service.

Baker A. 1991. Training as a management tool: creating the climate and maintaining the momentum. Proceedings of the American Association of Zoological Parks and Aquariums, pp. 563–568.

Beck K, Loomis M, Lewbart G, Spelman L, Papich M. 1995. Preliminary comparison of plasma concentrations of gentamycin injected into the cranial and caudal limb musculature of the eastern box turtle (*Terrapene carolina carolina*). *Journal of Zoo and Wildlife Medicine* 26:265–268.

Bernal D, Dickson KA, Shadwick RE, Graham JB. 2001. Review: analysis of the evolutionary convergence for high performance swimming in laminid sharks and tunas. *Comparative Biochemistry and Physiology. A, Comparative Physiology* 129:695–726.

Bernal D, Sepulveda C, Mathieu-Costello O, Graham JB. 2003. Comparative studies of high performance swimming in sharks I. Red muscle morphometrics, vascularization and ultrastructure. *The Journal of Experimental Biology* 206:2831–2843.

Bernal SD, Graham JB. 2001. Water-tunnel studies of heat balance in swimming mako sharks. *The Journal of Experimental Biology* 204:4043–4054.

Bone Q. 1999. Microscopical anatomy, physiology and biochemistry of elasmobranch muscle fibers. In: *Sharks, Skates, and Rays. The Biology of Elasmobranch Fishes* (WC Hamlett, ed.), pp. 115–143. Baltimore: Johns Hopkins University Press.

Bone Q, Chubb AD. 1983. The retial system of the locomotor muscle in the thresher shark. *Journal of the Marine Biological Association of the United Kingdom* 63:239–241.

Brown EA, Franklin JE, Pratt E, Trams EG. 1972. Contributions to the pharmacology of quinaldine (uptake and distribution in the shark and comparative studies). *Comparative Biochemistry and Physiology. A, Comparative Physiology* 42(1):223–231.

Butler PJ. 1999. Respiratory system. In: *Sharks, Skates, and Rays: The Biology of Elasmobranch Fishes* (WC Hamlett, ed.), pp. 174–195. Baltimore: John Hopkins University Press.

Carey FG, Teal JM, Kanwisher JW, Lawson KD, Beckett JS. 1971. Warm-bodied fish. *Integrative and Comparative Biology* 11(1):137–143.

Carey FG, Casey JG, Pratt HL, Urquhart D, McCosker JE. 1985. Temperature, heat production and heat exchange in laminid sharks. *Memoirs of the Southern California Academy of Sciences* 9:92–108.

Carrier JC, Musick JA, Heithaus MR, eds. 2004. *Biology of Sharks and Their Relatives*. Boca Raton: CRC Press.

Carrier JC, Musick JA, Heithaus MR, eds. 2011. *Sharks and Their Relatives II: Biodiversity, Adaptive Physiology and Conservation*. Boca Raton: CRC Press.

Cavin J, Smolowitz R, Lewbart GA, Cavin RM. 2007. The effects of propofol and ketamine/medetomidine in the spiny dogfish (*Squalus acanthias*). Proceedings of the International Association for Aquatic Animal Medicine, Lake Buena Vista, FL, p. 123.

Chapman CA, Renshaw GM. 2009. Hematological responses of the grey carpet shark (*Chiloscyllium punctattum*) and epaulette shark (*Hemiscyllium ocellatum*) to anoxia and re-oxygenation. *Journal of Experimental Zoology. Part A, Comparative Experimental Biology* 311:422–438.

Clauss T, Berliner A, Brainard B. 2011. Chemical restraint in bonnethead sharks (*Sphyrna tiburo*): pilot studies with select sedatives and anesthestics. Proceedings of the International Association for Aquatic Animal Medicine, Las Vegas, NV, p. 121.

Cliff G, Thurman GD. 1984. Pathological and physiological effects of stress during capture and transport in the juvenile dusky shark, *Carcharhinus obscurus*. *Comparative Biochemistry and Physiology. A, Comparative Physiology* 78:167–173.

Compagno LJV. 1999. Systematics and body form. In: *Sharks, Skates, and Rays: The Biology of Elasmobranch Fishes* (WC Hamlett, ed.), pp. 1–42. Baltimore: John Hopkins University Press.

Daly J, Gunn I, Kirby N, Jones R, Galloway D. 2007. Ultrasound examination and behavior scoring of captive broadnose sevengill sharks, *Notorynchus cepedianus* (Peron, 1807). *Zoo Biology* 26(5):383–395.

Davie PS, Franklin CE, Grigg GC. 1993. Blood pressure and heart rate during tonic immobility in the black tipped reef shark (*Carcharhinus melanoptera*). *Fish Physiology and Biochemistry* 12:95–100.

Davis MR, Mylniczenko ND, Storms TN, Raymond F, Dunn JL. 2006. Evaluation of intramuscular ketoprofen and butorphanol as analgesics in chain dogfish (*Scyliorhinus retifer*). *Zoo Biology* 25:491–500.

Dunn RF, Koester DM. 1990. Anesthetics in elasmobranchs: a review with emphasis on halothane-oxygen-nitrous oxide. *Journal of Aquaculture and Aquatic Sciences* 5:44–52.

Frick LH, Reina RD. 2009. The physiological response of Port Jackson sharks and Australian swellsharks to sedation, gill-net capture, and repeated sampling in captivity. *North American Journal of Fisheries Management* 29:127–139.

Garcia-Parrage D, Alvaro T, Valls M, Malabia A. 2007. Tiletamine-Zolazepam injectable anesthesia: an easy technique to handle fish in large volume aquaria. Proceedings of the International Association for Aquatic Animal Medicine, pp. 25–27.

Gilbert PW, Kritzler H. 1960. Experimental shark pens at the Lerner Marine Laboratory. *Science* 140:424.

Gilbert PW, Wood FG. 1957. Method of anesthetizing large sharks and rays safely and rapidly. *Science* 126:212–213.

Graham JB, Dickson KA. 2000. The evolution of thunniform locomotion and heat conservation in scombrid fishes: new insights based on the morphology of *Allothunnus fallai*. *Zoological Journal of the Linnean Society* 129:419–466.

Graham JB, Dickson KA. 2001. Anatomical and physiological specializations for endothermy. *Fish Physiology* 19:121–165.

Graham JB, Koehrn FJ, Dickson KA. 1983. Distribution and relative proportions of red muscle in scombrid fishes: consequences of body size and relationships to locomotion and endothermy. *Canadian Journal of Zoology* 61:2087–2096.

Greenwell MG, Sherrill J, Clayton LA. 2003. Osmoregulation in fish: mechanisms and clinical implications. *The Veterinary Clinics of North America. Exotic Animal Practice* 6:169–189.

Greer-Walker M, Pull G. 1975. A survey of red and white muscle in marine fish. *Journal of Fish Biology* 7:295–300.

Grogan ED, Lund R. 2004. The origin and relationships of early Chondrichthyes. In: *Biology of Sharks and Their Relatives* (JC Carrier, JA Musick, MR Heithaus, eds.), pp. 3–31. Boca Raton: CRC Press.

Gruber SH, Keyes RS. 1981. Keeping sharks for research. In: *Aquarium Systems* (AD Hawkins, ed.), pp. 373–402. London: Academic Press.

Grusha DS 2005. Investigation of the life history of the cownose ray (*Rhinoptera* bonasus). In fulfillment of a Master of Science at The College of William and Mary in Virginia. http://web.vims.edu/library/Theses/Grusha05.pdf (accessed January 27, 2014).

Hamlett WC, ed. 1999. *Sharks, Skates, and Rays: The Biology of Elasmobranch Fishes*. Baltimore: Johns Hopkins University Press.

Hammerschlag N. 2006. Osmoregulation in elasmobranchs: a review for fish biologists, behaviourists and ecologists. *Marine and Freshwater Behaviour and Physiology* 39:209–228.

Harms CA. 1999. Anesthesia in fish. In: *Zoo and Wild Animal Medicine, Current Therapy 4* (ME Fowler, RE Miller, eds.), pp. 158–163. Philadelphia: W.B. Saunders.

Harvey B, Denny C, Kaiser S, Young J. 1988. Remote intramuscular injection of immobilizing drugs into fish using a laser-aimed underwater dart gun. *The Veterinary Record* 122:174–177.

Henningsen A. 1994. Tonic immobility in 12 elasmobranchs: use as an aid in captive husbandry. *Zoo Biology* 13:325–332.

Hoffmayer ER, Parsons GR. 2001. The physiological response to capture and handling stress in the Atlantic sharpnose shark, *Rhizoprionodon terraenovae*. *Fish Physiology and Biochemistry* 25:277–285.

Holmgren S, Nilsson S. 1999. Digestive System. In: *Sharks, Skates, and Rays: The Biology of Elasmobranch Fishes* (WC Hamlett, ed.), pp. 144–173. Baltimore: Johns Hopkins University Press.

Holz PH. 1999. The reptilian renal portal system: a review. *Bulletin of the ARAV* 9:4–9.

Holz PH, Burger JP, Pasloske K, Baker R, Young S. 2002. Effect of injection site on carbenicillin pharmacokinetics in the carpet python, *Morelia spilot. Journal of Herpetological Medicine and Surgery* 12:12–16.

Hseu J-R, Yeh S-L, Chu Y-T, Ting Y-Y. 1995. The use of 2-phenoxyethanol as an anesthetic in the transport of black porgy Acanthopagrus schlegeli. *Journal of the Fisheries Society of Taiwan* 3(1): 11–18 (in Chinese with English abstract).

Hseu J-R, Yeh S-L, Chu Y-T, Ting Y-Y. 1996. Effects of anesthesia with 2-phenoxyethanol on the hematological parameters of four species of marine teleosts. *Journal of the Fisheries Society of Taiwan* 23:43–48.

Hseu J-R, Yeh S-L, Chu Y-T, Ting Y-Y. 1997. Different anesthetic effects of 2-phenoxyethanol on four species of teleost. *Journal of the Fisheries Society of Taiwan* 24:185–191.

Idler DR, Truscott B. 1966. 1α-Hydroxycorticosterone from cartilagenous fish: a new adrenal steroid in blood. *Journal of the Fisheries Research Board of Canada* 23:615–619.

Idler DR, Truscott B. 1967. 1α-Hydroxycorticosterone: synthesis in vitro and properties of an interrenal steroid in the blood of cartilagenous fish (Genus *Raja*). *Steroids* 9:457–477.

Idler DR, Truscott B. 1968. 1α-hydroxycorticosterone and testosterone in body fluids of a cartilaginous fish (*Raja radiata*). *Journal of Endocrinology* 42:165–166.

Idler DR, Truscott B. 1969. Production of 1α-hydroxycorticosterone in vivo and in vitro by elasmobranchs. *General and Comparative Endocrinology* 2(Suppl.):325–330.

Karsten AH, Rice CD. 2004. c-Reactive protein levels as a biomarker of inflammation and stress in the Atlantic sharpnose shark (*Rhizoprionodon terraenovae*) from three southeastern USA estuaries. *Marine Environmental Research* 58:747–751.

Lacy E, Reale E. 1999. Urinary System. In: *Sharks, Skates, and Rays: The Biology of Elasmobranch Fishes* (WC Hamlett, ed.), pp. 353–397. Baltimore: Johns Hopkins University Press.

Larid LM, Oswald RL. 1975. Benzocaine (ethyl p-aminobenzoate) as a fish anesthetic. *Fisheries Management* 64:92–93.

Latas PJ. 1987. The use of azaperone in the spiny dogfish (*Squalus acanthias*). Proceedings of the International Association for Aquatic Animal Medicine, pp. 157–165.

Lécu A, Herbert R, Coulier L, Murray MJ. 2011. Removal of an intracoelomic hook via laparotomy in a sandbar shark (*Carcharhinus plumbeus*). *Journal of Zoo and Wildlife Medicine* 42: 256–262.

Lewbart GA. 2001. Clinical examination. In: *Manual of Oranamental Fish*, 2nd ed. (WH Wildgoose, ed.), pp. 85–89. Gloucester: BASVA.

Li X, Keith DE, Evans CJ. 1986. Multiple opioid receptor-like genes are identified in diverse vertebrate phyla. *FEBS Letters* 397:25–29.

Lorenz RG, Tyler AN, Faull KF, Makk G, Barchas JD, Evans CJ. 1986. Characterization of endorphins from the pituitary of the spiny dogfish (*Squalus acanthias*). *Peptides* 7(1):119–126.

Mandelman JW, Farrington MA. 2007. The physiological status and mortality associated with otter-trawl capture, transport, and captivity of an exploited elasmobranch, *Squalus acanthias*. *ICES Journal of Marine Science* 64:122–130.

Mandelmann JW, Skomal GB. 2009. Differential sensitivity to capture stress assessed by blood acid-base status in five carcharinid sharks. *Journal of Comparative Physiology. B, Biochemical, Systemic, and Environmental Physiology* 179:267–277.

Manire C, Hueter R, Hull E, Spieler R. 2001. Serological changes associated with gill-net capture and restraint in three species of sharks. *Transactions of the American Fisheries Society* 130:1038–1048.

Manire CA, Rasmussen LEL, Maruska KP, Tricas TC. 2007. Sex, seasonal, and stress-related variations in elasmobranch corticosterone concentrations. *Comparative Biochemistry and Physiology. A, Comparative Physiology* 148:926–935.

Manning AM. 2002. Oxygen therapy and toxicity. *The Veterinary Clinics of North America. Small Animal Practice* 32:1005–1020.

Maren TH, Embry R, Broder LE. 1968. The excretion of drugs across the gill of the dogfish, *Squalus acanthias*. *Comparative Biochemistry and Physiology. A, Comparative Physiology* 26: 853–864.

Marshall H, Field L, Afiadata A, Sepulveda C, Skomal G, Bernal D. 2012. Hematological indicators of stress in longline-captured sharks. *Comparative Biochemistry and Physiology. A, Comparative Physiology* 162:121–129.

Miller SM. 2001. Surgical resolution of post-ovulatory egg stasis in a wobbegong shark. *Exotic DVM Magazine* 3(1):29–24.

Mitchell MA, Miller SM, Heatley JJ, Wolf T, Lapuz F, Smith A. 2001. Clinical and cardiorespiratory effects of propofol in the white spotted bamboo shark (*Chiloscyllium plagiosum*). *Veterinary Anesthesia and Analgesia* 29:97–112.

Moyes CD, Fragoso N, Musyl MK, Brill RW. 2006. Predicting postrelease survival in large pelagic fish. *Transactions of the American Fisheries Society* 135:1389–1397.

Mylniczenko ND. 2010. Medical management of rays. In: *Zoo and Wild Animal Medicine Current Therapy 7* (ME Fowler, RE Miller, eds.), pp. 170–176. St. Louis: Elsevier Saunders.

Mylniczenko ND, Curtis EW, Wilborn RE, Young FA. 2006. Differences in hematocrit of blood samples obtained from two venipuncture sites in sharks. *American Journal of Veterinary Research* 67:1861–1864.

Mylniczenko ND, Harris G, Wilborn RE, Young FA. 2007. Blood culture results from healthy captive and free-ranging elasmobranchs. *Journal of Aquatic Animal Health* 19:159–167.

Naples LM, Mylniczenko ND, Zachariah TT, Wilborn RE, Young FA. 2012. Evaluation of critical care blood analytes assessed with a point-of-care portable blood analyzer in wild and aquarium-housed elasmobranchs and the influence of phlebotomy site on results. *Journal of the American Veterinary Medical Association* 241(1):117–125.

Neiffer DL, Nolan EC, Wilson A 2009. Comparison of three immersion agents (tricaine methanesulfonate, Aqui-s(iso-eugenol), and eugenol for short duration immobilization of captive sSouthern stingrays (*Dasyatis americana*) from an open water system in the Bahamas. Proceedings of the American Association of Zoo Veterinarians, p. 170.

Oetinger MI, Zorzi GD. 1995. The biology of freshwater elasmobranchs. *Journal of Aquaculture and Aquatic Sciences* 7:1–162.

Olson KR. 1999. Rectal gland and volume homeostatis. In: *Sharks, Skates, and Rays: The Biology of Elasmobranch Fishes* (WC Hamlett, ed.), pp. 329–352. Baltimore: John Hopkins University Press.

Oswald RL. 1978. Injection anesthesia for experimental studies in fish. *Comparative Biochemistry and Physiology. C: Comparative Pharmacology* 60:19–26.

Penning M 2012. Immobilizing marine fish for transport or surgery: from angelfish to tiger sharks, whether individuals or multi-species groups. North American Veterinary Conference, January 18.

Piiper J, Baumgarten D. 1969. Blood lactate and acid-base balance in the elasmobranch *Scyliorhinus stellaris* after exhausting activity. *Pubblicazioni della stazione zoologica di Napoli* 37:84–94.

Raines JA, Clancy MM. 2009. Sedation by orally administered ketamine in goldfish, *Carassius auratus*; hybrid striped bass, *Morone saxatilis* x *M. chrysops*; and ocellated river stingray, *Potamotrygon motoro*. *Journal of the World Aquaculture Society* 40:788–794.

Randall DJ, Perry SF. 1992. Catecholamines. In: *Fish Physiology*, Vol. 12A (WS Hoar, DJ Randall, AP Farrell, eds.), pp. 255–300. San Diego: Academic Press.

Rasmussen LEL, Crow GL. 1993. Serum corticosterone concentrations in immature captive whitetip reef sharks, *Triaenodon obesus*. *The Journal of Experimental Zoology* 267:283–287.

Rasmussen LEL, Gruber SH. 1990. Serum levels of circulating steroid hormones in free-ranging carcharhinoid sharks. *NOAA Technical Report* 90:143–155.

Rasmussen LEL, Gruber SH. 1993. Serum concentrations of reproductively-related circulating steroid hormones in the free-ranging lemon shark, *Negaprion brevirostris*. *Environmental Biology of Fishes* 38:167–174.

Renshaw GM, Kutek AK, Grant GD, Anoopkumar-Dukie S. 2012. Forecasting elasmobranch survival following exposure to severe stressors. *Comparative Biochemistry and Physiology. A, Comparative Physiology* 162:101–112.

Rose JD. 2002. The neurobehavioral nature of fishes and the question of awareness and pain. *Reviews in Fisheries Science* 10:1–38.

Ross LG. 2001. Restraint, anesthesia and euthanasia. In: *Manual of Oranamental Fish*, 2nd ed. (WH Wildgoose, ed.), pp. 75–83. Gloucester: BSAVA.

Ross LG, Ross B. 2008. *Anaesthetic and Sedative Techniques for Aquatic Animals*. Oxford, UK: Blackwell Science.

Sabalones J, Walters H, Rueda CAB. 2004. Learning and behavioral enrichment in elasmobranchs. In: *The Elasmobranch Husbandry Manual: Captive Care of Sharks, Rays and Their Relatives* (M Smith, D Warmolts, D Thoney, R Hueter, eds.), pp. 169–182. Columbus: Ohio Biological Survey.

Sepulveda CA, Wegner NC, Bernal D, Graham JB. 2005. The red muscle morphology of the thresher sharks (Family Alopiidae). *The Journal of Experimental Biology* 208:4255–4261.

Skomal G, Bernal D. 2011. Physiologic responses to stress in sharks. In: *Sharks and Their Relatives II: Biodiversity, Adaptive physiology and Conservation* (JC Carrier, JA Musick, MR Heithaus, eds.), pp. 459–490. Boca Raton: CRC Press.

Skomal GB. 2007. Evaluating the physiological and physical consequences of capture on post-release survivorship in large pelagic fishes. *Fisheries Management and Ecology* 14:81–89.

Smith M, Warmolts D, Thoney D, Hueter R, eds. 2004. *The Elasmobranch Husbandry Manual: Captive Care of Sharks, Rays and Their Relatives*. Columbus: Ohio Biological Survey.

Snelson FF Jr, Rasmussen LEL, Johnson MR, Hess DL. 1997. Serum concentrations of steroid hormones during reproduction in the Atlantic stingray, *Dasyatis sabina*. *General and Comparative Endocrinology* 108:67–79.

Snow PJ, Plenderleith MB, Wright LL. 1993. Quantitative study of primary sensory neuron populations of three species of elasmobranch fish. *Journal of Comparative Neurology* 334:97–103.

Snyder SB, Richard MJ, Berzins IK, Stamper MA. 1998. Immobilization of sandtiger sharks (*Odontaspis taurus*) using medetomidine/ketamine. Proceedings of the International Association for Aquatic Animal Medicine 31, pp. 123–124.

Spotte S. 1992. *Captive Seawater Fishes*. New York: John Wiley and Sons.

Stoskopf MK. 1986. Preliminary notes on the immobilization and anesthesia of captive sharks. *Erkrankungen der Zootiere* 28: 145–151.

Stoskopf MK. 1993. Shark pharmacology and toxicology. In: *Fish Medicine* (MK Stoskopf, ed.), pp. 809–816. Philadelphia: WB Saunders.

Stoskopf MK, Smith B, Klay G. 1984. Clinical note: blood sampling of captive sharks. *Journal of Zoo and Wildlife Medicine* 15:116–117.

Sundh H, Olsen RE, Fridell F, Gadan K, Evensen O, Glette J, Taranger GL, Myklebust R, Sundell K. 2009. The effect of hyperoxygenation and reduced flow in fresh water and subsequent infectious pancreatic necrosis virus challenge in sea water, on the intestinal barrier integrity in Atlantic salmon, *Salmo salar* L. *Journal of Fish Diseases* 32(8):687–698.

Totland GK, Kryvi H, Bone Q, Flood PR. 1981. Vascularization of the lateral muscle of some elamobranchiomorph fishes. *Journal of Fish Biology* 18(2):223–234.

Truscott B, Idler DR. 1968. The widespread occurrence of a corticosteroid 1α-hydroxylase in the interrenals of Elasmobranchii. *Journal of Endocrinology* 40:515–526.

Truscott B, Idler DR. 1972. Corticosteroids in plasma of elasmobranchs. *Comparative Biochemistry and Physiology. A, Comparative Physiology* 42:41–50.

Tuttle AD, Dunn JL. 2003. Evaluation of intramuscular use of medetomidine (alpha-2 adrenergic agonist) as an alternative to tricaine methane sulfonate (MS-222, Finquel) for sedation and anesthesia in teleosts and elasmobranchs. Proceedings of the International Association for Aquatic Animal Medicine 34, pp. 43–44.

Tyler P, Hawkins AD. 1981. Vivisections, anaesthetics and minor surgery. In: *Aquarium Systems* (AD Hawkins, ed.), pp. 248–278. London: Academic Press Inc.

Vaughan DB, Penning MR, Christison KW. 2008. 2-phenoxyethanol as anaesthetic in removing and relocating 102 species of fishes representing from Sea World to uShaka Marine World South Africa. *Onderstepoort Journal of Veterinary Research* 75:189–198.

Vogelnest L, Spielman DS, Ralph HK. 1994. The imobilisation of spotted sevengill sharks (*Notorynchus cepedianus*) to facilitate transport. *Drum and Croaker* 25(5–6):30–32.

Walker MD. 1972. Physiologic and pharmacologic aspects of barbiturates in elasmobranchs. *Comparative Biochemistry and Physiology. A, Comparative Physiology* 42:213–221.

Wells RMG, McIntyre RH, Morgan AK, Davie PS. 1986. Physiological stress responses in big gamefish after capture: observations on plasma chemistry and blood factors. *Comparative Biochemistry and Physiology. A, Comparative Physiology* 84:565–571.

Wendelaar Bonga SE. 1997. The stress response in fish. *Physiological Reviews* 77:1–39.

Williams TD, Rollins M, Block BA. 2004. Intramuscular anesthesia of bonito and Pacific mackerel with ketamine and medetomidine and reversal of anesthesia with atipamezole. *Journal of the American Veterinary Medical Association* 225:417–421.

Wright KN, Whitaker BR. 2001. Pharmocotherapeutics. In: *Amphibian Medicine and Captive Husbandry* (KN Wright, BR Whitaker, eds.), pp. 309–330. Malabar: Krieger Publishing Co.

Zimmerman DM, Armstrong DL, Curro TG, Dankoff SM, Vires KW, Cook KK, Jaros ND, Papich MG. 2006. Pharmacokinetics of florfenicol after a single intramuscular dose in white-spotted bamboo sharks (*Chiloscyllium plagiosum*). *Journal of Zoo and Wildlife Medicine* 37(2):165–173.

PERSONAL COMMUNICATIONS

Boylan, Shayne. 2011. South Carolina Aquarium, Charleston, SC 29401, USA

Cavin, Julie and Innis, Charlie. 2011. New England Aquarium, Central Wharf, Boston, MA 02110, USA

Davis, Ray. 2002. Sea World, Orlando, FL 32821, USA

Harvey, Brian. 2012. Fugu Fisheries Ltd., Victoria, BC

Ito, Takaomi. 2011. Osaka Aquarium KAIYUKAN in Osaka, Japan

Larson, Karthy. 2011. Ocean Park, Aberdeen, Hong Kong

McEwan, Tony. 2002. The Scientific Centre, Salmiya, 22036, Kuwait

Mulican, Timothy. 2002. The Newport Aquarium, Newport, KY 41071, USA

Naples, Lisa. 2011. John G. Shedd Aquarium, Chicago, IL 60605, USA

Penning, Mark. 2012. Disney's Animals, Science & Environment, Lake Buena Vista, FL. 36830

Yanagisawa, Makio. 2011. Okinawa Churaumi Aquarium in Okinawa, Japan

Walsh, Michael. 2002. Sea World, Orlando, FL 32821, USA.

17 Amphibians

Eric Baitchman and Mark Stetter

INTRODUCTION

Amphibians are native to all continents, except Antarctica, and are routinely maintained in captive situations as pets, in laboratories, and in zoos. They reside in a wide variety of habitats including aquatic, semi-aquatic, and terrestrial. Amphibians are found from the equatorial rainforest to Canada, where they may remain frozen through the winter. There are more than 6000 species, including frogs, toads, salamanders, newts, and caecilians (IUCN 2008). There is significant concern about worldwide amphibian declines and its implications for global ecosystem health.

Veterinarians are most likely to be involved with captive anurans (frogs and toads) or caudates (salamanders and newts). It is not uncommon for amphibians to require sedation or anesthesia for diagnostics, surgery, or research.

ANATOMY AND PHYSIOLOGY

Amphibians have several unique and clinically relevant anatomical characteristics. The first is they go through metamorphosis and change from strictly aquatic larval forms (i.e., tadpoles) to terrestrial adults. These metamorphoses include dramatic anatomical changes; growth of legs, loss of gills, resorption of tails (anurans), and formation of lungs. As a completely aquatic tadpole with gills, they have very similar respiration to fish.

The respiratory physiology of amphibians is unlike that of any other animal taxa. Four different types of respiration are employed, including branchial, cutaneous, pulmonary, and buccopharyngeal. All species utilize branchial respiration (gills) as larvae, and some pedomorphic species, such as axolotl (*Ambystoma mexicanum*), mudpuppies (Proteidae), and sirens (Sirenidae),

retain gills as adults (Duellman & Trueb 1994). All adult amphibians utilize cutaneous respiration to varying degrees that can account for a significant portion of the animals' total oxygen exchange. The largest family of salamanders, the Plethodontidae or lungless salamanders, perform nearly all of their respiration via cutaneous gas exchange (Duellman & Trueb 1994). In species that possess lungs, however, the majority of oxygen intake is usually via pulmonary exchange, while the cutaneous route still accounts for the majority of carbon dioxide exchange (Duellman & Trueb 1994; Hillman et al. 2009). Lungs are inflated by positive pressure ventilation achieved through buccal pumping. Small amounts of gas exchange may also occur across buccopharyngeal mucus membranes. Central respiratory drive to increase respiratory frequency, or tidal volume is stimulated by either decrease in PO_2 or increase in PCO_2 (Branco & Glass 1995; Fonseca et al. 2012; Hillman et al. 2009).

Amphibian skin is highly permeable and well vascularized. In addition to respiratory gas exchange, it is the primary route of water exchange and also actively participates in electrolyte balance. Smooth-skinned animals, adapted to moister environments, have higher permeability and are susceptible to dehydration through insensible water loss. In most species, the ventral pelvic region, often referred to as the pelvic patch or drink patch, is the area of highest water uptake. It is especially well developed in terrestrial species, showing increased surface area and vascularity in this region (Fig. 17.1).

VASCULAR ACCESS

Vascular access is limited by animal size. Fine-gauge needles or catheters (24 gauge or smaller) work best in

---

Zoo Animal and Wildlife Immobilization and Anesthesia, Second Edition. Edited by Gary West, Darryl Heard, and Nigel Caulkett.
© 2014 John Wiley & Sons, Inc. Published 2014 by John Wiley & Sons, Inc.

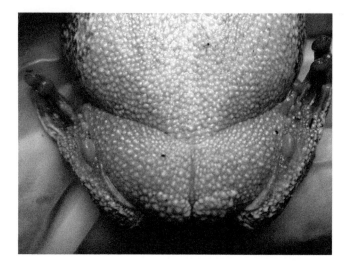

Figure 17.1. Ventral pelvic region of a gray tree frog, *Hyla versicolor*. Note the verrucae hydrophilicae, or granular sculpturing of the skin, providing increased surface area for water absorption. This region can have application for drug absorption as well.

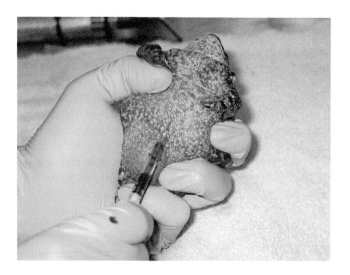

Figure 17.2. Collecting blood from the ventral abdominal vein in a western toad, *Anzxyrus boreas*.

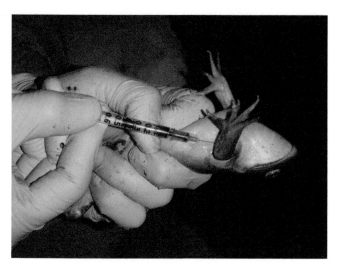

Figure 17.3. Collecting blood from the axillary plexus in a bullfrog, *Rana catesbeiana*.

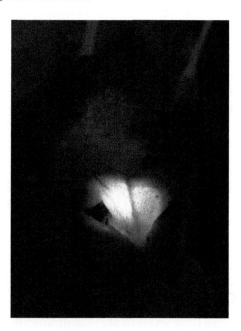

Figure 17.4. Transillumination technique highlighting the ventral abdominal vein in a Borneo eared frog, *Polypedates otilophus*.

animals that are large enough. Useful sites include the ventral abdominal vein on the caudal ventral midline (Fig. 17.2), femoral vein behind the stifle, axillary venous plexus (Fig. 17.3), sublingual plexus, and ventral tail vein in caudates. Other sites may be possible, such as the brachial vein or lateral abdominal veins in larger species. Transillumination is a useful technique for highlighting the pathways of major vessels (Fig. 17.4).

GENERAL ANESTHETIC CONSIDERATIONS

The aquatic nature and skin permeability of amphibians makes topical use of anesthetic agents a convenient means of achieving systemic effects. Amphibian anes-

thesia is very similar to fish anesthesia in methodology and drugs used (Stetter 2001). The anesthetic compounds are most commonly delivered in water and absorbed across the animal's skin or gills. Inhalant anesthetic agents may be used either topically or in solution. When gas anesthetics are delivered into a chamber or bubbled through water, induction can be prolonged or unsuccessful. Some amphibians can be intubated awake and administered an inhalant anesthetic for induction. Parenteral or injectable anesthetics are often unreliable, have a very low margin of safety, may be associated with a prolonged recovery, and dosages are very species specific (Crawshaw 2003; Stetter 2001; Wright & Whitaker 2001).

Aquatic amphibians can be kept out of water for extended periods of time if the skin is kept moist to prevent damage or dehydration, and ensure dermal respiration is maintained (Wright & Whitaker 2001). When working with entirely aquatic species (e.g., African clawed frog, *Xenopus laevis*), tank water from the animal's environment is used. This reduces exposure to abrupt environmental changes (i.e., temperature and pH). All water used for anesthesia is tested using standard reagent test kits to ensure there are no elevated deleterious variables, such as ammonia (Wright & Whitaker 2001). Toxin-free (dechlorinated) water within the animal's preferred body temperature range (usually 15–23°C, 59–73°F) is used (Wright & Whitaker 2001). Bottled spring water at room temperature is often a convenient standard for use, or amphibian Ringer's solution may be prepared.

Whatever container is used for an anesthetic chamber must be thoroughly cleaned and rinsed. Since amphibians absorb chemicals across their skin, cleaning solutions or other chemicals left in a container can be toxic. In addition, some amphibians secrete toxins from their skin, and it is important to rinse containers well between patients. Sealable plastic bags are an efficient container for anesthetic bath induction chambers and can be discarded when administration is complete. Other potential induction chambers include small plastic containers with lids, or small fish aquariums. Many amphibians exhibit an excitement phase during induction, making it important to have an enclosed container to prevent the patient leaping out and the interior should be smooth and padded if possible, to prevent injury (Crawshaw 2003; Stetter 2001; Wright & Whitaker 2001). When a water bath is being used for anesthetic application, there should be an interface with the air at the surface (i.e., do not fill the container completely to the lid). Animals with lungs are removed from the water after induction and positioned with nostrils elevated to ensure against aspiration.

When using a bath solution to induce anesthesia, the induction dose received is dependent on the surface area of the animal. That is, smaller animals with greater surface area are being exposed to larger amounts of anesthetic than larger animals with smaller surface area relative to body size. Consideration should be given to adjusting solution concentrations based on body size (Goulet et al. 2010, 2011).

Moistened gloves are worn when handling amphibians, to protect their skin, as well as to protect the handler from potentially toxic secretions in some species (Crawshaw 2003; Stetter 2001; Wright & Whitaker 2001). Rinsed nonlatex, nonpowdered gloves are recommended for handling adults, due to potential species sensitivities, and only washed vinyl gloves have been found safe for handling amphibian larvae. Mortality was seen in tadpoles exposed to latex, nitrile, and unwashed vinyl gloves (Cashins et al. 2008; Gutleb et al. 2001).

Amphibians are not commonly fasted prior to anesthesia. Their larynx remains tightly closed even under general anesthesia and the chance of aspiration is very low (Wright & Whitaker 2001). Regurgitation or gastric prolapse, however, has been reported in studies using isoflurane or eugenol in *X. laevis* or eugenol in *Rana pipiens* (Goulet et al. 2011; Lafortune et al. 2001; Smith & Stump 2000). While no lasting adverse effects were appreciated in those animals, consideration might be given to fasting for 24 hours when feasible, particularly if the amphibian's diet includes large prey items or if the anesthetic procedure is to include celomic surgery.

Respiratory ventilation is usually reduced or absent during amphibian anesthesia. The dermis is kept moist to allow for efficient dermal respiration. Cutaneous oxygen exchange, however, may be low in some species (Hillman et al. 2009), and supplemental oxygen should be considered to avoid hypoxemia and acidemia (Andersen & Wang 2002). While some amphibians can sustain anoxia for long periods, reoxygenation is a significant stress and risks free-radical injury to tissues (Bickler & Buck 2007). For long surgical procedures, the patient can be placed in a shallow water bath with oxygen bubbled into it. Intubation is also a safe option to provide supplemental oxygen (G. Crawshaw and D. Mader, pers. comm., 2013). Small species may be intubated with modified intravenous catheters or noncuffed Cole tubes may be used in larger species. The larynx is usually tightly closed, even in anesthetized animals, and the tube may need to be gently forced (G. Crawshaw, pers. comm.). The trachea is very short and the tube is placed just past the larynx (Stetter 2001). Amphibian lungs are composed of thin-walled membranes and manual or mechanical ventilation is done gently. Larger species can be ventilated at a pressure of 5 cm H_2O, with a breath every 10 seconds (D. Mader, pers. comm.).

MONITORING

The skin under the mandible and along the ventral cervical region is the gular region; movement in this area is a primary means of respiration. As a patient becomes anesthetized, gular respirations decrease, and there is a diminished withdrawal reflex (Crawshaw 2003; Stetter 2001; Wright & Whitaker 2001). Light anesthesia is associated with loss of righting reflex and an absence of abdominal respirations. Surgical anesthesia is indicated by a loss of withdrawal reflex and cessation of gular respiration (Crawshaw 2003; Stetter 2001; Wright & Whitaker 2001). When the patient has ceased movement and appears to be anesthetized, the animal may be placed on to dorsal recumbency to see if the amphibian has lost its righting reflex. For procedures requiring light anesthesia (e.g., blood sampling, radiographs, and physical examinations), the patient is removed from the container and quickly rinsed with anesthetic-free water before the procedure begins. If surgical anesthesia is required, an aggressive toe pinch of the rear leg will help determine if there is loss of the withdrawal reflex and nociception.

Anesthetized amphibians usually become apneic; abdominal and gular respirations cease. This can be very disconcerting for the anesthetist who relies on respiratory rate for assessing anesthesia. Consideration should be given to intubation or other means of supplementing oxygen, as discussed above.

Heart rate is a more useful indicator for anesthetic monitoring (Crawshaw 2003; Wright & Whitaker 2001). In most anesthetized patients in dorsal recumbency, the heart is seen contracting on the midline just caudal to the shoulders. Direct visualization, a Doppler monitor, or ultrasound is used to measure heart rate (Crawshaw 2003; Stetter 2001; Wright & Whitaker 2001). Although normal heart rates for species are not extensively published, a significant decrease in baseline heart rate is of concern and indicates excessive anesthetic depth. Pulse oximetry has not been validated in amphibians, but may show trends in hemoglobin saturation for long procedures and can assist with monitoring pulse (Fig. 17.5). Intermittently monitoring withdrawal reflex will determine if the patient is transitioning from surgical to light anesthesia. A patient that regains its withdrawal reflex, or gular respirations, requires supplementation if a surgical plane of anesthesia is still required. For supplementation, a 50% concentration of the induction solution is applied topically via syringe or partial water bath. When the animal reaches an adequate level of anesthesia, the application is discontinued.

During recovery, animals should be kept moist and well oxygenated, preferably at the preferred optimal temperature for the species. Full recovery is considered when the animal is responsive, respiring normally, and has regained all reflexes (Wright & Whitaker 2001).

ANALGESIA

Excellent discussions on nociception in amphibians can be found in Machin (1999), and Stevens (2011). Amphibians share the same array of nociceptive afferent nerves, spinal cord neurotransmitters, and endogenous opioid peptides as mammals. While the perception of pain in an amphibian is unknown, all of the same nociceptive pathways are conserved as in higher phylogenetic classes of vertebrates. Analgesia should be considered for any noxious procedures in amphibians. Drugs and dosages are summarized in Table 17.1.

Opioids

All mammalian opioid receptors: mu, delta, and kappa, are present in the central nervous system of amphibians. While receptor selectivity is less than in mammals, the relative analgesic potency mu > delta > kappa, is the same (Stevens 1996, 2004). Dosages tend to be much

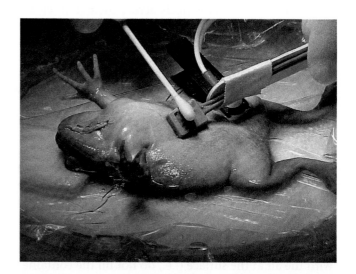

Figure 17.5. A tomato frog, *Dyscophus insularis*, under surgical anesthesia in a liquid anesthetic bath, being monitored by Doppler and pulse oximetry. Note the nostrils are elevated above the water line with gauze pads.

Table 17.1. Analgesic drug dosages for amphibians

Drug	Dosage	Route	Duration	Comments
Fentanyl	0.3–0.8 mg/kg	SC	>4 hours	ED_{50} = 0.5 mg/kg in *Rana pipiens*[a]
Morphine	18–33 mg/kg	SC	>4 hours	ED_{50} = 25 mg/kg in *Rana pipiens*[a]
Buprenorphine	27–79 mg/kg	SC	>4 hours	ED_{50} = 50 mg/kg in *Rana pipiens*[a]
	50 mg/kg	IC	NE	Shortened time to normal behavior following surgery in *Notophthalmus viridescens*[b]
Butorphanol	0.5 mg/L	72-hour bath	NE	Shortened time to normal behavior following surgery in *Notophthalmus viridescens*[b]
Dexmedetomidine	120 μg/kg	SC	>8 hours	*Rana pipiens*[c]
Meloxicam	0.1 mg/kg	IM	NE	Reduced PGE2 in *Rana catesbeiana*; analgesic effect not examined[d]

[a]Stevens et al. (1994) (ranges based on 95% confidence interval of ED_{50}).
[b]Koeller (2009).
[c]Brenner et al. (1994).
[d]Minter et al. (2011).
ED_{50}, effective dose in 50% of test subjects; NE, not examined.

higher in amphibians compared with mammals and onset to peak analgesic effect is longer at 60 minutes or greater when given systemically (Stevens et al. 1994). Planning analgesia for procedures should take this delay of onset in to account.

α-2 Adrenegric Agonists

Administration of α-2 adrenergic agonists to amphibians provides analgesia without sedation. Normal movement, including righting, corneal, and hind limb withdrawal reflexes, all remain intact. Onset of effect is rapid and long lasting, with peak effect occurring by 60 minutes and lasting for 6–8 hours or more (Brenner et al. 1994).

Nonsteroidal Anti-Inflammatory Drugs (NSAIDs)

Little good data exist using NSAIDs as analgesia in amphibians. Flunixin meglumine is reported to provide significant analgesia. The dosages used in two studies, however, are extremely high (25 mg/kg) compared with typical doses in other taxa, and one animal that died during the trial had histopathologic evidence of renal congestion and inflammation (Coble et al. 2011). Meloxicam reduced circulating prostaglandin E2 in *Rana catesbeiana*, implying it can suppress the inflammatory response and may, therefore, provide an analgesic effect (Minter et al. 2011). No significant effect was seen, however, when using meloxicam in analgesic trials with *X. laevis* (Coble et al. 2011). Mild analgesia is reported from a study with two uncommon NSAIDs, indomethacin and ketorolac (Stevens et al. 2001).

ANESTHETIC DRUGS

Anesthetic drugs and dosages are summarized in Table 17.2.

Tricaine Methanesulfonate (MS-222 or Finquel®)

This is the most commonly used anesthetic for amphibians (Cooper 2003; Crawshaw 2003; Downes 1995; Stetter 2001; Wright & Whitaker 2001). It is effective

in all species, with all developmental stages of amphibians, and it has a wide margin of safety. It is also the only FDA-approved anesthetic in fish and can be acquired through aquaculture distributors (Wright & Whitaker 2001).

Tricaine methanesulfonate is a white powder that easily dissolves in water. Its mechanism of action, similar to other local anesthetics, is as a sodium channel blocker inhibiting nerve conduction. Used systemically, it creates anesthesia via central nervous system depression (Cakir & Strauch 2005). In aqueous solution, it is very acidic, especially at higher concentrations and with waters that have a low buffering capacity (Crawshaw 2003; Downes 1995; Stetter 2001; Wright & Whitaker 2001). This acidic solution is not only irritating to the patient, but the drug is also in a more ionized form and, therefore, less effective as an anesthetic at low pH levels. It is important to buffer the solution to keep the pH at 7.0–7.4 (Crawshaw 2003; Downes 1995; Stetter 2001; Wright & Whitaker 2001). This is easily accomplished by adding sodium bicarbonate to the mixture. Common baking soda (powdered sodium bicarbonate) is added to the solution until saturation (powder no longer dissolves) is achieved. Because the patient is being induced in an anesthetic water bath, rather than a dosage based on body weight, the anesthetic solution concentration is determined by the level of sedation or anesthesia required along with relative life stage (larvae vs. adult) or species of amphibian (Crawshaw 2003; Downes 1995; Stetter 2001; Wright & Whitaker 2001). In general, much lower concentrations are required for younger larval stages, species with external gills, and for the more aquatic frogs compared with the terrestrial toads. Refer to Table 17.1 for general recommendations of concentrations.

For a desired volume of solution, the exact amount of tricaine methanesulfonate is weighed out, dissolved in water, and the buffer is added until neutral pH is achieved. The solution is not stable over long periods of time and is discarded after each use. A portion of anesthetic solution is added to the induction chamber (a sealed plastic bag or container) at a level sufficient to cover approximately half of the patient's body. A

Table 17.2. Anesthetic drug dosages for amphibians

Drug	Dosage	Route	Comments
Tricaine methanesulfonate			Add buffer until neutral pH whenever using tricaine
	0.2–0.5 g/L	Bath	Larvae and paedomorphic species
	1.0–2.0 g/L	Bath	Adults
Eugenol	350 μL/L	Bath	Using 99% pure eugenol oil; see chapter text for comments using clove oil
Isoflurane	2–3 mL/L	Bath	
	0.025–0.035 mL/g BW	Topical gel	3 mL isoflurane, 1.5 mL water, 2.5 mL water-based gel
	0.03–0.06 mL/g BW	Liquid	Use absorbent pad with plastic backing to apply to dorsum
Benzocaine	0.2–0.3 g/L	Bath	Pure benzocaine will require dissolution in ethanol first, up to 1% ethanol in final solution.

BW, body weight.

further portion of the remainder of solution can be diluted to half the induction concentration, to be used as a maintenance solution to drip on the patient as needed for longer procedures.

Although induction times are variable, initial effects can be seen within a few minutes, with surgical plane of anesthesia in up to 30 minutes. General comments in the earlier sections apply to induction and monitoring in tricaine anesthesia. Loss of gular respiration is expected at a surgical plane of anesthesia and excessive anesthetic depth will cause cardiac depression on a dose-dependent basis (Cakir & Strauch 2005).

Eugenol

Eugenol is the active compound in clove oil, wherein eugenol concentration can vary widely, from 47% to 88% (Chaieb et al. 2007). It is worth noting that when dosing clove oil, the percentage of eugenol may not be known, nor is the possible composition of other active or inactive compounds present. Interpretation of published dosages of clove oil as an anesthetic should take this variability in to consideration. Simple side-by-side comparison of protocols using clove oil is not straightforward. Purified eugenol can be obtained for use as an anesthetic, which has the advantage of a known single concentration for more accurate and consistent dosing. As more published reports using purified eugenol are produced, species and dosage comparisons can be made more easily. The terms "clove oil" and "eugenol" are not used interchangeably in this chapter.

Eugenol has been used as a topical anesthetic in humans, as well as a general anesthetic in invertebrates, fish, and amphibians. Its mechanism of action is as a local anesthetic, creating analgesia and anesthesia by blocking sodium voltage-gated channels as well as vanilloid receptor TRPV1 and activating inhibitory GABA$_A$ receptors (Goulet et al. 2010).

Eugenol or clove oil induction is most effective via an immersion bath solution, as with tricaine methanesulfonate, and is prepared in a similar manner. Eugenol solutions do not need to be buffered. Surgical anesthesia has been reliably achieved in multiple reports with *R. pipiens* and *X. laevis*. Regurgitation or gastric prolapse has been observed in these studies as a fairly common side effect during induction or recovery, though apparently without adverse consequence (Goulet et al. 2011; Guenette et al. 2007; Lafortune et al. 2001). Clove oil anesthesia has been reported in one caudate species, *Ambystoma tigrinum*, where a surgical plane of anesthesia was achieved in 67% (8/12), at a higher dose than required for *R. pipiens* (Mitchell et al. 2009).

Toxicity studies in *Xenopus* indicate that smaller animals have a higher incidence of toxic effect. Smaller animals have a higher surface area and, therefore, likely absorb anesthetic at a higher dosage per body weight relative to larger animals in the same bath concentration. Smaller *Xenopus* are also less mature than larger animals, so the mechanism of toxicity could be either dose or age dependent (Goulet et al. 2010, 2011). Histopathologic findings in small animals (28.2 ± 13.7 g) 24 hours after receiving anesthetic doses (350 µl/L) of eugenol included apoptosis of distal tubular cells in the renal medulla, followed by regeneration 1 week after anesthesia. Animals that received daily anesthesia for three consecutive days had tubular apoptosis ranging from mild to severe, followed by tubular regeneration, massive hepatic necrosis, and hemorrhage of celomic fat bodies 1 week later (Goulet et al. 2011). Large female *Xenopus* (111.7 ± 18.3 g) showed no histopathologic abnormalities 24 hours after anesthesia in the same bath concentration (Guenette et al. 2007). Cardiovascular depression is also seen with smaller animals in a surgical plane of anesthesia, but not in larger animals (Goulet et al. 2010; Guenette et al. 2007). Cutaneous necrosis has been reported with topical application in *Xenopus* at eugenol concentrations of 60 mg/mL or greater (Ross et al. 2006).

Isoflurane

Isoflurane is a safe and effective anesthetic in amphibians and may be familiar and useful to the practitioner who does not keep tricaine methanesulfonate in stock (Stetter 2001). Topical applications of liquid isoflurane or bath immersion in isoflurane solution are the most reliable means of induction. Isoflurane gas can also be delivered in the traditional vaporized form via a chamber or by bubbling vaporized isoflurane and oxygen from an anesthetic system into a water bath (Crawshaw 2003; Stetter 2001; Wright & Whitaker 2001). In both cases, a sealed container is used to minimize human exposure and increase isoflurane concentrations in the air chamber. While these methods can be effective in some cases, they are associated with slow induction times and rapid recoveries once the patient is removed from the chamber. Frogs in a gas induction chamber can cease ventilation, thereby significantly increasing induction times (Barter et al. 2007). The aquatic frog *Xenopus* was not anesthetized by bubbling vaporized isoflurane in to a water chamber (Smith & Stump 2000). Intubation and maintenance of large amphibian patients with isoflurane gas may be performed with an uncuffed endotracheal tube (Wright 2006).

The most effective and longest lasting methods of isoflurane anesthesia are application of concentrated liquid isoflurane to the skin or immersion in an isoflurane bath solution (Stetter 2001). For the immersion bath, a syringe is used to add the liquid isoflurane directly into the water through a needle. The needle tip is placed below the surface of the water and the isoflurane liquid is injected and mixed into the bath. A concentration of 2–3 mL/L is most commonly used (Crawshaw 2003; Stetter 2001).

When applying concentrated liquid isoflurane directly to the skin, a carrier solution or barrier is created to increase dermal contact time prior to the isoflurane evaporating. A gel mixture is created using 3 mL of liquid isoflurane, 1.5 mL of water, and 3.5 mL of K-Y® Jelly (Stetter 2001). These three items are placed into a 10 mL empty serum vial and vigorously shaken until a uniform gel is established. This isoflurane gel can now be administered to the patient's dorsum at dosages of 0.025–0.035 mL/gram body weight (Stetter 2001). Lower dosages are used for more aquatic species and higher dosages for thicker skinned terrestrial species (e.g., toads). After the isoflurane gel is mixed in the vial, the indicated volume is withdrawn through a syringe and needle and the gel deposited on the patient's dorsum. Once applied, the patient is placed in a small sealed container until induction is complete. After induction, the anesthetic gel preparation should be rinsed from the patient's skin. Patients anesthetized with topical isoflurane gel will remain under anesthesia for 45–80 minutes. Shorter anesthetic times with a more rapid recovery are seen with the liquid isoflurane in water method (Stetter 2001), or the isoflurane and water solution can be dripped on the skin at a rate needed to maintain anesthetic depth, similar to the method for maintenance with tricaine methanesulfonate.

Topical application of concentrated isoflurane liquid was successful for anesthetizing *Xenopus* frogs using an absorbent pad with a plastic backing. Isoflurane at 0.03–0.06 mL/gram body weight is used to saturate the absorbent pad, cut to size to cover the animals' dorsum, and placed against the skin with the plastic backing facing up (Smith & Stump 2000).

It is possible sevoflurane can be used in amphibians, but no anesthetic studies have been published. Sevoflurane liquid mixed with either sterile lubricant or pluronic/lecithin organogel have shown good absorption across frog skin in *in vitro* experiments (Ardente et al. 2008).

Adverse complications are few when using isoflurane by the earlier-described methods. *Xenopus* frogs fed within 1 day of isoflurane induction tended to regurgitate. Injectable administration of isoflurane (intracelomic, subcutaneous, or intramuscular) is not recommended due to variable results and high mortality (Smith & Stump 2000).

Human exposure to vaporized isoflurane is of concern during protocols involving isoflurane liquid. Procedures should be performed within a fume hood or beneath an active scavenging system.

Miscellaneous Topical Anesthetic Drugs

A variety of drugs traditionally used for local analgesia in mammals have been evaluated for general anesthetic use in amphibians. Benzocaine has been used most widely with good results in a variety of anuran and caudate amphibians (Andersen & Wang 2002; Cakir & Strauch 2005; Crawshaw 2003; Wright & Whitaker 2001). Benzocaine powder is not readily soluble in water and should be dissolved in ethanol first. The volume of ethanol in final anesthetic solution should not exceed 1% (Wright & Whitaker 2001). A commercially available topical gel product, Orajel®, containing 10–20% benzocaine has been successfully utilized in caudates and anurans topically in its original form and in solution as an immersion bath (Brown et al. 2004; Cecala et al. 2007; Guenette & Lair 2006). At least one study found unexpected mortality in *Bufo fowleri* with a 1 g/L Orajel® bath (equivalent to 0.2 g/L benzocaine; Cecala et al. 2007). No mortality, however, was seen in another bufonid, *Bufo marinus*, using 1 g/L pure benzocaine dissolved in ethanol and water (Andersen & Wang 2002).

A topical xylocaine spray (10% solution) produced satisfactory anesthesia in two *Rana* species (Garcia Aguilar et al. 1999). High mortality was seen in *R. pipiens* exposed to a commercial product containing lidocaine 2.5% and prilocaine 2.5% cream (Guenette & Lair 2006).

Injectable Anesthetic Drugs

Propofol is a short-acting intravenous anesthetic in mammals and reptiles that potentiates γ-aminobutyric acid (GABA) receptors. In amphibian species, intravenous administration is a challenge, and its effects when given by alternate routes are highly variable. In *R. pipiens*, 10 mg/kg perivascularly in the sublingual plexus produced brief and light anesthesia following a short induction time (Lafortune et al. 2001). *Xenopus laevis* were induced to a brief light anesthesia in an 88 mg/L immersion bath, while all animals died when exposed to bath concentrations of 175 mg/L or higher (Guenette et al. 2008). Surgical anesthesia was not achieved in either of these studies. Intracelomic administration of 35 mg/kg in *Ambystoma tigrinum* did produce very brief surgical anesthesia after prolonged induction times (Mitchell et al. 2009). Given the variability of reported dosages and routes of administration, and potential mortality at higher concentrations, specific recommendations for its use in amphibians are not possible. Differences in GABA receptor density between species may introduce further variability of propofol effect among amphibians (Guenette et al. 2008).

Another GABA agonist anesthetic, alfaxalone, is described for surgical anesthesia in a single case report with an axolotl. Induction in a 5 mg/L immersion bath was followed with maintenance by irrigation of the external gills with the same solution, supplemented as necessary with additional drops of 10 mg/L solution (McMillan & Leece 2011).

Alpha-2 adrenergic agonists, such as medetomidine and dexmedetomidine, do not produce sedation in amphibians. A related drug, etomidate, did produce anesthesia in *Xenopus laevis* tadpoles (Paris et al. 2007).

A variety of other injectable anesthetic agents, including ketamine, tiletamine/zolazepam, and various barbiturates, have been used. These agents are not rec-ommended, as they are less reliable than the topical and inhalant anesthetic agents. They are associated with large species variability in effect and produce significantly higher mortality rates.

REFERENCES

Andersen J, Wang T. 2002. Effects of anaesthesia on blood gases, acid-base status and ions in the toad *Bufo marinus*. *Comparative Biochemistry and Physiology. Part A, Molecular and Integrative Physiology* 131:639–646.

Ardente A, Barlow B, Burns P, Goldman R, Baynes R. 2008. Vehicle effects on in vitro transdermal absorption of sevoflurane in the bullfrog, *Rana catesbeiana*. *Environmental Toxicology and Pharmacology* 25:373–379.

Barter L, Mark L, Smith A, Antognini J. 2007. Isoflurane potency in the Northern leopard frog *Rana pipiens* is similar to that in mammalian species and is unaffected by decerebration. *Veterinary Research Communications* 31:757–763.

Bickler P, Buck L. 2007. Hypoxia tolerance in reptiles, amphibians, and fishes: life with variable oxygen availability. *Annual Review of Physiology* 69:145–170.

Branco L, Glass M. 1995. Ventilatory responses to carboxyhaemo-globinaemia and hypoxic hypoxia in *Bufo paracnemis*. *The Journal of Experimental Biology* 198:1417–1421.

Brenner G, Klopp A, Deason A, Stevens C. 1994. Analgesic potency of alpha adrenergic agents after systemic administration in amphibians. *Journal of Pharmacology and Experimental Therapeutics* 270:540–545.

Brown H, Tyler H, Mousseau T. 2004. Orajel® as an amphibian anesthetic: refining the technique. *Herpetological Review* 35:252.

Cakir Y, Strauch S. 2005. Tricaine (MS-222) is a safe anesthetic compound compared to benzocaine and pentobarbital to induce anesthesia in leopard frogs (*Rana pipiens*). *Pharmacological Reports* 57:467–474.

Cashins S, Alford R, Skerratt L. 2008. Lethal effect of latex, nitrile, and vinyl gloves on tadpoles. *Herpetological Review* 39:298–301.

Cecala K, Price S, Dorcas M. 2007. A comparison of the effectiveness of recommended doses of MS-222 (tricaine methanesulfonate) and Orajel® (benzocaine) for amphibian anesthesia. *Herpetological Review* 38:63–66.

Chaieb K, Hajlaoui H, Zmantar T, Kahla-Nakbi A, Rouabhia M, Mahdouani K, Bakhrouf A. 2007. The chemical composition and biological activity of clove essential oil, *Eugenia caryophyllata* (*Syzygium aromaticum* L. myrtaceae): a short review. *Phytotherapy Research* 21:501–506.

Coble D, Taylor D, Mook D. 2011. Analgesic effects of meloxica, morphine sulfate, flunixin meglumine, and xylazine hydrochloride in African clawed frogs (*Xenopus laevis*). *Journal of the American Association for Laboratory Animal Science* 50:355–360.

Cooper J. 2003. Urodela (Caudata, Urodela): salamanders, sirens. In: *Zoo and Wild Animal Medicine*, 5th ed. (M Fowler, R Miller, eds.), pp. 33–40. St. Louis: W.B. Saunders.

Crawshaw G. 2003. Anurans (Anura, Salienta): frogs, toads. In: *Zoo and Wild Animal Medicine*, 5th ed. (M Fowler, R Miller, eds.), pp. 22–33. St. Louis: W.B. Saunders.

Downes H. 1995. Tricaine anesthesia in amphibia: a review. *Bulletin of the Association of Reptilian and Amphibian Veterinarians* 5:11–16.

Duellman W, Trueb L. 1994. *Biology of Amphibians*. Baltimore: Johns Hopkins University Press.

Fonseca E, da Silva G, Fernandes M, Giusti H, Noronha-de-Souza C, Glass M, Bícego K, Gargaglioni L. 2012. The breathing pattern and the ventilatory response to aquatic and aerial hypoxia and hypercarbia in the frog *Pipa carvalhoi*. *Comparative Biochemistry and Physiology. Part A, Molecular and Integrative Physiology* 162:281–287.

Garcia Aguilar N, Palcios Martinez C, Ross L. 1999. Controlled anaesthesia of *Rana catesbeiana* (Shaw) and *Rana pipiens* (Schreber 1792) using xylocaine delivered by spray. *Aquaculture Research* 30:309–311.

Goulet F, Helie P, Vachon P. 2010. Eugenol anesthesia in African clawed frogs (*Xenopus laevis*) of different body weights. *Journal of the American Association for Laboratory Animal Science* 49:460–463.

Goulet F, Vachon P, Helie P. 2011. Evaluation of the toxicity of eugenol at anesthetic doses in African clawed frogs (*Xenopus laevis*). *Toxicologic Pathology* 39:471–477.

Guenette S, Lair S. 2006. Anesthesia of the leopard frog, Rana pipiens: a comparative study between four different agents. *Journal of Herpetological Medicine and Surgery* 16:38–44.

Guenette S, Helie P, Beaudry F, Vachon P. 2007. Eugenol for anesthesia of African clawed frogs (*Xenopus laevis*). *Veterinary Anaesthesia and Analgesia* 34:164–170.

Guenette S, Beaudry F, Vachon P. 2008. Anesthetic properties of propofol in African clawed frogs (*Xenopus laevis*). *Journal of the American Association for Laboratory Animal Science* 47:35–38.

Gutleb A, Bronkhorst M, van den Berg J, Murk A. 2001. Latex laboratory gloves: an unexpected pitfall in amphibian toxicity assays with tadpoles. *Environmental Toxicology and Pharmacology* 10:119–121.

Hillman S, Withers P, Drewes R, Hillyard S. 2009. *Ecological and Environmental Physiology of Amphibians*. New York: Oxford University Press.

IUCN, Conservation International, and NatureServe. 2008. An analysis of amphibians on the 2008 IUCN Red List. http://www.iucnredlist.org/amphibians (accessed January 17, 2014).

Lafortune M, Mitchell M, Smith J. 2001. Evaluation of medetomidine, clove oil, and propofol for anesthesia of leopard frogs, *Rana pipiens*. *Journal of Herpetological Medicine and Surgery* 11(4):13–18.

Koeller CA. 2009. Comparison of buprenorphine and butorphanol analgesia in the eastern red-spotted newt (*Notophthalmus viridescens*). *Journal of the American Association for Laboratory Animal Science* 48(2):171–175.

Machin K. 1999. Amphibian pain and analgesia. *Journal of Zoo and Wildlife Medicine* 30:2–10.

McMillan M, Leece E. 2011. Immersion and branchial/transcutaneous irrigation anaesthesia with alfaxalone in a Mexican axolotl. *Veterinary Anaesthesia and Analgesia* 38:619–623.

Minter L, Clarke E, Gjeltema J, Archibald K, Posner L, Lewbart G. 2011. Effects of intramuscular meloxicam administration on prostaglandin E2 synthesis in the North American bullfrog (*Rana catesbeiana*). *Journal of Zoo and Wildlife Medicine* 42:680–685.

Mitchell M, Riggs S, Singleton C, Diaz-Figueroa O, Hale L. 2009. Evaluating the clinical and cardiopulmonary effects of clove oil and propofol in tiger salamanders (*Ambystoma tigrinum*). *Journal of Exotic Pet Medicine* 18:50–56.

Paris A, Hein L, Brede M, Brand P, Scholz J, Tonner P. 2007. The anesthetic effects of etomidate: species specific interaction with α-2 adrenoceptors. *Anesthesia and Analgesia* 105:1644–1649.

Ross A, Guenette S, Helie P, Vachon P. 2006. Case of cutaneous necrosis in African clawed frogs *Xenopus laevis* after the topical application of eugenol. *The Canadian Veterinary Journal. la Revue Veterinaire Canadienne* 47:1115–1117.

Smith J, Stump K. 2000. Isoflurane anesthesia in the African clawed frog (*Xenopus laevis*). *Contemporary Topics in Laboratory Animal Science* 39:39–42.

Stetter M. 2001. Fish and amphibian anesthesia. *The Veterinary Clinics of North America. Exotic Animal Practice* 4:69–82.

Stevens C. 1996. Relative analgesic potency of mu, delta, and kappa opioids after spinal administration in amphibians. *Journal of Pharmacology and Experimental Therapeutics* 276: 440–448.

Stevens C. 2004. Opioid research in amphibians: an alternative pain model yielding insights on the evolution of opioid receptors. *Brain Research. Brain Research Reviews* 46:204–215.

Stevens C. 2011. Analgesia in amphibians: preclinical studies and clinical applications. *The Veterinary Clinics of North America. Exotic Animal Practice* 14:33–44.

Stevens C, Klopp A, Facello A. 1994. Analgesic potency of mu and kappa opioids after systemic administration in amphibians. *Journal of Pharmacology and Experimental Therapeutics* 269: 1086–1093.

Stevens C, Maciver D, Newman L. 2001. Testing and comparison of non-opioid analgesics in amphibians. *Contemporary Topics in Laboratory Animal Science* 40:23–27.

Wright K. 2006. Overview of amphibian medicine. In: *Reptile Medicine and Surgery*, 2nd ed. (D Mader, ed.), pp. 947–949. St. Louis: Saunders Elsevier.

Wright K, Whitaker B, eds. 2001. *Amphibian Medicine and Captive Husbandry*. Malabar: Krieger Publishing.

18 Crocodilian Capture and Restraint

Kent A. Vliet

INTRODUCTION

Anesthesia and chemical immobilization of crocodilians usually requires some form of confinement and physical restraint for safe drug administration and to prevent them from seeking refuge in their aquatic environment. Anesthesia and immobilization are discussed in Chapter 20. The following is a description of capture and restraint techniques that minimize the potential for injury to handlers and animals.

Crocodilians are dangerous; they are capable of injuring, scarring, maiming, and even killing handlers. This is not to imply they are bad, loathsome, or evil. It is simply the result of being large, tremendously powerful, predatory, agile, and adaptable. No one can safely work with these animals until this is fully comprehended. Further, you must remind yourself of this every time you work with them; complacency is our greatest threat.

There are many ways to safely capture and restrain even very large crocodilians. There are a greater number of incorrect ways. Each capture is different and always has the potential to go wrong. There are many variables that must be taken into account in successfully capturing and restraining a crocodilian.

Ultimately, no amount of detail in this chapter, training, or experience will guarantee no harm to those working with these animals. If you cannot personally accept this liability, you should neither attempt any of the techniques discussed in this chapter nor should you work with crocodilians. Accepting this liability is part of the commitment necessary to work with these magnificent animals.

For larger captive crocodilians, the trend is to reduce contact with the keeper staff by providing shift enclosures and training the animals to use them. This is much preferred over physically capturing and restraining an animal. While the former (shifting) is strongly encouraged, the latter (capture and restraint) will form the body of this chapter.

Few publications describe techniques for the safe capture, restraint, and handling of captive crocodilians. Most descriptions are of free-living species: for example, the American alligator (*Alligator mississippiensis*) (Chabreck 1963; Forster 1991; Joanen & Perry 1972; Jones 1965; Jones & Hayes-Odum 1994; Murphy & Fendly 1974; Wilkinson 1994); the American crocodile (*Crocodylus acutus*) (Mazzotti & Brandt 1988); the Nile crocodile (*Crocodylus niloticus*) (Hutton et al. 1987; Kofron 1989; Pooley 1984); and the saltwater crocodile (*Crocodylus porosus*) (Walsh 1987; Webb & Messel 1977). While useful insights and methods are gleaned from these articles, most describe traps that are of little practical application in the captive environment. A detailed list of equipment and techniques used in alligator research is found in McDaniel and Hord (1990). Fowler (1978) makes brief mention of restraint of smaller captive crocodilians. Almandarz (1986) describes physical restraint techniques of reptiles, including crocodilians. The most comprehensive reference is that of Wise (1994). This article contains many pertinent and useful insights that serve as a valuable reference for anyone interested in developing the skills necessary to safely work with these animals. The following discussion builds on and expands the contributions of the earlier-mentioned references.

This chapter does not detail all of the possible techniques for capture and restraint. The author has included those he is experienced with, accustomed to, and which he believes provide enhanced safety. The author has had the opportunity to capture all 23 crocodilian species during several thousand captures over 20

Zoo Animal and Wildlife Immobilization and Anesthesia, Second Edition. Edited by Gary West, Darryl Heard, and Nigel Caulkett.
© 2014 John Wiley & Sons, Inc. Published 2014 by John Wiley & Sons, Inc.

Table 18.1. Suggested standard list of materials used for crocodilian capture and restraint

1. Capture ropes (different diameters relative to animal sizes)
2. Restraint ropes
3. Jaw ropes
4. Defensive poles
5. Catchpoles
6. Mouth poles
7. Tape
   A. Duct tape
   B. Electrical tape
8. Rubberized shelf mat
9. Cable straps
10. Eye cloth
11. Eye covers (gauze or paper towel)
12. Hooks
   A. Stump ripper
   B. Livestock hook
   C. Python hook
13. Restraint equipment (ladder, crate, etc.)
14. Knives and wire cutters
15. Trauma kit

years, in both captive and free-living situations. Techniques evolve, and new, better practices come into use. Others may have different, and even better, methods than those presented here.

CAPTURE EQUIPMENT

Crocodilians frequently damage and destroy capture equipment. Consequently, restraint is either an expensive exercise or one develops sets of equipment that are easy and inexpensive to manufacture. The latter allows an adequate supply of equipment to always be available. The standard equipment the author and the staff of the St. Augustine Alligator Farm and Zoological Park use for crocodilian capture and handling is described in Table 18.1.

Ropes

Capture Ropes Ropes are essential for most captures; they are used to gain a hold on, to restrain, and for the safe release of animals. Several ropes are always available for any capture. The size used depends on the crocodilian to be captured. Smaller specimens require smaller diameter ropes, while larger animals necessitate thicker and stronger ropes. Too small ropes may cinch too tightly on the animal or burn into a keeper's hands during a struggle. Ropes of too great a diameter will not close tightly enough over the neck or jaws, allowing the animal to work itself free.

For adult animal captures, the author uses either 1.3 cm (1/2 in) or 1.6 cm (5/8 in) ropes. They can be sisal (hemp), nylon, cotton, or a mixture. Ropes have different tensile strengths; it must be adequate for the size and mass of the animal to prevent breakage and animal escape. Nylon ropes are generally the strongest.

Cotton and sisal work well for many purposes, but rot if not allowed to dry after use. This leads to problems during captures of large animals; the rope may separate under tension, allowing the animal to go free and the keepers to fall back and possibly injure one another. Woven or braided ropes are less likely to kink or fail than twisted ropes. Many ropes float on the water surface preventing their placement under the head of a submerged crocodilian. Consequently, ropes are assessed before purchase and use for their ability to sink when soaked. The best ropes the author has used are those designed for arborists. They are soft and pliable yet strong, and they do not tend to "burn" hands when jerked by a crocodilian. However, they are also expensive.

Rope length depends on the intended use. Excessive length makes it difficult to gather and control during hectic moments in captures. The author frequently lassos crocodilians from a distance. For large crocodilians, several people are needed to pull a roped animal from the water or to a position where it can be safely secured. For these purposes, the author uses 8–9 m (25–30 ft) ropes.

Restraint Ropes Smaller diameter and shorter ropes are ideal for restraint. Ropes of 0.6 (1/4) or 1 cm (3/8 in) diameter are used to tie the legs off of the ground to prevent movement, or tie down an animal to a ladder or platform.

Jaw Ropes Jaw ropes are used to tie the jaws shut or remove the tape off of an animal's jaws as it is being released. These are generally small diameter, 0.3 (1/8) to 0.5 cm (3/16 in), and shorter, 3 (10) to 3.7 m (12 ft), ropes. Cotton clothes line works well for this purpose.

Poles

Defensive The primary use of a defensive pole is for protection of the handler(s). They must be of sufficient diameter and heft to maintain a safe distance between the holder and crocodilian during capture. When charged or lunged at by an overly enthusiastic animal, block the animal's advance and move to the other side of the pole.

These poles serve many other purposes. Animals can be discouraged from advancing toward a handler by lightly laying the pole on the soft tissues of its nostrils, or against its earflap. Similarly, animals are encouraged to move out of the way, allowing access to a particular animal for capture. In addition, the pole is used after capture to manipulate and position the animal (e.g., move legs, lift jaws, and force the jaws shut) without getting too close.

Defensive poles are generally wooden; if they are bitten by an animal they do not cause significant damage to the teeth. The author uses a heavy, large diameter length of bamboo approximately 1.5 (5) to 1.8 m (6 ft) in length.

Poles greatly increase safety while working in close proximity to crocodilians. However, care must be taken when using them with larger crocodilians. Poles can become dangerous to personnel if grabbed and held in the crocodilian's jaws. When the animal swings its head from side to side, the pole may strike and injure a person. Care must also be taken when recovering a pole from a crocodilian.

Catch A variety of catchpoles are used to grab and hold. They all include a long rod with a noose or snare at one end. For larger animals (>2 m), poles are designed so the noose and rope attachment separates from the rod. Commercial catchpoles are used when no other poles are available. They are sturdy and give very good control over the animal. However, even relatively small crocodilians (≥1.5 m) roll or spin violently enough during capture to twist and kink the cable snare, thereby destroying it. Further, during a struggle, the metal rotating cuff adjacent to the snare will push into the animal's head and neck and cause injury. Frequent use of commercial catchpoles is not recommended because of initial purchase cost, and the expense and time of repeated repair and maintenance.

Alternatively, it is easy, quick, and very inexpensive to make catchpoles. There are three commonly used, simple designs. The preferred is a "break-away" rope noose secured to the end of a pole with electrical tape. Once the rope is placed over the head and neck of the animal, the pole is pulled free and removed from the capture area. Recommended poles for this design are long (3–5 m), 3- to 4-cm (1 1/2 in) diameter wooden rods or lightweight aluminum electrical conduit. Swimming pool net poles also can be used; they are lightweight, long, and extensible.

Schedule 40 PVC pipes can also be used to make other catchpoles. Snares are made of twisted metal cable and affixed to the end (Fig. 18.1). The snare is attached by a metal swivel coupled to an eyebolt through an end cap. The cap is glued onto the end of the PVC pole (Fig. 18.1). An advantage of this design is that snares of different diameter, or that have become damaged during a capture, can be rapidly exchanged during a capture. A small wire is attached to the snare base to keep it open until in place on the animal. Surprisingly, jacketed cables with plastic coverings cause more skin damage than exposed metal cables.

The simplest homemade catchpole for animals ≤2–3 m (8 or 9 ft) consists of a nylon or cotton rope run through a length of 1.5–2 cm (1/2 to 3/4 in) PVC pipe (Fig. 18.2). The rope is secured through a hole drilled in the pipe wall close to the end, then run out of the pipe and back in again, to form the noose, and then down the length of the PVC. When the noose is placed around the animal, the rope extending from the

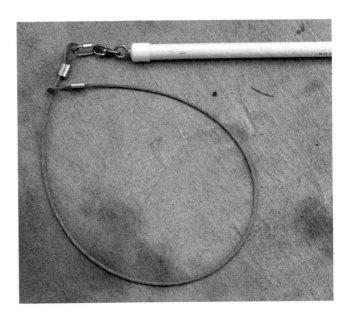

Figure 18.1. A homemade cable snare used for catching small-to medium-sized crocodilians. The catchpole is made of PVC piping.

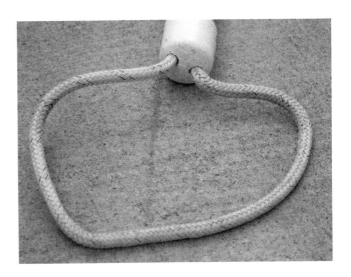

Figure 18.2. A homemade rope snare used for catching small-to medium-sized crocodiles. It can also be used as a jaw noose; the rope is placed around the upper and lower jaws and either twisted or the rope pulled at the distal end to tighten. The pole is made of PVC piping.

back end of the pole is pulled tight and bent back against the pole for added friction. PVC pipes bend and fracture if they are used to lift animals. Once secured with the noose, the restrainer pulls back in line with the direction of the pipe to pull the animal for positioning and restraint.

Mouth A short version of the noose design works exceedingly well as a mouth pole for closing and securing the jaws of captured crocodilians prior to taping or tying. The noose is placed over the jaws and tightened. Once the jaws are shut, the pole is twisted several times to add more tension to the noose. A person then steps in to quickly secure the jaws.

Tape

Tape is essential after capture and during restraint; jaws can be safely secured and heavier tapes are used to immobilize legs to prevent movement. The most commonly used are silver duct and black PVC electricians tape. Always have a sufficient amount on-hand.

Cable Straps

Nylon cable straps (zip ties) are very useful for securing the jaws of some crocodilians (i.e., narrow-jawed species) even before one captures the animal. These come in various lengths and tensile strengths; the largest can resist a force of 100 kg.

Shelf Mat: Rubberized

Shelf mats are made of rubber-coated, woven fabric. They are used as non-skid shelf coverings and are readily purchased. The mats are cut into 5 to 10 cm (2 to 4 inch) wide strips to wrap around the snout or the entire head. They are used for this purpose because they do not slip in a wet environment. The crocodile jaws are held shut with a mouth pole or by hand, wrapped with the mat and then taped over. The sponginess of the mat prevents the tape from binding too tightly. Also, the nonslip nature of this material prevents jaw tape from slipping forward and covering the nostrils during transport.

Eye Cloth

The eyes are covered before or after capture with a cloth, towel, burlap bag, or an old T-shirt. This has a calming effect on the animals and likely reduces stress during the capture period. The blinded crocodilian is much less likely to avoid capture and to struggle following capture. Additionally, if the animal does attempt to strike, it is undirected and less likely to injure. Eye cloths are safely and gently placed over the eyes using a hook. The cloth is soaked before placement so it will more completely cover the eyes of the partially submerged crocodilian.

Eye clothes are secured with a couple of wraps of duct tape. Crocodilian eyes can be voluntarily withdrawn down into the skull, but some caution must be used when taping the eye cloth. Do not press the eyes too hard or apply too much pressure with the tape. If the eyes are to be covered for an extended period, gauze pads or a folded paper towel are placed over them before taping.

Hooks

Hooks are absolutely essential tools when working with crocodilians. They facilitate work around the animals by allowing placement of ropes, manipulation of legs, and so on, without bringing human appendages within striking range. Several different hook types have been used by the author. Heavy snake hooks (e.g., python hooks) are sufficiently robust for positioning ropes around a crocodilian's head, lifting legs, lifting the jaws, and so on. Hooks are also useful for removing and retrieving ropes during release.

The author also uses long, very lightweight fiberglass hooks designed for livestock showing (Fig. 18.2). These break fairly easily, but are also inexpensive. They are not substantial enough to manipulate an animal, but are excellent for rope noose placement and positioning. When capturing a submerged crocodilian, it is often possible to carefully position a rope noose over and around the head with these hooks without disturbing the animal and causing it to move.

Restraint and Transport Devices

Once captured and the jaws secured, there are many ways to confine or restrain a crocodilian (e.g., bags, buckets, ice chests, shipping crates, ladders, platforms, and cargo nets or marine mammal slings). The restraint technique and equipment selected depends on (1) animal size, (2) duration of confinement, and (3) distance to be transported. A more detailed discussion of these devices is given later.

Knives and Other Tools

Cutting implements are always available during a capture. Knives are used to cut tape, frayed rope, and so on. Wire cutters are used to cut through cable straps when used on the snouts of some specimens.

Trauma Kit

If the capture techniques described in this chapter are followed, the risks to personnel are minimized. However, the capture team should always be prepared for someone being injured during restraint. This includes having a well stocked trauma kit on hand to provide immediate aid.

TO CATCH A CROCODILIAN

As described above, crocodilians can be massive, powerful and often react violently to physical restraint. During capture safety of personnel is paramount, followed closely by the welfare of the animals. The techniques favored by this author restrain the animals completely to limit the possibility of self-injury to the animal and personnel injury. The essential components of successful capture are planning, communication, caution, and knowledge of the animals.

Planning and Preparation

Capture and restraint of small specimens is usually routine and does not necessitate much planning or preparation. This is absolutely not the case when attempting to capture and restrain a larger specimen (i.e., ≥2 m, 6 ft in total length). Preparation includes careful planning, discussion, and oversight. One person (the team or crew leader) is designated "in charge," and he or she directs everyone else what to do, where to be, and so on. Each person's role or roles is discussed and clearly understood before the operation commences.

However, many plans are quickly rendered moot if the capture subject is uncooperative. Each capture experience is different; it is not possible to foresee all of the variables likely to be encountered. Flexibility and strategy, the ability to change capture plans in mid-course while still maintaining a safe working environment, are essential. As handlers become more experienced with captures, they develop a greater repertoire of techniques to apply to specific situations.

Communication is essential before, during, and after a capture to insure the safety of the staff and the animal. Each team member must listen for, and continue to receive instructions from, the team leader throughout the procedure. The team leader must also continually look out for crew safety, make sure staff is in their proper positions, performing their assigned roles, everyone is outside of the strike zone of the animal, and escape routes are kept clear at all times.

Environmental Assessment
The first stage of preparation is assessment of the capture environment. If the animal is in a simple off-exhibit enclosure, this may be fairly straightforward. However, an animal on display in a complex habitat full of obstacles and possibly with other enclosure mates requires more forethought. It is important to answer several questions when assessing the capture environment.

Where Are the Escape Routes? This is perhaps the most important question. More than one route is preferred, but often not available. All team members must be aware of these routes, and they are left clear at all times during the capture.

What Is Physically Possible? The geography of an enclosure will determine access and the capture technique used. For example, low overhanging vegetation, large amounts of vegetation, and logs or rocks in a pool make it difficult to get a rope on an animal.

Is the Animal Trained to Shift? Many institutions provide off-exhibit shift areas, similar to those used for mammalian carnivores or large hoofed stock. Crocodilians can be rapidly trained with food to utilize these shifts, and even to move into transport crates. This training facilitates working with these animals and reduces the need for stressful and potentially injurious captures.

Will the Animal Be Caught in Water or on Land? The habitat is assessed to determine whether staging the capture on land or in the water is best and safe. In many enclosures, land surface is insufficient or too crowded with vegetation and furniture to allow a well-coordinated capture. Similarly, some water features make it difficult to gain access to the animal. If the plan is to catch in the water, will the staff be on shore or down in the pool or both?

The characteristics of any water feature must be known to make a proper assessment of its utility in catching an animal. Important variables to know include total pool area, the water depth, whether the water can be lowered without emptying the pool, the slope of pool sides, and whether staff can easily get out of it.

Land capture requires sufficient space for both the team and the animal, and must allow the staff to stay safely outside the strike zone. If the animal is on land, the plan should include a contingency for capturing it in the water. Unless caught immediately, crocodilians will seek refuge in water. If either land or water offer ample opportunity for capture, consider choosing to catch in the water. On land, crocodilians feel threatened and cornered. Water is a natural refuge and they often lay more passively, allowing easier placement of the rope and positioning of personnel.

Where Will the Animal Be Restrained? In some situations, the crocodilian is removed from the enclosure to provide enough space to safely work around the animal. In other situations, the jaws are secured while the animal is in the exhibit, then it is removed from the habitat before full restraint or loading into a crate.

Are There Other Animals Present? Other crocodilians obstruct access or pose a significant and potentially serious threat to staff and the animal to be captured. If possible, these animals are shifted out of the way before beginning. Additional staff may be needed to fend them off during capture; these animals may become involved as the animal and catch team move about the enclosure. The heightened stress or anxiety in the enclosure associated with the capture may cause these animals to strike out. Care is taken to avoid injury to the animal being caught up and the staff members involved.

Animal Assessment
Not all techniques are appropriate for all species or size class. It is useful to have knowledge of the animal to be captured; crocodilian species are known for differences in temperament and their capabilities. Saltwater crocodiles (*C. porosus*) and Cuban crocodiles (*Crocodylus rhombifer*) are especially dangerous; they may charge and are powerful and agile jumpers. However, this does not imply other species are less dangerous. There are

also individual animal differences; some usually mild-mannered species can be unexpectedly belligerent. Ideally, all crocodilians are approached with the same degree of caution. There must be a healthy understanding and respect for the physical abilities of these animals.

Other aspects of the animal's biology, particularly snout morphology, are also considered when preparing for a capture. Slender-snouted species are more prone to serious snout damage during capture than are species with broader, more robust snouts. As a result, special precautions are necessary in preparing for capture of these more fragile species. Protecting the jaws prior to capture with cable straps may reduce disfiguring injuries. Conversely, exceptionally robust or broad-snouted species (e.g., the broad-snouted caiman, *Caiman latirostris*) are often difficult to safely secure because there is relatively little purchase area for hands or mouth-poles.

The "toothiness" of the animal to be captured is noted. Protruding teeth cause damage, or even serious injury, when accidentally caught on a hand or arm or forcefully slammed into a team member during a struggle. This danger persists even after the jaws have been secured. Many captive crocodilians have abnormal tooth development, resulting in misaligned teeth protruding from the jaws. In some species (e.g., the false gharial, *Tomistoma schlegelii*), the teeth are long, slender, sharp, and naturally interdigitate, making them very difficult to handle. In these animals, it is necessary to wrap the entire jaw line in tape, or with a bath towel, rubberized shelf mat, or other material to prevent injury.

CAPTURE AND HANDLING BASICS

Strike Zones

The crocodilian head is its most dangerous part. Many people unfamiliar with these animals believe the tail is the main area to be avoided. While it is true the tail can cause injury, it is the head that has a mouth full of 70–80 teeth and a very high bite force.

The stocky body form and heavily ossified skin of crocodilians limits their flexibility. However, they can and will strike sideways with exceptional speed. In most crocodilians lying on the ground, the strike zone is defined by the arc of the head swinging from side to side. It is, therefore, much safer to approach an animal, secured by a rope around its neck, from the front than the side.

In the process of swinging its large, massive head rapidly to the side, a crocodilian generally swings or slaps with its tail. The tail is solid and strong and can knock a person off his or her feet or knock them toward the jaws. Consequently, the tail arc must also be avoided by catch personnel.

Roping

Captures generally begin with the securing of a snare or rope noose to the animal. There are two basic variations of this procedure.

Neck Noosing This technique involves placing the rope over the head and cinching it around the neck. It is usually used for alligator, caiman, and heavy-bodied crocodiles. These animals have fairly large jowls at the back of the head behind that the rope noose can take hold. Crocodilian necks are thick, heavily muscled, and usually capable of enduring without injury the forces that occur during struggling. In captivity, where it is often possible to carefully place the rope before closing the noose, some prefer to also hook the noose under one forelimb so it does not cinch tight around the neck. This technique is necessary in very large, heavy specimens that have to be pulled up and over a steep bank or the lip of a pool. This is to prevent too much force being applied to the neck and spine.

Top Jaw Noosing Top-jaw noosing is used in species with body profiles too slim to allow a neck noose. The rope is caught in the teeth and held firmly. It is of a narrower diameter (≤1.3 cm, 1/2 in) allowing it to bind more closely around the upper jaw.

A clear advantage of this technique is the greater control of the head, since there is restraint of the snout. However, a major disadvantage is that when the crocodile jerks, twists, or shakes, which they do with tremendous force and speed, all of the force is transmitted through the rope into the hands of the holder. Those who use top-jaw noosing usually secure the jaws with a narrow rope. Two people stand on either side of the head, outside of the strike zone, with the rope stretched between them. This is placed under the lower jaw, and then the ends of the jaw rope are wrapped around one another and exchanged. As the rope is pulled, the jaws are forced together. One person then steps in and holds the knot while the second ties a securing knot. A safer alternative is the use a mouth pole.

Securing the Jaws

Depending in part upon the size of the crocodilian, the jaws can be secured with a variety of materials.

Tape Once the jaws have been closed (by hand in very small specimens or a mouth pole in larger animals), their jaws are usually taped. The standard used on larger crocodilians is silver, fabric duct tape. It has reasonably good adhesion to itself, but animals otherwise unrestrained are usually able to work it off of their jaws within a few hours. A major advantage is it has very little stretch, making it difficult to apply too tightly.

This author uses black PVC electrician's tape to secure the jaws of crocodilians ≤3 m (10 ft) for short periods of time. It is very quick to apply and sticks well to itself. Most other tapes do not adhere well to crocodilians, especially when wet. During application, the tape must be wrapped around the snout and taped to itself to provide a good hold. A general rule is one wrap of electrical tape for each foot (0.3 m) of animal (i.e., for a 5-ft or 1.6-m alligator, wrap the tape five times around the snout).

Do not leave a crocodilian taped for more than a few hours. Electrical tape has a lot of stretch and can be applied with enough force to block blood flow to the skin. If it remains in place for too long, it will cause ischemic skin damage resulting within a few days in scabbing, sloughing, and scarring.

The author has also used the heavy, bright red, tape used for drywall seams. This has excellent adhesive force and a small amount of stretch. However, it does not tear readily, making it necessary to cut with a knife. The great advantage of this tape is that it is highly visible, making it immediately obvious when an animal has thrown its tape and its jaws are unsecured. This is an added safety measure, especially when transporting several animals at once.

Always create a tab when taping an animal; fold back the end so that it is easy to see and grasp. This facilitates removal of the tape during the release.

Cable Straps Cable straps (zip ties) are frequently used on slender-snouted species (e.g., *Tomistoma*, *Gavialis*, *Crocodylus intermedius*, and *Crocodylus johnsoni*). There is an increased risk they will damage or even break their snout/lower jaw during capture. This often happens when the animal bites on something in the exhibit and then rolls, applying torsion to the jaws. Securing the jaws shut before a capture reduces the chances of injury. The captures also move more rapidly; staff can restrain the animal in a shorter period of time, further reducing chances of injury.

To use cable strap, first make a noose by inserting the tip of the strap through the locking mechanism. Then, drill or punch a small hole through the tip of the strap and thread a string, wire, or monofilament line through and tie it. The string and the tip of the cable strap noose are then run through a length of 0.6 (1/4) to 1.3 cm (1/2 inch) PVC pipe to serve as a catchpole. The noose can be accurately placed over the jaws without touching them. A rapid tug on the string will close the noose and pin the jaws shut, often without disturbing the animal. Alternatively, the cable strap noose is suspended from the string and lowered into a position around the jaws. A swift jerk tightens the strap around the jaws.

This technique is also used with other crocodilian species, but it is more difficult to zip-tie the jaws of broad-snouted species. However, in many species, there is a notch or depression in the jaw (e.g., behind an enlarged tooth) into which the cable strap can take hold and tighten down onto the snout.

Caution must be used with nylon straps. Do not trust them; they often are not affixed tightly and can easily slip, releasing the jaws. They also become more brittle with time and prone to breakage; buy new ones before each capture.

Other Binds Less frequently, jaws are bound with rubber bands or heavy cord. Strong, heavy, rubberbands made by cutting tire inner tubes into rings can be used for animals ≤3 m (10 ft) in length.

Eye Coverage
Cover the eyes whenever restraining a crocodilian. Use an eye cloth or, if the animal is fully restrained, cover with your hand. During a capture, drop an eye cloth in place with a hook. This prevents the animal from seeing your movements, makes it less likely the animal will become unruly and prevents the animal from directing a strike toward a capture team member. Covering the eyes also keeps the animal quieter and may reduce the stress of the experience for the animal.

Go to the Bathroom
There is no delicate way to state this and it seems an odd thing to mention in a discussion of catching crocodiles but, before beginning any major catch up operation, make sure each person on the catch team has visited the restroom. These operations can be time consuming and can be tense for the staff involved. The necessities of bodily functions can arise making a team member uncomfortable and distracted. This can result in actions being rushed or mistakes being made.

CAPTURE AND RESTRAINT
Hatchling/Juvenile (≤1 m)
Hatchling and small juvenile-sized crocodilians can still inflict a painful bite, so caution is still necessary when working with these animals. Biting a keeper is also stressful to the animal and may damage teeth or jaw structures. Also, the animals are small enough that no matter where you grab them, you're never very far from the mouth.

This size animal is easily grasped by hand. Approach from behind and grab and hold firmly by the neck, over the shoulders or on the front half of the torso (Fig. 18.3). To reduce the chance of a bite, use a hook, a small stick or rod, or even a broom to push the head away from the hand and block as the animal is picked up. Pillstrom tongs, a standard tool for most herpetologists (Chapter 21), do not work well with crocodilians. The bony armor on the neck and dorsum prevents the tongs from gaining a firm purchase and the animals can twist, roll, and wrest themselves free. There is also a natural tendency to squeeze the tongs more firmly to prevent this resulting in injury to the animal.

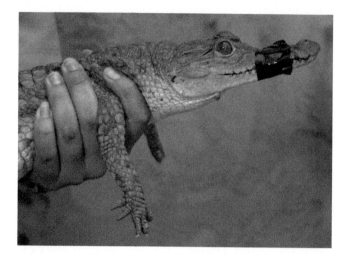

Figure 18.3. Physical restraint of a small crocodilian (*Crocodylus mindorensis*). Note the electrician tape placed around the jaws and the hand grasping the neck and forelimbs.

Once the animal is in hand the jaws must be secured. The animal is held firmly around the neck with one hand, and the other hand is advanced from behind, keeping it close to the body. It is placed around the neck and slowly slid forward while gently squeezing. As it moves up onto the head, it will slowly close the jaws. The eyes are covered and the head held with this hand. The jaws are then secured shut with tape (even transparent tape will work on this-sized animal, a rubber band, or a short length of cotton clothesline) (Fig. 18.3).

Subadults (≤2 m)

Subadult crocodilians or the adults of smaller species (e.g., Chinese alligator, *Alligator sinensis*; African dwarf crocodile, *Osteolaemus tetraspis*; both species of the caiman genus *Paleosuchus*) are perhaps the most difficult size class to capture and handle safely. These animals are large and powerful enough to provide a large struggle, yet still agile and quick enough to turn rapidly and snap.

The tool of choice for these animals is the catchpole made by running a loop of rope through a length of PVC pipe. The loop is placed over the animal's head and around the neck and pulled tight. The rope is bent back against the PVC pipe for added friction. PVC does have some flexion so the animal is not completely controlled. However, the animal can easily be dragged and positioned with this device. Greater control of the animal is achieved if a second person grabs the tip of the tail and pulls the animal. This stretches the animal between the catchpole and the second handler. Maintaining pressure on the tail prevents the animal from twisting or turning to bite. A mouth pole is used to close and secure the jaws. With the animal still controlled by the catchpole, the mouth-pole is placed over the snout and the rope pulled tight. It is preferable to stand at the side and slightly behind the animal's head when doing this. The jaws are closed with pressure applied by pulling the rope. When the jaws are completely shut, the mouth pole is twisted several times to add pressure to the jaws. When the jaws are secure and the mouth pole is holding, another crew member steps in and tapes the jaws.

Adult (≥2 m)

Capture and restraint of larger crocodilians is as much a matter of manpower and logistics as it is of proper procedure and safety. A sufficient number of staff is a necessity for a safe and efficient operation. Two people are plenty for a 2-m (6-ft) specimen. Generally, it is best to have at least three or four team members for a 2.5–3 m (8–9 ft) animal. Four or even more people are needed for specimens greater than 3 m (10 ft).

Not to belabor the point, it is ideal for working with these large specimens that they be trained to shift and, even better, into a crate. This provides substantial daily or weekly safety benefits to keeper staff and removes most of the trauma and anxiety of a physical capture. If this is not an option, or if the animal fails to shift when needed, than one may have to proceed with a capture.

As described earlier, before beginning capture of a large crocodilian, make sure ropes that are not frayed or worn and have been soaked are available. Wet ropes not only sink better to position them around an animal, but they do not burn the skin of the animal as dry ropes often will during a struggle.

Catching Adult Crocodilians in Water If the plan is to catch the crocodilian in the pool, the following are some suggestions for techniques to use. If it is possible to lower the water, drop it to a level that just covers the back of the animal (approximately 25 cm, 10 in). This depth limits the animal's mobility within the water feature while still allowing it to submerge its head. It also provides better visibility of the animal and any obstacles. It is important to keep enough water in the pool for the animal to remain submerged. As long as it can keep its eyes underwater, it is much less likely to become violently defensive.

There are various means of securing an animal in this situation. Most commonly, a rope is placed around the head and neck, and possibly one of the forelimbs. Hooks greatly facilitate safe rope placement and positioning of the noose. Alternatively a wide lasso is thrown over the head, or a break-away noose or a cable snare catchpole are used to get a line on the animal. If the animal is slender-snouted, or if there are many obstacles in the environment on which the animal might injure itself, the jaws are first secured with a cable strap.

If the team is familiar with the temperament of the animal and it is not reacting violently, it is often possible to manipulate the animal when the water is shallow. Large nets or marine mammal slings may be used to slide under the animal, envelop it, and lift it out of the pool area, greatly reducing the animal's struggles and chances for injury. Animals may also be able to be pushed or herded into a crate or a large-diameter PVC pipe that has been placed in the pool (Saumure et al. 2002).

A common disadvantage of catching in the water is most pools are hard-sided. They are generally constructed of concrete or gunite and readily damage the side of the head of a struggling crocodilian. Attempt to keep the animal away from the pool sides as it struggles, and move it past these structures as rapidly as possible. Sealed foam rubber gym mats or other shock-absorbing materials can be placed against the side of a pool to protect the animal.

Catching Adult Crocodilians on Land Once the rope is placed on a crocodilian on land, there will be a struggle. They are able to generate a tremendous amount of resistance with their short legs forced into the ground. It is best to have sites already identified where one can tie off the rope (fence posts, trees, etc). Trees must be of sufficient diameter to resist the force of the animal; larger crocodilians will uproot a small tree. Tying off the rope restricts the animal's movements, facilitates repositioning of the handlers to provide further restraint and, perhaps most importantly, saves energy. Tired or exhausted catch crews are more likely to make mistakes. Successful techniques used for capture of crocodilians on land include the following sections.

The use of a rope to secure a hold on the animal is most common. Rope lassos can be tossed over the head or the rope is placed with a hook or catchpole. Once the rope is secure, the crocodilian is pulled to the designated work area. The animal is tied to a tree or post. Most carefully prepared capture plans unravel when the crocodilian begins to roll. This tangles ropes, scatters equipment, moves the animal into areas that compromise it or the catch staff and, generally, messes up an otherwise well-organized process. Catch leaders must recognize and concede when a plan has been disrupted. Most often, it is best to pause momentarily, regroup, reorganize, and then begin again. Once an animal is tied off, it may be possible to cinch a second rope to the tail. Stretch the animal and tie off the second line. This may help prevent the animal from rolling. Once the animal is restrained, a mouth pole is used to close and secure the jaws.

If there is a tree or post within the area, try to pull the animal up to it so that the head is pulled up against the tree. This acts as a stubbing post and can greatly restrict the movement of the head, making it safer to work around the animal.

Most crocodilians, when roped, will pull against the rope in an attempt to escape. A few may be more bold or aggressive and lunge at the staff on the other end of the rope. If this appears to be a potential, either control the animal by catching it up with a rigid catchpole, or place a second rope over the head and stretch the animal between them.

Mounting There are situations in which it is necessary to straddle over or "mount" a large crocodilian. With caution, procedure, and experience, this is a fairly safe technique. However, the level of security it offers personnel is much less than that of other methods recommended in this chapter (i.e., shifting, working at a distance with hooks and poles, or physical restraint on a backboard). If any of these other methods satisfy the purpose, use them instead.

Mounting allows one person to control the animal and its head, take blood or other samples, and facilitates measurement. Once in position on top of the animal, the handler is relatively safe. Even with vigorous twists from side to side, the animal should be unable to bite. Care is taken to prevent the animal from rolling. The best technique to prevent this is for other catch crew to keep the tail straight and pull the hind limbs back and off the ground. Some species (especially caiman) are quite capable of and prone to snapping their heads straight up as a handler leans over them. This is extremely dangerous and can cause serious injury; sit up straight while straddled on the animal.

To attain this position, the handler must move into the animal's strike zone, hence the danger of this technique. To do this safely, the animal must be tightly roped and the rope tied securely in front of the head. This prevents the animal from twisting back on the restrainer. The handler moves up along the axis of the animal's body, essentially straight up the tail and the back. Stay as close to the body as possible. If the animal thrashes unexpectedly, this will reduce the impact and help maintain your balance. The author finds it useful to nudge the animal with his foot before he proceeds. This tests whether the animal is ready to burst into a struggle. When ready to mount, move forward quickly and deliberately. Place one foot against the base of the tail just behind a hind limb. Move forward rapidly, place the other foot against the other side of the torso at midbody, and quickly drop into a seated position on its back, with knees planted behind the forelimbs of the animal. Cover the eyes with your hand, and keep your other hand on the top of the head and snout. Do not let fingers trail off the side of the face as this might elicit a snap to the side.

When ready to "dismount," make sure the path behind is clear and quickly step back off of the animal in the same manner you approached; place your feet against the body and step back along the body axis.

RESTRAINT AND TRANSPORT

Once the crocodilian is captured and the jaws safely secured, the techniques for safely and efficiently move it vary. The method of transport depends, obviously, on the size of the specimen and the distance it must be transported. For transport within the institution, smaller specimens are simply carried or placed in a bag, pillow case, duffel bag, bucket, or ice chest. However, even small crocodilians can deliver a painful slap with the tail. This is prevented by placing the tail underneath the arm while holding the animal around the neck and supporting its weight on your arm.

Larger specimens can be heavy, at least unwieldy if not often combative, and difficult to lift and carry. There is a natural tendency to try to lift these specimens by their legs. This can be injurious and must be avoided. The shoulder and hip joints of crocodilians are relatively shallow. It is not difficult to pull a limb out of the joint when lifting its leg. If an animal must be lifted, reach underneath and support it from below the torso and tail. However, crocodilians are not accustomed to being off of the ground; they will often struggle, twist, and attempt to roll. The head must always be controlled. Even with the jaws taped shut, it is dangerous. Always keep it directed away from others and keep your head away from it.

Ideally, larger crocodilians are either placed into a shipping crate or strapped to a backboard, platform, or aluminum ladder for transport (Fig. 18.4). They must

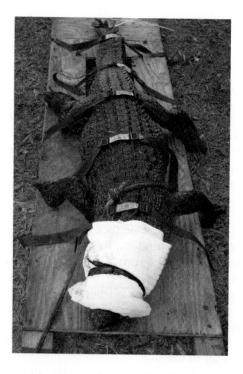

Figure 18.4. Physical restraint of large crocodilian (*Crocodylus novaeguinae*) with a restraint board. Cargo straps are used to tie the animal to the board. A towel covers the eyes to reduce struggling.

be thoroughly restrained to prevent them from struggling to free themselves and potentially injure themselves or the capture team. Although harsh, it has many benefits to the animal as well as to personnel. Some crocodilians will continue to struggle for long periods after capture. This increases their stress and exhausts them. Very large saltwater crocodiles (*C. porosus*) are known to struggle to such an extent that they build up dangerously high levels of lactic acid in their bloodstream (Seymour et al. 1987). This can result in severe acidosis and death. Crocodilians that are completely restrained on a board or platform usually cease to resist. Without the continued struggle, there is little chance of the animal seriously compromising itself physiologically.

Restraint can be in the form of nylon cable straps (for smaller specimens), ropes, or cargo straps. The platform can be lifted easily and can be placed on a cart or truck for transport. Straps are placed in several places along the body: over the neck, across the shoulders just behind the forelimbs, across the center of the torso, just in front of the hind limbs, on the base of the tail just past the pelvis, and one or more wraps across the anterior half of the tail (Fig. 18.4). The head is also secured. If the animal is restrained on an aluminum ladder, it is possible to run the rope through the hollow rungs of the steps to completely secure it to the structure. Cargo straps can be purchased in a variety of widths and strengths. It is best to use those that have a wrenching action to tighten the strap after it is attached.

It is possible to physically restrain even the largest of crocodilians in this manner assuming the platform and straps are sufficiently strong. However, it can be difficult to release the grip on the buckle of very large cargo straps. A heavy hook is useful for this purpose. For transport to other institutions, crocodilians are generally confined to a shipping crate.

RELEASE TECHNIQUES

Releasing an animal that has been captured poses as many safety concerns as the initial capture. One must be concerned not only with the safety of the staff, but also with risks to the animal being released or its enclosure mates.

There is a real possibility the animal may attempt to turn and bite after its jaws have been unbound. Methods should be utilized to put distance between the catch personnel and the animal being released. One such method is the use of a jaw rope. A length of narrow rope is passed underneath the tape or rubber-band holding the jaws shut. It is passed from the front to the back so there is no danger of accidentally causing the binds to slip and release the jaws prematurely. The rope is then tied off so that it will grip the binds. With the animal in position, all other restraints are removed, taking care not to trip on or accidentally pull the jaw rope. When all restraints are free, and all personnel are well away from the animal, a hard tug on the jaw rope will pull the bindings from the jaws, freeing the animal.

In cases where the animal has been "top-jaw roped," it serves as the jaw rope. With the jaws still firmly taped or tied, the noose of the top-jaw rope is opened. The length of rope still firmly held in the crocodile's jaws is then used to make several wraps around the snout. This then serves to secure the jaws while the other bindings are removed. When all other restraints are removed and everyone is safely away, the top-jaw rope is unwrapped from the snout. The animal will open its mouth and release the rope.

A rope noose catchpole or mouth pole is ideal for assisting release. The animal is restrained by the catchpole while the jaw bindings are removed. The pole prevents the animal from moving toward the catch team member holding it. When everyone is safely back from the animal, the catchpole is removed.

Immediately after release, crocodilians may be highly agitated. If there are other enclosure mates, there is a possibility of displaced aggression, leading to injury of one or more of the other animals. Before releasing a crocodile, make sure it is positioned at a distance from others.

If it is suspected aggression will occur, it is possible to release an animal with its jaws still bound and remove the bindings later. Retape the jaws and insert a piece of rope or a metal ring under the tape. The rope should float and have a large loop tied in its free end. Once the animals have had sufficient time to calm down after release, a long-handled hook is used to catch the loop in the rope or the metal ring and pull the tape from the jaws.

REFERENCES

Almandarz E. 1986. Physical restraint of reptiles. In: *Zoo & Wild Animal Medicine* (ME Fowler, ed.), pp. 151–155. Philadelphia: W.B. Saunders.

Chabreck RH. 1963. Methods of capturing, marking, and sexing alligators. Proceedings of the Annual Conference of the Southeastern Association of Game and Fish Commissioners 17:47–50.

Forster DL. 1991. A new technique for the daytime capture of adult alligators. Proceedings of the Annual Conference of the Southeastern Association of Fish and Wildlife Agencies 45:198–200.

Fowler ME. 1978. *Restraint and Handling of Wild and Domestic Animals*. Ames: Iowa State University Press.

Hutton JM, Loveridge JP, Blake DK. 1987. Capture methods for the Nile crocodile in Zimbabwe. In: *Wildlife Management: Crocodiles and Alligators* (GJW Webb, SC Manolis, PJ Whitehead, eds.), pp. 243–247. Surrey Beatty and Sons: Chipping Norton.

Joanen T, Perry WG Jr. 1972. A new method for capturing alligators using electricity. Proceedings of the Annual Conference of the Southeastern Association of Game and Fish Commissioners 25:124–130.

Jones D, Hayes-Odum L. 1994. A method for the restraint and transport of crocodilians. *Herpetological Review* 25(1):14–15.

Jones FK Jr. 1965. Techniques and methods used to capture and tag alligators in Florida. Proceedings of the Annual Conference of the Southeastern Association of Game and Fish Commissioners 19:98–101.

Kofron CP. 1989. A simple method for capturing large Nile crocodiles. *African Journal of Ecology* 27:183–189.

Mazzotti FJ, Brandt LA. 1988. A method of live-trapping wary crocodiles. *Herpetological Review* 19(2):40–41.

McDaniel J, Hord L. 1990. Specialized equipment and techniques used in alligator management and research. In: *Crocodiles: Proceedings of the 12th Working Meeting of the Crocodile Specialist Group*, Volume 2, pp. 20–38. IUCN: The World Conservation Union, Gland, Switzerland.

Murphy TM, Fendly TT. 1974. A new technique for live trapping of nuisance alligators. Proceedings of the Annual Conference of the Southeastern Association of Game and Fish Commissioners 27:308–311.

Pooley AC 1984. Field notes on capturing crocodiles, pp. 42–47. Appendix 6B in Whitaker R. 1984. Preliminary survey of crocodile in Sabah, East Malaysia. Report to World Wildlife Fund Malaysia, Kuala Lumpur.

Saumure RA, Freiermuth B, Jundt J, Rowlett L, Jewell J. 2002. A new technique for the safe capture and transport of crocodylians in captivity. *Herpetological Review* 33(4):294–296.

Seymour RS, Webb GJW, Bennett AF, Bradford DF. 1987. Effect of capture on the physiology of *Crocodylus porosus*. In: *Wildlife Management: Crocodiles and Alligators* (GJW Webb, SC Manolis, PJ Whitehead, eds.), pp. 253–257. Chipping Norton: Surrey Beatty and Sons.

Walsh B. 1987. Crocodile capture methods used in the Northern Territory of Australia. In: *Wildlife Management: Crocodiles and Alligators* (GJW Webb, SC Manolis, PJ Whitehead, eds.), pp. 249–252. Chipping Norton: Surrey Beatty and Sons.

Webb GJW, Messel H. 1977. Crocodile capture techniques. *The Journal of Wildlife Management* 41(3):572–575.

Wilkinson PM 1994. A walk-through snare design for the live capture of alligators. In: *Crocodiles: Proceedings of the 12th Working Meeting of the Crocodile Specialist Group*, Volume 2, pp. 74–76. IUCN: The World Conservation Union, Gland, Switzerland.

Wise M. 1994. Techniques for the capture and restraint of captive crocodilians. In: *Captive Management and Conservation of Amphibians and Reptiles. Contributions to Herpetology*, Vol. 11 (JB Murphy, K Adler, JT Collins, eds.), pp. 401–405. Ithaca: Society for the Study of Amphibians and Reptiles.

19 Crocodilians (Crocodiles, Alligators, Caiman, and Gharial)

Gregory J. Fleming

INTRODUCTION

Crocodilians are one of the oldest living groups of reptiles and by their shear size and character are popular exhibit animals in zoos. Many of the 23 crocodilian species are endangered, and conservation programs, in both zoos and in situ, are increasingly making higher demands for safe and effective chemical immobilization and anesthesia.

PHYSIOLOGY AND ANATOMY

Crocodilians spend much of their time entirely submerged except for their eyes and nares. Each nostril acts as a waterproof valve that is closed with a muscular flap during submersion. This reflex may be obtunded by immobilizing agents that relax the muscles of the nostril, allowing water into the respiratory tract (Fleming 1996). An additional respiratory valve is formed by the soft palate and gular fold. The elongated soft palate presses down against the gular fold, which protrudes from the floor of the mouth. This seal allows the crocodilian to open its mouth underwater without water rushing into the internal nares and the glottis. The gular fold may need to be displaced to visualize the glottis for endotracheal intubation (Fig. 19.1).

Crocodilians possess a pair of well-developed lungs (Klide & Klein 1973). The primary respiratory muscle groups are the intercostal and two transverse membranes, the postpulmonary and posthepatic. These membranes are comprised primarily of fibrous tissue with a muscular component (Van der Merwe & Kotze 1993). The postpulmonary membrane separates the lungs from the liver, and the posthepatic membrane is attached to a sheet of muscle that inters at the ospubis. These two membranes act as a diaphragm. Ventilation is achieved by expanding the intercostal muscles, and then membranes pull the liver in a caudal direction, creating a negative pressure around the lungs. The lungs then expand and the air is drawn through the nostrils into the lungs. The glottic valve is then closed, holding the air in the lungs. Once the glottal valve relaxes, air in the lungs is expelled passively via the elastic recoil of the intercostal muscles and the postpulmonary/posthepatic membranes and lung tissue.

The air flow in the lungs of alligators has been shown to be unidirectional, passing through parabronchi similar to birds (Farmer & Sanders 2010). The significance for anesthesia is unknown.

Cardiovascular System

Crocodiles are the only reptiles that possess four-chambered hearts (Murphy 1996). The heart functions like a mammal's, with the exception of anatomical adaptations for an aquatic lifestyle. These include the foramen of Panizzi, an opening between the left and right ventricle, the subpulmonary conus situated in the pulmonary outflow tract of the right ventricle, and the aortic anastomosis that connect the two aortic arches just posterior to the heart (Axelsson 2001). In addition, crocodilians have a left aorta that arises from the right ventricle, which allows blood to bypass the lungs and be recirculated into the systemic circulation (Axelsson 2001).

The foramen of Panizza is a small window located between the intraventricular septum at the confluence of the left and right aortic arches (Millchamp 1988). It acts as a pressure valve allowing blood to flow between the venous and arterial systems. This flow from high pressure to low pressure results in venous admixture. When the animal is breathing, left ventricular pressure

Zoo Animal and Wildlife Immobilization and Anesthesia, Second Edition. Edited by Gary West, Darryl Heard, and Nigel Caulkett.
© 2014 John Wiley & Sons, Inc. Published 2014 by John Wiley & Sons, Inc.

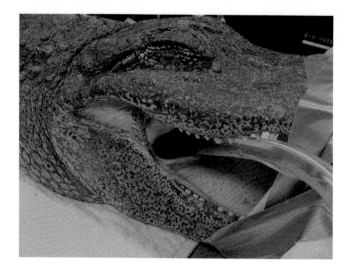

Figure 19.1. View of the gular fold of a Chinese alligator (*Alligator sinensis*) being depressed with a tongue depressor to access the epiglottis. Note the oral speculum constructed of a piece of PVC pipe wrapped with tape.

is greater, allowing a small amount of oxygenated blood to flow through the foramen of Panizza into the venous blood supply (Millchamp 1988). When the crocodilian submerges, air held in the lungs restricts blood flow through the pulmonary capillary beds, resulting in pulmonary hypertension, which increases right ventricular and pulmonary arterial pressures. As a result, blood flows from right to left through the foramen of Panizza. Deoxygenated blood is diverted away from the lungs through the left aortic arch to organs that are not sensitive to low levels of oxygen (e.g., liver and stomach) (Grenard 1991). Oxygenated blood is diverted to oxygen-sensitive organs (i.e., the heart and brain). A combination of blood shunting and anerobic metabolism may allow an inactive crocodilian to stay submerged for 5–6 hours (Lane 1996).

This right to left shunt through the foramen of Panizza may have clinical implications during anesthesia when the crocodilian does not have ventilatory support or is apneic. Shunting of blood away from the lungs will delay inhalant anesthetic uptake and removal. This emphasizes the importance of assisted ventilation.

Renal Portal System

Crocodilians possess a renal portal system composed of the renal portal vein arising from the epigastric and external iliac veins (Millchamp 1988). These vessels drain blood from the dorsal body wall, the cloaca, sex organs, and the bladder. Drugs injected into the caudal half of the body, base of the tail and hind legs, may be cleared by the kidneys prior to reaching the systemic circulation. In other reptile species, such as the red-eared slider, studies have showed a significant a hepatic first-pass effect following hind limb drug administra-

tion (Holz 1997). A study comparing front leg versus hind leg injections of buprenorphine resulted in a 70% decrease in the bioavailability of buprenorphine when injected in the hind end (Kummrow et al. 2008). Thus, care should be taken when administering nephrotoxic drugs in the hind legs, and when possible, inject anesthetic drugs in the front legs until further research can be completed on crocodilian vascular anatomy (Mosley 2011).

Physiologic Reference Ranges

Obtaining heart and respiratory rates is very difficult in awake crocodilians. In one study, juvenile American alligators (*Alligator mississippiensis*) and smooth-sided caimans (*Caiman sclerops*) were implanted with monitoring equipment and isolated from human contact for 12–20 hours before measuring cardiac and respiratory rates. Normal respiratory and heart rates at 22°C were 0.6 and 11.6 beats per minute, and 1.6 and 14.2 beats per minute, respectively. Following visual contact with humans, both heart and respiratory rates doubled to 30 beats per min and 6 breaths per min (Huggins et al. 1969). Consequently, most captured crocodilians are likely to be tachycardic and tachypneic. In general, heart and respiratory rates vary inversely with the size of the animal, but are affected by environmental temperatures. In Nile crocodiles (*Crocodylus niloticus*), heart rates increased as temperatures increased from 1 to 8 beats per minute at 10°C up to 24 to 40 beats per minute at 28°C. Prolonged exposure to high temperatures above 40°C will cause irreversible cardiac damage. Heart rates as high as 55 beats per min at 29°C have been recorded in Nile crocodiles caught in traps (Klide & Klein 1973; Loveridge 1979).

Thermoregulation

Crocodilians are poikilothermic, regulating their body temperatures by using external environmental heat sources. They also operate at a preferred optimum body temperature (POBT) similar to mammalian internal body temperatures. For captive crocodilians, a good range for environmental temperatures is 25–35°C (Bennet 1996). Given a selection of temperatures, they are able to select the POBT for their metabolic needs.

Temperatures below and above POBT interfere with digestion and immune function. American alligators take twice as long to digest food at 20 than 28°C, while smooth-fronted caimans digest food three times faster at 30 than 15°C (Coulson & Hernandez 1983; Diefenbach 1975). However, experimental infection of American alligators kept at 30°C demonstrated the greatest white blood cell response to infection and survival of the infection, while alligators held above the POBT at 35°C succumbed to infection in 3 weeks (Glassman & Bennet 1978).

Crocodilians under general anesthesia should be kept at temperatures near their POBT or around 29.5°C

(Bennet 1996). Environmental temperatures below POBT decrease metabolism and thereby prolong clearance of injectable drugs, resulting in delayed recoveries. Induction may also be prolonged because of slowed absorption and circulation times. For example, large Nile crocodiles induced with the neuromuscular blocker, gallamine, took twice as long to become recumbent at 14°C (40 minutes) than at 26°C (20 minutes) (Fleming 1996).

RESTRAINT TECHNIQUES

All crocodilians are capable of inflicting serious damage by ether biting or lashing out with tails. For this reason, a number of restraint techniques have been developed for wild and captive crocodilians (Loveridge & Blake 1972; Wallach & Hoessle 1970; Walsh 1987). The goal of physical restraint is to be able to administer injectable anesthetics quickly and safely.

Successful restraint must be safe for both the handlers and the crocodilian. Reported injuries associated with physical restraint include fractured bones, damaged eyes, and drowning (Walsh 1987). Prolonged struggling will result in marked lactic academia, with pH levels dropping to 6.6–6.8 (normal range 7.2 ± 0.2) (Seymore et al. 1987). Like other reptiles, crocodilians take a prolonged period of time to recover from elevations in lactic acid, which have been implicated fatalities post restraint (Webb & Messel 1977). Captured crocodilians may become unconscious and drown if not allowed to rest after prolonged physical restraint (Sedgwick 1986). A variety of capture techniques have been described using scoop nets, squeeze cages, tongs, harpoons, rope traps, snares, box traps, and tubes, all with varying success (Blake 1993; Fowler 1985, 1986; Jones & Hayes-Odum 1994; Wallach & Hoessle 1970). Physical restraint of crocodilians is described in Chapter 20.

DRUG DELIVERY

The goal of drug delivery is to get close enough to the animal to administer the anesthetics safely. In most cases, this entails using injectable agents.

Darts

Darting can be a satisfactory method of delivering immobilizing agents to crocodilians. However, they have several major disadvantages to their use in these animals: (1) it is difficult to get an accurate shot while the crocodilian is in the water; (2) it is difficult to determine if the dart has fully discharged; (3) the osteoderms covering most of the dorsal surfaces of crocodilians may deflect the dart; and (4) once the animal is darted, if unrestrained, they may submerge, become immobilized, and drown. In captivity, in controlled situations (i.e., a dry enclosure), a dart may be an appropriate way to deliver drugs remotely; however, in the field, darts are rarely used (Blake 1993; Flammard et al. 1992).

Hand Syringe

The hand syringe has the advantage that it can be accurately placed and the rate of injection can be controlled. However, the animal must be secured for safe injection. This technique can be used for smaller crocodilians that are hand-restrained and for administering reversal agents to larger specimens. Both intramuscular and intravenous routes can be used as described later.

Pole Syringe

The advantage of a pole syringe is that crocodilians can be injected while unrestrained in a shallow pool, net, or a snare. The main disadvantage is that the injector must be within 2.5 m of the animal, and injection volumes are limited to 10–15 mL. If the anesthetic agent is not administered fast enough, the pole syringe and handler may be damaged by the animal.

Injection Sites

The base of the tail just caudal to the hind legs has been a common area for intramuscular injections in crocodilians (Jacobson 1984). This area is composed of many layers of muscle, with the vertebrae located deep within the muscle, and there is no risk of injecting into any internal organs when using a pole syringe. The main disadvantage is in obese animals; there may be a layer of fat, which if injected, could delay drug absorption. Another factor to consider is the possibility of a significant hepatic first-pass effect following hind limb drug administration (Mosley 2011). When possible, IM injections into the front legs may be a more efficacious route of drug administration. In any case, care must be taken to direct the needle between the scutes to assure a complete drug delivery. Intravenous injections are best accomplished by accessing the lateral coccygeal vein or the ventral tail vein (Wellehan et al. 2004). This site can be used to obtain blood samples, inject intravenous drugs, or for intravenous catheter placement (Fig. 19.2).

Handling

Once the immobilizing drug has taken effect, it is prudent to use a pole or stick to stimulate the crocodilian a number of times to ensure there is no response. Once this is accomplished, the eyes should be covered with a damp towel and the jaw should be taped shut. Care must be taken to avoid taping the nostrils shut.

The crocodilian can then be rolled onto a stretcher or a large tarp. Care must be taken not to pull and tug on the legs of the animal. Large crocodilians may weigh up to 500 kg, and pulling on legs to move them or lift them may result in fractures or luxations (Blake 1993). To accommodate lifting a crocodilian out of shallow

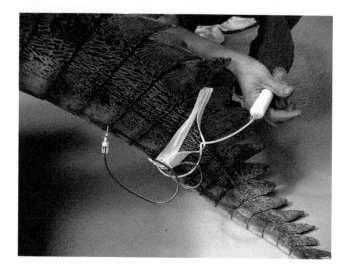

Figure 19.2. Intravenous blood draw via accessing the lateral coccygeal vein. The needle is inserted at a 90° angle at the lateral midline of the tail, just beneath the lateral spinus process of the vertebral body. This same approach may be used to complete intravenous injections of anesthetic drugs such as propofol.

water, 1 m lengths of flat 2-in commercial crane slinging can be placed under the chest and hind legs. By using the slings to lift, animals can easily be picked up and moved without pulling on the legs (Fleming 1996).

If the animal is to be intubated, a mouth gag, made of a steel ring, polyvinyl chloride (PVC) pipe, or a wood block should be used to prop open the mouth. Depending on the size of the animal, steel tubing (in varying diameter and width) can be cut and wrapped with several layers of tape or leather so as not to damage the teeth. A hole in the middle of the gag allows for the passage of anesthetic tubes or endoscopic equipment.

MONITORING

Physiologic monitoring can include the use of stethoscope, pulse oximeter, Doppler blood flow transducer, electrocardiography (ECG), ultrasound, or blood gas analysis. Anesthetic depth is evaluated using the withdrawal reflex of limbs, increasing or decreasing cardiac rates, righting response, bite and corneal reflexes (Bennet 1996; Heaton-Jones et al. 2002; Neill 1971).

The electrocardiogram and reference values have been described for the American alligator (Heaton-Jones 1996). The ECG leads are attached to 2.5-cm needles passed through the skin. Although pulse oximetry may be used to assess heart rate, it does not appear to accurately calculate oxygen saturation in reptiles (Mosley et al. 2004). Crocodilian skin thickness and pigmentation may further hamper measurement with the transmission probe, whereas a reflectance probe in the cloaca may improve the signal achieved. Blood gas measurement in crocodilians may be difficult to

interpret because numerous variables, such as temperature, feeding, and sample site (arterial, venous, or a combination of both), may influence the results. American alligators have the ability to reduce the affinity of hemoglobin to reduce blood oxygen affinity at certain pH levels. This allows for more oxygen to be released from the hemoglobin under certain condition, such as acidemia, increasing the total amount of oxygen available to tissues (Busk et al. 2000).

Doppler blood flow transducer appears to a very reliable method of obtaining heart rate (Bennet 1996; Neilson 1996). The probe is placed over the heart or a large blood vessel, such as the ventral coccygeal, brachial, or femoral artery. Blood flow in the optic arteries may be detected by placing the probe against the globe with the eye lid or third eye lid closed. Alternatively, a dorsally directed probe placed in the cloaca may detect arterial blood flow.

ANALGESIA

Information on the use of analgesics in reptiles and specifically crocodilians is limited. As is common in exotic animal medicine, extrapolation of drug doses from similar species is needed to develop effective analgesia. The use of butorphanol as an analgesic in reptiles has been promoted for years based on research in birds (Paul-Murphy et al. 1999). However, multiple studies in other reptilian species, such as green iguanas and red-eared sliders, revealed that butorphanol at higher doses may result in sedation, but does not itself result in analgesia (Baker et al. 2011; Fleming & Robertson 2006; Mosley 2011; Mosley et al. 2003; Sladky et al. 2007, 2008). Until further analgesic trials with butorphanol in crocodilians are completed, the author does not advocate its use as an analgesic.

The use of opioids such as morphine at (0.8 mg/kg) and meperidine (pethidine) (2 mg/kg) in juvenile saltwater crocodiles showed evidence of analgesia as measured with thermal antinociception (Kanui & Hole 1992). In red-eared sliders, using infrared thermal latency testing, morphine dosed at 1.5 and 6.5 mg/kg IM resulted in analgesia, but caused long-lasting respiratory depression at higher doses (Sladky et al. 2007). Using the same methodology, morphine at 10 and 20 mg/kg IM in bearded dragons resulted in analgesia, but was delayed until 8 hours after administration (Sladky et al. 2008). In a recent study in red-eared sliders, tramadol (5 mg/kg PO every 5 days) induced analgesia via both opioid and nonopioid pathways (Baker et al. 2011). The author has used tramadol in numerous reptilian species at 5 mg/kg PO with good anecdotal success.

The use of meloxicam (0.2 mg/kg PO, IM, IV) has been reported in reptiles, and administration either intravenously or orally resulted in the same bioavailability. (Hernandez-Divers et al. 2004; Wellehan 2006;

Whiteside & Black 2004). This author has used meloxicam (0.1 mg/kg orally once a day for 14 days) in two adult Nile crocodiles with traumatic foot lesions. The day following treatment, both crocodiles showed marked improvement in ambulation, with no evidence of lameness. After a single dose of ketoprofen at 2 mg/kg, IV and IM, in green iguanas, the terminal half-life was greater than that of dogs, suggesting dosing intervals for ketoprofen in reptiles should be longer than in mammals (i.e., >24 hours) (Tuttle et al. 2006).

TRANQUILIZERS AND SEDATIVES

Diazepam hydrochloride (0.22–0.62 mg/kg), administered 20 minutes prior to succinylcholine, resulted in a smoother induction and lower doses in American alligators (Loveridge & Blake 1972). Heart rates were decreased, respiration was maintained, and recovery for most was within 3 hours. Ketamine and diazepam have also been resulted in recovery times of 6 hours (Frye 1991). An alternative is zolazepam combined with tiletamine (Telazol).

Reversal/Recovery Reversal of benzodiazepine tranquilizers in mammals with flumazenil has been achieved in dogs at a ratio of 1:13, flumazenil to diazepam, or at 1:20, flumazenil to zolazepam (Lang 1987; Terpin et al. 1978). Without a reversal agent, recovery times of up to 6 hours in reptiles have been recorded (Frye 1991). Flumazenil is very expensive, making its routine use, particularly in larger reptiles, prohibitive.

LOCAL ANALGESIA

Local anesthetics are indicated for minor surgical procedures, such as skin lacerations or abscess removal (Burke 1986; Jacobson 1984). Toxic lidocaine doses have not been established for crocodilians.

A nerve locater can be used to assist in the accurate placement of local anesthetic around nerves (Wellehan 2006). Nerve locators use a pulsatile electric current passed through a needle in contact with the motor nerve (e.g., mandibular nerve) that innervates and thus stimulates an identifiable muscle (e.g., digastricus muscle). Local anesthetic (e.g., 2% mepivacaine, 1 mg/kg) injected down the needle blocks nerve conduction. This technique has been used to provide analgesia in the mandible of American alligators, dwarf crocodile (*Osteolaemus tetraspis*) and Yacare caiman (*Caiman yacare*) (Wellehan 2006).

IMMOBILIZING DRUGS
Muscle Relaxants

Muscle relaxants do not provide analgesia for painful procedures, and auditory, visual, and tactile stimulation must be minimal. (Huggins et al. 1969) They have

been utilized historically in Africa for transportation and capture of wild crocodilians (Fleming 1996).

Gallamine Triethiodide The short-acting nondepolarizing neuromuscular blocking agent gallamine triethiodide produces flaccid muscle paralysis (Loveridge 1979; Woodford 1972). Even though paralyzed, the crocodile is fully conscious and aware of auditory, visual, and tactile stimulation, which may result in increased heart and respiratory rates (Lloyd et al. 1994). The eyes of immobilized crocodilians should be covered and all external stimuli (i.e., noise) kept to a minimum. Gallamine may cause the mouth to open as the muscles relax, commonly referred to as the flaxidil reaction (Blake 1993). Gallamine has been the drug of choice in South Africa, where it has been used for immobilization of Nile crocodiles for over 25 years in both the field and in captivity (Loveridge 1979; Webb & Messel 1977).

A wide range of dosages have been reported, 0.6 mg/kg IM in a 312-kg Nile crocodile to 4 mg/kg IM in a 9.7-kg crocodile (Loveridge 1979). An additional study of 38 adult Nile crocodiles reported effective dosages of 1–2 mg/kg IM (Fleming 1996). Larger crocodiles over 3 m were immobilized with dosages of 1.1 mg/kg IM, while smaller crocodiles less than 3 m were immobilized with a dosage of 2 mg/kg IM. Gallamine overdosage may result in bradycardia, gastrointestinal hypermotility, increased salivation, mydriasis, and respiratory muscle paralysis and death (Blake 1993; Lloyd et al. 1994). Faster induction times (15–30 minutes) were reported with higher environmental temperatures (30°C). Cuban crocodiles have also been successfully immobilized, with gallamine at doses of 0.64 to 4 mg/kg IM (Lloyd 1999). Gallamine (1 mg/kg IM) has a low therapeutic index in American alligators and may cause death (Jacobson 1984). Deaths in false gharials (*Tomistoma schlegelii*) have also been reported (Frye 1991; Lang 1987).

Reversal/Recovery Crocodilians immobilized with gallamine recover within 12–24 hours without reversal. Recovery appears to be due to renal excretion of the unchanged drug (Flammard et al. 1992). Farmed Nile crocodiles are routinely left to recover without reversal in a shaded area with no access to water for 24 hours, until they walk (Flammard et al. 1992; Webb & Messel 1977). Accidental drowning may occur in partially recovered animals.

Neostigmine methylsulphate (0.03 to 0.06 mg/kg) antagonizes the effects of gallamine in the Nile crocodile (Flammard et al. 1992; Fleming 1996; Jacobson 1984). Recovery occurs within 5–40 minutes depending on dose and temperature. Redosing may rarely be necessary (Pleuger 1973). It is advisable to reverse the crocodile several meters from water and allow it to get up and walk into the water to assure that it has recovered (Fleming 1996). Side effects reported in mammals, but not crocodilians, include those of a cholinergic crisis (vomiting, diarrhea, salivation, and bradycardia) (Schumacher 1996).

Succinylcholine Chloride Succinylcholine, unlike the other muscle relaxants, produces depolarization before muscle relaxation. This depolarization can produce acute hyperkalemia, lactic academia, extreme muscle pain, and phallus prolapse in males. Since there are better alternatives to its use, it is not recommended for the immobilization of crocodilians.

Succinylcholine has been used alone and in combination with other drugs for many years in numerous crocodilian species (Blake 1993, Flammerd 1992; Jacobson 1984, Klide & Klein 1973, Loveridge & Blake 1972; Millchamp 1988; Spiegal et al. 1984). American alligators >1.5 m are immobilized at 0.4 mg/kg. Smaller alligators require a larger dose (1 mg/kg IM), with recumbency in 5 minutes and recovery in 1.5 hours (Jacobson 1984). Higher dosages (3–5 mg/kg IM) also produced rapid recumbency within 4 minutes, but prolonged recovery (up to 7–9 hours) may occur (Brisaben 1966). The combination of succinylcholine (0.37 mg/kg IM) and diazepam (0.24 mg/kg IM) successfully immobilized adult American alligators (Loveridge & Blake 1972). The diazepam, administered 20 minutes before the succinylcholine, reduced stress and the succinylcholine dose. All animals were completely recovered within 3 hours. Juvenile caiman (*Caimen crocodylus*) are immobilized at dosages of 0.33–2.2 mg/kg IM, with recovery in 5–40 minutes (Johnson 1991).

Both freshwater (*Crocodylus johnsoni*) and saltwater crocodiles (*Crocodylus porus*) have been immobilized successfully (Loveridge & Blake 1972). Saltwater crocodiles required a higher dosage of succinylcholine (2.2–5 mg/kg) than freshwater crocodiles (0.8 mg/kg to 0.3 mg/kg) at 5- and 35-kg, respectively. The dosage for both species was inversely related to weight. Immobilization was achieved at 5–7 minutes and up to three times the therapeutic dosage resulted in no deaths (Loveridge & Blake 1972).

Reversal/Recovery There is no reversal for succinylcholine; recovery is dependent on metabolism and renal excretion (Pleuger 1973). Severe liver disease will limit metabolism and prolong recovery. At preferred optimum body temperature, recovery takes 30 minutes to several hours depending on the dose administered (Jacobson 1984; Lloyd et al. 1994).

Atracurium Besylate In American alligators, atracurium besylate (15 mg/kg IM) 15 minutes after diazepam (0.4 mg/kg IM) induced loss of righting reflex within 40 minutes and recovery by 6 hours (Clyde et al. 1990). Five of eight animals became severely apneic (<1 breath/min), and were manually ventilated with room air for up to 5 hours. With safer, more effective drugs available, is use is not recommended in crocodilians.

Reversal/Recovery Neostigmine methylsulfate (0.05 mg/kg IM) and atropine sulfate (0.01–0.02 mg/kg IM) reversed the muscle relaxation induced by atracurium (Clyde et al. 1990).

Opioids

Etorphine Hydrochloride Effective etorphine dosage varies considerably between and within crocodilian species. For example, American alligators weighing 1.6–3.9 kg required a dose of 1.3–3.1 mg/kg, while larger alligators weighing 39.5–68.0 kg required only 0.03–1.3 mg/kg (Hinsch & Gandal 1969). American alligators administered 0.29–0.51 mg/kg IM were immobilized within 20–25 minutes and were recovered in 60–180 minutes with no reversal drug (Hinsch & Gandal 1969). A 0.11-kg caiman administered the larger dosage of 44 mg/kg was immobilized at 11 minutes and recovered by 40 minutes (Thurmon et al. 1996). Intraperitoneal administration is effective, reducing induction times while having a similar duration of effect compared with IM administration. However, in Nile crocodiles, dosages as high as 8 mg/kg IM were ineffective and only produced pupillary dilatation (Loveridge 1979).

Reversal/Recovery Without administration of reversal drugs, crocodilians recover within 1–3 hours (Lang 1987). There is no report of using either naloxone or naltrexone to reverse etorphine in crocodilians.

Dissociative Anesthetics

Ketamine Hydrochloride Ketamine alone has variable immobilization or anesthetic effect. It has been used to anesthetize spectacled caiman (44–50 mg/kg), juvenile American alligators (11–12 mg/kg) (1 hour induction) (Beck 1972; Stoskopf 1993), and adult American alligators (45–70 mg/kg) (20 minutes induction) (Stoskopf 1993). Additional trials in American alligators at 50 mg/kg were reported to be successful, whereas 30 mg/kg had variable results (Heaton-Jones 1996; Loveridge 1979). Ketamine at 18–45 mg/kg in Nile crocodiles had little effect, while doses at 59–110 mg/kg caused death in three animals (Loveridge 1979). Dosages of ketamine in the range of 110 mg/kg have caused bradycardia and respiratory arrest in other reptile species (Burke 1986).

Recovery/Reversal There is presently no reversal agent for ketamine and recovery times vary with dose, taking up to several hours.

Tiletamine and Zolazepam Tiletamine/zolazepam (15 mg/kg IM) in American alligators did not produce complete immobilization (Jacobson 1984). Palpebral reflexes were unaffected; hind limb withdrawal was slow, and episodes of paddling were noted. Righting reflex was achieved 3 hours post injection; however, with higher doses, reversal times may be prolonged.

Reversal/Recovery Partial reversal of tiletamine/zolazepam has been reported by using flumazenil at 1 mg per 20 mg of zolazepam (Lang 1987). Flumazenil has a high affinity for benzodiazapine receptors and competes with zolazepam resulting in a rapid reversal of the teletamine in 2–4 minutes in mammals (Neilson 1996). Flumazenil, however, is seldom indicated in partially reversing Telazol because it is very expensive, and reversing the zolazepam will leave the tiletamine on board, which may result in seizures.

Barbiturates

The first reported use of pentobarbital was an oral dose of 200 mg/kg, followed by 15 mg/kg IP, in a Nile crocodile for removal of a gastric foreign body (Page 1996). It was later demonstrated in this species a dose of 28 mg/kg had an induction time of 2 hours and a recovery of 12 days, and 53 mg/kg could cause death (Loveridge 1979). Pentobarbital administered to spectacled caiman at 8.8–15.4 mg/kg IM resulted in induction times of 30–45 minutes and recovery times of 1–5 days. The use of barbiturates in crocodilians for immobilization is, therefore, not recommended.

Alpha-2 Agonists

Xylazine has been used with variable success in Nile crocodiles. Used alone at 3–11 mg/kg it had no observable effect. A combination of xylazine at 1–2 mg/kg IM, followed 30 minutes later by 20 mg/kg IM of ketamine, resulted in effective surgical anesthesia for 50 minutes with a 3–4 hour recovery. (Idowu & Akinrinmade 1986)

Medetomidine has been used in American alligator at 131–220 μg/kg in combination with ketamine 7.5–10 mg/kg, with juvenile alligators requiring the higher dose (Heaton-Jones et al. 2002). Mean induction time for juveniles was 19.6 minutes, and in adults was 26.6 minutes. Total anesthesia times were 61–220 minutes, with any procedure over 120 minutes receiving supplemental inhalant anesthesia. Doses of medetomidine of 150 ug/kg resulted in bradycardia and bradypena (Smith et al. 1998a, 1998b, 1998c).

Relative high dosages (500–750 ug/kg IM) of medetomdine were required to immobilize juvenile (>3 kg) estuarine and freshwater crocodiles (Olsson & Phalen 2012a). The freshwater crocodiles required the higher dosage for immobilization.

Medetomidine (130–170 μg/kg) successfully immobilized four large (150–370 kg) estuarine crocodiles (*Crocodylus porosus*) (Olsson & Phalen 2012b) approximately 30 minutes after hand injection into the triceps muscle. The dosage appeared inversely related to body-weight. Reversal occurred within five minutes after IM administration of atipamezole.

Dexmedetomidine, an isomer of medetomidine, is approximately 1.6× as potent as medetomidine. Given the concentration of the commercially available formulation (0.5 mg/mL) and the high dosages required for immobilization, dexmedetomidine is only used in relatively small crocodilians.

Reversal/Recovery Yohimbine hydrochloric acid is used at a dose of 0.1 mg/kg IM to reverse the effects of xylazine. If reversal agents are not used, recovery times are variable, depending on dose, and may last 3–12 hours (Frye 1991; Lang 1987). Reversal of medetomidine in reptiles with atipamazole, a selective alpha-2 adrenergic antagonist, at five times the dose of the medetomidine given IM provides reversal. For reversal of dexmedetomidine, the dosage of atipamezole is 10 times. Reversal times vary with dose and body temperature, but in the earlier study with alligators, this was achieved in 35–37 minutes (Dennis & Heard 2002; Heaton-Jones et al. 2002).

OTHER INJECTABLE AGENTS

Tricaine Methanesulfonate (MS-222)

Tricaine methanesulfonate (MS-222) has been used at 88–99 mg/kg IM in juvenile American alligators, producing immobilization in 10 minutes and recovery in 9–10 hours (Brisaben 1966). A higher dosage of 150 mg/kg anesthetized an American alligator for 30 hours (Coulson & Hernandez 1983). Tricaine has also been used in spectacled caiman at 110–154 mg/kg IM with no effect (Johnson 1991). Unbuffered MS-222 is highly acidic and will cause tissue necrosis. There is also no commercially available approved parenteral form of MS-222. For reasons outlined earlier, it is not recommended for use in crocodilians.

Propofol

Propofol is an excellent induction agent and a single injection may give 15–25 minutes of surgical anesthesia, with righting reflexes returning after 25–40 minutes. It can be used as a continuous infusion to maintain surgical anesthesia (Divers 1996; Schumacher 1996). Its major disadvantage is that it must be injected IV, limiting its use in large crocodilians unless they are restrained. Dosages in reptiles from 10 to 15 mg/kg IV have been reported. It is the author's opinion, however, that dosages as low as 1–2 mg/kg in large animals may be enough to allow for intubation, while 5–6 mg/kg is appropriate for small or juvenile crocodilians (Dennis & Heard 2002). A butterfly needle, or extension set, may be used allowing the needle to be left in the vein for additional propofol to be titrated to effect. Due to its short duration of effect, propofol is best used in combination with an inhalant anesthetic for maintenance. Propofol is the author's most popular choice for induction of all reptilian species, including crocodilians, where IV access can be obtained. Even large crocodilians trained to station in a restraint box may be induced with an IV injection of propofol with little stress or danger to the animal or the handlers.

Alfaxalone

The short-acting steroidal alfaxalone was previously available commercially in combination with alfadolone and solubilized with cremophor EL, which produced sometimes severe allergic reactions in mammals. A new commercial preparation contains alfaxolone alone bound to cyclodextrine to provide water solubility. Although marketed for IV use, it has been used IM in small domestic mammals without evidence of pain or tissue damage. The low concentration (10 mg/mL) or the commercial preparation, however, precludes its IM use in medium to large animals due to volume.

Alfaxalone (4 mg/kg IV, dorsal cervical sinus) provided 40–60 minutes of surgical anesthesia for implantation of radiotransmitters in 5- to 10-kg Johnson River crocodiles (*Crocodylus johnstoni*) (Franklin et al. 2009). A similar dosage (3 mg/kg IV) was used in 0.5-kg estuarine crocodiles (*Crocodylus porosus*) (Seebacher & Franklin 2004). Respiratory support was provided using an endotracheal tube and Ambu bag.

INHALANT ANESTHESIA

Endotracheal intubation and assisted respiration are recommended for inhalant anesthesia (Schumacher 1996), since aquatic species are capable of long periods of apnea. Injectable anesthetics are used for induction to allow safe access for intubation. Crocodilians have complete tracheal rings and cuffed endotracheal tubes, if overinflated, may cause avascular necrosis of the mucosa. To place the endotracheal tube, the snout should be grasped with two hands and the head and neck flexed 90° into a dorsal position. The mandible and maxilla can then be separated and a block of wood, speculum, can be placed (Fig. 19.1).

Positive pressure ventilation (PPV) at a rate of two breaths per minute or less is adequate for crocodilians (Schumacher 1996). Once the surgical or painful part of the procedure is completed, PPV can be switched from oxygen to room air and an Ambu bag. This will negate the negative respiratory effect of 100% oxygen, and a decreased respiration rate will allow an increase in systemic CO_2 levels to stimulate breathing. In the author's experience, this works very well for all reptilian species. In large crocodilians, a double-demand valve (Horne et al. 2001) can be used with pressurized room air (scuba tank) to achieve the same results.

For crocodilians weighing <5 kg, a nonrebreathing system is indicated with a flow of 300–500 mL/kg/min. For crocodilians >5 kg, a circle system 1–2 L/min for maintenance is recommended (Bennet 1996). This may be lower than in mammals of comparative size, but

oxygen requirements for crocodilians is much lower (Coulson & Hernandez 1983; Coulson et al. 1989).

Isoflurane provides fast induction, good muscle relaxation, and rapid recovery. Isoflurane is not metabolized, but is eliminated exclusively by the lungs so it can be used in compromised patients (Bennet 1996; Schumacher 1996). Induction is accomplished at a rate of 4–5% at 2–4 L/min; maintenance rates of 1–4% will vary depending on the injectable pre-anethetic agent used. Recovery should take 10–60 minutes depending on the depth of anesthesia and type of premedication agent.

Halothane has also been used with good success in reptiles; however, induction and recovery times are prolonged when compared to isoflurane (Bonath 1979; Neilson 1996). Although the use of sevoflurane in crocodilians has not been reported, it has been used in a number of other reptilian species and does produce faster induction and recovery times than isoflurane with minimal cardiopulmonary effects (Bertelsen et al. 2005; Chittick et al. 2002; Rooney et al. 1999).

Nitrous oxide is an underutilized gas anesthetic and can be used in combination (1 part oxygen to 1–2 parts nitrous oxide) with isoflurane, sevoflurane or halothane (Neilson 1996). This gas is rapidly taken up and removed from the lungs, reduces inhalant anesthetic requirement, and produces added analgesia during painful procedures (Atkinson et al. 1977; Bertelsen et al. 2005).

ANESTHETIC PROTOCOLS

In designing an anesthetic protocol for a crocodilian, it is difficult to provide specific guidelines for each species and situation (Table 19.1). It is important to consider the species, medical condition, enclosure, temperature, staffing, and ultimate goal of the immobilization when formulating a plan. In the next section are a few of the author's suggestions for anesthetizing crocodilians. However, these drugs and dosages have not been evaluated in all crocodilian species, and some variability in response is inevitable.

Adult Crocodilian

1. Medetomidine 70–100 ug/kg and ketamine 7–10 mg/kg IM or IV, intubate, then isoflurane at 2–3% at 1–2 L/min via an endotracheal tube (circle system) with forced ventilation at 3–4 breaths/min should be used. While isoflurane reaches steady state, the medetomidine can be reversed with atipamezole at five times the medetomidine dose.
2. Nile crocodile: gallamine 1–2 mg/kg IM (diazepam 0.25 mg/kg IM optional). This may be sufficient for noninvasive procedures such as translocation. For invasive or painful procedures (surgery), maintenance with isoflurane at 2–3% at 1–2 L/min via an

Table 19.1. Commonly used drugs in crocodilians

Drug	Dosage	Species	Remarks	Reference
Analgesia				
Morphine	0.8 mg/kg IM	*Crocodylus porosus*		Kanui and Hole (1992)
Meperidine	1–2 mg/kg IM	*C. porosus*		Kanui and Hole (1992)
Meloxicam	0.1–0.2 mg/kg IM or PO SID for 5–7 days	Most species		Whiteside and Black (2004), Wellehan (2006)
Tramadol	5 mg/kg PO q 5 days	Most species		Baker et al. (2011)
Ketoprofen	2 mg/kg IM q 24–48 h	Most species		Tuttle et al. (2006)
Butorphanol			May cause sedation but not analgesia	Sladky et al. (2007); Sladky et al. (2008); Fleming and Robertson (2006); Mosley (2011)
Anesthesia				
Ketamine	11–110 mg/kg IM	Most species	Variable response when used alone	Frye (1991); Jacobson (1984); Loveridge and Blake (1972); Millichamp (1988);
Medetomidine	500–750 μg/kg IM	*C. porosus* and *C. johnstoni*	Juvenile crocodilians >3kg. *C. johnstoni* required higher dosage for immobilization.,	Olsson and Phalen (2012a)
Medetomidine	130–170 μg/kg IM triceps	*C. porosus* 150–370kg	Dosage inversely proportional to mass.	Olsson and Phalen (2012b)
Ketamine and medetomidine	10 mg/kg and 0.1 mg/kg IM	Most species	American alligator	Heaton-Jones et al. (2002); Smith et al. (1998a, 1998b, 1998c)
Ketamine and xylazine	7.5–10 mg/kg and 1–2 mg/kg IM	Most species		Idowu and Akinrinmade (1986)
Tiletamine/zolazepam	5–15 mg/kg IM	Most species	Start at low end of dose for intubation	Jacobson (1984)
Propofol	3–10 mg/kg IV	Most species		Divers (1996); Schumacher (1996)
Alfaxalone	3–5 mg/kg IV	Most species	Start at low end of dose for intubation	Franklin et al. (2009); Seebacher and Franklin (2004)
Diazepam	0.22–0.62 mg./kg IM	Most species	Poor IM absorption	Loveridge and Blake (1972)
Reversal agents				
Atipamezole	5 times the dose of medetomidine IM	Most species Most species		Heaton-Jones et al. (2002); Smith et al. (1998a, 1998b, 1998c)
Yohimbine	0.1 mg/kg IM	Most species		Lang (1987)
Flumazenil	1:13 or 1:20 times the dose of benzodiazepine IV	Most species		Lang (1987)
Naltrexone	100 times the dose of opioid	Most species		G.J. Fleming, pers. comm., 2011
Neostigmine	0.03–0.06 mg/kg IM	*Crocodylus niloticus*		Jacobson (1984); Flammard et al. (1992); Fleming (1996)
Inhalant agents				
Isoflurane	1–5%	Most species	2–3% for maintenance	Bennet (1996); Schumacher (1996)
Sevoflurane	1–5%	Most species	Higher than isoflurane for maintenance	Bertelsen et al. (2005); Chittick et al. (2002); Rooney et al. (1999)
Halothane	1–5%	Most species	Not recommended due to hepatotoxicity and cardiotoxicity	
Paralytics				
Gallamine	1–2 mg/kg IM	*C. niloticus*	No analgesia	Fleming (1996); Frye (1991); Jacobson (1984); Lang (1987); Loveridge (1979)
Succinlycholine	0.33–5 mg/kg IM	Most species	No analgesia	Blake (1993); Jacobson (1984); Millichamp (1988); Spiegal et al. (1984)

endotracheal tube (circle system) with forced ventilation at 3–4 breaths/min should be used. The gallamine may be reversed with neostigmine methylsulphate at a dose of 0.03 to 0.06 mg/kg IM. Reversal with IV injection is discouraged, as the crocodilian may become alert within a few minutes.

3. Telazol 4–8 mg/kg IM (this will not be sufficient to reach surgical anesthesia; however, intubation should be possible). Maintenance with isoflurane at 2–3% at 1–2 L/min via an endotracheal tube (circle system) with forced ventilation at 3–4 breaths/min. Long recovery of 4–8 hours many be encountered with using Telazol, care should be taken not to immerse the crocodilian in deep water during this period.

Juvenile or Restrained Adult Crocodilian

1. Propofol 3–5 mg/kg IV (caudal/ventral tail vein). Animal will have to be properly restrained, or behaviorally conditioned to achieve IV access. Additional propofol may have to be titrated to effect. Maintenance with Isoflurane at 2 to 3% at 300–500 mL/kg/min via an endotracheal tube (nonrebreathing system) with forced ventilation at 3–4 breaths/min.

REFERENCES

Atkinson RS, Rushman GB, Lee AJ. 1977. *A Synopsis of Anesthesia*, 8th ed. Chicago: John Wright and Sons.

Axelsson M. 2001. The crocodilian heart: more controlled than we thought? *Experimental Physiology* 86(6):785–789.

Baker BB, Sladky KK, Johnson SM. 2011. Evaluation of the analgesic effects of oral and subcutaneous tramadol administration in red-eared slider turtles. *Journal of the American Veterinary Medical Association* 238:220–227.

Beck CC. 1972. Chemical restraint of exotic species. *Journal of Zoo Animal Medicine* 3:3–66.

Bennet RA. 1996. Anesthesia. In: *Reptile Medicine and Surgery* (DR Mader, ed.), pp. 241–247. Philadelphia: W.B. Saunders.

Bertelsen MF, Mosely CAR, Crawshw GJ, et al. 2005. Anesthetic potency of sevoflurane with and without nitrous oxide in mechanically ventilated Dumeril monitors. *Journal of the American Veterinary Medical Association* 227(4):575–578.

Blake DK. 1993. The Nile crocodile (*Crocodylus niloticus*): capture, care, accommodation, and transportation. In: *The Capture and Care Manual* (AA McKensie, ed.), pp. 654–675. Pretoria: Wildlife Decision Support Services CC and The South African Veterinary Association.

Bonath K. 1979. Halothane inhalation anesthesia in reptiles and its clinical control. *International Zoo Yearbook* 19:112–115.

Brisaben LL. 1966. Reactions of the American alligator to several immobilizing drugs. *Copeia*:129–130.

Burke TJ. 1986. Reptile anesthesia. In: *Zoo and Wildlife Animal Medicine*, 2nd ed. (ME Fowler, ed.), pp. 153–155. Philadelphia: W.B. Saunders.

Busk M, Overgaard J, Hicks JW, et al. 2000. Effects of feeding on arterial blood gases in the American alligator, *Alligator mississippiensis*. *The Journal of Experimental Biology* 203:3117–3124.

Chittick EJ, Stamper MA, Ceasley JF, et al. 2002. Medetominidine, ketamine, and sevoflurane for anesthesia of injured loggerhead sea turtles: 13 cases (1996–2000). *Journal of the American Veterinary Medical Association* 221(7):1019–1025.

Clyde VL, Cardeilhac P, Jacobson E. 1990. Chemical restraint of American alligators (*Alligator mississipiensis*) with atracurium and tiletamine-zolazepam. Proceedings of the American Association of Zoo Veterinarians, p. 288. Denver, CO.

Coulson RA, Hernandez T. 1983. *Alligator Metabolism: Studies on Chemical Reactions in vivo*. London: Pergamon Press.

Coulson RA, et al. 1989. Biochemistry and physiology of alligator metabolism in vivo. *American Zoologist* 29:921.

Dennis PM, Heard DJ. 2002. Cardiopulmonary effects of medetomidine-ketamine combination administered intravenously in gopher tortoises. *Journal of the American Veterinary Medical Association* 220(10):1516–1519.

Diefenbach CO. 1975. Thermal preferences and thermoregulation in *Caiman crocodilius*. *Copeia* 3:530–540.

Divers SJ. 1996. The use of propofol in reptile anesthesia. Proceedings of the 1996 Association of Reptile and Amphibian Veterinarians, pp. 57–59. Tampa, FL.

Farmer CG, Sanders K. 2010. Unidirectional airflow in the lungs of alligators. *Science* 327:338–340.

Flammard JR, Rogers PS, Blake DK. 1992. Immobilization of crocodiles. In: *Use of Tranquilizers in Wildlife* (H Ebedes, ed.), pp. 61–65. Pretoria: Department of Agricultural Development.

Fleming GJ. 1996. Capture and chemical immobilization of the Nile crocodile (*Crocodylus niloticus*) in South Africa. Proceedings of the 1996 Association of Reptile and Amphibian Veterinarians, pp. 63–66. Tampa, FL.

Fleming GJ, Robertson S. 2006. Use of thermal threshold test response to evaluate the antinociceptive effects of butorphanol in juvenile green iguanas (*Iguana iguana*). American Association of Zoo Veterinarians, p. 279. Tampa, FL.

Fowler ME. 1985. *Restraint and Handling of Wild and Domestic Animals*. Ames: Iowa State University Press.

Fowler ME. 1986. Restraint. In: *Zoo and Wild Animal Medicine*, 2nd ed. (ME Fowler, ed.), pp. 37–51. Philadelphia: W.B. Saunders.

Franklin CE, Read MA, Kraft PG, et al. 2009. Remote monitoring of crocodilians: implantation, attachment and release methods for transmitters and data-loggers. *Marine and Freshwater Research* 60:284–292.

Frye FL. 1991. *Biomedical and Surgical Aspects of Captive Reptile Husbandry*, 2nd ed. Malabar: Krieger Publishing Company.

Glassman AB, Bennet CE. 1978. Response of the alligator to infection and thermal stress. In: *Energy and Environmental Stress in Aquatic Systems* (JH Throp, JW Gibbons, eds.), Washington, DC: Technical Information Center, U.S. Department of Energy.

Grenard S. 1991. *Handbook of Alligators and Crocodiles*. Malabar: Krieger Publishing.

Heaton-Jones TG. 1996. Development of anesthesia in crocodilians. Proceedings of the 1996 Association of Reptile and Amphibian Veterinarians, pp. 63–66. Tampa, FL.

Heaton-Jones TG, Ko JCH, Heaton-Jones BS. 2002. Evaluation of medetomidine-ketamine anesthesia with antipamazole reversal in American alligators (*Alligator mississippiensis*). *Journal of Zoo and Wildlife Medicine* 33(1):36–44.

Hernandez-Divers SJ, McBride M, Koch T, et al. 2004. Single-dose oral and intravenous pharmacokinetics of meloxicam in the green iguana (*Iguana iguana*). Proceedings of the Association of Reptile and Amphibian Veterinarians, p. 106.

Hinsch H, Gandal CP. 1969. The effects of etorphine (M-99), oxymorphone hydrochloride and meperidine hydrochloride in reptiles. *Copeia*: 404–405.

Holz P. 1997. The anatomy and perfusion of the renal portal sysem in the red-eared slider (*Trachemys scripta elegans*). *Journal of Zoo and Wildlife Medicine* 28(4):378–385.

Horne WA, Tchamba MA, Loomis MR. 2001. A simple method of providing intermittent positive-pressure ventilation to etorphine-immobilized elephants (*Loxodonta africana*) in the field. *Journal of Zoo and Wildlife Medicine* 32:519–522.

Huggins SE, Hoff HE, Pena RV. 1969. Heart and respiratory rates in crocodilian reptiles under conditions of minimal stimulation. *Physiological Zoology* 42:320–333.

Idowu AL, Akinrinmade JF. 1986. Xylazine and ketamine anesthesia in captive Nile crocodiles. *Tropical Veterinarian* 4:139.

Jacobson ER. 1984. Immobilization, blood sampling, necropsy techniques, and diseases of crocodilians: a review. *Journal of Zoo Animal Medicine* 15:38–45.

Johnson JH. 1991. Anesthesia, analgesia, and euthanasia of reptiles and amphibians. Proceedings of the American Association of Zoo Veterinarians, Calgary, pp. 132–138.

Jones D, Hayes-Odum L. 1994. A method for the restraint and transport of crocodilians. *Herpetological Review* 25(1):14–15.

Kanui TI, Hole K. 1992. Morphine and pethidine antinociception in the crocodile. *Journal of Veterinary Pharmacology and Therapeutics* 15(1):101–103.

Klide AM, Klein LV. 1973. Chemical restraint of three reptilian species. *Journal of Zoo Animal Medicine* 4:8–11.

Kummrow MS, Tseng F, Hesse L, et al. 2008. Pharmacokinetics of buprenorphine after single-dose subcutaneous administration in red-eared sliders (*Trachemys scripta elegans*). *Journal of Zoo and Wildlife Medicine* 39:590–595.

Lane TJ. 1996. Crocodilians. In: *Reptile Medicine and Surgery* (DR Mader, ed.), pp. 78–94. Philadelphia: WB Saunders.

Lang JW. 1987. Crocodilian behavior: implications for management. In: *Wildlife Management: Crocodiles and Alligators* (GJW Webb, SC Manolis, PJ Whitehead, eds.), pp. 273–294. Clipping Norton: Surrey Beatty and Sons Printing.

Lloyd M. 1999. Crocodilian anesthesia. In: *Zoo and Wild Animal Medicine*, 4th ed. (ME Fowler, RE Miller, eds.), pp. 205–216. Philadelphia: W.B. Saunders.

Lloyd ML, Reichard T, Odum RA. 1994. Gallamine reversal in Cuban Crocodiles (*Crocodylus rhombifer*) using neostigmine alone versus neostigmine with hyaluronidase. Proceedings American Association of Zoo Veterinarians, pp. 117–120.

Loveridge JP. 1979. The immobilization and anesthesia of crocodilians. *International Zoo Yearbook* 19:103–112.

Loveridge JP, Blake DK. 1972. Techniques in the immobilization and handling of the Nile crocodile (*Crocodylus niloticus*). *Arnoldia* 40:1–14.

Millichamp NJ. 1988. Surgical techniques in reptiles. In: *Contemporary Issues in Small Animal Practice: Exotic Animals* (ER Jacobson, GV Kollias, eds.), p. 49. New York: Churchill Livingstone.

Mosley C. 2011. Pain and nociception in reptiles. *The Veterinary Clinics of North America. Exotic Animal Practice* 14:45–60.

Mosley CAE, Dyson D, Smith D. 2003. Minimum alveolar concentration of isoflurane in green iguanas and the effect of butorphanol on minimum alveolar concentration. *Journal of the American Veterinary Medical Association* 222(11):1559–1564.

Mosley CAE, Dyson D, Smith D. 2004. The Cardiovascular dose-response effects of isoflurane alone and conbined with butorphanol in the green iguana. *Veterinary Anaesthesia and Analgesia* 31(1):64–72.

Murphy MJ. 1996. Cardiology and circulation. In: *Reptile Medicine and Surgery* (DR Mader, ed.), pp. 95–103. Philadelphia: W.B. Saunders.

Neill WT. 1971. *The Last of the Ruling Reptiles Alligators, Crocodiles, and Their Kin*. New York: Columbia University Press.

Neilson L. 1996. Chemical Immobilization of free-ranging terrestrial mammals. In: *Lumb and Jones Veterinary Anesthesia*, 3rd ed. (JC Thurmon, WJ Tranquilli, GJ Benson, eds.), p. 737. Baltimore: Williams and Wilkins.

Olsson A, Phalen D. 2012a. Preliminary studies of chemical immobilization of captive juvenile estuarine (*Crocodylus porosus*) and Australian freshwater (*C. johnstoni*) crocodiles with medeto-

midine and reversal with atipamezole. *Veterinary Anaesthesia and Analgesia* 39:345–356.

Olsson A, Phalen D. 2012b. Medetomidine immobilisation and atipamezole reversal in large estuarine crocodiles (*Crocodylus porosus*) using metabolically scaled dosages. *Australian Veterinary Journal* 90:240–244.

Page CD. 1996. Current reptilian anesthesia procedures. In: *Zoo and Wild Animal Medicine*, 3rd ed. (ME Fowler, ed.), pp. 140–143. Philadelphia: W.B. Saunders.

Paul-Murphy J, Brunson DB, Miletic V. 1999. Analgesic effects of butorphanol and buprenorphine in conscious African grey parrots (*Psittacus erithacus erithacus* and *Psittacus erithacus timneh*). *American Journal of Veterinary Research* 60:1218–1221.

Pleuger CA. 1973. Gastrotomey in a crocodile: a case report. *Journal of the American Veterinary Medical Association* 117:297–299.

Rooney MD, Levine G, Gaynor J, et al. 1999. Sevoflurane anesthesia in desert tortoises. *Gopherus agassizii*. *Journal of Zoo and Wildlife Medicine* 30:64–69.

Schumacher J. 1996. Reptiles and amphibians. In: *Lumb and Jones Veterinary Anesthesia*, 3rd ed. (JC Thurmon, WJ Tranquilli, GJ Benson, eds.), pp. 670–685. Baltimore: Williams and Wilkins.

Sedgwick C. 1986. Inhalation anesthesia for captive wild mammals, birds, and reptiles. In: *Zoo and Wild Animal Medicine*, 2nd ed. (ME Fowler, ed.), pp. 52–56. Philadelphia: W.B. Saunders.

Seebacher F, Franklin CE. 2004. Integration of autonomic and local mechanisms in regulating cardiovascular responses to heating and cooling in a reptile (*Crocodylus porosus*). *Journal of Comparative Physiology. B, Biochemical, Systemic, and Environmental Physiology* 174:577–585.

Seymore RS, Webb GJW, Bennett AF, et al. 1987. Effect of capture on the physiology of *Crocodylus porosus*. In: *Wildlife Management: Crocodiles and Alligators* (GJW Webb, SC Manolis, PJ Whitehead, eds.), pp. 253–257. Clipping Norton: Surrey Beatty and Sons Printing.

Sladky KK, Miletic V, Paul-Murphy J, et al. 2007. Analgesic efficacy and respiratory effects of butorphanol and morphine in turtles. *Journal of the American Veterinary Medical Association* 230:1356–1362.

Sladky KK, Kinney ME, Johnson SM. 2008. Analgesic efficacy of butorphanol and morphine in bearded dragons and corn snakes. *Journal of the American Veterinary Medical Association* 233:267–273.

Smith JA, McGuire NC, Mitchell MA. 1998a. Cardiopulmonary physiology and anesthesia in crocodilians. Annual Proceedings of the Association of Reptile and Amphibian Veterinarians, pp. 17–23.

Smith JA, Mitchell MA, Backhues TN, et al. 1998b. Immobilization of American alligators with medetomidine and its reversal with atipamazole. *Veterinary Surgery* 28:133.

Smith JA, Mitchell MA, Backhues TN, et al. 1998c. Sedative and cardiopulmonary effects medetomidine and atipamazole in American alligators. Proceedings of the Joint Conference of the American Association of Zoo Veterinarians and American Association of Wildlife, pp. 26–277.

Spiegal RA, Lane TJ, Larsen RE, et al. 1984. Diazepam and succinylcholine chloride for restraint of the American alligator. *Journal of the American Veterinary Medical Association* 185:11.

Stoskopf M. 1993. Anesthesia. In: *Aquaculture for Veterinarians, Fish Husbandry and Medicine*. (L Brown, ed.), pp. 161–168. New York: Pergamon Press.

Terpin KM, Dodson P, Spotila J. 1978. Observations on ketamine hydrochloride as an anesthetic for alligators. *Copeia* 1:147–148.

Thurmon JC, Tranquilli WJ, Benson GJ. 1996. Preanesthetics and aneshtetic adjunts. In: *Lumb and Jones Veterinary Anesthesia*, 3rd ed. (JC Thurmon, WJ Tranquilli, GJ Benson, eds.), pp. 187–232. Baltimore: Williams and Wilkins.

Tuttle AD, Papich M, Lewbart GA, et al. 2006. Pharmacokinetics of ketoprofen in the green iguana (*Iguana iguana*) following single intravenous and intramuscular injections. *Journal of Zoo and Wildlife Medicine* 37:567.

Van der Merwe NJ, Kotze SH. 1993. The topography of the thoracic and abdominal organs of the Nile crocodile (Crocodylus niloticus). *The Onderstepoort Journal of Veterinary Research* 60: 219–222.

Wallach JD, Hoessle C. 1970. M-99 as an immobilizing agent in poikilotherms. *Veterinary Medicine, Small Animal Clinician* 65: 163–167.

Walsh B. 1987. Crocodile capture methods used in the Northern territory of Australia. In: *Wildlife Management: Crocodiles and Alligators* (GJW Webb, SC Manolis, PJ Whitehead, eds.), pp. 249–252. Chipping Norton: Surrey Beatty and Sons Printing Ltd.

Webb JW, Messel H. 1977. Crocodile capture techniques. *The Journal of Wildlife Management* 41(3):572–575.

Wellehan JFX. 2006. The use of nervelocater in lizards and crocodilians. *Journal of Zoo and Wildlife Medicine* 37(3):405–408.

Wellehan JFX, Lafortune M, Gunkel CG, et al. 2004. Coccygeal vascular catherization of lizards and crododiians. *Journal of Herpetological Medicine and Surgery* 14(2):26–28.

Whiteside DP, Black SR. 2004. The use of meloxicam in exotic felids at the Calgary Zoo. The Proceedings of the American Association of Zoo Veterinarians, pp. 346–349. San Diego, CA.

Woodford MH. 1972. The use of gallamine triethiodide as a chemical immobilizing agent for the Nile crocodile (*Crocodylus niloticus*). *East African Wildlife Journal* 10:67–70.

20 Venomous Reptile Restraint and Handling

Frederick B. Antonio

INTRODUCTION

This chapter presents information and recommendations for the restraint of venomous reptiles in either a clinical environment or field conditions. For simplicity, a venomous reptile refers to venomous snakes. A section at the end of the chapter will review management of venomous lizards of the family Helodermatidae (Gila monsters and beaded lizards). Envenomation will be referred to as snakebite, although it is recognized helodermids can also inflict a serious bite.

It is intended that the employment of the techniques described in this chapter will greatly reduce the probability of snakebite. There is always some inherent risk, however, when handling and restraining venomous reptiles. The combination of planning, training, and gaining experience for the skills necessary for proper handling will significantly reduce the probability for error.

In recent years, captive venomous reptiles have increased in popularity in the private sector. They are the topics of numerous television series, and are portrayed as both exciting and dangerous, often by actors and commentators that inspire young viewers to engage in interactions with venomous species. Many private collectors, researchers, and zoo professionals have only a vague notion of the potential lethality of their charges. Their ignorance includes both the potential physiological effects of venoms and the behaviors that make venomous snakes difficult to restrain (Altimari 1998). Some states within the United States prohibit personal possession of venomous reptiles, while others lack any regulation. Florida annually issues over 500 venomous reptile permits for personal possession. Many private collections are "underground" and reptile clinicians should expect to examine virtually any species of native or exotic venomous reptile. Safe handling of these animals requires veterinarians, researchers, and support staff be familiar with and use proper methods. The following sections present current procedures and techniques designed to limit unrestrained contact with venomous reptiles and thereby promote safety during examinations, clinical procedures, and field work.

General Characteristics

Snake venoms evolved primarily to aid in prey acquisition and secondarily for defense. More than 2700 snake species are currently recognized within about 18 families and 420 genera (Greene 1997). Of these, 250–500 species may induce serious physiologic effects in humans. These belong primarily to the families Elapidae (cobras, kraits, mambas, coral snakes, and sea snakes) and Viperidae (true vipers and pit vipers).

Almost every colubrid snake family has at least one species whose venom has the potential to produce either morbidity or mortality in humans. These include (Fry 2006a) Colubridae (*Dispholidus* and *Thelatornis*), Dipsadidae (*Hydrodynastes*, *Xenodon*, and *Waglerophis*), Atractaspididae (*Atractapis* and *Homoroselaps*), Homalopsidae (*Cerberus*, *Enydris*, and *Homalopsis*), Natricidae (*Macropisthodon* and *Rhabdophis*), Psammophiidae (*Malpolon*, *Psammophis*, and *Rhamphiophis*), and Pseudoxyrhophiidae (*Leioheterodon* and *Madagascarophis*). Of these, the most commonly imported are the boomslang, *Dispholidus typus*; African twigsnake, *Thelotornis capensis*; Blanding's treesnake, *Boiga blandingi*; road guarder, *Conophis lineatus*; Japanese water snake, *Rhabdophis tigrinus*; and the false pitviper, *Xenodon* spp.

Evolution of reptilian venom systems (Fry et al. 2006b), demonstrates some extant "nonvenomous"

Zoo Animal and Wildlife Immobilization and Anesthesia, Second Edition. Edited by Gary West, Darryl Heard, and Nigel Caulkett.
© 2014 John Wiley & Sons, Inc. Published 2014 by John Wiley & Sons, Inc.

snake taxa and certain lizards of Varanidae (monitor lizards) and Iguania to have toxin-secreting oral glands. A thorough review of nonfront-fanged colubroid snakes (Weinstein et al. 2011) analyzes documented case reports of bites inflicted by approximately 100 species and discusses clinical management of medically significant species, most commonly referred to as "rear-fanged" snakes. Studies of this kind confirm toxic salivary secretions in extant reptiles, usually products of the Duvernoy's gland, that present a continuum of toxicity from mild to severe. Their presence and effects in human victims requires further study to build clinical evidence as to their potential severity. Thus, it is prudent for the clinician to treat suspect or unusual species, especially opisthoglyphs, with the same precautions as they do with recognized venomous species.

Venom delivery systems originate from modified salivary glands. These vary from mucous-producing oral glands to well-developed encapsulated glands with separate compressor musculature to express venom through a duct to individual hollow fangs. There are four dental patterns in snakes (Greene 1997): aglyphous, undifferentiated maxillary teeth, present in primitive snakes and some colubrids; opisthoglyphous, enlarged teeth (may be grooved to facilitate induction of salivary secretions) located on the posterior ends of the maxillary bones, present in rear-fanged snakes; proteroglyphous, enlarged true hollow fangs located on the anterior end of the maxillary bones that have restricted movement, present in elapids; and solenoglyphous, elongated hollow fangs located on highly movable maxillary bones, fangs are folded back along the roof of the mouth when not in use, present in vipers and pitvipers. These four basic dental morphologies represent a progression in efficiency for venom induction when biting.

One impressive variation in fang structure with management implications is found in the elapid species referred to as spitting cobras. Eye injuries by spitting snakes (Chippaux 2006) include African species (*Naja nigricollis, Naja katiensis, Naja mossambica, Naja pallida, Naja crawshayi,* and *Hemachatus hemachatus*) and some populations of Asian cobras (*Naja sputatrix*). These species have a fang structure and discharge orifice to defensively eject venom aimed at the eyes of an intruder. Target accuracy and the distance of ejection are from 1 to 5 m (Russell 1980). Full face shields (Fig. 20.1) are recommended at all times when working these species. If venom comes in contact with an eye, wipe remaining venom away from the eyes and begin immediate copious irrigation with sterile saline solution (Boyer & Murphy 1999). A long-sleeved lab coat or protective garment is recommended to shield skin. Venom may also be expressed on the inside of a restraint tube. Expelled venom must be treated with extreme caution during both the procedure and the cleanup process. Dried venom on glass can be aerosolized during

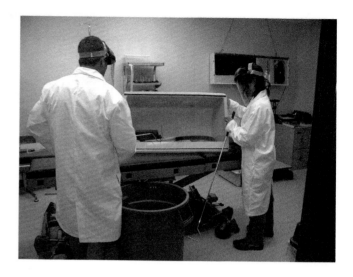

Figure 20.1. Full face shields and protective garments are recommended when working with all species of spitting cobras. Red-spitting cobra, *Naja pallida,* Central Florida Zoo and Botanical Gardens.

cleaning and cause injury to eyes and mucous membranes.

SNAKE BEHAVIOR

Handling and restraint should be approached every time as a novel experience that may be significantly different from previous procedures. Planning the procedure with the total focus of all persons involved is required. Complacency or a casual approach, no matter how experienced the handler, can result in an unexpected and disastrous outcome.

Every species exhibits different behaviors when manipulated. Defensive behaviors vary with the individual temperament of each snake, and the handler must observe and read these behaviors to adjust their response and modify techniques if needed. Altimari (1998) describes the temperaments of many captive venomous snake species. Viperids tend to defensively coil and may strike out in any direction. Elapids are more dangerous to manipulate and may initially attempt to flee. However, they can turn and strike at any time, or strike first then look for an escape route. Striking distances are approximately two-thirds of the total body length. For some species, however, when traveling and lunging while striking, it is difficult to determine a safe working distance in an open environment. Always over estimate the strike range.

Snakebite

In the United States prior to 1950, exotic venomous snakes were primarily found in zoos. Increased interesting in reptiles during the latter twentieth century has resulted in the United States as the major importer of reptiles, representing 80% of the world trade or approximately 2,000,000 reptiles imported annually (Keyler 2006). The vast majority of snakebites occur in private collections comprising a large variety of genera and species (Seifert 2006a). Of these nearly half are elapid bites. The incidence of nonnative envenomations has increased significantly over the past decade. Statistics on snakebite in clinical situations are difficult to obtain as many are not reported to data surveillance systems. Toxic Exposure Surveillance System (TESS) data for 2002 showed the number of exotic snakebites in the United States to be 125 (Keyler 2006), and around 100 exotic bites reported to the American Association of Poison Control Centers annually (Lai et al. 2006).

In a survey of 40 academic institutions that used venomous reptiles in research projects (Ivanyi & Altimari 2004), 18 facilities reported 42 envenomations and 6 dry bites from 20 species. The majority of these bites (87.5%) were the result of inappropriate capture techniques and inadequate restraint methods, including free handling snakes, pinning, handling with gloves, and improper use of restraint tubes. Card and Roberts (1996) surveyed North American zoos to determine the incidence of venomous reptile bites received by staff. Out of 30 reptile collections that maintained venomous reptiles, 21 zoos reported a staff member bitten during a 25-year period, with a total of 31 incidents. Of these, 15 envenomations occurred during routine handling, 5 during physical restraint, and 1 during a veterinary procedure. In a survey of 32 venom extraction facilities worldwide (Powell et al. 2006), envenomation averaged one per facility every 2 years. Although records of envenomation in veterinary medicine are lacking, the potential is ever present when a client presents a venomous reptile for examination and treatment. In many cases, this is a novel experience for the practitioner who lacks behavioral knowledge of the species, handling expertise, and proper equipment.

Antivenom

Antivenom is the only product recommended for treatment of snakebite. The goal of this immunotherapy is to neutralize venom components with antibodies and prevent them from reaching their sites of action. All snakebites are medical emergencies requiring effective response protocols and knowledgeable case approach by the treating physicians once the victim arrives in the Emergency Room. Treatment of snakebite is outside the scope of this chapter, but it remains the responsibility of the veterinary clinician or researcher to either possess the appropriate antivenin or know the nearest local source for the species to be restrained.

The appropriate foreign antivenom for exotic snake species should be present when working with these species as it is not stocked in hospital pharmacies. Ideally, it should be provided by the client and accompany the snake during transport to the clinician. Antivenom for native species is usually stocked at local hospitals for venomous species found in that region. It is recommended to contact local hospital pharmacies to periodically check on current inventories as antivenom can be difficult to obtain and supplies may be limited.

Treatment of envenomations is a challenge to physicians as most have never treated a snakebite victim. Case approach, the appropriate use of antivenom, and patient support have also been controversial. Locating and obtaining appropriate antivenom may be difficult, resulting in critical delays (Seifert 2006b). Species-specific antivenom should be sought unless there is evidence for cross-species efficacy. Most private collectors do not routinely maintain exotic antivenoms (Keyler 2006). Lack of sufficient appropriate antivenin can be a determining factor in choosing not to accept cases or engage in specific research projects that involves the handling of venomous snakes.

In the United States, foreign-manufactured antivenom can be imported by facilities or individuals under an Investigational New Drug license issued by the Food and Drug Administration, Department of Health and Human Services. These products may be species specific or polyvalent. Some antivenoms have shown cross-species neutralization (Minton 1999), but evidence must be available for cross-species efficacy before relying on this strategy. The appropriate antivenom should be provided by a responsible owner or researcher and travel with the snake to the clinic. If the owner does not have the appropriate antivenin, the nearest source should be located prior to arrival. For long-term studies, the acquisition and stocking of the appropriate antivenom is recommended.

An Online Antivenom Index (OAI), developed by the Association of Zoos and Aquariums (AZA) and the American Association of Poison Control Centers (AAPCC), lists specific antivenoms for treatment of exotic snakebite and their locations across the country. This antivenom inventory can be accessed by calling Poison Control (U.S. phone: 1-800-222-1222) to locate the nearest source for specific antivenom appropriate for the species. In most cases, the source is an AZA facility that logs their institutional inventory on the OAI site. Poison control centers have access to this information and should be consulted when locating a potential source of antivenom for projects or procedures involving venomous snakes.

An additional source for foreign antivenoms is the Miami-Dade Fire Rescue Antivenin Bank (formerly the Florida Antivenin Bank, Inc.) which stocks a significant inventory of antivenoms. Information on their holdings and procedures for requesting antivenom can be found on their website (http://www .venomousreptiles.org). A phone call can arrange an emergency response (Emergency Envenomation, phone 786-336-6600; nonemergency 786-331-4444) to arrange antivenom transport to the attending hospital.

This service can be a critical element in the treatment of snakebite when quantities of appropriate antivenom are lacking.

MANAGEMENT GUIDELINES

Strict protocols for handling venomous reptiles, routine husbandry, and staff training promote safety for staff and animals. Written protocols for snakebite response must be in place prior to receiving venomous reptiles. Snakebite protocols and case approach for attending physicians should be established with the local hospital and emergency room physicians to help insure swift and consistent treatment. A list of consulting physicians, that are experts in treating snakebite, should be readily available as a resource for local treating physicians, as few will be familiar with proper clinical management of snakebite.

The following venomous reptile handling protocols serves as a baseline for establishing best practices and may be expanded to incorporate unique aspects of facilities or research projects.

1. Venomous reptiles should not be handled by anyone except designated personnel.
2. Staff should be thoroughly trained, knowledgeable, and comfortable with handling procedures.
3. Always review techniques and procedures with staff. Set up the work space in advance and clear the area of unnecessary objects or obstacles. Have all appropriate tools readily available.
4. Never work venomous reptiles when in a hurry, mentally distracted, or on medication that may impair alertness, reflexes, or response time.
5. Two qualified personnel should always be present. Assistance is often needed and a second person is crucial should snakebite occur.
6. Cages should remain locked until they are ready to be opened. Always announce a cage is to be opened so the attention of support staff is immediately focused on the procedure.
7. All cages should be clearly marked "VENOMOUS." An additional label should state the name of the species (common and scientific name), the number of animals in the enclosure, type of antivenom to be administered, and the typical number of vials recommended for a moderate envenomation.
8. Never handle a reptile that appears dead directly with your hands. Always use a tong or snake hook to test for movement. The mouth of a dead specimen should be carefully taped closed to avoid unintentional contact with the fangs.

EQUIPMENT AND METHODS

Venomous reptiles can be managed safely by using the proper tools and techniques. Training and experience plays a significant role in developing expertise. A working knowledge of snake behavior and their reaction to stimuli will aid in strategizing the best methods to use for a particular procedure. An organized and methodical approach to handling and restraint increases control and is assuring to support staff that may be unfamiliar with working venomous reptiles. Equipment and methods described here are proven techniques. Innovations can produce further modifications for specific procedures. Historic methods, such as pinning a snake behind the head for manual restraint (Fig. 20.2), are a dangerous manipulation and should be discouraged.

Snake Hooks

The manipulation of venomous snakes using snake hooks (Fig. 20.3), as opposed to tongs, lowers the potential of injury to the animal. Reptiles have a single

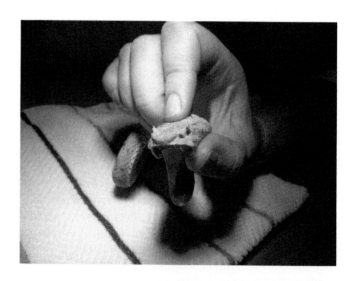

Figure 20.2. Pinning behind the head for manual restraint is not recommended. Snakes when struggling can move fangs independently while dislodging the mandible to succeed with envenomation. Eyelash viper, *Bothriechis schlegeli*, The Orianne Society.

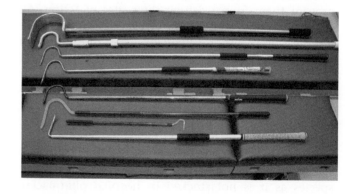

Figure 20.3. Snake hooks (top to bottom): Wide-blade "python hook," extension hook, double-handled hook, various styles, and "L hook" or pinning hook.

occipital condyle supporting their skulls upon the cervical spine. Rough handling or improper restraint can cause spinal injury (Frye 1991) when the snake twists or thrashes. Vertebral morphology and the limitations of movement by vertebrae and axial musculature reviewed are by Gasc (1976). Using tongs for restraint can also induce the snake to bite itself. This can result in self-inflicted fang penetration and envenomation. Although the effects of self-envenomation are usually minimal due to immunity, mechanical damage due to fang penetration can have a serious outcome.

Choice of snake hook is dependent on the size and species. Hooks come in a variety of sizes and configurations and can be "homemade" or purchased from specialty suppliers (e.g., Midwest Tongs, Greenwood, MO, http://www.tongs.com). Two main design aspects need to be considered when choosing the appropriate hook. First, the length of the hook handle must be longer than the striking distance to the hand. In most species, this is usually two-thirds the length of the snake or more! The second is the terminal end of the hook, which supports the snake, should be of sufficient diameter to comfortably hold the weight of the snake. Large, heavy animals require the wider support surface found on larger diameter hooks. "Python hooks" have wide flattened surfaces of 3–6 cm for added comfort to the snake during lifting. This results in a more consistent manipulation of large vipers (genus *Agkistrodon, Bitis, Crotalus, Lachesis,* and *Vipera*). The main disadvantage of "python hooks" is they usually lack sufficient shaft length for large specimens. A hook with a terminal "L-shaped" end is not recommended. The snake will slide down the shaft if it is lifted higher than the handle of the hook. Hooks are relatively simple tools that can be made and tailored to problematic species or individuals.

Basic steps when using a hook:

1. Always set up all required equipment first (transfer or holding containers, and a clear work area) and review with personnel the procedure steps. It is desirable to have a second potential handler with a hook should assistance be required.
2. Always open bags, containers, and cages using proper safety methods.
3. The hook tip is initially inserted under the anterior portion of the snake and slid caudally to the midpoint or its approximate center of gravity, on the body side facing the handler.
4. Once the hook is at the desired location, lift the snake in one motion, just high enough for the head and tail to clear the surface. This will induce the snake to hold and balance. If it is still moving and not balanced, gently set the animal down and repeat the process.
5. Once balanced, lift and move the snake to the desired location. Prevent the head and tail from touching objects during transfer. This will often startle the snake and induce it to come off the hook.
6. Gently set the snake down and remove the hook. Be prepared to use the hook to keep the snake under control or to further manipulate it for the intended procedure.

Longer handled hooks for larger and more agile snakes may have a second grip located above the base grip of the hook. Using two hands on the hook, with the second (anterior) grip as a pivot point, aids in lifting heavier specimens while increasing dexterity and control of the specimen. Care must always be taken that the position of the second grip (hand closest to the snake) is outside the striking range of the snake.

Some snakes require "double-hooking" to distribute their weight at two points. This includes very large, massive specimens where support on a single surface will cause discomfort or injury. Snakes with medical problems (e.g., fused vertebrae, or a recent surgery) are also supported this way. Active snakes and arboreal prehensile-tailed species are also handled with greater control when double-hooked.

The use of two snake hooks requires more finesse than one.

1. Hold a hook in each hand and insert them under the middle portion of the snake, on the same side of the body that faces the handler.
2. Move the hooks away from each other to points dividing the snake's length into thirds. While the hooks are being moved to these locations, each hook should be lifted slightly testing the snake's tendency to balance.
3. Once the hooks are appropriate for balance, lift the snake and determine if it is stable. If so, transfer the in a smooth, deliberate movement.
4. When lifting, outward pressure (away from the snake's midpoint) of the hooks will help keep tension on the snake and not draw the hooks together if the snake tries to progress forward.

This technique requires practice, but is not difficult. Each snake reacts differently to the double-hooking process. For specimens that benefit from double-hooking, this is an excellent technique and should be used routinely.

Tongs and Forceps

Various styles of snake tongs and forceps (Fig. 20.4) are available from reptile equipment dealers (e.g., Midwest Tongs). They should not be used as a primary method of restraint due to their potential to injure. Many snakes will thrash or bite the tongs when held tight enough for restraint. If tongs are used directly for restraint, the contacting surface of the tongs should be padded to create a firm but "soft" restraint. This style

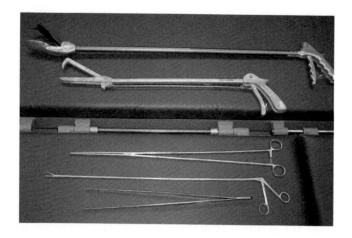

Figure 20.4. Tongs and forceps (top to bottom): Midwest Tong®, Pilstrom Tong®, hemostatic forceps, endoscopic forceps, and tissue forceps.

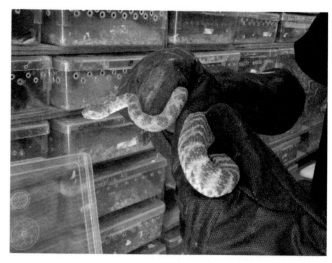

Figure 20.5. Puncture-resistant gloves can offer protection from snakebite of small- to medium-sized species. However, all handling precautions must be met as this method requires the handler to work in very close proximity to the snake. Tiger rattlesnake, *Crotalus tigris*, Glades Herp Farm.

of tong can be very useful when working in the field, primarily with small to medium-sized specimens. In captivity, tongs should only be used as a last resort or in an emergency. Their use is not an acceptable substitute for lack of training or skill with a snake hook (Altimari 1998).

Long-handled tongs are ideal when used for feeding, removing cage items, manipulating container lids, holding restraint tubes, and lifting holding bags. Tong length must always be longer than the maximum striking distance of the snake.

Elongated forceps (Fig. 20.4) are used for feeding small snakes, removing retained shed or ectoparasites, and assessing in judging the depth of anesthetized animals. Forceps length may range from 30 to 45 cm. They must be used cautiously when working in close proximity to the head, allowing for potential movement and strike ability.

Protective Gloves

Wearing protective gloves for handling venomous snakes (Fig. 20.5) has been used by a limited number of researchers. While this method does have its advocates, extreme caution must be used as it places the handler in close proximity to the snake. Defensive strikes may not only target the gloves, but also the handler's arms and body that are not protected. Some snakes appear not to recognize gloves as strike targets as they do bare fingers and hands. This gives the impression that the snake is tame and not prone to biting. That condition can change quickly and the snake should always be handled so that its strike range is limited to the padded/protective areas of the gloves. A popular brand, HexArmor® (HexArmor, Grand Rapids, MI, http://www.hexarmor.com) produces the Hercules™ R6E glove made with SuperFabric® that may offer sufficient protection for most small- to medium-sized

species. The company does not offer any guarantees in regard to protection from snakebite. The condition of the gloves with prolonged use needs to be monitored as the integrity of the material may break down over time (R. Keszey, pers. comm., 2011.).

Shift Boxes

Most snakes will enter boxes where they can seek visual and tactile security. Shift boxes are placed either inside the enclosure or attached to the outside. Box size need only be large enough for the snake to lie comfortably in a resting coil. Many snakes prefer to wedge into a tight fitting space for physical and tactile security. Normally, the snake's head when residing in a shift box is pointed toward the opening (entrance hole), awaiting the passing of potential prey. They will commonly strike out at any movement in front of the opening. Training some elapids to enter shift boxes (Kipp et al. 2006) is achieved with classical conditioning techniques. This is a very useful management tool for long-term captive animals requiring routine handling.

Shift boxes are most appropriate for large, swift elapids. They can be designed to attach directly to the cage (Fig. 20.6). In snake collections requiring multiple enclosures, the openings in cages, shift boxes, and the points of attachment are standardized so boxes can be interchanged. Cages are also designed with a center divider that allows the handler to shift the snake from one side to the other to facilitate safe servicing. The divider slide space should be sufficiently narrow to prevent escape when the divider is removed.

Shift boxes within a cage (Fig. 20.7) should be solid with a bottom and locking door (Rossi 1995). They are easily fabricated from plywood and sealed with poly-

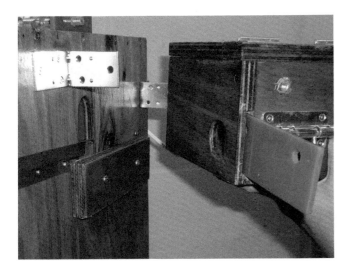

Figure 20.6. Shift box and interfacing cage for an arboreal snake. Not shown are transparent top and side panels of shift box. Used for Gold's tree cobra, *Pseudohaje goldii*, Central Florida Zoo and Botanical Gardens.

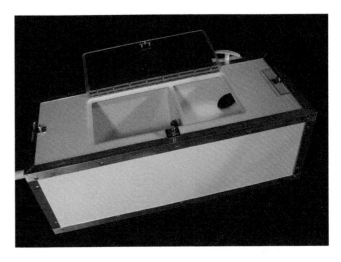

Figure 20.8. Shift box/squeeze box. Inner panel manually slides toward the entrance hole in the box for tube restraint or against transparent slotted end for injections (Dallas Zoo, courtesy of Habitat Systems Limited).

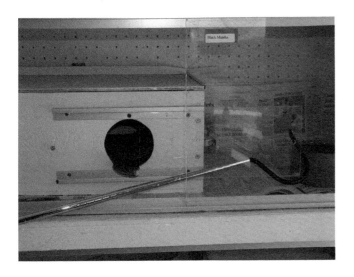

Figure 20.7. Shift box in cage. Shift box door can be slid close with a snake hook and locked. Black mamba, *Dendroaspis polylepis* (courtesy of Medtoxin Venom Laboratories).

urethane to facilitate cleaning. A horizontal sliding door is designed to be closed with a hook once the animal is enclosed. A locking pin or mechanism for the shift box door is secured prior to removing from the cage and when transporting the snake.

Many styles and designs for shift boxes that attach to the outside of enclosures have been used to facilitate safe cage servicing or to aid with restraint and immobilization for veterinary procedures. Historically in zoos and research facilities, boxes have been designed and fabricated "in house" to fit a specific enclosure for a designated species or individual. Shift boxes have primarily been used for shifting large elapids that are dangerous to work in an open environment using a

hook. However, any venomous species is a candidate for shifting to insure a safe and controlled procedure.

Shift boxes attached to enclosures need to incorporate the following design elements:

1. Appropriate comfortable size for the snake
2. Sturdy construction, able to endure dropping and long-term use
3. Secure method of attachment to the enclosure
4. Locking slide door that corresponds to the door on the cage
5. Large top opening access door (lockable)
6. Clear top and/or side section to view the snake
7. Adequate ventilation holes
8. Sealed surfaces to promote easy cleaning.

Variants on the above design combine a squeeze for restraint. An interior sliding wall (Fig. 20.8) is used to push the snake toward the opening and into the restraint tube. Care is taken to ensure restraint tube diameter matches the box opening so no gaps exist. Additionally, the tube and the box must be securely attached (usually manually braced) to prevent changes in restraint tube position. Once the snake enters the tube a safe distance, it is grabbed and restrained using a normal tube restraint grasp.

More advanced designs (Habitat Systems Limited, Des Moines, IA. http://www.habitatsystemsltd.com) combine features to aid in the husbandry and management of venomous snakes (Fig. 20.9). Optional elements include removable squeeze apparatus with a slotted end panel for injections, capped side ports with interchangeable openings of various diameters for tube restraint, enclosed top feeding chamber with sliding false floor (drops feed rodent into shift box without directly opening the box), and removable center dividers

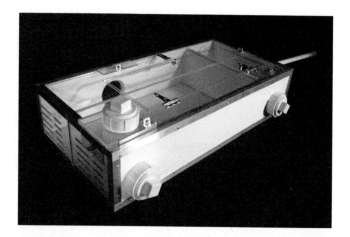

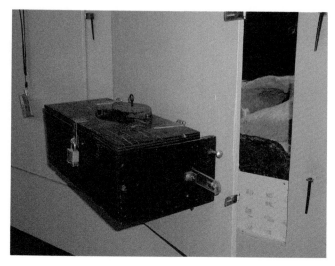

Figure 20.9. Shift box/squeeze box. Features include removable squeeze apparatus, slotted end for injections, two capped side ports for tube restraint, and top capped feeding chamber with sliding false floor for protected feeding. Not shown is removable center divider to create "U-maze" to facilitate total entry of long snakes. Jacksonville Zoo and Gardens, black mamba exhibit, *Dendroaspis polylepis* (courtesy of Habitat Systems Limited).

Figure 20.10. Traditional shift box. This simple design enables the snake to shift out of cage eliminating direct contact. Snake can then be transferred for anesthesia or other procedures.

to create a "U-maze" to facilitate total entry of long snakes. These features increase control while emphasizing safety.

Some boxes incorporate a built-in restraint shield or framed wire mesh panel that can be pushed down for temporary restraint. A common application of this design using a wire mesh top panel is for king cobras (*Ophiophagus hannah*) that frequently retain spectacles. This design is also helpful if treatment requires repeated intramuscular injections.

Shift box design is a function of intended use (Fig. 20.10). They can be used to accomplish tube restraint and anesthesia using the entrance hole of the box. Variations have been described (Bertram & Larsen 2004), but the basic design and function remains the same. When using shift boxes, the users must know how all doors operate (especially when removing the box and a second snake is in the cage!) along with corresponding locking and safety features. Some boxes are overdesigned, increasing the opportunity for an open or unsecured door. Doors and locks are always double checked visually and for movement prior to assessing if a snake is safely secured.

Unattended boxes that have been removed from the enclosure are placed in larger, secured, and labeled containers to alert staff to the presence of a venomous snake.

Restraint or "Squeeze" Box

These boxes are (Quinn & Jones 1974) used to restrain movement of a snake for examination, measurement, and radiography. They consist of a box and a clear shield to press the snake against the bottom of the box for temporary restraint (Fig. 20.11). Most have been made of wood, but acrylic boxes have the advantage of

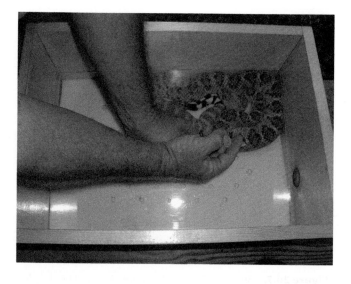

Figure 20.11. Traditional restraint box for clinical and field applications. Primarily used for injections and measuring. Western diamondback rattlesnake, *Crotalus atrox*.

being able to view the snake from all sides, including the ventrum (Krebs et al. 2006).

The size of the box is determined by the snake; it should enable the animal to lay coiled in a normal position. The open top of the box is fitted with 0.5 cm thick Plexiglas shield, with a center handle, that can be lowered to press the snake against a thick foam rubber or other soft material pad.

It is important the shield closely fits the sides of the box to prevent the snake from wedging its head through a gap. The shield is initially lowered using tongs, then secured by hand once safely in place. Holes are drilled into the shield to facilitate injections. Multiple holes are drilled across the shield since the position of the snake is random. Shields made of diamond mesh expanded sheet metal have also been used (M. Whitney, pers. comm.), but care must be taken to avoid the snake striking and injuring oral areas.

Measurement is accomplished using a dry-erase ink marker to draw a mid-dorsal line equaling the length of the snake. A thin wire is superimposed over the drawn line, then straightened and measured. Map measurers have also been used to trace line lengths.

If a restraint box is to be used for a period of time, holes are drilled through the sides to permit the passage of aluminum rods to hold down the shield (Fowler 1978). If a restraint box is used for radiology, it must have a locking mechanism for the top acrylic shield. Snakes secured in such a fashion should not be left unattended and placed in a secured, labeled container.

Restraint Tubes

Manual restraint and immobilization of venomous snakes has been described using a wide variety of techniques for a variety of applications. For many procedures, manipulation of venomous snakes without chemical immobilization is desirable for initial examination, medication, and simple procedures, including removal of adhered shed, palpation, blood sampling, and sex determination.

Techniques that employ restraint tools as the primary method of restraint such as nooses, tongs, strap sticks, bucket restraint (Gillingham et al. 1983), noose tube restraint (King & Duvall 1984), strap boards (Ward & Harrell 1983), and manual restraint following pinning with a snake hook are to be avoided. While used with some success by professional snake handlers in the venom extraction industry, these methods increase the risk of snakebite for the occasional handler and can injure the snake. Safer methods using clear tubes and shift, restraint, and anesthesia boxes are preferred. These remote handling methods require more time and equipment, but greatly reduce direct contact with the snake. All procedures should optimize protected contact and effective control, thereby insuring handler safety.

The standard for safe handling of venomous snakes is Plexiglas tube restraint (Murphy 1971). This method minimizes risk to the handler and potential injury to the snake. Clear, hollow tubes are available in a variety of acrylic materials. They can be purchased as individual tubes, usually sold in 2-m lengths, of various diameters (McMaster-Carr, Atlanta, GA, http://www.mcmaster.com). Sets of restraint tubes are also available from some reptile supply companies. Thin-wall, flexible tubes crack easily and, therefore, less safe than thicker-walled tubes. Polycarbonate hollow rods and PETG (a copolyester material) with a minimum wall thickness of 0.25 cm are best. These products are more durable and do not break if dropped.

The basic steps for tube restraint are as follows:

1. Choose a tube with an inside diameter that will not allow the snake to turn around (inside diameter less than the length of the snake's head or slightly larger than the snake's girth at mid-body).
2. Using a hook, place the snake on a smooth surface. Small and medium-sized specimens are worked within a container. This is usually a trash can or other open-top container large enough to facilitate movement by the handler to manipulate the snake into the tube. Large and more sedentary snakes are worked on the floor or the ground in field conditions. There must be ample open space for handlers to maneuver safely around the snake. Containers are preferred since they limit the range of motion and position of the snake.
3. Use tongs that are longer than the snake's striking range to hold the tube. Grasp the tube in the middle with the tongs in one hand (usually the left hand for a right-handed person) and slowly lower the open end of the tube toward the snake in a manner that will not induce the snake to strike at the tube. Snakes that strike the open end of the tube may incur oral lesions, primarily associated with the mucous membranes that cover the fangs.
4. Using a hook that is longer than the snake's striking range and held above that point, gently touch or hook the animal to manipulate it into the tube (Fig. 20.12). This is a combined maneuver moving the tube and the snake in a fashion that will entice it to enter the tube.

This procedure requires patience! Never hurry and always stay in control of the process.

1. The first goal is to get the snake's head inside the opening of the tube. This should be done quickly to reduce the chance of the snake striking.

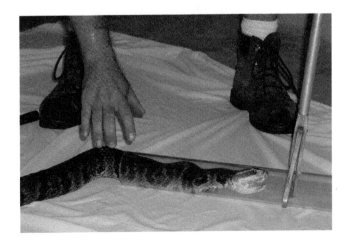

Figure 20.12. Tube restraint. Position of primary handler and snake in tube just prior to restraint. Florida cottonmouth, *Agkistrodon piscivorus*, Central Florida Zoo and Botanical Gardens.

2. Sometimes moving the snake backward with the snake hook will encourage it to move forward, entering the tube.
3. Once the snake starts to enter the tube, hold the tube motionless so as not to startle the snake.
4. More active snakes require the tube to be "worked down" the body following its undulating movements.
5. Once the snake has entered the tube, and is at least half way in (the tong grasp point on the tube if the tube is grasped in the middle) and still moving forward, lay the hook down (or hand it to an assistant), and with that hand quickly grasp the snake and the end of the tube in which the snake entered (Fig. 20.13). This secures the snake in the tube and prevents it from backing out. The other hand is used to grasp and support the animal.

Never over commit to the grab! If the snake begins to back out of the tube or quickly progresses to the end of the tube, abort the procedure and start over.

1. Once restrained, immediately visually check your grasp! Both the tube and the snake should be held firmly to keep the snake from progressing forward or backward.
2. Make sure there is not an opening between your fingers and the palm of the hand that could allow the snake to withdraw a body coil and withdraw from the tube.
3. With medium to large snakes, the assistant should immediately support and restrain the animal's body once it has been successfully restrained. This permits the primary handler to focus their attention on securing the snake while supporting the tube with their other hand.

4. If a snake has a large girth at mid-body and a relatively small head, a smaller-diameter tube is inserted inside the open end of the tube and over the snake's head to keep it from turning around.

Snakes that are anesthetized require a controlled release from the restraint tube in the following sequence:

1. The primary handler grasps the tube midway with the tongs while maintaining tube restraint with the other hand.
2. The snake and tube are placed in a container and angled vertically. The grip on the snake is released and the hand is withdrawn rapidly from the container (and snake's striking range).
3. The primary handler and the assistant pick up hooks for further handling.
4. The container is secured and labeled appropriately.

The primary handler and the assistant always review the steps before and during the process to ensure an understanding of roles and expectations.

Many large-bodied pitvipers will attempt to progress up the tube when released. This should be avoided to prevent the snake becoming stuck in the tube. While still maintaining manual restraint, these snakes should be pulled down the tube to a safe point near the end prior to release. When released, many snakes will quickly withdraw from the tube and immediately strike back at the handler. Alternatively, some species (i.e., elapids) will attempt to flee. Handlers need to be prepared to use hooks to keep the snake under control.

Tube restraint can also be accomplished directly from a shift box, facilitated by a squeeze apparatus adapted to the box (Fig. 20.14). The diameter of the restraint tube must match the hole in the shift box.

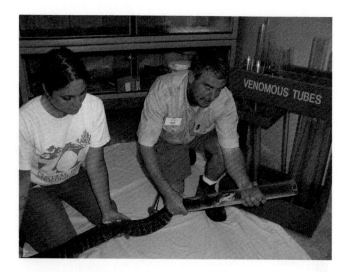

Figure 20.13. Tube restraint completed. With large specimens, the primary handler secures the snake and tube while the secondary handler supports and restrains the body. Florida cottonmouth, *Agkistrodon piscivorus conanti*, Central Florida Zoo and Botanical Gardens.

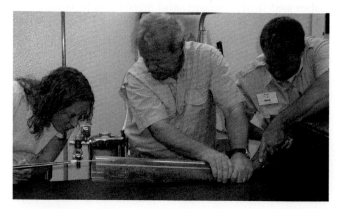

Figure 20.14. Tube restraint directly from a shift box containing a squeeze apparatus. In addition to tube restraint, the body of this 14' king cobra (*Ophiophagus hannah*) is also manually held in the shift box during examination to maintain control of the body (Central Florida Zoo and Botanical Gardens, photo credit Sarah Burke).

Tube restraint provides the handlers and clinicians a high degree of control during the examination. The snake is advanced to the end of the tube for cranial and oral examination. Various locations along the snake's body can also be examined. Care is taken to keep a significant portion of the anterior body in the tube. Restraint tubes are also used for administering oral medications and force-feeding (Radcliffe 1975). The major advantage of this technique is that the snake is restrained without grasping the head, and the animal is positioned in a relative straight line to facilitate examination, medication, tube-feeding, and anesthesia.

A variation of acrylic tube restraint (Mauldin & Engeman 1999) employs wire mesh cable holders as the restraint "tube". While this method can be used with some snakes, it is not recommended for venomous species since they will bite through openings in the mesh resulting in either envenomation of the handler or oral trauma to the snake.

Restraint Tube Modifications

Clear acrylic restraint tubes can be modified for the needs of the clinician. Tubes are cut to various lengths to facilitate safe handling (i.e., longer tubes for longer snakes). Tubes can be drilled to create access holes and elongate cut-outs are made for increased access for minor procedures. Appropriately sized PVC caps, rubber stoppers, or wooden corks are temporarily or permanently secured at one end to prevent the snake from progressing through the tube.

Care is taken when any opening is made along the length of the tube to prevent hands and fingers from crossing these openings. Many species are capable of biting and protruding a fang through these openings. Bite attempts on the inside of the tube will release venom that will run down the inside of the tube to the hand. Handlers should wear latex gloves to prevent venom contact with the skin that may lead to envenomation through microcuts. All tubes must be thoroughly washed and disinfected immediately after use.

Anesthesia Boxes

Full clinical examination and surgical procedures require chemical immobilization and anesthesia (See Chapter 20). This is essential when evaluating cranial features, such as the nostrils, infra-orbital pits, spectacle and eyes, oral cavity, glottis, and tongue. More general procedures, such as blood sampling, examination of the integument, removing adhered shed skin, removal of ectoparasites, cloacal examination and sampling, and palpation may be accomplished by tube restraint. Radiology may be performed on snakes in shift boxes, squeeze boxes (through a fixed acrylic shield) or through bags if the specimen is inactive. If an intended procedure presents a safety concern for personnel, full chemical immobilization is strongly recommended. Some snakes can be induced in restraint

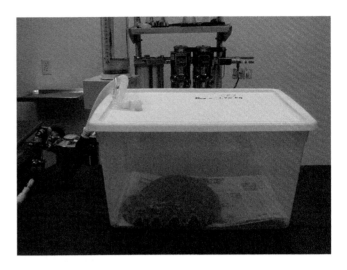

Figure 20.15. Anesthesia box. A clear plastic storage box with fitted with an adapter to receive the corrugated breathing tube from the anesthesia machine. The transparent container facilitates viewing to judge level of induction. Rhinoceros viper, *Bitis nasicornis*, Central Florida Zoo and Botanical Gardens.

tubes with propofol administered into the ventral coccygeal vessels (Chapter 20).

A variety of containers for venomous snakes can be used as inhalant anesthesia boxes. Large clear plastic Rubbermaid® or Sterilite® storage boxes (Fig. 20.15) are available from retail stores. Snakes are placed directly into these boxes only if the lids can be secured to prevent escape. Transparent containers allow observation of the snake during anesthetic induction. A snake contained in a cloth snake bag may be placed inside an anesthesia box. However, judging anesthetic level will depend on evaluating declining movement in the bag. When testing the movement of a snake inside a bag, always use instruments (forceps and tongs) and never manually palpate the bag.

A snake contained in a shift box or ventilated restraint box can also be placed in an anesthesia box. The anesthesia box, fitted with an adapter for the breathing system, allows for infusion of the inhalant anesthetic in oxygen from the machine. A shift box may also be enclosed in a plastic bag for administration of inhalation anesthetic through the opening. However, induction is very difficult to evaluate when the snake is enclosed in two containers.

Guidelines to assess whether a snake is safely anesthetized include lack of response to tactile stimulation, inhibition of tongue flicking, and lack of ability to right itself when turned over on its dorsum. Snakes can hold their breath for 15–20 minutes and anesthetic induction can be prolonged. Once anesthetized, a restraint tube is placed over the head and anterior portion of the body as a secondary safety precaution and the snake is then carefully removed from the box. For continued delivery of inhalant anesthetic, either a cover can be fitted over the open end of the restraint tube, a mask placed directly over the head if removed from a restraint tube, or direct endotracheal intubation, whereby a tube is inserted through the snake's glottis and into the trachea (Chapter 20).

Transport

Safe transport and receiving of venomous reptiles requires planning and setting up the appropriate equipment in advance. Securing the snake in a cloth bag and placing it in a ventilated locked box is recommended. The cloth bag should be of tight-woven, strong material that allows for good ventilation. Bags are examined for small holes that may be tested by the snake and enlarged, leading to escape. Bags are turned inside out so the seam is on the outside to avoid entanglement in loose threads. Only one animal should be contained in each bag to eliminate defensive striking and to facilitate removal. Bags should be long (deep) enough to be easily knotted at the open end and additionally secured with strong tape or plastic cable ties.

To place a snake in a bag, it is hung inside an empty container and secured in an open position using clips (clothes pins work well). Tongs are used by an assistant to hold the sides of the bag open. They are then used to close the bag after the snake is guided in by a hook. Commercially available "snake baggers," long-handled rods with an attached and removable bag, increase safety in the bagging process (Snake Bagger®, Midwest Tongs). Never be too anxious to manually close the top of the bag. Most snakes tend to climb upward after being dropped into the bag. Always visually know where the snake is. Use tongs to close and secure the bag, or twist and pull the neck of the bag under the shaft of a secured snake hook prior to knotting.

When knotting, first transfer the bagged snake to a flat surface. Place the shaft of the snake hook across the twisted neck of the bag, pull to secure the snake in the far end of the bag, and tie the neck of the bag. For additional security, the bag is secured with strong tape or cable ties on either side of the knot. This must be done away from the portion holding the snake. Bags are labeled to identify the snake species with a noticeable "VENOMOUS" notation made on the label. Red labels with the "skull and crossbones" symbolizing poison are most effective. Tongs are used to clamp the bag just under the knot for lifting. Bags should always be carried above the knot and away from the handler's body. Bagged snakes are placed in a suitable container or box while waiting for procedures or transport. Transport boxes containing more than one bagged snake have solid dividers to eliminate the potential for snakes biting each other.

Transport boxes are locked, well ventilated, and kept away from temperature extremes. Boxes are kept out of the sun and transported in air-conditioned vehicles to avoid hyperthermia. Boxes are clearly labeled "CAUTION: VENOMOUS SNAKES" and stored in locked rooms while awaiting transport.

The same level of caution used in bagging the snake must be used during removal from transport containers. Open the transport boxes using the level of caution as if the snake inside had escaped the containment bag. Keep fingers and hands away from openings (use tongs) and be prepared to hook a snake into a holding container. The bag is removed from the container using tongs. Snakes can bite through cloth bags, induced by limited visual capability or when the bag is touched. Bites through either bags or screened surfaces can result in significant envenomation. Under these circumstances, a snake's fangs can become momentarily hung up in the bag material, resulting in the expression of large quantities of venom.

Prior to untying the snake bag, place the bag on a flat surface and position the shaft of the snake hook across the neck of the bag below the knot, securing the snake in the end of the bag. All extremities are held safely away from this portion of the bag. Once untied, tongs are used to secure the open bag end. It is then picked up and lowered into a container. The snake is released by picking up the bottom end of the bag with the tongs. Bags with a hemline sewn across the bottom corners of the bag provide an area of material to grab without pinching the snake.

A field transport box (Birkhead et al. 2004) for carrying large numbers of venomous snakes combines both tube restraint and a modified transport container. In this design, 10 polyethylene restraint tubes, capped at both ends, are secured by spacers in a transport container. The advantage of this design is individual containment of each snake that is positioned for immediate manipulation or restraint.

The International Air Transport Association (IATA) publishes Live Animal Regulations that are adopted by most airline carriers. When shipping air freight, it is prudent to review these regulations in case airline employees question the design and features of the shipping crate and the methods by which the snakes are contained. IATA requirements (for snakes see Part 8, Container Requirement #44) are presented as examples to be adopted depending on the species and size of the snake. Specific suggestions in the IATA regulations include container rigidity, packing material, size and type of container, specification for snake bags, double-bagging snakes with a transparent mesh inner bag for inspection, wire-covered containers, and an abbreviated listing of venomous snakes and some colubrids that are considered venomous. It is the responsibility of the shipper to ensure materials and methods are appropriate for safe transport. It is rare that an airline employee will ask the shipper to open a container of venomous snakes for inspection. This is not the case for international shipments that are routinely inspected by wildlife customs agents charged with monitoring species covered under the Convention on International Trade in Endangered Species of Wild Fauna and Flora (CITES).

VENOMOUS LIZARD MANAGEMENT

Gila Monsters and Beaded Lizards (Helodermatidae)

Venomous lizards known to produce significant envenomation in humans are restricted to two species, the Gila monster (*Helododerma suspectum*) and the Mexican beaded lizard (*Heloderma horridum*). As studies continue on the evolution of reptilian venom systems (Fry et al. 2006b) additional "nonvenomous" lizard taxa will be recognized as having toxin-secreting oral glands. Currently, this is restricted to some species of monitor lizards (family Varanidae), especially the desert monitor (Ballard & Antonio 2001).

Helodermatids are large, stout-bodied lizards with large heads, powerful jaws, and short legs adapted to digging. They are easily recognized by their colorful, intricate skin patterns, and rounded tuberculate scales that give them a beaded appearance. Gila monsters average 36 cm as adults, while beaded lizards can reach 1 m in total length.

Helodermatids have evolved a "defensive venom" tailored to create significant pain to ward off predators. Bites are extremely painful and can have systemic effects, including a rapid drop in blood pressure that may result in hypotensive shock (Preston 1988). Unlike snakes, the venom glands of helodermids are mandibular and appear as a rounded swelling located midway on the lower jaw. The large triangular-shaped head is the result of well-developed musculature associated with biting and maintaining a vice-like grip. When biting, helodermatids exhibit a pumping action of the jaw musculature while embedding the enlarged, grooved, venom-conducting teeth, located above the venom glands. Accounts of severe gripping bites result in the use of pliers, crow bars, severing of jaw musculature, and decapitation to disengage the lizard from the bitten extremity. Severity of envenomation is a function of the amount of time the lizard is allowed to bite. Envenomation is treated symptomatically as there is no antivenom for helodermatids.

Helodermatids are deceptive, normally exhibiting slow movements and a sluggish behavior, but are capable of swift lateral and upward movements of the head and upper body when attempting to bite. Of 21 venomous bites received by zoo workers over a 25-year period (Card & Roberts 1996), four were inflicted by helodermatids. The authors concluded that because helodermatids are generally considered relatively benign captives, this assumption misleads individuals to handle them carelessly. No matter how much their owner professes its tameness; all helodermatids should be handled with the same caution as for venomous snakes.

Manual restraint of helodermatids requires first pinning the head down on a flat surface with a snake hook or pinning bar prior to restraint (Fig. 20.16). Once secured, they are picked up with a firm grip at the base of the head and a forelimb held between the fingers to maintain control of the upper body. Once elevated, the second hand is used to support and hold the body (Fig. 20.17). Locking hemostats (40–60 cm) have also be used to successfully pin helodermatids (Poulin & Ivanyi 2003) by using the interlocking base portion (area between the finger eyelets) as the pinning bar.

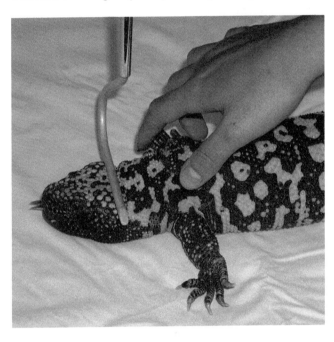

Figure 20.16. Prerestraint position for helodermatids. Head should be immobilized prior to manual restraint. Gila monster, *Heloderma suspectum*, Central Florida Zoo and Botanical Gardens.

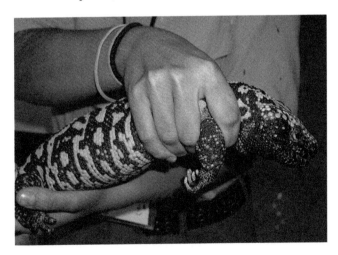

Figure 20.17. Helodermatids can be manually restrained by securing a firm grip at the base of the head with a forelimb held between the fingers to maintain control of the upper body. Once elevated, the second hand is used to support and hold the body. Gila monster, *Heloderma suspectum*, Central Florida Zoo and Botanical Gardens.

Helodermatids can be closely examined using manual restraint. Examination of the oral cavity using a hard rubber speculum has limited use since they will vigorously bite down on any object placed in its mouth.

Helodermatids can be anesthetized by administering an inhalant anesthetic into an induction chamber. Anesthetized helodermatids should again be pinned as described earlier before removal from the anesthetic chamber. One of the last reflexes to be lost is the defensive bite.

ACKNOWLEDGMENTS

For various courtesies and insights, I thank L.A. Antonio, S. Antonio, C. Barden, B. Breitbeil, J. Clark, J. Facente, D.J. Heard, G. Lepera, J. Montisano, C. Russo, J. Stabile, and G. Van Horn.

PRODUCTS MENTIONED IN THE TEXT

Habitat Systems Limited
4489 N.W. Second Avenue, Suite 3B
Des Moines, IA 50313
Phone: 888.909.5795
Web address: http://www.habitatsystemsltd.com

HexArmor
2000 Oak Industrial Drive NE
Grand Rapids, MI 49505
Phone: 877.692.7667
Web address: http://www.hexarmor.com

McMaster-Carr
6100 Fulton Industrial Blvd.
Atlanta, GA 30336-2852
Phone: 404.346.7000
Web address: http://www.mcmaster.com

Midwest Tongs
14505 S. Harris Road
Greenwood, MO 64034
Phone: 877.878.6647
Web address: http://www.tongs.com

REFERENCES

Altimari W. 1998. *Venomous Snakes: A Safety Guide for Reptile Keepers.* Danbury: Society for the Study of Amphibians and Reptiles. Herp. Circ. 26.

Ballard V, Antonio FB. 2001. Natural history notes: *Varanus griseus* (desert monitor); toxicity. *Herpetological Review* 32(4):261.

Bertram N, Larsen KW. 2004. Putting the squeeze on venomous snakes: accuracy and precision of length measurements taken with the "squeeze box." *Herpetological Review* 35:235–238.

Birkhead RD, Williams MI, Boback SM, Greene MP. 2004. The cottonmouth condo: a novel venomous snake transport device. *Herpetological Review* 35(2):153–154.

Boyer DM, Murphy JB. 1999. *Recommendations for Emergency Snakebite Procedures.* Silver Spring: Association of Zoos and Aquariums Antivenom Index.

Card W, Roberts DT. 1996. Incidence of bites from venomous reptiles in North American zoos. *Herpetological Review* 27(1): 15–16.

Chippaux J-P. 2006. *Snake Venoms and Envenomations.* Malabar: Krieger Publishing.

Fowler ME. 1978. *Restraint and Handling of Wild and Domestic Animals.* Ames: Iowa State University Press.

Fry BG. 2006a. The molecular evolution of lizard and snake venoms: clinical and evolutionary implications. *Journal of Medical Toxicology* 2(1):34–35.

Fry BG, Vidal N, Norman JA, Vonk F, Scheib H, Ramjan S, Kuruppu S, Fung K, Hedges S, Richardson M, Hodgson W, Ignjatovic V, Summerhayes R, Kochva E. 2006b. Early evolution of the venom system in lizards and snakes. *Nature* 439:584–588.

Frye FL. 1991. *Reptile Care, an Atlas of Diseases and Treatments.* Neptune City: TFH Publ.

Gasc JP. 1976. Snake vertebrae: a mechanism or merely a taxonomist's toy? In: *Morphology and Biology of Reptiles.* (Ad'A Bellairs, CB Cox, eds.), pp. 177–190. New York: Academic Press.

Gillingham JC, Clark DL, Teneyck GR. 1983. Venomous snake immobilization: a new technique. *Herpetological Review* 14(2):40.

Greene HW. 1997. *Snakes: The Evolution of Mystery in Nature.* Berkeley, CA: University of California Press.

Ivanyi C, Altimari W. 2004. Venomous reptile bites in academic research. *Herpetological Review* 35(1):49–50.

Keyler DE. 2006. Exotics in the homeland. *Journal of Medical Toxicology* 2(1):36.

King MB, Duvall D. 1984. Noose tube: a lightweight, sturdy, and portable snake restraining apparatus for field and laboratory use. *Herpetological Review* 15(4):109.

Kipp SL, Krebs J, Simmons LG. 2006. Venomous snake shift training at the Henry Doorly Zoo. *Journal of Medical Toxicology* 2:39–40.

Krebs J, Curro TG, Simmons LG. 2006. The use of a venomous reptile restraining box at Omaha's Henry Doorly Zoo. *Journal of Medical Toxicology* 2(1):40.

Lai MW, Klein-Schwartz W, Rodgers GC, Abrams JY, Haber DA, Bronstein AC, Wruk KM. 2006. 2005 Annual Report of the American Association of Poison Control Centers' national poisoning and exposure database. *Clinical Toxicology* 44:803–932.

Mauldin RE, Engeman RM. 1999. A novel snake restraint device. *Herpetological Review* 30(3):158.

Minton S. 1999. Antivenoms recommended for venomous snakes commonly displayed in zoos. Silver Spring: Association of Zoos and Aquariums, *Antivenom Index.*

Murphy JB. 1971. A method for immobilizing venomous snakes. *International Zoo Yearbook* 11:233.

Poulin S, Ivanyi CS. 2003. A technique for manual restraint of helodermatid lizards. *Herpetological Review* 34(1):43.

Powell RL, Sánchez EE, Pérez JC. 2006. Farming for venom: survey of snake venom extraction facilities worldwide. *Applied Herpetology* 3:1–10.

Preston CA. 1988. Hypotension, myocardial infarction, and coagulopathy following Gila monster bite. *The Journal of Emergency Medicine* 7:37–40.

Quinn H, Jones JP. 1974. Squeeze box technique for measuring snakes. *Herpetological Review* 5(2):35.

Radcliffe CW. 1975. A method for force-feeding snakes. *Herpetological Review* 6(1):18.

Rossi JV. 1995. *Snakes of the United States and Canada: Keeping Them Healthy in Captivity*, Vol. 2. Malabar: Krieger Publishing.

Russell FE. 1980. *Snake Venom Poisoning.* Philadelphia: J.B. Lippincot.

Seifert SA. 2006a. TESS-based characterization of non-native snake envenomation in the United States. *Journal of Medical Toxicology* 2(1):35–36.

Seifert SA. 2006b. Just a *Naja* envenomation. *Journal of Medical Toxicology* 2(1):30–31.

Ward RJ, Harrell EH. 1983. A restraining apparatus for anaesthetized snakes. *Herpetological Review* 9(4):139–140.

Weinstein SA, Warrell DA, White J, Keyler DE. 2011. *"Venomous" Bites from Non-Venomous Snakes.* Waltham: Elsevier.

21 Squamates (Snakes and Lizards)

Mads F. Bertelsen

INTRODUCTION

Sedation and anesthesia are essential components of veterinary care of lizards and snakes. These techniques are employed to enable surgery and other painful or invasive procedures, to facilitate handling and to enhance the quality or safety of diagnostic procedures while minimizing stress and discomfort. Within the field of reptilian anesthesia, there has been a gradual and continuing evolution from hypothermia and manual restraint to balanced, well-controlled anesthesia. Several excellent reviews on reptile anesthesia are available (Bennett 1998; Heard 2001; Malley 1997; Schumacher & Yelen 2005), while controlled clinical studies are still comparably scarce. Generally speaking, squamates are rather tough, and life-threatening anesthetic complications are rare.

TAXONOMY AND BIOLOGY

The nomenclature within the class Reptilia is undergoing continuous change, and taxonomy remains controversial. Briefly, the order Squamata consists of more than 50 families and 7700 species of lizards and snakes. While members of the group range from the tropics to the near-arctic, and vary in size from a few centimeters to 8 m, the basic anatomical and physiological features as well as reactions to anesthetic drugs are surprisingly uniform.

ANATOMY AND PHYSIOLOGY

Reptiles are ectothermic vertebrates with relatively low metabolic rates. Their pulmonary and cardiac anatomy, as well as their control of respiration, differs from those of mammals. Despite 200 years of study, many aspects of reptilian anatomy and, more notably, physiology remain poorly understood.

Cardiovascular System

All reptiles possess two atria divided by a complete atrial septum. Each opens into the ventricle by a separate atrio-ventricular ostium. The ventricle of noncrocodilian reptiles is incompletely divided by a horizontal septum-like muscular ridge. This ridge and an opposing thickening in the ventricular wall divide the ventricle into two subcompartments. The incomplete ventricular separation creates the potential for intracardiac mixing or shunting of blood. This may occur as a left-to-right (L-R) shunt or a right-to-left (R-L) shunt. A L-R shunt results in oxygenated pulmonary venous blood reentering pulmonary circulation, while a R-L shunt results in a fraction of deoxygenated systemic venous blood bypassing the lungs and returning into systemic circulation, resulting in alveolar to arterial gradients for respiratory gases. The reduction in arterial oxygen pressure in reptiles during R-L shunting is considerable and is well documented in turtles as well as lizards (Hicks & Comeau 1994; Hlastala et al. 1985; Hopkins et al. 1996; Wang & Hicks 1996).

The extent and direction of shunting is highly dependent on the degree of functional separation, determined by evolutionary adaptations. At one extreme, turtles, which have poorly developed ventricular separation and similar pulmonary and systemic arterial blood pressures, have large intracardiac shunts (Shelton & Burggren 1976; Wang & Hicks 1996; White et al. 1989). In contrast, varanid lizards have a very well-developed muscular ventricular septum, and a large difference between pulmonary and systemic pressures (similar to that seen in mammals) resulting in

Zoo Animal and Wildlife Immobilization and Anesthesia, Second Edition. Edited by Gary West, Darryl Heard, and Nigel Caulkett.
© 2014 John Wiley & Sons, Inc. Published 2014 by John Wiley & Sons, Inc.

only low grade shunting (Burggren & Johansen 1982; Heisler & Glass 1985; Heisler et al. 1983). In some species (e.g., varanids), the shunting patterns are essentially identical during apnea and ventilation (Heisler & Glass 1985). In other species, however, a clear relationship exists between cardiac shunting patterns and the stage of respiration. Breath holding is associated with decreased pulmonary perfusion, and large R-L intracardiac shunts, while periods of pulmonary ventilation are characterized by increased pulmonary blood flow leading to a reduction in the R-L shunt (Hicks & Krosniunas 1996). This is thought to stabilize oxygen content in the blood during respiratory pauses and to ration pulmonary oxygen by forcing periods of tissue hypoxia during diving.

Respiratory System

The squamate glottis is located at the base of the tongue, quite rostrally in the oral cavity. The glottis is closed during most of the respiratory cycle, opening only during inspiration and expiration. The trachea of the squamates has incomplete cartilaginous rings, while those of chelonians and crocodilians have complete tracheal rings (Davies 1981; Kardong 1972a, 1972b). Lizards and primitive snakes have two roughly symmetrical lungs, while in more advanced snakes, the left lung is reduced in size or absent. In general, gas exchange occurs in the cranial portion of the lung, while the caudal portion may be reduced to an air sac-like structure. The relative lung volume, as well as the compliance of the reptilian lung far exceeds that of mammals, but the surface available for gas exchange is smaller.

The basic pattern of respiration is an exhalation followed by an inspiration, followed by a nonventilatory period of varying length. Most reptiles exhibit an intermittent breathing pattern characterized by periods of apnea interrupted by brief ventilatory periods consisting of one to several breaths (Abe & Johansen 1987; Glass & Wood 1983; Templeton & Dawson 1963).

Reptiles, most notably freshwater turtles, are remarkably resistant to ambient hypoxia. While green iguanas can breath hold up to 4.5 hours (Moberly 1968), chelonians may survive complete environmental anoxia for hours or days at their normal body temperatures (Belkin 1963, 1968; Bickler 1992), and weeks to months at very low temperatures (Hicks & Farrell 2000; Ultsch & Jackson 1982). An increase in body temperature leads to increased metabolic oxygen consumption, and consequently to increased ventilation.

Implications for Inhalational Anesthesia

As described, the systemic arterial blood of reptiles may have gas tensions considerably different from the gas within the lung (Hicks & Comeau 1994; Wang & Hicks 1996). The main reasons for this gradient are functional intrapulmonary venous admixture, and R-L

intracardiac shunting. Of these two, ventilation/perfusion heterogeneity appears remarkably constant among species, whereas the degree of intracardiac shunting shows marked species differences (Powell & Hopkins 2004). For example, reported values for the pulmonary to arterial oxygen difference, when breathing 21% oxygen, range from only 13.6 mmHg in monitor lizards (Mitchell et al. 1981) to 60–70 mmHg in turtles (Burggren & Shelton 1979) and snakes (Seymour & Webster 1975). In comparison, the pulmonary to arterial difference created by a small physiological shunt in mammals and birds is minor. The consequence of R-L shunting may be that induction and recovery from inhalational anesthesia is slower and less predictable than in mammals and birds.

VASCULAR ACCESS SITES

The most reliable vascular access site is the ventral tail vessels, located immediately ventral to the coccygeal vertebrae. In snakes, these vessels are mostly approached from the ventral midline, but in many lizards, a lateral approach is often more convenient. The palatine veins may be accessed in larger anesthetized snakes. Indwelling catheters may be placed in the cephalic, femoral, abdominal, or ventral cervical vessels using cut-down techniques. Fluids and certain drugs may be administered by the intraosseus route. In lizards, intraosseus catheterization may be performed in the humerus, femur, or tibia following local analgesia of the cannulation site. Cardiac puncture for drug administration as well as for obtaining blood samples is an option in snakes, but although only minor damage to the myocardium following cardiac puncture has been documented in ball pythons (Isaza et al. 2004; McFadden et al. 2011), the procedure is likely stressful and this author sees the approach as a last resort.

PREANESTHETIC CONSIDERATIONS

Body weights vary markedly, and an accurate weight should be obtained prior to administering drugs to the reptilian patient. The hydration status of the subject should be assessed, and abnormalities corrected. Animals should be subjected to a physical examination prior to anesthesia, and if time, budget, and facilities allow, a blood sample for PCV, CBC, and plasma biochemistry profile, as well as ultrasonographic or radiographic imaging may aid in preanesthetic evaluation. Starving the animals prior to surgery is not generally indicated, but large quantities of feed in the stomach may theoretically impair pulmonary function. In infrequently feeding snakes, massive increases in oxygen consumption follow feeding (Overgaard et al. 1999), and heart as well as liver weight increases (Andersen et al. 2005; Secor & Diamond 1997). As these factors are all likely to increase the risk of anesthetic complications, elective procedures should be avoided in recently fed snakes. In a recent study, however, no effect on recovery times were found in garter snakes anesthetized 1, 2, 3, and 10 days post feeding (Preston et al. 2010).

MAINTAINING BODY TEMPERATURE

Induction time, anesthetic dose, and recovery time (Arena et al. 1988; Dohm & Brunson 1998; Green et al. 1981; Preston et al. 2010), as well as general metabolism, are all temperature dependent and maintaining the animal's body temperature within the preferred optimum zone (POZ) is crucial. This is achieved through the use of heating pads, circulating water blankets, water bottles, bean bags, and so on. For most temperate and tropical species, a body temperature of 25–35°C during induction, anesthesia, and recovery will be appropriate. In garter snakes anesthetized with methohexital, recovery time at 21°C was twice as long as at 31°C (Preston et al. 2010), and warming animals toward the high end of the POZ once the procedure is over may be attempted to obtain faster recoveries.

MONITORING PHYSIOLOGICAL FUNCTION

Most monitoring modalities used in domestic species may be applied to reptiles. Body temperature should be monitored with a cloacal thermometer or temperature probe able to measure low temperatures. Heart rate and rhythm may be monitored using ECG or Doppler flow detection units. Particularly, the latter offers simple audible monitoring. In snakes, the heart rate may usually be determined by visual inspection of the ventral scales approximately 25% of the snake's length from the head, while in many lizards, the heart rate may be visually observed in the jugular groove. The position of the heart in lizards varies between different species. For example, the heart in iguanids and agamids is located very close to the pectoral girdle, while in varanids and chameleons, it is located more caudally, almost to the middle of the coelomic cavity.

Blood pressure may be measured invasively only following cut-down procedures, limiting usefulness to research settings. Commercially available oscillometric devices applied to the tail of snakes or the femoral region of lizards unfortunately seem to have limited value, but may perhaps provide trend information (Chinnadurai et al. 2009, 2010)

Respiration may be assessed visually and in intubated animals main stream or side stream capnography provides useful information, although cardiac shunting and dilution as a consequence of excessive sampling rates of the devices used may give rise to erroneous readings (Hernandez-Divers et al. 2005). The use of pulse oximetry in reptiles remains controversial (Diethelm et al. 1998; Hernandez-Divers et al. 2005;

Mosley et al. 2004) as values obtained may not correlate with measured arterial oxygenation (Mosley et al. 2004). If monitored continuously, however, pulse oximetry may provide trends to assess oxygenation over time.

Arterial blood gas analysis can provide valuable information on oxygenation and acid-base status. Although cost-effective portable equipment is increasingly available, the difficulty of obtaining arterial blood samples reduces relevance in the clinical setting. Venous blood samples are readily available and may partly reflect arterial values. In anesthetized iguanas, for example, arterial and venous oxygen pressures may be almost identical, and carbon dioxide pressure only slightly different, which may suggest very low tissue metabolism and oxygen consumption during anesthesia (Mosley et al. 2004).

MONITORING DEPTH OF ANESTHESIA

The clinical signs associated with induction of general anesthesia in reptiles are fairly consistent. Generally, muscle relaxation in lizards starts at mid-body and moves forward, then backwards so that tail tone is lost last (Bonath 1977; Bonath & Zschege 1979). In varanids induced with inhalation anesthetics, the front limbs lose tone first, followed by the hind limbs and the neck approximately simultaneously. Then righting reflex is lost, and finally, the tail tone (Bertelsen et al. 2005b). The tongue retraction "reflex" in snakes and varanids persists beyond the loss of tail tone and righting reflex (Schumacher et al. 1997), and often is present at the surgical plane, as is the corneal reflex (Arena et al. 1988; Bertelsen & Sauer 2011). Loss of these reflexes may indicate excessive anesthetic depth. Animals retain the ability to react to painful stimuli even after the loss of righting reflex and tail tone, and the response to toe or tail pinching should be evaluated before deciding that surgical anesthesia has been achieved.

ENDOTRACHEAL INTUBATION

Due to the large oral cavities and rostral position of the glottis, lizards and snakes are easily intubated. The glottis is visualized at the bottom of the mouth, immediately caudal to the tongue (Fig. 21.1a,b). A noncuffed endotracheal tube of appropriate size is inserted and taped in place allowing positive pressure ventilation, either manually or using mechanical ventilators. Snakes and some lizards may be intubated awake, following the application of topical analgesics to the glottis. Endotracheal tubes are commercially available down to 1 mm ID, but for the smallest subjects, over-the-needle IV catheters (12–19 G) may be used.

A piece of rubber tubing, a folded gauze pad or a wooden mouth gags, depending on the size of the subject, may be used to prevent the animal from biting

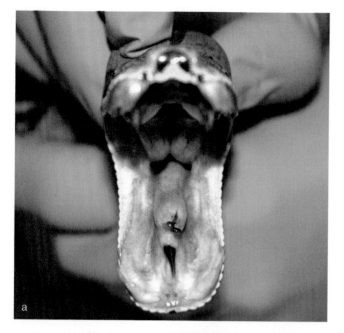

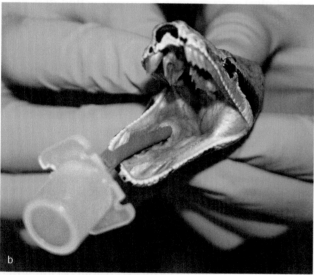

Figure 21.1. (a) The oral cavity of a boa constrictor (*Boa constrictor*). Note the rostral location of the partly open glottis. (b). The oral cavity of a boa constrictor showing the endotracheal tube within the glottis after intubation.

on the tube. In small reptiles, taping the animal, the endotracheal tube, and the breathing system to the table, a board, or a tongue depressor may prevent tube displacement and injury.

VENTILATION

The combination of very low metabolic rates and extreme resilience to hypoxemia allow anesthetized reptiles to experience long periods of apnea without deleterious effects. However, until more is known about the exact requirements, mechanical ventilation is recommended during deep or prolonged anesthesia. Apart

from preventing hypoxemia, mechanical ventilation ensures delivery and removal of inhalational anesthetics' anesthetic agents.

Following endotracheal intubation, mechanical ventilation may be achieved by manually "bagging" the animal or by means of a ventilator of appropriate size. For many species, specialized laboratory animal or very small animal equipment is necessary to avoid overventilation, and even with this equipment it may be hard to achieve respiratory rates that are low enough. When artificially ventilating lizards and snakes, the larger tidal volume and lower minute ventilation compared with mammals should be taken into consideration, and if available, capnography should be used to monitor the level of ventilation. A minute ventilation of 50–75 mL/kg and a frequency of 0.5–4 breaths/minute will be adequate in most species.

INHALATION ANESTHESIA

Inhalational anesthesia is commonly used for induction and maintenance of reptile anesthesia (Read 2004). As in other species, the advantages of inhalational anesthetics include superior control of anesthetic depth, wide safety margins, excellent muscle relaxation, faster recovery, and "built-in" oxygen supplementation. As mentioned earlier, induction and recovery times in reptiles tend to be longer and more variable than in mammals and birds, due to breath holding, intracardiac shunting, and slow circulatory time.

Anesthetic Potency

Minimum alveolar concentration or minimum anesthetic concentration (MAC) is the standard measure of potency of inhalational anesthetic agents (Quasha et al. 1980). MAC is defined as the anesthetic concentration that prevents gross purposeful movement in 50% of an anesthetized population subjected to a supramaximal noxious stimulus, traditionally a surgical incision. Apart from permitting comparison of anesthetic agent potency, the value allows standardization and comparison of various depths of anesthesia as multiples of MAC. Using MAC values also provides a way of assessing the synergism between two anesthetics. Other terms, essentially equivalent to MAC are sometimes reported in birds and reptiles (e.g., minimum anesthetic dose, effective dose 50, and minimum infundibular concentration). Generally, MAC for a given agent varies little across mammalian species (Quasha et al. 1980) and the limited number of reports available indicate that the same applies to reptiles, although evolutionary differences in cardiopulmonary performance may give raise to greater variability among reptiles (Bertelsen et al. 2005c).

As MAC only "accounts for" 50% of the population, vaporizer settings of 1.3 MAC are recommended to achieve surgical anesthesia. As a likely consequence of R-L intracardiac shunting, the equilibrium between inhaled substances and body occurs more slowly in reptiles. Consequently, effective MAC decreases over time in iguanas (and probably other reptiles) (Barter et al. 2006; Brosnan et al. 2006), indicating inhaled gas levels should be decreased toward the end of lengthy procedures.

Equipment

Inhalant anesthetics are delivered by agent-specific vaporizers using oxygen or a mix of oxygen and nitrous oxide as the carrier gas. Standard anesthetic machines fitted with nonrebreathing (Bain's) or circle systems are used, and for smaller specimens, laboratory animal equipment has great potential. Commercially available small animal face masks, as well as masks home made from plastic bottles or syringe cases work well.

Due to low metabolic rates, oxygen consumption is low (<1 mL/kg/min, Perry 1989), and flowrates may be reduced considerably compared with mammalian settings. In practice, the flow rate is often determined by the performance of flow meters and vaporizers and rates of 250–1000 mL/min will be appropriate for most reptiles.

Induction

Unlike chelonians, where inductions may be prohibitively prolonged, mask induction is feasible in lizards and snakes (Fig. 21.2). Animals may also be induced in chambers or plastic bags filled from a vaporizer at maximal setting, or simply by adding a small volume of the concentrated agent on a piece of cotton wool (e.g., approximately 1 mL isoflurane/L chamber volume). With the latter approach, close attention should be

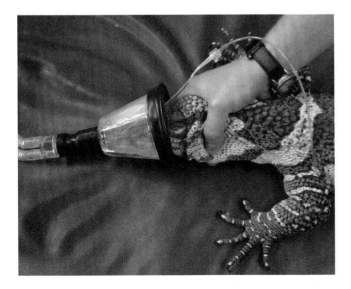

Figure 21.2. Mask induction of a monitor lizard with isoflurane. Note the use of a standard small animal face mask.

kept, as inductions may be quite rapid, and toxic levels could be reached if animals are left too long.

INHALATION ANESTHETICS

Early Inhalants

One of the first reports of anesthesia in reptiles is of John Tait describing the surgical removal of venom glands from rattlesnakes under chloroform anesthesia (Tait 1938). Later, prolonged induction and recovery periods were described in several snake species anesthetized with methoxyflurane (Burke & Wall 1970; Gandal 1966). There are no recent reports on the use of either agent, and the drugs have long been superseded by newer agents.

Ether anesthesia is associated with very long induction (40–60 minutes) and recovery periods in lizards and snakes (Bonath & Zschege 1979; Brazenor & Kaye 1953), and while still occasionally used in physiological research and venom production, the agent must be considered obsolete in a clinical setting. It is also flammable and potentially explosive and, therefore, a hazardous chemical to store and use.

Halothane

Halothane delivered at 3–6% results in moderate sedation to profound anesthesia in lizards and snakes. At halothane concentrations of 5.8% the mean induction time at 22–25°C has been reported to be 24 minutes in lizards ($n = 38$), and 35.3 minutes in snakes ($n = 12$) (Bonath 1977, 1979; Bonath & Zschege 1979). Shorter induction times (5–19 minutes) were reported using 5% halothane in a 3:1 nitrous oxide/oxygen mixture (Custer & Bush 1980). A transient initial excitement stage has been described in rattlesnakes at very high doses (Hackenbrock & Finster 1963).

In snakes, halothane significantly decreases respiration rate and tidal volume (Bonath 1977, 1979; Bonath & Zschege 1979; Custer & Bush 1980), leading to respiratory acidemia (Custer & Bush 1980), while heart rate decreases mildly or remains unchanged (Bonath 1977, 1979; Bonath & Zschege 1979; Custer & Bush 1980).

Recovery times following brief anesthetic events are relatively short (24–35 minutes), while recovery times from deeper anesthesia are reported to be much longer (Bonath 1977, 1979; Bonath & Zschege 1979).

No information exists on the potency of halothane in reptiles, and data on cardiopulmonary function during halothane anesthesia is limited to that described earlier. Halothane continues to be used in physiological research, but in the clinical setting has been replaced by isoflurane and sevoflurane.

Isoflurane

Isoflurane is used extensively in reptiles. In lizards, the time to initial relaxation and loss of righting reflex breathing 5% is typically 4–9 minutes (Hernandez-Divers et al. 2005; Mauthe von Degerfeld 2004; Schildger et al. 1993; Spelman et al. 1996), while the time to complete relaxation is 13–20 minutes depending on the species (Bertelsen et al. 2005b; Mosley 2000). In snakes, induction times with mask induction tend to be slightly longer (Schildger et al. 1993), but direct intubation of the awake snake followed by mechanical ventilation with the drug leads to rapid induction. As mentioned, faster inductions may be achieved using higher inspired concentrations by adding isoflurane directly to the induction chamber.

Isoflurane causes a moderate (approximately 25%) reduction in heart rate (Hernandez-Divers et al. 2005; Maas & Brunson 2002) and a severe reduction in respiratory rate (Maas & Brunson 2002) compared with values in manually restrained animals. It should be considered, however, that values in manually restrained subjects are significantly higher than in undisturbed animals (Bertelsen et al. 2005b). During anesthesia, a dose-dependent reduction in systemic blood pressure is observed (Chinnadurai et al. 2010; Mosley et al. 2004). At low concentrations animals continue breathing (Spelman et al. 1996), but at levels adequate for surgical anesthesia mechanical ventilation is usually necessary.

The minimum alveolar concentration at 30–35°C has been reported to be $1.9 \pm 0.59\%$ in rat snakes (Maas & Brunson 2002), $1.8 \pm 0.3\%$ to $2.1 \pm 0.6\%$ in iguanas (Barter et al. 2006; Mosley et al. 2003a), and $1.54 \pm 0.17\%$ in monitors (Bertelsen et al. 2005c), indicating that vaporizer settings of 2–2.5% will be appropriate to maintain surgical anesthesia in most subjects. As a likely consequence of R-L intracardiac shunting at the beginning of anesthesia, MAC decreases over time in iguanas (Barter et al. 2006), indicating that inhaled gas levels should be decreased toward the end of lengthy procedures. The MAC decreases with decreasing body temperature (Dohm & Brunson 1998). In an attempt to determine the cardiac anesthetic index, seven iguanas were subjected to up to 9.2% isoflurane without any apparent signs of cardiac arrest, suggesting a very wide margin of safety (Mosley et al. 2003b).

Recovery time depends on the depth and duration of anesthesia, and is relatively short (2–12 minutes), following brief, shallow anesthetic events (Schildger et al. 1993; Spelman et al. 1996), intermediate (30–40 minutes) following light surgical anesthesia, and more prolonged (50–70 minutes) following deep anesthesia (Bertelsen et al. 2005b; Mosley 2000). In general, recovery times appear longer and more variable in snakes than in lizards.

Sevoflurane

Induction times using sevoflurane are slightly shorter than with isoflurane (Bertelsen et al. 2005b; Hernandez-Divers et al. 2005). In lizards induced with 8%, the time

to initial relaxation and loss of righting reflex is around 6 minutes (Hernandez-Divers et al. 2005) while the time to complete relaxation is approximately 11 minutes (Bertelsen et al. 2005b). As for isoflurane, direct intubation of the awake animal followed by mechanical ventilation with the drug leads to rapid induction. The addition of 66% nitrous oxide will speed up inductions slightly (Bertelsen et al. 2005b).

Sevoflurane induction has been subjectively judged as smoother and associated with less breath holding than with isoflurane (Hernandez-Divers et al. 2005), but the respiratory rate during induction appears to be similar or even marginally lower with sevoflurane (Bertelsen et al. 2005b). Sevoflurane causes a moderate reduction in heart rate (Hernandez-Divers et al. 2005; Maas & Brunson 2002) and a severe reduction in respiratory rate (Maas & Brunson 2002) compared with values in manually restrained animals. The hemodynamic effects of sevoflurane in iguanas are similar to those with isoflurane (Barter et al. 2006).

The minimum alveolar concentration at 30–35°C has been reported to be $2.42 \pm 0.57\%$ in rat snakes (Maas & Brunson 2002), $2.51 \pm 0.46\%$ in monitor lizards (Bertelsen et al. 2005a), and $3.1 \pm 1.0\%$ in iguanas (Barter et al. 2006), indicating that vaporizer settings of 3–3.5% will be appropriate to maintain surgical anesthesia in most subjects. In a study of monitor lizards, the coadministration of 66% nitrous oxide resulted in a 25% reduction in sevoflurane MAC (Bertelsen et al. 2005a), and similar reductions are likely to occur in other species and with other inhalants.

With the modern inhalant anesthetics, the length of the recovery period appears to be influenced more by the duration and depth of anesthesia (and the extent of intracardiac shunting) than by the agent used (Brosnan et al. 2006). After short time, relatively superficial anesthesia sevoflurane will result in faster recoveries than isoflurane (Hernandez-Divers et al. 2005), but following prolonged, deep anesthesia, that difference is marginal (Bertelsen et al. 2005b).

Desflurane

Desflurane is the least soluble of the volatile anesthetics, and thus theoretically has the fastest inductions and recoveries. However, it may cause airway irritability, requires specialized heated vaporizers, and is rarely used in veterinary practice. The minimum alveolar concentration at 34–35°C has been reported to be $8.9 \pm 2.1\%$ in iguanas, with hemodynamic effects being similar to those of isoflurane and sevoflurane (Barter et al. 2006).

Nitrous Oxide

Nitrous oxide (N_2O) may be used as a supplemental anesthetic (at 50–66% with oxygen) during induction with inhalational agents (Bennett et al. 1999; Custer & Bush 1980), resulting in marginally shorter induction times (Bertelsen et al. 2005b). In monitor lizards, 66% N_2O delivered with sevoflurane reduced the sevoflurane requirement (MAC) with 25% (Bertelsen et al. 2005a). Assuming that a relationship of simple linear additivity between sevoflurane and nitrous oxide exists, the MAC for N_2O in varanids can be estimated to be 244%. Apart from reducing the concentration of the primary agent which may improve cardiopulmonary function, the use of N_2O likely provides improved analgesia over delivery in 100% oxygen.

Carbon Dioxide

Carbon dioxide (CO_2) is occasionally used for the immobilization of venomous snakes during venom extraction (Wang et al. 1993). Unconsciousness is thought to be mediated through central nervous system acidosis, and this procedure is not recommended in clinical practice. A mixture of 3–5% CO_2 in oxygen may be used during mechanical ventilation to achieve high oxygenation and delivery of inhalational agents while avoiding the respiratory acidemia seen during hyperventilation (T. Wang, pers. comm.), and the use of a 10% CO_2 mixture has been suggested to stimulate respiration during recovery (Malley 1997).

PARENTERAL ANESTHESIA

Numerous injectable anesthetics have been used in snakes and lizards with varying success. These include etorphine hydrochloride (Hinsch & Gandal 1969; Wallach & Hoessle 1970), pentobarbital sodium (Arena et al. 1988; Betz 1962; Karlstrom & Cook 1955), thiopental sodium (Karlstrom & Cook 1955), methohexital (Preston et al. 2010; Wang et al. 1977), MS-222 (Green & Precious 1978; Karlstrom & Cook 1955), urethane (Calderwood 1971), nicotine (Calderwood 1971), decamethonium iodide (Brazenor & Kaye 1953), tubocuraine chloride (Brazenor & Kaye 1953), and procaine hydrochloride (Livezey 1957). While still occasionally used in experimental settings, these agents must be considered obsolete in clinical practice.

Propofol

Provided vascular access can be gained, propofol is this author's agent of choice for anesthetic induction. Administered intravenously or intraosseously at dosages of 5–10 mg/kg, propofol will cause induction in 1–5 minutes (Anderson et al. 1999; Bennett et al. 1998; McFadden et al. 2011). Propofol administered perivascularly is ineffective, but unlike barbiturates does not cause tissue damage. Administration via the ventral tail vessels is generally feasible in patients larger than 250 g, although there are significant species differences.

In lizards and snakes, propofol causes a slight decrease in heart rate and a marked respiratory depression (Anderson et al. 1999; Bennett et al. 1998). The respiratory depression is dose dependent and appears to be affected by the duration of administration; low doses given slowly cause less apnea than high doses administered as a bolus.

The duration of anesthesia depends on the dosage; 5 mg/kg results in 20–30 minutes of anesthesia, while longer recovery times are seen following 10 mg/kg dosage. Anesthesia may be maintained by inhalation or by continuous propofol infusion. An infusion rate of 0.5 mg/kg/min proved excessive in green iguanas (Bennett et al. 1998), and rates of 0.2–0.4 mg/kg/min are likely more appropriate.

For most species, a dose of 5–10 mg/kg given slowly is appropriate for short procedures or as induction for inhalational anesthesia.

Alphaxalone

The steroid anesthetic alfaxalone is highly insoluble in water and historically was formulated in combination with alphadalone and the solubilizing agent cremaphor. This drug found some use in reptiles (Calderwood & Jacobson 1979; Lawrence & Jackson 1983), but its use was discontinued as cremaphor was associated with allergic reactions in domestic animals. More recently, alfaxalone has been solubilized with 2-hydroxypropylbeta-cyclodextrin (Estes et al. 1990). When given IV, this formulation has much the same effects as propofol. In veiled chameleons, a surgical plane of anesthesia lasting for 5–10 minutes was achieved 2 minutes following 5 mg/kg IV (Knotec et al. 2011a). In green iguanas, 5 mg/kg IV resulted in about 15 minutes of anesthesia with minimal effect on heart rate and respiratory rate (Knotec et al. 2011b). Interestingly, unlike propofol, alfaxalone is effective when administered intramuscularly at higher dosages. In iguanas, 10 mg/kg provides light sedation, 20 mg mg/kg provides a level suitable for minor procedures or for endotracheal intubation and supplementation with inhalational anesthesia, and 30 mg/kg provides an anesthetic plane suitable for surgical procedures of limited duration (up to 40 minutes) (Bertelsen & Sauer 2011). In iguanas, there is an initial dose-dependent depression of respiration followed by a significant increase in frequency over time (Bertelsen & Sauer 2011). In accordance to principles of metabolic scaling, smaller individuals require higher dosages. In an unpublished study in leopard geckos, 30–40 mg/kg of alfaxalone IM was required for heavy sedation, and 50 mg/kg IM is likely required for a surgical level. Unfortunately, at these dosages the low concentration of the commercially available formulation requires clinically excessive IM injection volumes.

Ketamine

Ketamine hydrochloride has been used extensively in reptiles, primarily snakes, since its discovery in the late 1960s (Glenn et al. 1972; Schumacher et al. 1997).

The effective dosage depends on the body temperature (Arena et al. 1988); at lower body temperatures, lower doses are required, but longer induction and recovery times are observed (Arena et al. 1988; Green et al. 1981). Effects are highly species dependent (Arena et al. 1988; Cooper 1974; Hill & Macklessy 1997; Ogunranti 1987; Schildger et al. 1993), but large individual variation is also observed (Cooper 1974; Hill & Macklessy 1997).

Recommended dosages range from 12–44 mg/kg for sedation (Bennett 1998; Glenn et al. 1972; Schildger et al. 1993; Spelman et al. 1996) to 55–88 mg/kg for surgical anesthesia (Bennett 1998; Glenn et al. 1972; Schildger et al. 1993). Even higher dosages (100–220 mg/kg) are occasionally reported (Arena et al. 1988; Harding 1977). The time to peak effect following intramuscular injection is approximately 30 minutes (Cooper 1974; Custer & Bush 1980; Glenn et al. 1972; Green et al. 1981).

In snakes and lizards, moderate ketamine dosages are associated with increased heart rates (Arena et al. 1988; Schumacher et al. 1997), hypertension (Schumacher et al. 1997), and respiratory depression (Arena et al. 1988; Ogunranti 1987; Schumacher et al. 1997), the latter peaking at 30–60 minutes (Arena et al. 1988; Ogunranti 1987). At increasing dosages, the drug will induce apnea, bradycardia (Cooper 1974; Custer & Bush 1980; Glenn et al. 1972; Green et al. 1981), and eventually death.

The main problem with ketamine anesthesia in reptiles is the extended recovery periods. Reported recovery times range from 6–24 hours at 15 mg/kg (Hill & Macklessy 1997) to 2–3 days at 40–80 mg/kg (Custer & Bush 1980; Glenn et al. 1972; Green et al. 1981) and 6–7 days at 100–130 mg/kg (Glenn et al. 1972).

Ketamine may be combined with sedatives, such as benzodiazepines and alpha-2-agonists, for better muscle relaxation, a reduction in required dose, and shorter recovery times (Bennett 1998; Heard 2001; Malley 1997). Due to the variable effects, long recovery periods and the availability of alternative protocols, the author rarely uses the dissociative agents.

Zolazepam-Tiletamine

The potent cyclohexamine tiletamine combined with the benzodiazepine zolazepam has found some use in reptile anesthesia (Boever & Caputo 1982; Gray et al. 1974; Read 2004), but very little published information exists. The onset of effects is faster than with ketamine (Mauthe von Degerfeld 2004), while cardiopulmonary effects are likely similar to those produced by ketamine. In early studies, dosages of 30–40 mg/kg administered to iguanas resulted in surgical anesthesia lasting 8–16 hours, while variable effects were seen with doses of up to 88 mg/kg in snakes (Boever & Caputo 1982). In Komodo dragons, dosages of 5.5 mg/kg caused repetitive head and neck movements 10–25 minutes before resulting in sedation (Spelman et al. 1996). In iguanas,

10 mg/kg resulted in a brief period of excitement followed by good relaxation (Mauthe von Degerfeld 2004). Despite its long duration of action and variable effects, low doses (2–5 mg/kg) may be useful for sedation prior to handling or intubation, particularly of larger animals.

Sedatives

Sedative and tranquilizing drugs such as benzodiazepines and alpha 2-agonists may be used in squamates, but studies to document their effects are lacking. Because of the difficulty in accessing the vascular system and airways in chelonians, there has been much more focus on the use of these drugs in turtles and tortoises, and as results may likely be extrapolated to snakes and lizards.

OTHER TECHNIQUES

Hypothermia, once used as a means of immobilizing reptiles (Calderwood 1971; Kaplan 1969), is considered an unacceptable clinical practice, as is electroanesthesia (Northway 1968).

RECOVERY

As mentioned earlier, recovery times in reptiles are prolonged compared to birds and mammals. Body temperature critically affects speed and quality of recovery so animals should be kept warm. If mechanical ventilation was used, animals should gradually be weaned off ventilation. The easiest way to do so is by manually ventilating every 1–5 minutes using an Ambu-bag or similar to allow buildup of CO_2. Periods of apnea of 5–10 minutes are unlikely to cause deleterious effects. Since hyperoxia may downregulate respiration in reptiles (Glass & Johansen 1976), and possibly promote R-L shunting, recovery in room air (21% oxygen) as opposed to 100% oxygen may be used. However, while faster recoveries were experienced when ventilating iguanas with 21% oxygen following short-time isoflurane anesthesia (Diethelm & Mader 1999), no difference could be demonstrated following longer anesthetic events (Bertelsen et al. 2005b).

COMPLICATIONS

Complications are relatively rare using the protocols suggested, but respiratory depression or apnea and prolonged recoveries are among those most commonly encountered (Read 2004). These problems may be reduced by providing adequate mechanical ventilation and by maintaining body temperature within physiological limits.

ANALGESIA

Since the first edition of this book, more attention has been given to pain perception and modulation in reptiles (Mosley 2011). Despite these efforts, reptilian analgesia is still an obscure subject, and solid recommendations are hard to give.

In anoles, the administration of the μ-receptor opioid morphine (5 mg/kg IM) caused a latency of the tail-flick response (Mauk et al. 1981). Similarly, morphine (10–20 mg/kg) increased thermal withdrawal latency in red-eared sliders (Sladky et al. 2007) and bearded dragons (Sladky et al. 2008), but appears to be ineffective in corn snakes at dosages up to 40 mg/kg (Sladky et al. 2008). Morphine is associated with severe respiratory depression, but another μ-receptor opioid tramadol appears to have similar effects on thermal withdrawal latency (10–15 mg/kg PO, SC) in turtles with much less respiratory depression (Baker et al. 2011). Similarly, another μ-receptor opioid hydromorphone (0.5 mg/kg IM) increased thermal withdrawal time in sliders (Mans et al. 2012). In contrast, the predominant κ-receptor opioid butorphanol (20 mg/kg SC) was ineffective in bearded dragons and sliders, but effectively increased thermal withdrawal latency in corn snakes (Sladky et al. 2007, 2008). Accordingly in iguanas, butorphanol (1 mg/kg IM) failed to decrease the minimum anesthetic dose of isoflurane (Mosley et al. 2003a), and did not provide demonstrable analgesia in a heat pad test (Fleming & Robertson 2012). These differences are likely associated with species differences in expression of the different classes of opioid receptors (Sladky et al. 2009), making extrapolation to other species very difficult. In contrast, nonsteroidal anti-inflammatory drugs would be expected to behave much the same across species, and although the role of the cyclooxygenase system in reptiles has not been studied, clinical evidence supports the efficacy of nonsteroidal anti-inflammatory drugs (NSAIDs) in reptiles (Hernandez-Divers 2006), and they appear widely used (Read 2004). A pharmacokinetic trial of meloxicam in iguanas showed excellent bioavailability following PO administration, and suggested administration of meloxicam at a dose of 0.2 mg/kg IV or PO results in plasma concentrations >0.1 μg/mL for approximately 24 hours (Divers et al. 2010). Further, daily administration of high doses (1 or 5 mg/kg) for 12 days did not induce any histologic changes in gastric, hepatic, or renal tissues (Divers et al. 2010). Similarly, daily administration of meloxicam (0.2 mg/kg IM for 10 days) in iguanas failed to demonstrate any significant clinical, biochemical or hematological abnormalities (Trnkova et al. 2007). In an attempt to evaluate the effect of meloxicam (0.3 mg/kg IM) and butorphanol (5 mg/kg IM), the postoperative physiological stress response in ball pythons was evaluated, failing to demonstrate an effect of any drug (Olesen et al. 2008). However, even in the saline-treated control group, there was only minimal measurable physiological response to surgery, questioning the validity of the model.

Despite the lack of documentation, analgesics should be part of any anesthetic regimen that involves potentially painful procedures. Opioids and NSAIDs are the most relevant candidates for successful treatment, and suggested dosages of selected drugs are given in Table 21.1.

As in any species, preemptive analgesia offers intraoperative as well as postoperative analgesia, and likely will reduce the amount of anesthetic needed. Local analgesics (e.g., lidocaine) are commonly used in reptiles. In small subjects, diluting the drugs (e.g., 1 : 10 in sterile water) prior to administration will help to avoid overdosing.

SELECTED PROTOCOLS

For most snakes and lizards, the author recommends one of three approaches (Table 21.2): induction with propofol (5–10 mg/kg, IV) or alfaxalone (5 mg/kg, IV; 20–30 mg/kg, IM) followed by isoflurane or sevoflurane anesthesia for longer duration; mask or chamber induction with isoflurane or sevoflurane; or direct

Table 21.1. Selected anesthetic, sedative and analgesic drugs used in snakes and lizards

Generic Name	Dosage (mg/kg)	Reversal Agent	Reference
Propofol	5–10	None	Anderson et al. (1999); Bennett et al. (1998); McFadden et al. (2011)
Alfaxalone	5–10 IV 20–40 IM	None	Knotec et al. (2011a, 2011b) Bertelsen and Sauer (2011)
Midazolam	1–2	Flumazenil	
Medetomidine	0.05–0.15	Atipamezole	
Ketamine	10–40[a]	None	Custer and Bush (1980); Glenn et al. (1972); Schumacher et al. (1997)
Zolazepam-Tiletamine	2–10	Flumazenil for zolazepam	Mauthe von Degerfeld (2004)
Meloxicam	0.1–0.3	None	Divers et al. (2010); Hernandez-Divers (2006)
Morphine[b]	10–15	Naltrexone, naloxone	Sladky et al. (2008)
Tramadol[b]	10–15	Naltrexone, naloxone	Baker et al. (2011)
Butorphanol[c]	0.5–2	Naltrexone, naloxone	Sladky et al. (2008)

[a]Dosages up to 220 mg/kg have been reported (Arena et al. 1988).
[b]In lizards.
[c]In snakes.

Table 21.2. Recommended anesthetic protocols for snakes and lizards

	Pre-Medication	Induction	Maintenance
Small snake	None	Propofol 5–10 mg/kg, IV Chamber induction with isoflurane or sevoflurane	Isoflurane or sevoflurane by endotracheal tube
Large snake	None or Alfaxalone 10 mg/kg, IM or Telazol 5–10 mg/kg, IM	Propofol 2–7 mg/kg, IV Direct intubation[a] followed by ventilation with isoflurane or sevoflurane Chamber-induction with isoflurane or sevoflurane	Isoflurane or sevoflurane by endotracheal tube
Venomous snake	None	Propofol 5–10 mg/kg, IV[b] Chamber-induction with isoflurane or sevoflurane	Isoflurane or sevoflurane by endotracheal tube
Small lizard	None	Propofol 5–10 mg/kg, IV Alfaxalone 20–40 mg/kg, IM Chamber-induction with isoflurane or sevoflurane	Isoflurane or sevoflurane by endotracheal tube
Large lizard	None or Telazol 5–10 mg/kg	Propofol 3–10 mg/kg, IV Mask with isoflurane or sevoflurane	Isoflurane or sevoflurane by endotracheal tube

Note: Please refer to chapter for details.
[a]Desentization of the glottis with a drop or spray of local analgesic recommended.
[b]If properly restrained.

intubation and induction with isoflurane or sevoflurane. For large and aggressive specimens, injection with low doses of ketamine (e.g., 5 mg/kg, IM) or tiletamine/zolazepam (e.g., 3 mg/kg, IM), with or without medetomidine (e.g., 100 µg/kg, IM) or midazolam (e.g., 1 mg/kg, IM), may be used to allow safe handling. Dosages of commonly used drugs are presented in Table 21.1.

FIELD TECHNIQUES

For field work, when equipment must be kept to a minimum, the protocols using parenteral drugs are recommended. Depending on the size of the animal and the invasiveness of the procedure, intramuscular alfaxalone (10–40 mg/kg) or intravenous propofol (5–10 mg/kg) may be employed. Liquid isoflurane or sevoflurane administred directly into a small airtight container or plastic bag containing the animal is another straight forward means of induction even in the field, but care should be taken to ensure effective breathing of the animals once removed from the container.

REFERENCES

Abe A, Johansen K. 1987. Gas exchange and ventilatory responses to hypoxia and hypercapnia in *Amphisbaena alba* (Reptilia: Amphisbaenia). *The Journal of Experimental Biology* 127: 159–172.

Andersen JB, Rourke BC, Caiozzo VJ, Bennett AF, Hicks JW. 2005. Physiology: postprandial cardiac hypertrophy in pythons. *Nature* 434:37–38.

Anderson N, Wack R, Calloway L, Hetherington T, Williams J. 1999. Cardiopulmonary effects and efficacy of propofol as an anesthetic agent in brown tree snakes, *Boiga irregularis*. *Bulletin of the Association of Reptile and Amphibian Veterinarians* 9:9–15.

Arena P, Richardson K, Cullen L. 1988. Anaesthesia in two species of large Australian skink. *The Veterinary Record* 123:155–158.

Baker BB, Sladky KK, Johnson SM. 2011. Evaluation of the analgesic effects of oral and subcutaneous tramadol administration in red-eared slider turtles. *Journal of the American Veterinary Medical Association* 238:220–227.

Barter LS, Hawkins MG, Brosnan RJ, Antognini JF, Pypendop BH. 2006. Median effective dose of isoflurane, sevoflurane, and desflurane in green iguanas. *American Journal of Veterinary Research* 67:392–397.

Belkin D. 1963. Anoxia: tolerance in reptiles. *Science* 139: 492–493.

Belkin D. 1968. Aquatic respiration and underwater survival of two freshwater turtle species. *Respiration Physiology* 4:1–14.

Bennett R. 1998. Reptile anesthesia. *Seminars in Avian and Exotic Pet Medicine* 7:30–40.

Bennett R, Schumacher J, Hedjazi-Haring K, Newell S. 1998. Cardiopulmonary and anesthetic effects of propofol administered intraosseously to green iguanas. *Journal of the American Veterinary Medical Association* 212:93–98.

Bennett R, Divers S, Schumacher J, Wimsatt J, Gaynor J, Stahl S. 1999. Anesthesia: roundtable. *Bulletin of the Association of Reptile and Amphibian Veterinarians* 9:20–27.

Bertelsen MF, Sauer CD. 2011. Alfaxalone anaesthesia in the green iguana (*Iguana iguana*). *Veterinary Anaesthesia and Analgesia* 38:461–466.

Bertelsen MF, Mosley CA, Crawshaw GJ, Dyson DH, Smith DA. 2005a. Anesthetic potency of sevoflurane with and without nitrous oxide in mechanically ventilated Dumeril monitors. *Journal of the American Veterinary Medical Association* 227: 575–578.

Bertelsen MF, Mosley CA, Crawshaw GJ, Dyson D, Smith DA. 2005b. Inhalation anesthesia in Dumeril's monitor (*Varanus dumerili*) with isoflurane, sevoflurane and nitrous oxide: effects of inspired gasses in induction and recovery. *Journal of Zoo and Wildlife Medicine* 36:62–68.

Bertelsen MF, Mosley CA, Crawshaw GJ, Dyson D, Smith DA. 2005c. Minimum alveolar concentration of isoflurane in mechanically ventilated Dumeril monitors. *Journal of the American Veterinary Medical Association* 226:1098–1101.

Betz T. 1962. Surgical anesthesia in reptiles, with special reference to the water snake, *Natrix rhimbifera*. *Copeia*:284–287.

Bickler P. 1992. Effects of temperature and anoxia on regional cerebral blood flow in turtles. *The American Journal of Physiology* 262:R538–R541.

Boever W, Caputo F. 1982. Telazol (CI 744) as an anesthetic agent in reptiles. *Journal of Zoo Animal Medicine* 13:59–61.

Bonath K. 1977. Narkose der Reptilien. In: *Narkose der Reptilien, Amphibien und Fische.* (K Bonath, ed.), pp. 9–62. Berlin: Verlag Paul Parey.

Bonath K. 1979. Halothane inhalation anaesthesia in reptiles and its clinical control. *International Zoo Yearbook* 19:112–125.

Bonath K, Zschege C. 1979. Experimentelle Untersuchungen zur klinischen Anwendung und Überwachung der Inhalationsnarkose bei Reptilien. *Zentralblatt für Veterinärmedizin [A]* 26:341–372.

Brazenor C, Kaye G. 1953. Anesthesia for reptiles. *Copeia:* 165–170.

Brosnan RJ, Pypendop BH, Barter LS, Hawkins MG. 2006. Pharmacokinetics of inhaled anesthetics in green iguanas (*Iguana iguana*). *American Journal of Veterinary Research* 67:1670–1674.

Burggren W, Johansen K. 1982. Ventricular haemodynamics in the monitor lizard *Varanus exanthematicus*: pulmonary and systemic pressure separation. *The Journal of Experimental Biology* 96:343–354.

Burggren W, Shelton G. 1979. Gas exchange and transport during intermittent breathing in chelonian reptiles. *The Journal of Experimental Biology* 82:75–92.

Burke T, Wall B. 1970. Anesthetic deaths in cobras (*Naja naja* and *Ophidophagus hannah*) with methoxyflurane. *Journal of the American Veterinary Medical Association* 157:620–621.

Calderwood H. 1971. Anesthesia for reptiles. *Journal of the American Veterinary Medical Association* 159:1618–1625.

Calderwood H, Jacobson E. 1979. Preliminary report on the use of saffan on reptiles. American Association of Zoo Veterinarians Annual Proceedings, pp. 23–26.

Chinnadurai SK, Wrenn A, DeVoe RS. 2009. Evaluation of noninvasive oscillometric blood pressure monitoring in anesthetized boid snakes. *Journal of the American Veterinary Medical Association* 234:625–630.

Chinnadurai SK, DeVoe R, Koenig A, Gadsen N, Ardente A, Divers SJ. 2010. Comparison of an implantable telemetry device and an oscillometric monitor for measurement of blood pressure in anaesthetized and unrestrained green iguanas (*Iguana iguana*). *Veterinary Anaesthesia and Analgesia* 37:434–439.

Cooper J. 1974. Ketamine hydrochloride as an anesthetic for East African reptiles. *The Veterinary Record* 95:37–41.

Custer R, Bush M. 1980. Physiologic and acid-base measures of gopher snakes during ketamine or halothane-nitrous oxide anesthesia. *Journal of the American Veterinary Medical Association* 177:870–874.

Davies P. 1981. Anatomy and physiology. In: *Diseases of Reptilia* (J Cooper, O Jackson, eds.), pp. 9–73. New York: Academic Press.

Diethelm G, Mader D. 1999. The effects of FIO2 on post anesthetic recovery times in the green iguana. Proceedings of the Association of Reptile and Amphibian Veterinarians, pp. 169–170.

Diethelm G, Mader D, Grosenbaugh D, Muir W. 1998. Evaluating pulse oximetry in the green iguana, *Iguana iguana.* Proceedings of the Association of Reptile and Amphibian Veterinarians. pp. 11–12.

Divers SJ, Papich M, McBride M, Stedman NL, Perpinan D, Koch TF, Hernandez SM, Barron GH, Pethel M, Budsberg SC. 2010. Pharmacokinetics of meloxicam following intravenous and oral administration in green iguanas (*Iguana iguana*). *American Journal of Veterinary Research* 71:1277–1283.

Dohm L, Brunson D. 1998. Effective dose of isoflurane for the desert iguana (*Diposaurus dorsalis*) and the effect of hypothermia on effective dose. Proceedings of the American College of Veterinary Anesthetists, p. 543.

Estes KS, Brewster ME, Webb AI, Bodor N. 1990. A non-surfactant formulation for alfaxalone based on an amorphous cyclodextrin: activity in rats and dogs. *International Journal of Pharmaceutics* 65:101–107.

Fleming GJ, Robertson SA. 2012. Assessments of thermal antinociceptive effects of butorphanol and human observer effect on quantitative evaluation of analgesia in green iguanas (*Iguana iguana*). *American Journal of Veterinary Research* 73:1507–1511.

Gandal C. 1966. A practical anesthetic technique in snakes, utilizing methoxyflurane. *Journal of the American Animal Hospital Association* 4:258–260.

Glass M, Johansen K. 1976. Control of breathing in *Acrochordus javanicus*, an aquatic snake. *Physiological Zoology* 49:328–340.

Glass M, Wood S. 1983. Gas exchange and control of breathing in reptiles. *Physiological Reviews* 63:232–260.

Glenn J, Straight R, Snyder C. 1972. Clinical use of ketamine hydrochloride as an anesthetic agent for snakes. *American Journal of Veterinary Research* 33:1901–1903.

Gray C, Bush M, Beck C. 1974. Clinical experience using CI-744 in chemical restraint and anesthesia of exotic specimens. *Journal of Zoo Animal Medicine* 5:12–21.

Green C, Precious S. 1978. Reptilian anaesthesia. *The Veterinary Record* 102:110.

Green C, Knight J, Precious S, Simpkin S. 1981. Ketamine alone and combined with diazepam or xylazine in laboratory animals: a 10 year experience. *Laboratory Animals* 15:163–170.

Hackenbrock C, Finster M. 1963. Fluothane: a rapid and safe inhalation anesthetic for poisonous snakes. *Copeia:*440–441.

Harding K. 1977. The use of ketamine anaesthesia to milk two tropical rattlesnakes (*Crotalus durissus terrificus*). *The Veterinary Record* 100:289–290.

Heard D. 2001. Reptile anesthesia. *The Veterinary Clinics of North America. Exotic Animal Practice* 4:83–117.

Heisler N, Glass M. 1985. Mechanisms and regulation of central vascular shunts in reptiles. In: *Cardiovascular Shunts: Phylogenetic, Ontogenetic, and Clinical Aspects* (K Johansen, W Burggren, eds.), pp. 334–353. Copenhagen: Munksgaard.

Heisler N, Neumann P, Maloiy G. 1983. The mechanism of intracardiac shunting in the lizard *Varanus exanthematicus. The Journal of Experimental Biology* 105:15–31.

Hernandez-Divers SJ. 2006. Meloxican and reptiles: a practical approach to analgesia. Proceedings of the North American Veterinary Conference, pp. 1637–1637.

Hernandez-Divers SM, Schumacher J, Stahl S, Hernandez-Divers SJ. 2005. Comparison of isoflurane and sevoflurane anesthesia after premedication with butorphanol in the green iguana (*Iguana iguana*). *Journal of Zoo and Wildlife Medicine* 36: 169–175.

Hicks J, Comeau S. 1994. Vagal regulation of intracardiac shunting in the turtle *Pseudemys scritpa. The Journal of Experimental Biology* 186:109–126.

Hicks J, Farrell A. 2000. The cardiovascular responses of the redeared slider (*Trachemys scripta*) acclimated to either 22 or 5 degrees celcius. *The Journal of Experimental Zoology* 203: 3765–3774.

Hicks J, Krosniunas E. 1996. Physiological states and intracardiac shunting in non-crocodilian reptiles. *Experimental Biology Online* 1:1–12.

Hill R, Macklessy S. 1997. Venom yields from several species of colubrid snakes and differential effects of ketamine. *Toxicon* 35:671–678.

Hinsch H, Gandal C. 1969. The effects of etorphine (M-99), oxymorphone hydrochloride and meperidine hydrochloride in reptiles. *Copeia:*404–405.

Hlastala M, Standaert D, Pierson D, Luchtel D. 1985. The matching of ventilation and perfusion in the lung of the tegu lizard, *Tupinambis nigropunctatus. Respiration Physiology* 60:277–294.

Hopkins S, Wang T, Hicks J. 1996. The effect of altering pulmonary blood flow on pulmonary gas exchange in the turtle *Trachemys (Pseudemys) scripta*. *The Journal of Experimental Biology* 199:2207–2214.

Isaza R, Andrews G, Coke R, Hunter R. 2004. Assessment of multiple cardiocentesis in ball pythons (*Python regius*). *Contemporary Topics in Laboratory Animal Science* 43:35–38.

Kaplan H. 1969. Anesthesia in amphibians and reptiles. *Federation Proceedings* 28:1541–1546.

Kardong K. 1972a. Morphology of the respiratory system and its musculature in different snake genera. I. Crotalus and Elaphe. *Gegenbaurs Morphologishe Jahrbuch* 117:285–302.

Kardong K. 1972b. Morphology of the respiratory system and its musculature in different snake genera. II. *Charina bottae*. *Gegenbaurs Morphologishe Jahrbuch* 117:364–376.

Karlstrom E, Cook S. 1955. Notes on snake anesthesia. *Copeia*: 57–58.

Knotec Z, Hrda A, Kley N, Knotkova Z. 2011a. Alfaxalon anesthesia in veiled chameleon (*Chameleo calyptratus*). Proceedings of the American Association of Reptile and Amphibian Veterinarians, pp. 179–181.

Knotec Z, Hrda A, Trnkova S. 2011b. Alfaxalon anesthesia in green iguanas (*Iguana iguana*). Proceedings of the Annual Meeting of the European College of Zoological Medicine, 68.

Lawrence K, Jackson O. 1983. Alphaxalone/alphadolone anaesthesia in reptiles. *The Veterinary Record* 112:26–28.

Livezey RL. 1957. Procaine hydrochloride as a killing agent for reptiles and amphibians. *Herpetologia* 13:280.

Maas A, Brunson D. 2002. Comparison of anesthetic potency and cardiopulmonary effects of isoflurane and sevoflurane in colubrid snakes. Proceedings of the American Association of Zoo Veterinarians, pp. 306–308.

Malley D. 1997. Reptile anaesthesia and the practicing veterinarian. *In Practice* 19:351–368.

Mans C, Lahner LL, Baker BB, Johnson SM, Sladky KK. 2012. Antinociceptive efficacy of buprenorphine and hydromorphone in red-eared slider turtles (*Trachemys scripta elegans*). *Journal of Zoo and Wildlife Medicine* 43:662–665.

Mauk MD, Olson RD, LaHoste GJ, Olson GA. 1981. Tonic immobility produces hyperalgesia and antagonizes morphine analgesia. *Science* 213:353–354.

Mauthe von Degerfeld M. 2004. Personal experiences in the use of association tiletamine/zolazepam for anaesthesia of the green iguana (*Iguana iguana*). *Veterinary Research Communications* 28(Suppl. 1):351–353.

McFadden MS, Bennett RA, Reavill DR, Ragetly GR, Clark-Price SC. 2011. Clinical and histologic effects of intracardiac administration of propofol for induction of anesthesia in ball pythons (*Python regius*). *Journal of the American Veterinary Medical Association* 239:803–807.

Mitchell G, Gleeson T, Bennett A. 1981. Pulmonary oxygen transport during activity in lizards. *Respiration Physiology* 43: 365–375.

Moberly W. 1968. The metabolic responses of the common iguana, *Iguana iguana*, to walking and diving. *Comparative Biochemistry and Physiology* 27:21–32.

Mosley C. 2011. Pain and nociception in reptiles. *The Veterinary Clinics of North America. Exotic Animal Practice* 14:45–60.

Mosley CA. 2000. Evaluation of isoflurane and buthorphanol in the green iguana (*Iguana iguana*). MSc Thesis, University of Guelph, Guelph.

Mosley CA, Dyson D, Smith DA. 2003a. Minimum alveolar concentration of isoflurane in green iguanas and the effect of butorphanol on minimum alveolar concentration. *Journal of the American Veterinary Medical Association* 222:1559–1564.

Mosley CA, Dyson D, Smith DA. 2003b. The cardiac anesthetic index of isoflurane in green iguanas. *Journal of the American Veterinary Medical Association* 222:1565–1568.

Mosley CA, Dyson D, Smith DA. 2004. The cardiovascular dose-response effects of isoflurane alone and combined with butorphanol in the green iguana (*Iguana iguana*). *Veterinary Anaesthesia and Analgesia* 31:64–72.

Northway R. 1968. Electroanesthesia of green iguanas (*Iguana iguana*). *Journal of the American Veterinary Medical Association* 155:1034.

Ogunranti J. 1987. Some physiological observations on ketamine hydrochloride anaesthesia in the agamid lizard. *Laboratory Animals* 21:183–187.

Olesen MG, Bertelsen MF, Perry SF, Wang T. 2008. Effects of preoperative administration of butorphanol or meloxicam on physiologic responses to surgery in ball pythons. *Journal of the American Veterinary Medical Association* 233:1883–1888.

Overgaard J, Busk M, Hicks JW, Jensen FB, Wang T. 1999. Respiratory consequences of feeding in the snake *Python molorus*. *Comparative Biochemistry and Physiology. Part A, Molecular and Integrative Physiology* 124:359–365.

Perry S. 1989. Structure and function of the reptilian respiratory system. In: *Lung Biology in Health and Disease. Comparative Pulmonary Physiology. Current Concepts*, Vol. 39 (C Lenfant, S Wood, eds.), pp. 216–217. New York: Marcel Dekker.

Powell FL, Hopkins SR. 2004. Comparative physiology of lung complexity: implications for gas exchange. *News in Physiological Sciences* 19:55–60.

Preston DL, Mosley CAE, Mason RT. 2010. Sources of variability in recovery time from methohexital sodium anesthesia in snakes. *Copeia*:496–501.

Quasha A, Eger EI, Tinker J. 1980. Determination and applications of MAC. *Anesthesiology* 53:315–334.

Read MR. 2004. Evaluation of the use of anesthesia and analgesia in reptiles. *Journal of the American Veterinary Medical Association* 224:547–552.

Schildger B, Baumgartner R, Häfeli W, Rübel A, Isenbügel E. 1993. Narkose und Immobilisation bei Reptilien. *Tierarztliche Praxis* 21:361–376.

Schumacher J, Yelen T. 2005. Anesthesia and analgesia. In: *Reptile Medicine and Surgery*, 2nd ed. (D Mader, ed.), pp. 442–452. Philadelphia: W.B. Sanders-Elsevier.

Schumacher J, Lillywhite H, Norman W, Jacobson E. 1997. Effects of ketamine HCl on cardiopulmonary function in snakes. *Copeia*:395–400.

Secor SM, Diamond J. 1997. Effects of meal size on postprandial responses in juvenile Burmese pythons (*Python molorus*). *The American Journal of Physiology* 272:R902–R912.

Seymour R, Webster M. 1975. Gas transport and acid-base balance in diving sea snakes. *The Journal of Experimental Zoology* 191:169–182.

Shelton G, Burggren W. 1976. Cardiovascular dynamics of the chelonia during apnoea and lung ventilation. *The Journal of Experimental Biology* 64:323–242.

Sladky KK, Miletic V, Paul-Murphy J, Kinney ME, Dallwig RK, Johnson SM. 2007. Analgesic efficacy and respiratory effects of butorphanol and morphine in turtles. *Journal of the American Veterinary Medical Association* 230:1356–1362.

Sladky KK, Kinney ME, Johnson SM. 2008. Analgesic efficacy of butorphanol and morphine in bearded dragons and corn snakes. *Journal of the American Veterinary Medical Association* 233:267–273.

Sladky KK, Kinney ME, Johnson SM. 2009. Effects of opioid receptor activation on thermal antinociception in red-eared slider turtles (*Trachemys scripta*). *American Journal of Veterinary Research* 70:1072–1078.

Spelman L, Cambre R, Walch T, Rosscoe R. 1996. Anesthetic techniques in komodo dragons (*Varanus komodoensis*). Proceedings of the American Association of Zoo Veterinarians, pp. 247–250.

Tait J. 1938. Surgical removal of the poison glands of rattlesnakes. *Copeia*:10–13.

Templeton J, Dawson W. 1963. Respiration in the lizard *Crotaphytus collaris*. *Physiological Zoology* 36:104–121.

Trnkova S, Knotkova Z, Hrda A, Knotek Z. 2007. Effect of non-steroidal anti-inflammatory drugs on the blood profile in the green iguana (*Iguana iguana*). *Veterinarni Medicina* 52: 507–511.

Ultsch G, Jackson D. 1982. Long-term submergence at 3°C of the turtle *Chrymys scripta bellii*, on normoxic and severely hypoxic water. I. Survival, gas exchange and acid-base status. *The Journal of Experimental Biology* 96:11–28.

Wallach J, Hoessle C. 1970. M-99 as an immobilizing agent in poikilothermes. *Veterinary Medicine* 65:163–167.

Wang RT, Kubie JL, Halperm M. 1977. Brevital sodium: an effective anesthetic agent for performing surgery on small reptiles. *Copeia*:738–743.

Wang T, Hicks J. 1996. The interaction of pulmonary ventilation and the right-left shunt on arterial oxygen levels. *The Journal of Experimental Biology* 199:2121–2129.

Wang T, Fernandes W, Abe A. 1993. Blood pH and O_2 homeostasis upon CO_2 anesthesia in the rattlesnake (*Crotalus durissus*). *The Snake* 25:21–26.

White F, Hicks J, Ishimatsu A. 1989. Relationship between respiratory state and intracardiac shunt in turtles. *The American Journal of Physiology* 256:R240–R247.

22 Chelonia (Tortoises, Turtles, and Terrapins)

Alessio Vigani

INTRODUCTION

Within the class Reptilia, the order Chelonia includes almost 300 species of tortoises, turtles, and terrapins. They inhabit many different habitats, from tropical rain forests to deserts, from freshwater swamps to oceans. The wide variety of environments, dietary preferences, and activity levels explains the substantial differences in metabolic rate among chelonian species. They also differ significantly in body size, from the 0.1-kg adult Cape tortoise (*Homopus* spp.) to the 1000-kg adult leatherback sea turtle (*Dermochelys coriacea*) (Raphael 2003). Most tortoises are generally shy, harmless animals, but there are differences in temperament among chelonians. Many aquatic species are natural predators and often respond with aggression to potential threats. These species can be dangerous and require caution when handled.

Interventions in the field for research purposes and the management of patients in the hospital setting represent the main conditions where sedation and general anesthesia are needed. It follows that the choice of the anesthetic protocol will depend on the invasiveness of the procedure and on the environment where it will take place. Collection of diagnostic samples in the field generally only requires mild to moderate sedation and, ideally, wild animals should return to the wild without the risk of any residual anesthetic effect. For this purpose, sedative protocols that include short-acting and reversible agents are particularly suitable.

Invasive surgical procedures, instead, should be performed under general anesthesia in the controlled environment of a veterinary hospital. The facility should be equipped with specific anesthesia equipment and monitoring devices. Prior to anesthesia, the patient should be thoroughly evaluated and acclimatized,

homeostasis should be restored, and thermoregulation should be supported in order to optimize the response of the patient to the anesthetic. Appropriate analgesia should be provided to any patient that is to undergo a painful procedure. New information on the ability of reptiles, chelonians included, to feel pain underlines the responsibility of every veterinarian to properly prevent and manage pain in these species.

Furthermore, independently from the operative setting, prerequisites to the design of a safe anesthetic protocol are a good knowledge not only of the anatomy and physiology, but also of the species-specific differences in response to anesthetic drugs and dosages. Multiple studies have evaluated the efficacy of a variety of single or combined anesthetic and analgesic drugs in different species of chelonians. Interesting pharmacokinetics data on some drugs, as well as information on their respiratory and cardiovascular effects in chelonians, are now available.

The perfect anesthetic agent does not exist for any species, including the chelonian. There is no anesthetic drug devoid of side effects and even the most recently marketed agents produce dose-related toxicity. For this reason, the use of combinations of small doses of multiple drugs has become popular in anesthesia. This anesthetic technique is referred to as *balanced anesthesia* and has been shown to be superior to single-agent anesthesia in humans and many veterinary species (Kushiro et al. 2005; Sanders et al. 2008). The explanation of its success is the use of small doses summates the advantages, but not the disadvantages, of the individual components of the mixture. It follows the safety of the anesthetic protocol largely depends on the right choice of drugs, used at the adequate dose for the patient. Excellent previous reviews on chelonian anesthesia are present in the literature and represent

Zoo Animal and Wildlife Immobilization and Anesthesia, Second Edition. Edited by Gary West, Darryl Heard, and Nigel Caulkett.

invaluable sources of information for the veterinarian. This chapter focuses on reviewing, to the best of the author's knowledge, the most current literature on anesthetic and analgesic techniques used in turtles, tortoises, and terrapins. The specific drugs, protocols, and dosages are reported with the sole goal to establish a database from which informed medical decisions can be independently made.

ANATOMY AND PHYSIOLOGY

Cardiovascular

The cardiovascular system is characterized by many morphological and functional peculiarities. The heart is three chambered and valentine shaped. It is located within the pericardial sac, at midline, above the cranial portion of the plastron, immediately cranial to the liver. The large right and left atria are distinct and open independently into an anatomically single but functionally divided ventricle. The right atrium receives deoxygenated blood from the systemic venous circulation via a preatrial muscular, thin-walled chamber called the *sinus venosum*. The latter represents the confluence site of blood from the left and right precaval veins, the postcaval vein, and the left hepatic vein.

The cardiac muscle constituting the *sinus venosum* acts also as the pacemaker of the heart. This electrical activity is detectable on the electrocardiogram by the presence of a "SV wave" preceding atrial depolarization.

The left atrium receives oxygenated blood from the pulmonary circulation via the left and right pulmonary veins. The ventricular muscle is internally organized in a series of ridges that divide the ventricle into three functional chambers: namely, *cavum pulmonale*, *cavum venosum*, and *cavum arteriosum*. Blood coming from the right atrium enters first the *cavum venosum* and then the *cavum pulmonale*, which has a direct pulmonary arterial output into the pulmonary trunk. Left atrial blood enters the *cavum arteriosum* and secondarily the *cavum venosum*, which opens into the systemic arterial systems via the left and right aortas (Farrell et al. 1998). It follows that the *cavum venosum* receives both deoxygenated (directly from right atrium) and oxygenated blood (indirectly from the left atrium), with the potential for mixing of the two.

The ventricular anatomy is such that in physiologic conditions of normal ventilation, there is a high degree of separation between the systemic and pulmonary circulations, with minimal mixing between venous and arterial blood. During ventilation, systemic ventricular output matches with the pulmonary ventricular output and intracardiac shunting is low. With the animal at rest, the nature of the physiological cardiac shunting in chelonian is bidirectional, with coexistence of right-to-left and a left-to-right components (Farrell et al. 1998).

The extraordinary adaptability of chelonians is fully displayed during apnea. The dive reflex induces complex physiologic changes, including modulation of intracardiac shunting (Hicks & Malvin 1992). During breath holding, arterial tension of oxygen progressively decreases. This induces vasoconstriction of the pulmonary arterial vasculature and causes a substantial decrease in pulmonary blood flow (Crossley et al. 1998). During apnea in turtles, the increased pulmonary arterial pressure causes the systemic venous return to be preferentially directed into the systemic circulation (R-L shunt), bypassing the lungs. This mechanism produces a oxygen sparing effect in the lungs (Jackson 2000). Aquatic, and to a lesser extent terrestrial chelonians, have been shown to develop right to left intracardiac shunting in hypoxic conditions (Hicks et al. 1996). During ventilatory periods, the cardiovascular changes are the reciprocals of those occurring during apnea: the heart rate increases, the pulmonary vascular resistance falls, and pulmonary blood flow is maximized. Blood flow measurements indicate a net formation of a left-to-right shunt during ventilation, which increases hemoglobin oxygen saturation of pulmonary arterial blood (Shelton & Burggren 1976). Low rates of elimination of inhalant anesthetics, such as isoflurane or sevoflurane, can be expected whenever cardiac shunting exists.

Hypoxemia and the subsequent R-L shunt trigger a generalized hypometabolic state (Hicks & Wang 1999). This hypometabolic condition significantly decreases the hepatic function, with a potential detrimental effect on the clearance of drugs (Platzack & Hicks 2001). Therefore, it is important to provide ventilation and oxygenation during anesthesia to maintain a steady cardiovascular and metabolic state. Once cardiac shunting is present, it may be difficult to provide oxygen supplementation.

The direction (right to left vs. left to right) and size of shunting in chelonians are influenced by multiple factors that control cardiac function. These include both adrenergic and cholinergic innervation. Stimulation of the vagus in tortoises results in an increase in pulmonary arterial pressure and net formation of R-L shunt (Hicks & Comeau 1994). In contrast, epinephrine or the stimulation of the cardiac sympathetic nerves abolish R-L shunting and induce vasodilation of the pulmonary vasculature. In *Trachemys scripta*, it has been shown that the infusion of epinephrine increases the blood flow in the pulmonary circulation (left-to-right shunt) and eliminates the systemic venous admixture in the aortic arches (Hicks & Malvin 1992).

An additional important factor that modulates cardiac shunting is thermoregulation. Variation of body temperature from the physiologic optimal conditions has major effects on the circulatory system (Krosniunas & Hicks 2003). At normal body temperature, the intracardiac shunting is relatively stable, with a small right to left shunt. Interestingly, both heating and cooling result in the development of an increased R-L intracardiac shunt (Galli et al. 2004). The ability to selectively shunt blood flow away from the pulmonary circulation is likely the cause of prolonged recoveries from inhalant anesthesia. Therefore, during anesthesia, the maintenance of steady physiologic thermal conditions is important to provide optimal gas exchange, including inhaled anesthetics.

The renal portal system (RPS) maintains sufficient blood flow to the renal tubules at times when a decreased effective circulating volume generates a low glomerular blood flow. The portal vein is a large vessel that enters the kidney and originates at the confluence of the *epigastric* and *external iliac* veins. It contains muscular valves capable of shunting blood from the caudal half of the body directly to the kidney. Hydration status seems to play a primary role in the activity of the RPS and affects the degree of shunting. Dehydration causes an increased diversion of blood. The blood in the RPS is exposed to the renal tubular surface and this may result in increased clearance of drugs normally excreted through the tubules into the urine. Angiographic studies have also shown that a large amount of venous blood from the hind limbs is directed to the liver (Holz et al. 1997b). Therefore, renal and hepatic levels of some drugs injected into the caudal limbs may be unpredictable. It has been demonstrated, however, that the injection site is unlikely to have any influence over the activity of most drugs and the caudal half of a chelonian is available for drug administration (Holz et al. 1997b). For example carbenicillin, a drug largely excreted by tubular secretion, was injected into the hind limbs of turtles. The systemic blood levels of the drug obtained were just slightly lower compared with the fore limb injection (Holz et al. 1997a). Whether the same scenario applies to drugs injected into the dorsal venous sinus of the chelonian tail remains unclear. In green iguanas (*Iguana iguana*), the venous flow from the tail was found to directly enter the kidney through the renal portal circulation (Benson & Forrest 1999). Until adequately investigated, it is advisable not to use the dorsal venous sinus for drug administration in dehydrated chelonians.

Respiratory System

Chelonians are obligate nasal breathers. Open mouth breathing indicates decreased airflow through the nasal cavities, possibly due to pathology. The external nares open into a keratinized vestibule divided symmetrically by a cartilaginous septum into right and left nasal chambers. The nasal chambers lay above the hard palate and extend aborally into the oropharynx through a ventral recess. Turbinates, sinuses, and soft palate are absent. The glottis is located at the base of the tongue, with species-specific differences in morphology. In aquatic species in particular, it is characterized by a strong muscular component needed to provide efficient sealing of the distal airways during immersion. The trachea is composed of complete rings, is relatively short, and bifurcates in paired bronchi at the level of the mid-cervical region (McArthur et al. 2004). It is, therefore, easy to unilaterally intubate most chelonians.

The lungs are located dorsally in the coelomic cavity, and their dorsal surface is attached to the carapace. All chelonians have multichambered lungs with paired unbranched intrapulmonary bronchi reinforced by cartilage over their entire length. In sea turtles, the intrapulmonary bronchi are supported by cartilaginous rings, are broad cranially and taper caudally. In other chelonians, the bronchi are uniform in diameter for their entire length, and the supporting cartilage forms a network instead of separate rings. Each bronchus opens into 3–11 chambers from which multiple sub-compartments, referred to as "niches", originate. The chelonian analogues of mammalian alveoli are termed "faveoli," "ediculae," and " trabeculae," and represent the parenchymal gas exchange units (Perry 1998).

The presence of the carapace impedes the costal component of ventilation; therefore, muscle induced movements of the viscera and limbs are responsible for alterations in intrapulmonary pressure. Chelonians do not possess a functional muscular diaphragm. A horizontal septum, or pseudodiaphragm, separate the lungs form other intracoelomic organs. In some chelonians, such as sea turtles, the horizontal septum is extensive and attaches the liver and stomach to the ventral surface of the lung. This attachment maximizes the transmission of the movement of the body wall and limb girdles through the visceral mass to the lungs. Limb movements stretch the septum downward, causing expansion of the lungs. The lung expansion generates a negative intrapulmonary pressure and facilitates the passive inflow of air during inspiration. The "muscle pump" mechanism is abolished by immobility; subsequently, ventilation is then profoundly depressed during anesthesia. Ventilatory artificial support by intermittent positive pressure ventilation (IPPV) is, therefore, always recommended in anesthetized chelonians. IPPV can be provided either manually or mechanically with a ventilator.

Chelonians are unable to cough and lack effective ciliary clearance of respiratory material. This explains why their ability at clearing secretions and foreign material from their lower respiratory tract is very poor. Consequently, inflammatory exudates tend to accumulate in dependent area of the lungs with severe effects on respiratory function and gas exchanges. The innate resilience of chelonians, however, allows them to withstand extreme physiologic perturbations, such as severe hypoxia or hypercapnia, and clinical signs of respiratory distress occur late in the course of the primary disease (McArthur et al. 2004).

Reptiles, compared with avian and mammalian species, have a relatively large lung volume in which is distributed a relatively small respiratory surface area. The multichambered lungs of chelonians, however, represent the advantage of a more complex surface elaboration compared with the single-chambered lungs of other reptiles. Studies in *T. scripta* showed the septa that divide the pulmonary chambers provide a 40% larger surface area used for gas exchanges compared with the outer wall of the lungs. This yields effective gas exchange to cover metabolic requirements (Perry 1998).

Respiration is characterized by intermittent breathing patterns with ventilatory periods alternated with nonventilatory pauses. The respiratory cycle in terrestrial species consists of a passive inspiratory followed by an active expiratory phase. The latter is reversed in aquatic species. These peculiarities, along with the high compliance values of chelonian lungs, produce a significantly lower work of breathing compared with mammals. In regard to anesthesia, however, the chelonian highly compliant lungs are extremely easy to inflate and hence highly sensitive to barotrauma (Herman et al. 1997). It is recommended, therefore, that low peak inspiratory pressures be used during IPPV.

The need to maintain low the energy requirements of ventilation is also reflected by the adaptive mechanisms that chelonians operate in response to increased metabolic stress. Increasing tidal volume is ineffective and represents a major energy expense in chelonians. This explains why most tortoises and turtles during activity increase their minute ventilation by increasing the respiratory rate and not by increasing tidal volume. In regard to the driving mechanisms of ventilation, hypoxia and hypercarbia affect the length of respiratory cycles differently. Hypoxia induces bradypnea, while hypercapnia causes tachypnea. The explanations of these opposite effects are oxygen preservation and the elimination of carbon dioxide, respectively. Converesely, both the artificial induction of hyperoxia or hypocapnia, independently from one another, cause persistent cessation of spontaneous ventilation (Wang et al. 1998). Therefore, the maintenance of blood gas variables within physiologic range is critical during anesthesia to avoid long lasting alteration of ventilatory function.

Many chelonians can perceive a low oxygen environment and develop a cardiorespiratory response similar to the dive reflex described in mammals. They become apneic, bradycardic, and convert to anaerobic metabolism. These physiological changes, combined with cardiac shunting, facilitate diving and hibernation, but complicate the use of inhaled anesthetic agents. The alterations in respiratory circulation typical of the chelonian dive reflex can affect the uptake and excretion rates of inhalant anesthetics.

Pain and Nociception

Pain and nociception are often mistakenly considered synonymous. Pain is inherently subjective, and in animals is defined as an unpleasant sensory and emotional experience associated with actual or potential tissue damage. Pain represents the interpretation by the cerebral cortex of a noxious stimulus, and consciousness, therefore, is a prerequisite to feel pain. Nociception instead, refers to the physiologic or neuroanatomical components necessary to sense and transmit the noxious stimuli to the brain (IASP 1994). Any organism that has developed these neuroanatomical structures is defined as sentient. In a sentient animal, therefore, nociception persists during unconsciousness and anesthesia unless analgesic interventions are provided (Giordano 2005).

Multiple studies in different reptile species have demonstrated the presence of the neuroanatomical apparatus for sentience and nociception (Liang & Terashima 1993; ten Donkelaar & de Boer-van Huizen 1987). It has been shown that environmental stimuli elicit impulse transmission from sensory receptors, through the spinal cord, to the animal's brain. Furthermore, the reptile cerebral structures are operationally sophisticated enough to convert the impulses into perceived sensations (Giordano 2005). The opioid receptor gene family is highly conserved across multiple vertebrate orders, and new information is now available on opioid receptors and their modulation in chelonians (Li et al. 1996; Reiner 1987). For example, μ and δ opioid receptors are located throughout the brain in aquatic turtles, with δ opioid receptors being more abundant than μ opioid receptors (Xia & Haddad 2001). With respect to endogenous opioid related neurotransmitters, proenkephalin and other neuropeptides (i.e., neuropeptide FF) are present in the brain of turtles with a distribution similar to that in mammals and birds (Munoz et al. 2008). New information is also now available on the role of the different opioid receptors in nociception and analgesia in chelonians (Sladky et al. 2009). For example, kappa (κ) opioid receptors are significantly less involved in nociception and pain compared with μ-opioid receptor. Kappa receptor agonists do not produce any detectable analgesic effect in turtles whereas agents with μ agonist activity significantly increase the nociceptive threshold (Wambugu et al. 2010).

In nonverbal species, suffering is expressed in the form of behavioral changes that are often not obvious to the observer (Holsti et al. 2008; Holton et al. 2001). Chelonians are not an exception. It follows, independently from the inability of these animals to show evident expressions of pain, that veterinarians should consider that chelonians are capable of suffering when a noxious stimulus in applied, and therefore they should be provided with appropriate analgesia.

PERIANESTEHTIC CONSIDERATIONS AND PATIENT MANAGEMENT

Preanesthetic Assessment

A complete history provides crucial information regarding the patient's environment, husbandry, and diet, and helps to determine duration and severity of clinical signs of the medical condition. The observation of the unstressed patient is important to determine the level of activity of the patient unbiased by any restraint.

Ideally, prior to anesthesia, the patient should be acclimatized to the new environment, and the room temperature and humidity should be set within the ideal range for the species. This obviously does not apply to emergency cases where immediate intervention is required. As with all ectotherms, chelonian body temperature is reliant on the environmental temperature. The preferred optimal temperature zone (POTZ) refers to the ideal environmental temperature range selected by a particular species. Each species has its own POTZ and it is only when the animal is in its POTZ that its physiology is functioning at its best. For most chelonians, data regarding optimal environmental temperature and humidity can be found in the literature. If the specific POTZ is uncertain, exposure to a room temperature range of 24–28°C during preanesthetic stabilization seems to be appropriate for most chelonian species (McArthur et al. 2004).

Body temperature should be measured prior to anesthesia. Oscillations in body temperature in ectothermic species are common, and it is important to identify and correct wide variations from the normal range. All chelonians have what is referred to as an "active temperature range" or "ATR." This is the body temperature range where they are capable of normal, voluntary activity. Each species has a different ATR (McArthur et al. 2004). Critically ill patients are often hypothermic and the prompt restoration of normothermia is of critical importance to maximize the chance of patient stabilization. On the other hand, overheating should also be carefully avoided. Hypothermia and hyperthermia have significant effects on metabolic rate (drug clearance), acid base status, intracardiac shunting (respiratory gas exchanges and inhalant anesthetic uptake and clearance), and inhalant agent potency (decreased minimum alveolar concentration [MAC] during hypothermia). Therefore, attention to maintaining normothermia in the perianesthetic period is a priority for the anesthetist.

The preanesthetic physical examination consists of the assessment of systems and organs and should include a preliminary visual examination aimed to determine body condition, nutritional and hydration status, and presence of trauma. Body weight must be recorded in order to ensure accurate dosing of anesthetics.

A basic assessment of the cardiovascular system of the patient should be performed prior to anesthesia. Heart rate and pulse rate and strength can be evaluated noninvasively with a Doppler flow detector. Pencil and flat probes are selected based on the size of the animal and the location where the probe must be placed. For cardiac auscultation, a pencil probe can be placed lateral to the neck at the level of the thoracic inlet. For pulse assessment, a flat probe can detect blood flow in vessels directly beneath the probe. Suitable arteries for pulse assessment are the carotid and femoral artery (McArthur 2007). Several formulas to determine the normal heart rate based on body weight in reptiles have been given by different authors. However, the absence of validation studies and the significant physiologic differences between species often make those equations clinically inadequate for predicting heart rate.

Baseline respiratory rate and depth are measured before induction. Identification of even mild signs of respiratory disease should be considered as an expression of potentially severe respiratory illness. Chronic respiratory disease is fairly common, and chelonians are able to withstand extensive injury to the respiratory system before showing signs of distress.

Ideally, when planning elective procedures, a venous blood sample should be collected prior to anesthesia for hematologic and plasma biochemical evaluation. Blood should be collected into lithium heparin tubes as EDTA causes lysis of reptilian erythrocytes. As a general rule, the sample size should not be larger than 1% of the body weight of the subject. Abnormalities in the laboratory variables of special interest for the anesthesiologist are represented by, but not limited to, the following: presence of anemia or hemoconcentration, hypoproteinemia, hypoglycemia, hyperuricemia, and electrolytes and acid-base imbalances. The presence of any of the earlier-mentioned abnormalities warrant further investigation to identify the underlying cause and properly treat prior to anesthesia.

The patient's hydration status should be assessed based on history, physical examination, and laboratory findings. At present, however, the evaluation of hydration status in is still somewhat subjective. Indications of dehydration are sunken eyes, reduced skin turgor, and hematological and plasma biochemical alterations, such as hemoconcentration and hyperproteinemia (McArthur 2004). Ion pump activation and significant fluid reabsorption by the lower urinary tract and digestive tract complicate the use of many variables as indicators of hydration. In most reptiles, approximately 75% of body weight is water. In chelonians, the presence of the carapace reduces the value closer to that found in mammals, which is approximately 66%. However, in contrast to mammals, the total body water is equally distributed between the intra- and extracellular fluid compartments, and 30% of the extracellular fluid volume exists in the intravascular space (Smits & Kozubowski 1985). These differences should be considered to accurately plan and administer fluids to chelonians.

Differences in response to various inhaled and injectable sedatives and anesthetics have also been shown between chelonian species. The drugs and doses effective and safe in one species may not apply to other chelonians.

Handling of Dangerous Chelonians

Chelonians generally do not need significant restraint during examination, and most herbivorous animals can be handled with no real risk of danger to the personnel. However, aggressive and potentially dangerous species represent exceptions. Snapping turtles (*Chelydra* spp.), softshell turtles (*Trionyx* spp.), and marine chelonians may show unpredictable, aggressive reactions, and these large animals can inflict serious injuries with their beaks and claws. These species should be handled with extreme caution. Wearing heavy-duty gloves is recommended, but serious bite injuries can still occur despite their use. These animals can be examined more safely after they have bitten or locked on nontraumatic objects, such as a PVC pipe. When working with aggressive species, the help of an assistant is often necessary.

Smaller marine, snapping, and softshell turtles can be held with a hand on either side of the carapace, with the head directed away from the operator and other people (Fig. 22.1). Turtles of the genera *Chelydra* and *Trionyx* are able to extend their head up to the level of their hindlimbs. It is important to determine the "safe zone" around the animal. Medium-sized (10 kg–40 kg) marine and snapping turtles are better controlled with one hand around the nuchal scute (cranial carapace above the neck) and the other on the caudal carapace (Fig. 22.2). Very large individuals of these species are capable of incredible strength, and stretchers or canvas slings should be used during maneuvering procedures. Marine chelonians should never be picked up by their flippers. This is due to the risk of causing luxations and fractures.

While necessary in some cases, chemical immobilization should be considered as a last resort in the simple physical examination procedure. Whenever sedation is used, an aquatic animal must not be reintroduced into water until it is fully recovered in order to avoid the risk of drowning.

Venipuncture and Intravenous Catheterization

Venipuncture and venous catheterization for phlebotomy and drug or fluids administration purposes are difficult. The diversity in morphology of turtles and tortoises precludes any single dependable venipuncture site for all species. Therefore, it is important to know the location of multiple potential sites and select the most appropriate for the individual species. Venipuncture sites previously described include the jugular veins, dorsal cervical sinus, subcarapacial (subvertebral) sinus, and the dorsal coccygeal vein (Lloyd & Morris 1999). Other peripheral venipuncture sites, where only small blood samples can be obtained, are the radio-humeral venous plexus and the femoral vein. These sites may be more yielding in larger animals.

It is recommended that blood collection be from the jugular veins when possible. Samples taken from the jugular site are least likely to be lymph diluted (Jacobson et al. 1992). On either side of the neck, external and internal jugular veins are present in many chelonian species. Either can be used for venipuncture. The external jugular vein is larger and located in a lateral

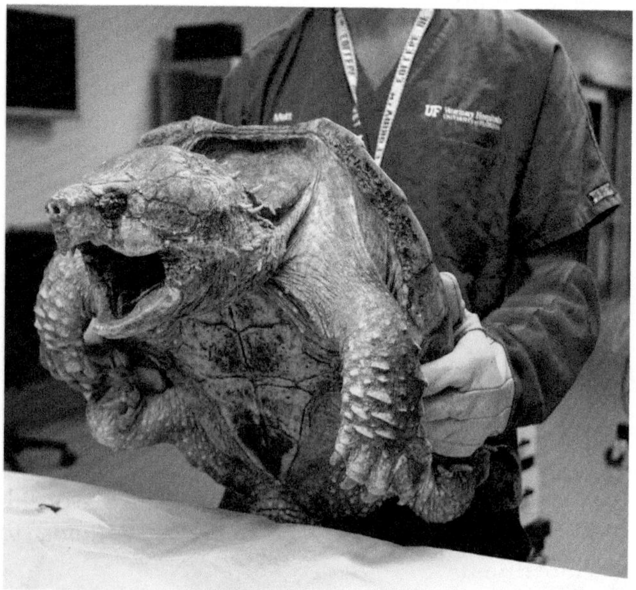

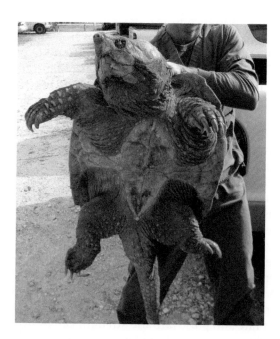

Figure 22.1. Appropriate physical restraint of a medium-size (15 kg) alligator snapping turtle (*Macrochelys temminckii*). Note the position of the hands on either side of the shell. The use of reinforced gloves provide additional protection from the claws.

Figure 22.2. Physical restraint of a large (30 kg) alligator snapping turtle (*Macrochelys temminckii*). The animal is controlled with one hand on the nucal scute and the other on the caudal carapace. The head of the animal is directed away from the operator.

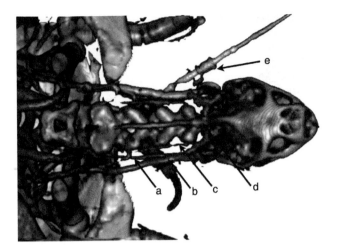

Figure 22.3. CT-scan 3D reconstruction of the neck of the Gopher tortoise (*Gopherus polyphemus*). The vascular structures are identified as follows: (a) carotid artery, (b) external jugular vein, (c) internal jugular vein, (d) occipital venous sinus. (e) Indicates a intravenous catheter placed in the left external jugular vein.

to dorsolateral position. It runs approximately in a line from the dorsal edge of the tympanic membrane parallel to the dorsal plane of the neck in the direction of the thoracic inlet (Fig. 22.3). Extension of the neck is needed to allow the jugular vein to be raised and seen. This is possible in many small chelonians, but in large individuals (>10 kg), or aggressive species such as snapping turtles, it is often impossible without adequate chemical restraint. Should the jugular site prove impractical, the subcarapacial sinus or the dorsal coccygeal vein may represent good alternatives, particularly for intravenous drug administration.

The subcarapacial venous sinus can be easily accessible in small chelonians (<10 kg) (Fig. 22.4). It is located under the carapace, on the dorsal midline, at the junction of the common intercostal and the caudal branch of the external jugular veins, just cranial to the eight cervical vertebra (Hernandez-Divers & Hernandez-Divers 2002). To the author's knowledge, the quality and reliability of diagnostic blood samples taken from this site has not been evaluated. It appears, however, to be a suitable site for intravenous injections.

The dorsal coccygeal vein is a safe and dependable venipuncture site in snapping turtles (Fig. 22.5). The dorsal coccygeal vein runs in the dorsal midline from the tip of the tail to the carapace. Blood samples from this site can be unpredictably lymphodiluted; therefore, when clear fluid is sampled, another attempt should be made at a different site. The vessel is occasionally more superficial than expected, and a needle that is inserted between the vertebrae too deep has the potential to enter the vertebral canal. Therefore, accurate disinfection of the skin of the tail is mandatory before attempting venipuncture.

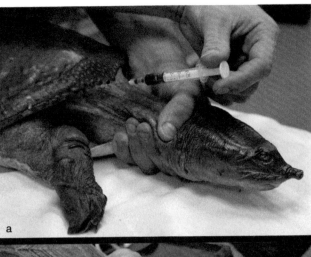

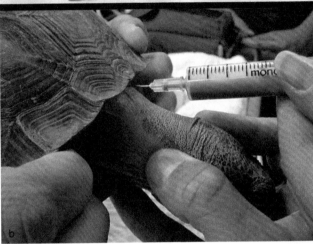

Figure 22.4. Use of the subcarapacial venous sinus for blood withdrawal (a) in a Florida softshell turtle (*Apalone ferox*), and for intravenous injection of propofol (b) in a gopher tortoise (*Gopherus polyphemus*). The needle is inserted on the midline of the neck, at the junction between the skin and the carapacial nucal scute. The needle is advanced caudally while maintaining gentle negative aspiration on the syringe until blood is flowing into the chamber.

In marine turtles, the dorsal cervical sinus is a reliable venipuncture site and it is popular with those working with these chelonians. It is useful both for blood withdrawal and intravenous injections. The paired sinuses are parallel to the midline and are located on either side, 0.5–1 cm away from the dorsal spinous processes of the proximal cervical vertebrae. They are found 0.5- to 3-cm deep depending upon the size of the animal.

Suitable anatomical locations for intravenous catheter placement are limited; the jugular veins are usually the only option. Jugular catheter placement can be performed with either a venous cut-down or percutaneously. Prior sedation is recommended and often necessary for a successful catheter placement. In general, over-the-needle, 22- to -auge, 2- to 4-cm long IV catheters can be used for short-term placement. When

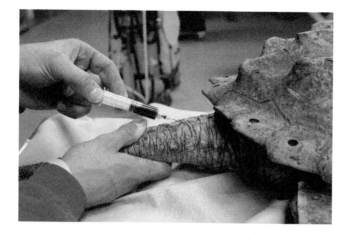

Figure 22.5. Venipunture in a alligator snapping turtle (*Macrochelys temminckii*) using the dorsal approach to access the dorsal coccygeal vein. The main advantage of this venipuncture site is represented by its location in the "safe zone" around the animal. For safety, an assistant should be restraining the animal during the venipuncture procedure.

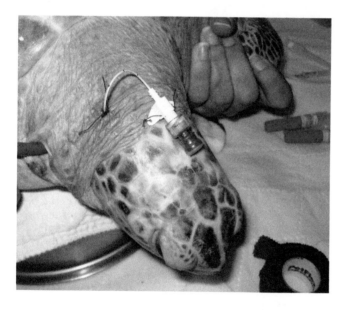

Figure 22.6. Single-lumen jugular catheter placed in the external jugular vein of a green sea turtle (*Chelonia mydas*). The catheter was inserted using a over-the-wire technique. The winged proximal portion is secured to the skin with sutures.

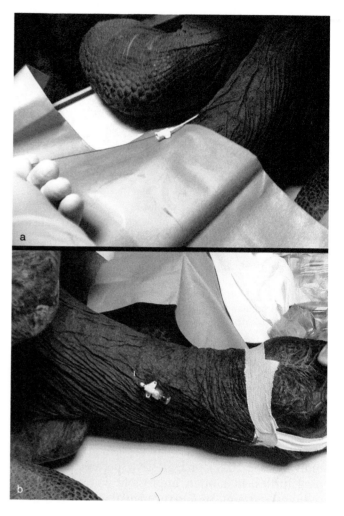

Figure 22.7. Placement of a long-term jugular catheter in an Aldabra tortoise (*Aldabrachelys gigantea*). In the anesthetized animal, the external jugular vein is identified by palpation of the dorsolateral aspect of either side of the neck. A hollow needle is advanced through the skin until blood is aspirated. The catheter is then inserted using the Seldinger technique: a blunt guidewire is passed through the needle (a), then the needle is removed. A dilating device may be passed over the guide wire to slightly enlarge the vessel. Finally, the central line itself is then passed over the guidewire, which is then removed. All the lumens of the line are aspirated and flushed. The catheter is finally secured with sutures to the skin (b).

long-term venous access is required, indwelling polyurethane or silicon central venous catheters should be used (Fig. 22.6). This author recommends the use of the standard Seldinger technique (over-the-wire) for percutaneous placement of long-term catheters (Fig. 22.7).

Fluid Therapy

When a fluid deficit is clearly identified or the hydration status of the patient is unknown, peri-anesthetic fluid therapy is indicated to replace the deficit in active circulating volume and restore tissue perfusion and homeostasis. Hypotonic fluids, such as 5% dextrose in water (D5W), generally diffuse primarily in the intracellular space whereas isotonic crystalloids contain a sodium concentration similar to that of the extracellular space, making them the ideal solution for replacing extracellular volume deficits.

There is still debate on the best type of fluids to administer to reptiles given their blood is hypotonic compared with birds and mammals. There are several guidelines for fluid replacement in reptiles, but most of the standard crystalloids, such as lactated or acetated Ringer's, and normal saline solutions can safely be used. Two recipes of isotonic solution are "diluted saline" (9 parts 0.9% NaCl and 1 part sterile water) and "reptile Ringer's" (2 parts 2.5% dextrose/0.45% saline with 1 part lactated Ringer's). It is generally accepted a rate of 25 mL/kg every 24 hours is appropriate as a rehydrating rate. In chelonians, total fluids given at one time should not exceed 2–3% of total body weight (Norton 2005). Constant rate infusion in preferable over intermittent boluses. Fluids can be administered orally, intravenously, or intracoelomically. Oral rehydration is recommended for clinically stable, mildly to moderately dehydrated patients; whereas the intravenous route is preferred in severely dehydrated patients. Intracoelomic fluids should be avoided in patients with present or suspected respiratory disease, intracoelomic space-occupying lesion, obstipation, and egg retention (McArthur 2004).

Traumatized patients that have suffered severe hemorrhage should be promptly fluid resuscitated. In these cases, the intravenous route is considered ideal for fluid administration. In these patients, however, the low intravascular volume and vasoconstriction often limit intravenous access.

In the presence of life threatening hypovolemia, the intravenous administration of hypertonic solutions(i.e., 7.5% NaCl) and colloids (hydroxyethyl starches and dextrans) is indicated to provide selective intravascular volume expansion. The recommended doses of hypertonic solutions and colloids in mammals are 2–4 mL/kg and 5–10 mL/kg, respectively. The safety of such indications has not been proved in chelonians. Thus, the author recommends to start with lower initial volumes (1–2 mL/kg) and then re-assess the response of the patient.

ANALGESIA

A recent survey of the use of analgesics by reptile veterinarians indicated analgesia is withheld in more than 50% of the patients by more that 60% of the responders (Read 2004). This finding may be partially explained by our inability to detect pain in reptiles due to lack of definitive information on behaviors proven to be pathognomonic of pain. Ultimately, pain assessment is made even more difficult by the evidence that reptiles seem to voluntarily suppress pain-related behaviors when they are observed (Fleming & Robertson 2006). Sadly, for all these reasons, pain control in reptiles has been largely overlooked. The current knowledge and better understanding of pain perception in reptiles support the importance of providing appropriate analgesia whenever an invasive procedure is performed. An excellent review of the current literature on pain assessment and analgesia in reptiles has been recently published (Mosley 2011).

Among opioid analgesics, morphine has been shown to provide analgesia in chelonians whereas butorpha-nol, even at dosages largely exceeding the mammalian therapeutic doses, did not have any effect on thermal threshold (Sladky et al. 2007). The analgesic action of morphine (1.5 mg/kg) in chelonians appears to have a time of onset of 2–8 hours postadministration and duration of more than 24 hours. Unfortunately this analgesic effect is coupled with a significant, long-lasting respiratory depression (Sladky et al. 2007). Meperidine, a synthetic μ pure agonist, induced significant decrease in the duration of limb retraction after formalin injection in Speke's hinged tortoise (*Kinixy's spekii*) at the dose of 20 mg/kg. This drug appears to provide a degree of analgesia equivalent to morphine (Wambugu et al. 2010). Pharmacokinetic data of buprenorphine in red-eared sliders (*Trachemys scripta elegans*) established the subcutaneous administration of 0.075–0.1 mg/kg every 24 hours is sufficient to maintain plasma drug concentrations considered analgesic for humans (Kummrow et al. 2008). The analgesic effect of buprenorphine in chelonians has not been evaluated. Tramadol, an atypical synthetic opioid, has been recently shown to provide long-lasting analgesia in chelonians with minimal respiratory depression. In red-eared sliders (*T.s. elegans*), the oral administration of 10–25 mg/kg increased thermal threshold for up to 96 hours (Baker et al. 2011). These dosages are much higher than those generally used in clinical practice (0.5–4 mg/kg).

Nonsteroidal anti-inflammatory agents (NSAIDs) are widely used in reptiles based on their proven potent analgesic activity in mammals. Interestingly, there is no proven scientific evidence of the analgesic activity of NSAIDs in chelonians or other reptiles. This could be due to our incapacity to effectively assess pain. To the author's knowledge a limited number of studies evaluated pharmacokinetics (PK) and pharmacodynamics (PD) of NSAIDs in chelonians. In green iguanas (*Iguana iguana*) the oral administration of meloxicam at 0.2 mg/kg resulted in plasma concentrations considered analgesic for mammals (Divers et al. 2010). In loggerhead sea turtles (*Careta careta*), it was shown the clearance of meloxicam was significantly higher than reported for the iguana suggesting the need for more frequent dose intervals to maintain effective plasma concentrations (Soloperto et al. 2012). This may not, however, correlate with analgesia because the plasma concentration of NSAIDs does not directly correlate with clinical effect.

The safety of the use of NSAIDs in reptiles has been evaluated in studies involving repeated daily administrations. No significant biochemical abnormalities or histopathological lesions were seen (Hernandez-Divers et al. 2004). Despite this, it is still possible NSAIDs can cause severe side effects as reported in mammals. Normal hydration status and renal function should always be ensured prior to NSAID administration. Although the clinical use of NSADs in reptiles does not appear to delay wound healing, it has been shown the administration of selective NSAIDs cyclooxygenase-2 inhibitors to geckos after tail amputation significantly retards the regenerative process (Sharma & Suresh 2008).

Local anesthesia represents an irreplaceable component of a multimodal anesthetic approach. Local anesthetics (LA) prevent the transmission of nerve impulses by interrupting the sodium influx into the neurons. In sensory nerve fibers, the signal from a noxious stimulus is then stopped at its origin and is prevented from reaching the central nervous system. LA agents vary in potency and duration of action. Lidocaine and bupivacaine represent the most commonly used agents in veterinary practice. Bupivacaine is more potent and longer acting compared with lidocaine, but the actual duration of action in reptiles is undetermined. In chelonians, the local injection of LA is useful for facilitating minor surgical interventions, but local anesthesia alone is not sufficient to provide analgesia for more invasive procedures. The infiltraton around the surgical site (local block) represents the most diffuse use of LA in chelonians, but more advanced techniques have also been described (Hernandez-Divers et al. 2009).

Lidocaine (2%) injected intrathecally at an approximate dose of 1 mL per 25 kg in hybrid Galapagos tortoises (*Geochelone nigra*) was sufficient to perform phallectomy (Rivera et al. 2011). The technique provided adequate analgesia, without need of supplemental systemic analgesics. The ambulatory function returned to normal within 60 minutes after administration in all the animals in the study. The short analgesic effect limits the single administration use of LA to the perioperative period. To provide prolonged analgesia using LA, repeated administrations are required. For this purpose, the placement of long-term intrathecal catheters is possible in chelonians and, in this author's experience, has been effective (Fig. 22.8).

It is suggested to not go over the dosages of LA described for mammals until specific toxicological information in chelonians is available. The analgesic agents for which PK and PD data are currently available in chelonians are listed in Table 22.1.

ANESTHETIC INDUCTION AND MAINTENANCE

Generally, induction and maintenance of anesthesia are relatively simple, but at times they can be particularly challenging and frustrating to the anesthetist.

Mask induction with inhaled anesthetics can be used, but is associated with pronged induction times. Aquatic species are well adapted to the episodic breathing pattern and able to stay apneic for very extensive periods of time, preventing the adequate delivery of inhaled anesthetic (Bienzle & Boyd 1992). Induction times may be reduced by inducing respiration by gently moving the forelimbs forwards and backwards.

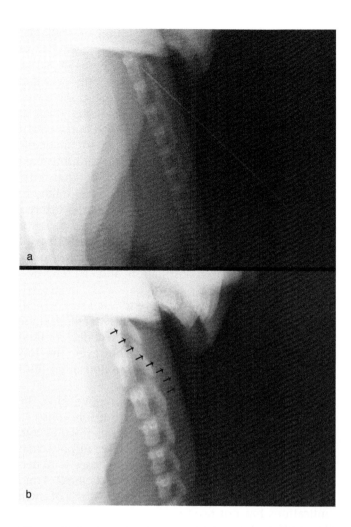

Figure 22.8.   Lateral radiographic views of the placement of a inthathecal catheter in a Galapagos tortoise (*Chelonoidis nigra*). A Tuohy needle is slowly advanced between the spinous processes of two consecutive coccygeal vertebrae and placed in the vertebral canal (a) into the intrathecal space (space between dura mater and leptomeninx). The catheter is threaded through the needle and advanced a few centimeters into the vertebral canal (b). The needle is then withdrawn over the catheter. The catheter is secured to the skin with sutures to prevent it becoming dislodged. The catheter can be used for repeated administrations of analgesics and local anesthetics. The small black arrows indicate the catheter placed into the intrathecal space.

Awake intubation and induction is more effective. The mouth is forcibly opened and the endotracheal tube inserted through the glottis. This allows controlled ventilation to deliver the inhaled anesthetic. Large tortoises, however, are unbelievably powerful animals and are impossible to forcibly intubate without sedation. Further, strong laryngeal sphincter muscles seal the glottis of aquatic species, making awake intubation difficult. Repeated attempts to force open the closed glottis are not recommended due to risk of causing severe tissue damage. Instead, gentle manipulation and patience in waiting for the animal to voluntarily open the glottis often facilitate the intubation. A short piece

Table 22.1. Analgesic agents with pharmacokinetic and pharmacodynamic data available in chelonian species

Drug	Dose (mg/kg)	Route	Analgesic Activity	Comments	Source
Buprenophine	0.075–0.1	IV, IM	Not established	Elevated drug plasma concentrations up to 24 hours	Kummrow et al. (2008)
Butorphanol	2.8–28	IM, IV	None	No analgesic effect even at high doses; at high doses prolonged respiratory depression	Sladky et al. (2007)
Lidocaine	0.8	Intrathecal	Good	Duration of analgesia up to 60 minutes; temporary paraparesis can occur	Rivera et al. (2011)
Lidocaine	1	SQ (local infiltration)	Moderate	Used alone not sufficient analgesia for celioscopy	Hernandez-Divers et al. (2009)
Meloxicam	0.2	SQ	Not established	Anecdotal evidence of clinical efficacy	McArthur (2004)
Meperidine	20	IV, IM	Good	Analgesic efficacy similar to morphine	Wambugu et al. (2010)
Morphine	1.5	IV, IM	Good	Dose-dependent respiratory depression	Sladky et al. (2007)
Tramadol	5–10	PO	Good	Long-lasting analgesic effect up to 96 hours	Baker et al. (2011)
Tramadol	10–25	SQ	Good	Slower onset and shorter duration of analgesia compared with PO administration	Baker et al. (2011)

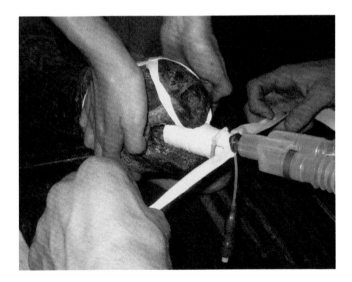

Figure 22.9. A piece of PVC pipe used as oral speculum facilitates intubation and protects the endotracheal tube. Both the mouth gag and the endotracheal tube are secured with tape to the head of the animal to prevent dislodgment.

of PVC pipe used as that mouth gag facilitates intubation and protects the endotracheal tube (Fig. 22.9).

Injectable sedative and anesthetic agents are commonly administered intramuscularly due to the difficulty of gaining intravenous access without previous sedation. Intramuscular administration of ketamine combined with benzodiazepines or α_2-adrenergic agonists often produce adequate sedation and muscle relaxation. The pectoral muscles are a preffered site for intramuscular injections. Reported parenteral drug combinations and dosages are given in Table 22.2.

In some species, the presence of easily accessible veins and venous sinuses facilitate direct intravenous administration of anesthetics. In sea turtles, the cervical venous sinus is an easily accessible site for injection (Moon & Hernandez Foester 2001). It is often used for induction, but limited information is available on the rate of distribution of anesthetics using this route. If the desired effect is not achieved at the recommended dosage of a drug, it is recommended not to repeat the administration to avoid overdosage (Wood et al. 1982).

The dorsal coccygeal vein is in this author's experience a safe and reliable site for IV injection in unsedated snapping turtles (*Chelydra* spp. and *Macrochelys temminckii*). The subcarapacial venous sinus is easily accessible for injections in small chelonians; however, extravasation of drug is likely when this access is used. The subcarapacial sinus runs close to the submeningeal space where the cervical vertebra join the carapace. Deaths in gopher tortoises (*Gopherus polyphemus*) have been associated with the inadvertent injection of propofol into this space while attempting subcarapacial injection (Quesada et al. 2010).

When the intravenous (IV) route is utilized, propofol titrated to effect is a good choice for induction of anesthesia. Used as a single agent, it requires doses between 4 and 8 mg/kg to produce anesthesia. Alternatively, the combination of ketamine (5 mg/kg) and medetomidine (0.05 mg/kg) given intravenously appears to be safe in many aquatic and terrestrial species. Alfaxalone/alfadolone at the dose of 24 mg/kg given intracoelomically was shown to produce surgical anesthesia in red ear sliders (Lawrence & Jackson 1983). A new formulation of alfaxalone (Alfaxan®) is now

Table 22.2. Selected sedative and anesthetic protocols used in chelonian species

Species	Protocol (Drug)	Dose (mg/kg)	Route	Onset (Minutes)	Reversal (Drug/Route)	Recovery (Minutes)	References
Aldabra tortoises *Aldabrachelys gigantea*	Medetomidine + Ketamine + Morphine	0.03 / 3 / 0.4	IM	30–45	Atipamezole IM / Naloxone IM	Up to 45	Vigani (2010)
Aldabra tortoises *Aldabrachelys gigantea*	Medetomidine + Ketamine	0.025–0.08 / 3–8	IV	45	Atipamezole IV	Up to 15	Lock et al. (1998)
Chinese box turtles *Cuora flavomarginata*	Medetomidine + Ketamine + Morphine	0.1 / 10 / 1.5	IM	30	Atipamezole IM / Naloxone IM	Up to 21	Hernandez-Divers et al. (2009)
Desert tortoises *Gopherus agassizii*	Medetomidine	0.15	IM	20	Atipamezole IM	30–60	Sleeman and Gaynor (2000)
Desert tortoises *Gopherus agassizii*	Sevoflurane	5% in O_2	Inhaled	5	Not administered	Up to 35	Rooney et al. (1999)
Florida softshell turtles *Apalone ferox*	Tricaine methanesulfonate (MS-222)	1g/L	Immersion	Not specified	Not administered	Not specified	Bagatto et al. (1997)
Galapagos tortoises *Chelonoidis nigra*	Medetomidine + Ketamine	0.1 / 10	IV	11	Not administered	Up to 70	Knafo et al. (2011)
Galapagos tortoises *Chelonoidis nigra*	Medetomidine + Ketamine + Morphine	0.02 / 2 / 0.4	IM	30	Atipamezole IM / Naloxone IM	Up to 60	Vigani (2010)
Gopher tortoises *Gopherus polyphemus*	Medetomidine + Ketamine	0.1 / 5	IV	Not specified	Atipamezole	Not specified	Dennis and Heard (2002)
Greek tortoises *Testudo greca*	Alphaxalone/Alphadolone	9–16	IM	25–40	Not administered	Up to 4 hours	Lawrence and Jackson (1983)
Kemp's ridley sea turtle *Lepidochelys kempi*	Medetomidine + Ketamine	0.015–0.03 / 2.5–3	IV	15	Not administered	200	Smith et al. (2000)
Leatherback sea turtles *Dermochelys coriacea*	Medetomidine + Ketamine	0.03–0.1 / 3–12	IV	20	Atipamezole IV	Up to 120	Harms et al. (2007)
Lepard tortoises *Geochelone pardalis*	Medetomidine + Ketamine	0.1 / 5	IV	16	Atipamezole IV	Up to 30	Lock et al. (1998)
Loggerhead sea turtle *Caretta caretta*	Propofol	5	IV	2	Not administered	Up to 170	MacLean et al. (2008)
Loggerhead sea turtle *Caretta caretta*	Medetomidine + Ketamine	0.05 / 5	IV	9	Atipamezole IV	Up to 84	Chittick et al. (2002)
Red-eared sliders *Trachemys scripta elegans*	Propofol	10–20	IV	2–4	Not administered	90–120	Ziolo and Bertelsen (2009)
Red-eared sliders *Trachemys scripta elegans*	Medetomidine + Ketamine	0.1–0.2 / 5–10	IM	Not specified	Atipamezole IM	60	Greer et al. (2001)
Red-eared sliders *Trachemys scripta elegans*	Midazolam	1.5	IM	6	Not administered	40	Oppenheim and Moon (1995)
Side-neck turtle *Podocnemis expansa*	Xylazine + Propofol	1.5 / 5–10	IM / IV	1–2	Not administered	156–198	Santos et al. (2008)
Snapping turtle *Chelydra serpentine*	Ketamine + Midazolam	20–40 / 2	IM	15	Not administered	210	Bienzle and Boyd (1992)
Softshell turtle *Pelodiscus sinensis*	Lidocaine	700mg/L	Immersion	6	Not administered	5	Park et al. (2006)
Yellow-footed tortoises *Geochelone denticulata*	Medetomidine + Ketamine	0.1 / 5	IV	16	Atipamezole IV	Up to 30	Lock et al. (1998)

available. It can be administered intravenously or intramuscularly for short surgical procedures, at the same dosages described for the previous mixture. The low concentration (10 mg/mL), however, precludes intramuscular injection in any animal larger than a kilogram.

Softshell aquatic turtles appear to possess an amphibian-like modality of fluid absorption across nonenteral surfaces (e.g., skin and mucous membranes beside the enteral mucosa) (Bagatto et al. 1997). In spiny and Florida softshell turtles (*Apalone apinifera* and *Apalone ferox*), tricaine methanesulfonate (MS-222) has been tested as an immersion anesthetic. A concentration of g/L provided a quick onset of surgical anesthesia. All the animals in the study survived and the technique was considered safe by the authors (Bagatto et al. 1997). Lidocaine-hydrochloride diluted in bicarbonate-buffered water was also used as anesthetic in softshelled turtle (*Pelodiscus sinensis*). Immersion at 700 mg/L produced anesthesia within 6 minutes after exposure. Recovery time was short, after removal of the animal from the anesthetic solution (Park et al. 2006).

Succinylcholine and other neuromuscular blocking agents alone have been used in the past for immobilization of chelonians. This class of drugs does not have any anesthetic or analgesic properties and the patient is completely conscious while paralyzed. The depolarization before muscle relaxation associated with succinylcholine also causes pain, lactic academia, and hyperkalemia. For these reasons, the use of neuromuscular blocking agents alone for immobilization is considered unacceptable.

Endotracheal intubation is facilitated by the use of a tongue depressor to better expose the glottis. In aquatic turtles, there is abundant soft tissue at the base of tongue, which can make visualization of the glottis difficult (Fig. 22.10).

Gentle upwards pressure on the skin surface between the mandibular branches helps to expose the glottis. The size of endotracheal tube can be estimated either by external palpation of the trachea or by visualizing the glottal diameter during inspiration. The glottal opening is usually smaller than the tracheal diameter. Cuffed endotracheal tubes can be used, but overinflation of the cuff can potentially cause tracheal injury. The trachea is relatively short, particularly in sea turtles, and the selective intubation of a bronchus is possibly if a long endotracheal tube is inserted too far.

Immobility has a substantial negative impact on ventilation due to the important role of limb movement for lung expansion (Gatten 1974b; Taylor et al. 2010). The respiratory drive is also depressed by the direct effect of anesthetic agents on the respiratory centers. This predisposes the patient to hypoxemia and hypercapnia. Also, hypoventilation prevents the constant delivery of anesthetic when inhalation anesthesia is used. Manual or mechanical intermittent positive

pressure ventilation (IPPV) are, therefore, recommended for general anesthesia. Tidal volumes are highly variable and influenced by species and body position. Sea turtles have much higher tidal volumes compared with terrestrial tortoises (Lutcavage & Lutz 1996). The lung compliance is also much lower in dorsal recumbency compared with ventral recumbency (Lutcavage et al. 1989). Concerns exist to the possible detrimental effect of positive pressure ventilation on the cardiovascular system. However, examination of the effect of artificially manipulating lung volume on blood flows and heart rate in the freshwater turtle (*Trachemys scripta elegans*), showed increases in lung volume have no effect on pulmonary blood flow (Herman et al. 1997). It is difficult to assess effective artificial ventilation in the clinical setting. Current recommendations for IPPV are two to six breaths per minute using tidal volumes ranging from 15 to 20 mL/kg, with peak airway pressures less than 10 cm H_2O.

For pronged procedures, anesthesia can be maintained by use of supplemental doses of the drug combination

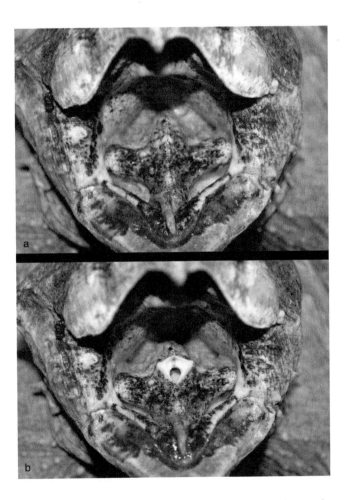

Figure 22.10. Glottal apparatus of an alligator snapping turtle (*Macrochelys temminckii*) during breath holding (a), and during inspiration (b). Note the perfect seal of the closed glottis. Waiting for the animal to voluntarily open the glottis facilitates the endotracheal intubation.

used for induction or more commonly by use of inhaled anesthetics. Gaining familiarity with multiple anesthetic agents and protocols in different species, allows prediction of the patient response and the duration of effect of each specific anesthetic agent or combination.

Important aspects of patient care during anesthesia include continuous patient monitoring, appropriate fluid therapy, maintenance of the species' preferred body temperature, appropriate analgesia, and lubrication of the eyes. In giant tortoises, the protection of the limbs and the phallus (frequently prolapsed in males during anesthesia) is also critical for avoiding severe crushing injuries caused by the weight of the anesthetized animal.

MONITORING

The extreme physiologic resilience of reptiles should never be considered an excuse to overlook constant assessment of an anesthetized patient. Information is now available on the application of several types of monitoring equipment in chelonian anesthesia (Bailey & Pablo 1998; Hernandez-Divers 2004; Mosley et al. 2004). The accuracy and reliability of much of this equipment, however, is only beginning to be determined and for the most part has not been validated. This underlines the importance of the role of the anesthesiologist in the constant direct assessment of anesthetic depth, cardiopulmonary function, body temperature, and other physiologic parameters.

Anesthetic Depth

The accurate assessment of anesthetic depth is challenging. Several authors have previously proposed guidelines for the assessment of the stage of anesthesia in chelonians (McArthur 2004). Stages 1 and 2 are associated with minimal muscle relaxation, persistence of head withdrawal reflex, and voluntary response to painful stimuli. These anesthetic stages are indicated for noninvasive or minimally invasive procedures.

Stage 3 (Surgical anesthetic stage) is characterized by immobility, absence of head withdrawal reflex, marked muscle relaxation occurring craniocaudally as anesthetic depth increases, and no voluntary muscle response to noxious stimulation. This is considered a suitable stage for performing invasive surgical or diagnostic procedures.

The deepest anesthetic stage (Stage 4) represents severe medullary depression due to anesthetic overdose. This stage is associated with life-threatening, severe cardiovascular depression and is clinically detected by the loss of all reflexes, including the vent and corneal reflexes.

In chelonians, hypoventilation and apnea are common during anesthesia even at lighter stages. Therefore, the assessment of respiration does not rep-

resent a good indicator of anesthetic depth, and ventilatory support should be provided to all anesthetized chelonians. Heart rate is influenced by multiple factors including temperature and oxygenation, making this an unreliable parameter for the assessment of anesthetic depth (Krosniunas & Hicks 2003; McArthur et al. 2004).

Cardiovascular Function

The main aim of cardiovascular monitoring is to assure adequate blood flow to the tissue. Monitored variables include heart rate and rhythm, pulse, and changes in intravascular volume caused by blood loss. It has been reported that baseline heart rate in reptiles, maintained within its preferred optimal temperature zone, can be estimated using the formula: $33.4 \times (Wt_{kg}^{-25})$ based on allometric scaling (Sedgwick 1991). However, insufficient data is available on the reliability of this calculation in chelonians. Further, given heart rate is highly affected by variations in body temperature, any kind of approximation is of limited significance and potentially misleading during anesthesia.

Direct auscultation of cardiac sounds is a simple method of basic assessment of heart rate and rhythm. In anesthetized patients, an esophageal stethoscope can be placed into the thoracic esophagus to the level of the heart for direct auscultation. Since it may cause reflux of gastric contents, the trachea should be intubated prior to its placement. The stethoscope tubing has to be slowly advanced until the maximal sound intensity is reached. It can be connected to a standard stethoscope headpiece for intermittent monitoring or to a portable amplified speaker for continuous assessment.

The electrocardiogram (ECG) detects the electrical activity of the heart. It should be noted the presence of normal electrical activity does not indicate normal cardiac function. Myocardial conduction can continue despite absence of myocardial contraction, which is referred to as pulseless electrical activity. Therefore, the monitoring of cardiovascular function should not rely solely on an ECG. The ECG can be used as a standard three-limb lead configuration, but the thick scaly skin limits its sensitivity in this configuration and requires the use of a hypodermic needle for effective lead attachment (Bailey & Pablo 1998). A base-apex ECG configuration represents a good alternative during anesthesia. Esophageal base-apex ECG lead configurations are commercially available in different sizes and are often combined on the same tubing with an esophageal stethoscope. For anesthetic monitoring, the ECG is usually viewed in lead II. The reptilian ECG tracing is comprised of three primary complexes: P wave, QRS complex, and T wave. An SV wave may precede the P wave and represents the depolarization of the sinus venosus (Fig. 22.11). As in mammalian species, the P wave and the QRS complex represent atrial depolarization

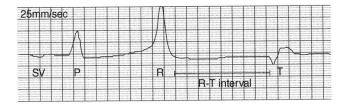

Figure 22.11. Electrocardiographic tracing of an anesthetized Galapagos tortoise (*Chelonoidis nigra*). On the tracing, the following waves are identified: (SV) sinus venosus depolarization, (P) atrial depolarization, (R) ventricular depolarization, and (T) ventricular repolarization. Note that systolic phase of the cardiac cycle is physiologically prolonged (R-T interval is approximately 1.6 seconds).

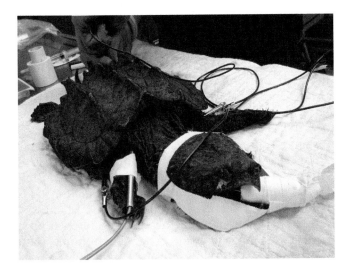

Figure 22.12. Cardiovascular monitoring of a juvenile alligator snapping turtle (*Macrochelys temminckii*) during anesthesia. A 8-Hz Doppler pencil probe is placed on the side of the neck with the detecting crystal directed toward the thoracic inlet. The ECG is used in a standard three limb lead configuration.

and ventricular depolarization, respectively. The T wave indicates ventricular repolarization. In chelonians, this repolarization phase is physiologically very prolonged (Holz & Holz 1995).

Due to the paucity of research, there is still limited understanding regarding ECG interpretation in chelonians and all reptiles in general (Kik & Mitchell 2005).

The use of an 8-Hz Doppler ultrasonic flow probe is a good alternative to direct auscultation to detect blood flow. It also allows the detection of pulse in major vessels. For these reasons, many authors promote the Doppler as the most useful and reliable cardiovascular monitoring device in reptiles (McArthur 2004; Schumacher 2007). Several types of probes are available, adult and pediatric flat probes and pencil probes. In chelonians, the pencil probe is most useful for the detection of cardiac blood flow. It is placed on either side of the neck on the ventral aspect of the thoracic inlet (Fig. 22.12). Flat probes can also be taped over the carotid

arteries (ventrolateral aspect of the neck), the coccygeal artery (base of the tail), and femoral arteries for continuous assessment of pulse rate and quality.

Pediatric probes are preferred over adult probes due to the higher sensitivity in detecting flow in small vessels.

Determination of peripheral pulse rate and rhythm can also be obtained with the use of a pulse oximeter. As discussed in the next section, pulse oximetry is more often used as a respiratory monitor. Unfortunately, the use of pulse oximetry in chelonians for detecting pulse is limited by placement sites for the probe. Reflectance probes placed in the oral cavity or the cloaca may be a better choice. Some pulse oximetry units are extremely sensitive, and the presence of a strong pulsatile signal does not necessarily correlate with adequate blood flow to the tissues. When the probe is correctly applied, less than 10% of normal blood flow is required for pulse oximeters to detect a pulse (Bailey & Pablo 1998).

During surgery hemorrhage is common and monitoring blood loss is always indicated to determine the need for intervention. In small patients (<1 kg), any detectable blood loss can produce a significant decrease in circulating blood volume and consequent deterioration of patient homeostasis.

Respiratory Function

The direct visualization of respiratory movements, such as thoracic excursions, can be difficult. The presence of respiratory movements does not indicate adequate ventilation. The use of respiratory monitoring, therefore, is essential.

Arterial blood gas analysis is the ideal method for assessment of respiratory gas exchange, directly measuring the degree of oxygenation (arterial oxygen concentration or PaO_2) and ventilation (arterial carbon dioxide concentration or $PaCO_2$). Unfortunately, the clinical applicability of blood gas analysis in chelonians is limited. Arterial blood sampling in chelonians is difficult and impractical. Additionally, multiple blood draws can represent a significant blood loss in very small patients. Reptiles tend to tolerate alterations in $PaCO_2$ and PaO_2 much more than mammals, and thus normal values for mammals may not be applicable (Hernandez-Divers 2004). In mammalian species, venous blood gas analysis can be used for assessing ventilation (venous CO_2 concentration approximates arterial concentration) but not oxygenation. However, the reliability of venous blood gas analysis in chelonians has not been demonstrated. For all of these reasons, the value of routine blood gas analysis in chelonians remains questionable. Other monitoring devices of respiratory function are capnometry and pulse oximetry.

Capnometry measures carbon dioxide concentration in expired gases (PetCO_2). In mammalian species, capnometry is a noninvasive monitoring tool for assessing ventilation due to the good correlation between the end tidal concentration of CO_2 and arterial CO_2 concentration. In chelonians this correlation is not consistent due to cardiac shunting. The absolute values of $PetCO_2$, therefore, may not be a reliable indicator of arterial CO_2 due to the unpredictable gradient between end-tidal and arterial carbon dioxide (Hernandez-Divers 2004). Capnometry is best used over time to assess trends and to identify potential anesthetic complications. For this purpose, devices with graphing capability (capnograph) that display a continuous waveform (capnogram) are more useful than standard capnometers. Any large, sudden decrease in $PetCO_2$ requires further investigation. These drops are commonly associated with obstruction or kinking of the endotracheal tube, but can also be indicative of an abrupt decrease in cardiac output.

Mainstream and sidestream capnometry devices are commercially available. Mainstream analyzers use a detecting window inserted into the anesthetic circuit. A sensor mounted on the detecting window measures $PetCO_2$. Sidestream analyzers continuously aspirate gas from the anesthetic circuit, and the sensor for the analysis is located away from the ventilator circuit. There are some concerns when capnometry is used in small species. Large detecting window (mainstream) or sampling chamber (sidestream) attached to the endotracheal tube add significant mechanical dead space. Pediatric connectors can reduce this added dead space. The sensor of mainstream devices may add an excessive amount of weight on the endotracheal tube, causing possible kinking. Sidestream devices require the continuous removal of gas from the circuit (100–200 mL per minute), and in very small animals, this sampling rate can be similar to or higher than the tidal volume of the patient. Relatively new veterinary designed sidestream capnometers, such as the Capnovet-10 (Vetronic Services, Devon, UK) use smaller sampling volumes and are suitable for use in patients weighing less than 100 g (Stanford 2004).

Pulse oximetry is used to noninvasively measure the oxygen saturation of arterial hemoglobin (SpO_2). A plethysmograph (to detect pulsatile blood flow) and a combined spectrophotometer (to measure changes in light absorbance) constitute the functional components of a pulse oximeter. Although pulse oximetry is one of the most commonly used anesthetic monitoring devices in reptiles, its technical limitations and high susceptibility to measurement errors and artifacts should be considered. Pulse oximetry has been designed for use in mammals, meaning it detects typical mammalian pulse, and is calibrated using the mammalian oxygen hemoglobin dissociation curve. In reptiles, the characteristics of these variables are markedly different when compared with mammals (Frische et al. 2001). In green iguanas, it was shown the absorbencies for oxyhemoglobin (660 nm) and deoxyhemoglobin (990 nm)

were in agreement with mammalian references, indicating that pulse oximetry could be reliable in certain reptile species (Diethelm et al. 1998). Unfortunately, the transmittance probes used in mammals do not provide consistent readings when applied to the skin of reptiles. Reflectance probes are more easily placed inside the esophagus or the cloaca to maximize the chance of reading. In the green iguana, a reflectance pulse oximeter probe placed in the esophagus and was inaccurate (Mosley et al. 2004). As for capnography, pulse oximetry is best used to look at the trends in measurements, rather than at the absolute saturation values.

Body Temperature

As in all ectothermic animals, normal thermoregulation in chelonians results from the direct interaction between the animal and the external environment. A series of behavioral patterns and modulations of the cardiovascular system tightly regulate the amount of heat derived from the environment (Galli et al. 2004). During anesthesia, all of these mechanisms are blunted or even abolished and hypothermia is a common occurrence. The direct effect on the cardiovascular system is a progressive decrease in cardiac output and an increase in intracardiac shunting (Krosniunas & Hicks 2003). The anesthetist, therefore, is responsible for appropriately monitoring and modulating body temperature in anesthetized chelonians. The aim is to minimize variations from the species' preferred body temperature range allowing better patient homeostasis (Gatten 1974a). Intraoperatively, this goal is accomplished by appropriately insulating and actively warming the patient (Fig. 22.13).

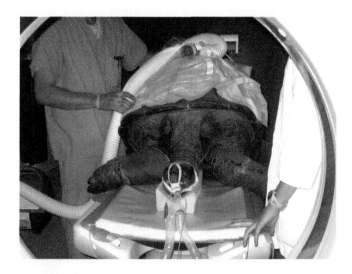

Figure 22.13.   Active warming the patient with a forced warm air blower (Bair Hugger®, Arizant Healthcare Inc., Eden Prairie, MN). The maintenance of the patient's temperature within the preferred body temperature range is an important aspect of patient care in chelonians. Unpredictable disarrangement of the chelonian's homeostasis can occur in response to sudden changes in body temperature.

Patient temperature can be continuously monitored using cloacal or esophageal probes. The patient should not be in direct contact with cold surfaces and should be covered with plastic drapes during prolonged surgical procedures to decrease the dispersion of internal heat. Warm water bottles, circulating warm water blankets, and forced warm air blowers, in ascending order of efficiency, also represent suitable tools for actively increasing and maintaining normothermia. When active warming is provided, attention should be paid not to overheat the patient. Increasing the temperature above the ATR increases oxygen consumption and the animal breathing room air (e.g., during the recovery period) may be unable to meet the increased oxygen demand. It should be noted body temperatures above 38°C are lethal for most chelonian species.

As mentioned in a previous section, the preferred body temperature or ATR in chelonians is species dependent. For example, many freshwater turtles will tolerate temperatures between 20 and 25°C, whereas sea turtles and land tortoises are better adapted to temperatures between 25 and 30°C (George 1996; McArthur et al. 2004).

Suboptimal temperatures are associated with decreased metabolic rate and consequent unpredictably prolonged clearance of anesthetic agents. When body temperature declines, recovery times are commonly prolonged while inhaled anesthetic requirements are reduced.

Blood Glucose

Monitoring blood glucose in juvenile patients and debilitated patients or during prolonged anesthesia is recommended to detect hypoglycemic episodes. However, the occurrence of hypoglycemia in anesthetized chelonians has not been documented and the need for repeated glucose checks is debatable.

RECOMMENDED SEDATIVES AND ANESTHETIC AGENTS

Injectable Drugs

Combinations of parenteral drugs belonging to different classes permit a reduction the required dosages of each agent, therefore reducing their potential side effects. It has been shown multiple drug combinations provide better sedation, muscle relaxation, and shorter induction and recovery times compared to the use of single agents. The administration of specific antagonists for some classes of sedatives makes it possible to modulate the duration of their effect.

α_2-**Adrenergic Agonists** Alpha$_2$-adrenergic agonists are extensively used sedatives in chelonian anesthesia (Holz & Holz 1994; Lock et al. 1998; Sleeman & Gaynor 2000). The rapid onset of action, the potent sedation, and the possibility to reverse their sedative effect with specific antagonists are the major advantages of α_2-agonists compared with other sedatives. Alpha$_2$ agonists are also characterized by a mild analgesic activity (Greer et al. 2001b). Alpha$_2$-adrenergic agonists are part of many anesthetic protocols owing to their synergistic effect with other agents, such as ketamine (Chittick et al. 2002; Greer et al. 2001b). Xylazine when combined with ketamine produced moderate sedation in freshwater turtles (*Trachemys*) (Holz & Holz 1994). Xylazine (1.5 mg/kg), administered intramuscularly, followed by intravenous induction with propofol (5 mg/kg), also produced moderate sedation for 2.5 hours in Amazonian turtles (*Podocnemis expansa*) (Santos et al. 2008). In loggerhead sea turtles (*Caretta caretta*), medetomidine (0.05 mg/kg) combined with ketamine (5 mg/kg) was shown to produce rapid induction (Chittick et al. 2002). Wild leatherback sea turtles (*Dermochelys coriacea*) were effectively immobilized for measurement of physiologic variables with a combination of medetomidine (0.03–0.08 mg/kg) and ketamine (3–8 mg/kg) (Harms et al. 2007). In Galapagos tortoises (*Ge. nigra*), medetomidine (0.1 mg/kg) and ketamine (10 mg/kg) given intravenously as a combination produced a surgical plane of anesthesia sufficient to perform celioscopy for about 45 minutes (Knafo et al. 2011). In adult Aldabra tortoises (*Aldabrachelys gigantea*), intramuscular medetomidine (0.02–0.03 mg/kg), ketamine (2–3 mg/kg), and midazolam (0.1 mg/kg), have been used by the author as an induction and maintenance anesthetic protocol for both diagnostic and minor surgical procedures.

Pronounced cardiopulmonary side effects, however, are common after administration of α_2-adrenergic agonists in chelonians and appear to be similar to those seen in mammals (Dennis & Heard 2002). The effect of alpha$_2$-adrenergic agonists on the cardiovascular system appears to be dose-unrelated. Bradycardia and hypoxemia were described in desert tortoises (*Gopherus agassizii*) sedated with medetomidine (0.15 mg/kg) (Sleeman & Gaynor 2000). Medetomidine (0.1 mg/kg) produced good sedation, but also moderate bradycardia in leopard tortoises (*Geochelone pardalis*) and yellow foot tortoises (*Geochelone denticulata*) (Lock et al. 1998). Similar effects were seen in Aldabra tortoises (*Aldabrachelys gigantea*) at the dose of 0.025–0.08 mg/kg (Lock et al. 1998). In gopher tortoises, the combination of medetomidine (0.1 mg/kg) and ketamine (5 mg/kg) produced moderate hypertension, hypercapnia, and hypoxemia (Dennis & Heard 2002). For these reasons, the use of supplemental oxygen is highly recommended when α_2-adrenergic agonists are used.

Severe cardiovascular changes can be also caused by the intravenous administration of reversal agents. The antagonist atipamezole (0.5 mg/kg) given IV was demonstrated to produce severe hypotension and even undetectable carotid pulse in gopher tortoises (*Gopherus polyphemus*) (Dennis & Heard 2002). Based on these findings, it is recommended to utilize the intramuscular route for injection of the reversal agent of α_2-agonist.

The stereoisomer dexmedetomidine is now commonly used in veterinary anesthesia. Its potency in mammals appears to be twice as high as that of medetomidine (Kuusela et al. 2001). There are no published studies on the sedative effect of dexmedetomidine in chelonians. Medetomidine is still commercially available as a compounded preparation at high concentrations (10–20–40 mg/mL). In large chelonians (>100 kg), these concentrated solutions are a good choice for intramuscular administration to significantly reduce the volume of injection.

Ketamine Ketamine is a dissociative anesthetic commonly utilized in many reported anesthetic protocols for chelonians. Ketamine has a large margin of safety due to its supportive cardiovascular effects and its lower respiratory depression when compared with other induction agents, such as barbiturates and propofol. Used alone, ketamine requires very high dosages to produce general anesthesia in chelonians (30–50 mg/kg), does not produce adequate muscle relaxation, and is associated with prolonged induction and recovery times of up to 24 hours (Holz & Holz 1994). The combination of ketamine with other sedatives produces a synergistic effect at reducing the doses of the single agents. Benzodiazepines and α_2-adrenergic agonists improve the anesthetic profile of ketamine, producing better muscle relaxation and making it possible to obtain a plane of anesthesia more suitable for surgical interventions (Chittick et al. 2002). Benzodiazepines are primarily added to produce muscle relaxation (Bienzle & Boyd 1992). Alpha$_2$-adrenergic agonists are often used to significantly decrease the ketamine dose and to achieve deeper anesthetic planes (Greer et al. 2001a; Harms et al. 2007; Lock et al. 1998). Medetomidine and xylazine, added to ketamine, are a very common induction protocol for both aquatic and terrestrial species. Several dosing regimens have been reported in different chelonians, showing significant interspecies variability in dose and sedative effect (see Table 22.2). Ketamine also has intrinsic analgesic properties, due to its antagonist effect on N-methyl-D-aspartate (NMDA) receptors. The presence of this type of receptor has been demonstrated in chelonians (Bickler et al. 2000). The analgesic effect of ketamine is mild and short-lived for treatment of surgical pain and superior analgesia is provided by the use of a multimodal approach. The addition of more potent systemic analgesics, such as opioids, and the use of LA are recommended for management of acute surgical pain.

Propofol Propofol is a fast-acting hypnotic agent formulated for intravenous injection only. Several reports describe the safety of propofol as induction agent in several chelonian species (McArthur 2007; Smith et al. 2000; Ziolo & Bertelsen 2009) (see Table 22.2). Propofol produces induction of general anesthesia within 1–2 minutes after injection (Santos et al. 2008). The duration of effect is usually 30–45 minutes at the typical dosages of 2–10 mg/kg. Large species appear to require lower doses compared with small chelonians (McArthur 2004). In a study in loggerhead sea turtles (*Caretta caretta*), propofol (5 mg/kg) produced an adequate plane of anesthesia for laparoscopic sex determination. The duration of effect lasted 30 minutes (MacLean et al. 2008). Prolonged apnea following induction with propofol is a common complication in chelonians and prompt intubation and manual ventilation are therefore required. Dose-dependent hypotension can be severe following rapid administration. Slow injection over 1 minute allows the anesthetist to titrate the administration to the desired effect, minimizing the cardiovascular depression. Propofol does not have any analgesic activity and it should always be combined with analgesics when performing surgical procedures. Propofol given as a constant rate infusion (0.2–0.4 mg/kg/min) or as incremental boluses (0.5–1 mg/kg) is suitable for maintenance of anesthesia in mammals, but the safety and the appropriate rates of infusion in reptiles have not been determined. The fast induction and recovery time and the possibility to modulate the effect by adjusting the dose, make propofol the author's anesthetic of choice whenever the intravenous route is accessible.

Midazolam

Midazolam is a benzodiazepine with similar potency to diazepam. Compared with diazepam, the more hydrosoluble molecule of midazolam produces more constant absorption and better bioavailability after intramuscular injection. Midazolam used alone, even at dosages 10 times higher than the therapeutic doses for mammals, was repeatedly shown not to produce significant sedation in some chelonian species (Harvey-Clark 1993). In sliders, 1.5 mg/kg IM provided moderate sedation with minimal cardiovascular and respiratory changes (Oppenheim & Moon 1995). In snapping turtles (*Chelydra serpentina*), the combination of midazolam and ketamine appeared to produce better sedation and muscle relaxation compared to use of single agents (Bienzle & Boyd 1992). General anesthesia, however, could not be achieved even at high dosages. The recommended dosages for chelonians range between 0.1 and 1 mg/kg. When midazolam is used in chelonian anesthesia, it is suggested to combine it with other agents, such as ketamine or propofol, to produce adequate anesthetic depth (Holz & Holz 1994; Wood et al. 1982). The sedative effect of midazolam can be reversed by the specific antagonist flumazenil (0.01–0.04 mg/kg).

Alfaxalone Alfaxalone is a neurosteroid that exerts its anesthetic effect by binding to GABA-receptors. It was originally introduced in the 1970s as a mixture with alfadolone for induction of anesthesia. The trade name of the compound in the veterinary market was Saffan®. This formulation was later withdrawn from the market because of the occurrence of lethal anaphylactoid reactions in small animals. These adverse effects were induced by the presence in the compound of Cremophor EL®, as a solubilizing agent.

Recently alfaxalone, as a new water-soluble formulation, has been reintroduced on the veterinary market under the brand name of Alfaxan®. Water solubility of this preparation is due to the binding of the alfaxalone molecule to a cyclodextrine molecule. This mixture does not cause histamine release unlike the old formulation.

Unlike propofol, alfaxalone can also be administered via the intramuscular route, providing a possible alternative of anesthetic induction when vascular access is not available. It should be noted, however, that the use of the intramuscular route requires higher dosages compared with the intravenous route. In chelonians, alphaxalone given IM produced anesthesia at the dosage of 10–20 mg/kg (Lawrence & Jackson 1983). Alfaxan is available at the concentration of 10 mg/mL and its use in large chelonians (>10 kg), therefore, may be limited by the very large volume of drug which then must be injected intramuscularly.

Neuromuscular Blocking Agents The use of nondepolarizing neuromuscular blocking agents (NNMBAs) has been recently described to facilitate endotracheal intubation in chelonians (Kaufman et al. 2003). Nondepolarizing neuromuscular blockers have a much safer toxicological profile compared with depolarizing agents such as succinylcholine. NNMBAs do not have any anesthetic or analgesic activity, therefore, they should never be utilized alone for immobilization. They must be considered only as complementary to a balanced anesthetic technique. Rocuronium is a NNMBA with rapid onset and intermediate duration of action. Rocuronium (0.2 mg/kg IM) has been shown to permit endotracheal intubation in Gulf Coast box turtles (*Terrapene carolina major*) and in Amazon turtles (*Podocnemis expansa*) within 15 minutes after administration (Kaufman et al. 2003; Scarpa Bosso et al. 2009). The effects of NNMBAs can be antagonized with neostigmine. In the studies mentioned earlier, recovery time (time to walking) from rocuronium occurred within 30 minutes after administration of neostigmine (0.04–0.07 mg/kg IM). Glycopyrrolate (0.01 mg/kg) can be coadministered with neostigmine to prevent its potential parasympathetic effects.

Inhaled Anesthetics

Currently, the inhalants isoflurane and sevoflurane are favored for maintenance of anesthesia in reptiles (Shaw et al. 1992). High concentrations of inhaled anesthetics and awake endotracheal intubation are required when these agents are used for induction. The potency of inhaled anesthetics is conventionally expressed as the < MAC. The values of MAC for isoflurane and sevoflurane in green iguanas (*Iguana iguana*) were 1.8% and 3.1%, respectively (Barter et al. 2006). Specific values of MAC for chelonian species have not been determined yet, but clinical evidence suggests the inspired concentrations required for surgical anesthesia are similar to the ones reported for other reptiles. Sevoflurane, by virtue of its low solubility in blood, is associated with faster anesthetic induction and recovery times when compared with isoflurane in mammals. Similar findings were shown in reptiles. In green iguanas (*Iguana iguana*), recovery time was significantly longer in animals anesthetized with isoflurane (35 ± 27 minutes) when compared with sevoflurane (7 ± 4 minutes) (Hernandez-Divers et al. 2005). Recovery times after 2 hours of anesthesia with 2% isoflurane averaged 4 hours in Kemp's ridley sea turtles, whereas prolonged anesthesia in desert tortoises, induced and maintained with sevoflurane, was associated with recovery times averaging 30 minutes (Moon & Stabenau 1996; Rooney et al. 1999). However, the high intracardiac shunting typical of aquatic chelonians may have contributed to these significant differences.

Interestingly, it has been shown in green iguanas that the MAC of inhalants tends to decrease over time, most likely reflecting limitations to anesthetic uptake and distribution. The progressive decrease in anesthetic requirements could also suggest that for any given end-tidal anesthetic concentration, the plane of anesthesia may deepen over time during prolonged procedures (Brosnan et al. 2006). For this reason, it is important to constantly monitor the depth of anesthesia and to titrate the concentration of inhalant to decrease the risk of overdose.

Chelonians can voluntarily breath-hold and successful use of inhaled anesthetics requires controlled ventilation for adequate drug uptake and elimination. Pure oxygen is the carrier gas usually utilized with inhalants. However, experimental evidence suggests hyperoxia depresses ventilation in both terrestrial and aquatic chelonians (Glass et al. 1978). Hypoxia, however, appears to be a common anesthetic complication in chelonians supporting the use of high inspired oxygen concentrations. Consequently, the ideal carrier gas mixture that would provide adequate oxygenation and maintain appropriate ventilation is still undetermined.

Inhalants do not provide any analgesic effect; therefore, appropriate addition of analgesics is required for any surgical procedure. Intraoperative pain management and use of balanced anesthetic techniques will also decrease the requirements of inhalant and hence side effects. For example, the cardiovascular depression associated with inhalant anesthesia in reptiles, as in mammals, has been shown to be dose dependent (Mosley et al. 2004). For this reason, the multimodal approach to chelonian anesthesia using injectable and inhaled agents has gained the favor of many investigators (Chittick et al. 2002; McArthur 2004; Moon & Hernandez Foester 2001; Shaw et al. 1992) (see Table 22.2).

RECOVERY

Recovery time from anesthesia appears to be prolonged in chelonians when compared with mammals exposed to the same anesthetic agent. This difference may be due to the lower efficiency of the metabolic pathways of reptiles (McArthur et al. 2004). Additionally, temperature significantly affects the metabolic rate and the cardiovascular physiology of chelonians (Krosniunas & Hicks 2003). Both represent critical factors affecting a timely and successful recovery from anesthesia. For instance, hypothermia is associated with a decrease in metabolic function, which could delay the clearance of many injectable agents. Additionally, the amplification of intracardiac shunting, occurring when body temperature is below the ATR, can decrease the elimination of inhaled anesthetics through the lungs. Warming the patient above the preferred temperature for the species is also discouraged owing to the risk of increased oxygen demand (Galli et al. 2004). Consequently, the maintenance of body temperature within the ATR is recommended. Respiratory depression also persists during the recovery period. Noticeably, chelonians can occasionally take spontaneous breaths in the early postoperative period, but these should not be misinterpreted as signs of complete recovery from anesthesia. It is recommended to maintain the patient intubated until consistent spontaneous ventilation and voluntary movements are present.

There is evidence that catecholamines modulate cardiac shunting in chelonians (Overgaard et al. 2002). Particularly in *Trachemys*, epinephrine was shown to increase pulmonary blood flow by directly reversing the presence of right to left shunting. Ongoing studies at the University of Florida are investigating the efficacy and safety of the administration of epinephrine in reducing recovery time after inhalant anesthesia in chelonians.

REFERENCES

Bagatto B, Blankenship EL, Henry RP. 1997. Tricaine methane sulfonate (MS222) anesthesia in spiny and Florida soft-shell turtles *Apalone spinifera* and *Apalone ferox*. *Bulletin of the Association of Reptilian and Amphibian Veterinarians* 7(2):9–11.

Bailey JE, Pablo LS. 1998. Anesthetic monitoring and monitoring Eqmpment: application in small exotic pet practice. *Seminars in Avian and Exotic Pet Medicine* 7(1):53–60.

Baker BB, Sladky KK, Johnson SM. 2011. Evaluation of the analgesic effects of oral and subcutaneous tramadol administration in red-eared slider turtles. *Journal of the American Veterinary Medical Association* 238(2):220–227.

Barter LS, Hawkins MG, Brosnan RJ, et al. 2006. Median effective dose of isoflurane, sevoflurane, and desflurane in green iguanas. *American Journal of Veterinary Research* 67(3):392–397.

Benson KG, Forrest L. 1999. Characterization of the renal portal system of the common green iguana (*Iguana iguana*) by digital subtraction imaging. *Journal of Zoo and Wildlife Medicine* 30(2): 235–241.

Bickler PE, Donohoe PH, Buck LT. 2000. Hypoxia-induced silencing of NMDA receptors in turtle neurons. *The Journal of Neuroscience* 20(10):3522–3528.

Bienzle D, Boyd CJ. 1992. Sedative effects of ketamine and midazolam in snapping turtles (*Chelydra serpentina*). *Journal of Zoo and Wildlife Medicine* 23(2):201–204.

Brosnan RJ, Pypendop BH, Barter LS, et al. 2006. Pharmacokinetics of inhaled anesthetics in green iguanas (*Iguana iguana*). *American Journal of Veterinary Research* 67(10):1670–1674.

Chittick EJ, Stamper MA, Beasley JF, et al. 2002. Medetomidine, ketamine, and sevoflurane for anesthesia of injured loggerhead sea turtles: 13 cases (1996–2000). *Journal of the American Veterinary Medical Association* 221(7):1019–1025.

Crossley D, Altimiras J, Wang T. 1998. Hypoxia elicits an increase in pulmonary vasculature resistance in anaesthetised turtles (*Trachemys scripta*). *The Journal of Experimental Biology* 201 (Pt 24):3367–3375.

Dennis PM, Heard DJ. 2002. Cardiopulmonary effects of a medetomidine-ketamine combination administered intravenously in gopher tortoises. *Journal of the American Veterinary Medical Association* 220(10):1516–1519.

Diethelm G, Mader DR, Grosenbaugh DA, et al. 1998. Evaluating pulse oximetry in the green iguana (Iguana iguana). Proceedings of the Association of Reptile and Amphibian Veterinarians, pp. 11–12.

Divers SJ, Papich M, McBride M, et al. 2010. Pharmacokinetics of meloxicam following intravenous and oral administration in green iguanas (*Iguana iguana*). *American Journal of Veterinary Research* 71(11):1277–1283.

Farrell AP, Gamperl AK, Francis ETB. 1998. Comparative aspects of heart morphology. In: *Biology of the Reptilia* (C Gans, AS Gaunt, eds.), pp. 375–424. Ithaca: Society for the Study of Amphibians and Reptiles.

Fleming GJ, Robertson SA. 2006. Use of thermal threshold test response to evaluate the antinociceptive effects of butorphanol in juvenile green iguanas (Iguana iguana). Annual Meeting American Association of Zoo Veterinarians, pp. 279–280.

Frische S, Bruno S, Fago A, et al. 2001. Oxygen binding by single red blood cells from the red-eared turtle *Trachemys scripta*. *Journal of Applied Physiology* 90(5):1679–1684.

Galli G, Taylor EW, Wang T. 2004. The cardiovascular responses of the freshwater turtle *Trachemys scripta* to warming and cooling. *The Journal of Experimental Biology* 207(Pt 9): 1471–1478.

Gatten RE Jr. 1974a. Effects of temperatures and activity on aerobic and anaerobic metabolism and heart rate in the turtles *Pseudemys scripta* and *Terrapene ornata*. *Comparative Biochemistry and Physiology. A, Comparative Physiology* 48(4):619–648.

Gatten RE Jr. 1974b. Percentage contribution of increased heart rate to increased oxygen transport during activity in *Pseudemys scripta*, *Terrapene ornata* and other reptiles. *Comparative Biochemistry and Physiology. A, Comparative Physiology* 48(4):649–652.

George RH. 1996. Health problems and diseases of sea turtles. In: *The Biology of Sea Turtles* (P Lutz, J Musick, eds.), pp. 363–385. New York: CRC Press Inc.

Giordano J. 2005. The neurobiology of nociceptive and antinociceptive systems. *Pain Physician* 8(3):277–290.

Glass M, Burggren WW, Johansen K. 1978. Ventilation in an aquatic and a terrestrial chelonian reptile. *The Journal of Experimental Biology* 72:165–179.

Greer LL, Jenne KJ, Diggs HE. 2001. Medetomidine-ketamine anesthesia in red-eared slider turtles (*Trachemys scripta elegans*). *Contemporary Topics in Laboratory Animal Science* 40 (3):8–11.

Harms CA, Eckert SA, Kubis SA, et al. 2007. Field anaesthesia of leatherback sea turtles (*Dermochelys coriacea*). *The Veterinary Record* 161(1):15–21.

Harvey-Clark C. 1993. Midazolam fails to sedate painted turtles, Chrysemys picta. *Bulletin of the Association of Reptilian and Amphibian Veterinarians* 3:7–8.

Herman J, Wang T, Smits AW, Hicks JW. 1997. The effects of artificial lung inflation on pulmonary blood flow and heart rate in the turtle Trachemys scripta. *The Journal of Experimental Biology* 200(Pt 19):2539–2545.

Hernandez-Divers SM, Hernandez-Divers SJ. 2002. Angiographic, anatomic and clinical technique descriptions of a subcarapacial venipuncture site for chelonians. *Journal of Herpetological Medicine and Surgery* 12(2):32–37.

Hernandez-Divers SJ, McBride M, Koch T, et al. 2004. Single-dose oral and intravenous pharmacokinetics of meloxicam in the green iguana (Iguana iguana). Proceedings of the Association of Reptilian and Amphibian Veterinarians, pp. 106.

Hernandez-Divers SJ, Stahl SJ, Farrell R. 2009. An endoscopic method for identifying sex of hatchling Chinese box turtles and comparison of general versus local anesthesia for coelioscopy. *Journal of the American Veterinary Medical Association* 234(6): 800–804.

Hernandez-Divers SM. 2004. Blood gas evaluation in the green iguana. *Bulletin of the Association of Reptilian and Amphibian Veterinarians*:45–46.

Hernandez-Divers SM, Schumacher J, Stahl S, et al. 2005. Comparison of isoflurane and sevoflurane anesthesia after premedication with butorphanol in the green iguana (*Iguana iguana*). *Journal of Zoo and Wildlife Medicine* 36(2):169–175.

Hicks J, Comeau S. 1994. Vagal regulation of intracardiac shunting in the turtle *Pseudemys scripta*. *The Journal of Experimental Biology* 186(1):109–126.

Hicks JW, Malvin GM. 1992. Mechanism of intracardiac shunting in the turtle *Pseudemys scripta*. *The American Journal of Physiology* 262(6 Pt 2):R986–R992.

Hicks JW, Wang T. 1999. Hypoxic hypometabolism in the anesthetized turtle, *Trachemys scripta*. *The American Journal of Physiology* 277(1 Pt 2):R18–R23.

Hicks JW, Ishimatsu A, Molloi S, Erskin A, et al. 1996. The mechanism of cardiac shunting in reptiles: a new synthesis. *The Journal of Experimental Biology* 199(Pt 6):1435–1446.

Holsti L, Grunau RE, Oberlander TF, et al. 2008. Is it painful or not? Discriminant validity of the Behavioral Indicators of Infant Pain (BIIP) scale. *The Clinical Journal of Pain* 24(1): 83–88.

Holton L, Reid J, Scott EM, et al. 2001. Development of a behaviour-based scale to measure acute pain in dogs. *The Veterinary Record* 148(17):525–531.

Holz P, Holz RM. 1994. Evaluation of ketamine, ketamine/ xylazine, and ketamine/midazolam anesthesia in red-eared sliders (*Trachemys scripta elegans*). *Journal of Zoo and Wildlife Medicine* 25(4):531–537.

Holz P, Barker IK, Burger JP, et al. 1997a. The effect of the renal portal system on pharmacokinetic parameters in the red-eared slider (*Trachemys scripta elegans*). *Journal of Zoo and Wildlife Medicine* 28(4):386–393.

Holz P, Barker IK, Crawshaw GJ, et al. 1997b. The anatomy and perfusion of the renal portal system in the red-eared slider (*Trachemys scripta elegans*). *Journal of Zoo and Wildlife Medicine* 28(4):378–385.

Holz RM, Holz P. 1995. Electrocardiography in anaesthetised red-eared sliders (*Trachemys scripta elegans*). *Research in Veterinary Science* 58(1):67–69.

IASP. 1994. Part III: pain terms, a current list with definitions and notes on usage. In: *Classification of Chronic Pain*, 2nd ed. (H Merskey, N Bogduk, eds.), pp. 209–214. Seattle: IASP Press.

Jackson DC. 2000. Living without oxygen: lessons from the freshwater turtle. *Comparative Biochemistry and Physiology. Part A, Molecular & Integrative Physiology* 125(3):299–315.

Jacobson ER, Schumacher J, Green M. 1992. Field techniques and clinical techniques for sampling and handling blood for haematologic and selected biochmical determinations in the desert tortoise. *Copiea* 1:237–241.

Kaufman GE, Seymour RE, Bonner BB, et al. 2003. Use of rocuronium for endotracheal intubation of North American Gulf Coast box turtles. *Journal of the American Veterinary Medical Association* 222(8):1111–1115.

Kik MJL, Mitchell MA. 2005. Reptile cardiology: a review of anatomy and physiology, diagnostic approaches, and clinical disease. *Seminars in Avian and Exotic Pet Medicine* 14(1):52–60.

Knafo SE, Divers SJ, Rivera S, et al. 2011. Sterilisation of hybrid Galapagos tortoises (*Geochelone nigra*) for island restoration. Part 1: endoscopic oophorectomy of females under ketamine-medetomidine anaesthesia. *The Veterinary Record* 168(2):47.

Krosniunas EH, Hicks JW. 2003. Cardiac output and shunt during voluntary activity at different temperatures in the turtle, *Trachemys scripta*. *Physiological and Biochemical Zoology: PBZ* 76 (5):679–694.

Kummrow MS, Tseng F, Hesse L, et al. 2008. Pharmacokinetics of buprenorphine after single-dose subcutaneous administration in red-eared sliders (*Trachemys scripta elegans*). *Journal of Zoo and Wildlife Medicine* 39(4):590–595.

Kushiro T, Yamashita K, Umar MA, et al. 2005. Anesthetic and cardiovascular effects of balanced anesthesia using constant rate infusion of midazolam-ketamine-medetomidine with inhalation of oxygen-sevoflurane (MKM-OS anesthesia) in horses. *The Journal of Veterinary Medical Science* 67(4):379–384.

Kuusela E, Raekallio M, Vaisanen M, et al. 2001. Comparison of medetomidine and dexmedetomidine as premedicants in dogs undergoing propofol-isoflurane anesthesia. *American Journal of Veterinary Research* 62(7):1073–1080.

Lawrence K, Jackson OF. 1983. Alphaxalone/alphadolone anaesthesia in reptiles. *The Veterinary Record* 112(2):26–28.

Li X, Keith DE Jr, Evans CJ. 1996. Mu opioid receptor-like sequences are present throughout vertebrate evolution. *Journal of Molecular Evolution* 43(3):179–184.

Liang YF, Terashima S. 1993. Physiological properties and morphological characteristics of cutaneous and mucosal mechanical nociceptive neurons with A-delta peripheral axons in the trigeminal ganglia of crotaline snakes. *The Journal of Comparative Neurology* 328(1):88–102.

Lloyd M, Morris P. 1999. Chelonian venipuncture techniques. *Bulletin of the Association of Reptilian and Amphibian Veterinarians* 9(1):26–29.

Lock BA, Heard DJ, Dennis P. 1998. Preliminary evaluation of medetomidine/ketamine combinations for immobilization and reversal with atipamezole in three tortoise species. *Bulletin of the Association of Reptilian and Amphibian Veterinarians* 8(4): 6–9.

Lutcavage ME, Lutz PL. 1996. Diving physiology. In: *The Biology of Sea Turtles* (PL Lutz, JA Musick, eds.), pp. 277–296. New York: CRC Press.

Lutcavage ME, Lutz PL, Baier H. 1989. Respiratory mechanics of the loggerhead sea turtle, *Caretta caretta*. *Respiration Physiology* 76:13–24.

MacLean RA, Harms CA, Braun-McNeill J. 2008. Propofol anesthesia in loggerhead (*Caretta caretta*) sea turtles. *Journal of Wildlife Diseases* 44(1):143–150.

McArthur S. 2004. Anesthesia, analgesia and euthanasia. In: *Medicine and Surgery of the Tortoises and Turtle*, 1st ed. (S McArthur, R Wilkinson, J Meyer, eds.), pp. 379–401. Oxford: Blackwell Publishing.

McArthur S. 2007. Chelonian anesthesia. Small animal and exotics. Proceedings of the North American Veterinary Conference 21:1574–1579. Orlando, FL.

McArthur S, Meyer J, Innis C. 2004. Anatomy and physiology. In: *Medicine and Surgery of the Tortoises and Turtle*, 1st ed. (S McArthur, R Wilkinson, J Meyer, eds.), pp. 35–72. Oxford: Blackwell Publishing.

Moon PF, Hernandez Foester S. 2001. Reptiles: aquatic turtles (chelonians). In: *Zoological Restraint and Anesthesia*. (D Heard, ed.). Ithaca: International Veterinary Information Service. http://www.ivis.org (accessed February 13, 2014).

Moon PF, Stabenau EK. 1996. Anesthetic and postanesthetic management of sea turtles. *Journal of the American Veterinary Medical Association* 208(5):720–726.

Mosley C. 2011. Pain and nociception in reptiles. *The Veterinary Clinics of North America. Exotic Animal Practice* 14(1):45–60.

Mosley CA, Dyson D, Smith DA. 2004. The cardiovascular dose-response effects of isoflurane alone and combined with butorphanol in the green iguana (*Iguana iguana*). *Veterinary Anaesthesia and Analgesia* 31(1):64–72.

Munoz M, Smeets WJ, Lopez JM, et al. 2008. Immunohistochemical localization of neuropeptide FF-like in the brain of the turtle: relation to catecholaminergic structures. *Brain Research Bulletin* 75(2–4):256–260.

Norton T. 2005. Chelonian emergency and critical care. *Seminars in Avian and Exotic Pet Medicine* 14(2):106–130.

Oppenheim Y, Moon P. 1995. Sedative effects of midazolam in red-eared slider turtles. *Journal of Zoo and Wildlife Medicine* 26:409–413.

Overgaard J, Stecyk JA, Farrell AP, et al. 2002. Adrenergic control of the cardiovascular system in the turtle *Trachemys scripta*. *The Journal of Experimental Biology* 205(Pt 21):3335–3345.

Park I, Cho SH, Hur J. 2006. Lidocaine hydrochloride–sodium bicarbonate as an anesthetic for soft-shelled turtle *Pelodiscus sinensis*. *Fisheries Science* 72:115–118.

Perry SF. 1998. Lungs: comparative anatomy, functional morphology, and evolution. In: *Biology of the Reptilia* (C Gans, AS Gaunt, eds.), pp. 1–92. Ithaca: Society for the Study of Amphibians and Reptiles.

Platzack B, Hicks JW. 2001. Reductions in systemic oxygen delivery induce a hypometabolic state in the turtle *Trachemys scripta*. *American Journal of Physiology: Regulatory Integrative and Comparative Physiology* 281(4):R1295–R1301.

Quesada RL, Aitken-Palmer C, Conley K, et al. 2010. Accidental submeningeal injection of propofol in gopher tortoises (*Gopherus polyphemus*). *The Veterinary Record* 167(13):494–495.

Raphael BL. 2003. Chelonians (turtles, tortoises). In: *Zoo and Wildlife Medicine*, 5th ed. (ME Fowler, RE Miller, eds.), pp. 48–58. St. Louis: Elsevier Science.

Read MR. 2004. Evaluation of the use of anesthesia and analgesia in reptiles. *Journal of the American Veterinary Medical Association* 224:547–552.

Reiner A. 1987. The distribution of proenkephalin-derived peptides in the central nervous system of turtles. *The Journal of Comparative Neurology* 259(1):65–91.

Rivera S, Divers SJ, Knafo SE. 2011. Sterilisation of hybrid Galapagos tortoises (*Geochelone nigra*) for island restoration. Part 2: phallectomy of males under intrathecal anaesthesia with lidocaine. *The Veterinary Record* 168:78.

Rooney MB, Levine G, Gaynor J, et al. 1999. Sevoflurane anesthesia in desert tortoises (*Gopherus agassizi*). *Journal of Zoo and Wildlife Medicine* 30(1):64–69.

Sanders RD, Ma D, Brooks P, Maze M. 2008. Balancing paediatric anaesthesia: preclinical insights into analgesia, hypnosis, neuroprotection, and neurotoxicity. *British Journal of Anaesthesia* 101(5):597–609.

Santos AL, Bosso AC, Alves Junior JR, et al. 2008. Pharmacological restraint of captivity giant Amazonian turtle *Podocnemis expansa* (Testudines, Podocnemididae) with xylazine and propofol. *Acta Cirurgica Brasileira* 23(3):270–273.

Scarpa Bosso A, Quagliatto Santos A, Machado Brito F, et al. 2009. The use of rocuronium in giant Amazon turtle *Podocnemis expansa* (Schweigger, 1812) (Testudines, Podocnemididae). *Acta Cirúrgica Brasileira* 24(4):311–315.

Schumacher J. 2007. Chelonia (turtles and tortoises). In: *Zoo Animal and Wildlife Immobilization and Anesthesia*, 1st ed. (G West, D Heard, N Caulkett, eds.), pp. 259–266. Hoboken: Blackwell Publishing.

Sedgwick CJ. 1991. Allometrically scaling the data base for vital sign assessment used in general anesthesia of zoological species. Proceedings of the American Association of Zoo Veterinarians, pp. 360–369.

Sharma P, Suresh S. 2008. Influence of COX-2-induced PGE2 on the initiation and progression of tail regeneration in northern house gecko, *Hemidactylus flaviviridis*. *Folia Biologica* 54(6): 193–201.

Shaw S, Kabler S, Lutz P. 1992. Isoflurane: a safe and effective anesthetic for marine and freshwater turtles. Proceedings of the International Wildlife Rehabilitation Council, pp. 112–119.

Shelton G, Burggren W. 1976. Cardiovascular dynamics of the chelonia during apnoea and lung ventilation. *The Journal of Experimental Biology* 64(2):323–343.

Sladky KK, Miletic V, Paul-Murphy J, et al. 2007. Analgesic efficacy and respiratory effects of butorphanol and morphine in turtles. *Journal of the American Veterinary Medical Association* 230(9): 1356–1362.

Sladky KK, Kinney ME, Johnson SM. 2009. Effects of opioid receptor activation on thermal antinociception in red-eared slider turtles (*Trachemys scripta*). *American Journal of Veterinary Research* 70(9):1072–1078.

Sleeman JM, Gaynor J. 2000. Sedative and cardiopulmonary effects of medetomidine and reversal with atipamezole in desert tortoises (*Gopherus agassizii*). *Journal of Zoo and Wildlife Medicine* 31(1):28–35.

Smith C, Turnbull B, Osborn A, et al. 2000. Bone scintigraphy and computed tomography: advanced diagnostic imaging techniques in endangered sea turtles. Proceedings of the American Association of Zoo Veterinarians and International Association for Aquatic Animal Medicine Joint Conference, pp. 217–221.

Smits AW, Kozubowski MM. 1985. Partitioning of body fluids and cardiovascular responses to circulatory hypovolaemia in the turtle, Pseudemys scripta elegans. *The Journal of Experimental Biology* 116:237–250.

Soloperto S, Di Bello A, Lai OR, et al. 2012. Pharmacokinetic behaviour of meloxicam in loggerhead sea turtle (Caretta caretta). 32nd International Sea Turtle Symposium.

Stanford M. 2004. Practical use of capnography in exotic animal anesthesia. *Exotic DVM* 6(3):57–60.

Taylor EW, Leite CA, McKenzie DJ, et al. 2010. Control of respiration in fish, amphibians and reptiles. *Brazilian Journal of Medical and Biological Research = Revista Brasileira de Pesquisas Medicas e Biologicas* 43(5):409–424.

ten Donkelaar HJ, de Boer-van Huizen R. 1987. A possible pain control system in a non-mammalian vertebrate (a lizard, *Gekko gecko*). *Neuroscience Letters* 83(1–2):65–70.

Vigani A. 2010. Development of a balanced anesthetic protocol in giant tortoises and interspecific differences. A case series. Proceedings of 8th Annual Symposium on the Conservation and Biology of Tortoises and Freshwater Turtles, p. 47. August 16–19, Orlando, FL.

Wambugu SN, Towett PK, Kiama SG, et al. 2010. Effects of opioids in the formalin test in the Speke's hinged tortoise (Kinixy's spekii). *Journal of Veterinary Pharmacology and Therapeutics* 33(4): 347–351.

Wang T, Smits AW, Burggren W. 1998. Pulmonary function in reptiles. In: *Biology of the Reptilia* (C Gans, AS Gaunt, eds.), Vol. 19, pp. 297–394. Ithaca: Society for the Study of Amphibians and Reptiles.

Wood FE, Critchley KH, Wood JR. 1982. Anesthesia in the green sea turtle, Chelonia mydas. *American Journal of Veterinary Research* 43(10):1882–1883.

Xia Y, Haddad GG. 2001. Major difference in the expression of delta- and mu-opioid receptors between turtle and rat brain. *The Journal of Comparative Neurology* 436(2):202–210.

Ziolo MS, Bertelsen MF. 2009. Effects of propofol administered via the supravertebral sinus in red-eared sliders. *Journal of the American Veterinary Medical Association* 234(3):390–393.

Section III
Bird Anesthesia

23 Avian Anatomy and Physiology

Ashley M. Zehnder, Michelle G. Hawkins, and Peter J. Pascoe

INTRODUCTION

When considering anesthetic procedures for avian patients, it is critical to be aware of their unique respiratory and circulatory physiology. By appreciating the ways in which birds differ from mammals, clinicians can approach anesthetic procedures with more confidence and can hopefully improve outcomes for their patients.

RESPIRATORY SYSTEM

The avian respiratory system is different from mammals in that it has separate ventilatory and gas exchange compartments, making it highly efficient compared with other vertebrates (James et al. 1976).

Ventilatory Compartment

This compartment includes the major airways, an air sac system, and the thoracic skeleton with its associated muscles. When the beak is closed, the choanal slit located on the dorsal palate of the oral cavity covers the glottis. This allows air flowing through the nares to be directed into the trachea. The epiglottis is absent from the upper respiratory tract. In most species, the glottis is easily visualized at the base of the tongue, which makes endotracheal intubation straightforward.

All bird species have complete tracheal rings making the trachea less susceptible to collapse. However, this can still occur during handling of smaller species. The presence of complete tracheal rings may also make birds more susceptible to the formation of tracheal membranes secondary to damage of the tracheal mucosa. This is discussed more thoroughly in the following chapter on cagebird anesthesia. There are a handful of species with notable anatomical variations of the upper respiratory tract. Male ruddy ducks and both sexes of emus have a tracheal sac-like diverticulum that can be confused for a ruptured trachea. (King 1989) In emus, this diverticulum arises as a slit-like opening through incomplete tracheal rings from the ventral surface of the caudal one-fourth of the extrathoracic trachea. The caudal end may extend almost to the sternum (King 1989). This sac allows for the booming call of the emu. In the ruddy duck, a pear-shaped sac opens from the dorsal tracheal wall just caudal to the larynx and extends between the esophagus and trachea (King 1989). This sac is only found in males and may be involved in the bill-drumming display. In both species, positive pressure ventilation will inflate the sac and some anesthetic gas may be sequestered, potentially affecting anesthetic depth. A bandage can be wrapped around the neck over this area to prevent inflation of the sac. A bullous enlargement of the trachea is found in some species of Anseriformes (King 1989). A median septum is present in the trachea of some penguins and petrels. This septum divides the trachea from the bronchial bifurcation cranially for variable distances depending upon the species. For example, the median septum of the rockhopper penguin is only 5 mm in length (King 1989), but still may allow for unilateral endobronchial intubation. The median septum of the jackass penguin extends to within 1 cm of the larynx allowing both unilateral endobronchial intubation and the potential for trauma during intubation (Zeek 1951). However, endotracheal tubes can be modified to allow bilateral intubation in species with median septa.

There is significant variation in tracheal length between species, which has important implications for anatomical dead space. The typical bird trachea is reported to be 2.7 times longer than that of a similarly sized mammal, but because it is approximately 1.3 times wider, the net effect is resistance to air flow is similar to mammals (King 1989). Tracheal dead space volume is approximately four times that of comparably sized mammals (King 1989). In some species (e.g., some swans, cranes, spoonbills, and curassows), convoluted loops and coils further increase dead space. Healthy, conscious birds compensate for this larger dead space with a larger tidal volume and lower respiratory frequency than mammals. This results in minute ventilation rates that are about 1.5–1.9 times those of mammals (Frappell et al. 2001; Powell & Whittow 2000). Anesthetic drugs will, however, depress ventilation and a greater percentage of minute ventilation becomes dead space ventilation (Ludders 1998; Ludders & Matthews 1996).

In most caged birds, there are four paired air sacs that extend throughout the coelomic cavity (cervical, cranial thoracic, caudal thoracic and abdominal) and one unpaired interclavicular air sac (Duncker 1971, 1972; Jaensch et al. 2002; McLelland 1989). There may also be diverticula that pneumatize the cervical vertebrae, some thoracic vertebrae, vertebral ribs, sternum, humerus, pelvis, and femur (Duncker 1971, 1972, 1974; Jaensch et al. 2002; James et al. 1976; McLelland 1989). The air sacs are poorly vascularized and function primarily as mechanical bellows providing airflow to the lungs during ventilation (Duncker 1971, 1974; Magnussen et al. 1976; Scheid 1979). Due to the lack of a muscular diaphragm, differing pressures do not occur between the thoracic and abdominal cavities (Duncker 1971, 1974; McLelland 1989; Scheid & Piiper 1989). Inspiration and expiration occur through movement of the sternum by contraction of the cervical, thoracic, and abdominal muscles (Duncker 1971; Scheid & Piiper 1987). Since both inspiration and expiration are active movements that require muscle activity, anything that depresses muscle function or impairs thoracic movement will decrease ventilation. The degree of muscle relaxation caused by anesthetic drugs depends upon the anesthetic(s) used, depth of anesthesia, and physical condition (Ludders 2001).

Restriction of movement of the sternum and thoracic muscles due to overexuberant physical restraint, and dorsal and ventral recumbency are reported to lead to hypoventilation (Curro 1998; Forbes 1999; Heard 1997; Jaensch et al. 2002; King & Payne 1964; Pettifer et al. 2002). It has been hypothesized that dorsally recumbent patients have their air sacs and lung openings (ostia) compressed by the internal organs, which may be exacerbated by increasing anesthetic duration (King & Payne 1962, 1964). This hypothesis has led to recommendations to avoid dorsal recumbency in anesthetized birds when possible. Until recently, the only studies of this effect have been in the domestic chicken. The chicken has a very well-developed pectoral musculature that may compress the thorax during respiration

in dorsal recumbency more so than lighter-bodied birds. Chickens and other domestic poultry also usually have large amounts of intracoelomic fat that reduces air sac volume. Additionally, chickens have a somewhat different gas exchange anatomy that may affect ventilation in dorsal recumbency. It was shown in a recent evaluation of air sac and lung volume in red-tailed hawks that even birds with significant coelomic fat did not demonstrate a reduction in lung volume, only air sac volume when in dorsal recumbency (Malka et al. 2009). In a recent study evaluating effects of positioning on spontaneous ventilation in red-tailed hawks during isoflurane anesthesia, no significant differences were found in minute ventilation, heart or respiratory rates, or arterial blood pressures when birds were placed in either dorsal or lateral recumbency. The PaO_2 was significantly higher in dorsal recumbency (Hawkins et al. 2013). Any adverse effect of positioning appears to be negated by assisted ventilation.

Gas Exchange

The parabronchial lungs are the primary tissues for gas exchange (Barnas et al. 1991; Duncker 1971, 1972; Scheid & Piiper 1970). The paired lungs are firmly attached to the ribs and vertebral column dorsally and extend from the thoracic inlet caudally to the level of the adrenals and the cranial division of the kidneys (Duncker 1971, 1972). Avian lungs are relatively smaller compared with mammalian and the parabronchi are nonexpandable. There are two types of parabronchial tissue and the ratio of these tissues varies with species. The paleopulmonic parabronchial tissue is found in all birds and comprises the majority of the lung volume in most species (Duncker 1971, 1972; McLelland 1989) (Duncker 1971, 1972; McLelland 1989). In this tissue, airflow is unidirectional throughout the respiratory cycle. Penguins and emu have only paleopulmonic parabronchi. The neopulmonic parabronchial tissue is also found in most species. However, it is only well developed in domestic poultry and songbirds, accounting for approximately 20–25% of total lung volume (Duncker 1972; Fedde 1980). Air flow through the neopulmonic parabronchi is bidirectional (Duncker 1971, 1972; McLelland 1989). Two complete cycles of inspiration and expiration are necessary to exchange the inhaled gas completely (Scheid & Piiper 1970, 1989). Most air from the first inspiration is directed to the caudal air sacs. That gas flows from the caudal air sacs into the lungs on the first expiration through a unique system of aerodynamic valving (Banzett et al. 1987; Powell & Scheid 1989). Air from the lungs moves into the cranial air sacs with the second inspiration and is moved out through the trachea into the environment on the second expiration. This two-breath cycle allows a continuous flow of air to the gas exchange surfaces, whereas the less efficient mammalian breathing cycle allows gas exchange to occur only at the end of inspiration. Due to this unique system of air flow, a bird with an upper respiratory obstruction can still be ventilated effectively if an air sac is cannulated through the body wall (Korbel et al. 1993, 1996; Korbel 1998; Mitchell et al. 1999; Piiper et al. 1970; Rode et al. 1990; Whittow & Ossorio 1970; Wijnberg et al. 1991). Additional information on air sac cannulation is provided in Chapter 24.

Gas exchange is extremely efficient and a cross-current model is used to describe the blood and gas association (Duncker 1972; Maina et al. 2010; Makanya et al. 2011; McLelland 1989; Powell & Whittow 2000; Scheid 1979; Scheid & Piiper 1970, 1987). As the gas flow through the majority of parabronchi (i.e., the paleopulmonic parabronchi) is unidirectional, the cross-current anatomy of the pulmonary vasculature allows for the continuous exchange of gases throughout the length of the parabronchi. This results in a more efficient oxygen and carbon dioxide exchange than in the mammalian alveolus (Gleeson & Molony 1989; King & Payne 1964; Powell & Whittow 2000). In addition, birds have a larger relative gas exchange surface area, longer capillary blood transit times, and thinner blood–gas barrier than mammals of comparable weights, resulting in greater gas exchange efficiency (Gleeson & Molony 1989; McLelland 1989; Maina et al. 2010; Powell & Scheid 1989; Powell & Whittow 2000). More recently, it has been described that pulmonary capillaries in avian lungs are much less susceptible to pressure changes than mammalian lungs, primarily due to epithelial bridges within avian pulmonary capillaries. This makes them less susceptible to collapse or expansion due to changes in blood pressure (Watson et al. 2008).

Allometric analyses have been used to predict the effect of body size on respiratory variables associated with gas exchange efficiency between mammals and birds (Frappell et al. 1992, 2001; Maloney & Dawson 1994). A study using 50 avian species found general agreement with the older allometric equations with some minor differences in coefficients. The variables determined in this study agree with anatomic data and clinical observations, suggesting that irrespective of body size, birds tend to breathe slower and deeper, have lower minute ventilation, and have a greater demand for oxygen when compared with mammals, making the avian respiratory system more highly efficient in terms of oxygen extraction (Table 23.1).

In mammals, the functional residual capacity (FRC) acts to buffer changes in oxygen partial pressures during the respiratory cycle. In the past, it has been suggested that there is little FRC in avian lungs and, therefore, birds have little mechanism for blunting the effects of apnea on PaO_2 and $PaCO_2$ (McLelland 1989). However, there is a significant reservoir of gas in the air sacs and unidirectional flow of gases through the avian lung may minimize the potential for significant

Table 23.1. Comparison of allometric equations for respiratory variables in birds and mammals

Variable	Birds	Mammals
Oxygen consumption (VO2)	$16.3M^{0.68}$	$12.9M^{0.73}$
Minute ventilation (VE)	$385M^{0.72}$	$518M^{0.74}$
Tidal volume (VT)	$22.9M^{1.08}$	$10.8M^{1.01}$
Breaths per minute (f)	$17M^{-0.34}$	$49.1M^{0.26}$

M, body mass.

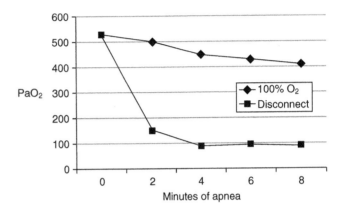

Figure 23.1. Change in oxygen tension during 8 minutes of apnea in six chickens anesthetized with isoflurane. In one treatment, the chickens were connected to an anesthetic circuit containing oxygen (100% O_2), and in the second, they were disconnected from the circuit at the onset of apnea (Disconnect).

fluctuations in blood gas tensions during short periods of apnea. For example, in chickens, 8 minutes of apnea after breathing 100% oxygen resulted in oxygen blood gas tensions that decreased at a similar rate to that seen in mammals (P.J. Pascoe, unpubl. obs.) (Fig. 23.1). Having a high concentration gradient (>95% O_2) and small distances to traverse allows for diffusion of oxygen through the lungs as the oxygen is being removed by the blood, accounting for this delayed onset of hypoxia. In a bird breathing room air, there is a very small diffusion gradient and, because oxygen consumption is higher in birds than mammals, any periods of apnea, however brief, must be treated immediately. Normal blood gas values for selected species are presented in Table 23.2. It should be noted that these values are obtained in awake birds on room air. Over a range of 19 species, PaO_2, $PaCO_2$, and pH were noted to average (SD) 91.6 (8.5), 31.4 (4.2), and 7.50 (0.03), respectively (Powell & Whittow 2000). From these data, it is clear that birds tend to have $PaCO_2$ tensions that are lower than many mammals.

Avian ventilation is controlled by both central and peripheral mechanisms. Respiration rates are lower, in some cases one-third of the mammalian rate, for a comparably sized animal (Powell & Whittow 2000; Scheid & Piiper 1989). The anatomical location of the central ventilatory controls appears to be in the pons

Table 23.2.   Published blood gas values for selected species of birds

Species	PaO2 (Torr)	PaCO2 (Torr)	PH	Reference
Pigeon	95	34	7.50	Bouverot (1978)
Female domestic fowl	87	29.2	7.52	Piiper et al. (1970)
Pekin duck	93.1–100	33.8–36.3	7.46–7.47	Bouverot et al. (1989)
Red-tailed hawk	108	27	7.49	Kollias and McLeish (1978)

Note: All values were obtained in awake, resting birds breathing room air.

and medulla oblongata, as in mammals, with facilitation and inhibition most likely coming from higher regions of the brain (Powell & Whittow 2000). Peripheral extrapulmonary chemoreceptors, specifically the carotid bodies, respond to changes in PO_2 and PCO_2 in the same manner as those observed in mammals (Scheid & Piiper 1989). The chemical drive on respiratory frequency and ventilatory duration also appears to depend on vagal afferent feedback from intrapulmonary receptors, as well as extrapulmonary chemoreceptors, mechanoreceptors, and thermoreceptors (Crank et al. 1980; Powell & Whittow 2000; Scheid & Piiper 1989; Scheid et al. 1978). Birds have a unique group of peripheral receptors, the intrapulmonary chemoreceptors (IPC). They are present in the lung and are exquisitely sensitive CO_2 receptors (Banzett & Burger 1977; Burger et al. 1974; Crank et al. 1980; McLelland 1989; Powell & Scheid 1989; Scheid & Piiper 1989; Scheid et al. 1978). The rate of action potential generation by IPCs is inversely proportional to PCO_2, as they are inhibited by increases in PCO_2. However, it is unclear whether low lung PCO_2 or high pH is the immediate stimulus for signal transduction in the IPCs (Bebout & Hempleman 1999). Compared with mammals, respiratory function in birds may be more sensitive to the effects of inhalant anesthetics because of their effect on the avian IPCs, depressing their ability to adjust ventilation in response to changes in PCO_2 (Ludders 2001). Studies have shown inhalants depress the responsiveness of a number of peripheral control mechanisms that can directly or indirectly affect ventilation (Bagshaw & Cox 1986; Molony 1974; Pizarro et al. 1990).

CARDIOVASCULAR SYSTEM

The cardiovascular system also exhibits significant adaptations to the high metabolic demands necessary for flight. The heart is four-chambered. Compared with mammals, birds have a proportionally larger heart, higher stroke volumes, cardiac output, and resting mean arterial pressures (Grubb 1983; Smith et al. 2000). Heart rates vary significantly among species, with resting rates ranging from 150 to 1000bpm. Such high frequencies make obtaining accurate heart rates difficult, and very few commercially available monitors are able to count greater than 250bpm.

The distribution of the Purkinje fibers within the ventricular myocardium allows for the fibers to completely penetrate the endocardium and through to the epicardium, facilitating synchronous beating at rapid heart rates (Keene & Flammer 1991). This pattern of fiber distribution is responsible for the QRS morphology of the avian ECG (Smith et al. 2000). The ventricles and atria receive a higher density of both sympathetic and parasympathetic nerve fibers compared with mammals (Smith et al. 2000). Endogenous catecholamines are released during stress and pain. They can have a significant impact during anesthesia because some inhalant anesthetics sensitize the myocardium to catecholamine-induced arrhythmias (Aguilar et al. 1995; Greenlees et al. 1990; Joyner et al. 2008; Ludders & Matthews 1996). Clinical observations suggest manipulation of fractured bones, especially the pectoral girdle, causes significant bradycardia and arrhythmias in some patients. However, it is unknown whether this is a vagotonic or baroreceptor effect. Hypercapnia, hypoxemia, and some anesthetics can depress cardiovascular function.

There is an increasing awareness of the need to monitor blood pressure in avian patients during anesthesia as techniques for monitoring improve. However, when direct blood pressure measurements are compared across a variety of species in different orders, there is significant variability (Table 23.3). This can make it difficult to determine what values are normal for a particular species. There appears to be a trend for Galliformes and pigeons to have lower pressures than Psittaciformes, which also appear to average lower than raptorial species, but this is based on a low number of species. Blood pressure is the result of cardiac output and peripheral vascular resistance. Both of these are affected by a number of factors, including autoregulatory control, humoral, hormonal, and neural influences (Smith et al. 2000). Very short-term adjustments are mainly the result of reflex responses within the small arteries and arterioles. Tissue production of metabolic products, including CO_2, pH, and others, may cause a functional hyperemia in local tissues (Smith et al. 2000). Circulating hormones, such as epinephrine, norepinephrine, and angiotensin II, also have significant effects on peripheral vascular resistance (Smith et al. 2000). There has not been sufficient research into the differences in the multitude of factors between species to know which is responsible for the differences in resting blood pressures noted clinically. This means that monitoring trends for a particular patient under

Table 23.3. Published direct blood pressure (DBP) ranges in avian species

Species	SAP ± SD	MAP ± SD	DAP ± SD	Experimental methods	Reference
Pigeon	93 ± 10	82 ± 14	72 ± 13	Isoflurane, SV	Touzot-Jourde et al. (2005)
	88 ± 11	75 ± 10	60 ± 11	Isoflurane, MV	Touzot-Jourde et al. (2005)
Chicken	99 ± 13	84 ± 13	69 ± 15	Sevoflurane, MV	Naganobu et al. (2000)
Pekin duck		128 ± 14		Baseline awake values	Goelz et al. (1990)
		120 ± 19		Halothane, SV, 15 minutes post induction	Goelz et al. (1990)
		119 ± 17		Isoflurane, SV, 15 minutes post induction	Goelz et al. (1990)
		122 ± 20[a]		Isoflurane, 1.0 MAC, SV	Ludders et al. (1990)
Sandhill crane		205 ± 29[a]		1× MAC isoflurane, MV	Ludders et al. (1989)
		133 ± 9[a]		1× MAC isoflurane, SV	Ludders et al. (1989)
Cockatoo		143 ± 4[a]		Isoflurane, SV	Curro et al. (1994)
Amazon		133 ± 10[a]		Isoflurane, MV (0 minutes)	Pettifer et al. (2002)
		122 ± 7[a]		Isoflurane, SV (0 minutes)	Pettifer et al. (2002)
	163 ± 18	155 ± 18	148 ± 18	Isoflurane, SV (wing values)	Acierno et al. (2008)
Great horned owl	232 ± 37	203 ± 28	178 ± 25	Baseline awake values	Hawkins et al. (2003)
	243 ± 26	203 ± 28	208 ± 22	After propofol CRI induction (0 minute)	Hawkins et al. (2003)
Red-tailed hawk	220 ± 51	187 ± 42	160 ± 45	Baseline awake values	Hawkins et al. (2003)[b]
	225 ± 53	185 ± 45	167 ± 54	After propofol CRI induction (0 minute)	Hawkins et al. (2003)[b]
	178 ± 27	159 ± 25	143 ± 24	Isoflurane anesthesia (average values)	Zehnder et al. (2009)[b]
	180 ± 41	141 ± 30	111 ± 25	Isoflurane anesthesia (0 minute)	Pavez et al. (2011)[b]
Bald eagle	194 ± 13[a]		158 ± 13[a]	Isoflurane, spontaneous ventilation	Joyner et al. (2008)
	146 ± 13[a]		135 ± 13[a]	Sevoflurane, spontaneous ventilation	Joyner et al. (2008)
Crested caracara	226 ± 18	201 ± 19	180 ± 18	Sevoflurane anesthesia Spontaneous ventilation	Escobar et al. (2009)

[a]Values reported are mean ± standard error.
[b]These studies utilized the same study population of animals, although the individual animals may vary.
CRI, constant rate infusion; MV, manual or controlled ventilation; SV, spontaneous ventilation.

anesthesia is more important than the actual blood pressure value. More information on techniques for measuring blood pressure under anesthesia is provided in Chapter 24.

The renal portal system consists of an arrangement of smooth muscles forming a valve within the external iliac vein at its junction with the efferent renal vein (King & McLelland 1984). This valve is controlled by both adrenergic and cholinergic stimulation. Epinephrine causes the valve to relax, allowing venous blood to be directed to the systemic circulation. Acetylcholine causes the valve to contract, allowing venous blood from the legs to perfuse the renal tubules (Akester 1967; Akester & Mann 1969; Burrows et al. 1983; Johnson 1979; Palmore & Ackerman 1985). The clinical significance of this valve is controversial. The renal portal system may play an important role in conditions where consistent blood levels of a drug, such as an antimicrobial, are required (Ludders & Matthews 1996). There have been few studies to examine the effects of the renal portal system on anesthetics. There was no difference in onset, duration, or recovery between injection of xylazine/tiletamine/zolazepam in ostriches into the thigh or muscles at the base of the wings (Carvalho et al. 2006). In great-horned owls, butorphanol injected into the medial metatarsal vein has a significantly smaller area under the curve than the same dose injected into the jugular vein, suggestive of increased excretion through the renal portal system (Riggs et al. 2008). Until additional studies have been performed, the authors recommend nephrotoxic drugs or drugs exhibiting high renal excretion be administered into the cranial half of the body.

THERMOREGULATION

Heat is lost via radiation, evaporation, convection, and conduction. The normal body temperatures of most caged birds range from 39 to 43°C (Dawson & Whittow 2000). Since many birds are small and have a high body-to-surface area ratio they radiate heat rapidly. Once anesthetized, the bird is immobile and relaxed so it will generate less heat from muscle contraction. It is also subject to evaporative loss from the respiratory tract (dry anesthetic gases), skin surfaces (surgical preparations solutions), and open-body cavities, conduction of heat via surface contact, and convection of warm gases from around the bird (Wessel et al. 1966). Anesthesia redistributes blood flow and depresses thermoregulatory response, further promoting heat loss. The core body temperature of pigeons with no external heat support dropped ≥8°C in ≤30 minutes of inhalant anesthesia (Harrison et al. 1985). Hypothermia has a number of adverse physiologic effects. It results in bradypnea, and decreased minute ventilation and tidal volume (Moon & Ilkiw 1993). Hypothermia decreases anesthetic requirement and metabolism and will prolong recovery (Ludders & Matthews 1996). Therefore, monitoring of core body temperature and providing thermal support are mandatory to reduce anesthetic morbidity and mortality in the anesthetized and recovering patient.

REFERENCES

Acierno MJ, da Cunha A, Smith J, et al. 2008. Agreement between direct and indirect blood pressure measurements obtained from anesthetized Hispaniolan Amazon parrots. *Journal of the American Veterinary Medical Association* 233(10):1587–1590.

Aguilar RF, Smith VE, Ogburn P, et al. 1995. Arrhythmias associated with isoflourane anesthesia in bald eagles (*Haliaeetus leucocephalus*). *Journal of Zoo and Wildlife Medicine* 26(4):508–516.

Akester AR. 1967. Renal portal shunts in the kidney of the domestic fowl. *Journal of Anatomy* 101(Pt 3):569–594.

Akester AR, Mann SP. 1969. Adrenergic and cholinergic innervation of the renal portal valve in the domestic fowl. *Journal of Anatomy* 104(Pt 2):241–252.

Bagshaw RJ, Cox RH. 1986. Baroreceptor control of heart rate in chickens (*Gallus domesticus*). *American Journal of Veterinary Research* 47(2):293–295.

Banzett RB, Burger RE. 1977. Response of avian intrapulmonary chemoreceptors to venous CO2 and ventilatory gas flow. *Respiration Physiology* 29(1):63–72.

Banzett RB, Butler JP, Nations CS, et al. 1987. Inspiratory aerodynamic valving in goose lungs depends on gas density and velocity. *Respiration Physiology* 70(3):287–300.

Barnas GM, Hempleman SC, Harinath P, et al. 1991. Respiratory system mechanical behavior in the chicken. *Respiration Physiology* 84(2):145–157.

Bebout DE, Hempleman SC. 1999. Chronic hypercapnia resets CO2 sensitivity of avian intrapulmonary chemoreceptors. *The American Journal of Physiology* 276(2 Pt 2):R317–R322.

Bouverot P. 1978. Control of breathing in birds compared with mammals. *Physiological Reviews* 58(3):604–655.

Bouverot P, Dougest D, Sebert P. 1989. Role of the arterial chemoreceptors in ventilatory and circulatory adjustments to hypoxia in awake Pekin ducks. *Journal of Comparative Physiology* 133:177–186.

Burger RE, Osborne JL, Banzett RB. 1974. Intrapulmonary chemoreceptors in *Gallus domesticus*: adequate stimulus and functional localization. *Respiration Physiology* 22(1–2):87–97.

Burrows ME, Braun EJ, Duckles SP. 1983. Avian renal portal valve: a reexamination of its innervation. *The American Journal of Physiology* 245(4):H628–H634.

Carvalho HS, Ciboto R, Cortopassi SRG 2006. Anatomical study of the renal portal system and its implications for the use of anesthetic agents in the restraint of ostriches (*Struthio camelus*). Proceedings of the 9th World Congress of Veterinary Anaesthesiology, Santos, Brazil, p. 212.

Crank WD, Kuhlmann WD, Fedde MR. 1980. Functional localization of avian intrapulmonary CO2 receptors within the parabronchial mantle. *Respiration Physiology* 41(1):71–85.

Curro TG. 1998. Anesthesia of pet birds. *Seminars in Avian and Exotic Pet Medicine* 7(1):10–21.

Curro TG, Brunson DB, Paul-Murphy J. 1994. Determination of the ED50 of isoflurane and evaluation of the isoflurane-sparing effect of butorphanol in cockatoos (*Cacatua* spp). *Veterinary Surgery* 23(5):429–433.

Dawson WR, Whittow GC. 2000. Regulation of body temperature. In: *Sturkie's Avian Physiology*, 5th ed. (GC Whittow, ed.), pp. 343–390. San Diego: Academic Press.

Duncker HR. 1971. *The Lung Air Sac System of Birds: A Contribution to the Functional Anatomy of the Respiratory Apparatus*. Berlin: Springer-Verlag.

Duncker HR. 1972. Structure of avian lungs. *Respiration Physiology* 14(1):44–63.

Duncker HR. 1974. Structure of the avian respiratory tract. *Respiration Physiology* 22(1–2):1–19.

Escobar A, Thiesen R, Vitaliano SN, et al. 2009. Some cardiopulmonary effects of sevoflurane in crested caracara (*Caracara plancus*). *Veterinary Anaesthesia and Analgesia* 36(5):436–441.

Fedde MR. 1980. Structure and gas-flow pattern in the avian respiratory system. *Poultry Science* 59(12):2642–2653.

Forbes NA. 1999. Anaesthesia and analgesia for exotic species (birds). In: *Manual of Small Animal Anaesthesia and Analgesia* (C Seymour, R Gleed, eds.), pp. 283–294. Cheltenham: BSAVA.

Frappell P, Lanthier C, Baudinette RV, et al. 1992. Metabolism and ventilation in acute hypoxia: a comparative analysis in small mammalian species. *The American Journal of Physiology* 262(6 Pt 2):R1040–R1046.

Frappell PB, Hinds DS, Boggs DF. 2001. Scaling of respiratory variables and the breathing pattern in birds: an allometric and phylogenetic approach. *Physiological and Biochemical Zoology* 74(1):75–89.

Gleeson M, Molony V. 1989. Control of breathing. In: *Form and Function in Birds* (AS King, J McLelland, eds.), pp. 439–484. New York: Academic Press.

Goelz MF, Hahn AW, Kelley ST. 1990. Effects of halothane and isoflurane on mean arterial blood pressure, heart rate, and respiratory rate in adult Pekin ducks. *American Journal of Veterinary Research* 51(3):458–460.

Greenlees KJ, Clutton RE, Larsen CT, et al. 1990. Effect of halothane, isoflurane, and pentobarbital anesthesia on myocardial irritability in chickens. *American Journal of Veterinary Research* 51(5):757–758.

Grubb BR. 1983. Allometric relations of cardiovascular function in birds. *The American Journal of Physiology* 245(4): H567–H572.

Harrison GJ, Christensen KA, Crawford JF, et al. 1985. A clinical comparison of anesthetics in domestic pigeons and cockatiels, pp. 7–22.

Hawkins MG, Wright BD, Pascoe PJ, et al. 2003. Pharmacokinetics and anesthetic and cardiopulmonary effects of propofol in red-tailed hawks (*Buteo jamaicensis*) and great horned owls (*Bubo virginianus*). *American Journal of Veterinary Research* 64(6):677–683.

Hawkins MG, Malka S, Pascoe PJ, et al. 2013. Evaluation of the effects of dorsal versus lateral recumbency on the cardiopulmonary system during anesthesia with isoflurane in red-tailed hawks (*Buteo jamaicensis*). *American Journal of Veterinary Research* 74(1):136–143.

Heard DJ. 1997. Anesthesia and analgesia. In: *Avian Medicine and Surgery* (RB Altman, SL Clubb, GM Dorrestein, eds.), pp. 807–828. Philadelphia: W.B. Saunders.

Jaensch SM, Cullen L, Raidal SR. 2002. Air sac functional anatomy of the sulfur-crested cockatoo (*Cacatua galerita*) during isoflurane anesthesia. *Journal of Avian Medicine and Surgery* 16(1): 2–9.

James AE, Hutchings G, Bush M, et al. 1976. How birds breathe: correlation of radiographic with anatomical and pathological studies. *Journal of the American Veterinary Radiology Society* 17:77–86.

Johnson OW. 1979. Urinary organs. In: *Form and Function in Birds* (A King, J McLelland, eds.), pp. 183–235. London; New York: Academic Press.

Joyner PH, Jones MP, Ward D, et al. 2008. Induction and recovery characteristics and cardiopulmonary effects of sevoflurane and isoflurane in bald eagles. *American Journal of Veterinary Research* 69(1):13–22.

Keene BW, Flammer K. 1991. ECG of the month. *Journal of the American Veterinary Medical Association* 198(3):408–409.

King AS. 1989. Larynx and trachea. In: *Form and function in Birds* (AS King, J McLelland, eds.), pp. 69–103. New York: Academic Press.

King AS, McLelland J. 1984. Urinary system. In: *Birds: Their Structure and Function* (AS King, J McLelland, eds.), pp. 175–186. Philadelphia: Bailliere Tindall.

King AS, Payne DC. 1962. The maximum capacities of the lungs and air sacs of *Gallus domesticus. Journal of Anatomy* 96:495–503.

King AS, Payne DC. 1964. Normal breathing and the effects of posture in *Gallus domesticus. The Journal of Physiology* 174 :340–347.

Kollias G, McLeish I. 1978. Effects of ketamine hydrochloride in red-tailed hawks (*Buteo jamaicensis*). I. Arterial blood gas and acid base. *Comparative Biochemistry and Physiology. C: Comparative Pharmacology* 60(1):57–59.

Korbel R, Milovanovic A, Erhardt W, et al. 1993. The aerosaccular perfusion with isoflurane in birds: an anaesthetic measure for surgery in the head region, pp. 9–42.

Korbel R, Burike S, Erhardt W, et al. 1996. Effect of nitrous oxide application in racing pigeons (*Columba livia gmel.*, 1979, var. dom: a study using the airsac perfusion technique. *Israel Journal of Veterinary Medicine* 51:133–139.

Korbel RT 1998. Air sac perfusion anesthesia (APA). An anaesthetic procedure for surgery in the head area and for ophthalmoscopy in birds: a practical guideline. *Veterinary Observer*, November.

Ludders JW. 1998. Respiratory physiology of birds: considerations for anesthetic management. *Seminars in Avian and Exotic Pet Medicine* 7(1):3–9.

Ludders JW. 2001. Inhaled anesthesia for birds. In: *Recent Advances in Veterinary Anesthesia and Analgesia: Companion Animals* (RD Gleed, JW Ludders, eds.). Ithaca: IVIS.

Ludders JW, Matthews N. 1996. Birds. In: *Lumb & Jones' Veterinary Anesthesia* (JC Thurmon, WJ Tranquilli, GJ Benson, eds.), pp. 645–669. Baltimore: The Williams and Wilkins Co.

Ludders JW, Rode J, Mitchell GS. 1989. Isoflurane anesthesia in sandhill cranes (*Grus canadensis*): minimal anesthetic concentration and cardiopulmonary dose-response during spontaneous and controlled breathing. *Anesthesia and Analgesia* 68(4): 511–516.

Ludders JW, Mitchell GS, Rode J. 1990. Minimal anesthetic concentration and cardiopulmonary dose response of isoflurane in ducks. *Veterinary Surgery* 19(4):304–307.

McLelland J. 1989. Anatomy of the lungs and air sacs. In: *Form and Function in Birds* (AS King, J McLelland, eds.), pp. 221–279. New York: Academic Press.

Magnussen H, Willmer H, Scheid P. 1976. Gas exchange in air sacs: contribution to respiratory gas exchange in ducks. *Respiration Physiology* 26(1):129–146.

Maina JN, West JB, Orgeig S, et al. 2010. Recent advances into understanding some aspects of the structure and function of mammalian and avian lungs. *Physiological and Biochemical Zoology* 83(5):792–807.

Makanya AN, El-Darawish Y, Kavoi BM, et al. 2011. Spatial and functional relationships between air conduits and blood capillaries in the pulmonary gas exchange tissue of adult and developing chickens. *Microscopy Research and Technique* 74(2): 159–169.

Malka S, Hawkins MG, Jones JH, et al. 2009. Effect of body position on respiratory system volumes in anesthetized red-tailed hawks (*Buteo jamaicensis*) as measured via computed tomography. *American Journal of Veterinary Research* 70(9):1155–1160.

Maloney SK, Dawson TJ. 1994. Ventilatory accommodation of oxygen demand and respiratory water loss in a large bird, the emu (*Dromaius novaehollandiae*), and a re-examination of ventilatory allometry for birds. *Journal of Comparative Physiology* 164B:473–481.

Mitchell J, Bennett RA, Spalding M. 1999. Air sacculitis associated with the placement of an air breathing tube, pp. 145–146.

Molony V. 1974. Classification of vagal afferents firing in phase with breathing in *Gallus domesticus. Respiration Physiology* 22 (1–2):57–76.

Moon PF, Ilkiw JE. 1993. Surface-induced hypothermia in dogs: 19 cases (1987–1989). *Journal of the American Veterinary Medical Association* 202(3):437–444.

Naganobu K, Fujisawa Y, Ohde H, et al. 2000. Determination of the minimum anesthetic concentration and cardiovascular dose response for sevoflurane in chickens during controlled ventilation. *Veterinary Surgery* 29(1):102–105.

Palmore WP, Ackerman N. 1985. Blood flow in the renal portal circulation of the turkey: effect of epinephrine. *American Journal of Veterinary Research* 46(7):1589–1592.

Pavez JC, Hawkins MG, Pascoe PJ, et al. 2011. Effect of fentanyl target-controlled infusions on isoflurane minimum anaesthetic concentration and cardiovascular function in red-tailed hawks (*Buteo jamaicensis*). *Veterinary Anaesthesia and Analgesia* 38(4): 344–351.

Pettifer GR, Cornick-Seahorn J, Smith JA, et al. 2002. The comparative cardiopulmonary effects of spontaneous and controlled ventilation by using the Hallowell EMC anesthesia workstation in Hispaniolan Amazon parrots (*Amazonia ventralis*). *Journal of Avian Medicine and Surgery* 16(4):268–276.

Piiper J, Drees F, Scheid P. 1970. Gas exchange in the domestic fowl during spontaneous breathing and artificial ventilation. *Respiration Physiology* 9(2):234–245.

Pizarro J, Ludders JW, Douse MA, et al. 1990. Halothane effects on ventilatory responses to changes in intrapulmonary CO_2 in geese. *Respiration Physiology* 82(3):337–347.

Powell FL, Scheid P. 1989. Physiology of gas exchange in the avian respiratory system. In: *Form and Function in Birds* (AS King, J McLelland, eds.), pp. 393–437. New York: Academic Press.

Powell FL, Whittow GC. 2000. Respiration. In: *Sturkie's Avian Physiology*, 5th ed. (GC Whittow, ed.), pp. 233–264. San Diego: Academic Press.

Riggs SM, Hawkins MG, Craigmill AL, et al. 2008. Pharmacokinetics of butorphanol tartrate in red-tailed hawks (*Buteo jamaicensis*) and great horned owls (*Bubo virginianus*). *American Journal of Veterinary Research* 69(5):596–603.

Rode JA, Bartholow S, Ludders JW. 1990. Ventilation through an air sac cannula during tracheal obstruction in ducks. *Journal of the Association of Avian Veterinarians* 4(2):98–102.

Scheid P. 1979. Mechanisms of gas exchange in bird lungs. *Reviews of Physiology, Biochemistry and Pharmacology* 86:137–186.

Scheid P, Piiper J. 1970. Analysis of gas exchange in the avian lung: theory and experiments in the domestic fowl. *Respiration Physiology* 9(2):246–262.

Scheid P, Piiper J. 1987. Gas exchange and transport. In: *Bird Respiration* (TJ Seller, ed.), pp. 97–129. Boca Raton: CRC Press.

Scheid P, Piiper J. 1989. Respiratory mechanics and air flow in birds. In: *Form and Function in Birds* (AS King, J McLelland, eds.), pp. 369–391. New York: Academic Press.

Scheid P, Gratz RK, Powell FL, et al. 1978. Ventilation response to CO2 in birds. II. Contribution by intrapulmonary CO2 receptors. *Respiration Physiology* 35(3):361–372.

Smith FM, West NH, Jones DR. 2000. The cardiovascular system. In: *Sturkie's Avian Physiology* (GC Whittow, ed.), pp. 141–231. San Diego: Academic Press.

Touzot-Jourde G, Hernandez-Divers SJ, Trim CM. 2005. Cardiopulmonary effects of controlled versus spontaneous ventilation in pigeons anesthetized for coelioscopy. *Journal of the American Veterinary Medical Association* 227(9):1424–1428.

Watson RR, Fu Z, West JB. 2008. Minimal distensibility of pulmonary capillaries in avian lungs compared with mammalian lungs. *Respiratory Physiology and Neurobiology* 160(2):208–214.

Wessel HU, James GW, Paul MH. 1966. Effects of respiration and circulation on central blood temperature of the dog. *The American Journal of Physiology* 211(6):1403–1412.

Whittow GC, Ossorio N. 1970. A new technique for anesthetizing birds. *Laboratory Animal Care* 20(4 Pt 1):651–656.

Wijnberg ID, Lagerweij E, Zwart P 1991. Inhalation anaesthesia in birds through the abdominal air sac, using a unidirectional, continuous flow. Proceedings of the 4th International Congress of Veterinary Anaesthesia, p. 80.

Zeek PM. 1951. Double trachea in penguins and sea lions. *The Anatomical Record* 111(3):327–343.

Zehnder AM, Hawkins MG, Pascoe PJ, et al. 2009. Evaluation of indirect blood pressure monitoring in awake and anesthetized red-tailed hawks (*Buteo jamaicensis*): effects of cuff size, cuff placement, and monitoring equipment. *Veterinary Anaesthesia and Analgesia* 36(5):464–479.

24 Cagebirds

Michelle G. Hawkins, Ashley M. Zehnder, and Peter J. Pascoe

INTRODUCTION

The anesthesia of caged (and other species) of birds is unique not only from the aspect of anatomy and physiology, but also due to unique requirements for anesthetic equipment, monitoring, and species-specific pharmacology. It is critical to understand the limitations of currently available technologies when dealing with small patients to plan safe anesthetic procedures.

PREANESTHETIC EVALUATION

The medical history and husbandry of the pet bird is essential for preanesthetic evaluation. History regarding diet, appetite, previous diseases, and drug therapy should always be collected. Examination of the bird's cage and its contents is useful to assess heavy metal exposure and the bird's droppings. The quantity and quality of the droppings will help determine whether the bird has been eating. Changes in color or consistency of the droppings suggest abnormalities in the gastrointestinal, hepatic, or urinary systems (Doneley et al. 2006).

Allowing time for acclimation to new surroundings will reduce stress and unmask clinical disease. A complete physical examination, including respiratory, cardiac, renal, and hepatic function, should always be performed and baseline values recorded for comparison during anesthesia. The bird should first be examined closely in its cage, paying particular attention to respiratory rate and effort. The resting respiratory rate is recorded prior to physical restraint for comparison with rates under anesthesia. The quality of respiration is evaluated by ausculting the air sacs ventrally and the lungs dorsally for evidence of harsh airway sounds or evidence of wheezing. The trachea is also ausculted and gently palpated for any abnormalities. The heart is ausculted carefully for murmurs and a baseline heart rate recorded for comparison during anesthesia. Pulse quality is assessed at either the median ulnar or medial metatarsal arteries, evaluating it for symmetry and strength. The body weight is recorded for calculating accurate fluid and medication dosages.

Accurate assessment of renal and hepatic function is difficult during the physical examination. Urine and urates in the droppings are evaluated for quantity and color. Red-tinged urine could be due to hematuria, but may be due to dietary colorings. Green or yellow urate discoloration may be biliverdinuria and a sign of hepatic dysfunction (Doneley et al. 2006). Coelomic palpation is performed to assess for organomegaly that may mechanically compress the air sacs and lungs.

Hydration status is evaluated, recorded, and dehydration corrected, if possible, prior to anesthesia. Compensatory mechanisms are blunted under anesthesia, exacerbating underlying hypotension and poor peripheral perfusion. Hydration assessment includes examination of the moistness of the cloacal and ocular mucous membranes and the elasticity of the skin at the eyelids and over the keel. Sunken eyes and cool extremities also indicate dehydration. The refill time after digital compression of the median ulnar vein should be immediate; venous refill times of >1 second have been suggested to correlate with >7% dehydration (Steinohrt 1999). The PCV will often be increased during dehydration. In pigeons, water deprived for 72 hours, the plasma urea nitrogen increased 6.5–15.3×, but the uric acid only showed a 1.4–2× increase (Lumeij 1987). Clinically, however, it appears uric acid does go up with moderate-to-severe dehydration, and will resolve with rehydration.

Zoo Animal and Wildlife Immobilization and Anesthesia, Second Edition. Edited by Gary West, Darryl Heard, and Nigel Caulkett.
© 2014 John Wiley & Sons, Inc. Published 2014 by John Wiley & Sons, Inc.

Ideally, a complete blood count and biochemical profile are performed prior to anesthesia. If one hematocrit tube of blood can be collected, a packed cell volume (PCV), whole blood smear for estimated white blood cell count and differential, blood glucose, and several other biochemistry tests can be obtained. There are several new tabletop biochemical analysis systems that require only a very small volume of blood to provide a complete biochemistry profile. Any anemias are characterized as either acute or chronic and regenerative or nonregenerative. Acute anemias are corrected prior to anesthesia as birds may not be able to compensate for lowered levels of oxygen delivery. Transfusion is indicated as in mammals if the PCV is <15–20% and the total solids are <3–3.5 g/dL. However, pet birds often have PCV ≥40% so if the blood loss is acute, the authors may perform a transfusion at a higher PCV. Also, avian total protein values are much lower than those in mammals (2–3 g/dL). There is a poor correlation between total solids measured by refractometer and protein values measured with the biuret method, making the former an inaccurate criterion for avian transfusion (Lumeij & de Bruijne 1985). The type of surgery to be performed and potential for blood loss are assessed so a fluid plan can be prepared. PCV may decrease 3–5% during anesthesia due to vascular hemodynamic changes associated with certain anesthetic drugs. Hypoglycemia (<200 mg/dL) is supplemented before anesthesia and glucose concentration monitored. Calcium gluconate is commonly administered in African gray parrots (50–100 mg/kg IM; diluted with saline 1 : 1) prior to induction to prevent hypocalcemia, a common problem in these species.

The gastrointestinal system has a very rapid transit time compared with most mammals. It is, therefore, important to carefully consider the nutritional plane of the patient. Prolonged anorexia will lead to a negative energy balance requiring nutritional support in the perianesthetic period. Other indications for additional nutritional support include reduced to absent fecal production and significant reduction in body weight. Nutritional requirements differ between species and classes. To calculate nutritional requirements for the critically ill patient, the basal metabolic rate (BMR) is first calculated: BMR (kcal/day) = K (BW$_{kg}^{0.75}$); K = 78 in nonpasserines; K = 129 in passerines. While these two K-factors provide a basic means of estimating avian BMR, many additional factors have been calculated for specific species. The authors refer the reader to appropriate avian nutritional texts for additional detail (Klasing 1998). The maintenance energy requirements (MER) are adjustments to the BMR based upon hypermetabolism associated with any disease processes. The most common adjustments are 1.2–1.5× BMR (range 0.5–2.0×) (McDonald 2006). The chosen diet depends upon the patient's nutritional needs. Foods can be blended to a liquid, or commercially available enteral products are used based upon the patient's protein, carbohydrate, and fat requirements. Total parenteral nutrition or partial enteral nutrition is not commonly utilized due to catheter-related complications, poor patient tolerance, and lack of appropriate formulations.

PREANESTHETIC SUPPORTIVE CARE

Fluid Support
Daily maintenance fluid rates are approximately 40–60 mL/kg/day. This range is based upon studies where drinking is the main route of water intake. Birds weighing ≥100 g drink approximately 5–8% of body mass/day. This increases at progressively smaller body masses to drinking rates as high as 50% for birds weighing 10–20 g (Bartholomew & Cade 1963; Skadhauge 1981; Zeigler et al. 1972). Estimation of fluid replacement is based upon body weight and dehydration percentage: Estimated dehydration (%) × body weight (gm) = fluid deficit (mL). One-fourth to one-half the deficit is given in the first 6–12 hours, then the remainder over the following 24 hours (Abou-Madi & Kollias 1992).

Oral (PO) fluids are only useful for mild dehydration and are contraindicated in head trauma, GI stasis, lateral recumbency, or seizuring. Subcutaneous (SC) fluids are commonly used for maintenance and mild-to-moderate dehydration. However, large volumes may not be absorbed due to the paucity of blood vessels in the subcutis and peripheral vasoconstriction. Volumes of up to 10–15 mL/kg/site can be injected into the inguinal folds, axilla, or dorsum. Overdistension of the SC site can result in compromise of the blood supply and decreased fluid absorption. Before each injection, the administration site is inspected for previous delays in absorption. Only isotonic or nonirritating fluids should be given SC. Dextrose solutions ≥2.5% are not given SC as equilibration between the SC fluids and the extracellular fluid will exacerbate preexisting electrolyte imbalances (Abou-Madi & Kollias 1992; Steinohrt 1999).

Fasting
Preanesthetic fasting duration is determined by species, size, and clinical status, with a goal of reducing regurgitation yet minimizing hypoglycemia (Harrison 1991). Fasting times between 2 and 4 hours have been recommended in medium-sized psittacines, whereas birds ≤100–200 g may not be fasted due to high metabolic rates and easily depleted glycogen stores. However, in broiler chickens and adult Japanese quail fasted 12 and 48 hours, respectively, blood glucose remained within clinically acceptable ranges (Lamosova et al. 2004; van der Wal et al. 1999). No studies have been performed evaluating the effect of fasting on psittacines. Scheduling procedures as early in the day as possible reduces fasting times. In species with high metabolic rates, clear

fluids high in carbohydrates may be provided to maximize calories while minimizing crop and stomach contents prior to anesthesia. The crop contents may be gently aspirated if anesthesia cannot be delayed.

EQUIPMENT

Endotracheal Intubation

The main advantages of tracheal intubation are that it provides a patent airway, reduces dead space, and allows easy application of positive pressure ventilation. The disadvantages are that it can be associated with trauma to the airway, it can significantly increase airway resistance and the tube can become occluded due to mechanical forces or because of secretions. These factors need to be carefully considered when deciding to intubate a patient. The increase in airway resistance is of greatest importance in very small patients since the resistance varies with the fourth power of the radius. For example, decreasing the radius from 5 to 3 mm would increase the resistance sevenfold, whereas a decrease from 3 to 1 mm would increase resistance >80 times. Since an increased resistance would require the patient to work harder to breathe, this effect can be minimized by providing positive pressure ventilation.

Despite the above cautions, the authors recommend that for any procedure that requires greater than 10 minutes of anesthesia, intubation should be performed. Many types of endotracheal tubes have been used in birds. Cole, noncuffed and cuffed tubes have all been used successfully in caged birds (Fig. 24.1). Cole tubes have a narrow tip that is static in diameter for a short distance then increases in diameter. The distal end is advanced into the trachea until the larger diameter abuts against the glottis, creating a seal. However, these tubes tend to plug with secretions easily.

Overinflation of the cuff on an endotracheal tube can cause tracheal mucosal epithelial trauma due to lack of expansion of the tracheal rings or, alternatively, the tracheal rings may rupture with severe overinflation. Inflammation of the tracheal epithelium may lead to fibrotic narrowing of the tracheal lumen with complete transtracheal membranes (Fig. 24.2). Cuffed tubes without the cuff inflated also have the potential to cause tracheal mucosal damage and inflammation due to the irregularity of the plastic surface of the cuff on the tracheal epithelium. Because this inflammatory process requires time, clinical signs of dyspnea associated with this type of tracheal trauma may not become evident for up to several weeks post intubation. There have been a small number of case reports and one multi-institutional review documenting tracheal stenosis or tracheal membrane formation in psittacines post intubation, as well as other species (blue-billed curasow) (de Matos et al. 2006; Evans et al. 2009; Jankowski et al. 2010; Sykes et al. 2013). These cases have been

managed with tracheal anastomosis with one bird having no respiratory signs for 2-year post resection (Jankowski et al. 2010). Various factors including ventilation techniques and endotracheal tube disinfection protocols have been suspected to contribute to this phenomenon, and these are factors that are associated with tracheal stenosis in humans (Wain 2009), but no definitive correlation with protocols or procedures has been identified to date.

Although noncuffed tubes are most commonly used, there are several disadvantages to their use. They do not provide a sealed airway, allowing escape of anesthetic

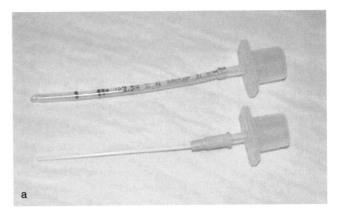

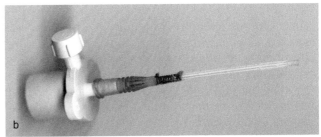

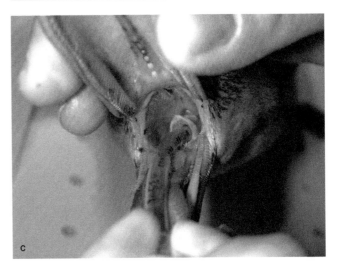

Figure 24.1. Various endotracheal tube types are used in avian clinical practice. Cole, noncuffed, and cuffed tubes have all been used successfully in caged birds (a). Catheters can be modified and used as ET tubes for very small patients (b). Intubation is straightforward as visualization of the glottis is not difficult in most caged birds (c).

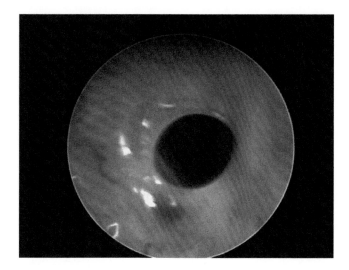

Figure 24.2. Transtracheal membrane occluding approximately 75% of the tracheal lumen in a double yellow-headed Amazon parrot. Note the significant vascularization of the membrane. These membranes have been reported most commonly in birds up to several weeks after intubation with both cuffed and non-cuffed endotracheal tubes. Various factors such as over-inflation of the cuff, ventilation techniques and endotracheal tube disinfection protocols have been evaluated but no definitive correlations have been identified to date.

gases. This increases the amount of anesthetic gas required and environmental contamination. Also, airway protection from aspiration of secretions or gastrointestinal contents is reduced. This makes it imperative that the oral cavity be clean prior to intubation and monitored throughout the procedure. Elevation of the head and neck may reduce regurgitation of gastrointestinal contents from the crop, proventriculus or ventriculus into the oral cavity. Cuffed tubes have been used in larger avian patients. The cuff is carefully inflated with just enough air to prevent leakage when 10–15 cm H_2O pressure is applied (Curro 1998; Ludders & Matthews 1996).

The patient size determines the endotracheal tube size used. The smallest commercial noncuffed tubes have an internal diameter (ID) of 1 mm. However, tubes <2 mm ID are often highly flexible and kink easily. The smallest-diameter cuffed tube is 2.5 mm ID. Very small birds may be intubated with teflon IV, red rubber, or urinary catheters. Care is taken to ensure that no sharp edges are present at the end. This is achieved by using a small piece of silicone tubing over the end of the catheter. Ends of catheters can be cut and adapted for use as endotracheal tubes if they are gently filed with an emery board to remove rough edges.

As stated previously, endotracheal tubes with small internal diameters impose significant resistance to gas flow, especially if mucus accumulates. During inhalant anesthesia, copious thick mucus production can occur due to the drying effects of the inspired cold, dry gases.

In the authors' experience, humidification of the gases reduces mucus plug formation. Commercially available endotracheal tube humidifiers are available (Humidi-vent Mini Agibeck Product, Hudson RCI, Temecula, CA). Disadvantages of their use include increased dead space and filter plugging with secretions. The use of an endotracheal tube with a Murphy eye, which has both side and end openings, decreases the likelihood of mucus occlusion.

Endotracheal tube obstruction is detected by monitoring the ventilatory pattern. As the airway occludes the expiratory phase duration becomes prolonged (Ludders & Matthews 1996). An anticholinergic (atropine and glycopyrrolate) reduces mucus production and mucus plug formation. However, it also increases mucus viscosity, making it harder to clear secretions from the tube. Some clinicians recommend that the endotracheal tube be removed and replaced after every hour of anesthesia for long procedures.

Extension of the neck, gentle traction on the tongue and pressure under the mandibular beak will push the glottis forward to aid in endotracheal tube placement. Psittacines have a thick, fleshy tongue that makes glottal visualization slightly more difficult. Some birds have very brisk glottal closure reflexes. Intubation in these patients can be facilitated by applying a very small amount of lidocaine to the larynx and waiting 60 seconds. If possible, the tube is secured to the mandibular beak to allow for monitoring the oral cavity during anesthesia. Any portion of the tube extending from the circuit to the glottis is dead space; cutting the tube as close as possible to its entry into the oral cavity will minimize this mechanical dead space.

Inhalant anesthetics can also be administered through a cannula inserted into an air sac for induction and maintenance in birds as small as zebra finches (Fig. 24.3) (Korbel R 1998; Korbel et al. 1993; Mitchell et al. 1999; Nilson et al. 2005; Piiper et al. 1970; Rode et al. 1990; Whittow & Ossorio 1970; Wijnberg et al. 1991). Air sac cannulation provides an airway when upper respiratory tract obstruction is present (e.g., syringeal foreign bodies or granulomas). It is also used for procedures involving the upper airway or cranium (Jaensch et al. 2001; Nilson et al. 2005; Piiper et al. 1970). It is also placed for acute life-threatening obstruction and can be left in place to provide longer-term respiratory support, but not generally for more than 3–5 days without replacing tubes, as inflammatory tissue and cells will accumulate on the tube tip (Korbel et al. 1996; Mitchell et al. 1999).

Materials used for air sac cannulas include sterile endotracheal tubes, large-gauge IV catheters (16–18 gauge), red rubber feeding tubes, and silastic tubing. If the bird is to breathe through the cannula, the tube diameter should be at least equal to the patient's tracheal diameter and short enough to minimize dead space and prevent coelomic soft tissue contusion.

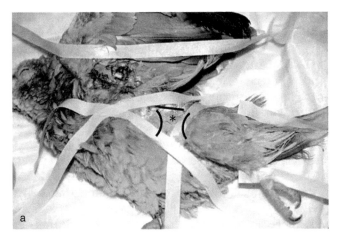

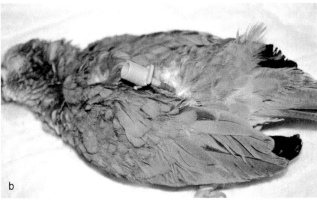

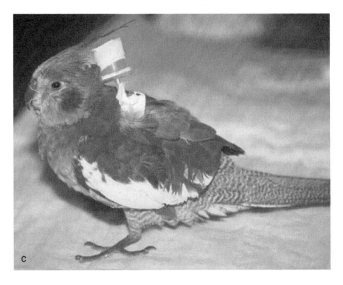

Figure 24.3. Placement of an air sac cannula. Strict asepsis should be observed when placing the cannula. Feathers over the site for cannulation should be gently plucked, contour feathers taped away from the cannula site and the area should be surgically prepared. The landmarks for air sac cannula placement are caudal to last rib, ventral to the vertebrae and, in most cases, cranial to hindlimb. The proper site for cannula insertion is marked with * (a). Once the cannula has been surgically placed, it is secured in place with suture (b). A piece of sterile gauze can be used as a filter to minimize contamination of the cannula with particulate matter (c).

Air sac catheters are usually placed in the left caudal thoracic or abdominal air sac to prevent trauma to the larger right liver lobe. However, catheter placement into the clavicular air sacs has also been reported (Rode et al. 1990; Rosskopf & Woerpel 1989). In sulfur-crested cockatoos (*Cacatua galerita*) caudal thoracic air sac intubation provided stable isoflurane anesthesia without significant respiratory functional changes. Even though caudal thoracic air sac PCO_2 decreased to 12.7 ± 7.9 mm Hg, spontaneous respiration was still present (Jaensch et al. 2001). Clavicular air sac catheterization was also evaluated, but was not successful at either maintaining anesthesia or providing ventilation. In a separate study, clavicular air sac PO_2 and PCO_2 were significantly lower than in the cranial thoracic air sacs suggesting, at least in sulfur-crested cockatoos, ventilation of this air sac is less than the cranial and caudal thoracic air sacs (Jaensch et al. 2002).

Air sac cannula placement is a relatively simple surgical procedure (Fig. 24.3). For placement into the left caudal thoracic or abdominal air sac, the landmarks are the last rib, the cranial aspect of the femur and the flexor cruris medialis muscles. Following removal of overlying feathers and aseptic preparation of the skin, a skin incision is made over the desired site. The underlying muscle and air sac membrane are bluntly dissected with a hemostat. The tip of the sterile catheter is grasped with the hemostat and passed into the air sac. The muscle and skin are closed securing the catheter in place. In an emergency, gas flow and ventilation are provided through an IV catheter placed at the same site and connected to an oxygen source. Care is taken not to advance the catheter needle too far and to limit oxygen flow to prevent hypocapnia. In apneic 1- to 1.7-kg chickens, a flow of 500 mL/min reduced PCO_2 to ≤ 20 mm Hg (Pascoe, unpubl. obs., 1992) so with a small catheter and flow through ventilation the O_2 flow should probably be <250 mL/kg. Oxygen and anesthetic gases from the cannulated site exit the trachea unless intubated with an occluded endotracheal tube. It is possible to scavenge waste gases by placing a mask or tube over the bird's head and connecting it to an active anesthetic scavenging system.

The most common adverse effects reported with air sac cannulation are apnea, subcutaneous emphysema, plugging of the tube, and bacterial contamination with associated coelomitis (Jaensch et al. 2001; Mitchell et al. 1999). Ensure meticulous cleaning/inspection of the tube to prevent plugging. Cleaning is performed with a sterile cotton tip applicator or Dacron swab. A filter can be designed from small weave gauze (i.e., from the inside of a Hepa-filtered mask) and placed over the end of tube to prevent particulate matter from entering. Although most birds tolerate air sac cannulas, an Elizabethan collar may be required for some. Following cannula removal, the body wall is closed to prevent subcutaneous emphysema.

Breathing Systems

Many nonrebreathing systems (e.g., Ayre's T-piece, Mapleson systems, Magill, Jackson-Rees, Norman elbow, and Bain) have and can be used for avian anesthesia. These systems require a relatively high fresh gas flow rate to remove carbon dioxide. These higher flow rates have the added benefit of providing rapid equilibration in inhalant concentration with changes in vaporizer setting. Nonrebreathing systems were traditionally viewed as ideal for small patients because of lower airflow resistance and reduced dead space. Circle systems were believed to have higher airflow resistance because they contain one way valves and soda lime canisters. However, the primary source of resistance is most likely the endotracheal tube. Studies in infants ≤10 kg (Rasch et al. 1988) and cats (Suter et al. 1989) have shown that resistance was insignificant compared with that produced by the endotracheal tube alone. Circle systems are heavier and bulkier, which predisposes to accidental extubation and difficulty working around the head. For this reason, a nonrebreathing system, such as the Bain breathing system, is recommended in small birds due to its lightweight design.

Specific flow rates for avian patients have not been defined. As in mammals, 2–3× minute ventilation appears appropriate when using the T-piece or Norman elbow, but in the Bain circuit, a lower flow rate of 150–200 mL/kg/min is effective (Ludders & Matthews 1996; Paul-Murphy & Fialkowski 2001). The removal of waste gases from the circuit occurs during the pause between expiration and inspiration. If the respiratory rate is high (shorter pause and therefore more mixing of inspired and expired gases), a higher flow rate is used (e.g., RR >40 increase the flow rate to 300 mL/kg/min).

Ventilators

Both injectable and inhalant anesthetics cause dose-dependent respiratory depression. Sick or debilitated birds may not be able to accommodate these physiologic changes, requiring intermittent positive pressure ventilation (IPPV). In mammals, IPPV is associated with reduced cardiac output and hypotension (Steffey & Howland 1977, 1980). In cranes anesthetized with isoflurane, spontaneous ventilation was associated with elevations in $PaCO_2$, hypotension and acidemia compared with controlled ventilation (Ludders et al. 1989a). Similarly, there was a significantly reduced $PaCO_2$-$PETCO_2$ gradient and no significant difference in mean arterial blood pressure in Hispaniolan parrots (*Amazona ventralis*) ventilated using IPPV compared with birds breathing spontaneously (Pettifer et al. 2002). It is possible that reduced cardiovascular performance associated with IPPV may not be a concern in birds. However, it is still recommended that cardiovascular variables be monitored closely during IPPV.

Ventilators must cope with the range of tidal volumes in the species of interest. In very small birds, this may be ≤1 mL, while in a large ostrich, it might be ≥2 L. Modern ventilators are usually pneumatic, but control mechanisms may be either pneumatic or electric. If electronically controlled, an auxillary power source is required if the bird is moved or power fails. The three variables controlled by a ventilator are tidal volume, rate of tidal volume delivery, and respiratory frequency. The method of control varies between ventilators. In volume-limited ventilators, tidal volume is set on the machine with the expectation that it will deliver the volume regardless of moderate changes in resistance. Even if the circuit is disconnected, the ventilator continues to cycle with no alteration in tidal volume or timing. Some ventilators allow the upper limit for inspired pressure to be set with an alarm. In pressure-limited ventilators, the end-inspiratory pressure is set. The ventilator will push gas into the bird until it reaches the set pressure, when the inspiratory phase will terminate and the ventilator allows for passive exhalation. A disconnect or large hole in an air sac is indicated by prolonged inspiration because the preset pressure is not reached. A third method is to set inspiratory time and achieve different tidal volumes by altering inspiratory flow rate. This is a form of volume-limited ventilation. The respiratory rate and tidal volume are determined by the gas flow rate. Hence, it is necessary to set a faster flow rate for a larger tidal volume. On some ventilators this is set by altering the knob labeled "I : E ratio." This is the inspiratory versus expiratory time and the setting will depend on the number of breaths per minute. If you want inspiration to take 1.5 seconds, the I : E ratio would need to be 1 : 3 for 10 breaths per minute (6 seconds per breath, 1.5 seconds for inspiration : 4.5 seconds for expiration) or 1 : 1 for 20 breaths per minute (3 seconds per breath : 1.5 seconds each for inspiration and expiration). The number of breaths per minute is mostly set by altering a timing device that begins a new inspiration after a set period of time.

When ventilating birds, it is essential to have a ventilator that can deliver small tidal volumes slowly to give an acceptable inspiratory time. During anesthesia, the ventilator should initiate the breath, not the bird, to control the PCO_2. In assisted ventilation mode, the bird initiates the breath when its PCO_2 reaches the point set by the central controllers of ventilation in the brain. Since the latter are depressed by anesthetics, assisted ventilation is not likely to decrease PCO_2.

The authors recommend initial inspiratory pressures of 8–10 cm H_2O and rates of 6–10 breaths per minute. Thoracic excursions are assessed as soon as the ventilator is started. The tidal volume is adjusted to achieve an appropriate thoracoabdominal expansion. The minute volume is lower than mammals (Frappell et al. 2001) and inspiratory times can be longer. At six breaths per minute, the I : E ratio could be set to 1 : 2 to 1 : 3 (inspiration occurring over 3.3 to 2.5 seconds). During coelomic surgery, when the air sacs have been opened, anesthetic will be pushed by the ventilator into the air being breathed by the surgeons. It is important to avoid or minimize personnel exposure to inhaled agents. In some cases, injectable anesthetics are used if the concerns about using inhalant anesthetics are great.

During positive pressure ventilation, it is possible the direction of gas flow within the lung is reversed. However, the crosscurrent exchange system is not dependent upon direction of flow and does not significantly affect gas exchange (Ludders & Matthews 1996; Piiper et al. 1970). If a mechanical ventilator is not available, hand ventilation delivered from the reservoir bag provides assisted ventilation.

THERMAL SUPPORT

Body temperature is monitored continuously throughout anesthesia. Prevention of heat loss is essential in the anesthetized patient and supplemental heat sources are used regardless of procedure length. Electronic thermometers and temperature probes provide accurate readings. Cloacal temperatures have been correlated with thoracic esophageal readings, suggesting core temperature may be indirectly monitored (Phalen et al. 1996). However, as cloacal musculature relaxes, peripheral temperature readings are lowered. Esophageal temperature probes provide consistent readings when placed at the level of the heart in the thoracic esophagus. Care is taken to ensure the crop is not damaged during placement and the probe does not back out resulting in incorrect temperature readings.

Since most heat is lost via radiation, the most effective technique to prevent heat loss is to minimize the temperature gradient between the bird and the room. Options include increased room temperature, insulating the patient with clear, plastic drapes, and wrapping nonsurgical fields. The surgical time and the amount of time that the body cavities are open are minimized, as are feather plucking and alcohol use for skin preparation. Latex gloves, empty fluid bags, or plastic bottles can be filled with water, warmed in a hot water bath or microwave and placed next to the bird. Water bottles are always wrapped in a towel to prevent burns. Circu-

lating warm water blankets insignificantly diminish rate of heat loss in birds (Phalen et al. 1996; Rembert et al. 2001). Radiant heat lamps are effective at maintaining core body temperature, but the optimal distance between the heat source and the patient differs with patient size, heat lamp strength, and the heat setting (Phalen et al. 1996; Rembert et al. 2001). Forced air warmers (Bair® Hugger) are more effective at minimizing hypothermia during anesthesia than other methods (Borms et al. 1994; Machon et al. 1999; Rembert et al. 2001). They are particularly effective when set up to have warm air rising around the patient either by wrapping the patient in the blanket or by using a perforated table. The patient's eyes are well lubricated to prevent corneal ulceration due to drying from the warm air.

Further reductions in heat loss are achieved by warming fluids and reducing respiratory cooling. In pigeons anesthetized for 90 minutes, there was no significant difference in heat loss between either a circle system with mechanical ventilator producing heated air, a nonrebreathing system with mechanical ventilator producing nonheated air and a Bain nonrebreathing circuit (Boedeker et al. 2005). This is in contrast to humans, cats, and rabbits in which heated, humidified anesthetic gases reduce or prevent the development of hypothermia (Haskins & Patz 1980; Newton 1975; Shanks 1974; Tausk et al. 1976). In intubated anesthetized ring-necked doves (*Streptopelia risoria*) without thermal support, hypothermia was not lessened by humidification and heating of inspired gases (Phalen et al. 1996). However, in anesthetized pigeons maintained on a facemask, heated inspired gas did minimize hypothermia (Jenkins 1988).

EMERGENCIES

Emergencies during anesthesia should be planned for and anticipated. Many can be averted by careful monitoring of respiratory and heart rates, and body temperature. Emergency equipment (i.e., endotracheal tubes, oxygen, IV catheters and materials for securing them, ventilatory support, and emergency drugs) should always be close by and prepared for use. It is recommended that emergency drug dosages be calculated and that 1–2 doses be predrawn before induction (Table 24.1).

Table 24.1. Avian emergency drug doses

Drug	Dosage	Route	Comments
Atropine	0.01–0.02 mg/kg	SC, IM, IV	Most species/Preanesthetic
	0.04–0.1 mg/kg	SC, IM, IV, IO, IT	Bradycardia
	0.5 mg/kg	IM, IV, IO, IT	CPR
Glycopyrrolate	0.01–0.02 mg/kg	IM, IV	Slower onset than atropine Most species/preanesthetic
	0.04 mg/kg	IV	Ratites
Epinephrine (1 : 1000)	0.05–0.5 mg/kg	IM, IV, IO, IT	CPR, bradycardia

Respiratory depression and arrest are treated by turning off the anesthetic and controlling ventilation. Cardiac arrest is usually a result of myocardial hypoxemia and inotropic and chronotropic anesthetic drug effects. Although treatment is often unrewarding, administration of epinephrine IV, intratracheal or by intracardiac injection, is recommended. Cardiac massage is nearly impossible due to the heart's anatomical location dorsal to the large bony sternum, but should be attempted. Severe bradycardia is treated with atropine, assuming it is due to increased parasympathetic tone. In very small birds, it is possible to see spontaneous ventricular defibrillation as the mass of the heart is small enough that it cannot maintain a fibrillatory pattern.

ANESTHESIA

Restraint

Correct restraint is essential to minimize patient stress and time required for anesthetic induction. Stressed birds may die from physical restraint, and this risk is magnified in sick or debilitated patients. Appropriate means of physical restraint must be assessed for each patient and appropriate stabilization and supportive care prepared prior to handling. Paper towels, wash cloths, hand towels, large bath towels, or blankets may be used based on the patient size. Hooding calms some species (e.g., raptors and ratites), but care must be taken to ensure adequate air flow. Leather gloves will not protect handlers from the crushing bite of a large parrot. Nets are used to capture birds in larger enclosures or escapees. They should be sized appropriately for the patient to minimize iatrogenic trauma. Once netted, the bird is gently removed to avoid trauma to the wings, legs, or toes. Ear protection for the handler (e.g., cotton balls or ear plugs) can be used when handling large psittacines (e.g., cockatoos and macaws). Face shields or goggles are used when handling birds likely to inflict ocular damage with the tip of their beaks (e.g., Ciconiiformes).

It is preferable for caged birds to be captured from within their travel cage or hospital enclosure to reduce the chance for injury and reduce stress induced by escape attempts in a room. All perches, toys, and food and water dishes are removed to facilitate capture and minimize trauma and ambient noise should be reduced. If a patient must be captured from a larger area, this should ideally be done in a small area that is free of windows and doors leading to the outdoors. Alternately, windows can be covered to minimize self-induced trauma if an escape occurs and doors are locked. Some methods to aid capture from a room include placing the bird on the floor or turning off lights, as this will often reduce the excitement level of the patient. Regardless of the physical restraint technique employed, care should be taken not to compromise thoracic cage movement or the ability of the anesthetist to monitor the patient. Movement with the bird in hand should be quiet and calm to reduce fright and stress. The capture is performed expeditiously to minimize stress. If a bird should escape and needs to be recaptured or is unduly excited, delay anesthesia until the bird has calmed down.

Once the bird is in hand, a towel is initially placed over the dorsum, then gently wrapped around the wings to restrict flapping and prevent damage to the wings and feathers. Once adequately restrained by the handler, birds are removed from the towel if possible to prevent hyperthermia that can occur subsequent to prolonged restraint. Small birds (e.g., passerines) are restrained with the head between thumb and forefinger, and the body within the palm. Alternatively, in smaller psittacines, the head is restrained using a "three point" technique, with thumb and middle finger supporting the mandible and the index finger on top of the head. Bruising of the face is possible in large macaws and only the minimum pressure necessary to restrict movement is applied. Gentle extension of the bird's neck further limits head movement. Large parrots are strong and will inflict severe wounds if the head and beak are not immediately controlled. Some prefer to encircle the birds neck with their fingers for restraint. A third technique places the thumb under the intermandibular space while the other fingers are placed over the top of the head. This is the author's choice for maintaining full control of the head during restraint. The other hand is placed on the dorsum to secure the wings and legs.

Preoxygenation

Preoxygenation is performed whenever possible and when hypoxemia may occur (i.e., upper respiratory obstruction, cardiac, pulmonary, or air sac disease). It replaces nitrogen in the respiratory system and can produce an oxygen reservoir 4–5× normal in the air sacs. The benefits are achieved in ≤1 minute of high inspired oxygen concentration in the healthy bird, but may take ≥5 minutes in a bird with compromised respiratory function. Preoxygenation is accomplished with an oxygen cage or an induction chamber in the unrestrained bird, or a facemask in the physically restrained bird. Levels rise slower in an unprimed oxygen cage or induction chamber than a tight-fitting facemask with minimal deadspace. If the bird is allowed to breathe room air, the parabronchial oxygen levels can fall precipitously if the bird becomes apneic.

Mask or Chamber Induction

Inhalant anesthesia induction is often performed with either a mask or induction chamber. Commercially available veterinary inhalant masks can be used for many species. However, differences in beak anatomy and location of nares require unique masks to be formed from syringe cases, plastic soda bottles, or other materi-

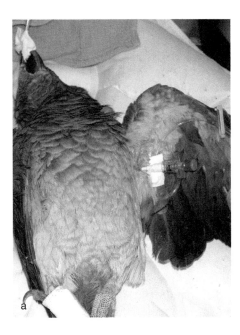
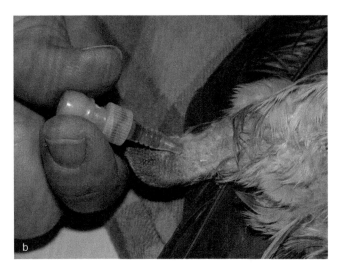

Figure 24.4. Sites for intravenous (IV) catheters include the ulnar (basilic) vein (a), medial metatarsal vein (b) or jugular vein. Small bore over-the-needle catheters (24 gauge or smaller) are most often necessary for avian patients.

als. The mask is as small as possible and the entire head of the patient is placed inside the mask. To minimize waste gas release, a seal is developed using a disposable latex glove placed over the mask with a central hole cut for the bird's neck. Although some have suggested that this seal can be used for positive pressure ventilation, it is not recommended by these authors. In addition to increased waste gas release, this technique will introduce gas into the gastrointestinal tract. Facemask induction in some birds (i.e., waterfowl) is associated with apnea and bradycardia that may last for 3–5 minutes (Ludders & Matthews 1996). This response may even occur from placing a facemask snugly onto the face and beak without inhalant anesthetic. This response is a stress response that appears to be mediated by stimulation of trigeminal nerve receptors in the beak and nares of diving ducks (Butler 1988; Jones et al. 1988; Woakes 1988). Premedication with a benzodiazepine may avert this response. If this response occurs, discontinue inhalation anesthesia, remove the mask, and provide 100% oxygen until bradycardia resolves.

Commercially available induction chambers sized for mice up to small dogs can be utilized for birds as small as hummingbirds. Advantages of these chambers are reduced waste gas and shorter induction times. In stressed birds, the chamber is covered with a towel to darken the chamber. Alternatively, an animal carrier or the front of a hospital cage is sealed with a plastic bag and inhalant anesthetic administered for induction of large or stressed patients. Disadvantages of induction chambers include the inability to auscult the patient, gas pollution when the chamber is opened, and trauma due to flapping during the excitement phase of anes-

thesia. The latter is reduced by padding the induction chamber and minimizing chamber size to reduce movement. Gas flow rates are adjusted to chamber size to provide an optimum rate of rise of the anesthetic concentration. This might be as low as 0.5 L/min for a 1 L up to 15 L/min for a 60-L chamber. The efficiency of the respiratory system makes high inhalant induction concentrations unnecessary. For example, isoflurane vaporizer settings rarely need exceed 3%. The bird is promptly removed after the righting reflex is lost. The final phase of the induction is accomplished using a mask to facilitate monitoring.

Vascular Support

During anesthesia or emergencies, intravenous (IV) or intraosseous (IO) fluids are used to provide replacement fluids. Sites for IV catheters include the basilic (ulnar), medial metatarsal, or jugular veins (Fig. 24.4). Small-bore over-the-needle catheters (≤24 gauge) are used. If blood is to be repetitively collected from the catheter, it should be placed in either the jugular (small patients) or a large peripheral vessel. The increased fragility of avian blood vessels, the lack of soft tissue support and patient temperament make catheter maintenance difficult. The catheter site is gently plucked and aseptically prepared. Catheters are secured with a bandage tape butterfly and sutured with an everting mattress pattern. The catheter site is bandaged for additional security. Complications of long-term, indwelling catheterization include infection and possibly fatal hemorrhage. Jugular catheters require 24-hour monitoring because fatal hemorrhage can occur if the bird pulls or chews on the catheter and damages the vessel.

Intraosseous catheterization is used in smaller patients or during cardiovascular collapse (Aguilar et al. 1993; Lamberski & Daniel 1992; Ritchie et al. 1990; Valverde et al. 1993). IO catheter maintenance is easier to achieve due to stability in the medullary cavity. Products that can be utilized include 18- to 24-gauge, 2- to 5-cm spinal needles, or 18- to 25-gauge 2-cm hypodermic needles. The length of the catheter should be long enough to extend 1/3 to 1/2 the length of the medullary cavity. A wire stylet may be necessary with hypodermic needles to reduce the potential for a bone core. Most commonly used sites include the distal ulna and proximal tibiotarsus. Pneumatic bones (i.e., the humerus and femur) are avoided. Feathers are gently plucked and the site surgically prepared. Wearing gloves, the sterile IO catheter is positioned at the center of the cnemial crest of the tibiotarsus or slightly ventral to the dorsal condyle of the distal ulna and parallel to the bone. The bone is held firmly with one hand while the other applies firm pressure combined with slight rotation (Fig. 24.5). Once the cortex is penetrated, the catheter should advance easily with little resistance. If there is further resistance, the opposite cortex has most likely been penetrated. The cannula is flushed with heparinized saline and should flow easily. Fluids will be seen flowing through the basilic vein when the cannula is correctly placed in the distal ulna. The insertion site is covered with antibiotic ointment and the cannula secured with a bandage tape butterfly at the exit point in the skin and sutured. A bandage can be placed over the cannula site for additional security to prevent trauma or damage to the catheter. Although IO catheters are reported to remain patent for 72 hours without flushing (Ritchie et al. 1990), it is recommended that the catheter be gently flushed with heparinized saline twice daily.

Complications associated with IO catheterization include penetration of both cortices, failure to properly enter the medullary cavity, and extravasation of fluids with associated pain. Extravasation has been observed even with proper catheter placement after 1–2 days of use (Steinohrt 1999). Intraosseous catheterization is contraindicated in septic patients and those with metabolic bone disease. Osteomyelitis may occur due to duration or placement of the IO catheter (Steinohrt 1999). Administration of alkaline or hypertonic solutions may also contribute to osteomyelitis and will cause pain and transient microscopic changes in the bone marrow (Lamberski & Daniel 1992; Ritchie et al. 1990). These solutions are, therefore, diluted prior to administration and the catheter is flushed with heparinized saline after any drug injection.

Crystalloid fluids (e.g., 0.9% NaCl [Baxter, Deerfield, IL], lactated Ringer's [Abbott Laboratories, North Chicago, IL], Normosol-R [CEVA Laboratories, Overland Park, KS], and Plasmalyte-A [Baxter]) are commonly used for IV volume support, maintenance, and rehydration. Fluids are warmed to body temperature (38–39°C) to prevent hypothermia.

Fluid rates of 10 mL/kg/h are recommended for healthy anesthetized patients. This rate is based on studies in human patients. While this is a starting point, it is recognized that rates in very small patients may need to be considerably higher, but caution should be exercised to not fluid overload small patients. Each patient is assessed individually for their fluid needs. Fluid boluses of 10–20 mL/kg over 5–7 minutes are well tolerated (Abou-Madi & Kollias 1992). For severe hemorrhage, whole blood transfusion (volume for volume) should be provided. If this is not available, it has been recommended to provide crystalloid fluids at 3× the volume of blood loss. However, this recommendation is based on mammals where the interstitial space is 2× the vascular volume. In birds, the interstitial space is 4× plasma volume (Skadhauge 1981). Replacement fluid volumes may need to be greater than 3× blood loss. Dextrose solutions are added to fluids for treatment of hypoglycemia. Parenteral dextrose use is minimized to prevent compartmental shifts in electrolytes and water leading to hypovolemia (Abou-Madi & Kollias 1992).

Hypertonic fluids (e.g., 7.5% NaCl) are used to expand intravascular volume during resuscitation following acute severe hemorrhage. Hypertonic saline has been evaluated in birds primarily for studying renal sodium excretion and the role of osmotic thirst in the control of normal drinking. In several studies, plasma osmolality increased after bolus infusion (Leary et al. 1998; Yeomans & Savory 1988). The major benefit of hypertonic saline is intravascular volume expansion at one-fourth the volume of isotonic solutions. The mammalian dosage (4 mL/kg) given over 10 minutes is used in birds. However, due to osmotic diuresis and rapid redistribution of sodium cations, the intravascular effect is transient (<30 minutes) and additional fluid therapy with a crystalloid or colloid must be used. Hypertonic fluids are contraindicated in dehydration, hypernatremia, and head trauma with intracranial hemorrhage. The sustained use of hypertonic saline is not recommended because hypernatremia and hyperchloremic acidemia, increased bleeding, and exacerbation of underlying cardiac and pulmonary disease due to fluid overload may occur.

Small patient size and species diversity often preclude the use of natural colloids, such as homologous or heterologous plasma. The indications for the use of synthetic colloids (e.g., hetastarch 6%, Hextend and hemoglobin-based oxygen carriers) are the same as hypertonic saline although the benefits last longer. All are cleared through the kidneys so they are used with caution in patients with cardiac or renal impairment. They do not provide albumin, thrombocytes, or coagulation factors. Potential adverse effects include anaphylactoid reactions and blood coagulation abnormalities. In critically ill raptors, boluses of hetastarch (10–15 mL/

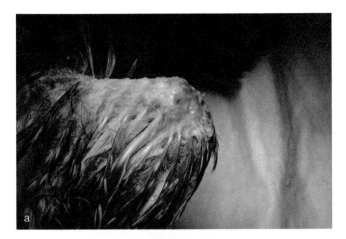
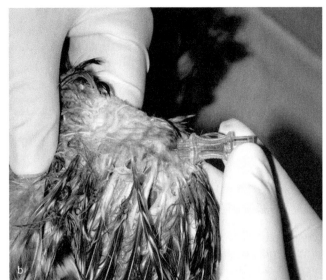
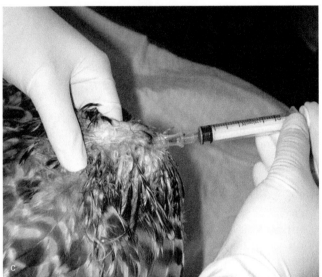
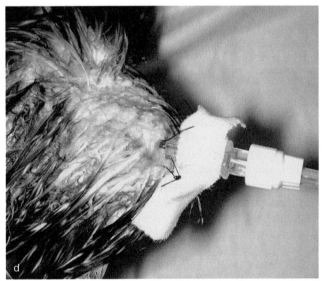
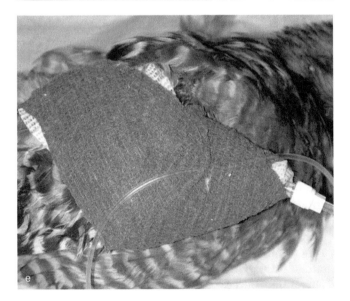

Figure 24.5. Intraosseous (IO) catheter placement in the distal ulna of a bird. Strict asepsis should be observed when placing the catheter. Feathers over the site should be gently plucked and the site should be surgically prepared (a). Wearing sterile gloves, the sterile catheter is positioned slightly ventral to the dorsal condyle of the distal ulna and parallel to the bone (b). The bone is held firmly with one hand while the hand other applies firm pressure combined with slight rotation (c). The cannula should be flushed with heparinized saline and should flow easily (d). The insertion site should be covered with an antibiotic ointment and the cannula should be secured with a bandage tape butterfly at the exit point in the skin and suture (d). A bandage can be placed over the cannula site for additional security and to prevent possible trauma or damage to the catheter (e).

kg 6%, q 8 h) for four or more treatments were well tolerated (Stone & Redig 1994). Alternatively, dosages ≤20 mL/kg/d are suggested.

Reported circulating blood volume % based on body weight varies considerably (Campbell et al. 1994): 5% in ring-necked pheasants (Campbell et al. 1994), 7.5 ± 1.5% in quail (Takei & Hatakeyma 1987), 16.3–20.3% in the racing pigeon (Campbell et al. 1994), 10.6 ± 2.9% in the galah (Jaensch & Raidal 1998), and 5.4 ± 10.5% and 13.1 ± 2.3% in two strains of chickens) (Makinde et al. 1986). Hemorrhage is better tolerated than in mammals. However, when severe (>30% blood volume) or the PCV <20%, whole blood transfusion is indicated. Heterologous blood cells (e.g., from pigeon, chicken) transfused into parrots last only 12 hours, causing a significant metabolic drain on the recipient as the body utilizes energy to destroy the foreign cells (Finnegan et al. 1997; Sandmeier et al. 1994). The half-life of homologous and autologous blood transfusions were 8.5 and 9.9 days in conures (*Aratinga* spp.), (Degernes & Crosier 1999), 12.5 and 12.2 days in cockatiels (*Nymphicus hollandicus*), (Degernes et al. 1999), and 7.1 and 26.8 days in pigeons, respectively (Sandmeier et al. 1994). In pigeons, PCV and total solids were elevated for ≥102 hours following homologous transfusion. (Finnegan et al. 1997)

The storage of whole blood or blood products has been little studied to date (Morrisey et al. 1997), and transfusions with fresh whole blood are recommended. The anticoagulants citrate phosphate dextrose adenine (CPDA-1) and acid citrate dextrose (ACD) are used most commonly at a ratio of 1 : 9 whole blood : anticoagulant. If given rapidly, the citrate can decrease ionized calcium and decrease myocardial contractility. It may be necessary to give calcium gluconate or chloride to the patient to reverse this effect. Donors are screened for infectious diseases. A major/minor crossmatch is performed prior to transfusion. Sixty-six percent of major crossmatches performed between different species were positive for agglutination or hemolysis, whereas between the same species, they were all negative (Stauber et al. 1996). Mammalian protocols are presently followed for blood collection and administration. Pediatric blood filters have been evaluated for their ability to cause hemolysis in chicken blood and an 18-μM filter did not cause hemolysis compared with nonfiltered control (Jankowski & Nevarez 2010).

There is little published information available on the safety and efficacy of hemoglobin-based oxygen carriers (HBOC). Evaluation of the effects of fluid resuscitation in an acute blood loss (60% blood volume) model in ducks (*Anas platyrhnychos*) showed decreased mortality in birds receiving HBOC combined with crystalloid fluids. The comparison groups received hetastarch combined with crystalloid fluids and crystalloid fluids alone (Lichtenberger et al. 2003). HBOC has a short half-life in mammals (30–40 hours). Adverse

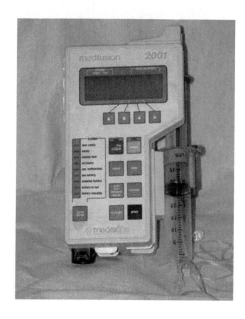

Figure 24.6. In order to provide accurate infusion rates for small avian patients, fluid infusion pumps and syringe pumps are most commonly required.

effects in mammals include discolored mucous membranes, sclera, and urine, affecting patient monitoring (Antinoff 2003; Lichtenberger 2004). Rapid bolus infusion (5-mL/kg HBOC and 10-mL/kg crystalloid fluids over 1 minute) has been given in patients with acute blood loss without any adverse effects (Lichtenberger et al. 2001, 2002, 2003).

Standard micro-drip fluid sets used in small animal veterinary practice (60 drops/mL) will not allow appropriate infusion rates in very small patients. Instead, fluid infusion and syringe pumps are used for accurate fluid administration (Fig. 24.6).

PREANESTHETICS

Parasympatholytics

Several authors question the necessity of routine medication with parasympatholytics (Table 24.2). Atropine and glycopyrrolate reduce mucus production and plug formation, but increase viscosity (Ludders & Matthews 1996). Additionally, some practitioners avoid using anticholinergics in birds because they increase heart rate, cardiac work, and myocardial oxygen demand. Therefore, the use of these agents should be weighed against their potential side effects.

Sedatives and Tranquilizers

Sedatives and tranquilizers are used to decrease anxiety and fear during induction. However, most tranquilizers lack analgesia. Additionally, most require injection and the handling and restraint may be as much as required for anesthetic induction. The merits of premedication must be weighed against this additional stress.

Table 24.2. Injectable premedication/emergency, sedative, tranquilizer, and anesthetic drugs used in cagebirds

Drug	Dosage (mg/kg)	Route	Indication(s)	Comments	References
Benzodiazepines					
Diazepam	0.2–2.0	IM, IV	Most species. Premedication, sedation, anticonvulsant, appetite stimulant	IM administration may cause severe muscle irritation and absorption may be delayed 0.25–0.5 mg/kg has been used as an appetite stimulant and to improve acceptance to novel captive diets for raptors and wild passerines Reversal with flumazenil	Abou-Madi (2001); Samour (2000); Clyde & Paul-Murphy (1999); Rupiper & Ehrenberg (1994); Suarez (1993); Massey (2003)
	2.5–4.0	PO	Most species/sedation		Ritchie et al. (1994)
	7.3–8.0	IN	Canaries	Dose divided into each nare and given slowly. Dorsal recumbency for approx. 35 minutes.	Vesal and Eskandari (2006); Vesal and Zare (2006)
Midazolam				In larger macaws, the author's have noted regurgitation after doses of >0.3–0.5 mg/kg IM. Water soluble; does not cause muscle irritation with IM use. Reversal with flumazenil	
	0.1–2.0	IM, IV	Most species/ premedication, sedation, appetite stimulant	IM onset 5–15 minutes. Higher dosages may cause profound sedation.	Abou-Madi (2001); Day and Roge (1996)
	2.0–6.0	IM	Quail, sedation	High dosages give greatest sedation without cardiopulmonary effects, but adequate sedation also found with lower dosages, just shorter duration of sedation.	Day and Roge (1996)
	2.0	IM	Canada geese/sedation	For 15–20 minutes	Valverde et al. (1990)
	2.0	IN	Hispaniolan Amazon parrots	Mild-to-moderate sedation in 3 minutes; reduced vocalizations, struggling and defensive behaviors for 15 minutes; reversed with IN flumazenil	Mans et al. (2010)
	7.3–8.0	IN	Canaries, ring-necked parakeets.	Dose divided into each nare and given slowly. Dorsal recumbency for approximately 17 minutes. Flumazenil reduced time to recovery.	Vesal and Eskandari (2006); Vesal and Zare (2006)
Flumazenil	0.02–0.10	IM, IV	Most species.	Benzodiazepine reversal agent.	Abou-Madi (2001); Day and Roge (1996); Machin and Caulkett (1998)
	0.05	IN	Mallard ducks		Machin and Caulkett (1998b)
	0.13–0.15	IN	Canaries, ring-necked parakeets.	Dose divided evenly between nares and given slowly.	Vesal and Eskandari (2006)

(Continued)

Table 24.2. (Continued)

Drug	Dosage (mg/kg)	Route	Indication(s)	Comments	References
α-2 Adrenergic agonists					
Detomidine	0.3	IM	Rock partridges	Marked sedation/significant decrease in HR, RR, decrease in cloacal temperature, prolonged recoveries (260 ± 18 minutes)	Uzun et al. (2006)
	12	IN	Ring-necked parakeets	Dose divided into each nare and given slowly; sedation <3 minutes but did not allow dorsal recumbency or manipulation; reversal with atipamezole significantly reduced time to recovery	Vesal and Eskandari (2006)
	12–15	IN	Canaries	Dose divided into each nare and given slowly; higher dose prolonged sedation but could not place in dorsal recumbency; prolonged duration of effect (258 ± 2 minutes) but completely reversed with yohimbine IN	Vesal and Zare (2006)
Dexmedetomidine	0.025	IM	Common buzzards	Use half the recommended dose of medetomidine. Reversal with same dose of atipamezole Adequate restraint to prevent reaction to handling, but did not allow for intubation. Completely reversed with atipamezole. Mean times to loss of righting reflex = 3.5 ± 1 minutes in common buzzards. No arrhythmias noted on ECG. No excitement or major adverse effects observed in either group.	Santangelo et al. (2009)
	0.075	IM	Common kestrels	Adequate restraint to prevent reaction to handling, but did not allow for intubation. Completely reversed with atipamezole. Mean times to loss of righting reflex = 7 ± 1.2 minutes in common kestrels.	Santangelo et al. (2009)
Medetomidine	0.2–2	IM	Pigeon, yellow-crowned Amazon	0.08–2mg/kg IM associated with inadequate sedation. Profound respiratory depression may occur. Much higher dosages appear to be required in some avian spp. when compared with mammals.	Pollock et al. (2001); Sandmeier (2000)
	0.25–0.35	PO	Chickens	Sedation	James et al. (1999)
Xylazine	1.0–10.0	IM, IV	Most species, tranquilization. In combination with ketamine for anesthesia.	Not recommended by itself for tranquilization and seldom used in pet birds due to adverse effects—excitement, convulsions, bradycardia, arrhythmias, bradypnea, hypoxemia, hypercarbia, and death when used alone; most useful in ratites Adequate sedation often with <4 mg/kg, in smaller psittacines dosages up to 10mg/kg may be required.	Clyde and Paul-Murphy (1999); Carpenter (2000); Huckabee (2000); Ludders et al. (1989a); Samour (2000)

Drug	Dose (mg/kg)	Route	Species	Comments	References
α₂ Adrenergic antagonists					
Atipamezole				α₂ adrenergic antagonist; 1 : 1 volume reversal of dexmedetomidine/medetomidine is general rule; although the same effects would be expected as with medetomidine, there are no data available on the efficacy of atipamezole reversal of dexmedetomidine in birds	
	0.25–0.5	IM	Psittacines, pigeons, raptors, geese	Righting reflex regained 2–10 minutes after administration	Machin and Caulkett (1998a); Samour (2000); Pollock et al. (2001); Santangelo et al. (2009)
	1.3–1.6	IV	Chickens		James et al. (1999)
	0.18–0.28	IV	Mallard ducks		Machin and Caulkett (1998a)
	6.0	IN	Ring-necked parakeets	Dose divided evenly between nares and given slowly, significantly reduced recumbency time after detomidine administration	Vesal and Eskandari (2006)
Yohimbine	0.1–0.2	IV	Psittacines, raptors, waterfowl, ratites	Reversal for xylazine.	Carpenter (2000); Heard (1997); Jensen et al. (1992); Keffen (1993); Raath et al. (1992); Samour (2000)
	1.0	IV	Most species including psittacines, guinea fowl		Teare (1987)
	0.1–0.2	IM, IV	Raptors		Huckabee (2000)
	0.11–0.275	IM	Budgerigars		Heaton and Brauth (1992)
	0.1–1.0	IM	Most species		Abou-Madi (2001)
Dissociative anesthetics					
Ketamine	20–50	SC, IM, IV	Psittacines, pigeons, ratites, poultry, waterfowl. Restraint 30–60 minutes	Usually combined with an alpha-2 adrenergic or with a benzodiazepine to improve relaxation, depth of anesthesia. Not recommended as a sole anesthetic agent due to reports of poor muscle relaxation, myoclonic contractions, opisthotonus and violent recoveries. Smaller sp require a higher dose, large birds tend to recover more slowly.	Beynon et al. (1996); Fowler (1995); Heard (1988); Jensen et al. (1992); Lawton (1996); Samour (2000)
	50	IO	Pigeons	Provided effective analgesia	Kamiloglu et al. (2008)
	5–30	PO	In bait, for ducks		Forbes (1991)
	50–100	PO	In bait for raptors		Samour (2000)

(Continued)

413

Table 24.2. (Continued)

Drug	Dosage (mg/kg)	Route	Indication(s)	Comments	References
Ketamine/diazepam	(K) 5–30 + (D) 0.5–2.0	(K) IM, (D) IM, IV	Most species	Ketamine should be given 5–15 minutes after diazepam for adequate muscle relaxation.	Cubas (2001)
	(K) 20 + (D) 1.0	IV	Toucans	For short procedures (15–20 minutes), give slowly.	
	(K) 75 + (D) 2.5	(K) IM, (D) IV	White leghorn cockerels	Diazepam administered 5 minutes before ketamine for typhlectomy; smooth induction/recovery; some limb contracture, hypothermia, hypoxia, hypercapnia	Maiti et al. (2006)
Ketamine/midazolam	(K) 10–40 + (M) 0.2–2.0	SC, IM	Most species including psittacines		Mandelker (1988); Marx and Roston (1996)
	(K) 40–50 + (M) 3.65	IN	Ring-necked parakeets	Dose divided into each nare and given slowly; onset of action <3 minutes, dorsal recumbency for 71 ± 47 minutes, recovery times reduced with flumazenil IN	Vesal and Eskandari (2006)
	(K) 50 + (M) 2.0	(K) IV, (M) IM	White leghorn cockerels	Midazolam administered 5 minutes before ketamine for typhlectomy; hypoxia, hypercapnia, torticollis, dyspnea, salivation noted; prolonged recovery (92–105 minutes)	Maiti et al. (2006)
Ketamine/xylazine/diazepam (K) Ketamine (X) xylazine (D) diazepam	(K) 25 + (X) 3.0 + (D) 4.0	K, X, D-IM	Roosters	Use with caution—significant decreases in HR, RR, cloacal temperatures, and prolonged recoveries (up to 4 hours)	Mostachio et al. (2008)
Ketamine/xylazine/midazolam (K) Ketamine (X) xylazine (M) midazolam	(K) 15 + (X) 2.5 + (M) 0.3	K, X, M-IM	Guinea fowl	Midazolam improved anesthetic quality	Ajadi et al. (2009)
Propofol	2.9–4.7 (induction); 0.4–0.55 (mg/kg/min) (maintenance)	IV	Red-tailed hawks and great horned owls	Minimal blood pressure effects, but ventilation was significantly reduced. Prolonged recoveries with moderate-to-severe excitatory CNS signs may occur in these species with an infusion	Hawkins et al. (2003)
	5.0 (induction); 1.0 (mg/kg/min) (maintenance)	IV	Hispaniolan Amazon parrots	Recovery times (15.4 ± 15.2 minutes) were prolonged when compared with isoflurane; 6/10 birds had agitated recoveries. Light anesthetic plane in 8/10 birds	Langlois et al. (2003)
	5.0 (induction); 0.5 (mg/kg/min) (maintenance)	IV	Wild turkeys		Schumacher et al. (1997)
	8–10 (induction); 1–4 as bolus PRM	IV	Mallard ducks, canvasback ducks		Machin and Caulkett (1998b, 1999)
	8.0 (induction); 0.8–0.9 (mg/kg/min) (maintenance)	IV CRI	Mute swans	Smooth inductions, minimal excitation on recovery	Muller et al. (2011)

Notes: These are suggested dosages based upon published information and the author's clinical experience. Species and individual variation in response to a given drug can be uncertain so the dosage should be adjusted depending upon the clinical response of the animal.

414

Benzodiazepines Diazepam may cause excitement, tachycardia, and tachypnea in birds if given IV. Uptake of diazepam from IM or SC injection is erratic. Midazolam (0.2–2.0 mg/kg IM) has been used as a sole sedative for minor, nonpainful procedures (i.e., radiographs) (Valverde et al. 1990). Low doses are most often used for preanesthetic sedation. In pigeons, midazolam (14–16 mg/kg IM) induced profound sedation and reduced isoflurane MAC by approximately ⅓ (Smith & Muir 1992; Smith et al. 1993). In quail, midazolam (2–6 mg/kg IM) produced chemical restraint and 40–60 minutes of sedation at the higher doses (Day & Roge 1996). In ring-necked parakeets (*Psittacus krameri*), midazolam administered intranasally alone or in combination with ketamine produced sedation that allowed dorsal recumbency and adequate sedation for minor procedures (Vesal & Eskandari 2006). Intranasal administration of midazolam (0.5 mg/kg) has been used by clinicians to facilitate beak trimming and sample collection in macaws (D. Heard, pers. comm. May 28, 2012). Sedation duration is significantly reduced after flumazenil administration. The authors recommend titrating the dose to avoid the reversal of the beneficial anxiolysis, sedation, and muscle relaxation.

Midazolam IM did not produce major alterations in cardiopulmonary function in Canada geese (Valverde et al. 1990), quail, (Day & Roge 1996), and racing pigeons (Smith & Muir 1992; Smith et al. 1993). Midazolam/ketamine IV produced anesthesia with full recovery in 23 minutes in ducks (Machin & Caulkett 1998b). Two authors (MGH/AMZ) have observed midazolam (0.25–1.0 mg/kg IM) associated regurgitation in larger macaws and cockatoos. Some animals did not stop until after flumazenil administration. Benzodiazepines should either be avoided in these species, or a lower midazolam dose be used and the patient closely monitored for regurgitation.

Alpha-2 Adrenergic Agonists Xylazine and medetomidine are most commonly reported alpha-2 adrenergic agonists in birds. However, as the use of dexmedetomidine supplants that of medetomidine, more information on the use of this newer agent will be available. Since 2007, dexmedetomidine has been approved for veterinary use in the United States. This drug is the dextro-enantiomer of medetomidine and has twice the potency of the racemic mixture, medetomidine, since levomedetomidine has no action at alpha-2 receptors. To aid dosing for practitioners, dexmedetomidine (0.5 mg/mL) is supplied at half the concentration of medetomidine (1.0 mg/mL), and dosing charts are available for dogs and cats. One study has examined the use of dexmedetomidine in two raptor species at a dose of approximately 25 μg/kg for common buzzards (*Buteo buteo*) and 75 μg/kg for common kestrels (*Falcon tinnunculs*) (Santangelo et al. 2009). The authors noted loss of righting in both species within approximately 8

minutes and sedation was sufficient to allow handling. In the study mentioned earlier, atipamezole was used for reversal at a total dose of 250 μg and provided rapid reversal of sedation. It should be noted atropine was administered in conjunction with dexmeditomidine in this study, which has been reported to cause increases in mean arterial blood pressure, heart rate, and the occurrence of cardiac arrhythmias in dogs and is not recommended for coadministration with dexmedetomidine (Congdon et al. 2011).

The major advantage of these agents is they can be reversed with atipamezole, yohimbine, or tolazoline. Alpha-2 adrenergic agonists can have profound cardiopulmonary effects, including respiratory depression, second-degree heart block, bradyarrhythmias, and increased sensitivity to catecholamine-induced cardiac arrhythmias (Altman 1980; Paul-Murphy & Fialkowski 2001; Ludders & Matthews 1996; Machin & Caulkett 1998b; Maiti et al. 2006; Varner et al. 2004). When used alone at high doses, xylazine is associated with respiratory depression, excitement, and seizure activity (Machin & Caulkett 1998b; Paul-Murphy & Fialkowski 2001; Ludders & Matthews 1996; Varner et al. 2004) and is not recommended for sedation. In Pekin ducks, xylazine produced significant respiratory depression, resulting in hypoxemia and hypercapnia and behavioral changes (i.e., moving, paddling, and picking at their enclosures) that lasted ≤45 minutes (Ludders et al. 1989b). In mallard ducks, xylazine/ketamine/midazolam IV resulted in cyanotic membranes and apnea in three; two died and the surviving animal was reversed with atipamezole (Machin & Caulkett 1998a). Xylazine (10 mg/kg) in rock partridges produced profound sedation only 2–5 minutes post administration and marked hypoventilation, but did not produce a significant decrease in heart rate (Uzun et al. 2006). In roosters undergoing typhlectomy, xylazine (3 mg/kg) induced a loss of righting response in 3–4 minutes. When diazepam (4 mg/kg) and ketamine (25 mg/kg) were given subsequently, significant decreases in heart rate, respiratory rate and cloacal temperature were observed. A lack of response to painful stimulus was maintained for approximately 1 hour (Mostachio et al. 2008). Xylazine was also evaluated in guinea fowl in combination with ketamine. The addition of midazolam to the combination appeared to improve the duration and quality of analgesic effect (Ajadi et al. 2009).

Much higher dosages of medetomidine appear to be required compared with mammals. In pigeons and yellow-crowned Amazon parrots, medetomidine (2 mg/kg IM) alone did not induce reliable sedation (Sandmeier 2000). Similarly, in pigeons, medetomidine (0.2 mg/kg) alone produced only moderate sedation, but significant bradycardia and bradypnea (Pollock et al. 2001). Also in pigeons, a medetomidine (0.2 mg/kg), butorphanol, ketamine combination produced profound sedation. However, significant bradycardia, bradypnea, and hypothermia were observed (Atalan et al. 2002). Arrhythmias in 3/8 pigeons resolved after atipamezole reversal.

In mallard ducks, medetomidine/midazolam/ketamine provided anesthesia and analgesia for 30 minutes duration when given IV, but not IM (Machin & Caulkett 1998a). Also in ducks, medetomidine/midazolam/ketamine IV produced respiratory depression, apnea, and acidemia; 1 of 12 died and 3 required assisted ventilation (Machin & Caulkett 1998a). Very high medetomidine dosages (≤10 mg/kg) in mallard ducks did not increase sedation over 0.2 mg/kg (Machin & Caulkett 1998a). One clinician reported seizures in canvasback ducks with medetomidine IV (N. Caulkett, pers. comm. May 28, 2012).

Since medetomidine appears to require combination with other injectable drugs for reliable effect, the advantages of rapid and smooth reversal with atipamezole are negated. Although the mammalian dosage of atipamezole (5× the medetomidine dose) has been shown to exhibit excellent reversal in some birds (Machin & Caulkett 1998b), a lower ratio (2.5×) also produces effective reversal (Machin & Caulkett 1998b; Sandmeier 2000). Based upon the many adverse effects and disadvantages reported for this class of drugs in birds, it is recommended they be used with great caution. It should also be noted that doses provided in this chapter for medetomidine can be used at half the value if using dexmedetomidine.

INJECTABLE ANESTHETICS

There are several situations in which injectable anesthetics are preferable to inhalants (Table 24.3). Surgeries involving the beak, mouth, glottis, or trachea are complicated by the presence of an endotracheal tube. Surgery within the coelomic cavity, respiratory system, or pneumatic bones exposes personnel to high levels of inhalant anesthetics. It is also more difficult to maintain a consistent plane of anesthesia using injectable agents. Injectable anesthetics are more commonly used in the field due to the ease of transport compared with inhalant anesthetic delivery equipment.

Many injectable drugs are highly variable in their effects between species and individuals (Machin & Caulkett 1998b; Samour et al. 1984). Some of these effects may include poor induction, inadequate muscle relaxation, cardiopulmonary depression, and prolonged or violent recoveries (Langlois et al. 2003; Ludders & Matthews 1996; Samour et al. 1984). Different delivery routes also affect efficacy and dosage. For example, in mallard ducks, IM administration of many anesthetics is not effective, suggesting poor drug uptake from the pectoral musculature. Also, no effect was identified when evaluating many drugs given intranasally to mallard ducks (Machin & Caulkett 1998b). Elimination of injectable anesthetics depends upon

drug distribution, and hepatic and/or renal biotransformation and excretion (Paul-Murphy & Fialkowski 2001). Due to the potential for side effects, patients must be weighed accurately and monitored closely.

Dissociative Anesthetics

Ketamine alone is not recommended due to poor muscle relaxation, myoclonic contractions, opisthotonus, and violent recoveries. It is usually combined with an alpha-2 adrenergic agonist or benzodiazepine to improve relaxation and anesthetic depth (Muir 1988). Ketamine may produce convulsions, excitation, and salivation in vultures, but these signs are rarely observed in other species (Muir 1988; Salerno & van Tienhoven 1976). Ketamine/alpha-2 adrenergic and ketamine/benzodiazepine combinations are used for short procedures (i.e., physical examination and minimally painful diagnostics) or induction as part of balanced anesthesia (Borzio 1973; Boever & Wright 1975; Kollias & McLeish 1978; Machin & Caulkett 1998b; McGrath et al. 1984; Raffe et al. 1993; Redig & Duke 1976; Vesal & Eskandari 2006).

Intramuscular (IM) administration of ketamine induces immobilization within 5–10 minutes and lasts for 5–20 minutes, with recovery in 40–100 minutes. These times are dependent upon size, dose given, body temperature, and health status (Paul-Murphy & Fialkowski 2001). In mallard ducks, midazolam/ketamine IV produced anesthesia with recovery in 23 minutes (Machin & Caulkett 1998b). In chickens, ketamine (120 mg/kg IM) produced no significant change in respiratory rate, but did induce bradycardia (Salerno & van Tienhoven 1976). As noted earlier, ketamine (15 mg/kg IM) in combination with xylazine (2.5 mg/kg IM) produced lateral recumbency in 3 minutes that lasted approximately 56 minutes in guinea fowl. The duration of recumbency was significantly longer (91 minutes) with the addition of midazolam (0.3 mg/kg IM) (Ajadi et al. 2009). In red-tailed hawks (*Buteo jamaicensis*), ketamine (30 mg/kg IM) produced no significant effect, compared with awake birds, in arterial blood gas, or acid-base values, but did produce mild hyperventilation (Kollias & McLeish 1978). The effects of IO versus IM administration of ketamine were compared in domestic pigeons and both the onset of anesthesia and recovery times were found to be shorter with IO administration. Heart rate decreased significantly in both groups (Kamiloglu et al. 2008).

Propofol

In pigeons (Fitzgerald & Cooper 1990) and chickens (Lukasik et al. 1997), propofol had a very narrow margin of safety and respiratory depression. However, at much lower dosages in turkeys (Schumacher et al. 1997) and mallard ducks (Machin & Caulkett 1998b), propofol is effective and safe if cardiopulmonary function is monitored and ventilatory support provided. Further research

Table 24.3. Analgesic drug dosages commonly used in birds

Drug	Dosage (mg/kg)	Route	Frequency	Species	Comments	References
OPIOID and OPIOID-like medications						
Butorphanol	0.5	IM, IV	Single	Red-tailed hawks; great horned owls	Very short $T_{1/2}$ by both IM and IV administration (approximately 1–2 hours). Shorter when given in m. metatarsal v. compared with m. ulnar v.	Riggs et al. (2008)
	2.0	IV	Single	Domestic chickens	Remained above minimum effective concentration for analgesia in mammals for approximately 2 hours.	Singh et al. (2011)
	1.0–5.0	IM	Single	Hispaniolan Amazon parrots; African gray parrots	Withdrawal thresholds to electrical stimuli reduced after 2 mg/kg IM for 2 hours	Guzman et al. (2011); Paul-Murphy et al. (1999); Sladky et al. (2006)
	20–50 μg/kg/min	IV	CRI		MAC reduction in psittacines with 3-mg/kg loading dose	
Buprenorphine	0.01	IM	Single	African gray parrots	May not achieve plasma concentrations at this dose; no change in withdrawal response to noxious stimuli	Paul-Murphy et al. (1999, 2004)
	0.25–0.50	IM	Single	Domestic pigeons	Decreased withdrawal from noxious stimulus for 2 hours (0.25 mg/kg) and 5 hours (0.5 mg/kg)	Gaggermeier et al. (2003)
Fentanyl	0.02–0.2	SC	Single	Cockatoos	Affected withdrawal threshold in some birds, hyperactivity noted	Hoppes et al. (2003)
	0.2–0.5 μg/kg/min	IV	CRI	Red-tailed hawks	Reduced isoflurane MAC 31–55% in a dose-related manner, without significant effects on HR, blood pressure, $PaCO_2$, or PaO_2	Pavez et al. (2011)
Nalbuphine	12.5	IM	Single		Excellent IM bioavailability; 12.5 mg/kg produced 3 hours analgesia; higher doses did not increase analgesic time	Keller et al. (2011); Sanchez-Migallon Guzman et al. (2011, 2013a)
Tramadol	7.5	PO	Single	Peafowl	Maintained human therapeutic concentrations for 12–24 hours (M1 metabolite)	Black et al. (2010)
	15.0	PO	q12h	Red-tailed hawks	Based on 11 mg/kg single dose	Souza et al. (2011)
	5.0	PO	q12h	American bald eagles	PO bioavailability high, based on 11-mg/kg single dose	Souza et al. (2009)
	30	PO	Single	Hispaniolan Amazon parrots	Reduced thermal withdrawal response for approximately 6 hours	Sanchez-Migallon Guzman (2012)

(Continued)

Table 24.3. (Continued)

Drug	Dosage (mg/kg)	Route	Frequency	Species	Comments	References
NSAIDs						
Carprofen	1.0	IM	Single	Chickens	Use caution in Gyps vultures	Cuthbert et al. (2007)
					Improved locomotion of lame birds 1 hour post treatment	McGeowen et al. (1999)
	30.0	IM	Single	Chickens	Painful behaviors (arthritis) reduced for 1 hour	Hocking et al. (2005)
	3.0	IM	Q12h	Hispaniolan Amazon parrots	Arthritis pain partially reduced for <12 hours	Paul-Murphy et al. (2009b)
Ketoprofen					Avoid in Gyps vultures; mortalities associated with clinical doses	Naidoo et al. (2010)
	2.0	IV, IM, PO	Single	Quail	Low IM, PO bioavailability	Graham et al. (2005)
	12	IM	Single	Chickens	Painful behavior reduced for 1 hour	Hocking et al. (2005)
	5.0	IM	Single	Mallard ducks	12-hour activity noted	Machin et al. (2001)
Meloxicam	0.1–0.5	IV	Single	Chickens, ostrich, ducks, turkeys, pigeons	Half-life in chickens and pigeons was three times as long as for ostrich, ducks and turkeys	Baert and De Backer (2003)
	2.0	IM, then PO	q 12 h	Pigeons	Provided analgesia postosteotomy for 9 days	Desmarchelier et al. (2012)
	1.0	IM	q 12 h	Hispaniolan amazon parrots	Improved weight bearing on arthritic limbs	Cole et al. (2009)
Piroxicam	2.0	IM, PO	Single	Cape Griffon vultures	Short $T_{1/2}$ less than 45 minutes	Naidoo et al. (2008)
	0.5–0.8	PO	q 12 h	Whooping cranes	Used for acute myopathy and chronic arthritis	J. Paul-Murphy, pers. comm. May 28, 2012
Sodium salicylate	100–200	IM	Single	Chickens	Arthritis painful behaviors partially reduced for 1hr	Hocking et al. (2005)
	25	IV	Single	Chickens, ostrich, ducks, turkeys, pigeons	Rapid clearance except long $T_{1/2}$ in pigeons	Baert & De Backer (2003)
Local anesthetics						
Bupivacaine	2–8	Peri-neural		Mallard ducks	Variable effectiveness for brachial plexus nerve block	Brenner et al. (2010)
Lidocaine	1–3	Local		Most species	Incision site infusion	Toxic effects have been documented in birds at doses of 2.7–3.3mg/kg
Ropivacaine	7.5	Peri-neural		Chickens	Successful brachial plexus block in 15 minutes, approximately 110 minutes of anesthesia	Cardozo et al. (2009)

Notes: These are suggested dosages based upon published information and the author's clinical experience. Species and individual variation in response to a given drug can be uncertain so the dosage should be adjusted depending upon the clinical response of the animal.

418

has confirmed it produces a rapid and smooth anesthetic induction. However, respiratory depression and significant apnea are common (Hawkins et al. 2003; Langan et al. 2000; Langlois et al. 2003; Machin & Caulkett 2000). In mute swans, propofol provided as a CRI was compared with multiple boluses for short procedures. The overall dose provided by boluses was lower, but the anesthesia was less predictable and the birds were prone to sudden awakening. On recovery, about 50% of the birds in both groups demonstrated a few minutes of excitement. Notably, these birds were maintained on room air, but did not experience a significant change in SpO₂ (Muller et al. 2011). However, ventilatory support is recommended for any bird anesthetized with propofol, regardless of whether bolus or constant rate infusion (CRI) techniques are utilized. Prolonged recovery, with or without moderate-to-severe CNS excitatory signs, has been reported, particularly after the use of a CRI (Hawkins et al. 2003; Langan et al. 2000; Langlois et al. 2003). However, one study evaluating its use in the field showed smoother recoveries than with isoflurane anesthesia (Machin & Caulkett 2000). The need for ventilatory support and the potential for excitatory and/or prolonged recoveries limit its use as a sole anesthetic. However, it has been proposed balanced anesthesia may produce propofol-sparing effects that may reduce these disadvantages (Langlois et al. 2003). The authors suggest a calculated propofol dose be given in 1/4 increments each administered over 30–60 seconds. This will allow more accurate dosing and minimize apnea and hypotension.

Inhalant Anesthetics
Inhalant anesthetics offer rapid induction and recovery, the ability to rapidly change anesthetic depth, and their use does not require an accurate body weight. Very little of the agent is metabolized, reducing the impact on hepatic and renal function, and recovery is independent of either. Disadvantages include pollution of the work environment and the expense of the anesthetic and associated equipment.

The minimum anesthetic concentration (MAC) necessary to prevent purposeful movement in response to a noxious stimulus in 50% of the patients is used as a measure of inhalant anesthetic potency. MAC for many species is very similar; most birds require approximately the same concentration of inhaled anesthetic for an equivalent amount of stimulation as mammals.

Halothane Halothane sensitizes the myocardium to catecholamine-induced arrhythmias in birds as it does in mammals (Naganobu et al. 2001). These arrhythmias occur especially during induction and recovery when catecholamine release is high. Halothane depresses the responsiveness of the avian IPC to CO₂. Thus, halothane anesthetized birds may have a depressed ability to adjust ventilation in response to changes in PCO₂

(Pizarro et al. 1990). Hypercapnia, ECG abnormalities, and hypothermia were more marked in galahs (*Eolophus roseicapillus*) anesthetized with halothane than with isoflurane (Wijnberg et al. 1991). Ducks anesthetized with halothane had a higher tendency for hypoventilation than did chickens, but heart rates were maintained in the ducks. This suggests some mechanism other than the dive response may be involved in this hypoventilation (Ludders 1992).

Isoflurane Isoflurane causes less cardiovascular depression than halothane (Jaensch et al. 1999; Ludders 1992; Ludders et al. 1990; Miller 2005). In mammals, it produces peripheral vasodilation and negative inotropic effects, possibly explaining the dose-dependent hypotension it induces in birds (Goelz et al. 1990; Greenlees et al. 1990; Ludders et al. 1989a; Ludders et al. 1990). When isoflurane was compared with sevoflurane and desflurane in red-tailed hawks, isoflurane caused a lower respiratory rate than desfluane. However, EtCO₂ did not change and the difference in respiratory rate is unlikely to be clinically significant (Granone et al. 2012). The MAC is 1.32% in chickens, 1.30% in Peking ducks, 1.34% in sandhill cranes, but only 1.07% in thick-billed parrots, demonstrating some significant species-specific variation (Ludders et al. 1989a; Ludders et al. 1990; Mercado et al. 2008). The isoflurane concentration required to produce apnea in ducks was 1.65× MAC and in cranes 2× MAC (Ludders et al. 1989a; Ludders et al. 1990). These values are less than those in dogs, cats, and horses (Miller 2005). If surgical anesthesia is achieved in 95% of patients at 1.3× MAC, isoflurane anesthesia has a low safety margin for apnea.

In addition to cardiopulmonary depression, inhalant anesthetics may cause cardiac arrhythmias. Cardiac arrhythmias have been noted in 35–75% of bald eagles (*Haliaeetus leucocephalus*) anesthetized with isoflurane (Aguilar et al. 1995; Joyner et al. 2008). In both of those studies, second-degree heart block was the most prevalent arrhythmia. In one study, they occurred during induction and recovery in 80% of the cases (Aguilar et al. 1995). Catecholamine release was suspected to be the cause. Cardiac arrhythmias are also commonly detected in other species (Aguilar et al. 1995; Goelz et al. 1990; Korbel et al. 1996), but in the authors' experience arrhythmias are most common in raptors. Cardiac stability is a perceived advantage of isoflurane anesthesia in birds compared with halothane. However, where an electrical fibrillation model was used to investigate myocardial irritant effects of isoflurane and halothane, the former had a lower threshold for electrical fibrillation than halothane (Greenlees et al. 1990). Clinically, arrhythmias appear to be uncommon, but do occasionally occur and warrant vigilant monitoring.

Sevoflurane Sevoflurane has better solubility than isoflurane or halothane. Low solubility allows for faster induction and recovery, as well as more rapid changes in anesthetic depth (Miller 2005; Thurmon et al. 1996). In pigeons, induction and recovery times were more rapid than with isoflurane (Korbel R 1998). This trend was also noted in bald eagles, with faster recovery times compared with isoflurane. A similar number of arrhythmias were noted with each agent (Joyner et al. 2008). In red-tailed hawks, only the time to visual tracking was faster with sevoflurane (and desflurane) compared with isoflurane. Induction time and time to extubation did not vary significantly. All recoveries were noted to be excellent or good (Granone et al. 2012). Sevoflurane administered at 3.5% provided adequate anesthetic plane in crested caracaras (*Caracara plancus*), with significant decreases in respiration rate (RR), arterial blood pressure (BP), cloacal temperature, and blood pH (Escobar et al. 2009). Time to induction and time to recovery were not recorded. Additionally, in several psittacine species, recovery times (time to extubation, sternal, and standing) were not significantly different between the two agents, but the birds subjectively appeared less ataxic (Quandt & Greenacre 1999). The time to intubation was longer with sevoflurane (≥4.4 minutes) than isoflurane. However, this was attributed to administration of sevoflurane below the suspected MAC in birds. In Hispaniolan parrots, the time to intubation (38 ± 2 seconds) was rapid with sevoflurane, which was attributed to the higher concentration used during induction. The time to extubation was also rapid (2.3 ± 0.4 minutes) (Klaphake et al. 2006).

In chickens, the MAC of sevoflurane was found to be 2.21% ± 0.32%, which is within the mammalian range (Naganobu et al. 2000). At this concentration, heart rate did not change significantly and cardiac arrhythmias were not observed up to 2× MAC (Naganobu et al. 2000). In another study in chickens, hypotension was observed during both spontaneous and controlled ventilation; dose-dependent hypotension was observed only during controlled ventilation (Naganobu et al. 2003). Tachycardia occurred during spontaneous ventilation while the heart rate remained unchanged during controlled ventilation. However, in Hispaniolan parrots, bradycardia was observed after 25 minutes using controlled ventilation (Klaphake et al. 2006). Increases in $PaCO_2$ (≤86 mm Hg) occurred with increased sevoflurane concentration during spontaneous ventilation. Hypercapnia-induced increases in sympathetic tone were suggested to account for the maintenance of the arterial blood pressures and heart rate in the spontaneously ventilated birds (Naganobu et al. 2003). In both chickens and Hispaniolan parrots, a significant bradypnea was observed (Klaphake et al. 2006; Naganobu et al. 2003).

Sevoflurane has a less irritating smell than other inhalants. In human pediatric patients, it is routinely used for mask induction to prevent struggling due to smell. While the agent cost is much higher than isoflurane, many practitioners use sevoflurane for induction then switch to the more cost-effective isoflurane for maintenance.

LOCAL ANESTHESIA

There are few studies evaluating local anesthetics in birds. In chickens, successful brachial plexus nerve blocks using lidocaine 2% or levobupivicaine were observed for 30–60 minutes in the majority of birds evaluated (D/Otaviano de Castro Vilan et al. 2006). Another investigator compared local blocks using lidocaine and bupivicaine in chickens and noted a longer duration of sensory blockade in the chickens treated with bupivicaine, but this difference was not statistically significant due a large amount of variation (Figueiredo et al. 2008). Brachial plexus blocks using ropivicaine (7.5 mg/kg) provided sensory and motor blockade for approximately 2 hours (Cardozo et al. 2009). However, attempts to perform brachial plexus block in mallard ducks with lidocaine and bupivicaine resulted in no consistent alteration in compound nerve action potentials (CNAP) or sensory nerve conduction velocities (SNCV), suggesting ineffective nerve blockade (Brenner et al. 2010).

Birds may be more sensitive to the toxic effects of local anesthetics than mammals. Toxic effects have been documented in birds at overall lower total doses of lidocaine (2.7–3.3 mg/kg) than in dogs (Hocking et al. 1997). Toxic effects are similar to those reported in mammals and seizures and cardiac arrest have been reported with higher dosages in birds (Ludders 1994). Other adverse effects include depression, drowsiness, muscle tremors, vomiting, hypotension, and arrhythmias, as well as CNS signs, such as ataxia and nystagmus.

Appropriate lidocaine dosing is difficult in the small avian patient, but toxicity can be prevented by using appropriate concentrations and volumes. This often requires the commercial lidocaine solution (2%; 20 mg/mL) be diluted 1 : 10, and total dosages not exceeding 2.5 mg/kg (Hocking et al. 1997; Ludders 1994). It is unknown whether this dilution allows either appropriate tissue drug levels for analgesia or the expected duration of analgesia to occur (Farley et al. 1994).

Bupivacaine is used conservatively due to concerns that its toxic effects may take longer to resolve. In mammals, the maximum recommended dosage of bupivicaine is 2 mg/kg. In mallard ducks (*Anas platyrhynchos*), bupivicaine (2 mg/kg SC) was shorter acting than in mammals (Machin 2001), and showed a faster absorption versus elimination rate. In addition, sequestration and redistribution suggested by increases in plasma concentrations at 6 and 12 hours, may make toxicity delayed. A 1 : 1 mixture of bupivicaine and dimethyl sulfoxide (DMSO) applied to amputated chicken beaks immediately after amputation improved feed intake (Glatz et al. 1992). Intraarticular bupivacaine (3 mg in 0.3-mL saline), was effective for treating arthritic pain in 1.5 kg chickens (Hocking et al. 1997).

EMLA is an acronym for "eutectic mixture of local anesthetic" and is a mixture of 2.5% lidocaine and 2.5% prilocaine for topical use. The depth of penetration of EMLA cream is dependent upon contact time with the skin. In humans, toxicity from EMLA cream is associated with improper administration (i.e., application to large surface areas, prolonged contact time, and application to damaged skin or mucous membranes). Common side effects in humans include skin blanching and local erythema. Less common side effects include methemoglobinemia or neurologic signs, generally when EMLA is applied to a large surface area for a prolonged time. Optimal use in humans requires application and occlusion for 1 hour prior. However, shorter times appear to be effective. There have been no studies evaluating shorter contact times in animals with thin skin as in birds. The maximum dosage must be calculated prior to administration to prevent toxicity. Systemic uptake may be increased after feather plucking due to skin damage and exposed feather follicles.

MONITORING

Due to the rapid rate at which birds may decompensate under anesthesia, monitoring is the most important aspect of avian anesthesia. Additionally, many monitors are not built for the small size and rapid heart rate of avian patients and may be more unreliable than in dogs and cats. This means having one person dedicated to consistent, hands-on monitoring and ensuring the anesthetist has a clear view of the patient are critically important.

Cardiovascular

Heart rate is widely variable between individuals and species. Knowledge of expected species values is important, but trends in rate during anesthesia are of more significance. Sudden bradycardia is an indication to decrease anesthetic depth and provide supportive care, such as fluid boluses

Heart rate and rhythm are monitored by an external or an esophageal stethoscope, ECG, or peripheral pulse rate. Peripheral pulse rates are determined at the brachial, medial metatarsal artery, or the carotid artery by direct palpation or with a Doppler ultrasonic probe. The Doppler probe is placed against the palatine artery on the dorsal palate of some species (Fig. 24.7).

ECG limb leads are placed close to the body. Due to the delicate nature of avian skin, the alligator clips are attached to needles or stainless steel suture passed through the skin, rather than directly attaching to the skin. Heart rate and presence of an ECG trace are insensitive indicators of anesthetic depth.

Blood pressure may be subjectively assessed by palpating the pulse at the median ulnar or medial metatarsal artery. Changes in pulse pressure and velocity are also reflected in sound volume changes when using a Doppler ultrasonic probe. Direct arterial pressure monitoring can also be performed. The most common sites include the brachial and carotid arteries (Fig. 24.8). The catheters are usually placed percutaneously, but a cut-down procedure is sometimes required to confirm arterial location. Significant arteriospasm may occur in some species. In this author's experience, cutaneous application of a small amount of EMLA 30 minutes prior to percutaneous arterial catheterization reduces arteriospasm. Alternatively, diluted 2.5% lidocaine is applied directly over the artery during a cut-down procedure. Occasionally, a profound bradycardia is associated with catheterization of a brachial artery.

Indirect blood pressure (iBP) monitoring is performed using a Doppler ultrasonic probe to detect arterial flow, a pressure cuff for occlusion, and a sphygmomanometer to measure pressure (Fig. 24.9). Recently, there have been several publications investigating the accuracy and precision of iBP monitoring in multiple avian species. In Hispaniolan Amazon parrots, iBP measurements obtained with a size 1 neonatal cuff (30–40% of limb diameter) did not provide adequate correlation with direct arterial measurements (Acierno et al. 2008). In red-tailed hawks, iBP measurements were found to more closely approximate MAP measurements over a range of blood pressures, and values obtained with a cuff 40–50% of the limb diameter did not differ significantly between wing or leg placement (Zehnder et al. 2009). A study evaluating the precision of multiple iBP measurements in awake psittacines found significant variability between repeated measurements when iBP cuffs were applied multiple times to the same limb (Johnston et al. 2011). Oscillometric devices have demonstrated high failure rates and unreliable measurements in avian patients and are not recommended for iBP monitoring (Acierno et al. 2008; Zehnder et al. 2009). From the studies that have been done, it seems that an appropriately sized cuff and sphygmomanometer can be used to evaluate trends in iBP during an anesthetic episode, but that repeated sampling that involves different cuff placements (as in different hospital visits) may be unreliable.

Respiratory

Respiratory rate and character should be closely monitored throughout anesthesia as this may be the first indication of problems and is a good sign for early intervention. Ventilation is assessed by observing the frequency and range of sternal motion and reservoir bag movement. Substituting balloons for regular reservoir bags will facilitate visualization of movement in

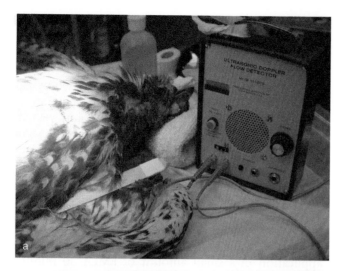
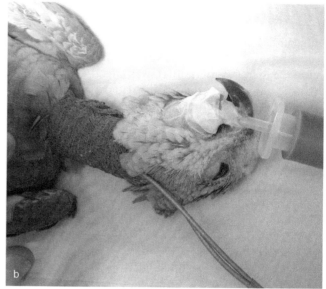
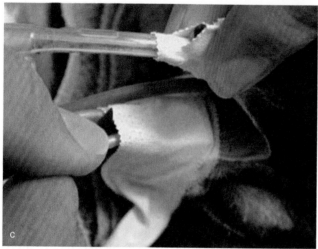

Figure 24.7. Peripheral pulse rates can be determined in many birds at the brachial artery (a), the medial metatarsal artery, or the carotid artery (b) either by direct pressure assessment or with a Doppler ultrasonic probe. Heart rate can also be detected by placement of the Doppler ultrasonic probe over the palatine artery (c) on the dorsal palate of some species of raptors and waterfowl.

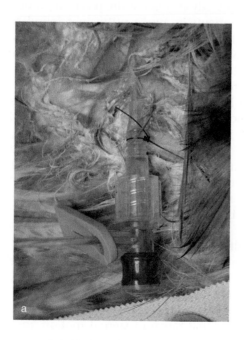
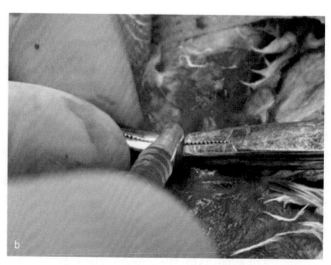

Figure 24.8. Arterial catheterization of the brachial artery in a bird. The brachial (a) and carotid arteries are the most common sites for arterial catheterization in birds. Percutaneous placement is utilized most commonly, but sometimes a surgical cut-down procedure is required to confirm the location of the artery (b).

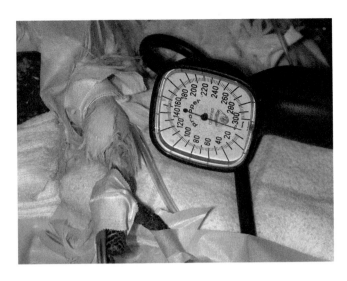

Figure 24.9. Indirect blood pressure monitoring can be performed using a Doppler ultrasonic probe to detect the arterial flow, a pressure cuff to occlude arterial blood flow and a sphygmomanometer to measure pressures.

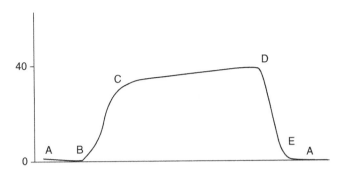

Figure 24.10. Avian capnogram.

patients with small tidal volumes. However, assessment of adequacy of ventilation by these methods in birds is inaccurate. A sudden change in respiratory pattern involving increased respiratory effort may indicate obstruction of the endotracheal tube, a particular concern in very small patients. Normal ventilation is associated with little to no respiratory tract noise. Whistling, wheezing, or harsh sounds may also indicate obstruction. Many birds (e.g., ducks) will normally have an expiratory syringeal noise during IPPV. Apnea ≥10–20 seconds is an indication to decrease anesthetic depth and provide assisted ventilation. The time between respiratory and cardiac arrests may be ≤1–2 minutes. Respiratory monitors that detect gas flow increase mechanical dead space.

End-tidal carbon dioxide ($PETCO_2$) monitoring is used to determine ventilatory efficacy. Ideally, the sampling port is located inside the endotracheal tube, but it should not increase airway resistance. Side-stream capnographs draw samples at a rate of 50–200 mL/min. This rate is usually fixed, but some allow alteration. In small birds, even this low flow may exceed minute ventilation so care should be taken to account for this removal of gas by the monitor.

There is relatively good correlation between $PETCO_2$ and $PaCO_2$, with $PETCO_2$ slightly exceeding $PaCO_2$ (Edling et al. 2001; Hawkins et al. 2003; Pettifer et al. 2002). In a study evaluating the accuracy of $PETCO_2$ in multiple raptor species, the authors found that side-stream PETCO2 overestimated $PaCO_2$ at low levels with the reverse trend at higher levels (Desmarchelier et al. 2007). This can occur in the avian parabronchus, but is impossible in alveolar gas exchange (Powell &

Whittow 2000). Carbon dioxide diffusion occurs across the length of the parabronchus, with a higher diffusion rate at the inspiratory, and a lower rate at the expiratory, end. Since arterialized blood returning to the heart is a mix of capillary blood draining the entire length of the parabronchus, $PaCO_2$ can be less than $PETCO_2$ in ideal cross current exchange. The capnogram provides important information regarding trends in $PETCO_2$ (Fig. 24.10).

Pulse oximetry has not been validated in birds. The absorption characteristics of oxygenated and deoxygenated avian and human hemoglobin are different resulting in underestimation of hemoglobin saturation (Schmitt et al. 1998). In pigeons, hemoglobin saturation trends were consistent, but values did not correlate with those derived from blood gas analyses and calculation (Schmitt et al. 1998). However, these monitors are often used to provide a pulse rate and some monitors have been adapted to count pulses up to 400 bpm.

Anesthetic Depth
The cere, beak, head, cloaca, and digits are used to assess response to pain. Surgical incisions and needle pricks evoke less response under anesthesia than for mammals. Withdrawal reflexes include toe pinch, stimulation of the interdigital tissue, pinching the scaly areas of the skin, cloacal pinch and feather plucking. Slight corneal and palpebral reflexes are maintained at a surgical plane; their absence may indicate excessively deep anesthesia. In raptors anesthetized with propofol contour feather plucking did not initiate a response in any bird at any time period during the CRI (Hawkins et al. 2003). Rather, toe clamping was a better guide to anesthetic depth.

Glucose
Blood glucose is monitored when possible, particularly during prolonged procedures. In auklets, the values determined by four handheld human glucose monitors were comparable with Chemstrip BG. However, values

for all systems were 33% less than those determined by a reference chemistry laboratory (Lieske et al. 2002). Blood storage in heparin was preferable to ethylenediaminetetraacetic acid (EDTA). Stored blood glucose values were stable for 4 hours.

Recovery

Recovery complications are usually associated with long anesthetic procedures (≥0.5–1.0 hours). This emphasizes the importance of minimizing anesthetic time. The vaporizer is turned off at the end of the procedure and circle breathing systems flushed with oxygen. This flushing is unnecessary with a nonrebreathing system. The patient remains connected to the breathing system and oxygen as long as possible. Signs of recovery include muscle fasciculations, then wing and leg movement. Once beak tone returns, the bird is extubated to prevent severing the endotracheal tube. Once extubated, an anesthetic face mask with or without the rubber diaphragm is placed over the bird's head to continue oxygen supplementation. Most are placed loosely in a towel and held upright to minimize self trauma and regurgitation. Respiration is monitored during towel restraint to ensure adequate sternal movement. Once recovered, the bird is placed in a warm, well-oxygenated environment for continued recovery. A quiet dark environment minimizes stress and movement.

ANALGESIA

Pain Recognition

Pain recognition is critical for providing timely analgesic selection. It requires consideration of age, sex, and species differences, as well as individual behavior and environmental factors. Birds either hide painful or exhibit different behaviors outside their home cage. Pain assessment must also account for different types and sources of pain (i.e., acute, chronic, visceral, and somatic). In lieu of species-specific pain scores, the use of a generic pain scale of 1–10 to evaluate a bird's pain and the response to treatment may be useful. A study evaluating pain in pigeons following orthopedic surgery used a detailed numeric rating scale plus a simple 1–10 pain scale and there was significant correlation between both methods (J. Paul-Murphy, pers. comm., March 20, 2013) Developing objective means to quantitate pain will aid clinicians in choosing analgesic therapies for their patients.

The observer must be familiar with normal and abnormal behavior to assess pain. Social species exhibit pain behaviors dependent upon the group social dynamics (Clyde & Paul-Murphy 1999). Predatory species exhibit abnormal behaviors more readily than prey species. Painful behaviors attract unwanted attention from predators, requiring masking to survive. The clinician is viewed as a potential predator.

Many clinical signs are associated with pain including change in temperament (either aggressive or passive), restlessness, reduced mobility or reluctance to stand or perch, lethargy, hunched appearance, sleep deprivation, tachypnea, and lameness. Reduced food consumption may occur, and bodyweight should be monitored. Animals with abdominal pain can exhibit tensing with a "tucked up" or "hunched" appearance. Birds may either avoid a painful body area or bite/chew it. Decreased or overgrooming (feather-picking) may occur at a painful site. Vocalization and writhing occur rarely during acute or severe pain. Owners often describe reduced vocalization in birds with traumatic injuries.

Few physiologic variables are consistent indicators of pain. In chickens during feather plucking, heart rates and respiratory rates were variable, but increased blood pressure was a reliable indicator (Gentle & Tilston 1999). Catecholamines are well-recognized humoral indicators of stress, but vary between individuals and species because of differences in adrenal content (Harvey et al. 1984). Corticosterone significantly increases in birds following pain, but it also increases with handling (Heatley et al. 2000). The use of noxious stimuli (primarily thermal) as well as induced pain models (Paul-Murphy et al. 2009a) will allow researchers to more objective evaluate the use of analgesics in birds.

A set of universal questions are used to determine if a patient is in pain:

1. Would the lesion or procedure be painful to any species?
2. Is the lesion or procedure damaging to tissues in any species?
3. Does the patient display any abnormal behavioral responses?

If the answer to any of these questions is yes, then the veterinarian must assume that the patient is in pain and an analgesic plan should be developed.

Opioids

Most opioid analgesics are used parenterally because of their overall poor oral bioavailability associated with the first pass effect. Analgesia is species and intraspecies variable at equipotent dosages. In pigeons, regional distribution of μ, κ, and δ receptors in the forebrain and midbrain were similar to mammals (Reiner et al. 1989). However, the κ and δ receptors were more prominent in the pigeon forebrain and midbrain than μ, and 76% were κ (Mansour et al. 1988). However, in 1-day-old chicks, receptor distribution was markedly different, suggesting either age or species effect (Csillag et al. 1990). Birds may not possess distinct μ and κ-receptors or the receptors have similar functions. This would explain why chickens are unable to discriminate μ and κ agonists and the isoflurane-sparing effects of μ and κ agonists appear similar to mammals. (Concannon et al. 1995)

Morphine at high dosages (200 mg/kg) produced analgesia in chicks (Schneider 1961). In another study, it produced a similar, but variable level of analgesia at dosages approximating those recommended in other species (Hughes 1990, 1990b). Variable morphine response has been detected between chicken breeds (Fan et al. 1981). Analgesic effects were observed in one breed, but two others exhibited hyperalgesia at the same dosage (Hughes 1990b). In a domestic fowl arthritis model, intraarticular injection of morphine (1–3 mg) showed no significant antinociception. However, it is unclear whether synovial fluid pH differences may have affected drug activity (Gentle et al. 1999).

Hydromorphone is primarily a μ -agonist, which is not frequently used in birds; however, it has been evaluated at doses of 0.1, 0.3, and 0.6 mg/kg in American kestrals (*Falco sparverius*) and was found to increase the foot withdrawal threshold to a thermal stimulus at all doses evaluated (Guzman et al. 2013). Fentanyl is a short-acting opioid that is uncommonly used in avian patients. One study in white cockatoos demonstrated no reduction in withdrawal thresholds following 0.02 mg/kg SC. A dose of 0.2 mg/kg did produce analgesia, but also hyperactivity (Hoppes et al. 2003). Fentanyl administered as an IV CRI in red-tailed hawks (*Buteo jamaicensis*) to target plasma concentrations of 8–32 ng/mL reduced the MAC of isoflurane 31–55% in a dose-related manner, without statistically significant effects on heart rate, blood pressure, or PaO$_2$. (Pavez et al. 2011)

In Hispaniolan parrots anesthetized with sevoflurane, preoperative butorphanol administration did not show significant anesthetic (including time to intubation and extubation) or cardiopulmonary effects. This suggests it is useful as part of a preemptive analgesic protocol with minimal adverse cardiopulmonary effects (Klaphake et al. 2006). Pharmacokinetic and pharmacodynamic data suggest 2–4 hours dosing intervals are appropriate in mammals. Butorphanol (1 mg/kg) produced an isoflurane-sparing effect in cockatoos and African gray parrots, but less in blue-fronted Amazons (Curro 1994; Curro et al. 1994; Paul-Murphy et al. 1999). In African gray parrots, butorphanol (1–2 mg/kg) showed an increased withdrawal threshold in response to electrical stimuli (Paul-Murphy et al. 1999). In red-tailed hawks and great-horned owls, butorphanol (0.5 mg/kg IV) had a half-life of 0.93 (0.94 IM) and 1.78 hours (1.84 IM), respectively (Riggs et al. 2008). In Hispaniolan parrots administered butorphanol (5 mg/kg SC), serum concentrations were undetectable at 2 and 12 hours (Sladky et al. 2006). More recently, the IV, IM, and PO pharmacokinetics of butorphanol were evaluated in Hispaniolan Amazon parrots (Guzman et al. 2011). Oral administration had very limited bio-

availability and is not recommended. The t$_{1/2}$ of IM and IV administration was very similar at 0.51 and 0.49 hours, respectively. The authors of that study recommend dosing every 2–3 hours (Guzman et al. 2011). Pharmacokinetics of butorphanol (2 mg/kg IV) in chickens demonstrated an elimination half-life of 69 minutes (Singh et al. 2011). In comparison with mammals, these studies indicate very frequent (impractical) butorphanol dosing is required to attain analgesic drug levels, and that the dosing seems to be very species-specific. In Hispaniolan parrots, a long-acting liposome-encapsulated, butorphanol tartrate formulation was safe and effective for up to 5 days following SC administration (Sladky et al. 2006). Dosing of 15 mg/kg with this formulation restored weight-bearing in an induced arthritis model of pain in Hispaniolan Amazon parrots and green-cheeked conures (Paul-Murphy et al. 2009a, 2009b). Unfortunately, this formulation is not commercially available.

There are few published reports of the use of buprenorphine. In a domestic fowl, arthritis model buprenorphine (0.05–1.0 mg) administered intraarticularly found no significant antinociception (Gentle et al. 1999). Early anecdotal reports suggesting buprenorphine (0.01–0.05 mg/kg IM) is effective in birds (Jenkins 1993; Schaeffer 1994) is contradicted by more recent studies. In African gray parrots, a high dose (0.1 mg/kg IM) achieved plasma concentrations in the human analgesic range for 2 hours (Paul-Murphy et al. 2004), and it affected withdrawal response to an electrical stimulus (Paul-Murphy et al. 1999).

Nalbuphine hydrochloride (HCl) is a semi-synthetic opioid that has recently been investigated for its use in psittacines. It is primarily a κ-receptor agonist and is a partial antagonist at the μ-receptor, similar to butorphanol. It is used in the treatment of moderate to severe pain in humans and has a relatively lower incidence of respiratory depression that does not appear to be dose dependent. Nalbuphine HCl was rapidly cleared after both IM and IV dosing of 12.5 mg/kg to Hispaniolan Amazon parrots and had excellent bioavailability following IM administration, with little sedation and no adverse effects (Keller et al. 2011). This dosage increased thermal foot withdrawal threshold values in this species for up to 3 hours while higher dosages (25 and 50 mg/kg IM) did not significantly increase thermal foot withdrawal threshold values (Sanchez-Migallon Guzman et al. 2011). A longer-lasting experimental formulation (*Nalbuphine decanoate*) was administered at 33.7 mg/kg IM to Hispaniolan Amazon parrots and thermal withdrawal threshold values were increased for up to 12 hours, four times longer than the standard formula (Sanchez-Migallon Guzman et al. 2013b). Additionally, this formulation resulted in prolonged plasma concentrations after IM administration in the Hispaniolan Amazon parrots, compared with nalbuphine HCl, maintaining plasma concentrations that may be antinociceptive for 24 hours when administered at 37.5 mg/kg (Sanchez-Migallon Guzman et al. 2013c). Unfortunately, as with the liposome-encapsulated butorphanol, nalbuphine decanoate is not currently commercially available. Based upon the receptor activity of this drug, and its reportedly few side effects, nalbuphine warrants further investigation as an analgesic for avian patients.

There have been limited investigations of tramadol, a centrally acting μ-agonist with some weak κ and δ activity, in birds. One of its 26 metabolites, O-desmethyltramadol(M1) is a more potent μ agonist than the parent compound (1/30th—M1 vs. 1/6000th—tramadol as potent as morphine). Tramadol also inhibits the reuptake of norepinephrine and serotonin so it has further analgesic actions via the descending inhibitory pathways. In red-tailed hawks treated with 11 mg/kg PO, analegesic thresholds for humans were maintained for approximately 4 hours with a $T_{1/2}$ of 1.3 ($\pm$0.6) hours (Souza et al. 2011). Based on the pharmacokinetic profile, the recommended dose is 15 mg/kg PO q 12h, although the analgesic threshold for birds is not known. The same authors investigated tramadol given IV or PO in bald eagles (Souza et al. 2009). Oral bioavailability was found to be high (97.9%) and authors recommended a dose of 5 mg/kg PO q 24 h. In Hispaniolan Amazon parrots, doses of 10 or 20 mg/kg orally did not result in significant antinociception to thermal stimuli, and human analgesic thresholds were only reached after dosing with 30 mg/kg orally or 5 mg/kg IV (Sanchez-Migallon Guzman et al. 2012). Transient bradycardia was noted after IV administration. In adult peafowl gavaged with 7.5 mg/kg, levels of tramadol remained over the human analgesic threshold for approximately 1 hour in 2/6 birds. However, the levels of M1 metabolite remained above the human therapeutic threshold for 12 hours in 5/6 birds and >24 hours in 3/6 birds. (Black et al. 2010). This underscores the importance of assaying for pharmacologically active metabolites in these studies.

Nonsteroidal Anti-Inflammatory Drugs (NSAIDs)

Ketoprofen is most commonly used parenterally because of limited oral pharmacokinetic data and difficulty in accurately dosing in small species. In Japanese quail (*Coturnix japonica*), ketoprofen (2 mg/kg PO, IM, IV) showed very low oral (24%) and IM (54%) bioavailability and the shortest half-life reported for any species (Graham et al. 2005). Additional studies are needed to determine whether drug formulation or interspecies physiologic differences account for these differences. In mallard ducks, ketoprofen (5 mg/kg IM) decreased blood thromboxane B_2 levels for approximately 12 hours (Machin et al. 2001).

Carprofen given SC improved the locomotion of lame domestic fowl significantly in a dose-dependent manner (McGeowen et al. 1999) and lame birds self-selected food containing carprofen (Danbury et al. 2000). Carprofen administered at 3 mg/kg IM q 12 h was insufficient to restore weight-bearing in induced arthritis in Hispaniolan parrots (Paul-Murphy et al. 2009b). The author (MGH) has used this NSAID (1–4 mg/kg PO, SC and IM q 12–24 h) short-term (<7 days) in many species. In pigeons, doses of 2, 5, and 10 mg/kg given IM once daily over 7 days resulted in significant increases in ALT, AST, and a mild decrease in total protein (primarily globumin) (Zollinger et al. 2011). Additionally, small intestinal vascular congestion was noted grossly and hepatic necrosis, renal congestion, and myoregeneration of the pectoral muscles were noted histologically, and the effects were significantly associated with dosing (Zollinger et al. 2011). While not significant, hepatic lipidosis was also noted and the frequency increased with dose. The authors speculate this may be secondary to decreased food consumption noted in pigeons within the highest dosing group (Zollinger et al. 2011). Additional research is needed to determine the appropriate dosing and frequency of dose-limiting side effects in birds.

Meloxicam, like carprofen, is a selective COX-2 antagonist. In ring-necked parakeets, oral meloxicam bioavailability approached 100% (Wilson et al. 2004). A significant variation in meloxicam half-life has been reported in birds. In ostriches, meloxicam IV had a very short half-life (0.5 hours) compared with ducks, turkeys, pigeons, and chickens (Baert & De Backer 2002, 2003). Dosing of meloxicam at 1.0 mg/kg IM q 12 h was found to return weight-bearing in an induced arthritis model in Hispaniolan Amazon parrots (Cole et al. 2009). In pigeons, a dose of 2 mg/kg q 12 h for 9 days was found to improve weight-bearing postosteotomy with no evidence of toxicity on hematologic or histopathologic assessment (Desmarchelier et al. 2012).

Celecoxib (10 mg/kg PO q 24 h) has been used in birds with clinical proventricular dilatation disease (PDD) (Dahlhausen et al. 2002). Treatment durations of 6–12 weeks are recommended. Clinical improvement is observed within the first 7–14 days with gradual resolution of clinical signs over the course of therapy. Premature treatment cessation may result in recrudescence of clinical signs. However, in some birds clinical improvement resumed with additional medical therapy.

Recently, massive mortalities in three vulture species on the Asian subcontinent lead to banning of the NSAID diclofenac (DF) on the Indian subcontinent. Common findings of diffuse visceral gout and proximal convoluted tubular damage indicated that the site of toxicity was the kidneys or the renal supportive vascular system (Meteyer et al. 2005; Naidoo & Swan 2009; Oaks et al. 2004; Swan et al. 2006). The association of DF with vulture mortalities led to several investigations to establish the mechanism of toxicity for DF and other NSAIDs in several avian species. The effect of DF on inhibition of renal prostaglandins and subsequent closure of the renal portal valves was proposed to cause severe renal ischemia and nephrotoxicity (Meteyer et al. 2005). Recent studies, however, determined vulture susceptibility to DF results from a combination of an increased reactive oxygen species (chemically reactive molecules containing oxygen, such as oxygen ions and peroxide), interference with uric acid transport, and the duration of exposure (Naidoo & Swan 2009). Both DF and meloxicam were found to be toxic to renal tubular epithelial cells following 12 hours of cell culture exposure, due to an increase in production of reactive oxygen species, although in cultures incubated with either drug for only 2 hours, meloxicam showed no toxicity in contrast to DF (Naidoo & Swan 2009). DF also decreased the transport of uric acid, by interfering with the *p*-aminohippuric acid channel. Additionally, the half-life of DF in vultures (14 hours) is much longer than chickens (2 hours) thus exposing vultures to toxic effects of DF for prolonged time periods.

Balanced or Multi-Modal Analgesia

Combinations of drugs acting at different points in the nociceptive system are more effective and less toxic than either drug given alone. For example, opioids act centrally to limit nociceptive input, whereas NSAIDS act peripherally to decrease inflammation, limiting nociceptive information that enters the CNS. Synergy has been demonstrated in laboratory animals (Malmberg & Yaksh 1993) and is being tested in the clinical environment.

APPENDIX

Humidi-vent Mini Agibeck Product®, Hudson RCI, Temecula, CA
0.9% saline, Baxter, Deerfield, IL
Lactated Ringer's solution, Abbott Laboratories, N. Chicago, IL
Normosol-R, CEVA Laboratories, Overland Park, KS
Plasmalyte-A, Baxter, Deerfield, IL
Hetastarch 6%, Braun Medical Inc., Irvine, CA
Hextend BioTime Inc., Emeryville, CA
Oxyglobin®, Biopure, Cambridge, MA

REFERENCES

Abou-Madi N. 2001. Avian anesthesia. *The Veterinary Clinics of North America. Exotic Animal Practice* 4:147–167.
Abou-Madi N, Kollias GV. 1992. Avian fluid therapy. In: *Kirk's Current Veterinary Therapy XI: Small Animal Practice* (RW Kirk, JD Bonagura, eds.), pp. 1154–1159. Philadelphia: W.B. Saunders.
Acierno MJ, da Cunha A, Smith J, Tully TN, Guzman DS, Serra V, Mitchell MA. 2008. Agreement between direct and indirect blood pressure measurements obtained from anesthetized Hispaniolan Amazon parrots. *Journal of the American Veterinary Medical Association* 233(10):1587–1590.
Aguilar RF, Johnston GR, Callfos CJ, Robinson H, Redig PT. 1993. Osseous-venous and central circulatory transit times of technetium-99m pertechnetate in anesthetized raptors following intraosseous administration. *Journal of Zoo and Wildlife Medicine* 24:488–497.
Aguilar RF, Smith VE, Ogburn P, Redig P. 1995. Arrhythmias associated with isoflourane anesthesia in bald eagles (*Haliaeetus leucocephalus*). *Journal of Zoo and Wildlife Medicine* 26(4):508–516.
Ajadi RA, Kasali OB, Makinde AF, Adeleye AI, Oyewusi JA, Akintunde OG. 2009. Effects of midazolam on ketamine-xylazine anesthesia in guinea fowl (*Numida meleagris galeata*). *Journal of Avian Medicine and Surgery* 23(3):199–204.
Altman RB. 1980. Avian anesthesia. *Compendium on Continuing Education for the Practising Veterinarian* 2:38–42.
Antinoff N. 2003. Use of blood transfusions and blood replacement products in clinical practice. *Journal of Avian Medicine and Surgery* 17(3):156–159.
Atalan G, Uzun M, Demirkan I, Yildiz S, Cenesiz M. 2002. Effect of medetomidine-butorphanol-ketamine anaesthesia and atipamezole on heart and respiratory rate and cloacal temperature of domestic pigeons. *Journal of Veterinary Medicine. A, Physiology, Pathology, Clinical Medicine* 49(6):281–285.
Baert K, De Backer P. 2002. Disposition of sodium salicylate, flunixin, and meloxicam after intravenous administration in ostriches (*Struthio camelus*). *Journal of Avian Medicine and Surgery* 16(2):123–128.
Baert K, De Backer P. 2003. Comparative pharmacokinetics of three non-steroidal anti-inflammatory drugs in five bird species. *Comparative Biochemistry and Physiology. Toxicology and Pharmacology* 134(1):25–33.
Bartholomew GA, Cade TJ. 1963. The water economy of land birds. *Auk* 80:504–539.
Beynon P, Forbes NA, Harcourt-Brown N. 1996. *Manual of Raptors, Pigeons, and Waterfowl*. Ames: Iowa State University.
Black PA, Cox SK, Macek M, Tieber A, Junge RE. 2010. Pharmacokinetics of tramadol hydrochloride and its metabolite O-desmethyltramadol in peafowl (*Pavo cristatus*). *Journal of Zoo and Wildlife Medicine* 41(4):671–676.
Boedeker NC, Carpenter JW, Mason DE. 2005. Comparison of body temperatures of pigeons (*Columba livia*) anesthetized by three different anesthetic delivery systems. *Journal of Avian Medicine and Surgery* 19(1):1–6.
Boever WJ, Wright W. 1975. Use of ketamine for restraint & anesthesia of birds. *Veterinary Medicine, Small Animal Clinician* 70(1):86–88.
Borms SF, Engelen SL, Himpe DG, Suy MR, Theunissen WJ. 1994. Bair hugger forced-air warming maintains normothermia more effectively than thermo-lite insulation. *Journal of Clinical Anesthesia* 6(4):303–307.
Borzio F. 1973. Ketamine hydrochloride as an anesthetic for wildfowl. *Veterinary Medicine, Small Animal Clinician* 68(12):1364–1365.
Brenner DJ, Larsen RS, Dickinson PJ, Wack RF, Williams DC, Pascoe PJ. 2010. Development of an avian brachial plexus nerve block technique for perioperative analgesia in mallard ducks (*Anas platyrhynchos*). *Journal of Avian Medicine and Surgery* 24(1):24–34.
Butler PJ. 1988. The exercise response and the "classical" diving response during natural submersion in birds and mammals. *Canadian Journal of Zoology* 66:29–39.
Campbell TW, Ritchie BW, Harrison GJ, Harrison LR. 1994. Hematology. In: *Avian Medicine: Principles and Applications* (Ritchie BW, Harrison GJ, Harrison LR, eds.), pp. 176–198. Lake Worth: Wingers Publishing.
Cardozo LB, Almeida RM, Fiuza LC, Galera PD. 2009. Brachial plexus blockade in chickens with 0.75% ropivacaine. *Veterinary Anaesthesia and Analgesia* 36(4):396–400.
Carpenter NA. 2000. Anseriform and galliform therapeutics. *The Veterinary Clinics of North America. Exotic Animal Practice* 3(1):1–17.

Clyde V, Paul-Murphy J. 1999. Avian Analgesia. In: *Zoo and Wild Animal Medicine: Current Therapy 4*. (M Fowler, R Miller, eds.), pp. 309–314. Philadelphia: WB Saunders.

Cole GA, Paul-Murphy J, Krugner-Higby L, Klauer JM, Medlin SE, Keuler NS, Sladky KK. 2009. Analgesic effects of intramuscular administration of meloxicam in Hispaniolan parrots (*Amazona ventralis*) with experimentally induced arthritis. *American Journal of Veterinary Research* 70(12):1471–1476.

Concannon KT, Dodam JR, Hellyer PW. 1995. Influence of a mu- and kappa-opioid agonist on isoflurane minimal anesthetic concentration in chickens. *American Journal of Veterinary Research* 56(6):806–811.

Congdon JM, Marquez M, Niyom S, Boscan P. 2011. Evaluation of the sedative and cardiovascular effects of intramuscular administration of dexmedetomidine with and without concurrent atropine administration in dogs. *Journal of the American Veterinary Medical Association* 239(1):81–89.

Csillag A, Bourne RC, Stewart MG. 1990. Distribution of mu, delta, and kappa opioid receptor binding sites in the brain of the one-day-old domestic chick (*Gallus domesticus*): an in vitro quantitative autoradiographic study. *The Journal of Comparative Neurology* 302(3):543–551.

Cubas Z. 2001. Medicine: family Rhamphastidae (toucans). In: *Biology, Medicine, and Surgery of South American Wild Animals* (M Fowler, Z Cubas, eds.), pp. 188–199. Ames: Iowa State University.

Curro TG. 1994. Evaluation of the isoflurane-sparing effects of butorphanol and flunixin in psittaciformes. Proceedings of the Association of Avian Veterinarians, pp. 17–19.

Curro TG. 1998. Anesthesia of pet birds. *Seminars in Avian and Exotic Pet Medicine* 7(1):10–21.

Curro TG, Brunson DB, Paul-Murphy J. 1994. Determination of the ED50 of isoflurane and evaluation of the isoflurane-sparing effect of butorphanol in cockatoos (*Cacatua* spp.). *Veterinary Surgery* 23(5):429–433.

Cuthbert R, Parry-Jones J, Green RE, Pain DJ. 2007. NSAIDs and scavenging birds: potential impacts beyond Asia's critically endangered vultures. *Biology Letters* 3(1):90–93.

Dahlhausen RD, Aldred S, Colaizzi E. 2002. Resolution of clinical proventricular dilatation disease by cyclooxygenase 2 inhibition. Proceedings of the Association of Avian Veterinarians, pp. 9–12.

Danbury TC, Weeks CA, Chambers JP, Waterman-Pearson AE, Kestin SC. 2000. Self-selection of the analgesic drug carprofen by lame broiler chickens. *The Veterinary Record* 146(11):307–311.

Day TK, Roge CK. 1996. Evaluation of sedation in quail induced by use of midazolam and reversed by use of flumazenil. *Journal of the American Veterinary Medical Association* 209(5):969–971.

Degernes LA, Crosier ML. 1999. Autologous, homologous, and heterologous red blood cell transfusions in Conures of the genus Aratinga. *Journal of Avian Medicine and Surgery* 13:10–14.

Degernes LA, Crosier ML, Harrison LD. 1999. Autologous, homologous, and heterologous red blood cell transfusions in cockatiels (*Nymphicus hollandicus*). *Journal of Avian Medicine and Surgery* 13:2–9.

de Matos REC, Morrisey JK, Steffey M. 2006. Postintubation tracheal stenosis in a blue and gold macaw (*Ara ararauna*) resolved with tracheal resection and anastomosis. *Journal of Avian Medicine and Surgery* 20(3):167–174.

Desmarchelier M, Rondenay Y, Fitzgerald G, Lair S. 2007. Monitoring of the ventilatory status of anesthetized birds of prey by using end-tidal carbon dioxide measured with a microstream capnometer. *Journal of Zoo and Wildlife Medicine* 38(1):1–6.

Desmarchelier M, Troncy E, Fitzgerald G, Lair S. 2012. Analgesic effects of meloxicam administration on postoperative orthopedic pain in domestic pigeons (*Columba livia*). *American Journal of Veterinary Research* 73(3):361–367.

Doneley B, Harrison GJ, Lightfoot TL. 2006. Maximizing information from the physical examination. In: *Clinical Avian Medicine* (GJ Harrison, TL Lightfoot, eds.), pp. 153–211. Palm Beach: Spix Publishing.

D/Otaviano de Castro Vilan RG, Montiani-Ferreirra F, Lange RR, Samonek JFV. 2006. Brachial plexus block in birds. *Exotic DVM* 8(3):86–91.

Edling TM, Degernes LA, Flammer K, Horne WA. 2001. Capnographic monitoring of anesthetized African grey parrots receiving intermittent positive pressure ventilation. *Journal of the American Veterinary Medical Association* 219(12):1714–1718.

Escobar A, Thiesen R, Vitaliano SN, Belmonte EA, Werther K, Nunes N, Valadao CA. 2009. Some cardiopulmonary effects of sevoflurane in crested caracara (*Caracara plancus*). *Veterinary Anaesthesia and Analgesia* 36(5):436–441.

Evans A, Atkins A, Citino SB. 2009. Tracheal stenosis in a blue-billed currasow (*Crax alberti*). *Journal of Zoo and Wildlife Medicine* 40(2):373–377.

Fan S, Shutt AJ, Vogt M. 1981. The importance of 5-hydroxytryptamine turnover for the analgesic effect of morphine in the chicken. *Neuroscience* 6(11):2223–2227.

Farley J, Hustead R, Becker KJ. 1994. Diluting lidocaine and mepivacaine in balanced salt solution reduces the pain of intradermal injection. *Regional Anesthesia* 19(1):48.

Figueiredo JP, Cruz ML, Mendes GM, Marucio RL, Ricco CH, Campagnol D. 2008. Assessment of brachial plexus blockade in chickens by an axillary approach. *Veterinary Anaesthesia and Analgesia* 35:511–518.

Finnegan MV, Daniel GB, Ramsay EC. 1997. Evaluation of whole blood transfusions in domestic pigeons (*Columba livia*). *Journal of Avian Medicine and Surgery* 11:7–14.

Fitzgerald G, Cooper JE. 1990. Preliminary studies on the use of propofol in the domestic pigeon (*Columba livia*). *Research in Veterinary Science* 49:334–338.

Forbes NA. 1991. Birds of prey. In: *BSAVA Manual of Exotic Pets* (P Beynon, JE Cooper, eds.), pp. 212–220. Ames: Iowa State University.

Fowler M. 1995. *Restraint and Handling of Wild and Domestic Animals*. Ames: Iowa State University.

Frappell PB, Hinds DS, Boggs DF. 2001. Scaling of respiratory variables and the breathing pattern in birds: an allometric and phylogenetic approach. *Physiological and Biochemical Zoology* 74(1):75–89.

Gaggermeier B, Henke J, Schatzmann U. 2003. Investigations on analgesia in domestic pigeons (*C. livia*, Gmel., 1789, var. dom.) using buprenorphine and butorphanol, pp. 70–73.

Gentle MJ, Tilston VL. 1999. Reduction in peripheral inflammation by changes in attention. *Physiology and Behavior* 66(2):289–292.

Gentle MJ, Hocking PM, Bernard R, Dunn LN. 1999. Evaluation of intraarticular opioid analgesia for the relief of articular pain in the domestic fowl. *Pharmacology, Biochemistry, and Behavior* 63(2):339–343.

Glatz PC, Murphy LB, Preston AP. 1992. Analgesic therapy of beak-trimmed chickens. *Australian Veterinary Journal* 69(1):18.

Goelz MF, Hahn AW, Kelley ST. 1990. Effects of halothane and isoflurane on mean arterial blood pressure, heart rate, and respiratory rate in adult Pekin ducks. *American Journal of Veterinary Research* 51(3):458–460.

Graham JE, Kollias-Baker C, Craigmill AL, Thomasy SM, Tell LA. 2005. Pharmacokinetics of ketoprofen in Japanese quail (*Coturnix japonica*). *Journal of Veterinary Pharmacology and Therapeutics* 28(4):399–402.

Granone TD, de Francisco ON, Killos MB, Quandt JE, Mandsager RE, Graham LF. 2012. Comparison of three different inhalant anesthetic agents (isoflurane, sevoflurane, desflurane) in red-tailed hawks (*Buteo jamaicensis*). *Veterinary Anaesthesia and Analgesia* 39(1):29–37.

Greenlees KJ, Clutton RE, Larsen CT, Eyre P. 1990. Effect of halothane, isoflurane, and pentobarbital anesthesia on myocardial irritability in chickens. *American Journal of Veterinary Research* 51(5):757–758.

Guzman DS, Flammer K, Paul-Murphy JR, Barker SA, Tully TN Jr. 2011. Pharmacokinetics of butorphanol after intravenous, intramuscular, and oral administration in Hispaniolan Amazon parrots (*Amazona ventralis*). *Journal of Avian Medicine and Surgery* 25(3):185–191.

Guzman DS, Drazenovich TL, Olsen GH, Willitis NH, Paul-Murphy JR. 2013. Evaluation of thermal antinociceptive effects after intramuscular administration of hydromorphone hydrochloride to American kestrels (*Falco sparverius*). *American Journal of Veterinary Research* 74(6):817–822.

Harrison GJ. 1991. Pre-anesthetic fasting recommended. *Journal of the Association of Avian Veterinarians* 5:126.

Harvey S, Phillips JG, Rees A, Hall TR. 1984. Stress and adrenal function. *The Journal of Experimental Zoology* 232:633–645.

Haskins SC, Patz JD. 1980. Effect of inspired-air warming and humidification in the prevention of hypothermia during general anesthesia in cats. *American Journal of Veterinary Research* 41(10):1669–1673.

Hawkins MG, Wright BD, Pascoe PJ, Kass PH, Maxwell LK, Tell LA. 2003. Pharmacokinetics and anesthetic and cardiopulmonary effects of propofol in red-tailed hawks (*Buteo jamaicensis*) and great horned owls (*Bubo virginianus*). *American Journal of Veterinary Research* 64(6):677–683.

Heard DJ. 1988. IME: overview of avian anesthesia. *AAV Today* 2:92–94.

Heard DJ. 1997. Anesthesia and Analgesia. In: *Avian Medicine and Surgery* (RB Altman, SL Clubb, GM Dorrestein, eds.), pp. 807–828. Philadelphia: W.B. Saunders.

Heatley JJ, Oliver Jack W, Hosgood G, Columbini S, Tully Thomas N. 2000. Serum corticosterone concentrations in response to restraint, anesthesia, and skin testing in Hispaniolan Amazon parrots (*Amazona ventralis*). *Journal of Avian Medicine and Surgery* 14(3):172–176.

Heaton JT, Brauth SE. 1992. Effects of yohimbine as a reversing agent for ketamine-xylazine anesthesia in budgerigars. *Laboratory Animal Science* 42(1):54–56.

Hocking PM, Gentle MJ, Bernard R, Dunn LN. 1997. Evaluation of a protocol for determining the effectiveness of pretreatment with local analgesics for reducing experimentally induced articular pain in domestic fowl. *Research in Veterinary Science* 63(3):263–267.

Hocking PM, Robertson GW, Gentle MJ. 2005. Effects of non-steroidal anti-inflammatory drugs on pain-related behaviour in a model of articular pain in the domestic fowl. *Research in Veterinary Science* 78(1):69–75.

Hoppes S, Flammer K, Hoersch K, Papich M, Paul-Murphy J. 2003. Disposition and analgesic effects of fentanyl in white cockatoos (*Cacatua alba*). *Journal of Avian Medicine and Surgery* 17(3):124–130.

Huckabee JR. 2000. Raptor therapeutics. *The Veterinary Clinics of North America. Exotic Animal Practice* 3(1):91–116, vi.

Hughes RA. 1990. Codeine analgesia and morphine hyperalgesia effects on thermal nocicpetion in domestic fowl. *Pharmacology, Biochemistry, and Behavior* 35:567–570.

Hughes RA. 1990b. Strain-dependent morphine-induced analgesic and hyperalgesic effects on thermal nociception in domestic fowl (*Gallus gallus*). *Behavioral Neuroscience* 104:619–624.

Jaensch SM, Raidal SR. 1998. Blood volume determination in galahs (*Eolophus roaseicapillus*) by indocyanine green clearance. *Journal of Avian Medicine and Surgery* 12(1):21–24.

Jaensch SM, Cullen L, Raidal SR. 1999. Comparative cardiopulmonary effects of halothane and isoflurane in galahs (*Eolophus roseicapillus*). *Journal of Avian Medicine and Surgery* 13:15–22.

Jaensch SM, Cullen L, Raidal SR. 2001. Comparison of endotracheal, caudal throacic air sac, and clavicular air sac administration of isoflurane in sulphur-crested cockatoos (*Cacatua galerita*). *Journal of Avian Medicine and Surgery* 15(3):170–177.

Jaensch SM, Cullen L, Raidal SR. 2002. Air sac functional anatomy of the sulfur-crested cockatoo (*Cacatua galerita*) during isoflurane anesthesia. *Journal of Avian Medicine and Surgery* 16(1):2–9.

James S, Sheppard C, Arland M. 1999. *The use of medetomidine as an oral sedative in galliformes*. Proceedings of the Annual Conference of the American Association of Zoological Veterinarians, pp. 293–294.

Jankowski G, Nevarez J. 2010. Evaluation of a pediatric blood filter for whole blood transfusions in domestic chickens (*Gallus gallus*). *Journal of Avian Medicine and Surgery* 24(4):272–278.

Jankowski G, Nevarez JG, Beaufrere H, Baumgartner W, Reed S, Tully TN, Hedlund C, Hennig G, Huck J. 2010. Multiple tracheal resections and anastomoses in a blue and gold macaw (*Ara ararauna*). *Journal of Avian Medicine and Surgery* 24(4):322–329.

Jenkins JR. 1988. Evaluation of thermal support for the avian surgical patient. Proceedings of the Association of Avian Veterinarians, pp. 153–157.

Jenkins JR. 1993. Postoperative care. *Seminars in Avian and Exotic Pet Medicine* 2(2):97–102.

Jensen JM, Johnson JH, Weiner ST (1992). *Husbandry and Medical Management of Ostriches, Emus, and Rheas*. College Station: Wildlife and Exotic Animal TeleConsultants.

Johnston MS, Davidowski LA, Rao S, Hill AE. 2011. Precision of repeated, Doppler-derived indirect blood pressure measurements in conscious psittacine birds. *Journal of Avian Medicine and Surgery* 25(2):83–90.

Jones DR, Furilla RA, Heieis MRA, Gabbott GRJ, Smith F. 1988. Forced and voluntary diving in ducks: cardiovascular adjustments and their control. *Canadian Journal of Zoology* 66:75.

Joyner PH, Jones MP, Ward D, Gompf RE, Zagaya N, Sleeman JM. 2008. Induction and recovery characteristics and cardiopulmonary effects of sevoflurane and isoflurane in bald eagles. *American Journal of Veterinary Research* 69(1):13–22.

Kamiloglu A, Atalan G, Kamiloglu NN. 2008. Comparison of intraosseous and intramuscular drug administration for induction of anaesthesia in domestic pigeons. *Research in Veterinary Science* 85(1):171–175.

Keffen R. 1993. The ostrich: capture, care, accomodation, and transportation. In: *Capture and Care Manual* (A McKenzie, ed.), pp. 634–652. Pretoria: Wildlife Decision Services.

Keller D, Sanchez-Migallon Guzman D, Kukanich B, Klauer JM, Paul-Murphy J. 2011. Pharmacokinetics of nalbuphine hydrochloride in Hispaniolan Amazon parrots (*Amazona ventralis*). *American Journal of Veterinary Research* 72:741–745.

Klaphake E, Schumacher J, Greenacre C, Jones MP, Zagaya N. 2006. Comparative anesthetic and cardiopulmonary effects of pre- versus postoperative butorphanol administration in hispaniolan amazon parrots (Amazona ventralis) anesthetized with sevoflurane. *Journal of Avian Medicine and Surgery* 20(1):2–7.

Klasing KC. 1998. *Comparative Avian Nutrition*. New York: Cabi Publishing.

Kollias GV Jr, McLeish I. 1978. Effects of ketamine hydrochloride in red-tailed hawks (*Buteo jamaicensis*) 1: arterial blood gas and acid base. *Comparative Biochemistry and Physiology* 60C:57–59.

Korbel R. 1998. Comparative investigations on inhalation anesthesia with isoflurane (Forene) and sevoflurane (sevorane) in racing pigeons (*Columba livia* Gmel., 1789, var. domestica) and presentation of a reference anesthesia protocol for birds. *Tierarztliche Praxis. Ausgabe K, Kleintiere* 26(3):211–223.

Korbel R, Milovanovic A, Erhardt W, Burike S, Henke J. 1993. The aerosaccular perfusion with isoflurane in birds: an anaesthetic measure for surgery in the head region, Proceedings of the Association of Avian Veterinarians. pp. 9–42.

Korbel R, Burike S, Erhardt W, Henke J, Petrowicz O. 1996. Effect of nitrous oxide application in racing pigeons (*Columba livia gmel.*, 1979, var. dom): a study using the airsac perfusion technique. *Israel Journal of Veterinary Medicine* 51:133–139.

Korbel RT. 1998. Air sac perfusion anesthesia (APA). An anaesthetic procedure for surgery in the head area and for ophthalmoscopy in birds: a practical guideline. *Veterinary Observer*, November.

Lamberski N, Daniel GB. 1992. Fluid dynamics of intraosseous fluid administration in birds. *Journal of Zoo and Wildlife Medicine* 23(1):47–54.

Lamosova D, Macajova M, Zeman M. 2004. Effects of short-term fasting on selected physiological functions in adult male and female japanese quail. *Acta Veterinaria* 73:9–16.

Langan JN, Ramsay EC, Blackford JT, Schumacher J. 2000. Cardiopulmonary and sedative effects of intramuscular medetomidine-ketamine and intravenous propofol in ostriches (*Struthio camelus*). *Journal of Avian Medicine and Surgery* 14(1):2–7.

Langlois I, Harvey RC, Jones MP, Schumacher J. 2003. Cardiopulmonary and anesthetic effects of isoflurane and propofol in Hispaniolan Amazon parrots (*Amazona ventralis*). *Journal of Avian Medicine and Surgery* 17(1):4–10.

Lawton MPC. 1996. Anaesthesia. In: *BSAVA Manual of Raptors, Pigeons and Waterfowl* (P Beynon, NA Forbes, N Harcourt-Brown, eds.), pp. 79–88. Ames: Iowa State University.

Leary AM, Roberts JR, Sharp PJ. 1998. The effect of infusion of hypertonic saline on glomerular filtration rate and arginine vasotocin, prolactin and aldosterone in the domestic chicken. *Journal of Comparative Physiology. B, Biochemical, Systemic, and Environmental Physiology* 168(4):313–321.

Lichtenberger M. 2004. Transfusion medicine in exotic pets. *Clinical Techniques in Small Animal Practice* 19(2):88–95.

Lichtenberger M, Orcutt C, DeBehnke D. 2002. Mortality and response to fluid resuscitation after acute blood loss in mallard ducks (*Anas platyrhynnchos*). Proceedings of the Association of Avian Veterinarians, pp. 65–67.

Lichtenberger MK, Rosenthal K, Brue R 2001. Administration of oxyglobin and 6% hetastarch after acute blood loss in psittacine birds. Proceedings of the Association of Avian Veterinarians, pp. 15–18.

Lichtenberger MK, Chavez W, Cray C. 2003. Mortality and response to fluid resuscitation after acute blood loss in mallard ducks. Proceedings of the Association of Avian Veterinarians, pp. 7–10.

Lieske CL, Ziccardi MH, Mazet JAK, Newman SH, Gardner IA. 2002. Evaluation of 4 handheld blood glucose monitors for use in seabird rehabilitation. *Journal of Avian Medicine and Surgery* 16(4):277–285.

Ludders JW. 1992. Minimal anesthetic concentration and cardiopulmonary dose-response of halothane in ducks. *Veterinary Surgery* 21(4):319–324.

Ludders JW. 1994. Avian anesthesia for the general practitioner. Proceedings of the North American Veterinary Conference, pp. 791–793. Gainesville: Eastern States Veterinary Association.

Ludders JW, Matthews N. 1996. Birds. In: *Lumb & Jones' Veterinary Anesthesia* (JC Thurmon, WJ Tranquilli, GJ Benson, eds.), pp. 645–669. Baltimore: The Williams and Wilkins Co.

Ludders JW, Rode J, Mitchell GS. 1989a. Isoflurane anesthesia in sandhill cranes (*Grus canadensis*): minimal anesthetic concentration and cardiopulmonary dose-response during spontaneous and controlled breathing. *Anesthesia and Analgesia* 68(4):511–516.

Ludders JW, Rode J, Mitchell GS, Nordheim EV. 1989b. Effects of ketamine, xylazine, and a combination of ketamine and xylazine in Pekin ducks. *American Journal of Veterinary Research* 50(2):245–249.

Ludders JW, Mitchell GS, Rode J. 1990. Minimal anesthetic concentration and cardiopulmonary dose response of isoflurane in ducks. *Veterinary Surgery* 19(4):304–307.

Lukasik VM, Gentz EJ, Erb HN, Ludders JW, Scarlett JM. 1997. Cardiopulmonary effects of propofol anesthesia in chickens (*Gallus gallus domesticus*). *Journal of Avian Medicine and Surgery* 11:93–97.

Lumeij JT. 1987. Plasma urea, creatinine and uric acid concentration in response to dehydration in the racing pigeon. *Avian Pathology: Journal of the W.V.P.A* 16:377–382.

Lumeij JT, de Bruijne JJ. 1985. Evaluation of the refractometer method for the determination of total protein in avian plasma or serum. *Avian Pathology: Journal of the W.V.P.A* 14:441–444.

Machin KL. 2001. Plasma bupivicaine levels in mallard ducks (Anas platyrhyncos) following a single subcutaneous dose, Proceedings of the Association of Avian Veterinarians. pp. 159–163.

Machin KL, Caulkett NA. 1998a. Cardiopulmonary effects of propofol and a medetomidine-midazolam-ketamine combination in mallard ducks. *American Journal of Veterinary Research* 59:598–602.

Machin KL, Caulkett NA. 1998b. Investigation of injectable anesthetic agents in mallard ducks: a descriptive study. *Journal of Avian Medicine and Surgery* 12(4):255–262.

Machin KL, Caulkett NA. 1999. Cardiopulmonary effects of propofol infusion in canvasback ducks (*Aythya valisineria*). *Journal of Avian Medicine and Surgery* 13(3):167–172.

Machin KL, Caulkett NA. 2000. Evaluation of isoflurane and propofol anesthesia for intraabdominal transmitter placement in nesting female canvasback ducks. *Journal of Wildlife Diseases* 36(2):324–334.

Machin KL, Tellier LA, Lair S, Livingston A. 2001. Pharmacodynamics of flunixin and ketoprofen in mallard ducks (*Anas platyrhynchos*). *Journal of Zoo and Wildlife Medicine* 32(2):222–229.

Machon RG, Raffe MR, Robinson EP. 1999. Warming with a forced air warming blanket minimizes anesthetic-induced hypothermia in cats. *Veterinary Surgery* 28(4):301–310.

Maiti SK, Tiwary R, Vasan P, Dutta A. 2006. Xylazine, diazepam and midazolam premedicated ketamine anaesthesia in white Leghorn cockerels for typhlectomy. *Journal of the South African Veterinary Association* 77(1):12–18.

Makinde MO, Fatunmbi OO, Oyewale JO. 1986. Determination of plasma and blood volumes in two strains of domestic fowl in Ibadan. *Bulletin of Animal Health and Production in Africa* 34:296–298.

Malmberg AB, Yaksh TL. 1993. Pharmacology of the spinal action of ketorolac, morphine, ST-91, U50488H, and L-PIA on the formalin test and an isobolographic analysis of the NSAID interaction. *Anesthesiology* 79(2):270–281.

Mandelker L. 1988. Avian anesthesia part 2: injectable agents. *Companion Animal Practice* 2:21–23.

Mans C, Sanchez-Migallon Guzman D, Lahner LL, Paul-Murphy J, Sladky KK. 2010. Intranasal midazolam for conscious sedation in Hispaniolan Amazon parrots (*Amazona ventralis*). Proceedings of the Annual Conference of the American Association of Zoological Veterinarians, p. 160. San Padre, TX.

Mansour A, Khachaturian H, Lewis ME, Akil H, Watson SJ. 1988. Anatomy of CNS opioid receptors. *Trends in Neurosciences* 11(7):308–314.

Marx K, Roston M. 1996. *The Exotic Animal Drug Compendium: An International Formulary*. Trenton: Veterinary Learning Systems.

Massey JG. 2003. Diseases and medical management of wild passeriformes. *Seminars in Avian and Exotic Pet Medicine* 12(1):29–36.

McDonald D. 2006. Nutritional considerations section I: nutrition and dietary supplementation. In: *Clinical Avian Medicine* (GJ Harrison, TL Lightfoot, eds.), pp. 86–107. Palm Beach: Spix Publishing.

McGeowen D, Danbury TC, Waterman-Pearson AE, Kestin SC. 1999. Effect of carprofen on lameness in broiler chickens. *The Veterinary Record* 144(24):668–671.

McGrath CJ, Lee JC, Campbell VL. 1984. Dose-response anesthetic effects of ketamine in the chicken. *American Journal of Veterinary Research* 45(3):531–534.

Mercado JA, Larsen RS, Wack RF, Pypendop BH. 2008. Minimum anesthetic concentration of isoflurane in captive thick-billed parrots (*Rhynchopsitta pachyrhyncha*). *American Journal of Veterinary Research* 69(2):189–194.

Meteyer CU, Rideout BA, Gilbert M, Shivaprasad HL, Oaks JL. 2005. Pathology and proposed pathophysiology of diclofenac poisoning in free-living and experimentally exposed oriental white-backed vultures (*Gyps bengalensis*). *Journal of Wildlife Diseases* 41(4):707–716.

Miller RD. 2005. *Miller's Anesthesia*, 5th ed. (Miller RD, ed.), Philadelphia: Churchill Livingstone.

Mitchell J, Bennett RA, Spalding M. 1999. Air sacculitis associated with the placement of an air breathing tube, pp. 145–146.

Morrisey JK, Hohenhaus AE, Rosenthal K, Giger U. 1997. Comparison of three media for the storage of avian whole blood, pp. 279–280.

Mostachio GQ, de-Oliveira LD, Carciofi AC, Vicente WR. 2008. The effects of anesthesia with a combination of intramuscular xylazine-diazepam-ketamine on heart rate, respiratory rate and cloacal temperature in roosters. *Veterinary Anaesthesia and Analgesia* 35(3):232–236.

Muir WW. 1988. Cardiopulmonary and anesthetic effects of ketamine and its enantiomers in dogs. *American Journal of Veterinary Research* 49(4):530–534.

Muller K, Holzapfel J, Brunnberg L. 2011. Total intravenous anaesthesia by boluses or by continuous rate infusion of propofol in mute swans (*Cygnus olor*). *Veterinary Anaesthesia and Analgesia* 38(4):286–291.

Naganobu K, Fujisawa Y, Ohde H, Matsuda Y, Sonoda T, Ogawa H. 2000. Determination of the minimum anesthetic concentration and cardiovascular dose response for sevoflurane in chickens during controlled ventilation. *Veterinary Surgery* 29(1):102–105.

Naganobu K, Hagio M, Sonoda T, Kagawa K, Mammoto T. 2001. Arrhythmogenic effect of hypercapnia in ducks anesthetized with halothane. *American Journal of Veterinary Research* 62(1):127–129.

Naganobu K, Ise K, Miyamoto T, Hagio M. 2003. Sevoflurane anaesthesia in chickens during spontaneous and controlled ventilation. *The Veterinary Record* 152(2):45–48.

Naidoo V, Wolter K, Cromarty AD, Bartels P, Bekker L, McGaw L, Taggart MA, Cuthbert R, Swan GE. 2008. The pharmacokinetics of meloxicam in vultures. *Journal of Veterinary Pharmacology and Therapeutics* 31(2):128–134.

Naidoo V, Swan GE. 2009. Diclofenac toxicity in Gyps vulture is associated with decreased uric acid excretion and not renal portal vasoconstriction. *Comparative Biochemistry and Physiology. Toxicology and Pharmacology* 149(3):269–274.

Naidoo V, Venter L, Wolter K, Taggart M, Cuthbert R. 2010. The toxicokinetics of ketoprofen in Gyps coprotheres: toxicity due to zero-order metabolism. *Archives of Toxicology* 84(10):761–766.

Newton DE. 1975. Proceedings: the effect of anaesthetic gas humidification on body temperature. *British Journal of Anaesthesia* 47(9):1026.

Nilson PC, Teramitsu I, White SA. 2005. Caudal thoracic air sac cannulation in zebra finches for isoflurane anesthesia. *Journal of Neuroscience Methods* 143(2):107–115.

Oaks JL, Gilbert M, Virani MZ, Watson RT, Meteyer CU, Rideout BA, Shivaprasad HL, Ahmed S, Chaudhry MJ, Arshad M, Mahmood S, Ali A, Khan AA. 2004. Diclofenac residues as the cause of vulture population decline in Pakistan. *Nature* 427(6975):630–633.

Paul-Murphy J, Fialkowski J. 2001. Inhaled anesthesia for birds. In: *Recent Advances in Veterinary Anesthesia and Analgesia: Companion Animals* (RD Gleed, JW Ludders, eds.). Ithaca: IVIS. http://heckyeahruroken.tumblr.com/post/76592052823/by (date accessed February 14, 2013).

Paul-Murphy J, Brunson DB, Miletic V. 1999. Analgesic effects of butorphanol and buprenorphine in conscious African grey parrots (*Psittacus erithacus erithacus* and *Psittacus erithacus timneh*). *American Journal of Veterinary Research* 60(10):1218–1221.

Paul-Murphy J, Hess J, Fialkowski JP. 2004. Pharmokinetic properties of a single intramuscular dose of buprenorphine in African grey parrots (*Psittacus erithacus erithacus*). *Journal of Avian Medicine and Surgery* 18(4):224–228.

Paul-Murphy JR, Krugner-Higby LA, Tourdot RL, Sladky KK, Klauer JM, Keuler NS, Brown CS, Heath TD. 2009a. Evaluation of liposome-encapsulated butorphanol tartrate for alleviation of experimentally induced arthritic pain in green-cheeked conures (*Pyrrhura molinae*). *American Journal of Veterinary Research* 70(10):1211–1219.

Paul-Murphy JR, Sladky KK, Krugner-Higby LA, Stading BR, Klauer JM, Keuler NS, Brown CS, Heath TD. 2009b. Analgesic effects of carprofen and liposome-encapsulated butorphanol tartrate in Hispaniolan parrots (*Amazona ventralis*) with experimentally induced arthritis. *American Journal of Veterinary Research* 70(10):1201–1210.

Pavez JC, Hawkins MG, Pascoe PJ, DiMaio Knych HK, Kass PH. 2011. Effect of fentanyl target-controlled infusions on isoflurane minimum anaesthetic concentration and cardiovascular function in red-tailed hawks (*Buteo jamaicensis*). *Veterinary Anaesthesia and Analgesia* 38(4):344–351.

Pettifer GR, Cornick-Seahorn J, Smith JA, Hosgood G, Tully TN. 2002. The comparative cardiopulmonary effects of spontaneous and controlled ventilation by using the hallowell EMC anesthesia workstation in Hispaniolan amazon parrots (*Amazonia ventralis*). *Journal of Avian Medicine and Surgery* 16(4):268–276.

Phalen DN, Mitchell ME, Cavazos-Martinez ML. 1996. Evaluation of three heat sources for their ability to maintain core body temperature in the anesthetized avian patient. *Journal of Avian Medicine and Surgery* 10(3):174–178.

Piiper J, Drees F, Scheid P. 1970. Gas exchange in the domestic fowl during spontaneous breathing and artificial ventilation. *Respiration Physiology* 9(2):234–245.

Pizarro J, Ludders JW, Douse MA, Mitchell GS. 1990. Halothane effects on ventilatory responses to changes in intrapulmonary CO_2 in geese. *Respiration Physiology* 82(3):337–347.

Pollock CG, Schumacher J, Orosz SE, Ramsay EC. 2001. Sedative effects of medetomidine in pigeons (*Columba livia*). *Journal of Avian Medicine and Surgery* 15:95–100.

Powell FL, Whittow GC. 2000. Respiration. In: *Sturkie's Avian Physiology*, 5th ed. (GC Whittow, ed.), pp. 233–264. San Diego: Academic Press.

Quandt JE, Greenacre CB. 1999. Sevoflurane anesthesia in psittacines. *Journal of Zoo and Wildlife Medicine* 30(2):308–309.

Raath JP, Quandt SK, Malan JH. 1992. Ostrich (*Struthio camelus*) immobilisation using carfentanil and xylazine and reversal with yohimbine and naltrexone. *Journal of the South African Veterinary Association* 63(4):138–140.

Raffe MR, Mammel M, Gordon M, et al. 1993. Cardiorespiratory effects of ketamine-xylazine in the great horned owl. In: *Raptor Biomedicine* (PT Redig, JE Cooper, JD Remple, et al., eds.), pp. 150–153. Minneapolis: University of Minnesota Press.

Rasch DK, Bunegin L, Ledbetter J, Kaminskas D. 1988. Comparison of circle absorber and Jackson-Rees systems for paediatric anaesthesia. *Canadian Journal of Anaesthesia* 35(1):25–30.

Redig PT, Duke GE. 1976. Intravenously administered ketamine HCl and diazepam for anesthesia of raptors. *Journal of the American Veterinary Medical Association* 169(9):886–888.

Reiner A, Brauth SE, Kitt CA, Quirion R. 1989. Distribution of mu, delta, and kappa opiate receptor types in the forebrain and midbrain of pigeons. *The Journal of Comparative Neurology* 280 (3):359–382.

Rembert MS, Smith JA, Hosgood G, Marks SL, Tully TN. 2001. Comparison of traditional thermal support devices with the forced-air warmer system in anesthetized hispaniolan amazon parrots (*Amazona ventralis*). *Journal of Avian Medicine and Surgery* 15(3):187–193.

Riggs SM, Hawkins MG, Craigmill AL, Kass PH, Stanley SD, Taylor IT. 2008. Pharmacokinetics of butorphanol tartrate in red-tailed hawks (*Buteo jamaicensis*) and great horned owls (*Bubo virginianus*). *American Journal of Veterinary Research* 69(5):596–603.

Ritchie BW, Otto CM, Latimer KS, Crowe DT. 1990. A technique of intaosseous cannulation for intravenous therapy in birds. *Compendium on Continuing Education for the Practising Veterinarian* 12(1):55–58.

Ritchie BW, Harrison GJ, Harrison LR. 1994. Formulary. In: *Formulary* (Ritchie BW, Harrison GJ, Harrison LR, eds.), pp. 457–479. Lake Worth: Wingers Publishing.

Rode JA, Bartholow S, Ludders JW. 1990. Ventilation through an air sac cannula during tracheal obstruction in ducks. *Journal of the Association of Avian Veterinarians* 4(2):98–102.

Rosskopf WJ, Woerpel RW. 1989. Abdominal air sac breathing tube placement in psittacine birds and raptors: Its use as an emergency airway in cases of tracheal obstruction. Proceedings of the Association of Avian Veterinarians. pp. 215–216.

Rupiper DJ, Ehrenberg M. 1994. Introduction to pigeon practice, Proceedings of the Association of Avian Veterinarians, pp. 479–497.

Salerno A, van Tienhoven A. 1976. The effect of ketamine on heart rate, respiration rate and EEG of white leghorn hens. *Comparative Biochemistry and Physiology* 55C:69–75.

Samour J. 2000. Pharmaceutics commonly used in avian medicine. In: *Avian Medicine* (J Samour, ed.), pp. 388–418. Philadelphia: Mosby.

Samour JH, Jones DM, Knight JA, Howlett JC. 1984. Comparative studies of the use of some injectable anaesthetic agents in birds. *The Veterinary Record* 115(1):6–11.

Sanchez-Migallon Guzman D, KuKanich B, Keuler NS, Klauer JM, Paul-Murphy JR. 2011. Antinociceptive effects of nalbuphine decanoate in Hispaniolan Amazon parrots (*Amazona ventralis*). *American Journal of Veterinary Research* 72(6):736–740.

Sanchez-Migallon Guzman D, Souza MJ, Braun JM, Cox SK, Keuler NS, Paul-Murphy JR. 2012. Antinociceptive effects after oral administration of tramadol hydrochloride in Hispaniolan Amazon parrots (*Amazona ventralis*). *American Journal of Veterinary Research* 73(8):1148–1152.

Sanchez-Migallon Guzman D, Kukanich B, Keuler N, Klauer JM, Paul-Murphy J. 2013a. Antinociceptive effects of nalbuphine hydrochloride in Hispaniolan Amazon parrots (*Amazona ventralis*). *American Journal of Veterinary Research* 74:196–200.

Sanchez-Migallon Guzman D, Braun JM, Steagall PV, Keuler NS, Heath TD, Krugner-Higby LA, Brown CS, Paul-Murphy JR. 2013b. Antinociceptive effects of long-acting nalbuphine decanoate after intramuscular administration to Hispaniolan Amazon parrots (*Amazona ventralis*). *American Journal of Veterinary Research* 74(2):196–200.

Sanchez-Migallon Guzman D, Kukanich B, Heath TD, Krugner-Higby LA, Barker SA, Brown CS, Paul-Murphy JR. 2013c. Pharmacokinetics of long-acting nalbuphine decanoate after intramuscular administration to Hispaniolan Amazon parrots (*Amazona ventralis*). *American Journal of Veterinary Research* 74(2):191–195.

Sandmeier P. 2000. Evaluation of medetomidine for short-term immobilization of domestic pigeons (*Columba livia*) and amazon parrots (Amazona species). *Journal of Avian Medicine and Surgery* 14(1):8–14.

Sandmeier P, Stauber EH, Wardrop KJ, Washizuka A. 1994. Survival of pigeon red blood cells after transfusion into selected raptors. *Journal of the American Veterinary Medical Association* 204(3):427–429.

Santangelo B, Ferrari D, Di Martino I, Belli A, Cordella C, Ricco A, Troisi S, Vesce G. 2009. Dexmedetomidine chemical restraint in two raptor species undergoing inhalation anaesthesia. *Veterinary Research Communications* 33(Suppl. 1):S209–S211.

Schaeffer DO. 1994. Miscellaneous species: analgesia and anesthesia. In: *Research Animal Anesthesia, Analgesia, and Surgery* (A Smith, M Swindle, eds.), pp. 129–136. Greenbelt: Scientists Centre for Animal Welfare.

Schmitt PM, Gobel T, Trautvetter E. 1998. Evaluation of pulse oximetry as a monitoring method in avian anesthesia. *Journal of Avian Medicine and Surgery* 12(2):91–99.

Schneider C. 1961. Effects of morphine-like drugs in chicks. *Nature* 191:607–608.

Schumacher J, Citino SB, Hernandez K, Hutt J, Dixon B. 1997. Cardiopulmonary and anesthetic effects of propofol in wild turkeys. *American Journal of Veterinary Research* 58:1014–1017.

Shanks CA. 1974. Humidification and loss of body heat during anaesthesia. II: effects in surgical patients. *British Journal of Anaesthesia* 46(11):863–866.

Singh PM, Johnson C, Gartrell B, Mitchinson S, Chambers P. 2011. Pharmacokinetics of butorphanol in broiler chickens. *The Veterinary Record* 168(22):588.

Skadhauge E. 1981. *Osmoregulation in Birds*. New York: Springer-Verlag.

Sladky KK, Krugner-Higby L, Meek-Walker E, Heath TD, Paul-Murphy J. 2006. Serum concentrations and analgesic effects of liposome-encapsulated and standard butorphanol tartrate in parrots. *American Journal of Veterinary Research* 67(5):775–781.

Smith J, Muir WW. 1992. Cardiopulmonary effects of midazolam and flumazenil in racing pigeons. *Veterinary Surgery* 21:499.

Smith J, Mason DE, Muir WW. 1993. The influence of midazolam on the minimum anesthetic concentration of isoflurane in racing pigeons. *Veterinary Surgery* 22(6):546–547.

Souza MJ, Martin-Jimenez T, Jones MP, Cox SK. 2009. Pharmacokinetics of intravenous and oral tramadol in the bald eagle (*Haliaeetus leucocephalus*). *Journal of Avian Medicine and Surgery* 23(4):247–252.

Souza MJ, Martin-Jimenez T, Jones MP, Cox SK. 2011. Pharmacokinetics of oral tramadol in red-tailed hawks (*Buteo jamaicensis*). *Journal of Veterinary Pharmacology and Therapeutics* 34(1):86–88.

Stauber E, Washizuka A, Wilson E, Wardrop J. 1996. Crossmatching reactions of blood from various avian species. *Israel Journal of Veterinary Medicine* 51(3/4):143.

Steffey EP, Howland D Jr. 1977. Isoflurane potency in the dog and cat. *American Journal of Veterinary Research* 38(11):1833–1836.

Steffey EP, Howland D Jr. 1980. Comparison of circulatory and respiratory effects of isoflurane and halothane anesthesia in horses. *American Journal of Veterinary Research* 41(5):821–825.

Steinohrt LA. 1999. Avian fluid therapy. *Journal of Avian Medicine and Surgery* 13(2):83–91.

Stone E, Redig PT. 1994. Preliminary evaluation of hetastarch for the management of hypoproteinemia and hypovolemia. Proceedings of the Association of Avian Veterinarians, pp. 197–199. St. Paul, MN.

Suarez D. 1993. Appetite stimulation in raptors. In: *Raptor Biomedicine* (PT Redig, JE Cooper, JD Remple, eds.), pp. 225–228. Minneapolis: University of Minnesota.

Suter CM, Pascoe PJ, McDonell WN. 1989. Resistance and work of breathing in the anesthetized cat: comparison of a circle breathing circuit and a coaxial breathing system. Proceedings of the Annual Conference of American College of Veterinary Anesthesiology, p. 18.

Swan GE, Cuthbert R, Quevedo M, Green RE, Pain DJ, Bartels P, Cunningham AA, Duncan N, Meharg AA, Oaks JL, Parry-Jones J, Shultz S, Taggart MA, Verdoorn G, Wolter K. 2006. Toxicity of diclofenac to Gyps vultures. *Biology Letters* 2(2):279–282.

Sykes JM 4th, Neiffer D, Terrell S, Powell DM, Newton A. 2013. Review of 23 cases of postintubation tracheal obstructions in birds. *Journal of Zoo and Wildlife Medicine* 44:700–713.

Takei Y, Hatakeyma I. 1987. Changes in blood volume after hemorrhage and injection of hypertonic saline in the conscious quail (*Coturnix coturnix japonica*). *Zoological Science* 4:803–811.

Tausk HC, Miller R, Roberts RB. 1976. Maintenance of body temperature by heated humidification. *Anesthesia and Analgesia* 55(5):719–723.

Teare JA. 1987. Antagonism of xylazine hydrochloride-ketamine hydrochloride immobilization in guineafowl (*Numida meleagris*) by yohimbine hydrochloride. *Journal of Wildlife Diseases* 23:301–305.

Thurmon JC, Tranquilli WJ, Benson GJ. 1996. Preanesthetics and anesthetic adjuvants. In: *Lumb and Jones' Veterinary Anesthesia*, 3rd ed. (Thurmon JC, Tranquilli WJ, Benson GJ, eds.), pp. 183–209. Baltimore: Williams and Wilkins.

Uzun M, Onder F, Atalan G, Cenesiz M, Kaya M, Yildiz S. 2006. Effects of xylazine, medetomidine, detomidine, and diazepam on sedation, heart and respiratory rates, and cloacal temperature in rock partridges (*Alectoris graeca*). *Journal of Zoo and Wildlife Medicine* 37(2):135–140.

Valverde A, Honeyman VL, Dyson DH, Valliant AE. 1990. Determination of a sedative dose and influence of midazolam on cardiopulmonary function in Canada geese. *American Journal of Veterinary Research* 51(7):1071–1074.

Valverde A, Bienzle D, Smith DA, Dyson DH, Valliant AE. 1993. Intraosseous cannulation and drug administration for induction of anesthesia in chickens. *Veterinary Surgery* 22(3):240–244.

van der Wal PG, Reimert HG, Goedhart HA, Engel B, Uijttenboogaart TG. 1999. The effect of feed withdrawal on broiler blood glucose and nonesterified fatty acid levels, postmortem liver pH values, and carcass yield. *Poultry Science* 78(4):569–573.

Varner J, Clifton KR, Poulos S, Broderson JR, Wyatt RD. 2004. Lack of efficacy of injectable ketamine with xylazine or diazepam for anesthesia in chickens. *Lab Animal* 33(5):36–39.

Vesal N, Eskandari MH. 2006. Sedative effects of midazolam and xylazine with or without ketamine and detomidine alone following intranasal administration in ring-necked parakeets. *Journal of the American Veterinary Medical Association* 228(3):383–388.

Vesal N, Zare P. 2006. Clinical evaluation of intranasal benzodiazepines, alpha-agonists and their antagonists in canaries. *Veterinary Anaesthesia and Analgesia* 33(3):143–148.

Wain JC Jr. 2009. Postintubation tracheal stenosis. *Seminars in Thoracic and Cardiovascular Surgery* 21(3):284–289.

Whittow GC, Ossorio N. 1970. A new technique for anesthetizing birds. *Laboratory Animal Care* 20(4 Pt 1):651–656.

Wijnberg ID, Lagerweij E, Zwart P. 1991. Inhalation anaesthesia in birds through the abdominal air sac, using a unidirectional, continuous flow. Proceedings of the 4th International Congress of Veterinary Anesthesia, p. 80.

Wilson G, Hernandez-Divers S, Budsberg S, Latimer K, Grant K, Pethel M. 2004. Pharmacokinetics and use of meloxican in psittacine birds. Proceedings of the Association of Avian Veterinarians, pp. 7–9. New Orleans, LA.

Woakes AJ. 1988. Metabolism in diving birds: studies in the laboratory and the field. *Canadian Journal of Zoology* 66:138.

Yeomans MR, Savory CJ. 1988. Intravenous hypertonic saline injections and drinking in domestic fowls. *Physiology and Behavior* 42(4):307–312.

Zehnder AM, Hawkins MG, Pascoe PJ, Kass PH. 2009. Evaluation of indirect blood pressure monitoring in awake and anesthetized red-tailed hawks (*Buteo jamaicensis*): effects of cuff size, cuff placement, and monitoring equipment. *Veterinary Anaesthesia and Analgesia* 36(5):464–479.

Zeigler HP, Green HL, Siegel J. 1972. Food and water intake and weight regulation in the pigeon. *Physiology and Behavior* 8(1):127–134.

Zollinger TJ, Hoover JP, Payton ME, Schiller CA. 2011. Clinicopathologic, gross necropsy, and histologic findings after intramuscular injection of carprofen in a pigeon (*Columba livia*) model. *Journal of Avian Medicine and Surgery* 25(3):173–184.

25 Penguins

Kate Bodley and Todd L. Schmitt

INTRODUCTION

The order Sphenisciformes (the penguins) consists of 18 species representing six genera. All occur in the Southern Hemisphere and are dependent upon nutrient-rich, cool to coldwater currents for their food sources. Most species are found in the northern cool temperate region of the Southern Ocean, up to latitude 30°S (Shirihai 2007). Several species are found in coastal and nearby waters of South Africa, South America, Australia, and New Zealand, and the most northerly species, the Galapagos penguin, occurs close to the equator. Two species live and breed on the Antarctic continent: the emperor penguin and the Adélie penguin (Table 25.1).

ANATOMY AND PHYSIOLOGY

Penguins are flightless birds that possess highly specialized anatomical and physiological features suitable for their pelagic lifestyle. Most penguin species spend >50% of their lives at sea. Many species make frequent, rapid, and prolonged dives while foraging. Emperor penguins may dive to depths greater than 500 m and remain submerged for more than 20 minutes (Meir & Ponganis 2009). Many species are exposed to extremely low environmental temperatures while on land, during their breeding and molting periods. The Magellanic penguin and the Galapagos penguin, however, must tolerate high environmental temperatures while on land, and then forage in cool ocean currents.

Penguins demonstrate remarkable development of various anatomical and physiological adaptations that allow them to forage and breed in such extreme environments. These adaptations are of potential significance during procedures involving restraint and anesthesia.

Penguins may be at greater risk of developing hyperthermia during restraint procedures than other avian species. Penguin feathers are not laid down in pterylae, rather they are densely packed over the entire skin surface. The lance-shaped contour feathers are very stiff and short, and have an attached downy afterfeather that provides insulation. Feathers are flattened during swimming, but feather shafts may be held erect while on land, providing a thick, air-filled, windproof coat (Dawson et al. 1999). During the premolting period, when most species gain significant body mass, a subcutaneous fat layer provides further insulation.

One thermoregulatory adaptation is the humeral arterial plexus, a vascular counter-current heat exchanger that limits heat loss through the flipper. Evidence for development of this structure arose in the fossil record during the late Cenozoic era, 49 million years ago, and it is believed to be a key adaptive feature that allowed penguins to successfully forage in cool and cold environments (Thomas et al. 2011). In addition, a postorbital *rete mirabile* reduces heat loss from the head, and multiple-vein arteriovenous associations in the legs facilitate countercurrent heat exchange and assist heat retention (Frost et al. 1975). Penguins may be relatively overinsulated while on land, particularly when they live in warm terrestrial environments. The feet and flippers will function to dissipate excess heat at high temperatures, via a general increase in blood flow to these structures and the bypassing of the countercurrent heat exchange systems. When African penguins are heat stressed, blood is shunted through a large marginal vein located in the axilla, which allows the axilla to be used as an efficient heat dissipator (Frost et al. 1975). Heat loss is also facilitated by panting and postural changes.

Zoo Animal and Wildlife Immobilization and Anesthesia, Second Edition. Edited by Gary West, Darryl Heard, and Nigel Caulkett.
© 2014 John Wiley & Sons, Inc. Published 2014 by John Wiley & Sons, Inc.

Table 25.1. Species of penguins

Genus	Species	Common Name	Habitat
Pygoscelidae	*Pygoscelis adeliae*	Adelie penguin	Circumpolar Antarctica
	Pygoscelis antarctica	Chinstrap penguin	Circumpolar Antarctica
	Pygoscelis papua	Gentoo penguin	Antarctica and sub-Antarctic islands
Aptenodyptidae	*Aptenodytes forsteri*	Emperor penguin	Circumpolar Antarctica
	Aptenodytes patagonicus	King penguin	Antarctica and sub-Antarctic islands
Eudyptidae	*Eudyptes moseleyi*	Northern rockhopper penguin	Sub-Antarctic and south temperate islands
	Eudyptes chrysocome	Southern rockhopper penguin	Sub-Antarctic and south temperate islands
	Eudyptes chrysolophius	Macaroni penguin	Antarctica and sub-Antarctic islands
	Eudyptes pachyrhynchus	Fiordland penguin	New Zealand
	Eudyptes schllegeli	Royal penguin	Sub-Antarctic islands
	Eudyptes robustus	Snares Island penguin	New Zealand
	Eudyptes sclateri	Erect-crested penguin	New Zealand
Megadyptidae	*Megadyptes antipodes*	Yellow-eyed penguin	New Zealand
Spheniscidae	*Spheniscus demersus*	African penguin	South Africa and Namibia
	Spheniscus humboldti	Humboldt penguin	Peru and Chile
	Spheniscus magellanicus	Magellanic penguin	Chile and Argentina, Falkland Islands
	Spheniscus mendiculus	Galapagos penguin	Galapagos Islands
Eudypotulidae	*Eudyptula minor*	Little penguin	Australia and New Zealand

Little penguins are restricted to a relatively narrow range of distribution in the temperate zone around Australia and New Zealand. They come ashore at night to nest in burrows, where they are not subjected to considerable heat loads, and mean sea temperatures are >10°C within their range (Stahel & Nichol 1982). Studies have demonstrated that this species differs from other birds in that it lacks a typical panting response. Little penguins are therefore less able to withstand heat stress than other species, and have limited ability to maintain body temperature in water <5°C (Stahel & Nichol 1988).

The upper respiratory tract contains several anatomical features of potential significance during anesthesia. The cricoid cartilage has a median ventral crest (the crista ventralis), which projects dorsally into the laryngeal lumen (McLelland 1989a). It forms an incomplete septum, and may reduce the diameter of the endotracheal tube used during anesthesia. A median septum that divides part of the trachea into right and left channels has also been observed in some penguin species. Its physiological significance is not known. The septum extends cranially from the bronchial bifurcation, and each tracheal tube is completely encircled by a cartilaginous ring. In African penguins, the septum terminates only a few centimeters short of the larynx; however, in rockhopper penguins, it is only 5-mm long (McLelland 1989a). In general, the septum is long in the Aptenodytes, short in the Eudyptes, and of intermediate length in the Pygoseles. Its length is variable within the Spheniscus. It is therefore possible to insert an endotracheal tube such that it enters only one side of the tracheobronchial tree.

The network of secondary bronchi and paleopulmonic parabronchi in penguins permits unidirectional airflow only, and neopulmonic anastomoses are poorly

developed (McLelland 1989b). They have a well-developed cervical air sac, which reaches from anterior to the clavicle to the level of the lung hilus. The abdominal air sac, in contrast, is very poorly developed and the skeleton is poorly pneumatized (McLelland 1989b).

Several penguin species have been found to have physiological adaptations that facilitate diving. Emperor penguins use a range of strategies to manage body oxygen stores while submerged, for example, hyperventilation and tachycardia during the predive period improves ventilation–perfusion matching during the dive, and arteriovenous shunts allow isolation of skeletal muscle from the circulation during a dive (Meir & Ponganis 2009; Ponganis et al. 2003). Additionally, wild diving emperor penguins demonstrate true diving bradycardia to maximize respiratory oxygen uptake and prolong the dive (Meir et al. 2008). In emperor penguins, the myoglobin concentration in the pectoral muscle is among the highest measured in any vertebrate (Ponganis et al. 2010). Emperor, Adélie, gentoo, and chinstrap penguins are known to possess hemoglobin with enhanced oxygen affinity compared with other birds. This increases their available oxygen when blood oxygen partial pressure is low during a dive (Meir & Ponganis 2009).

Most penguin species undergo periods of fasting during breeding, and all penguins will fast during their molt. Prolonged periods of fasting involve marked decreases in body mass. During the breeding fast, body mass loss averages 36–40% in macaroni penguins; during the molting fast, this species has total body mass loss of 45–50% (Williams 1995). During the molt, there is increased energy requirement for heat production and for the breakdown of stored proteins to provide amino acids for synthesis of feathers. This results in an increase in metabolic rate. Recent studies have demonstrated that there is a tradeoff between molting and the immune response in house sparrows (Moreno-Rueda 2010). The duration of the two fasting periods (the breeding fast and the molting fast) is greatest in the two largest penguin species: the emperor penguin and the King penguin (Williams 1995). Mazarro et al. (2007) determined that behavior and appetite of captive African penguins remained constant during seven handling events (weighing and blood collection under manual restraint) during molting; however, a molt-related anemia was detected. Heat loss in molting little penguins is about 1.6 times higher than in nonmolting birds (Williams 1995).

CAPTURE AND PHYSICAL RESTRAINT

Most penguin species may be captured by hand. Smaller species may be easily captured by hand from the burrow (Wallace et al. 1995) or while standing on land. Larger species may be caught by hand (Thil & Groscolas 2002a) or an appropriately sized hoop net may be used (Keymer et al. 2001). A metal rod, bent and covered with rubber at one end to form a hook, has been used to grasp the tarsometatarsus of free-ranging rockhopper penguins and draw them toward handlers, who would then restrain the birds (Karesh et al. 1999). A remote injection device has been used to administer intramuscular ketamine to free-ranging Humboldt penguins (Luna-Jorquera et al. 1996).

Penguins are relatively robust and can tolerate periods of restraint for noninvasive procedures; however, procedures must be planned so that they are performed quickly and efficiently, in order to reduce the risk of development of hyperthermia. Most penguins in captive environments will require placement in a carrier or crate for transport to the examination site. Penguins weighing less than 7 kg can be placed easily in a large, plastic dog kennel. For polar penguins, flat ice blocks are placed in the bottom of the kennel to aid with temperature regulation. Polar penguins larger than 7 kg require specially built wood or plastic transport crates that can accommodate flat ice blocks that are covered with a towel. Transport crates that have two folding doors opposite one another will provide adequate exposure to the penguin for restraint. The transport vehicle and receiving examination room must be air-conditioned, to prevent extreme temperature fluctuations and subsequent overheating.

The beak is large and sharp, so restraining the head is very important. Many institutions housing King penguins include safety glasses as standard personal protection equipment during handling.

Penguins are best approached from behind, so that the base of the head is grasped quickly and firmly. Penguin wings are powerful and may inflict injury during handling. The wings should not be grasped as

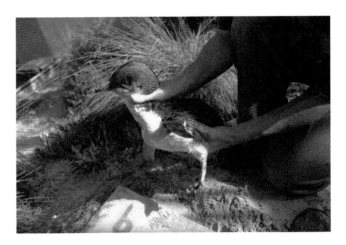

Figure 25.1. Restraint technique for a penguin less than 5 kg (little penguin). The animal is grasped behind the head and then held around the body caudal to the wings.

the initial point of restraint, as they may suffer significant injury (e.g., humeral fracture or joint injury). The wings should be held firmly against the body to avoid excessive flapping. If wing movement must then be controlled, a second hander may be required.

Penguins less than 5 kg body mass may be quickly restrained by hand. The rear of the head is grasped firmly at the base and then the limbs/body may be restrained. Very small penguins are grasped behind the head and then held around the body caudal to the wings (Fig. 25.1).

Most often, the larger penguin species can be guided into a smaller enclosure and loaded into a carrier for transport prior to a procedure. Larger penguins may be tucked under the handler's elbow, facing caudally. The handler kneels, facing the bird, and pulls it toward them, tucking its head under the elbow and against the body. The bird's head will sit under the handler's hip, the bird lies along the thigh, and the elbow secures the head. The handler then holds the feet secure. This level of restraint is suitable for minor procedures such as nail clipping (Fig. 25.2).

Restraint for induction of anesthesia generally requires more controlled restraint of the head and neck. The penguin is approached from behind. The handler wraps their arms around the body of the bird and presses the wings tightly against the body. The body of the penguin may be tucked between the knees, such that the handler has both hands free to position the head and neck (Fig. 25.3).

Procedures that require the bird to be immobile (e.g., venipuncture and anesthetic induction using a facemask) will generally require two or more handlers. Safe restraint of penguins larger than 10 kg generally requires two handlers. One handler controls the body, and the other controls the head by firmly grasping the back of the head and top or bottom of the bill base

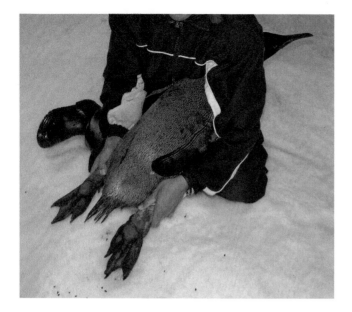

Figure 25.2. Restraint technique for a large penguin (King penguin) (courtesy of Village Roadshow Theme Parks).

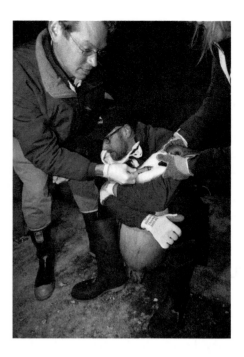

Figure 25.4. Emperor penguin: restraint for venipuncture (courtesy of SeaWorld San Diego).

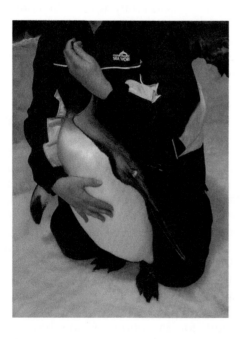

Figure 25.3. Restraint technique for a large penguin (King penguin) (courtesy of Village Roadshow Theme Parks).

(refer to Fig. 25.4). Penguins may be hooded to reduce stress during restraint procedures (Thil & Groscolas 2002a).

VASCULAR ACCESS

The medial metatarsal vein is easily accessible in penguins, but may be small, and the wound site is easily contaminated by fecal pathogens from unsanitary conditions in a rookery. It is located just above the medial

claw (Redrobe 2000) and is the least preferable venipuncture site. In smaller species, the brachial or jugular veins may be more useful for collection of diagnostic blood samples.

The cutaneous ulnar or basilic vein is not discernable in the wing of penguins; however, the brachial vein can be raised via pressure in the axilla, and lies parallel to the distal 1/3 of the humerus (Samour et al. 1983). It is readily accessible in the anesthetized penguin. In the conscious patient, the brachial vein is more difficult to access and may be difficult to occlude following venipuncture.

The jugular vein may be palpated along the right and left side of the neck. It is most easily accessible when the neck is extended and curved slightly away from the operator (Fowler & Fowler 2001; Redrobe 2000). Pressure is applied just anterior to the thoracic inlet, and the vein may be palpated ventral to the cervical muscles and dorsal to the trachea. A straight needle of size 22- to 19-gauge may be used for venipuncture for penguins <7 and >10 kg, respectively. Butterfly needles or scalp catheters, 25–21 gauge, may also be used but require more dexterity for successful blood draw. Samour et al. (1983) commented that penguins became stressed when the jugular vein was punctured, and considered the brachial vein a preferable venipuncture site in conscious birds. The jugular vein is readily occluded following venipuncture to prevent hematoma formation.

Specially designed penguin restraint devices have been used to facilitate venipuncture without anesthesia. Keymer et al. (2001) described a device made to hold free-ranging penguins on the Falkland Islands, including Magellanic penguins, rockhopper penguins, and gentoo penguins. Birds were held in a plastic tube, with a slit in the side that enabled exposure of the flipper and access to the brachial vein.

In the captive setting, training of aviculturists to restrain penguins for jugular venipuncture is paramount. For penguins <7 kg, most birds require the primary handler to restrain the body and the secondary handler to restrain the head. The primary handler can either kneel on the ground or sit on a chair or stool with the penguin (facing away from them) pinned/restrained using their knees. The secondary person gently and firmly grasps the top of the bill and back of head to extend the bird's head right or left over the primary restrainer's leg to allow venous access. Penguins larger than 10 kg require the primary handler to approach the bird from behind and wrap their arms, and sometimes legs, around the penguin. The secondary handler can restrain the bill and back of head firmly, and gently direct it over the primary handler's shoulder, allowing jugular venous access. Sometimes, a third person is required to maintain restraint of the penguin by aiding the primary handler (Fig. 25.4).

Intravenous catheters have been successfully maintained in the brachial vein and the medial metatarsal vein in several penguin species (Bradford et al. 2008; Wallace & Walsh 2005). Intraosseous fluid administration is difficult due to the dense, poorly pneumatized bones. Breitweiser (1994) described a technique for repeated administration of large volumes of intracelomic fluids to gentoo and rockhopper penguins that was well tolerated by conscious birds. The needle was placed just caudal to the keel and slightly left of the midline, and warmed fluids were administered into the celomic cavity, between the body wall and the distal end of the proventriculus. Subcutaneous fluids, whether indicated for maintenance or treatment of deficits, are administered using a 19- or 20-gauge needle with a standard fluid administration set. The skin behind the nape of the neck or dorsal scapular region is tented and the needle is inserted into the subcutaneous tissue space. Fluid volumes of 250–300 mL per site can be administered for penguins <7 kg. Fluid boluses 500 mL–1 L can be safely and efficiently administered in king and emperor penguins. Most penguins need only to be restrained briefly for placement of the needle and then can be allowed to roam in a confined space as the fluids are delivered.

ENDOTRACHEAL INTUBATION

The technique for endotracheal intubation is as for other birds. The presence of the crista ventralis may necessitate selection of an endotracheal tube with a smaller external diameter. The median septum of the trachea may result in unilateral intubation and/or tra-

cheal mucosal trauma. Some authors prefer to maintain penguins using a facemask because of the presence of the septum (Cranfield 2003). The point of separation of the two channels is generally distant enough from the glottis to allow insertion of a Cole endotracheal tube (Stoskopf & Kennedy-Stoskopf 1986).

Endotracheal tubes with the appropriate diameter should be selected. In the author's experience (KB), little penguins require endotracheal tube sizes 2.5–3.5 mm. The largest penguin species, emperor penguins, have been intubated using 9.0-mm endotracheal tubes (Kooyman et al. 1992). Inflation of the endotracheal tube cuff has not been shown to be harmful to the tracheal mucosa in the authors' experience, and may be required to prevent possible exposure to refluxed gastric fluid. Care must be taken not to over-inflate the cuff and cause subsequent tracheal membrane damage.

Laryngeal masks (LMA) have also been used to deliver anesthetic gases in penguins. Use of LMA is believed to reduce risk of postintubation trauma to the crista ventralis and tracheal mucosa (J. Sykes, pers. comm., Wildlife Conservation Society, Bronx, NY, August 2012). As laryngeal masks are designed for human pediatric patients, the airway should be repetitively evaluated during a procedure to ensure correct placement and patency.

PREANESTHETIC CONSIDERATIONS

In the zoological setting, it is preferable to obtain a complete history, physical examination, and blood analysis of the penguin to formulate a safe and efficient anesthetic protocol. Clinical history of the patient is reviewed to prepare for additional testing, monitoring, and/or avoid unnecessary anesthetic complications. Physical examination should include evaluation of: weight, body condition, hydration, nutritional status, and systematic evaluation of body organs. Apart from true emergencies, most anesthetic procedures should be conducted on stable patients. The clinical history and examination may identify physiological risks (ie. respiratory disease) or therapeutic needs of the patient prior to anesthesia. A preanesthetic blood analysis should include a cell blood count (CBC), hematocrit, total protein, albumin, globulins, glucose, uric acid, creatinine, aspartate aminotransferase (AST), calcium, phosphorous, and electrolytes (sodium, chloride, and potassium). Significant clinical pathology abnormalities should be corrected prior to anesthesia. Elective procedures should be postponed until the underlying condition is treated to alleviate risk of complications. Hydration status should be corrected prior to anesthesia, and the patient should be held in an environment where the temperature is appropriate for the species (e.g., using air-conditioning). The desired temperature range for polar to temperate species is approximately 5–18°C, respectively.

Capture and immobilization of wild penguins should be carried out in areas where there is no opportunity for escape into water. Where possible, fasting for a minimum of 8 hors is recommended, to empty the stomach prior to anesthesia.

Thil and Groscolas (2002a, 2002b) repeatedly anesthetized King penguins with tiletamine-zolazepam during their breeding (nonmolting) fast, and did not detect significant differences between induction time, duration of immobilization, and measured parameters (including heart rate [HR], cloacal temperature, and respiratory rate) during anesthesia carried out at different stages of the fast. However, anesthetic procedures conducted during periods of physiological stress, particularly molting, may carry greater risk of compromise for the patient. Vleck et al. (2000) determined that Adélie penguins that had fasted up to 40 days during courtship and early incubation showed no increase in corticosterone or heterophil : lymphocyte ratio with length of fasting, but in birds that had fasted more than 50 days, corticosterone levels increased. Such periods will be less nutritionally and environmentally stressful in penguins maintained under controlled conditions in captivity than in free-ranging birds. Breeding fasting and molting, however, will still occur in captivity and should be taken into consideration.

Penguin chicks are brooded by their parents, as they are unable to maintain constant body temperature. Adélie penguins are poikilothermic from hatching to approximately 9 days old (Williams 1995). Nonincubating adult birds (particularly during the period immediately prior to the molt) will have a thick subcutaneous fat layer. In King penguins, intramuscular administration of drugs requires injection to at least 2 cm depth (Thil & Groscolas 2002a, 2002b).

Positioning in dorsal recumbency adversely impacts respiratory function. Thil and Groscolas (2002a, 2002b) observed King penguins in dorsal recumbency developed tracheal obstruction due to accumulation of salivary secretions, and the birds lifted their heads to facilitate swallowing. They found penguins immobilized and placed in ventral recumbency had a reduced incidence of apnea and "head lifting" compared with those in dorsal recumbency. In addition, duration of immobilization was significantly prolonged in dorsally immobilized penguins. Penguins maintained with inhalant anesthesia can be manually or mechanically ventilated to compensate for the effects of dorsal recumbency.

INDUCTION AND MAINTENANCE PROTOCOLS

Inhalation anesthesia, using isoflurane or sevoflurane, is most frequently used for induction and maintenance in penguins. Anesthetic induction may be achieved by administration of 0.5–4% isoflurane and 3–8% sevoflurane via facemask. Maintenance of isoflurane is commonly 2.5–3%, whereas sevoflurane is 3–4.5%, depending on species and whether assisted ventilation is used.

Apnea and bradycardia can develop during mask induction, and have been ascribed to the cardiorespiratory "dive response." These changes, however, may be elicited as part of the defensive response to stress (Jones et al. 1988). This stress response may be ameliorated by the use of premedicants, such as benzodiazepines (Ludders & Matthews 2007). Intubation may be attempted when there is reduced jaw tone, reduced menace or palpebral reflex, and recumbency. It is not uncommon for penguins to continue "swimming" with wings beating during the initial phase of anesthesia; this excitement phase will abate as anesthetic depth increases. Wing beating may persist if the penguin is hypoventilating. Assisted ventilation, two to three breaths per minute, may be necessary to obtain a smoother induction of anesthesia (Wallace & Walsh 2005).

Use of sevoflurane for anesthetic induction, +/− maintenance has been reported in a number of penguin species (Bradford et al. 2008; Ponganis et al. 2001; Wallace & Walsh 2005). Sevoflurane has the potential for more rapid induction and recovery, due to its lower solubility than isoflurane. Its less pungent odor may reduce stress experienced during a facemask induction.

Midazolam 1.5 mg/kg, given intramuscularly, has been used to sedate little penguins, yellow-eyed penguins, and Fjordland penguins for noninvasive procedures, such as radiology (J. Ward, pers. comm., New Zealand Wildlife Health Center, Massey University, April 2011). Peak sedative effect generally occurred in 5–10 minutes, and duration of action was approximately 1–3 hours. Premedication with midazolam (using the same dose rate) also facilitated smoother and more rapid anesthetic inductions using isoflurane in oxygen via facemask. Gradually increasing isoflurane concentration from 0.5% has been used as a means of avoiding breath-holding during mask induction of little penguins (J. Ward, pers. comm.).

Tiletamine and zolazepam (5 mg/kg IM) produced safe immobilization of free-ranging adult King penguins (Thil & Groscolas 2002a, 2002b). Induction time (time to sternal recumbency) averaged 4 minutes, and duration of immobilization was approximately 1 hour (mean = 69.3 ± 2.2 minutes). Transitory apnea (maximum duration 1.5 minutes) was noted in 30% of bird anaesthetized. The level of anesthesia was sufficient for noninvasive procedures. Preliminary trials suggested a higher dose rate (10 mg/kg IM) is suitable for immobilization for surgical adipose tissue biopsies (Thil & Groscolas 2002b). Five- to seven-month-old fasting chicks were immobilized for 80 minutes after receiving a 4 mg/kg dosage.

Administration of ketamine (2.0–7.5 mg/kg IM) resulted in sedation of free-ranging Humboldt penguins (Luna-Jorquera et al. 1996). Ketamine (5 mg/kg

IM) facilitated handling for attachment of data loggers, but did not result in anesthesia. Birds recovered after 40–45 minutes. Higher dosages (7.5 mg/kg) resulted in salivation, muscular rigidity, reduced consciousness, and more prolonged recovery. Higher ketamine dosages (5–10 mg/kg IM), administered to nesting African penguins, resulted in prolonged anesthetic recovery (Wilson & Wilson 1989).

MONITORING

The mean deep body temperature in little penguins in their thermoneutral zone in air was 38.4 ± 0.8°C (Stahel & Nichol 1982). Core temperature in male emperor penguins incubating eggs must be maintained at 37.6–38.5°C during the Antarctic winter, via metabolic heat production and huddling behavior (Williams 1995). Deep body temperature measured in free-ranging emperor penguins during nocturnal rest (i.e., when birds were not diving) ranged from 36.0 to 38.7°C (Ponganis et al. 2001).

Esophageal probes may provide a more accurate measure of core temperature during anesthesia: the temperature taken 5 cm inside the cloaca represented core temperature in little penguins, whereas cloacal temperatures taken 3 cm from the vent were considerably lower (Stahel & Nichol 1982).

Mild hypothermia has been observed in King penguins undergoing prolonged anesthesia (duration approximately 75 minutes) using tiletamine-zolazepam in the field. This was addressed by placing the birds on insulative covers during the procedures (Thil & Groscolas 2002a, 2002b). Prolonged inhalant anesthetic procedures can cause hypothermia due to inhalation of dry cold oxygen; therefore, constant temperature monitoring is required. The presence of the highly insulative feathers will limit the effectiveness of contact heating methods.

In general, hyperthermia is considered a more likely adverse effect than hypothermia during restraint and anesthesia of penguins, due to the presence of an insulative subcutaneous fat layer and densely packed feathers. The anatomical adaptations that allow rapid cooling when penguins are exposed to high environmental temperatures may be utilized during anesthesia. In the field, application of snow to the underside of flippers and the feet has been used to cool penguins at risk of hyperthermia. In the captive setting, frozen ice blocks are initially placed on the feet and under the flippers to lower risk of hyperthermia (Fig. 25.5).

Respiratory rate and character should be constantly monitored during anesthesia, by observation of thoracic movements, and by those of the rebreathing bag during gaseous anesthesia. Pulmonary auscultation is best achieved over the dorsum.

The HR of a medium-sized penguin should be between 85 and 120 bpm (Stoskopf & Kennedy-Stoskopf

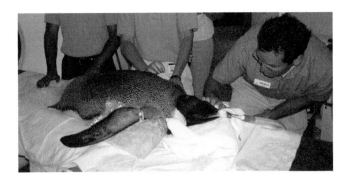

Figure 25.5. Maintenance of gaseous anesthesia in the emperor penguin. To prevent hyperthermia, ice is placed around the wings and feet (courtesy of SeaWorld San Diego).

1986). Sinus arrhythmia is not a common feature during cardiac auscultation (Stoskopf & Beall 1980). The HR of adult King penguins anesthetized using tiletamine-zolazepam was 99–115 bpm (Thil & Groscolas 2002b). HR and rhythm should be monitored throughout anesthesia, either by external auscultation near the ventral pectoral girdle or by using an esophageal stethoscope. HR during anesthesia may also be monitored using a Doppler probe placed over the brachial artery. A standardized technique for lead placement and electrocardiographic monitoring of HR and rhythm has been reported (Stoskopf & Kennedy-Stoskopf 1986). Heart rhythm must be monitored so that abnormal rhythms, such as AV block, tachycardia, or bradycardia will be noted and corrected (by administering appropriate treatment or by ending the procedure). Pulse oximetry will allow continuous assessment of trends in pulse rate and oxygenation in stationary birds; however, the oxygen saturation values in birds do not correlate well with arterial saturation derived from blood gas analyses (Schmitt et al. 1998). At the same oxygen saturation, the high absorption ratio in birds compared with humans results in a low saturation value on the human calibration curve used by pulse oximeters. It is notable that the oxygen-hemoglobin dissociation curve determined in gentoo, chinstrap, Adélie, and emperor penguins is significantly left-shifted when compared with most other birds. In these penguin species, the partial pressure of oxygen at which hemoglobin is 50% saturated (P_{50}) lies within the mammalian range rather than the avian (Meir & Ponganis 2009).

RECOVERY

Gaseous anesthetic agents generally result in a more rapid recovery from anesthesia than injectable agents. A rapid anesthetic recovery is preferable, particularly in free-ranging penguins, as prolonged interruption of normal behaviors may result in negative effects, such as disturbance of breeding and nest abandonment.

Signs of recovery include "swimming" or flapping of the flippers, leg, and head movement. Recovering penguins should be supported upright to prevent regurgitation or trauma to the flippers. Mild gastric reflux is not uncommon and should be managed by close observation and gently swabbing of the oropharynx with gauze to prevent aspiration of fluid. The endotracheal tube can be removed when the penguin displays a cough reflex and appears to swallow. Once extubated, penguins should not be allowed access to water until they have completely recovered from the effects of anesthetic agents. Free-ranging penguins can be housed inside portable temporary enclosures, situated close to the colony, until they have completely recovered. They must be protected from extremes of temperature and closely monitored while they are still demonstrating effects from anesthetic agents.

FIELD ANESTHESIA

Field anesthesia techniques should be chosen carefully. The environmental conditions and the physiological status and behavioral features of the species concerned must be evaluated. Planning immobilization procedures must include consideration of the potential detrimental impacts that the intervention produces. Living in an extreme environment is energetically costly, and stressful interventions may compromise survivorship and/or reproductive success.

Use of injectable agents will facilitate remote delivery of immobilizing drugs, potentially reducing stress induced by capture and manipulation. When remote delivery techniques are used, anesthetic drug delivery is less precise and adjustments in dose rate are not possible. The use of inhalational anesthetic agents to induce and maintain anesthesia allows the operator greater control over anesthetic depth and duration than the use of injectable agents for this purpose. Precision vaporizers must be housed in insulated containers when environmental temperatures are low, as they function efficiently only within a limited temperature range (Gales et al. 2005). Therefore, the apparatus used to deliver gaseous anesthetic agents may prove cumbersome and difficult to deploy under the environmental conditions encountered in sub-Antarctic and Antarctic habitats. Use of injectable anesthetic agents may be logistically preferable in such circumstances.

POSTANESTHETIC CHALLENGES

There have been no studies investigating the pharmacokinetic basis of analgesic drug doses in penguin species. Empirical use of butorphanol (1 mg/kg IM) has been reported for postsurgical analgesia (Bradford et al. 2008). In the author's experience (TS), tramadol (2–4 mg/kg, SID to BID, PO) has provided postoperative analgesia for medium and large penguins.

Use of the non-steroidal anti-inflammatory drug (NSAID), ibuprofen (3–5 mg/kg SID-BID), has been reported (Wallace & Walsh 2005). The author (KB) has used orally administered meloxicam (0.1–0.2 mg/kg SID-BID) in little penguins, and behavioral observations suggested an anti-inflammatory/analgesic effect. However, dosage and administration of NSAIDs should be carefully considered prior to their use. A clinical study by Baert and De Backer (2003) compared the plasma clearance rates of three NSAIDs in five bird species. Between species, the difference in protein binding alone was so great that the authors recommended the pharmacokinetics of each NSAID should be independently assessed for each target avian species. Adverse effects (such as renal tubular necrosis, visceral gout, and mortality) may occur following NSAID use.

REFERENCES

Baert K and De Backer P. 2003. Comparative pharmacokinetics of three non-steroidal anti-inflammatory drugs in five bird species. *Comparative Biochemistry and Physiology C: Toxicology and Pharmacology* 134(1):25–33.

Bradford C, Bronson E, Kintner L, Schultz D, McDonnell J. 2008. Diagnosis and attempted surgical repair of hemivertebrae in an African penguin (*Spheniscus demersus*). *Journal of Avian Medicine and Surgery* 22(4):331–335.

Breitweiser BA. 1994. Fluid therapy in penguins. *Penguin Conservation* 7(1):6–8.

Cranfield MR. 2003. Chapter 11: Sphenisciformes (Penguins). In: *Zoo and Wild Animal Medicine*, 5th ed. (ME Fowler, RE Miller, eds.), pp. 103–110. Philadelphia: W.B. Saunders.

Dawson C, Vincent JFV, Jeronimidis G, Rice G, Forshaw P. 1999. Heat transfer through penguin feathers. *Journal of Theoretical Biology* 199:291–295.

Fowler GS, Fowler ME. 2001. Chapter 6: Order sphenisciformes (penguins). In: *Biology, Medicine and Surgery of South American Wild Animals* (ME Fowler, ZS Cubas, eds.), pp. 53–64. Ames: Iowa State University Press.

Frost PGH, Siegfried WR, Greenwood PJ. 1975. Arterio-venous heat exchange systems in the Jackass penguin *Spheniscus demersus*. *Journal of Zoology* 175:231–241.

Gales N, Barnes J, Chittick B, Gray M, Robinson S, Burns J and Costa D. 2005. Effective, field-based inhalation anesthesia for ice seals. *Marine Mammal Science* 21(4):717–727.

Jones DR, Furilla MR, Heieis MRA, Gabbott GRJ, Smith FM. 1988. Forced and voluntary diving in ducks: cardiovascular adjustments and their control. *Canadian Journal of Zoology* 66:75–83.

Karesh WB, Uhart MM, Frere E, Gandini P, Braselton WE, Puche H, Cook RA. 1999. Health evaluation of free-ranging rockhopper penguins (*Eudyptes chrysocomes*) in Argentina. *Journal of Zoo and Wildlife Medicine* 30(1):25–31.

Keymer IF, Malcolm HM, Hunt A, Horsley DT. 2001. Health evaluation of penguins (Sphenisciformes) following mortality in the Falklands (South Atlantic). *Diseases of Aquatic Organisms* 45:159–169.

Kooyman GL, Ponganis PJ, Castellini MA, Ponganis EP, Ponganis KV, Thorson PH, Eckert SA, LeMayo Y. 1992. Heart rate and swim speeds of emperor penguins diving under sea ice. *The Journal of Experimental Biology* 165:161–180.

Ludders JW, Matthews NS. 2007. Chapter 34: Birds. In: *Veterinary Anesthesia and Analgesia*, 4th ed. (W Tranquilli, JC Thurmon, KA Grimm, eds.), pp. 841–868. Blackwell Publishing Professional, Ames Iowa USA, NJ: Wiley-Blackwell.

Luna-Jorquera G, Culik B, Aguilar R. 1996. Capturing Humboldt penguins *Spheniscus humboldti* with the use of an anaesthetic. *Marine Ornithology* 24:47–50.

Mazarro LM, Meegan J, Sarran D, Dunn L. 2007. Changes in hematologic parameters in molting African penguins (*Spheniscus demersus*). Proceedings of the 38th IAAAM Conference, Orlando FL, pp. 234–235.

McLelland J. 1989a. Chapter 2: Larynx and trachea. In: *Form and Function in Birds* (AS King, J McLelland, eds.), pp. 69–103. London: Academic Press.

McLelland J. 1989b. Chapter 5. Anatomy of the lungs and air sacs. In: *Form and Function in Birds* (AS King, J McLelland, eds.), pp. 221–279. London: Academic Press.

Meir JU, Ponganis PJ. 2009. High-affinity hemoglobin and blood oxygen saturation in diving emperor penguins. *The Journal of Experimental Biology* 212:3330–3338.

Meir JU, Stockard TK, Williams CL, Ponganis KV, Ponganis PJ. 2008. Heart rate regulation and extreme bradycardia in diving emperor penguins. *The Journal of Experimental Biology* 211: 1169–1179.

Moreno-Rueda G. 2010. Experimental test of a trade-off between moult and immune response in house sparrows *Passer domesticus*. *Journal of Evolutionary Biology* 23:2229–2237.

Ponganis PJ, Van Dam RP, Knower T, Levenson DH. 2001. Temperature regulation in emperor penguins foraging under sea ice. *Comparative Biochemistry and Physiology. Part A, Molecular and Integrative Physiology* 129:811–820.

Ponganis PJ, Van Dam RP, Levenson DH, Knower T, Ponganis KV, Marshall G. 2003. Regional heterothermy and conservation of core temperature in emperor penguins diving under sea ice. *Comparative Biochemistry and Physiology. Part A, Molecular and Integrative Physiology* 135:477–487.

Ponganis PJ, Welch TJ, Welch LS, Stockard TK. 2010. Myoglobin production in emperor penguins. *The Journal of Experimental Biology* 213:1901–1906.

Redrobe SP. 2000. Blood sampling techniques in penguins. Proceedings of the 31st Annual IAAAM Conference, pp. 616–617. New Orleans, LA.

Samour HJ, Jones DM, Pugsley S, Fitzgerald AK. 1983. Blood sampling techniques in penguins (Sphenisciformes). *The Veterinary Record* 113:340.

Schmitt PM, Gobel T, Tratvetter E. 1998. Evaluation of pulse oximetry as a monitoring method in avian anesthesia. *Journal of Avian Medicine and Surgery* 12(2):91–99.

Shirihai H. 2007. *A Complete Guide to Antarctic Wildlife, the Birds and Marine Mammals of the Antarctic Continent and the Southern Ocean.* London: A and C Black.

Stahel CD, Nichol SC. 1982. Temperature regulation in the little penguin, *Eudyptula minor*, in air and water. *Journal of Comparative Physiology. B, Biochemical, Systemic, and Environmental Physiology* 148:93–100.

Stahel CD, Nichol SC. 1988. Ventilation and oxygen extraction in the little penguin (*Eudyptula minor*), at different temperatures in air and water. *Respiration Physiology* 71:387–398.

Stoskopf MK and Beall FB. 1980. The husbandry and medicine of captive penguins. Proceedings of the Annual Conference of the American Association of Zoo Veterinarians, pp. 81–96. Washington, DC.

Stoskopf MK, Kennedy-Stoskopf S. 1986. Chapter 23: aquatic birds (Sphenisciformes, Gaviiformes, Podicipediformes, Procellariiformes, Pelecaniformes and Charadriiformes). In: *Zoo and Wild Animal Medicine* (ME Fowler, ed.), pp. 293–313. Philadelphia: W.B. Saunders.

Thil M, Groscolas R. 2002a. The use of Zoletil® to immobilize king penguins in the field. Proceedings of the European Association of Zoo and Wildlife Veterinarians (EAZWV), pp. 1–5. Paris.

Thil M, Groscolas R. 2002b. Field immobilization of king penguins with tiletamine-zolazepam. *Journal of Field Ornithology* 73:308–317.

Thomas DB, Ksepka DT, Fordyce RE. 2011. Penguin heat-retention structures evolved in a greenhouse Earth. *Biology Letters* 7:461–464.

Vleck CM, Vertalino N, Vleck D, Bucher TL. 2000. Stress, corticosterone, and heterophil to lymphocyte ratios in free-living Adélie penguins. *Condor* 102:392–400.

Wallace R, Walsh M. 2005. Chapter 6: Health. In: *Penguin Husbandry Manual*, 3rd ed., pp. 86–103. Silver Spring: American Zoo and Aquarium Association.

Wallace RS, Teare JA, Diebold E, Michael M, Willis MJ. 1995. Hematology and plasma chemistry values in free-ranging Humboldt penguins (*Spheniscus humboldti*) in Chile. *Zoo Biology* 14:311–316.

Williams TD. 1995. Chapter 7: Physiology. In: *Bird Families of the World: The Penguins Spheniscidae*, pp. 107–126. Oxford: Oxford University Press.

Wilson RP, Wilson MTJ. 1989. A minimal-stress bird-capture technique. *The Journal of Wildlife Management* 53(1):77–80.

26 Ratites

Jessica Siegal-Willott

INTRODUCTION

Ratites belong to the avian orders Struthioniformes (ostriches), Casuariformes (emus and cassowaries), Rheiformes (rheas), and Apterygiformes (kiwis) (Smith 2003). Depending on the classification system, Tinaniformes (tinamous) may also be included.

Taxonomy and Biology

Ostriches (*Struthio camelus*) are the largest living birds (Table 26.1). There are several recognized subspecies confined to Africa and portions of the Middle East. Ostriches are sexually dimorphic; males are generally larger and have distinctive black feathers and wing plumes.

The common (*Rhea americana*) and Darwin's or lesser (*Rhea pterocnemia*) rhea are endemic to the grasslands of South America. The emu (*Dromaius novaehollandiae*) is confined to Australia. Emus are second in size to the ostrich, with the females slightly larger than males. There are three cassowary species, the double-wattled (*Casuarius casuarius*), single wattled (*Casuarius unappendiculatus*), and the Dwarf cassowary (*Casuarius bennetti*), all native to the Australasian rainforests. The three species of kiwi are confined to New Zealand; the great spotted (*Apteryx haastii*), the little spotted (*Apteryx owenii*), and the brown (*Apteryx australis*). Tinamous are small flighted ground-dwelling birds from the forests of South America. There are 47 recognized species, and they are either classified as, or are considered the closest avian relatives to the ratites described above.

Anatomy and Physiology

The term "ratite" refers to the flat raft-like sternum lacking a keel bone for attachment of the large flight muscles. All have elongated necks and relatively long, muscular legs, but little pectoral muscle development. All possess elongated toenails for aggression or defense, and are strong and rapid runners. Ostrich toenails are blunted, whereas those of other ratites are sharp. Rheas can abruptly change direction when running, and both rheas and cassowaries are powerful swimmers.

As with other birds, ratites lack a diaphragm. They possess much reduced air sacs compared with flighted birds. Respiration requires movement of the sternum down and forward, with the ribs expanding outwards. This is inhibited when weight, such as from a person straddling the bird, is applied from above. Death of birds thus restrained has been attributed to hypoxemia. Only the femur is pneumatized in ostriches and emus (Fowler 1996).

The normal respiratory rate of an adult ostrich is 6–12 breaths/min (bpm), but may increase up to 40–60 bpm during periods of hyperthermia. Normal body temperature (38–40°C) is maintained during thermal stress using evaporative cooling from the trachea, air sacs, and pharynx (Fowler 1996). The ratite glottis is simple with a large opening, an adaptation proposed to facilitate inhalation of air during strenuous exercise (Fig. 26.1). The trachea is composed of complete cartilaginous rings.

Ratites possess a renal-portal system, similar to other birds. Although theoretically it might enhance excretion of renally eliminated drugs, in ostriches administered xylazine/tiletamine/zolazepam, there was no significant difference between injection in the thigh or muscles at the base of the wings in onset, duration, or recovery (Carvalho et al. 2006). The physiologic role of the renal-portal system is poorly understood; care is used when potentially nephrotoxic drugs or those primarily eliminated by the kidneys (i.e., ketamine) are

Zoo Animal and Wildlife Immobilization and Anesthesia, Second Edition. Edited by Gary West, Darryl Heard, and Nigel Caulkett.
© 2014 John Wiley & Sons, Inc. Published 2014 by John Wiley & Sons, Inc.

Table 26.1. Reported weight and height ranges for ratites and tinamous

Species	Height	Weight
Ostrich	2.1–3.0 m	≤160 kg[b]
Emu	1.5–1.9 m	30–55 kg[a]
Cassowarys		
Double wattled	1.3–1.7 m	♂ 29–34 kg
Single wattled	1.5–1.8 m	♀ ≤58 kg
Dwarf	1.0–1.1 m	NR
		17.6–25 kg
Rheas		
Greater	1.2–1.7 m	20–25 kg[b]
Darwin's	1.0–1.1 m	10–25 kg[b]
Kiwis	0.35–0.55 m	0.67–4 kg[a]
Tinamous	NR	0.04–2.3 kg[a]

[a]Females larger than males.
[b]Males larger than females.
NR, not reported.

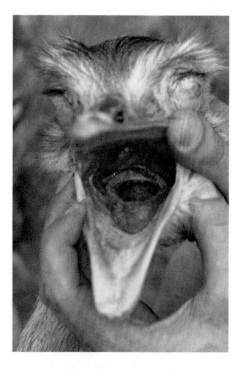

Figure 26.1. The glottis of most ratites, as in this rhea, is large and readily visible at the base of the tongue.

administered into the thigh musculature or medial metatarsal vein.

The ostrich is the largest living bird, with some males weighing as much as 160 kg (Table 26.1). Both male and female emus possess a ventral midline tracheal sac, approximately 10–15 cm cranial to the thoracic inlet.

The kiwi nares are located close to the beak tip; this location is thought to facilitate scent location of food among forest leaf litter. The kiwi egg is the largest proportionately of any living bird. Prior to oviposition, it occupies a large proportion of the coelomic cavity with a consequent reduction in air sac space. Further com-

promise to respiration due to pulmonary compression will occur if the animal is turned on her back. Kiwis also have lower body temperature (36.6–40.3°C) and metabolic rate than most other birds (Smith 2003).

PHYSICAL RESTRAINT

Young ratites (chicks and small juveniles) weighing ≤6 kg are manually restrained by supporting under the body and allowing the legs to hang or be folded. Birds weighing 6–15 kg are restrained with a hand around the abdomen, leaving the legs free. Care is taken during catching or handling to prevent damage to the legs. Chicks can also be wrapped in a towel for restraint or travel.

Juveniles and adult ratites require experienced handlers for restraint. These birds are large and strong, and possess large claws on the toes often used for defense. Emus and cassowaries in particular have large nails on the medial digit. Male ostriches are especially dangerous during the breeding season. Ratites jump, kick, and slash in a forward direction, and thus are approached from behind or the side to minimize risk of injury to the handler. Emus can also kick sideways, and rheas can kick in any direction. Gloves and protective clothing are often useful in preventing trauma from the distal limbs during restraint. Assuming a flat (prone) position on the ground will prevent trauma from kicking if escape from the bird is not possible.

Physical restraint of adult ratites by experienced handlers involves straddling the bird, with its legs in front of the holder. The wings should be grasped at the level of the humerus; the bird may also be restrained by a hand over the breast plate. Emus should not be restrained at the humerus, as the wings are reduced in size and may fracture. Emus accustomed to handling, and gently restrained from behind, may allow collection of blood or injection of anesthetics into the right jugular vein. The bird will, however, respond violently if the upper neck or head is grabbed.

Alternatively, in ostriches, the head may be grasped and quickly lowered below the level of the body. This prevents the ratite from kicking above its head level, minimizing the risks to the handler. This method of restraint is often used to place a hood, and possibly injection of medications.

Padded chutes, boards, alleyways, and stanchions are useful in the movement, separation, and isolation of individual animals for restraint and anesthetic procedures. Dim lighting (emus, rheas, cassowaries, and ostriches) and/or hooding (ostriches only) to decrease visual stimuli are useful for restraint. Hoods should cover the eyes without occluding the nostrils, and extend ~1/3 of the distance down the neck (Cornick-Seahorn 1996) (Fig. 26.2). Hooks are not recommended for catching or restraint as they may result in lacerations of the neck and/or trachea, and possibly death of

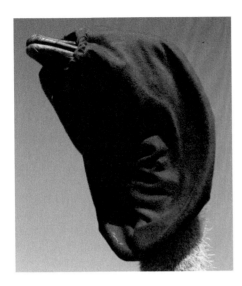

Figure 26.2. A hood reduces excitement and struggling in ostriches; it is not recommended in other ratites.

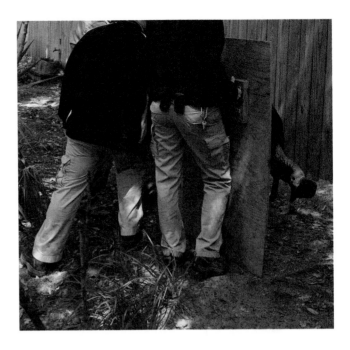

Figure 26.3. Wooden shields are used to protect handlers when approaching partially anesthetized ratites.

the bird if not used appropriately (Raines 1998). However, in some situations, this is the only way to catch the head for hood placement. Proper construction and application of hooks are described by Fowler (1995).

Emus present special challenges. Their skin is thin and easily lacerated. The head and long neck are vulnerable to injury because of the lack of significant muscle or soft tissue covering. The trachea is also easily collapsed. These birds are readily stressed, with subsequent respiratory or circulatory collapse, exertional rhabdomyolysis (Chapter 13), self-trauma, and hyperthermia (Chapter 5). Lastly, emus are capable of jumping high distances (≤2 m), and will attempt escape. Juvenile emus are more tractable, requiring only an experienced handler. One hand is placed between the legs and on to the sternum, leaving the other hand free to immobilize the head and neck (Mouser 1996).

Cassowaries are aggressive, requiring sedation or anesthesia for most handling procedures; hooding or covering the eyes is not adequate for safe restraint. During the very short period of sexual receptivity, captive females may be approached and allow examination and blood collection.

If possible, physical restraint occurs in secure areas, with solid, nonslip surfaces, free of large, deepwater sources, obstacles that may injure the bird or handler (hooks, nails, ledges, holes, wire, machinery, etc.), and at a suitable ambient temperature. Capture enclosures are designed to minimize risks to the patient and handlers, with easily accessible exit routes. Padded equine recovery stalls, with lights that can be dimmed, are excellent areas for restraint, induction, and recovery. Heavy foam pads, when used as shields, protect handlers and are used to compress birds in a confined space

for IM or IV injections. These pads are cleaned and disinfected between uses. Wooden shields are also useful to protect handlers when approaching lightly anesthetized animals (Fig. 26.3).

VASCULAR ACCESS

Intravenous injections and phlebotomy are performed using either the right jugular (14–22 g), brachial, or medial metatarsal vein. The medial metatarsal vein is not accessible in the awake adult. In emus, the basilic vein is small (although still able to be catheterized) as a result of vestigial wing development (Fig. 26.4). The wings are also prone to fracture during manual restraint (Cornick-Seahorn 1996).

Intravenous fluids are administered to anesthetized ratites at 5–10 mL/kg/h. Fluids commonly used include lactated Ringer's solution, Ringer's solution, and 0.9% sodium chloride. Fluid supplementation with dextrose may be warranted in young and/or debilitated birds. If IV access is not possible, intraosseous (IO) catheters may be placed in juvenile birds. The ulna and tibiotarsus are commonly used for IO access (Chapter 23).

ENDOTRACHEAL INTUBATION

Noncuffed endotracheal (ET) tubes are used to prevent pressure necrosis of the tracheal mucosa, although some authors prefer cuffed tubes to minimize the risk of aspiration, and ensure effective mechanical ventilation. The glottis is large and easily visualized for

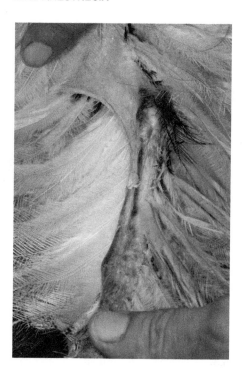

Figure 26.4. The wings of emus and most ratites are small and can be fractured if used to restrain an animal. The basilic vein on the medial surface of the wing can be used for blood collection in sedated or anesthetized animals, and for catheterization for fluid administration under anesthesia.

insertion of the ET tube (Fig. 26.1). Light bandaging around the neck of emus prevents air from distending the subcutaneous air sac during positive pressure ventilation.

The head and neck are positioned to prevent kinking of the ET tube, and to minimize risk of regurgitation and aspiration. Tube internal diameter varies with bird size, ranging from 4 to 18 mm. Intubation and positive pressure ventilation are recommended for all prolonged (≥10 minutes) or surgical procedures. Ventilatory support aims to achieve a tidal volume of 10–20 mL/kg, respiratory rate of 6–12 breaths per minute, and a peak inspiratory pressure of 10- to 15-cm water (Cornick-Seahorn 1996; Fowler 1996).

ANALGESIA

Use of analgesics is based on experience in other avian species (see also Chapter 7). Limited work has been done to establish dosage ranges in ratites. Fentanyl and butorphanol have been used as adjuncts to general anesthesia for pain control (Cornick-Seahorn 1996).

CHEMICAL RESTRAINT AND ANESTHESIA

Drugs used for chemical restraint in ratites are summarized in Table 26.2. Intramuscular administration is routine; the cranial and caudal thigh muscles and lum-

bosacral area (in nonobese birds) are used, since the pectoral muscles are not developed (Fig. 26.5). Injections into larger, more proximal thigh musculature may be more effective than those at more distal locations (Cushing & McClean 2010). The role of the renal-portal system in drug elimination following administration into caudal musculature has not been fully elucidated. Intravenous drug administration offers the most rapid method of immobilization; in intractable animals, IM sedation may be required prior to IV access.

Fasting times vary based on age and size of the bird, with little to no fasting in those <6 months old to prevent hypoglycemia. Adult ratites are fasted for 12–24 hours prior to induction (Cornick-Seahorn 1996; Lin et al. 1997).

Chemical immobilization is conducted in safe, secure areas with escape routes available for all personnel involved. Successful chemical immobilization varies with age and species, as well as experience level of the handlers and anesthetist(s).

Premedications

Anticholinergics are not commonly used, as they increase the viscosity of respiratory secretions, potentially leading to airway obstruction (Gilsleider 1998). Bradycardia is not commonly encountered during ratite anesthesia. In ostriches, anticholinergic therapy is indicated if heart rate falls below 30–35 bpm (Cornick & Jensen 1992). However, anticholinergic therapy is not consistently effective in treating bradycardia (Cornick & Jensen 1992). Many instances of bradycardia are likely due to hypertension and therefore refractory to anticholinergics.

Tranquilization and sedation have been achieved using acepromazine, azaperone, diazepam, midazolam, xylazine, detomidine, ketamine, and medetomidine, allowing for blood collection, minor procedures, and facilitation of induction of anesthesia (Table 26.2). These medications are usually administered IM; oral diazepam has been used successfully to sedate ostriches and cassowaries (Fowler 1995; N. Kapustin, pers. comm.).

Xylazine is commonly used, either alone or in combination with ketamine. Caution is warranted when using this alpha-2 agonist, as it has significant cardiorespiratory depressant effect. Onset of action is usually within 10 minutes, and may provide up to 30 minutes of sedation (Gilsleider 1998). High doses of xylazine IM allowed for IV ketamine induction 20 minutes later in adult ostriches (Al-Sobayil et al. 2009). Low dose medetomidine allowed for safe approach and limited handling in adult captive and free-ranging cassowaries, and was fully reversed with atipamezole administration (Westcott & Reid 2002). Higher doses produced heavy sedation adequate for full examination (Westcott & Reid 2002). Juvenile (<1 year) cassowaries were heavily

Table 26.2. Anesthetic agents used in adult ratites

Agent	Ostrich	Emu	Rhea	Cassowary	Comments	Reference
Sedation						
Azaperone	0.5–2					Jensen (1990)
	0.55					Gilsleider (1998)
Acepromazine	0.25					Ciboto et al. (2006)
Detomidine	1.5					Jensen (1990)
Diazepam	0.05	$5^{a,e}$	$5^{a,e}$	1 q 18 h	For recovery	Tully et al. (1996b)
	0.3–0.5					Smith (2003); Cornick-Seahorn (1996)
	$0.1–0.2^a$					Cornick-Seahorn (1996)
	$0.1–0.3^a$					Ramsey (1991)
	0.3^a					Gilsleider (1998)
	$0.33^{a,b}$					Lin et al. (1997)
	0.5–1					Cornick-Seahorn (1996)
	5^e PO					Fowler (1995)
Medetomidine	0.1				Light sedation	Van Heerden and Kefren, (1991)
	0.26–0.31				Heavy sedation	Westcott and Reid (2002)
	0.38–0.54					Westcott and Reid (2002)
Medetomidine/ ketamine				$0.09–0.13/3.4–4.3^b$	Heavy sedation	$Citino^g$
Medetomidine, medetomidine/ midazolam				0.12–0.13	1st dart	$Citino^g$
				$0.04/0.2^b$	2nd dart combo	
Midazolam	0.15^d					Cornick and Jensen (1992)
	$0.15^{a,b}$					Lin et al. (1997)
Telazol/diazepam		$3.3/0.13^b$				Tully (1996b)
Xylazine	0.2–2					Gilsleider (1998)
	0.4–0.9					Cornick and Jensen (1992)
	0.5–1					Fowler (1995)
	1					Ciboto et al. (2006)
	4					Al-Sobayil et al. (2009)
Xylazine/butorphanol			2.26–2.75/0.12–0.2			Lin et al. (1997)
Immobilization						
Carfentanil	3.3^e					Fowler (1995)
Carfentanil/ketamine	$3/200^e$					Fowler (1995)
Carfentanil/midazolam/ ketamine				$0.04–0.06/0.1–0.2/2.5–4.9^h$	Stormy induction possible	$Citino^g$
Etorphine	$1.5–6^{e,i}$				Variable	Fowler (1995)
Etorphine/ acepromazine	$2.5–3/50^{b,e}$				Excitement	Stoskopf et al. (1982)
	$3.6/15^{b,e}$				Moderate sedation	Samour et al. (1990)

(Continued)

Table 26.2. (*Continued*)

Agent	Ostrich	Emu	Rhea	Cassowary	Comments	Reference
Etorphine/acepromazine/xylazine	6/25/200^e					Samour et al. (1990)
Etorphine/ketamine	2–6^c/150–200^e			0.1/6.5 5(ket)^c 7–12^e/100–300^e	Reverse etorphine with diprenorphine Long, smooth recoveries	Ensley et al. (1984) Stoskopf et al. (1982)
Etorphine/medetomidine	8–9/4–8^{e,i}					Langan et al. (2000)
Medetomidine/ketamine	0.08/2^b 0.05–0.15/3–7				Bradycardia	Fowler (1995) Van Heerden and Kefren, (1991)
Metomidate/azaperone	20/6.6^b 10/3.3^b				Apnea; respiratory side effects; salivation, regurgitation at higher dose	Van Heerden and Kefren, (1991)
Telazol	5–20^b					Jensen (1993); Fowler (1995)
Xylazine	1–2.2					Smith et al. (2005)
Ketamine			12.5			Cushing and McClean (2010)
Thiafentanil/medetomidine Induction		0.175/0.09				Cullen et al. (1995)
Alphaxalone/alphadolone	2.41–4.8^a				Poor induction; apnea	Honnas et al. (1991)
Carfentanil	0.03^a 0.3					Cornick and Jensen (1992) Cornick-Seahorn et al. (1995)
Diazepam/telazol	0.1/4.4					Tully et al. (1996a)
Diazepam/ketamine	0.22/4.4^{a,d} 0.2–0.3^a/2–10^a 0.1/8 0.24/4.75^a 0.25^a/5^a 0.22^a/4.4^a	0.5/8^a			Bradycardia; Hypercapnia; poor induction	Honnas et al. (1991) Gilsleider (1998) Fowler (1995) Burba et al. (1996) Ciboto et al. (2006) Cornick and Jensen (1992)
Isoflurane	5%	5%	5%		Juveniles (<6mo)	Al-Sobayil et al. (2009)
Ketamine	8^a				Given 20 minutes post xylazine	Cornick-Seahorn (1996)
Ketamine/xylazine/guaifenesin		15/3/0.1% K/0.05% X/5% G			Induce with K/X; maintain on K/X/G IV at 2–4mL/kg/h	Langan et al. (2000) Langan et al. (2000)
Propofol	3^b 0.2mg/kg/min^f 10^a 4^a				Apnea may occur	Pye (2007) Ciboto et al. (2006)
Telazol	3.7^a 3^a 3.7^a 2.3–4.9^a 4.35 5	2.3–4.9^a	2.3–4.9^a		Poor/rough recovery; apnea After sedation with diazepam	Honnas et al. (1991) Ciboto et al. (2006) Cornick and Jensen (1992) Lin et al. (1997) Tully et al. (1996b) Gilsleider (1998)

Agent	Dose (mg/kg)				Comments	References
Xylazine/alphaxalone/alphadolone	1.13–1.85/1.66–3.53[a]					Cullen et al. (1995)
Xylazine/butorphanol/telazol	1.06–2.03/0.10–0.14/2.3–4.0[a]	1.06–2.03/0.10–0.14/3.4–4.9[a]	2.12–2.75/0.12–0.55/3.0–5.8[a]		Higher doses needed in rheas	Lin et al. (1997)
Xylazine/carfentanil	0.5/0.015[a]				Apnea	Honnas et al. (1991)
	0.5/0.15[a,d]				Reverse with yohimbine/naltrexone	Cornick and Jensen (1992)
	150 mg[e]/3 mg[e]					Raath et al. (1992)
Xylazine/diazepam/ketamine	0.44/0.15/2.8[a]					Honnas et al. (1991)
Xylazine/diazepam/ketamine	0.44/0.15/2.8[a]				Poor induction	Cornick and Jensen (1992)
Xylazine/ketamine	0.45/25					Matthews et al. (1991)
	2.2/2.2–3.3					Fowler (1995)
	0.5–1/2–10[a]					Gilsleider (1998)
Xylazine/ketamine/alphaxalone-alphadolone	1/5/12–17.1[a,b]					Gandini et al. (1986)
Analgesia						
Butorphanol	0.02				Supplemental A-A needed for prolonged procedures	Cornick-Seahorn (1996); Cornick-Seahorn et al. (1995)
	0.02–0.05[a]					
Ketoprofen	0.5–1					Pye (2007)
	1–2					Pye (2007)
Reversals						
Atipamezole	5–20[a,e]	0.2[a]				Ostrowski and Ancrenaz, (1995); Cushing and McClean (2010)
Diprenorphine	2× Etorphine dose (mg)		2× etorphine dose (mg)			Stoskopf et al. (1982)
Naltrexone	90–125 mg : 1 mg carfentanil	50x thiafentanil dose (mg)				Raath et al. (1992); Cushing and McClean (2010)
Yohimbine	0.11					Lin et al. (1997)
Emergency drugs						
Atropine	0.035					Fowler et al. (1987)
Doxapram	5[a]					Ostrowski and Ancrenaz, (1995)
Epinephrine	0.02–0.2[a]					Cornick-Seahorn (1996)
Glycopyrrolate	0.011[a]					Cornick and Jensen (1992)
Lidocaine	1–2[a]				For ventricular arrythmias	Cornick-Seahorn (1996)

Notes: Doses are based on mg/kg basis. All agents administered intramuscularly (IM) unless stated otherwise.

[a]Intravenous administration.
[b]Juvenile animal.
[c]Supplemental drug needed on mg/kg basis.
[d]Supplemental isoflurane needed for intubation.
[e]Total mg per bird.
[f]Constant rate infusion of propofol used to maintain a light plane of anesthesia in juvenile ostrich.
[g]Personal communication.
[h]Supplemental ketamine needed for transportation.
[i]Free ranging.
K, ketamine; X, xylazine; G, guaifenesin.

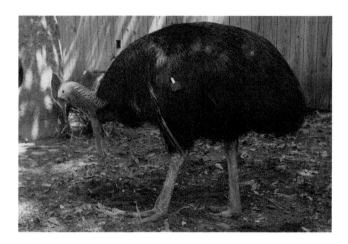

Figure 26.5. Intramuscular injections are administered into the upper thigh. This is done with either remote or hand injection.

sedated using medetomidine/ketamine combination; degree of sedation was somewhat variable, and supplemental M/K was occasionally necessary for some procedures (S.B. Citino, pers. comm., 2006). Intramuscular medetomidine, followed by medetomidine/midazolam IM, in these same cassowaries produced mild sedation adequate for crate loading (S.B. Citino, pers. comm., 2006).

Acepromazine is useful for muscle relaxation, but is contraindicated in debilitated animals, and is not a preferred method of tranquilization. Safer drugs for healthy and ill birds include diazepam and midazolam. Azaperone is useful for transport of animals, as it provides little muscle relaxation, but adequate tranquilization for up to 24 hours (Cornick-Seahorn 1996; Gilsleider 1998).

Immobilization

Opioid Combinations Carfentanil and etorphine have been used with limited and variable success. Carfentanil produces rapid recumbency, but has been associated with excitatory activity (frenzied running, circling, and walking backwards) (Cornick & Jensen 1992; S.B. Citino, pers. comm., 2006. In severe cases, this excitatory phase results in exertional rhabdomyolysis or trauma. Etorphine has been used in combination with acepromazine, acepromazine and xylazine, ketamine, and with medetomidine. In each case, satisfactory muscle relaxation and sedation were achieved, and use of medetomidine allowed for complete immobilization. In ostriches, etorphine combined with medetomidine produced recumbency in <10 minutes in most cases (Ostrowski & Ancrenaz 1995). Risks with these combinations include regurgitation, aspiration, myopathy, and death (Cornick-Seahorn 1996).

In juvenile ostriches (<1 year), etorphine/acepromazine had no or variable effect, from mild sedation to profound immobilization. Etorphine/ketamine

showed similar, but more reliable immobilization and recovery when administered to adult ostriches (Stoskopf et al. 1982). Some of the variability may have been due to dart failure. Manual restraint was used to assist the adults into sternal recumbency following adequate tranquilization. In contrast, lower dosages of etorphine/acepromazine administered via blow dart produced moderate sedation for 10–20 minutes in juvenile birds, with some ataxia and excitement during the initial immobilization (Samour et al. 1990). In adult ostriches, higher dosages of etorphine/acepromazine, in combination with xylazine, improved sedation and allowed manual restraint for diagnostic procedures. Initial effects were similar to those noted earlier (Samour et al. 1990). Ostriches appear resistant to high etorphine dosages (Samour et al. 1990; Stoskopf et al. 1982). Given the unpredictable effects of etorphine/acepromazine combinations, alternative immobilizing and induction agents should be considered first.

In adult cassowaries, etorphine (≤10 mg) did not produce immobilization (Stoskopf et al. 1982). However, a combination of etorphine/ketamine produced immobilization within 25 minutes in most birds, but was associated with long, rough recoveries (Stoskopf et al. 1982). A similar etorphine/ketamine combination (6/400 mg) was used to successfully induce a cassowary for surgical removal of a mass (Ensley et al. 1984). This combination produced recumbency within 5 minutes; however, supplemental ketamine was necessary for safe handling and administration of general anesthesia (Table 26.2). Adult cassowaries have been immobilized with a carfentanil/midazolam/ketamine combination. Animals were recumbent within 10 minutes, and occasionally exhibited an excitatory phase. Supplemental ketamine was given in some instances to allow for safe transport (S.B. Citino, pers. comm., 2006).

In adult emus, thiafentanil/medetomidine administration via Pneudart produced recumbency within 10 minutes in most cases; supplemental ketamine was necessary in three cases. Risks with this combination included respiratory acidosis and bradypnea, treated with IV atipamezole and supplemental orotracheal oxygen administration. Recovery following reversal and midazolam administration was rapid and smooth (Cushing & McClean 2010).

Other Combinations In ostrich chicks undergoing four different anesthetic combinations, only metomidate/azaperone IM produced satisfactory anesthesia and analgesia with relatively few side effects (Van Heerden & Kefren 1991). In the same chicks, tiletamine/zolazepam, metomidate, and metomidate/azaperone IM produced successful immobilization; an adult ostrich given a similar dose of tiletamine/zolazepam exhibited violent kicking and self-trauma, and insufficient immobilization (Van Heerden & Kefren 1991). The immobilization times were dosage dependent and most combinations did not fully eliminate voluntary movements. Medetomidine alone (0.1 mg/kg) did not produce immobilization (Van Heerden & Kefren 1991). In contrast, juvenile ostriches (9–11 months old) were successfully immobilized with a medetomidine/ketamine (0.08 mg/kg; 2 mg/kg) combination, although recumbency was not achieved in all cases (Langan et al. 2000). Tiletamine/zolazepam in combination with diazepam has also been used to immobilize a juvenile emu (Tully et al. 1996b), and ketamine alone has been used to immobilize an adult rhea, though quality of immobilization was not reported (Smith et al. 2005).

Induction

In young (≤6 months) and easily restrained animals (including kiwis and tinamous) induction may be accomplished using isoflurane alone; large subadult to adult birds require parenteral anesthetics. Inhalant induction is accomplished by starting at a high concentration (such as 5%), then decreasing to maintenance levels. This technique allows for rapid and smooth induction, and is the preferred method for ratites.

A variety of parenteral anesthetics alone or in combination (e.g., xylazine, ketamine, carfentanil, and tiletamine/zolazepam) (Table 26.2) have been investigated and used for induction. Selection is based on age, health status, and species. Known preexisting disease conditions are also considered.

Opioid Combinations Carfentanil has been used alone and in combination with xylazine for both immobilization and induction of anesthesia (Cornick & Jensen 1992; Honnas et al. 1991). Common complications include apnea, hypercapnia, excitability, agitation, and frenzied activity (Cornick & Jensen 1992). Naloxone, or preferably naltrexone, are used to reverse the effects of carfentanil, and tolazoline or atipamezole may be used to reverse the xylazine, making this a fully reversible combination. The addition of midazolam (0.1 mg/kg) to the C/X combination (0.025/1 mg/kg) allowed for smooth induction and recovery in an adult ostrich; midazolam was not reversed (S.B. Citino, pers. comm. 2006).

Other Combinations Tiletamine/zolazepam IV produced rapid and smooth induction with sternal recumbency in adult ostriches, and allowed for endotracheal intubation in juvenile ostriches (Ciboto et al. 2006; Gilsleider 1998; Honnas et al. 1991; Lin et al. 1997). Intravenous administration was facilitated by prior xylazine/butorphanol (X/B), xylazine, or acepromazine administration in adults; rheas required higher dosages of X/B than emus and ostriches to achieve the same level of sedation (Ciboto et al. 2006; Lin et al. 1997). Despite excellent induction, tiletamine/zolazepam IM is often associated with prolonged "rough" recoveries.

These effects are lessened by diazepam before or after tiletamine/zolazepam administration (Cornick & Jensen 1992; Tully et al. 1996b). Midazolam IM would be expected to produce similar effects as diazepam; benzodiazepine administration is encouraged when using tiletamine/zolazepam combinations. Finally, tiletamine/zolazepam IV may result in apnea, necessitating assisted ventilation (Cornick & Jensen 1992).

Immobilization with medetomidine/ketamine, followed by IV propofol, allowed for safe, smooth induction and recovery of anesthesia in juvenile ostriches (Langan et al. 2000). Transient apnea occurred but spontaneously resolved; all birds were bradycardic throughout the procedure. Light anesthesia was maintained with a constant rate infusion of propofol; higher doses are necessary for a surgical plane of anesthesia (Table 26.2). Successful sedation with IM acepromazine, followed by propofol IV has been reported in ostriches with minimal side effects, though volume to administer was reportedly large (Ciboto et al. 2006).

Ketamine alone is not recommended due to excitation during induction and recovery, and possible convulsions. Rather, it is combined with other drugs (e.g., diazepam, midazolam, medetomidine, or xylazine) (Al-Sobayil et al. 2009; Burba et al. 1996; Ciboto et al. 2006; Cornick & Jensen 1992; Langan et al. 2000; Tully et al. 1996a). High dosage diazepam/ketamine and other combinations result in "rough," unpredictable inductions, but smooth recoveries (Cornick & Jensen 1992). Diazepam (0.3–0.5 mg/kg IM) premedication facilitates induction with ketamine/diazepam IV (Cornick-Seahorn 1996). Xylazine combined with carfentanil (X/C) or ketamine (X/K) has resulted in successful induction in healthy ratites. However, rough recoveries were noted in some birds with X/K along with bradycardia and apnea (Cornick & Jensen 1992; Fowler 1995; Gilsleider 1998; Matthews et al. 1991). Xylazine/ketamine is not recommended in debilitated birds because of cardiopulmonary depression.

Pharmacokinetics in ostrich chicks premedicated with romifidine and induced with IM ketamine revealed rapid absorption and elimination half-life of K, similar to that of mammals (De Lucas et al. 2007). However, there is considerable variation in effectiveness of anesthetic agents used for induction. This variability may be related to dosage, route of administration, species, age and metabolic rate, degree of excitation, or individual variation (De Lucas et al. 2007). In general, diazepam appears to improve induction and recovery regardless of the other drugs used.

Maintenance

Isoflurane is the inhalant anesthetic of choice for chicks and juveniles, and lengthy procedures in adult birds. However, halothane, methoxyflurane, and nitrous oxide have also been used successfully. Significant decreases in respiratory rate and blood pressure have been recorded with isoflurane following X/K combinations in ostriches (Al-Sobayil et al. 2009).

Nonrebreathing systems are used in birds ≤7 kg, with an oxygen flow rate of 200 mL/kg/min. Circle rebreathing systems are used in larger birds (≥50 kg), with a flow rate of 20–30 mL/kg/min.

Injectable protocols have not provided adequate maintenance anesthesia for prolonged periods. Some success is possible using ketamine and xylazine for induction, followed by IV infusion of ketamine, xylazine, and guaifenesin (Cornick-Seahorn 1996) (Table 26.2). Repeated IV administration of ketamine (5 mg/kg) at 10–15 minute intervals can be used to prolong and/or maintain immobilization (Bruning & Dolensek 1986).

Intravenous pentobarbital is not recommended, as it has been associated with regurgitation and prolonged recoveries (Cornick-Seahorn 1996). Propofol may be a useful alternative for extended anesthetic procedures; clinical and research evaluation of its use in ratites is limited, but promising (Langan et al. 2000).

RECOVERY

Birds should be recovered in a dark, quiet, well-padded area to minimize stress and trauma. Use of diazepam (0.13–0.41 mg/kg IV) or midazolam (0.15 mg/kg IV) to produce a calming effect during the recovery period may help minimize self-trauma (Cornick & Jensen 1992; Cushing & McClean 2010). Alternatively, manual restraint of the bird in sternal recumbency until it is able to stand without assistance can be used. Some clinicians will restrain the bird in a towel or tarpaulin using tape or cargo straps until the bird is able to support itself. If this method of restraint is used, quick-release holding straps are recommended. Commercially available wraps are available for use in ratites (Raines 1998). An alternative method involves recovering the bird in sternal recumbency surrounded by hay bales, with a tent of bales over the top of the bird. The bird is not released from this enclosure until fully alert (D. Heard, pers. comm. 2006).

Reversal agents available include yohimbine, atipamezole, naloxone, naltrexone, diprenorphine, and flumazenil (Table 26.2). Reversal agents, such as yohimbine for antagonism of xylazine, are not commonly employed in ratite anesthesia protocols. Atipamezole is used for reversal of alpha-2 adrenergic agonists (xylazine, detomidine, and medetomidine), and flumazenil is used for reversal of the benzodiazepines. Flumazenil was not routinely used in the past because of associated costs and lack of necessity (Cornick-Seahorn 1996); recent reductions in flumazenil cost may allow for increased use for benzodiazepine reversal. Intramuscular injection of diprenorphine has been used to reverse the effects of etorphine. Intravenous naloxone administration followed by diprenorphine IM was noted to allow for smoother recovery following carfentanil administration than naloxone alone (Cornick & Jensen 1992).

In some cases, clinicians may prefer intramuscular administration of reversal agents instead of intravascular administration to allow for a more gradual recovery. Extubation is not recommended until the bird is swallowing on its own, and able to maintain its head in a normal position. The oral cavity should be examined prior to extubation to ensure excess secretions, blood, or debris is removed to maintain a clear airway. Renarcotization has not been reported, but birds should be monitored closely following reversal administration.

FIELD ANESTHETIC TECHNIQUES

There is presently no ideal technique for immobilization or anesthesia of ratites. Field immobilization is complicated by large drug volumes, and "rough" induction and recovery periods. There are also only limited reported investigations of field techniques. Both blowpipes and carbon dioxide-powered guns have been used, in combination with plain or barbed darts, for remote drug injection (Chapter 12). Ideally, reversible anesthetic regimens are used.

Administration of medications using darts delivered by CO_2-powered pistol has had mixed success for immobilization of cassowaries and ostriches (Fig. 26.5). Pole syringe use is hampered by difficulty in gaining proximity and access to injection sites (Stoskopf et al. 1982). Blowpipes and nonbarbed darts have also been used to deliver drugs to the thigh or lumbosacral muscles (Samour et al. 1990) (Fig. 26.5). For successful dart injection, a perpendicular trajectory path into the muscle is required. Darts projected at an angle are likely to bounce out of the muscle prior to full delivery of medications (Samour et al. 1990; Stoskopf et al. 1982). Ratites accumulate fat over the pelvis and paralumbar musculature, and in obese captive birds, this area is avoided for IM injection.

Evaluation of metodomidate/azaperone in captive ostrich chicks resulted in successful immobilization; although recommended for field use, it was not evaluated in adult ostriches or non-captive settings (Van Heerden & Kefren 1991). Etorphine and Etorphine/medetomidine combinations have been used to capture adult ostriches (Fowler 1995; Ostrowski & Ancrenaz 1995). Based on investigations in captive ratites, high dosage ketamine/xylazine combinations may produce field capture and restraint; supplemental IV ketamine is necessary to prolong immobilization (Bruning & Dolensek 1986).

Carfentanil may cause induction excitement; this is lessened when combined with xylazine (Raath et al. 1992). This combination otherwise produced minimal to no adverse side effects, and was reversed with naltrexone and yohimbine without complication. Carfentanil/ketamine combinations have also been recommended (Fowler 1995).

Exertional rhabdomyolysis (capture myopathy) may occur in chemically immobilized ratites (Chapter 13); field procedures are conducted by experienced personnel and at appropriate ambient temperatures. If excessive stress, excitement, or activity occurs prior to darting, it is prudent to abort the procedure. Medications and supplies necessary for treatment of exertional myopathy should be available during immobilization procedures.

MONITORING

Depth of anesthesia is assessed using heart rate and rhythm, respiratory rate and character, arterial blood pressure, wing and/or neck tone, and assessment of pedal, palpebral, and corneal reflexes. Continuous cardiac monitoring is achieved using an electrocardiogram or manual auscultation. Esophageal stethoscopes are used in chicks or small ratites. The brachial, medial metatarsal, or digital arteries are used for pulse assessment. Heart rates of 45–80 beats per minute are considered normal in anesthetized adults. The respiratory rate in an anesthetized adult ratite ranges from 25 to 40 (Gilsleider 1998).

Direct arterial blood pressures are measured by inserting catheters at the arterial sites listed earlier (Cornick & Jensen 1992; Lin et al. 1997). Additional arterial sites include the craniolateral aspect of the tibiotarsal bone, and parallel to the mandibular beak within the oral cavity (Cornick-Seahorn 1996). Indirect blood pressure monitoring has met with mixed success (Al-Sobayil et al. 2009; Cushing & McClean 2010). Based on information from mammalian species, a mean arterial pressure ≥60–70 mmHg is desirable. However, based on research it is proposed that ostriches normally have a higher arterial blood pressure than mammals (Cornick & Jensen 1992; Lin et al. 1997). Different drug combinations in different species and age animals are expected to affect the mean, systolic, and diastolic blood pressure; the limited ranges reported in the literature may serve as a rough guideline for acceptable values in ratites (Cornick & Jensen 1992; Lin et al. 1997; Matthews et al. 1991) (Table 26.3). Arterial blood gases and pH can also be monitored, although normal values are limited or nonexistent. Venous blood gas samples have been used to monitor acid-base status during anesthesia (Cushing & McClean 2010), and may be affected by age and sex of the bird (Bouda et al. 2009).

Additional monitoring includes capnography to assess ventilation, cloacal temperature, and pulse oximetry. The pulse oximetry probe can be applied at the wing web, tongue, intermandibular tissue, or tibiotarsal area. Juvenile birds in particular are susceptible to hypothermia, while adults may experience hyperthermia; frequent assessments of the cloacal temperature are recommended.

COMPLICATIONS

Complications associated with physical restraint either pre or post anesthesia include: wing fractures; tibiotarsal fractures; tarsometatarsal joint luxation; lacerations caused by hooks or other restraint devices; cervical vertebrae dislocation or fracture; compression injury of the trachea; hypoxemia; peroneal nerve damage; and capture myopathy.

Anesthetic complications noted in the literature include: hypothermia (especially very young and very thin birds); hyperthermia; regurgitation (especially in cases with preexisting gastrointestinal disease); hypoglycemia; neuropathy and myositis (due to insufficient padding during anesthesia); tracheal occlusion due to poor neck positioning; apnea; premature ventricular contractions (cause undetermined; Matthews et al. 1991); bradycardia; cardiac arrest; hypertension (Matthews et al. 1991); voluntary movement; self-trauma during recovery; excessive oral and respiratory secretions; hypocapnia (possibly related to excessive intermittent positive pressure ventilation); hypercapnia (Cornick & Jensen 1992; Cushing & McClean 2010); secondary fungal/yeast infections (Matthews et al. 1991) and rupture of great vessels (Cullen et al. 1995; Honnas et al. 1991).

Doxapram (5 mg/kg IV) can be used in cases of apnea, and hypotension can be treated using increased IV fluid administration, decreasing anesthetic depth, IV dobutamine (2–5 μg/kg/minute), or IV dopamine (5 μg/kg/minute). Epinephrine (0.02–0.2 mg/kg IV or intratracheal) can be used in cases of cardiac arrest, in conjunction with cardiac compression applied to the lateral aspect of the bird (Cornick-Seahorn 1996). Voluntary movement may be avoided by using butorphanol (0.02–0.05 mg/kg IV) to control pain, or by using ketamine intraoperatively (0.2 mg/kg IV). Bradycardia has been arbitrarily defined in the literature as heart rate <30 beats/min. Anticholinergic agents, such as glycopyrrolate or atropine, have met with variable success in treatment of bradycardia in ratites (Cornick-Seahorn 1996). Xylazine administration is thought to be associated with bradycardia in ratites, but conclusive evidence is lacking at this time.

Myopathy is treated with supportive care (IV fluids with bicarbonate, dextrose, corticosteroids, vitamin E-selenium, calcium, antibiotics, and flunixin meglumine) and possibly dantrolene for muscle relaxation.

DISEASES OF CONCERN

Procedures requiring general anesthesia in the ratite include: laceration repair; evaluation of traumatic injuries; evaluation and treatment of exertional myopathy (Smith et al. 2005; Tully et al. 1996a); sequestra removal (Tully et al. 1996b); castration (Pye 2007); removal of retained or infected yolk sacs; esophagostomy tube

Table 26.3. Systolic (SBP), mean (MAP), and diastolic (DAP) arterial blood pressures (mmHg) reported for anesthetized ratites

Drugs	Species	SBP		MAP		DAP		Reference
		Minimum	Maximum	Minimum	Maximum	Minimum	Maximum	
X/B	R	68–72	82–120	49–56	60–99	32–51	52–91	Lin et al. (1997)
I	E, R	55–105	121–222	37–84	99–168	30–79	84–147	Lin et al. (1997)
	O	102–150	148–198	92–140	142–175	84–128	130–170	Cornick and Jensen, (1992)
	O	145	206	118	171	90	147	Cornick and Jensen (1992)
TZ	E, R, O	47–178	186–232	44–126	135–210	39–103	122–192	Lin et al. (1997)
X/B/TZ	E, R, O	72–124	131–203	44–80	81–147	36–70	65–124	Lin et al. (1997)
D/K	O	160	254	126	212	85	198	Cornick and Jensen, (1992)
X/D/K	O	162	275	134	232	104	200	Cornick and Jensen, (1992)
X/C	O	160	185	132	158	90	122	Cornick and Jensen, (1992)
X/K	O	136	175	82	105	52	60	Cornick and Jensen, (1992)
	O	168–206	228	108–165	145–191	77–126	120–153	Matthews et al. (1991)
X/K/G	E	99	146	60	109	43	66	Cornick and Jensen (1992)

O, ostrich; E, emu; R, rhea; C, cassowary; X, xylazine; B, butorphanol; I, isoflurane; TZ, telazol (tiletamine/zolazepam); D, diazepam; K, ketamine; C, carfentanil; G, guaifenesin.

placement; proventriculotomy or ventriculotomy for foreign body removal; egg binding; orthopedic procedures, including correction of congenital or acquired musculoskeletal disorders; tumor removal; and impaction of the gastrointestinal tract (Burba et al. 1996; Cornick & Jensen 1992; Ensley et al. 1984; Gilsleider 1998; Honnas et al. 1991). Conditions causing a distended ventriculus or proventriculus (i.e., foreign body) necessitate rapid induction and intubation to minimize the risk of regurgitation and subsequent aspiration (Cornick-Seahorn 1996; Honnas et al. 1991).

REFERENCES

Al-Sobayil FA, Ahmed AF, Al-Wabel NA, Al-Thonayian AA, Al-Rogibah FA, Al-Fuaim AH, Al-Obaid AO, Al-Muzaini AM. 2009. The use of xylazine, ketamine, and isoflurane for induction and maintenance of anesthesia in ostriches (Struthio camelus). Journal of Avian Medicine and Surgery 23:101–107.

Bouda J, Nunez-Ochoa L, Avila-Gonzalez E, Doubek J, Fuente-Martinez B, Aguilar-Bobadilla J. 2009. Blood acid-base and plasma electrolyte values in healthy ostriches: the effect of age and sex. Research in Veterinary Science 87:26–28.

Bruning DF, Dolensek EP. 1986. Ratites. In: Zoo and Wild Animal Medicine, 2nd ed. (ME Fowler, ed.), pp. 277–291. Philadelphia: W.B. Saunders Co.

Burba DJ, Tully TN, Pechman RD, Cornick-Seahorn JL. 1996. Phalangeal amputation for treatment of osteomyelitis and septic arthritis in an ostrich (Struthio camelus). Journal of Avian Medicine and Surgery 10:19–23.

Carvalho HS, Ciboto R, Cortopassi SRG. 2006. Anatomical study of the renal portal system and its implications for the use of anesthetic agents in the restraint of Ostriches (Struthio camelus). Proceedings of the 9th World Congress of Veterinary Anaesthesiology, p. 212. Santos, Brazil.

Ciboto R, Cortopassi SRG, Lopes MAE, Carvalho RC, Baitelo CG. 2006. Comparison of chemical restraint techniques in ostrich (Struthio camelus). Brazilian Journal of Poultry Science 8:119–123.

Cornick JL, Jensen J. 1992. Anesthetic management of ostriches. Journal of the American Veterinary Medical Association 200:1661–1666.

Cornick-Seahorn JL. 1996. Anesthesiology of ratites. In: Ratite Management, Medicine, and Surgery (TN Tully, SM Shane, eds.), pp. 79–94. Malabar: Kreiger Publishing.

Cornick-Seahorn JL, Martin GS, Tully TN, Morris JM. 1995. Tourniquet-induced hypertension in an ostrich. Journal of the American Veterinary Medical Association 207:344–346.

Cullen LK, Goerke MA, Swan RA, Clark WT, Nandapi D, Colbourne C. 1995. Ostrich anaesthesia: xylazine premedication followed by alphaxalone/alphadolone and isoflurane. Australian Veterinary Journal 72:153–154.

Cushing A, McClean M. 2010. Use of thiafentanil-medetomidine for the induction of anesthesia in emus (Dromaius novaehollandiae) within a wild animal park. Journal of Zoo and Wildlife Medicine 41:234–241.

De Lucas JJ, Rodriguez C, Marin M, Gonzalez F, Ballesteros C, San Andres MI. 2007. Pharmacokinetics of intramuscular ketamine in young ostriches premedicated with romifidine. Journal of Veterinary Medicine 54:48–50.

Ensley PK, Launer DP, Blasingame JP. 1984. General anesthesia and surgical removal of a tumor-like growth from the foot of a double-wattled cassowary. Journal of Zoo Animal Medicine 15:35–37.

Fowler JD, Bauck L, Cribb PH, Presnell KR. 1987. Surgical correction of tibiotarsal rotation in an emu. Companion Animal Practitioner 1:26–30.

Fowler ME. 1995. Birds. In: Restraint and Handling of Wild and Domestic Animals, 2nd ed. (ME Fowler, ed.), pp. 304–316. Ames: Iowa State University Press.

Fowler ME. 1996. Clinical anatomy of ratites. In: Ratite Management, Medicine, and Surgery (TN Tully, SM Shane, eds.), pp. 1–30. Malabar: Kreiger Publishing.

Gandini GCM, Keffen RH, Burroughs REJ, Ebedes H. 1986. An anaesthetic combination of ketamine, xylazine and alphaxalone-alphadolone in ostriches (Struthio camelus). The Veterinary Record 118:729–730.

Gilsleider EF. 1998. Anesthesia and surgery of ratites. In: Veterinary Clinics of North America: Food Animal Practice (TN Tully, SM Shane, eds.), pp. 503–523. Philadelphia: W.B. Saunders.

Honnas CM, Jensen J, Cornick JL, Hicks K, Kuesis BS. 1991. Proventriculotomy to relieve foreign body impaction in ostriches. Journal of the American Veterinary Medical Association 199:461–465.

Jensen J. 1990. Ratite anesthesia and surgery. Proceedings, Ostrich Medicine Seminar for Veterinarians, pp. 6–7.

Jensen JM. 1993. Ratite restraint and handling. In: *Zoo and Wild Animal Medicine: Current Therapy 3* (ME Fowler, ed.), pp. 198–200. Philadelphia: W.B. Saunders.

Langan JN, Ramsay EC, Blackford JT, Schumacher J. 2000. Cardiopulmonary and sedative effects of intramuscular medetomidine-ketamine and intravenous propofol in ostriches (*Struthio camelus*). *Journal of Avian Medicine and Surgery* 14:2–7.

Lin H, Todhunter PG, Powe TA, Ruffin DC. 1997. Use of xylazine, butorphanol, tiletamine-zolazepam, and isoflurane for the induction and maintenance of anesthesia in ratites. *Journal of the American Veterinary Medical Association* 210:244–248.

Matthews NS, Burba DJ, Cornick JL. 1991. Premature ventricular contractions and apparent hypertension during anesthesia in an ostrich. *Journal of the American Veterinary Medical Association* 198:1959–1961.

Mouser D. 1996. Restraint and handling of the emu. In: *Ratite Management, Medicine, and Surgery* (TN Tully, SM Shane, eds.), pp. 41–45. Malabar: Kreiger Publishing Company.

Ostrowski S, Ancrenaz M. 1995. Chemical immobilization of red-necked ostriches (*Struthio camelus*) under field conditions. *The Veterinary Record* 136:145–147.

Pye GW. 2007. Intestinal entrapment in the right pulmonary ostium after castration in a juvenile ostrich (*Struthio camelus*). *Journal of Avian Medicine and Surgery* 21:290–293.

Raath JP, Quandt SKF, Malan JH. 1992. Ostrich (*Struthio camelus*) immobilization using carfentanil and xylazine reversal with yohimbine and naltrexone. *Journal of the South African Veterinary Association* 63:138–140.

Raines AM. 1998. Restraint and housing of ratites. In: *Veterinary Clinics of North America: Food Animal Practice* (TN Tully, SM Shane, eds.), pp. 387–399. Philadelphia: W.B. Saunders.

Ramsey E. 1991. Ratite restraint, immobilization, and anesthesia. Avian/Exotic Animal Medicine Symposium, pp. 176–178.

Samour JH, Irwin-Davies J, Faraj E. 1990. Chemical immobilization in ostriches (*Struthio camelus*) using etorphine hydrochloride. *The Veterinary Record* 127:575–576.

Smith DA. 2003. Ratites: tinamiformes (tinamous) and struthioniformes, rheiiformes, cassuariformes (ostriches, emus, cassowaries, and kiwis). In: *Zoo and Wild Animal Medicine*, 5th ed. (ME Fowler, RE Miller, eds.), pp. 94–102. St. Louis: Saunders.

Smith KM, Murray S, Sanchez C. 2005. Successful treatment of suspected exertional myopathy in a rhea (*Rhea americana*). *Journal of Zoo and Wildlife Medicine* 36:316–320.

Stoskopf MJ, Beall FB, Ensley PK, Neely E. 1982. Immobilization of large ratites: blue necked ostrich (*Struthio camelus austrealis*) and double wattled cassowary (*Casuarius casuarius*) with hematologic and serum chemistry data. *Journal of Zoo Animal Medicine* 13:160–168.

Tully TN, Hodgin C, Morris JM, Williams J, Zebreznik B. 1996a. Exertional myopathy in an emu (*Dromaius novaehollandiae*). *Journal of Avian Medicine and Surgery* 10:96–100.

Tully TN, Martin GS, Haynes PF, Cornick-Seahorn J, Pechman RD. 1996b. Tarsometatarsal sequestration in an emu (*Dromaius novaehollandiae*) and an ostrich (*Struthio camelus*). *Journal of Zoo and Wildlife Medicine* 27:550–556.

Van Heerden J, Kefren RH. 1991. A preliminary investigation into the immobilizing potential of a tiletamine/zolazepam mixture, metomidate, a metomidate and azaperone combination and medetomidine in ostriches (*Struthio camelus*). *Journal of the South African Veterinary Association* 62:114–117.

Westcott DA, Reid KE. 2002. Use of medetomidine for capture and restraint of cassowaries (*Casuarius casuaris*). *Australian Veterinary Journal* 80:150–153.

27 Raptors

Patrick T. Redig, Michelle Willette, and Julia Ponder

INTRODUCTION

The raptors or birds of prey are an assemblage of avian species representing convergent evolution from diverse lineages, as opposed to distinct taxonomic relationships among major orders. All are completely carnivorous birds, acquiring their food by active hunting and/or scavenging. The major orders of raptors are the Strigiformes (owls), Falconiformes (falcons), Accipitriformes (hawks and eagles), and the vultures. The taxonomic grouping of the vultures is not completely established. Two major groups exist, the so-called Old World vultures (order Falconiformes) and the New World vultures (order uncertain; possibly Falconiformes, or Accipitriformes, or Ciconiiformes [storks] or Cathartiformes [*Incertae sedis*]). There are approximately 280 species in various orders worldwide. Ravens (Passeriformes: Corvidae) are sometimes included among the raptors due to similarity in life history habits and a strong tendency to carnivory.

Average or representative weights for raptors range from the diminutive elf and Saw-whet owls (40–85 g) to the large eagles of the Amazon and Philippine rain forest (harpy eagle 5–9 kg M : F; Philippine eagle 4–6 kg M : F) and the condors (California and Andean 9–12 kg, respectively). In all species, except the New World vultures and ravens, reverse sexual dimorphism is expressed with females ranging from 10% to 30% larger than the males. With few exceptions, plumage characteristics are not dimorphic and there is substantial overlap in weights between males and females, hence sexual determination is not a definitive process except at the extremes of the size ranges.

ANATOMY AND PHYSIOLOGY

All raptors possess strong hooked beaks that are capable of inflicting mild to serious damage to handlers and can also damage anesthesia equipment, such as masks and hoses, if not properly restrained. Additionally, except for vultures, all have very strong grasping feet armed with sharp, curved talons, rendering the need for proper restraint to be of paramount concern. The mouth of nearly all is large and wide; the glottis is clearly visible at the base of the tongue.

Across species of raptors, the anatomy of the respiratory system does not vary appreciably except in size, and it exhibits the basic avian anatomy and physiology of lungs and air sacs as found in other avian groups (Heard 1997; Ludders 1998). As with other avian species, it is important to remember the tracheal rings are complete and cuffed intubation tubes should not be used.

Procedures involving anesthesia in raptors are regularly conducted in dorsal, lateral, and sternal recumbency without marked overt differences in ventilation or manner of managing the anesthetic episode. Studies involving air sac volumes by computed tomography (CT) of isoflurane-anesthetized red-tailed hawks demonstrated that subjects had the greatest lung and air sac volumes in sternal recumbency compared with lateral or dorsal positioning (Malka et al. 2009). There were no changes in ventilatory rate as a function of position, and other respiratory variables were not evaluated. Dorsal recumbency has long been regarded as reducing ventilatory function owing to increased effort to raise the sternum and pressure from viscera against the abdominal air sacs. While this theoretical possibility is recognized, these differences appear to be minor in day-to-day use of anesthesia. For long orthopedic procedures, however, sternal recumbency is recommended by the authors and is usually concordant with the principal surgical approaches to avian long bones (Redig & Roush 1978).

The digestive tract of raptors is typical of carnivorous birds with some variations. Falcons, hawks, eagles, and vultures have a crop, a varying saccular or expandable portion of the esophagus that stores food. Owls do not possess a true crop; rather, the mid-cervical esophagus is freely expansible and functions as a site of temporary food storage. All have a proventriculus (glandular stomach) positioned as a bell-shaped structure on the anterior aspect of the ventriculus. The latter is the site of chemical digestion and pellet formation. Pellets are formed from nondigestible food residues that are egested at the completion of the digestion cycle. The intestinal tract is relatively short and has rapid transit times. Owls have ceca, while falconiformes do not. The functional significance of ceca is poorly understood. When the gastrointestinal tract is full of food or contains an as-yet unegested pellet, there can be considerable enteric expansion and concomitant reduction in airspace in the abdominal air sacs. A 12- to 24-hour fast is generally recommended prior to anesthesia in all but the smallest raptors, where a small amount of "clean meat" (devoid of bones, feathers, or fur) may be fed up to a couple of hours before anesthesia without complication.

CAPTURE AND RESTRAINT

Many raptors are maintained in captivity, some in very close association with humans, as in the sport of falconry or trained and bonded to handlers for use in educational programs; this bonding necessitates different approaches to handling for restraint than for their wild counterparts. Most raptors are armed "front and back," and even relatively, tame, docile birds will often strike with the beak or talons when being restrained; caution and protection are strongly advised in all situations. That said, puncture wounds from talons are much more serious injuries than bite wounds. An injury to the handler's face from either is also often serious. Proper restraint ultimately requires control of the legs and the head; covering the latter with a towel or a properly fitting hood after the bird is restrained will greatly reduce the tendency for the bird to struggle.

The overall goals of handling are to maintain safety of the patient, the handler, and the clinician, to provide proper positioning for medical procedures, to protect feathers from bending and breakage, and to minimize stress. The major hazards to clinician and handler safety include talon wounds, beak wounds, and wing slapping, especially from eagles. The latter have been known to cause people black eyes and even to break their glasses. Personal protective gear, consisting of gloves of appropriate thickness and gauntlet length and safety glasses, are recommended. When handling eagles, the use of welder's leather cape, which protects the arms and shoulders from bites wounds, is further recommended.

To protect the bird and to avoid precipitating struggling and to prevent unintended injuries, it is important to cover the head of the patient with a hood or a towel to block out visual stimuli, to use slow, smooth continuous movements, and to establish good communication between the handler and the clinician so that who has control over the legs and head of the bird at any given time is never in doubt.

Capture of Untrained, Wild Birds

For wild birds being handled for rehabilitation or untrained display birds, "capture" is essentially the first component of the restraint procedure. On the one hand, the goal is capture with a minimum of risk to patient and the handler, with less concern about stress or psychological trauma to the bird; on the other hand, achieving firm control on a strong, struggling patient. Capture can be accomplished in any number of ways, depending on the demeanor of the bird and skill of the handler. Effective means include a dip net, or approaching the perched bird in the dark, using a light source that is quickly clicked off and on to provide the handler with a brief window of light to observe where the bird is and allow approach, or covering the bird with a large towel. Some species, great horned owls in particular, will sit on a perch giving a vivid threat display, but, in most cases, not make any attempt to escape or attack; these can be grabbed quite easily by the legs. Regardless of how the bird is approached, the objective is to bring ones hands in close proximity to the legs, one on either side. As the hands are moved closer slowly, there will come a point where the bird's personal space has been invaded (usually within about 3–5 in of the legs) and, instead of looking directly at the person approaching them, they will divert their gaze momentarily in the direction they intend to flee. In that moment, a quick grasping of each leg and lifting the bird off its perch will accomplish the capture portion. At that point, the wings are folded into the body and the bird is laid flat on a table or the floor, both legs are grasped in one hand with the index finger between the legs, and the other hand is used to grasp or cover the head (Fig. 27.1a,b).

These methods work "to a point" with most raptors up to about 5–6 Kg, which includes most species—the average handler can readily overcome their muscle strength. The very large eagles (harpy and Philippine) along with the large vultures demand greater skill and respect when being captured. The eagles have very large and powerful legs that require the handler to have

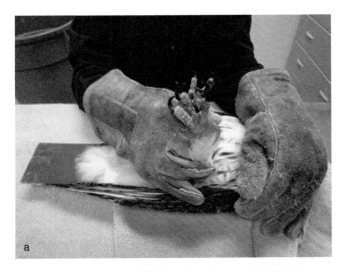

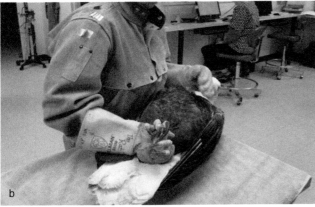

Figure 27.1. (a) Safely restrained raptor (red-tailed hawk) on the examination table. (b). Properly restrained large raptor (bald eagle). Notice protective gear worn by the handler, including leather welder's vest, gauntleted gloves, and safety glasses.

considerable strength and attention to detail in order to overcome their efforts to struggle free.

Vultures, both Old and New World, will defend themselves during capture by regurgitating. The material ejected is malodorous and difficult to remove from clothing.

Capture of Trained Raptors

For trained birds in which a bond of trust has been established, restraint is best accomplished without the drama of a capture episode. Though strictly manual methods are mostly used, chemical sedation can positively impact the process (see later). For manual restraint, if the subject is perched on a handler's gloved fist, it can be slowly approached (use of darkness is again helpful, but less necessary) from the front and the legs gently grasped by one hand with an index finger in between them. Control of the wings is gained as the bird is gently lifted off the fist and placed on a table and the head covered. Alternatively, the bird may be grasped over the wings from behind and firmly, but

gently lifted off the fist and laid on a table. Many falconry birds will have a hood on their head and this renders each of these methods that much easier. Another useful and relatively stress-free method for restraint of a hooded falcon is to place an oversized anesthesia face mask over the head of the bird and flow isoflurane for a few minutes until the bird is unstable, gently catching them when they fall backwards off the perch, and continue with induction.

Many of the issues of restraint of trained birds may be avoided by the use of small volumes of chemical restraint agents injected with a very small (27-gauge) needle into the pectoral muscle or given via the mouth or nares. An injected mixture of ketamine and dexmedetomidine (previously medetomidine) has been shown to be highly effective (Molero et al. 2007) and safe in large falcons and others (Table 27.1). This approach induced ataxia and general loss of response in 3–4 minutes that readily allowed further induction with low concentrations of isoflurane (2% induction and 1% maintenance). Upon cessation of isoflurane and intramuscular administration of the antagonist, atipamezole (0.15 mg/kg), smooth, uneventful recovery occurred within 10 minutes. The metabolism of ketamine while the bird was under isoflurane allowed recovery without the uncontrolled wing-flapping and other movements associated with recovery from ketamine anesthesia. Other injectable agents, especially midazolam, have been used in a similar manner (Table 27.1).

ANCILLARY ASPECTS OF ANESTHESIA IN RAPTORS

Intubation and Air Sac Cannulation

Intubation is not undertaken for short procedures, up to 20–30 minutes, and not at all in raptors weighing less than approximately 150 g, especially sharp-shinned hawks. In these, the inside diameter of the tube that would fit inside the trachea becomes too small and too prone to blockage by mucous. Appropriately sized tubes should be available, however, in order to provide a means for rapid intubation and ventilation should the bird become apneic.

Intubation of raptors is a straightforward procedure and recommended to provide a means of ventilatory support for any procedures that exceed 20–30 minutes. Mask administration is generally adequate for procedures of shorter duration; however, it is recommended to have appropriate-sized intubation tubes readily available should apnea occur. An uncuffed tracheal tube that slides easily into the trachea is selected; it is inserted only sufficiently to prevent the tip from slipping easily out of the trachea. Pieces of white adhesive tape are used to affix the tube to the beak or the head to prevent its being dislodged (Fig. 27.2). Intubation should be conducted only in birds that have been previously taken to a plane of surgical anesthesia via mask

Table 27.1. Reported dosages of more commonly used injectable anesthetics in raptors

Agent	Red-Tailed Hawk	Bald Eagle	Golden Eagle	Great Horned Owl	Falcons	Others	Comment	Reference
Ketamine	x						Multiple species, dosed at 5–20mg/kg, variable results, difficult recoveries	Samour et al. (1984)
Xylazine							Multiple species, 8–10mg/kg IM and 2–8mg/kg IV; generally inconsistent results and unfavorable levels of sedation; reversed with yohimbine (0.2mg/kg)	Freed and Baker (1989)
Ketamine/diazepam				x	x		10–30mg/kg + 1.5mg/kg K:D	Redig and Duke (1976)
Ketamine/xylazine							10–15mg/kg + 2mg/kg IM (K + X) For owls, response variable in *Bubo spp.*[a]	Carpenter (2013)
							Multiple species, dosage recommendations reflecting species variations in response using a 5:1 combination of ketamine and xylazine; largely superseded by ketamine/medetomidine procedures	Redig (1998)
Ketamine/xylazine/yohimbine	x						Yohimbine administered 20 minutes after induction with a 2:1 combination of ketamine and xylazine; yielded a dose-related reversal response and smooth recovery; xylazine superseded as earlier	Degernes et al. (1988)
Midazolam/butorphanol (for sedation)						x (Psittacines[b])	0.5mg/kg midazolam/1–3mg/kg butorphanol—IM 2mg/kg direct installation into nares	Lennox (2011) Mans et al. (2011)
Medetomidine[c]							60–85ug/kg as a preanesthetic agent for isoflurane 150–350ug/kg IM	Lawton (2008) Carpenter (2013)
Dexmedetomidine					x	Common buzzard (*Buteo buteo*)	Dosed at 25ug/kg and 75ug/kg for buzzards and kestrels, respectively. Reported better sedation than with medetomidine; smooth reversal with atipamezole	Santangelo et al. (2009)
Medetomidine/butorphanol							Medetomidine: 5–20ug/kg/butorphanol: 0.1–0.3mg/kg	Carpenter (2013) BSAVA Small Animal Formulary Appendix
Ketamine/medetomidine					x		Administered as pre-anesthetic to isoflurane in Saker falcons, reversed with atipamezole after Isoflurane anesthesia. Dosage schedule: 3mg/kg–60ug/kg–0.15mg/kg ketamine-medetomidine-atipamezole	Molero et al. (2007)
							2–4mg/kg + 25–75ug/kg IV (K + M); 3–5mg/kg + 50–100ug/kg IM (K + M)	Carpenter (2013)
Ketamine/medetomidine/butorphanol						x (Psittacines[b])	3mg/kg + 40ug/kg + 1mg/kg IM (K + M + B) premed or supplement to isoflurane	Carpenter (2013)
Fentanyl	x				x		Fentanyl produced a dose-related reduction in isoflurane MAD	Pavez et al. (2010)
Fentanyl/lidocaine (brachial plexus blocks)					x		A combination of fentanyl:lidocaine (50ug/kg:5mg/kg) was effective for brachial plexus nerve block—required use of a nerve locator	d'Ovidio et al. (2011)
Propofol	x			x			Induction and CRI rates assessed in hawks and owls (4.48mg/kg and 0.48mg/kg/min for hawks and 3.36mg/kg and 0.56mg/kg/min for owls; hypoventilation, prolonged and variable recovery, moderate-to-severe excitation observed	Hawkins et al. (2003)

[a]Author's experience.

[b]Author's opinion that this combination would be effective and safe in raptors.

[c]Medetomidine is no longer available at time of writing; has been replaced by dexmedetomidine; may be obtained by compounding.

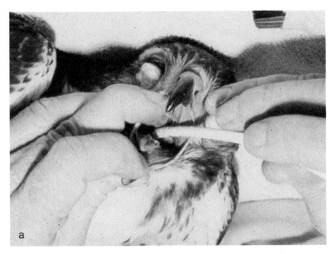

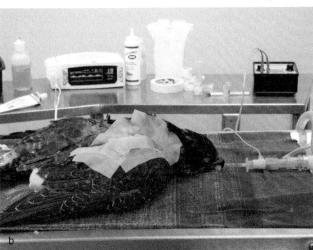

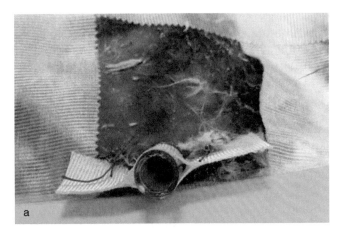

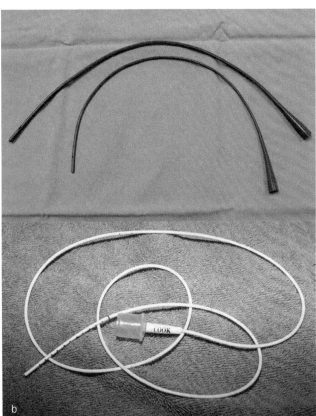

Figure 27.2. Insertion of intubation tube in a falcon (a) and intubated raptor (gyrfalcon) (b) prepped for orthopedic surgery. Note capnography and Doppler unit included in monitoring equipment array. While the latter may have limited utility for monitoring blood pressure, it serves as a useful means of audible monitoring of heart rate.

Figure 27.3. (a) Large-diameter air sac cannula in place for use as a breathing tube. (b) Small-diameter (8–12 Fr; 2.7–4.0 mm) air sac cannula made from red rubber tube (top) and commercially available dedicated air sac cannula tube (bottom) for use in administering gas anesthesia. Note added length to provide maneuverability without dislodging the tube from its insertion site (see Fig. 27.4c).

induction—attempts to intubate an awake bird are extremely stressful and should not be attempted. In some birds, insertion of the endotracheal tube will induce a period of apnea. This can be preempted by topically applying a small volume of 2% lidocaine to the rim of the glottis a few minutes prior to tube insertion.

Raptors are also amenable to air sac cannulation and this is a very useful modality for relieving dyspnea associated with upper airway obstruction or for administering gas anesthesia in instances where the presence of an endotracheal tube would interfere with manipulations about the head and mouth. Caudal thoracic air sac cannulation takes advantage of the normal physiologic direction of airflow from caudal to cranial to enter the lungs for gas exchange. Depending on the reason for cannulation, two scenarios for tube size are

considered. Where relief of dyspnea from upper airway blockage is the goal, a tube should be selected that is similar in size or slightly larger than the trachea itself to provide a low resistance pathway for air movement during spontaneous breathing (Fig. 27.3b). Where the cannula is intended for anesthesia administration, a smaller diameter tube that is more flexible (8–12 French red rubber tube or silicon) and of sufficient length

(50–100 cm typ.) to allow attachment of the anesthetic machine tubing at some distance from the patient is desirable (Fig. 27.3b).

Insertion of the air sac cannula is relatively simple and can be accomplished following mask induction. The tube is inserted on either the right or left side. The site is prepared for surgical approach and a stab incision made in the last intercostal space midway between the attachment point of the ribs on the vertebral column and the intercostal joint (Fig. 27.4a–c) and extended slightly by blunt dissection with a hemostat. The tube is inserted between the ribs arriving in the posterior thoracic air sac. Successful placement of the tube can be assessed by holding a small feather over the open end of the tube, or by looking for condensation from expired air on the wall of a clear breathing tube. Once proper placement has been determined, adhesive tape "wings" are applied to the tube at the level of exit through the skin, and sutured to the body wall with two small sutures (Fig. 27.4b). Breathing tubes may be left in place for several days to allow time for management and relief of the source of dyspnea.

Positive Pressure Ventilation

Intermittent positive pressure ventilation is essential for ventilator support during extended anesthetic periods (>30 minutes). Despite leakage from the loose fitting nature of the intubation tube, manual ventilation can be achieved by compression of a rebreathing bag attached to the open anesthesia circuit or by an ambu bag. Because of leakage as well as little risk of overinflation given the compliance of the air sacs and coelomic wall, pressures and volumes used for ventilation can be judged by watching the excursions of the sternum in the dorsally recumbent bird or elevations of the base of the tail in the ventrally recumbent bird. Rate of ventilation for the nonspontaneously breathing raptor is generally 6–12 respirations per

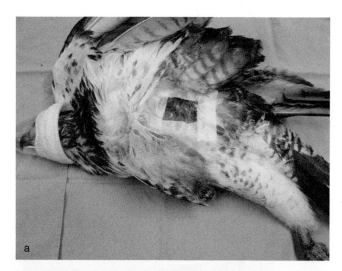
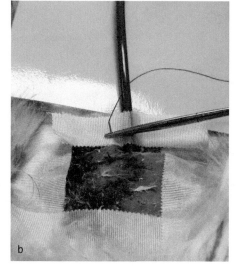
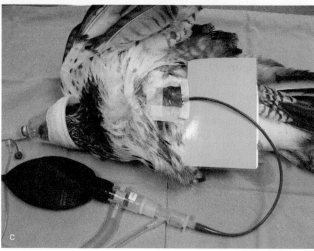

Figure 27.4. (a). Positioning of patient and preparation of insertion site in last intercostal space for air sac cannula: arrow indicates site. (b) Anchoring the air sac cannula in place by suturing tape wings to body wall. (c) Air sac cannula installed and attached to anesthesia administration tubing.

minute. Provision of intermittent positive pressure ventilation in the spontaneously breathing, anesthetized bird during a prolonged anesthetic episode is important; a rate of two cycles per minute is sufficient to maintain blood gases in a suitable range (Aguilar et al. 1995) for extended time periods. Though not commonly used, mechanical ventilators have been used to great effect by some clinicians (Hawkins & Pascoe 2007).

VASCULAR ACCESS

The sites for vascular access in general include the right jugular (in some cases, the left is sufficiently large to permit needle or catheter insertion), the basilic vein on the ventral aspect of the humerus, the cutaneous ulnar vein where it crosses the ventral aspect of the elbow, and the medial metatarsal vein, just proximal to the hock joint. The latter is somewhat variable. In addition, in raptors weighing less than 100 g, the cutaneous ulnar vein may be too small to access, except in falcons, where even in the case of kestrels and merlins, it is sufficiently large to allow venipuncture.

INJECTABLE DRUGS FOR (SEDATION) AND ANESTHESIA

While inhalant anesthetic agents are the workhorse of avian anesthesia and presently are highly recommended over injectable agents, there is a historical (Cooper 1974; Cooper & Frank 1974; Redig & Duke 1976) as well as increasing contemporary interest in the role of injectable agents as stand-alone short-term, reversible anesthetic agents, as sparing agents for isoflurane and other inhalant agents, and for sedation and analgesia (Table 27.1).

Analgesia is an important component of surgical anesthesia, and gas anesthetics alone are generally insufficient. Pain management is best accomplished through a multimodal approach where combinations of injectable drugs to address various pain pathways are used, thereby allowing lower concentrations of gas anesthetic and more effective pain management.

The recognized disadvantages of injectable agents are the interspecies variation and the general lack of research on a species-by-species basis to establish optimal dosing schedules and knowledge about pharmacological effects, not only for raptors, but for most avian species (Chapter 25). Some injectable drugs commonly used for minor procedures or as a preanesthetic for gas agents are discussed later. Prior to use of any injectable agents, the patient should be weighed to the nearest 10 g and the dose calculated accordingly.

Sedative Agents and Protocols

Benzodiazepines, such as diazepam (0.2–0.5 mg/kg IM) and midazolam (0.1–0.5 mg/kg IM), have been used

successfully for short nonpainful procedures or preanesthetic sedation. These drugs have sedative and antianxiety effects, as well as providing good muscle relaxation. However, they provide minimal analgesia. Recent reports in psittacines suggest use of midazolam directly instilled in the nares for sedation (2 mg/kg—Mans et al. 2011) or intramuscularly in combination with butorphanol (midazolam 0.25–0.5 mg/kg:butorphanol 1–3 mg/kg—Lennox 2011); limited experimentation in the clinic at The Raptor Center with bald eagles and a few other species suggests these protocols may have utility and should be researched further. Reversal of midazolam with flumazenil (0.05 mg/kg) is a further enhancement to its use.

Adrenergic agonists, such as xylazine (Freed & Baker 1989), medetomidine (Lawton 2008), and dexmedetomidine (Santangelo et al. 2009), may be used for general sedation or as a preanesthetic to inhalant anesthesia (Table 27.1). They have the advantages of requiring very small volumes and of being reversible with yohimbine or atipamezole. Lawton (2008) recommends the usage of medetomidine dosed at 60–85 μg/kg. Reported dosage ranges for the more potent dexmedetomidine ranged from 25 μg/kg in common buzzards (*Buteo buteo*) to 75 μg/kg in common kestrels (*Falco tinunculus*) (Santangelo et al. 2009). As adrenergic agonists, these agents may have some effect in countering hypotensive conditions associated with isoflurane anesthesia (Aguilar et al. 1995; Goelz et al. 1990; Schellbacher et al. 2011). Their use as immobilizing agents for anything other than minor surgical procedures is not recommended. These may have utility for conducting procedures in the field, such as a means of low stress restraint for transmitter attachment or blood collection (see later for use with opioids for analgesia).

These drugs are adequate for short procedures or can be utilized as a preanesthetic for inhalant anesthesia where they have a significant MAC-sparing and analgesic effects. Their use can cause notable bradycardia and respiratory depression. Xylazine has been used by some as a short-term sedative, but it is regarded as unreliable (though still useful with caution), owing to the cardiorespiratory effects and the possibility of hyperexcitability (Freed & Baker 1989; Lawton 2008).

Short-Term Anesthesia with Injectable Agents

Ketamine, a dissociative anesthetic, produces a dose-related unconsciousness and analgesia, but with highly variable species specific results and recoveries characterized by uncontrolled movements (Samour et al. 1984). Dosing varies between 10 and 200 mg/kg, according to the bird's size (the larger the bird, the smaller the per kilogram dose used; however, there is much species variability). We regard the upper end of this dosage range as excessively high and dangerous by a factor of 10. This drug should never be used alone. Despite indications of use in older literature (Redig &

Duke 1976), ketamine can be safely used only up to a dose of 20 mg/kg in raptors; lower doses are recommended, and these can be achieved by combining it with an adrenergic agonist.

Combinations of ketamine and alpha$_2$. adrenergic agonists (e.g., xylazine, medetomidine, and dexmedetomidine) or benzodiazepenes (diazepam and midazolam) have utility in anesthesia of raptors. A mixture of ketamine and diazepam was one of the original protocols utilized in raptors, but was found to be inferior to subsequent combinations of agents (Redig & Duke 1976). A combination of ketamine and xylazine (5:1 ratio) was extensively used at one time with varying degrees of success and marked species dependency as to results (Redig 1998). A combination of ketamine and xylazine in a 2:1 ratio was shown to be reversible with yohimbine and suggested to have utility for short procedures owing to the rapid metabolism of the ketamine (Degernes et al. 1988). Further study on xylazine alone as a sedative by Freed and Baker (1989) in a variety of raptors showed generally poor sedation, but good reversibility with yohimbine. For the most part, all uses of xylazine have been superseded by medetomidine or dexmedetomidine (Ramsey 2012).

Butorphanol (1–3 mg/kg IM q4–6h) is the most commonly used opioid for pain management in birds and is very effective for control of surgical pain at lower doses. Butorphanol, in combination with alpha$_2$ agonists (notably medetomidine), provides a useful protocol for short-term anesthesia (Ramsey 2012). Used as preoperative medication or a constant rate infusion (CRI) intraoperatively, butorphanol is inhalant-sparing. It is typically dosed at 1 mg/kg preanesthesia; however, doses as low as 0.3 mg/kg are effective as a preanesthetic agent; owing to its short half-life (1–q 2 hours), it may be repeated for long procedures (Hawkins & Pascoe 2007). Another opioid, fentanyl, has been demonstrated to reduce the minimum anesthetic dose (MAD) for isoflurane in red-tailed hawks (Pavez et al. 2010).

Propofol, a nonbarbiturate anesthetic, has been used as a bolus (1.33 mg/kg IV, titrate to effect) for induction and/or used as a CRI for maintenance of anesthesia. Propofol provides a rapid induction, but some species are reported to have extended recoveries and excessive excitement. A study in red-tailed hawks and great horned owls (Hawkins et al. 2003) utilizing propofol for induction by direct intravenous injection at 1 mg/kg/min followed by maintenance with CRI at predetermined doses (0.48 mg/kg/min for red-tailed hawks and 0.56 mg/kg/min for great horned owls) induced a light plane of anesthesia accompanied by transient CNS signs during recovery (Table 27.1). Respiratory depression and apnea were noted necessitating the recommendation that ventilatory support be provided in all phases of its use. The authors concluded this agent was of limited utility in these raptor species.

LOCAL AND REGIONAL ANESTHESIA (NERVE BLOCKS)

Regional anesthesia for perioperative anesthesia using nerve blocks have received scant attention and initial attempts involving blind injection of local anesthetics (lidocaine/bupivicaine) have yielded variable results in achieving brachial plexus nerve block (Brenner et al. 2010; Figueiredo et al. 2008). A significant improvement in efficacy has been reported by incorporating fentanyl with lidocaine (fentanyl 50 mcg/kg : lidocaine 15 mg/kg) and injecting it with the aid of a nerve locator. This approach was successful in providing analgesia and an isoflurane sparing effect in the repair of a humeral fracture in a peregrine falcon (d'Ovidio et al. 2011). While this appears to be a valuable approach to improving overall anesthesia for orthopedic procedures, clearly more work needs to be done to establish effective procedures across a variety of species and situations.

INHALANT ANESTHESIA

The halogenated hydrocarbons (isoflurane, sevoflurane, and desflurane) have been used successfully in wide variety of raptors (Table 27.2) and have replaced completely the use of halothane or methoxyfluorane. Each has its own characteristics of solubility in blood that affect the manner in which they are used. Isoflurane is the most utilitarian providing a suitably short induction time accompanied by little excitation, a sufficient downtime after mask removal to allow some short procedures, and a rapid recovery. It has been in use for raptors since the 1980s (Clutton 1986). Isoflurane has been shown to be arrhythmogenic in bald eagles (Aguilar et al. 1995). In addition, a Doppler echocardiography-based study showed that isoflurane, in addition to reducing heart rate, also reduced blood flow velocity; however, there was nonconcordant species variability in these measures (Straub et al. 2003). In contrast, sevoflurane and desflurane, while having shorter induction times and lesser cardiac and ventilatory impacts (Joyner et al. 2008), had very much more rapid recovery times, making it nearly impossible to conduct any examination or minor procedures with the mask removed before the bird began to recover (Granone et al. 2011). One study of sevoflurane in crested caracaras showed that while it caused mild reduction in various cardiopulmonary parameters, it was not arrhythmogenic (Escobar et al. 2009).

A study comparing isoflurane to sevoflurane was conducted in bald eagles (*Haliaeetus leucocephalus*) (Joyner et al. 2008). Sevoflurane produced more rapid induction and recovery than isoflurane, caused a lower increase in blood pressure, heart rate, and temperature over time, and had a slightly lesser occurrence of cardiac arrhythmias, though they were seen with both

Table 27.2. Inhalant anesthetics in raptors

Agent	Red-Tail	Bald Eagle	Golden Eagle	Great Horned Owl	Falcons	Other	Comment	Reference
Isoflurane		x					Reported incidence of arrhythmias	Aguilar et al. (1995)
Isoflurane/ sevoflurane		x					Showed decrease occurrence of arrhythmias with sevoflurane in bald eagles	Joyner et al. (2008)
Sevoflurane						Caracara	Moderate cardiovascular and respiratory depression	Escobar et al. (2009)
Isoflurane						Multiple species	Procedural methods for administering and monitoring isoflurane with observations on species variations in response	Redig (1998)
								Lawton (2008)
Various inhalants						Broad applications	General review of literature on use of inhalants	Fitzgerald and Blais (1993)
Isoflurane			x					Clutton (1986)
Isoflurane						Common buzzard (*Buteo buteo*)	Doppler-derived responses to isoflurane indicating alterations in blood flow velocity	Straub et al. (2003)
Isoflurane							Fentanyl administration resulted in reductions in isoflurane MAD without impact on blood gases or cardiovascular functions	Pavez et al. (2010)
Isoflurane					x			Molero et al. (2007)
Isoflurane			x				Among first reported uses of isoflurane in raptors—in 2:1 nitrous oxide:oxygen gas—difficulties with apnea, hypothermia, and inadequate immobilization at vaporizer setting of 1–1.5%	Clutton (1986)
Isoflurane/ sevoflurane/ desflurane	x						Compared three agents for induction, recovery parameters	Granone et al. (2011)

agents. Sevoflurane had higher MAC values than iso-flurane and was less likely to induce hypotension.

Preanesthetic Preparation

The goal of preanesthetic evaluation and preparation is to minimize the risk of anesthesia. While not always possible in emergency situations, taking the time to evaluate and prepare the patient can reduce the risk of an adverse event during anesthesia.

Fasting recommendations vary from none in small birds (use clean meat) with high metabolic rates to 12–24 hours in larger raptors (e.g., >500 g). If fasting is not an option, removing crop contents will reduce the risk of regurgitation and aspiration during recovery.

In addition to fasting, it is helpful to allow birds to acclimate in a quiet environment prior to anesthesia. This will allow for a decreased stress level and may reveal clinical symptoms previously hidden.

For raptors undergoing anesthesia for surgical procedures, fluids are routinely administered preoperatively during surgical preparation. Crystalloid (saline, lactated Ringers—up to 50 mL/kg) subcutaneously in the inguinal area or intravenous colloidal preparations (hetastarch—7 mg/kg) or combinations thereof may be used depending on circumstances. Crystalloids are generally sufficient to maintain vascular volume in the face of inhalant agent-induced vasodilatation (Steffey & Mama 2007). Colloids, however, may be indicated in providing prolonged vascular support if the there is a need to enhance colloidal osmotic pressure and arterial blood pressure, for instance, in hypoproteinemic patients. Insensible loss of fluids associated with the administration of 100% oxygen can be counteracted by incorporating an in-line bubbler vessel (Fig. 27.5) in the system to provide humidification of the airstream.

Pain Management and Inhalation Agent Sparing

Inhalation agents are regarded as having generally inadequate analgesia properties and therefore additional pain control is desirable. Utilization of this also reduces the amount of isoflurane necessary for a procedure. Butorphanol is the drug of choice, although this is based on limited information derived from pigeons. While dosage recommendations range from 1 to 3 mg/kg, our experience is doses as low as 0.3 mg/kg are effective. Typical surgical candidates (e.g., fracture patients) will have been placed on meloxicam (0.5–1.0 mg/kg) prior to surgical preparation, and this effectively reduces the amount of butorphanol required.

Atropine is avoided as it does not effectively dry up oral and pharyngeal secretions, tending instead to make them more viscous (Fitzgerald & Blais 1993).

Dyspnea

Even when severe or arising from severe air sac disease (e.g., aspergillosis), dyspnea is not usually regarded as

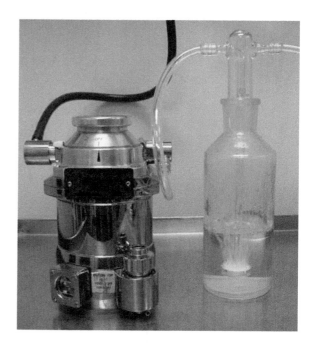

Figure 27.5.   In-line bubbler bottle for humidification of transport and anesthetic gases.

a contraindication to inhalant anesthesia. Between the state of unconsciousness, analgesia, and the 100% oxygen stream in which the gas is administered, dyspnea is almost always immediately lessened or relieved allowing relatively normal anesthesia to proceed. If possible, the cause of the dyspnea can be evaluated and sometimes alleviated (e.g., foreign body in the trachea).

Administration of Inhalant Agents

Induction   While sedative and preanesthetic agents are recommended in situations where restraint is difficult or undesirable, most inductions are undertaken by direct mask administration of the gaseous agent. An advantage of the highly efficient avian respiratory system is that it is very easy to rapidly induce anesthesia through a face mask. Anesthesia is typically induced with 4–5% isoflurane (or sevoflurane at 5–8%) in oxygen (1–2 L/min, depending on size of the patient) using a face mask and a nonrebreathing (Ayres T-piece or Bain) system. As soon as the bird begins to relax and the involuntary nictating membrane response slows, the vaporizer setting should be reduced to 2–3% and adjusted as necessary to maintain desired plane of anesthesia. For procedures lasting longer than 20–30 minutes, birds should be intubated as described earlier and in any case, intubation tubes should be available for emergencies. As many birds will keep their eyelids partially open during anesthesia, it is recommended to install ophthalmic ointment to prevent corneal drying.

Owls respond well to induction at lower concentrations of isoflurane, typically 1–2% with increasing concentrations as the animal begins to succumb to the agent. Use of higher levels results in a too rapid induction that increases the difficulty for equilibrating at a surgical plane without going into a dangerously deep level. Accipiters (especially sharp-shinned and sparrow hawks—goshawks and coopers hawks to a lesser extent) and merlins also benefit from a similar low dose approach to induction.

Maintenance Most raptors can be maintained at 1.5–2.5% isoflurane or 2–4% sevoflurane (lower concentrations if premedicated with analgesics or sedatives) with an oxygen flow rate of 1–2 L/min. Golden eagles and gyrfalcons require higher maintenance concentrations of isoflurane, usually at 3.5% or 4%. Anesthetic agents depress ventilation to a greater extent in birds than in mammals (Edling et al. 2001) and, therefore, hypoventilation should be presumed in all anesthetized birds. Intermittent positive pressure ventilation (2–4 times per minute) (Aguilar et al. 1995) manually administered is recommended to support the anesthetized patient. Since the avian patient can rapidly change condition during anesthesia, the patient should be constantly monitored by a person dedicated to this role. Key variables to monitor are respiratory rate and character (slow, even cycles being the desired condition), heart rate and rhythm, physical reflexes (especially corneal reflex), temperature, and blood pressure. Importantly, corneal and palpebral reflexes are slowed, but not eliminated during anesthetic episodes.

MONITORING

The following variables are routinely used for monitoring inhalation anesthesia: respiratory rate and character, nictating membrane response, toe pinch, heart rate, and muscle relaxation (neck or limb). In addition, monitoring body temperature through an esophageal or rectal thermometer is important to guard against both hyper- and hypothermia. In the intubated bird, end-tidal capnography using a side-stream sampling system (Fig. 27.6) is very effective for routine monitoring of ventilation (Desmarchelier et al. 2007; Edling et al. 2001). In such application, ventilation is managed so as to keep end-tidal CO_2 between 25 and 35 mmHg, effectively avoiding respiratory acidemia from inadequate ventilation, but not leading to respiratory alkalemia.

Respiratory Rate and Ventilation

As stated above, respiratory variables are the most important means of monitoring anesthesia. Respiratory patterns should be deep, even, and at a moderate rate—typically 12–20 cycles per minute. This rate, however, is highly variable depending on the size of the bird

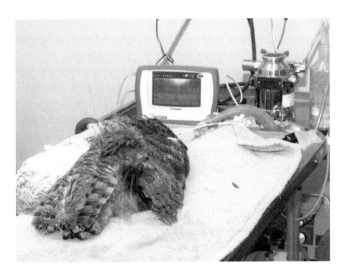

Figure 27.6. Capnographic unit in use. Note that there are collocated esophageal stethoscope and pulse oximeter transducers (not visible in this image).

with larger patients having slower respiratory rates. The character and pattern over the duration of the episode is more important than the absolute rate. Since changes in respiratory rate typically precede cardiac changes, respiration is probably the single most important factor to monitor.

It has been held in the past that because of their lack of alveoli, birds do not have a functional residual volume of air in their lungs to buffer changes in PaO_2 and $PaCO_2$ (Edling et al. 2001; McLelland 1989), and gas exchange does not occur unless there is movement of air through the air capillaries; this would suggest apnea could be immediately serious. Experience, however, has shown this not to be the case, and it has been argued (Hawkins & Pascoe 2007) birds contain a large reservoir of air in the air sacs, and when maintained on a 100% O2 supply, there is sufficient movement of gas across short diffusion distances to maintain O2 levels for a short period of time. This observation is consistent with our experience in anesthesia of thousands of raptors, and while not dismissing the risks of apnea, nonetheless, it moderates the reaction to it. Conversely, if apnea occurs in a bird breathing room air (e.g., if anesthetized with an injectable agent), apnea would be a considerably more serious issue requiring aggressive response. Potential causes of apnea include placement of an endotracheal tube, poor ventilation, dive response in waterfowl (trigeminal nerve response), hypothermia, and respiratory depression secondary to anesthetic drugs. The most important monitoring system for avian anesthesia is an alert technician who recognizes changes in respiratory patterns, evaluates the underlying causes, and corrects them. Should apnea occur, anesthetic gases should be turned off, the delivery system purged, oxygen flow reestablished and the patient manually ventilated. Oftentimes, manipulation or insertion (if not previously intubated) of the endotracheal tube or stimulation of the tongue, or the abdomen caudal to the sternum will reinitiate spontaneous breathing. If such stimulation is not effective, attach an ambu bag or other means of delivering air into the endotracheal tube (by mouth if necessary) and ventilate at 10–12 cycles per minute until respiration is restored. Gas delivery will need to be resumed at this point or the bird is likely to begin showing signs of recovery.

Heart Rate and Rhythm

In addition to a stethoscope (direct or esophageal), a Doppler monitor or EKG machine can be used to monitor heart rate and rhythm. Rates vary inversely with size of the bird. Small raptors will have rates >200bpm and generally too rapid to count. Mid-size birds (200–600g) will maintain heart rates between 180 and 250, while eagles will have heart rates of 80–150. Maintenance of an even, steady rhythm in the range of an acceptable rate for a given species is more important than an absolute number. Cardiac complications can be minimized by proper fluid therapy, oxygenation, ventilation, and appropriate anesthetic depth. Decreased heart rate should prompt a reduction of anesthetic gas concentration, evaluation and treatment of hypotension, and review of the patient's surgical situation (pain, tissue trauma, and positioning). Atropine administered intratracheally or via vascular access will often eliminate pain-related bradycardia. Hypotension is countered by crystalloid or colloid fluid administration. Cardiac arrest is typically preceded by apnea; however, on rare occasions it can occur without warning and largely for unknown reasons—underlying pathology is seldom found. Unfortunately, cardiac arrest is typically not successfully reversed.

Arrhythmias, primarily A-V blocks, have been reported to occur in a high percentage of bald eagles anesthetized with isoflurane (Aguilar et al. 1995; Joyner et al. 2008). However, it is not accompanied by cardiac arrest or other complications. Their causes are not apparent. As a practical matter, in our application in thousands of anesthetic episodes of anesthesia in eagles, they do not appear to present undue risk of morbidity or mortality.

Reflexes

Anesthetic depth can be evaluated by standard reflexes, such as palpebral, corneal, and pedal withdrawal, with corneal reflex being the most useful. For nonpainful procedures, a light plane of anesthesia will correlate with loss of voluntary motion, but with presence of all three monitored reflexes. At a surgical plane of anesthesia, the palpebral and withdrawal reflexes will be absent and the corneal reflex will be present, but slow.

Complete absence of a corneal reflex indicates a very deep state of anesthesia and is avoided.

Temperature

Monitoring and maintaining body temperature is critical in anesthetized raptor. Small raptors may quickly lose body heat as a result of impaired thermoregulation due to their small body mass relative to surface area. Large species and northern owl species that have a very heavy insulating down feather coats may become hyperthermic. In addition to impaired thermoregulation, the use of room temperature fluids, alcohol during surgical preparation, cool anesthetic gases, and removal of feathers can contribute to hypothermia. Difficulty maintaining an even anesthetic plane can be seen with either hypothermia or hyperthermia as a result of changes in ventilation. Monitoring body temperature can be done with an esophageal thermometer or a cloacal probe. Heat loss can be mitigated by providing a heat source such as a forced-air warming system (Bair Hugger®) or a circulating warm water blanket, or a conventional heating pad maintained on a low setting and usually turned off after a procedure has begun. The use of clear plastic surgical drapes may be beneficial in small birds as they provide both insulation for the patient as well as visualization of the patient. However, they are good insulators and will result in hyperthermia in larger raptors. Hyperthermia can be prevented or reversed by placing ice packs alongside the body of the patient.

VASCULAR SUPPORT

Prior to anesthesia, patients should be given a subcutaneous bolus of fluids (5mL/100g). For long surgical procedures or in critical patients, it is recommended to insert an indwelling catheter in an accessible vein shortly after induction, and provide a slow drip of an intravenous solution. This provides ready access to an injection port in the event antibradycardic (atropine) or emergency drugs need to be administered. Routinely, crystalloid fluids (saline or LRS) should be given at a rate of 10mL/kg/h for the first 2 hours, and then reduced to 5mL/kg/h for routine maintenance. Colloidal support may be added as deemed necessary, replacing a portion of the volume of crystalloids. Blood pressure assessment may be useful (Lloyd et al. 2007). When used with an appropriately sized blood pressure cuff, a Doppler unit may provide both heart rate and blood pressure information (Hawkins & Pascoe 2007); however, while useful for the former, high variability in blood pressure results diminish the usefulness of this method for routine monitoring (Zehnder et al. 2009). Alternatively, monitoring strength of pulse on a peripheral artery and the capillary refill time can be used as acceptable surrogates for actual blood pressure monitoring.

RECOVERY

Recovery is a critical phase of the anesthetic episode. Recovery is generally rapid once the gas anesthetic is removed, occurring gradually over several minutes (Joyner et al. 2008). The vaporizer should be turned off and the endotracheal tube briefly disconnected while the system is purged, then reattached so the bird can be maintained on oxygen during the recovery process and be prepared for assisted mechanical ventilation in the event of apnea. A brief excitatory phase will be experienced as the anesthetic plane lightens that may be accompanied by regurgitation. Extubation is done when the bird begins to make head movements. At the time of extubation and periodically during recovery, the oral cavity should be checked for signs of regurgitation or airway obstruction and any offending material removed with cotton-tipped applicators. It is critical not to impair the respiratory movements of the keel, as well as to be able to continue to monitor respiration. Gentle physical stimulation by moving the wings and legs can increase the rate/depth of respiration and help awaken the bird.

Once the bird is capable of upholding its head, it should be placed on a donut ring made from a towel and laid in a warm, dark, quiet environment to complete its recovery. Most birds are fully recovered in 30 minutes from inhalation anesthetic. Administration of butorphanol for intraoperative analgesia will typically cause the bird to sleep quietly for an extended time when left alone after recovery from the inhalant gases.

ANESTHETIC ADMINISTRATION THROUGH AN AIR SAC CANNULA

Gas flow rates need to be reduced relative to those that would be used for maintenance of a bird with either a face mask or an open system (0.5–1 L/min) (Fitzgerald & Blais 1993) or 2–3 times minute volume (Hawkins & Pascoe 2007) to prevent alkalemia from overventilation. Isoflurane and sevoflurane vaporizers have been shown to deliver anesthetics with acceptable precision and accuracy at flow rates as low as 0.05 L/min (50 mL/min), and some flow meters will allow accurate assessment of flow rate at levels as low as 0.05 L/min (Ambrisko & Klide 2006). Use of an in-line bubbler system not only humidifies the carrier gas, visualization of the stream of bubbles allows a further assessment of flow rate (Fig. 27.5). At this point, no guidelines exist for optimizing flow rates. As a practical matter, flow rates between 500 mL and 1 L/min are used; if there is a need to reduce ventilation, a smaller-diameter cannula size is used to reduce the rate of gas presentation into the air sac. Respiration movements cease entirely and monitoring is done by assessment of heart rate and corneal reflexes. Future refinements on this

methodology should include capnographic monitoring of exhaled gases and optimization of gas flows. A bird maintained with an air sac cannula will typically start to exhibit respiratory movements within less than a minute of the removal of the tube.

SPECIAL CONSIDERATIONS

Special attention needs to be applied when administering anesthetics to accipiter species of raptors (goshawks, Cooper's hawks, sparrowhawks, and sharp-shinned hawks). Injectable agents should be avoided entirely except as preanesthetic agents. It is advised that induction of these species start at low concentrations of isoflurane (1–2%) and be increased gradually over 2–3 minutes. A higher level of attention is paid to hydration status, pain reduction, and use of inhalant gas-sparing agents during anesthetic episodes. They are prone to sudden cardiac arrest, especially during recovery. The causes are not apparent (catecholamine-mediated?), but it appears to be associated with return of consciousness and visual awareness of their surroundings.

Additional use of pain management as an adjunct to isoflurane anesthesia is required for owls and golden eagles, and for most raptors when surgical procedures are being conducted on their feet (e.g., bumblefoot treatment). In general, this need can be met by dosing butorphanol at 1–3 mg/kg and repeating it every few hours during and after the surgical procedure, supplanting it with tramadol or meloxicam in the ensuing days.

REFERENCES

Aguilar RF, Smith VE, Ogburn P, Redig PT. 1995. Arrhythmias associated with isoflurane anesthesia in bald eagles (*Haliaeetus leucocephalus*). *Journal of Zoo and Wildlife Medicine* 26:508–516.
Ambrisko TD, Klide AM. 2006. Evaluation of isoflurane and sevoflurane vaporizers over a wide range of oxygen flow rates. *American Journal of Veterinary Research* 67:936–940.
Brenner JD, Larsen RS, Dickinson PJ, Wack RF, Williams, DC and Pascoe PJ. 2010. Development of an avian brachial plexus nerve block technique for perioperative analgesia in mallard ducks (*Anas platyrhynchos*). *Journal of Avian Medicine and Surgery* 24:24–34.
Carpenter JW. 2013. *Exotic Animal Formulary*, 4th ed. St. Louis: Elsevier-Saunders.
Clutton RE. 1986. Prolonged isoflurane anesthesia in the golden eagle. *Journal of Zoo Animal Medicine* 17:103–105.
Cooper JE. 1974. Metomidate anaesthesia of some birds of prey for laparotomy and sexing. *The Veterinary Record* 94:437–439.
Cooper JE, Frank LG. 1974. Use of the steroid anaesthetic CT 1341 in birds. *Raptor Research* 8:20–28.
Degernes LA, Kreeger TJ, Mandsager R, Redig PT. 1988. Ketamine-Xylazine anesthesia in red-tailed hawks with antagonism by yohimbine. *Journal of Wildlife Diseases* 24:322–326.
Desmarchelier M, Rondenay Y, Fitzgerald G, Lair S. 2007. Monitoring of the ventilatory status of anesthetized birds of prey by using end-tidal carbon dioxide measured with a microstream capnometer. *Journal of Zoo and Wildlife Medicine* 38:1–6.

d'Ovidio D, Noviello E, Nocerino M. 2011. Combination of fentanyl and lidocaine for brachial plexus block in a peregrine falcon. Proceedings of the European Association of Avian Veterinarians, pp. 394–396.

Edling TM, Degernes LA, Flammer K, Horne WA. 2001. Capnographic monitoring of anesthetized African grey parrots receiving intermittent positive pressure ventilation. *Journal of the American Veterinary Medical Association* 219:1714–1718.

Escobar A, Thiesen R, Vitaliano SN, Belmonte EA, Werther K, Nunes N, Valadao CAA. 2009. Some cardiopulmonary effects of sevoflurane in crested caracara (*Caracara plancus*). *Veterinary Anaesthesia and Analgesia* 36:436–441.

Figueiredo JP, Cruz ML, Mendes GM, Marucio RL, Ricco CH, Campagnol D. 2008. Assessment of brachial plexus blockade in chickens by an axillary approach. *Veterinary Anaesthesia and Analgesia* 35:511–518.

Fitzgerald G, Blais D. 1993. Inhalation anesthesia in birds of prey. In: *Raptor Biomedicine* (PT Redig, JE Cooper, JD Remple, DB Hunter, eds.), pp. 128–135. Minneapolis: University of Minnesota Press.

Freed D, Baker B. 1989. Antagonism of xylazine hydrochloride sedation in raptors by yohimbine chloride. *Journal of Wildlife Diseases* 25:136–138.

Goelz MF, Hahn AW, Kelley ST. 1990. Effects of halothane and isoflurane on mean arterial blood pressure, heart rate, and respiratory rate in adult Pekin ducks. *American Journal of Veterinary Research* 51:458–460.

Granone TD, Nicolas O, Killos MB, Quandt JE, Graham LF. 2011. Comparison of three different inhalant anesthetic agents (isoflurane, sevoflurane, desflurane) in red-tailed hawks (*Buteo jamaicensis*). Master's Thesis, University of Minnesota, College of Veterinary Medicine.

Hawkins MG, Pascoe PJ. 2007. Cagebirds. In: *Zoo Animal and Wildlife Immobilization and Anesthesia*, 1st ed. (G West, DJ Heard, N Caulkett, eds.), Ames: Wiley InterScience-Blackwell (online service).

Hawkins MG, Wright BD, Pascoe PJ, Kass PH, Maxwell LK, Tell LA. 2003. Pharmacokinetics and anesthetic and cardiopulmonary effects of propofol in red-tailed hawks (*Buteo jamaicensis*) and great horned owls (*Bubo virginianus*). *American Journal of Veterinary Research* 64:677–683.

Heard DJ. 1997. Avian respiratory anatomy and physiology. *Seminars in Avian and Exotic Pet Medicine* 6:172–179.

Joyner PH, Jones MP, Ward D, Gompf RE, Zagay N, Sleeman JM. 2008. Induction and recovery characteristics of cardiopulmonary effects of sevoflurane and isoflurane in bald eagles. *American Journal of Veterinary Research* 69:13–22.

Lawton MPC. 2008. Anesthesia and soft tissue surgery. In: *Avian Medicine*, 2nd ed. (J Samour, ed.), pp. 137–154. Philadelphia: Mosby-Elsevier.

Lennox AM. 2011. Sedation as an alternative to general anaesthesia in birds. Proceedings European Association Avian Veterinarians, pp. 250–253.

Lloyd C, Hebel C, Padrtova R. 2007. Non-invasive indirect blood pressure measurements in falconiformes. *Falco* 30:20–21.

Ludders JW. 1998. Respiratory physiology of birds: considerations for anesthetic management. *Seminars in Avian and Exotic Pet Medicine* 7:3–9.

Malka S, Hawkins MG, Jones JH, Pascoe PJ, Kass PH, Wisner ER. 2009. Effect of body position on respiratory system volumes in anesthetized red-tailed hawks (*Buteo jamaicensis*) as measured via computed tomography. *American Journal of Veterinary Research* 70:1155–1160.

Mans C, Guzman DSM, Lahner L, Paul-Murphy JR, Sladky KK. 2011. Intranasal midazolam causes conscious sedation in Hispaniolan Amazon Parrots (*Amazona ventralis*). Proceedings Association Avian Veterinarians, pp. 95–96.

McLelland J. 1989. Anatomy of the lungs and air sacs. In: *Form and Function in Birds*, Vol. 4 (AS King, J McLelland, eds.), pp. 221–279. New York: Academic Press.

Molero C, Bailey TA, Di Somma A. 2007. Anaesthesia of falcons with a combination of injectable anaesthesia (ketamine-medetomidine) and gas anaesthesia (isoflurane). *Falco* 30: 17–19.

Pavez JC, Pascoe P, Knych HKD, Kass PH, Hawkins MG. 2010. Effect of fentanyl target-controlled-infusions on isoflurane MAD for red-tailed hawks. Proceedings of the Association of Avian Veterinarians, p. 29.

Ramsey I, ed. 2012. *BSAVA Small Animal Formulary*, 7th ed. Gloucester: Wiley.

Redig PT. 1998. Recommendations for anesthesia in raptors with comments on trumpeter swans. *Seminars in Avian and Exotic Pet Medicine* 7:22–29.

Redig PT, Duke GE. 1976. Intravenously administered ketamine HCl and diazepam for anesthesia of raptors. *Journal of the American Veterinary Medical Association* 169:886–888.

Redig PT, Roush JC. 1978. Surgical approaches to the long bones of birds of prey. In: *Zoo and Wildlife Medicine*, 1st ed. (ME Fowler, ed.), pp. 246–253. Philadelphia: W.B. Saunders.

Samour J, Jones DM, Knight JA, Howlett JC. 1984. Comparative studies of the use of some injectable anaesthetic agents in birds. *The Veterinary Record* 114:6–11.

Santangelo B, Ferrari D, Di Martino I, Belli A, Cordella C, Ricco A, Troisi S, Vesce G. 2009. Dexmedetomidine chemical restraint of two raptor species undergoing inhalation anaesthesia. *Veterinary Research Communications* 33(Suppl. 1):S209–S211.

Schellbacher RW, DaCuhna A, Beaufrere H, Nevarez J, Tully TN. 2011. The effects of adrenergic agonists as a treatment for isoflurane-induced hypotension in Hispanioloan Amazon parrots (*Amazona ventralis*). Proceedings of the European Association of Avian Veterinarians, p. 67.

Steffey EP, Mama KR. 2007. Inhalation anesthetics. In: *Lumb and Jones' Veterinary Anesthesia and Analgesia*, 4th ed. (WJ Tranquilli, JC Thurman, KA Grimm, eds.), pp. 355–393. Ames: Blackwell Publishing.

Straub J, Forbes NA, Thielebein J, Pees M, Krautwald-Junghanns ME. 2003. The effects of isoflurane anaesthesia on some Doppler-derived cardiac parameters in the common buzzard (*Buteo buteo*). *Veterinary Journal (London, England: 1997)* 166:273–276.

Zehnder AM, Hawkins MG, Pascoe PJ, Kass PH. 2009. Evaluation of indirect blood pressure monitoring in awake and anesthetized red-tailed hawks (*Buteo jamaicensis*): effects of cuff size, cuff placement, and monitoring equipment. *Veterinary Anaesthesia and Analgesia* 36:464–479.

28 Galliformes and Columbiformes

Darryl Heard

INTRODUCTION

The order Galliformes contains the megapodes, guans, chachalacas, currasows, pheasants, grouse, junglefowl, and peafowl. Most galliformes are robust ground-dwelling birds, but are able to fly. The order Columbiformes includes pigeons and doves. The typical columbiforme has a short bill, small head, compact body, and short legs (Baptista et al. 1997).

Several species from these two orders are important for food production. For example, the domestic chicken, derived from the jungle fowl, is used for both meat and egg production. Many are also displayed in zoos and kept as pets. Some are highly endangered (Baptista et al. 1997; del Hoyo et al. 1994). The chicken and the rock dove (*Columba livia*), or pigeon, are commonly used in avian research. The latter is also a ubiquitous urban inhabitant.

ANATOMY AND PHYSIOLOGY

Avian anatomy and physiology relevant to anesthesia is described in Chapter 24. Columbiforme species range in size from the 30-g common ground dove (*Columbina passerina*) to the 2-kg crowned pigeons of New Guinea (Baptista et al. 1997). One of the largest galliformes is the wild turkey (*Meleagris gallopavo*), weighing up to 8–10 kg. The currasows and guans have markedly elongated tracheas relative to body size (Fitch 1999). This is thought to be an evolutionary adaptation to exaggerate the apparent size of a vocalizing bird.

PHYSICAL RESTRAINT

Both columbiformes and galliformes are relatively easy to handle. The main threat to the human restrainer is the large spurs present in some galliformes species. Galliformes will often sit still in the presence of a perceived threat. When given the opportunity, however, they use their powerful leg and flight muscles to explosively propel themselves into the air. In the process, many will shed feathers (fright molt) to prevent a predator or human grabbing hold. The feather loss can be extensive and aesthetically unpleasant, especially for zoo display animals and private pets. Rapid acceleration into the air can also propel the animal into a ceiling, cage top, or wire, causing severe trauma to the animal. Loss of skin on the skull can be extensive and potentially life-threatening. To reduce injury in aviaries, a false soft ceiling can be constructed to allow for absorption of the impact force. Similarly, when temporarily housing these birds, they should be kept in a quiet dark environment. Even short periods of struggling may lead to hyperthermia. This will be exacerbated in birds adapted to a cold environment (e.g., grouse and ptarmigan). Many galliformes are also excellent runners and readily escape a human pursuer. Camouflaged plumage sometimes makes detection in vegetation very difficult.

Pigeons can be gently held in the hand. One hold can incorporate the tail and legs in one grip. Similar to galliformes, however, they can launch themselves explosively into the air and escape.

Many food production species are obese and may have hepatic lipidosis. The author has seen spontaneous liver rupture and fatal hemorrhage in quail during handling related to the latter problem.

VASCULAR ACCESS

Vascular access is as in other birds (Chapter 25) and includes the external jugular, the basilic and the medial tarsometatarsal or saphenous vein. The external jugular veins of pigeons are difficult to identify because they are usually made up of a plexus rather than a distinct vessel. Intraosseous catheters are placed in the humerus, tibiotarsus, or femur. Intraosseous catheters have been used for administration of propofol in pigeons (Guimarães et al. 2006; Lopez et al. 1994). In large galliformes, the medial saphenous vein is a useful site to administer parenteral anesthetics in physically restrained animals.

ENDOTRACHEAL INTUBATION

Endotracheal intubation is usually simple. Columbiformes and galliformes can sometimes produce copious amounts of tracheal mucous. This may obstruct the tube or produce a "flapper valve" effect that allows air into the respiratory system with positive pressure ventilation, but not out. In these species, the patient needs to be monitored carefully to prevent hyperinflation. Clear endotracheal tubes are preferred to visualize any respiratory discharge, and periodic extubation to assess for blockage may be necessary during prolonged procedures.

As discussed earlier, the convoluted tracheal anatomy of currasows and guans may cause problems if secretions increase in response to intubation or the bird aspirates gastric reflux under anesthesia. Some clinicians prefer not to intubate these species because of the potential for tracheal obstruction or stenosis postoperatively (Evans et al. 2009). This, unfortunately, precludes supportive ventilation. If fluid accumulation is suspected (i.e., increased respiratory noise), it must be removed with suction. A long suction tube is placed as far down the trachea through the endotracheal tube and aspiration performed as the tube is pulled out. If this fails to relieve the problem, then either endoscopy or radiographic evaluation must be performed. If the obstruction cannot be immediately corrected, an air sac cannula will need to be placed for recovery (Chapters 25 and 28).

PRE-ANESTHETIC CONSIDERATIONS

As with all patients, physical examination is indicated prior to anesthesia. This may, however, be difficult in some galliformes because of stress and struggling. Prolonged struggling may lead to hyperthermia and potential myopathy (Spraker et al. 1987). Species adapted to cold (e.g., grouse) or high montane (e.g., some species of pheasant and tragopan) environments are more likely to develop these problems.

Both galliformes and columbiformes possess large complex crops. Depending on the physiological status of the bird, fasting for 4 or more hours may reduce the amount of food in the crop. Fluids should also be removed in animals that are likely to drink excessively.

The body condition of the bird should be assessed. As mentioned previously, many domestic species bred for food production are obese and have substantial intracoleomic fat accumulation. This fat decreases air-sac volume and may contribute to lung compression in dorsally recumbent birds. Both effects may be additive to anesthetic-induced hypoventilation and explain the apparent increased anesthetic morbidity and mortality seen in these species. Similarly, birds bred for egg production are more likely to have egg-yolk coelomitis, which can lead to fibrosis, fluid accumulation, and debilitating systemic infection and illness. A high fat to total body ratio may also be associated with abnormal drug distribution and accumulation resulting in delayed induction and recovery.

LOCAL AND REGIONAL ANESTHESIA

Local anesthetics can be used as in other avian species (Chapter 25). Care must be taken to ensure accurate calculation and administration of local anesthetics to prevent intoxication.

Brachial plexus blockade has been used experimentally in chickens with variable success (Cardozo et al. 2009; Figueiredo et al. 2008). Figueiredo et al. (2008) dissected chicken cadavers to determine anatomical landmarks for correct catheter placement. They then sedated adult female chickens (midazolam 1 mg/kg, butorphanol 1 mg/kg IM) and after 15 minutes restrained the birds in lateral recumbency with their heads covered. The wing to be blocked was abducted at a 90° angle to the thorax, and the apex of the axilla (proximal condyle of the humerus, proximal region of the coracoid and scapula) was palpated. A 20-SWG 50-mm catheter electrode (Braun Melsungen AG, Melsungen, Germany), teflon-coated except at the tip, was attached to a peripheral nerve stimulator (2–5 Hz, 0.12 mA; S48 stimulator; Grass, Warwick, RI). The catheter extension was filled and connected to a 3-mL syringe containing either lidocaine (20 mg/mL, 1 mL/kg) with epinephrine or bupivacaine (5 mg/mL, 1 mL/kg). The catheter was inserted at a 45° angle to the skin just below the apex of the axilla. It was advanced through the pectoralis muscle and fascia toward the chest wall in to the region around the first rib. The appropriate muscle response was confirmed when there was muscle contraction and flexion of the wing. Proximity to the brachial plexus was assessed as when the strongest abduction of the humerus and flexion of the wing occurred. After localization of the brachial plexus by the nerve stimulator, the local anesthetic solution was injected in 0.5-mL aliquots into the plexus sheath over 60 seconds. Onset of sensory denervation was 3–5 minutes, and duration of blockade was 60–90 minutes. The researchers, however, observed a relatively high failure rate of 33% with this technique. Cardozo et al. (2009) had more success using ropivacaine (0.75%, 1 mL/kg of the). The onset and duration of effect was approximately 15 and 115 minutes, respectively.

ANALGESIA

Analgesia is covered in Chapter 7. NSAIDs, opioids, and tramadol have been used and studied in these and other birds. In birds, NSAID pharmacokinetics and therapeutic index is highly variable, making safe drug selection difficult (Baert & De Backer 2003). Of the presently available NSAIDs, this author prefers using meloxicam (0.2–0.5 mg/kg sid to bid, PO or IM). Regardless of the drug and species, each analgesic regimen should be tailored to the individual and the type and severity of pain (Chapter 7). A multi-modal approach may be necessary, especially for severe and chronic pain. Although birds appear to respond best to κ opioid agonists (i.e., butorphanol 0.3–2.0 mg/kg bid to tid), there are a few papers indicating μ opioid agonists (morphine and fentanyl) are appropriate in some species and situations (Chapter 7; Concannon et al. 1995; Evrard & Balthazart 2002). For example, in Japanese quail (*Cortunix japonica*), morphine at relatively high dosages (10 and 20 mg/kg IM) significantly altered response latency and threshold in the hot water and foot pressure quantitative nocioception tests (Evrard & Balthazart 2002). These effects were blocked by naloxone.

Baert and De Backer (2003) studied the pharmacokinetics of a single intravenous dose of sodium salicylate (25 mg/kg), meloxicam (0.5 mg/kg), and flunixin (1.1 mg/kg) in five bird species, including chickens, turkeys, and pigeons. Chickens had a half-life (5.5 hours) approximately 10-fold as long as the other species for flunixin. The half-life of chickens (3.2 hours) and pigeons (2.4 hours) was threefold as long as the other bird species for meloxicam, and, for salicylic acid, the half-life in pigeons (14.9 hours) was at least three- to fivefold longer than in the other bird species. Once again, this study emphasizes the variability in response to NSAIDs in birds and the potential for toxicity.

Meloxicam (0.5 mg/kg IM) was ineffective in minimizing postoperative orthopedic pain in pigeons (Desmarchelier et al. 2012). A higher dosage (2.0 mg/kg IM), however, provided quantifiable analgesia that appeared safe in experimental conditions (Desmarchelier et al. 2012). In pigeons, carprofen (2–10 mg/kg IM once daily for seven days) was associated with increased aspartate aminotransferase and alanine aminotransferase enzyme concentrations, gross lesions in muscle injection sites and liver, and histologic lesions in liver and muscle (Zollinger et al. 2011). Meloxicam (5 mg/kg SC) and carprofen (25 mg/kg) improved gait function in a group of mildly lame broiler chickens (Caplen et al. 2013). The effects and safety of repetitive dosing were not evaluated.

Hussain et al. (2008) investigated the toxicopathological effects of diclofenac sodium (0, 0.25, 2.5, 10 and 20 mg/kg PO for 7 days) in broiler chicks (15 days old), pigeons (3 months old), and Japanese quail (4 weeks old). Dose-dependent clinical signs in all included depression, somnolence, decreased body weight, and mortality. Severity of clinical disease was most severe in broiler chicks, followed by pigeons and Japanese quail. Broiler chicks and pigeons developed visceral gout at the higher dosages (10 and 20 mg/kg), but not Japanese quail. The kidneys and liver were enlarged in all and the kidneys showed acute renal necrosis. The livers also showed fatty change and necrosis of hepatocytes.

Tramadol appears useful for managing postoperative as well as chronic pain associated with degenerative joint disease. This drug is metabolized to an active metabolite, O-desmethyltramadol (Black et al. 2010). Although relatively high dosages (≥5–10 mg/kg once to twice a day PO) are being recommended in birds based on some pharmacokinetic studies (Black et al. 2010; Souza et al. 2009, 2011, 2012) and a pain response study in Hispaniolan parrots (Guzman et al. 2012), this author has seen good responses in some birds with degenerative joint disease at lower dosages (1–5 mg/kg once to twice a day PO). Further research is necessary to define blood levels associated with analgesia in birds, rather than using human levels. The main observed side effects are anorexia, ataxia and dysphoria, and vomiting. These effects may be seen at high dosages or after repetitive dosing. There also appears to be some individual variation in response, possibly due to variable metabolism to the active form.

INDUCTION AND MAINTENANCE PROTOCOLS

Sedative and parenteral anesthetic dosages are summarized in Table 28.1.

Sedation

All birds are relatively resistant to the effects of alpha-2-adrenergic agonists. In pigeons, xylazine (16 mg/kg IM) or detomidine (1.4 mg/kg IM) produced only minor to moderate sedation adequate for handling and sample collection (Durrani et al. 2008, 2009). Similarly, in pigeons, medetomidine (0.08–2.0 mg/kg IM) produced inadequate sedation for handling and minor diagnostic procedures accompanied by moderate bradypnea and bradycardia (Pollock et al. 2001; Sandmeier 2000). At the lower end of the dosage range, it only produced ataxia to sternal recumbency with retention of the righting reflex (Pollock et al. 2001). In chickens, and presumably other birds, xylazine inhibits ventricular activity (Park & Park 1988). The duration of this effect is dose dependent, and reversible with either yohimbine or 4-aminopyridine.

Table 28.1. Parenteral anesthetics used in domestic galliformes and columbiformes

Species	Ketamine (K)	Xylazine	Medetomidine (M)	Detomidine	Diazepam (D)	Midazolam	Butorphanol (B)	Comments	Reference
Chicken rooster	25 IM	3 IM			4 IM			Xylazine given 15 minutes before other drugs. Adequate anesthesia for typhylectomy, but associated with hypothermia, cardiopulmonary depression, and prolonged recovery.	Mostachio et al. (2008)
Chicken white leghorn cockerel	10 IV	2 IV						Drugs combined in single injection. Induction and recovery approximately 2 and 70 minutes, respectively. Adequate anesthesia for typhylectomy. Bradycardia and bradypnea.	Maiti et al. (2006)
Chicken white leghorn cockerel	75 IM				2.5 IV			Ketamine given 5 minutes after diazepam. Induction and recovery approximately 9 and 80 minutes, respectively. Adequate anesthesia for typhylectomy. Hypothermia.	Maiti et al. (2006)
Chicken white leghorn cockerel	50 IV					2 IM		Ketamine given 5 minutes after midazolam. Induction and recovery approximately 18 and 100 minutes, respectively. Adequate anesthesia for typhylectomy.	Maiti et al. (2006)
Chicken layer	15 IM							Approx. 30 minutes between loss of righting to sternal recumbency. Adequate anesthesia for typhylectomy.	Eyarefe and Oguntoye (2012)
Chicken layer	15 IM							Combined with lidocaine 4 SC infiltrated along midline incision. Duration of recumbency approximately 100 minutes. Mild bradycardia, bradypena, and hypothermia relative to ketamine alone.	Eyarefe and Oguntoye (2012)
Guinea fowl	15 IM	2.5 IM						No apparent analgesia in response to clamping of skin and toes.	Ajadi et al. (2009)
Guinea fowl	15 IM	2.5 IM				0.3 IM		Duration of analgesia 37 ± 24 minutes. Midazolam prolonged recumbency, but was associated with some regurgitation and bradypnea.	Ajadi et al. (2009)
Guinea fowl	25 IM	1.0 IM						Rapid onset and good surgical anesthesia. Yohimbine 1.0 IV 40 minutes after XK administration shortened recovery.	Teare (1987)
Pigeon	60 IM							Light sedation and anesthesia/analgesia. Hyperthermia and rough recovery. Not recommended for use alone.	Durrani et al. (2008)
Pigeon				1.4 IM				Light sedation and anesthesia/analgesia. Bradypnea, bradycardia, and hypothermia. Safe for handling and least painful procedures.	Durrani et al. (2008)

Species	Dose	Dose	Dose	Comments	Reference
Pigeon	60 IM		1.4 IM	Rapid onset of action (approximately 2 minutes). Prolonged deep anesthesia and recovery with bradypnea, bradycardia, and hypothermia. Can be used for major surgical procedures.	Durrani et al. (2008)
Pigeon	100 IM	0.2 IM	0.2 IM	Ketamine given 15 minutes after MB. M reversed with atipamezole 60 minutes after K. Effective anesthesia for approx. 90% pigeons. Bradypnea, bradycardia, arrhythmias, and hypothermia.	Atalan et al. (2002)
Pigeon	120 IM	0.2 IM	0.2 IM	K 10 minutes after M. Deep anesthesia 15–60 minutes associated with initial tachypnea then bradypnea, profound bradycardia and progressive hyperthermia. Prolongation of P-R and R-R intervals on ECG.	Uzun et al. (2003)
Pigeon	30 IM	0.125 IM	0.125 IM	M reversed with atipamezole 0.065 IM at first sign of recovery. Deeper anesthesia and analgesia than D-K. Recovery rapid and smooth. Clinically, level of anesthesia unreliable and associated with wing flapping.	Lumeij and Deenik (2003)
Pigeon	60 IM		2 IM	Prolonged recovery.	Lumeij and Deenik (2003)
Pigeon	10 IM		0.2 IM	Sedation and muscle relaxation without loss of consciousness.	Azizpour and Hassani (2012)
Pigeon	75–150 IM	16 IM		Extensor rigidity, salivation, dose-dependent hypoxemia, respiratory academia, and hypercapnia.	Neal et al. (1981)
Pigeon	60 IM			Light sedation/anesthesia. Safe for handling and less painful procedures.	Durrani et al. (2009)
Pigeon	30 IM	8 IM		Light sedation/anesthesia and rough recovery. Not recommended.	Durrani et al. (2009)
Pigeon				Rapid onset (2 minutes). Deep anesthesia/analgesia with prolonged recovery. Suitable for painful procedures ≤90 minutes.	Durrani et al. (2009)
Pigeon	0.08–0.20 IM			Ataxia to sternal recumbency, but righting response retained.	Pollock et al. (2001)
Pigeon	5 IM	0.08 IM		Variable effects; mild to moderate sedation.	Pollock et al. (2001)
Pigeon	0.08 IM		0.5 IM	Variable effects; mild to moderate sedation.	Pollock et al. (2001)

Note: Dosages are in mg/kg.

477

Intranasal pipette administration of either xylazine (30 mg/kg), diazepam (6 mg/kg), or midazolam (6 mg/kg) provided fast reliable sedation in pigeons (Moghadam et al. 2009). Unlike the benzodiazepines, however, xylazine failed to produce adequate sedation for dorsal recumbency, and sedation was prolonged. The onset of action of midazolam was more rapid than diazepam.

In rock partridges (*Alectoris graeca*), xylazine (10 mg/kg IM), medetomidine (0.15 mg/kg IM), detomidine (0.3 mg/kg IM), or diazepam (6 mg/kg IM) produced variable sedation adequate to allow handling and for radiography (Uzun et al. 2006). Duration of effect and time to recovery were prolonged, especially for diazepam and detomidine. The greatest sedation was observed with xylazine, but as would be expected, it produced profound respiratory depression. All drugs were associated with decreased cloacal temperatures over time.

Parenteral Anesthesia

Ketamine and ketamine combinations have either been evaluated or used clinically in both galliformes and columbiformes (Table 28.1). The adverse effects are the same as in other avian species. Ketamine alone is not recommended because of increased salivation, muscle rigidity, and rough, sometimes prolonged recoveries associated with wing flapping and struggling. The addition of a benzodiazepine (i.e., diazepam or midazolam) provides improved muscle relaxation and sedation, but not analgesia. The addition of an alpha-2-adrenergic agonist (i.e., xylazine, detomidine, medetomidine) is also associated with improved muscle relaxation, as well as surgical analgesia. They are, however, more likely to produce cardiopulmonary depression, hypothermia and prolonged recovery. Atipamezole, administered IM when birds first show signs of recovery, can be used to reverse medetomidine, detomidine and xylazine.

In guinea fowl, yohimbine (1.0 mg/kg IV) shortened recovery from a combination of xylazine (1.0 mg/kg IM) and ketamine (25 mg/kg IM) (Teare 1987). Butorphanol added to the ketamine combinations further enhances surgical analgesia, but will also further depress cardiopulmonary function (Atalan et al. 2002).

The short-acting anesthetic propofol has been evaluated in pigeons (Fitzgerald & Cooper 1990; Guimarães et al. 2006), wild turkeys (Schumacher et al. 1997), and chickens (Lukasik et al. 1997). Propofol administration using the medial saphenous vein facilitates induction of large birds. In turkeys, propofol (5 mg/kg IV) administered over 20 seconds produced a rapid induction, but was associated with a short period of apnea, then bradypnea, hypercarbia, hypoxemia, and hypotension (Schumacher et al. 1997). Anesthesia was successfully maintained with a constant rate infusion of 0.5 mg/kg/min. Recovery was rapid and smooth once the infusion was discontinued. Propofol does not produce analgesia,

and must be used with other drugs for painful surgical procedures.

In pigeons, propofol (14 mg/kg IV) produced smooth rapid induction and good muscle relaxation (Fitzgerald & Cooper 1990). The duration of effect was 2–7 minutes and associated with marked respiratory depression. A very narrow safety margin was observed when ventilation was not assisted.

In chickens, propofol (4.5–9.7 mg/kg IV), followed by a constant rate infusion (0.5–1.5 mg/kg/min) for 20 minutes produced rapid induction and general anesthesia (Lukasik et al. 1997). As in other species, sometimes, marked cardiopulmonary depression was observed. Single or multiple runs of premature ventricular complexes were also observed in many birds. One bird required lidocaine (0.5 mg/kg IV) for ventricular tachycardia. Propofol at three times the induction dosage was fatal in all birds, indicating it has a low therapeutic index (Lukasik et al. 1997).

Intubation and ventilation, preferably with oxygen, is recommended when parenteral anesthetics are used for surgery and prolonged anesthesia. Administration of balanced electrolyte solutions either IV or IO will also ameliorate some of their hypotensive effects.

Inhalation Anesthesia

Isoflurane and sevoflurane are the most commonly used inhalant anesthetics in clinical practice. Their physiological effects and potencies in galliformes and columbiformes are the same as in other avian orders (Korbel 1998; Naganobu & Hagio 2000; Naganobu et al. 2000). Sevoflurane is associated with a more rapid recovery (Korbel 1998). As described previously, many domestic species have large stores of intracoelomic fat that impair ventilation, potentially prolonging inhalant anesthetic equilibration and recovery.

In chickens, both the μ opioid receptor agonist morphine and the κ agonist U50488H decreased isoflurane MAC in a dose-dependent (1–3 mg/kg IV) manner without significant effects on heart rate and blood pressure (Concannon et al. 1995). Compared with halothane or pentobarbital, isoflurane anesthesia resulted in a significantly lower threshold for electrical fibrillation of the chicken heart (Greenlees et al. 1990). In isoflurane-anesthetized pigeons, controlled ventilation delivered by a pressure-limited device was not associated with clinically important adverse cardiopulmonary changes but may be associated with respiratory alkalemia and cardiovascular depression when air sac integrity has been disrupted (Touzot-Jourde et al. 2005).

Although not an anesthetic or analgesic, the nondepolarizing, short-acting muscle relaxant atracurium besylate (0.15–0.45 mg/kg IV) can be used as an adjunct to inhalation anesthesia (Nicholson & Ilkiw 1992). Muscle relaxation is monitored with a nerve stimulator, and reversed with edrophonium (0.5 mg/kg IV). In chickens, the effective dosage of atracurium to result in

95% twitch depression in 50% of birds was 0.25 mg/kg, whereas the dosage to result in 95% twitch depression in 95% of birds was 0.46 mg/kg (Nicholson & Ilkiw 1992). The duration of effect at 0.25 mg/kg was approximately 35 minutes; at the highest dosage (0.45 mg/kg), 50 minutes. The cardiopulmonary effects of atracurium and edrophonium were clinically insignificant.

MONITORING

Monitoring is the same as in other birds (Chapter 25), and similar to mammals (Chapter 3). The bispectral index has been successfully used and validated to monitor brain electrical activity and level of unconsciousness in chickens during isoflurane anesthesia (Martin-Jurado et al. 2008).

End-tidal carbon dioxide concentration ($ETCO_2$), an indirect measure of $PaCO_2$, is inaccurate in pigeons and probably other avian species (Touzot-Jourde et al. 2005). This is particularly so during celioscopy, when the air sacs are perforated (Touzot-Jourde et al. 2005). Similarly, in chickens, $ETCO_2$ was not accurate in predicting $PaCO_2$ values in birds ventilated using air sac cannulation (Paré et al. 2013).

FIELD IMMOBILIZATION (WILD CAPTURE)

Physical trapping and capture techniques are well described by Bub et al. (1996). As mentioned previously, the main problems associated with wild galliformes in particular, and columbiformes to a lesser degree, is self-trauma, "fright" molting, and hyperthermia with associated capture myopathy (Spraker et al. 1987). Inhalation anesthesia using a precision vaporizer, when available, is preferred for induction because it is rapid and likely to minimize struggling. Intranasal midazolam (1–2 mg/kg) may achieve rapid sedation and decrease struggling and stress-induced injury.

Alpha-chlorolose has been used for sedation and capture of wild turkeys and doves (Bergman et al. 2007; Martin 1967). It is administered orally, has a prolonged effect, and can be associated with mortality. When used for capture of birds that may later be killed for food, local rules and regulations must first be reviewed.

REFERENCES

Ajadi RA, Kasali OB, Makinde AF, Adeleye AI, Oyewusi JA, Akintunde OG. 2009. Effect of midazolam and ketamine-xylazine anesthesia in Guinea fowl (*Numida meleagris galeata*). *Journal of Avian Medicine and Surgery* 23:199–204.

Atalan G, Uzun M, Demirkan I, Yildiz S, Cenesiz M. 2002. Effect of medetomidine-butorphanol-ketamine anaesthesia and atipamezole on heart and respiratory rate and cloacal temperatures of domestic pigeons. *Journal of Veterinary Medicine Series A* 49:281–285.

Azizpour A, Hassani Y. 2012. Clinical evaluation of general anaesthesia in pigeons using a combination of ketamine and diazepam. *Agricultural Journal* 7:101-105.

Baert K, De Backer P. 2003. Comparative pharmacokinetics of three non-steroidal anti-inflammatory drugs in five bird species. *Comparative Biochemistry and Physiology. C: Comparative Pharmacology* 134:25–33.

Baptista LF, Trail PW, Horblit HM. 1997. Family columbidae (pigeons and doves). In: *Handbook of the Birds of the World. Vol.4. Sandgrouse to Cuckoos* (J del Hoyo, A Elliott, J Sargatal, eds.), pp. 60–243. Barcelona: Lynx Edicions.

Bergman D, Wakeling BF, Veenendaal TB, Eisemann JD, Seamans TW. 2007. Current and historical use of alpha-chlorolose on wild turkeys. USDA National Wildlife Research Center:Staff Publications. Paper 754.

Black PA, Cox SK, Macek M, Tieber A, Junge RE. 2010. Pharmacokinetics of tramadol hydrochloride and its metabolite O-desmethyltramadol in peafowl (*Pavo cristatus*). *Journal of Zoo and Wildlife Medicine* 41:671–676.

Bub H, Hamerstrom F, Wuertz-Schaefer K. 1996. *Bird Trapping and Bird Banding: A Handbook for Trapping Methods all Over the World.* Ithaca: Cornell University Press.

Caplen G, Colborne GR, Hothersall B, Nicol CJ, Waterman-Pearson AE, Weeks CA, Murrell JC. 2013. Lame broiler chickens respond to non-steroidal anti-inflammatory drugs with objective changes in gait function: a controlled clinical trial. *Veterinary Journal (London, England: 1997)* 196:477–482.

Cardozo LB, Almeida RM, Fiúza LC, Galera PD. 2009. Brachial plexus blockade in chickens with 0.75% ropivacaine. *Veterinary Anaesthesia and Analgesia* 36:396–400.

Concannon KT, Dodam JR, Hellyer PW. 1995. Influence of a mu- and kappa-opioid agonist on isoflurane minimal anesthetic concentration in chickens. *The American Journal Veterinary Research* 56:806–811.

del Hoyo J, Elliott A, Sargatal J, eds. 1994. *Handbook of Birds of the World. Volume 2. New World Vultures to Guineafowl.* Barcelona: Lynx Edicions.

Desmarchelier M, Troncy E, Fitzgerald G, Lair S. 2012. Analgesic effects of meloxicam administration on postoperative orthopedic pain in domestic pigeons (*Columba livia*). *American Journal of Veterinary Research* 73:361–367.

Durrani UF, Khan MA, Ahmad SS. 2008. Comparative efficacy (sedative and anesthetic) of detomidine, ketamine and detomidine-ketamine cocktail in pigeons (*Columba livia*). *Pakistan Veterinary Journal* 28:115–118.

Durrani UF, Ashraf M, Khan MA. 2009. A comparison of the clinical effects associated with xylazine, ketamine, and a xylazine-ketamine cocktail in pigeons (*Columba livia*). *Turkish Journal of Animal and Veterinary Science* 33:413–417.

Evans A, Atkins A, Citino SB. 2009. Tracheal stenosis in a blue-crowned currasow (*Crax alberti*). *Journal of Zoo and Wildlife Medicine* 40:373–377.

Evrard HC, Balthazart J. 2002. The assessment of nociceptive and non-nociceptive skin sensitivity in the Japanese quail (*Coturnix japonica*). *Journal of Neuroscience Methods* 116:135–146.

Eyarefe OD, Oguntoye CO. 2012. A randomized trial of low-dose ketamine and lidocaine infiltration for laparo-caecectomy in layer chickens. *International Journal of Animal and Veterinary Advances* 4:252–255.

Figueiredo JP, Mariângela LC, Guilherme MM, Marucio RL, Ricco CH, Campagnol D. 2008. Assessment of brachial plexus blockade in chickens by an axillary approach. *Veterinary Anaesthesia and Analgesia* 35:511–518.

Fitch WT. 1999. Acoustic exaggeration of size in birds via tracheal elongation: comparative and theoretical analyses. *Journal of Zoology, London* 248:31–48.

Fitzgerald G, Cooper JE. 1990. Preliminary studies on the use of propofol in the domestic pigeon (*Columba livia*). *Research in Veterinary Science* 49:334–338.

Greenlees KJ, Clutton RE, Larsen CT, Eyre P. 1990. Effect of halothane, isoflurane, and pentobarbital anesthesia on myocardial irritability in chickens. *American Journal of Veterinary Research* 51:757–758.

Guimarães LD, Natalini CC, Flores FN, Camargo SF, Bopp S, Pippi NL. 2006. Evaluation of two intraosseous constant rate infusions of propofol in domestic pigeons. *Acta Scientiae Veterinariae* 34:325–329.

Guzman S-M, Souza MJ, Braun JM, Cox SK, Keuler NS, Paul-Murphy JR. 2012. Antinociceptive effects after oral administration of tramadol hydrochloride in Hispaniolan Amazon parrots (*Amazona ventralis*). *American Journal of Veterinary Research* 73:1148–1152.

Hussain I, Khan MZ, Khan A, Javed I, Saleemi MK. 2008. Toxicological effects of diclofenac in four avian species. *Avian Pathology* 37:315–321.

Korbel R. 1998. Comparative investigations on inhalation anesthesia with isoflurane (Forene) and sevoflurane (sevorane) in racing pigeons (*Columba livia* Gmel., 1789, var. domestica) and presentation of a reference anesthesia protocol for birds. *Tierärztliche Praxis Ausgabe K, Kleintiere/Heimtiere* 26:211–223.

Lopez J, Cruz JI, Pascual R, Burzaco O, Falceto MV. 1994. Pilot study and clinical observations on the use of propofol by the interosseous route in pigeons. *Journal of Veterinary Anaesthesia* 24:46.

Lukasik VM, Gentz EJ, Erb HN, Ludders JW, Scarlett JM. 1997. Cardiopulmonary effects of propofol anesthesia in chickens (*Gallus gallus domesticus*). *Journal of Avian Medicine and Surgery* 11:93–97.

Lumeij JT, Deenik JW. 2003. Medetomidine-ketamine and diazepam-ketamine anesthesia in racing pigeons (*Columba livia domestica*): a comparative study. *Journal of Avian Medicine and Surgery* 17:191–196.

Maiti SK, Tiwary R, Vasan P, Dutta A. 2006. Xylazine, diazepam, and midazolam premedicated ketamine anesthesia in white leghorn cockerels for typhylectomy. *Journal of the South African Veterinary Association* 77:12–18.

Martin LL 1967. Comparison of methoxymol, alpha-chlorolose, and two barbiturates for capturing doves. Proceedings of the 21st Annual Conference of the South-Eastern Association of Game and Fish Commissioners. pp 193–200.

Martin-Jurado O, Vogt R, Kutter APN, Bettschart-Wolfensberger R, Hatt J-M. 2008. Effect of inhalation of isoflurane at end-tidal concentrations greater than, equal to, and less than the minimum anesthetic concentration on bispectral index in chickens. *American Journal of Veterinary Research* 69: 1254–1261.

Moghadam AZ, Sadegh AB, Sharifi S, Habibian S. 2009. Comparison of intranasal administration of diazepam, midazolam and xylazine in pigeons: clinical evaluation. *Iranian Journal of Veterinary Science and Technology* 1:19–26.

Mostachio GQ, de Oliveira LD, Carciofi AC, Vicente WRR. 2008. The effects of anesthesia with a combination of intramuscular xylazine-diazepam-ketamine on heart rate, respiratory rate and cloacal temperature in roosters. *Veterinary Anaesthesia and Analgesia* 35:232–236.

Naganobu K, Hagio M. 2000. Dose-related cardiovascular effects of isoflurane in chickens during controlled ventilation. *The Journal of Veterinary Medical Science* 62:435–437.

Naganobu K, Fujisawa Y, Ohde H, Matsuda Y, Sonoda T, Ogawa H. 2000. Determination of the minimum anesthetic concentration and cardiovascular dose response for sevoflurane in chickens during controlled ventilation. *Veterinary Surgery* 29: 102–105.

Neal LA, Custer RS, Bush M. 1981. Ketamine anesthesia in pigeons (*Columba livia*): arterial blood gas and acid-base status. *Journal of Zoo Animal Medicine* 12:48–51.

Nicholson A, Ilkiw JE. 1992. Neuromuscular and cardiovascular effects of atracurium in isoflurane-anesthetized chickens. *American Journal of Veterinary Research* 53:2337–2342.

Paré M, Ludders JW, Erb HN. 2013. Association of partial pressure of carbon dioxide in expired gas and arterial blood at three different ventilation states in apneic chickens (*Gallus domesticus*) during air sac insufflation anesthesia. *Veterinary Anaesthesia and Analgesia* 40:245–256.

Park KS, Park JH. 1988. Effect of xylazine hydrochloride, yohimbine hydrochloride, and 4-aminopyridine on gizzard motility in chicken. *Korean Journal of Veterinary Research* 28:37–47.

Pollock CG, Schumacher J, Orosz SE, Ramsay EC. 2001. Sedative effects of medetomidine in pigeons (*Columba livia*). *Journal of Avian Medicine and Surgery* 15:95–100.

Sandmeier P. 2000. Evaluation of medetomidine for short-term immobilization of domestic pigeons (*Columba livia*) and Amazon parrots (*Amazona* species). *Journal of Avian Medicine and Surgery* 14:8–14.

Schumacher J, Citino SB, Hernandez K, Huff J, Dixon B. 1997. Cardiopulmonary and anesthetic effects of propofol in wild turkeys. *American Journal of Veterinary Research* 58:1014–1017.

Souza MJ, Martin-Jimenez T, Jones MP, Cox SK. 2009. Pharmacokinetics of intravenous and oral tramadol in the bald eagle (*Haliaeetus leucocephalus*). *Journal of Avian Medicine and Surgery* 23:247–252.

Souza MJ, Martin-Jimenez T, Jones MP, Cox SK. 2011. Pharmacokinetics of oral tramadol in red-tailed hawks (*Buteo jamaicensis*). *Journal of Veterinary Pharmacology and Therapeutics* 34:86–88.

Souza MJ, Sanchez-Migallon Guzman D, Paul-Murphy JR, Cox SK. 2012. Pharmacokinetics after oral and intravenous administration of a single dose of tramadol hydrochloride to Hispaniolan Amazon parrots (*Amazona ventralis*). *American Journal of Veterinary Research* 73:1142–1147.

Spraker TR, Adrian WJ, Lance WR. 1987. Capture myopathy in wild turkeys (*Meleagris gallopavo*) following trapping, handling and transportation in Colorado. *Journal of Wildlife Diseases* 23:447–453.

Teare JA. 1987. Antagonism of xylazine hydrochloride-ketamine hydrochloride immobilization in guinea fowl (*Numida meleagris*) by yohimbine hydrochloride. *Journal of Wildlife Diseases* 23:301–305.

Touzot-Jourde G, Hernandez-Divers SJ, Trim CM. 2005. Cardiopulmonary effects of controlled versus spontaneous ventilation in pigeons anesthetized for coelioscopy. *Journal of the American Veterinary Medical Association* 227:1424–1428.

Uzun M, Yildiz S, Atalan G, Kaya M, Sulu N. 2003. Effects of medetomidine-ketamine combination anaesthesia on electrocardiographic findings, body temperature, and heart and respiratory rates in domestic pigeons. *Turkish Journal of Veterinary and Animal Science* 27:377–382.

Uzun M, Onder F, Atalan G, Cenesiz M, Kaya M, Yildiz S. 2006. Effects of xylazine, medetomidine, detomidine, and diazepam on sedation, heart and respiratory rates, and cloacal temperature in rock partridges (*Alectoris graeca*). *Journal of Zoo and Wildlife Medicine* 37:135–140.

Zollinger TW, Hoover JP, Payton ME, Schiller CA. 2011. Clinicopathologic, gross necropsy, and histologic findings after intramuscular injection of carprofen in a pigeon (*Columba livia*) model. *Journal of Avian Medicine and Surgery* 25:173–184.

29 Free-Living Waterfowl and Shorebirds

Daniel M. Mulcahy

INTRODUCTION

Waterfowl (ducks, geese, and swans) are aquatic birds within the family Anatidae, order Anseriformes. They vary greatly in body mass, from several 100 g to greater than 13 kg (Olsen 1994). Shorebirds belong to the order Charadriiformes, of which three species of the family Scolopacidae will be discussed.

The introduction of isoflurane to avian medicine in the 1980s made general anesthesia safe enough to permit long surgical procedures. Several articles pertinent to waterfowl and shorebird anesthesia and analgesia have been published recently (Abou-Madi 2001; Clyde & Paul-Murphy 1999; Gunkel & Lafortune 2005; Hawkins & Paul-Murphy 2011; Heard 1993, 1997; Ludders 2008; Machin 2004, 2005a, 2005b; Machin & Caulkett 1998a; Paul-Murphy & Ludders 2001).

Birds feel pain in much the same physiochemical ways as do mammals, which means the principles of anticipating and treating pain in mammals are applicable (see Chapter 7). Sufficient progress in avian anesthesia has been made so there is no excuse for not using appropriate regimens for surgery in birds (Mueller 1982). Compared with poultry, pigeons (*Columba livia*), quail (*Coturnix* sp.), and psittacines, waterfowl pain has received little attention (Machin et al. 2001). Almost no information is published for shorebird anesthesia and analgesia. Species and individual variation is to be expected; a routine "one dose fits all" approach should be avoided.

THE PATIENT

The influence of body condition on anesthetic morbidity has received little attention. Obesity, a very common problem in domestic waterfowl, reduces tidal volume due to air sac compression. This can lead to hypercapnia, respiratory acidemia, and possibly death (Phalen et al. 1996). Free-living birds have increased intracoelomic fat at times during their life cycle and similar complications should be expected. Shorebirds (e.g., bar-tailed godwits, *Limosa lapponica*) may have a fat mass of 41% of their body weight at the beginning their very long migrations (Gill et al. 2005).

Birds at different stages of their life cycle have different anesthetic risks. Brooding hens trapped on the nest, and birds at the end of a long migration, are often dehydrated and in poor body condition. Overwintering birds and those caught after storms may be suffering nutritional stress. Harlequin ducks (*Histrionicus histrionicus*) caught during the winter had more anesthetic complications and deaths than those caught in the fall (Stoskopf et al. 2010). Harlequin ducks caught after a storm lasting 3 days or longer also exhibited more anesthetic complications and deaths than those caught during good weather or after storms lasting less than 2 days (Stoskopf et al. 2010). The ducks caught after the 3-day-long storm were hypoglycemic and hypokalemic, probably owing to higher exertion and reduced feeding opportunities during the storm, but the deficits were made up within a day. Ideally, avian blood glucose levels are ≥200 mg/dL before anesthesia. Inexpensive (about $100), over-the-counter blood glucose monitors require little blood, give rapid results, and are relatively accurate (Lieske et al. 2002).

To reduce acute stresses capture and handling are done quickly and competently; the bird is handled gently and anesthetic induction is begun as soon as possible. All equipment and supplies are readied before removing the bird from the holding container. A highly

Zoo Animal and Wildlife Immobilization and Anesthesia, Second Edition. Edited by Gary West, Darryl Heard, and Nigel Caulkett.
This chapter is in the public domain. Published 2014 by John Wiley & Sons, Inc.

stressed bird is more likely to resist anesthetic induction than a less stressed bird.

FASTING

Fasting before anesthesia and surgery has been both recommended and discouraged. A fast of 3–12 hours is recommended to empty the crop to reduce regurgitation and aspiration (Curro 1998; Harrison 1991; Redig 1998). In wild-caught waterfowl, a preinduction fast of an hour is sufficient for ingested food to clear (D. Mulcahy, unpubl. data, 2000). As a precaution, the anesthetized bird is laid on a foam pad or other platform slightly elevated (3–5 cm) above the anesthetic table. The bird's head is positioned on the table lower than the rest of its body. This lessens aspiration of refluxing esophageal or gastric contents.

ANESTHETIC ENVIRONMENT

Patient stress and anesthetist distractions are minimized during the perianesthetic period. The awake or recovering birds are caged in an area that is quiet and protected from the elements. Wild-caught birds are housed outdoors in containers placed where human traffic is minimal and where they cannot be inadvertently kicked or shoved. Lightly anesthetized birds are roused by loud noises (e.g., laughter, motor noises, and raised voices), stimuli that should be avoided.

PHYSICAL RESTRAINT

Physical restraint is used in captive and wild birds if the procedure is of short duration, causes minimal pain or distress, and the holder is experienced. Of paramount importance is bird and handler safety. The main goal is completion of the desired procedure in the minimum time required, with the least stress on the bird. However, restraint may not always be minimal or even gentle; wild birds are especially alert for a relaxed grip. They will then make an explosive attempt to escape or inflict harm upon the restrainer and person performing the procedure. A firm grip and proper technique minimize the potential for injury to all species involved. Fortunately, restraint of waterfowl, shorebirds, and seabirds is much less riskier than some other avian groups (e.g., raptors, psittacines, and large ratites).

Covering the eyes with a hood or a stocking reduces stress during transportation and handling. However, these covers are sometimes dislodged by the bird shaking its head. Ducks and geese are picked up for short periods by grasping the base of both wings in one hand and supporting the feet and body with the other (Fig. 29.1). This places considerable stress on the wings and is used only with additional support and not for fractious birds that may fracture a wing bone. It is a useful technique for controlling birds as they are removed from a transport container.

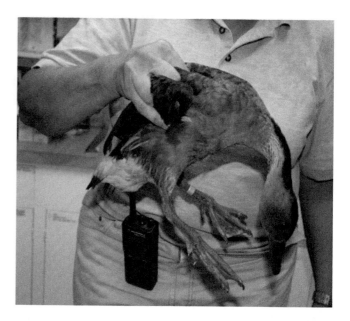

Figure 29.1. Restraint technique used for ducks and small geese. The humeri are grasped with the fingers of one hand. For heavier birds, the other hand should be placed under the feet to support the weight of the bird. Using this technique, birds should not be held for more than a minute or two to avoid damage (photograph courtesy of Scott Larsen).

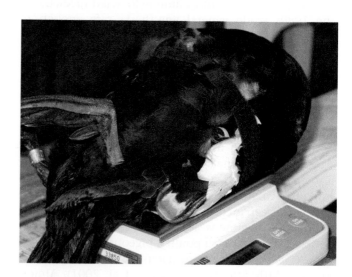

Figure 29.2. Temporary restraint of a male surf scoter (*Melanitta perspicillata*), here used to weigh the bird on a scale, by tucking the head under a wing and wrapping the bird snugly with "hook-and-loop" strapping. Care is taken to avoid interference with respiratory excursions of the keel and the duration of such restraint should be measured in seconds (photograph courtesy of Dan Esler).

Ducks and some geese are conveniently held by tucking their heads under a wing, which appears to cause mild sedation. For additional brief restraint, "hook-and-loop" strapping is wrapped snugly around the bird incorporating both folded wings. Care is taken not to restrict respiration. Restrained birds can then be weighed on a scale (Fig. 29.2).

For anesthetic induction, the bird is removed from the holding container and placed on a table. It is manually restrained by holding the folded wings and exerting slight downward pressure. Most birds will not struggle if the restraint does not vary. Handling during capture and processing can cause significant hyperthermia, which is exacerbated by environmental temperature (Davenport et al. 2004; Phalen et al. 1996). Plumage provides superb heat retention, especially in waterfowl and other species adapted for life in the cold water. Excess heat is lost by evaporation through panting, transdermally in featherless areas, and through the feet where blood circulation is under partial voluntary control.

RESPIRATORY CONTROL

Waterfowl have been used extensively in avian respiratory studies. A physiologic feature in waterfowl and other birds is the presence of intrapulmonary chemoreceptors that respond to pCO_2. They interface respiratory control and gas exchange by being more responsive to alterations in pCO_2 than pO_2 (Fedde et al. 1974; Hempleman & Burger 1984; Hempleman et al. 1986). These receptors provide feedback control to ventilation and match respiration with metabolism (Shoemaker & Hempleman 2001). Intrapulmonary chemoreceptors are afferent vagal neurons sensitive to pCO_2 tension variation in different parts of the avian lung (Hempleman & Bebout 1994; Hempleman et al. 2000, 2003). Receptor response is actually to H^+ from CO_2 hydration, and the receptors are inhibited rather than excited (Adamson & Burger 1986; Bebout & Hempleman 1999; Powell et al. 1978). Intrapulmonary receptors are located within the parabronchial gas exchange area (Nye & Burger 1978; Scheid et al. 1974). More than 95% of receptors are located in the caudal lung, an area that experiences marked CO_2 fluctuations during respiration (Scheid et al. 1974). Intrapulmonary chemoreceptors are part of a reflex arc that inhibits respiration when intrapulmonary pCO_2 decreases (Burger & Estavillo 1978).

MONITORING

Monitoring begins as soon as a bird is placed in front of the anesthetist, with observation of respiration and attitude. It ends when the bird is fully recovered and returned to its source. As is often stated, there is no better monitoring technique or device than a trained, experienced, and attentive anesthetist to assure the greatest patient stability and safety. Changes in anesthetic depth, body temperature, and cardiopulmonary status occur quickly in birds and must be identified and responded to just as quickly. In field work, a biologist is often drafted as anesthetist and given on the job training. To assure maximum efficacy, it is preferable

to concentrate acquisition of anesthesia experience in one person, rather than rotate the responsibility between multiple biologists. A trusted anesthetist allows the surgeon to concentrate on their job, contributing to quality work and reduced anesthesia time.

There are several schemes for staging anesthetic depth (Korbel 1998; Sandmeier 2000). In practice, most are too complicated, especially for relatively short procedures, and only serve to divert the attention of the anesthetist away from directly observing the patient. A simpler scheme for field work with a biologist anesthetist is given in Table 29.1 (Curro 1998; Rosskopf & Woerpel 1996). Successful induction has occurred when the legs and wings can be extended without being withdrawn and in most cases, this signals readiness for intubation.

Once intubated, the appropriate monitoring instrumentation is applied. Respiratory monitors, stethoscopes, electrocardiographs, capnographs, blood gas analyzers, blood pressure monitors, and cloacal and esophageal temperature probes have been used to assess anesthetic status of waterfowl (Fig. 29.3). Deciding the

Table 29.1. Simplified anesthesia levels of birds. The stages are continuous

Induction	Muscle relaxation, lowered head, drooping eyelids, wings and legs can be extended without being withdrawn.
Light	No response to positional change; corneal, palpebral and pedal withdrawal reflexes present; no volitional movement.
Medium	Respirations slow and deep; palpebral reflex absent; corneal and pedal reflexes sluggish or absent.
Deep	Respirations very slow and progressively shallow; reflexes absent.

Source: After Curro (1998).

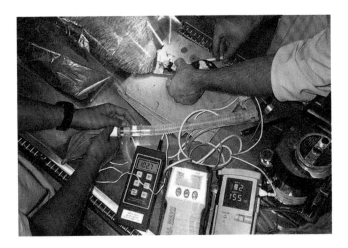

Figure 29.3. A lesser Canada goose (*Branta Canadensis*) anesthetized with isoflurane with anesthetic circuit shown. The patient, prepared for surgery, is being electronically monitored with a digital thermometer, capnograph, and pulse oximeter, and a blood sample is being drawn from the jugular vein for blood gas determination.

instrumentation to use depends on practicality and procedure length. It is contrary to the best interests of the patient to significantly extend anesthetic duration in order to place additional monitoring sensors and instruments. The anesthetist must understand that no electronic or mechanical monitor is to be blindly trusted.

The essential physiologic variables to monitor include heart rate and rhythm, respiration rate and depth, and body temperature. Reference values for cardiopulmonary variables vary between species and conditions; representative values are given in Table 29.2.

Respiration is evaluated by observation. Depth is judged by the extent of sternal movement. Movement of the rebreathing bag does not reliably reflect occurrence and depth of respiration, as the cuffless endotracheal tube may not form a sufficient seal. Arterial blood gas analysis is the definitive means of evaluating ventilation, but is rarely done in the field.

Tracheal secretions tend to be very thick. Clicking or gurgling noises indicate partial tracheal or endotracheal blockage; the endotracheal tube is withdrawn and cleaned if necessary. Sometimes, the plug is located in the trachea instead of the tube. Complete tracheal obstruction (as from a plug) is suggested by marked inspiratory and expiratory efforts with little to no air movement. In many cases, the anesthetist can force air past the obstruction with positive pressure, but the material then reobstructs the tube. End-tidal CO_2 readings will be low, despite assisted ventilation. If this occurs, the tube is removed immediately and either replaced or cleaned and reinserted. Tracheal mucous plugs are sometimes removed by inserting a longer, smaller diameter endotracheal tube, rotating, then withdrawing with the mucus plug attached. Obstructions occur more often with dehydration, which thickens secretions. Wild birds held for hours prior to surgery are assumed to be dehydrated, as they will rarely drink water provided in a holding container.

Electronic monitors are available that connect to the endotracheal tube to monitor respiratory activity (see Chapter 6). These instruments also display a calculated respiratory rate, but this should not be uncritically accepted. Manipulations of the bird's body can cause excursions of air through the trachea that are not part of the respiratory cycle. Observation of the graphic wave form of a capnograph can confirm observed respiration rates that reflect a true respiratory cycle (Fig. 29.3). However, not every capnograph is accurate at small tidal volumes (see Chapter 3). Capnography is considered accurate only during positive pressure ventilation (Sap et al. 1993). The end-tidal partial pressure of CO_2 slightly underestimates the arterial partial pressure of CO_2 (Edling et al. 2001). When monitoring with a capnograph, manual or positive pressure ventilation is adjusted to keep end-tidal CO_2 partial pressures at 30–45 mmHg (Edling et al. 2001).

The purpose of cardiovascular monitoring includes assuring that the heart is beating and the blood is circulating. Pulses are palpable at the tibiotarsal or elbow (cubital) joints, if the hands of the anesthetist and extension of a leg or wing will not disturb the procedure. A stethoscope, esophageal stethoscope, electrocardiograph, or Doppler flow detector is used for cardiovascular monitoring. In practice, only a single electronic monitor is used.

Pulse oximetry can be undependable due to motion artifact, inaccuracy, lack of calibration to avian hemoglobin, and discontinuity of values during surgical emergencies (Schmitt et al. 1998). Pulse oximeters are calibrated for human blood, and will give a lower saturation value for avian blood (Schmitt et al. 1998). For routine monitoring, the relative inaccuracy of oxygen saturation is not critical, and the pulse oximeter can be used to monitor trends in heart rate and oxygen saturation. Relying solely on pulse oximetry to monitor birds anesthetized with isoflurane in 100% oxygen is inadequate as they may be poorly ventilated despite adequate oxygenation (Edling et al. 2001).

Some commercial pulse oximeters measure very rapid heart rates, but it is advisable to query oximetry manufacturers about the possibility of modifying a unit to assure that function. Having a display of heart rate and oxygen saturation levels is valuable for monitoring avian anesthesia. It is often difficult to find a suitable site for placing the pulse oximeter probe. The interdigital webbing of the feet is used, but the presence of pigment may make the site unsuitable for a transmittance probe. Similarly, clamp probes are placed on the tip of the upper bill of ducks with lightly pigmented bills (Fig. 29.4). Reflectance probes are placed into either the esophagus or cloaca. Maintaining a constant, proper position with reflectance probes is a problem; the anesthetist may have to make frequent adjustments to assure adequate tissue surface contact.

Auscultation of the heart is a simple and direct means for monitoring heart rate and rhythm. The large pectoral muscle mass of waterfowl reduces transmission of cardiac sounds; the stethoscope diaphragm is placed on the dorsal thorax, lateral thorax, or thoracic inlet. However, placing a stethoscope under the surgical drape may be disruptive to the surgeon. The easiest cardiac monitor to use is an electronically amplified, battery powered, esophageal stethoscope (Audio Patient Monitor®, A.M. Bickford, Inc., Wales Center, NY). The sensor is a hollow plastic tube with multiple openings at the distal end, covered with a plastic cuff. Sensor tubes are available in a variety of diameters; the largest tube compatible with the esophagus is used for the best signal. The tube is inserted to the level of the heart (Fig. 29.3). Positioning is evaluated by listening to the volume and clarity of the signal. The long necks of waterfowl and shorebirds facilitate intraoperative adjustments without disturbing the surgeon. An audible

Table 29.2. Mean cardiopulmonary and blood gas values with SD (±) or range (–) for normal waterfowl

Species	Heart Rate (beats/min)	Respiration Rate (breaths/min)	Body Temperature (°C)	Systolic Blood Pressure (mmHg)	Diastolic Blood Pressure (mmHg)	Mean Blood Pressure (mmHg)	pHa	PaO$_2$ (mmHg)	PaCO$_2$ (mmHg)	HCO$_3$	Reference
Canada goose (*Branta canadensis*)	133 ± 8.4	18.7 ± 1.3	40.2 ± 0.58	194 ± 10.4	128 ± 7.0	155 ± 11.6	7.445 ± 0.001	87.6 ± 3.0	29.3 ± 2.3		Valverde et al. (1990)
Pekin duck (*Anas platyrhynchos*)	213 ± 8		41.3 ± 0.2			130.4 ± 5.4	7.473 ± 0.006	101.9 ± 1.6	31.1 ± 0.5	21.8 ± 0.5	Ludders et al. (1989b)
Pekin duck			41.6 ± 0.2				7.458 ± 0.011	101.3 ± 2.0	32.5 ± 0.8	21.8 ± 0.6	Ludders et al. (1990)
Pekin duck	190 ± 17	19 ± 4				128 ± 14					Goelz et al. (1990)
Pekin duck		7 (6–13)					7.42 (7.36–7.50)	86 (74–99)	30 (27–41)	18 (15–26)	Seaman et al. (1994)
Pekin duck	218 ± 32	17 ± 4	40.9 ± 0.4			124 ± 13	7.40 ± 0.04	84.4 ± 11.5	40.3 ± 2.7	23.7 ± 1.1	Rode et al. (2003)
Pekin duck							7.445 ± 0.0007	98.1 ± 0.8	30.5 ± 0.2		Mitchell et al. (2001)
Pekin duck		15.8 ± 1.5					7.45 ± 0.02	99.7 ± 2.4	30.1 ± 0.6		Shams et al. (1990)
Canvasback duck	158 ± 48	21 ± 3	39.0 ± 0.8	176 ± 26	127 ± 25	147 ± 24	7.42 ± 0.02	92.0 ± 2.5	30.2 ± 3.4		Machin and Caulkett (1999)

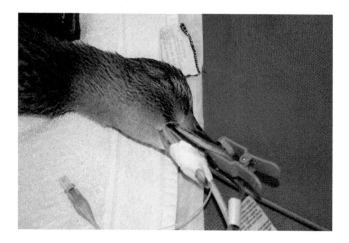

Figure 29.4. Placement of a pulse oximeter transmittance probe on the bill of a female mallard duck (*Anas platyrhynchos*). This technique works when there is little or no pigment on the bill (photograph courtesy of Scott Larsen).

signal of the heartbeat allows everyone involved in the surgery to monitor the patient. The sensor tube is placed immediately after intubation. Sometimes, respiratory sounds are also heard. Diminished or no heart sounds are usually due to inadvertent displacement of the sensor. However, the anesthetist must not spend too much time adjusting the sensor before raising the alarm about potential cardiac abnormalities.

An ultrasonic Doppler flow detector (Parks Medical®, Parks Medical Electronics Inc., Aloha, OR; Minidop®, Jorgensen Laboratories, Inc., Burlington, WI) is most commonly used for cardiac monitoring. The ultrasound probe is commonly taped over the cranial tibial artery, but the superficial ulnar artery at the distal humerus, and the carotid artery, are also used (Lichtenberger 2005; Zantop & Bowles 2000). The Doppler flow detector allows indirect monitoring of systolic blood pressures, using the appropriate pressure cuff size (40% of appendage circumference) around the leg proximal to the probe. Reference blood pressure values have been determined for a few species of waterfowl (Table 29.1). Diastolic, and therefore mean, blood pressure cannot be obtained with this method. Birds with systolic blood pressures ≤90 or ≥145 mmHg are evaluated for causes of hypotension and hypertension, respectively (Lichtenberger 2005). Hypovolemia is treated with bolus administration of crystalloids (10–20 mL/kg) or colloids (5 mL/kg) until systolic pressures are restored (Lichtenberger 2004). For immediate effect, fluids are given IV or intraosseously (Valverde et al. 1993).

Digital thermometers are more useful than traditional thermometers because their displays are easier to read. Digital thermometers are placed in either the cloaca or deep in the esophagus (Fig. 29.3). Cloacal sensors are taped in place, but the tape is easily dislodged by fecal fluid and the thermometer is difficult

to read if covered by a surgical drape. Digital thermometers with long, flexible extension sensors (e.g., Electrotherm Model 99A, Cooper Instrument Corporation, Middlefield, CT) are preferred for esophageal placement. To read core temperature, the sensor is inserted until it is past the thoracic inlet. Normal body temperature in waterfowl is 40–42°C, but tends to decline during anesthesia.

MAINTENANCE OF BODY TEMPERATURE

Body temperature maintenance within a normal range begins with a patient that is dry, clean, and minimally stressed. Hypothermia is more likely to occur in a patient with feathers wetted during capture and handling or fouled by feces and urine during transportation. Conversely, a bird severely stressed during capture, transported in a poorly ventilated container, and held for hours before a procedure at high environmental temperatures is very likely to be hyperthermic. In the author's experience with Arctic waterfowl and shorebirds, hyperthermia occurs more commonly than hypothermia, which is fortunate as it is more easily treated.

During normal respiration, the turbinates warm and humidify inspired air (Schmidt-Nielsen et al. 1970). The efficiency of evaporative heat exchange by the turbinates is such that the nasal surface temperature may be less than that of the ambient air (Jackson & Schmidt-Nielsen 1964). During exhalation, water and heat losses are minimized by the air being cooled and supersaturated as it passes over the turbinates. The reduction in evaporative water loss ranges from 55% to 71% in birds (Geist 2000). Exhaled air temperature at the external nares averaged 19.6°C lower than core temperature, while oropharyngeal temperature measured only 3.5°C lower, indicating the trachea is minimally involved in heat exchange (Geist 2000). The condensed moisture and heat recovered at the turbinates are returned to the body. In the intubated bird during anesthesia, breathing is shifted from nasopharyngeal to oropharyngeal, bypassing the countercurrent heat exchange and moisture recovery mechanisms in the nasal cavity. This accelerates heat and moisture loss. The type of breathing system used for avian anesthesia has little effect on body temperature loss. Pigeons anesthetized with three different systems had lost about 1.7°C by 45 minutes and 2.7°C at 90 minutes (Boedeker et al. 2005).

Correction of abnormal body temperatures is begun as soon as it is recognized. Hyperthermia is treated by wetting the unfeathered legs and feet with isopropyl alcohol. The feet of waterfowl efficiently control body temperature due to the presence of the *rete tibiotarsale*, a vascular network (Midtgård 1980). In severe hyperthermia, rapid correction requires other concerns be ignored. It may be helpful to also wet the axilla with alcohol, despite the risk of removing waterproofing of the feathers.

Correction of hypothermia is more difficult, and is best avoided. If body temperature decreases suddenly, dislodgment of the temperature sensor from within the thorax is suspected first. To treat a hypothermic bird, external heat is applied to the exposed skin of the feet and lower legs. Bags of water or saline heated up to 43°C, or chemical heat packs wrapped in a layer of cloth are placed on the feet. Leaks in the bags are avoided to prevent feather wetting that will exacerbate hypothermia. Waterfowl reduce heat loss by decreasing blood flow to their hind limbs, making external heat application to the feet less efficient. Hypothermic birds recover very slowly from anesthesia. They are held wrapped in a towel to conserve body heat during recovery. It is best to correct the body temperature abnormality during anesthesia rather than to expect the postanesthetic patient to recover on its own. Hypothermic birds are recovered and rewarmed with caution and with constant observation. Rewarming reverses peripheral vasoconstriction and increases metabolic demand for glucose (Heard 2000). Deaths of hypothermic birds that occur within several hours of the end of anesthesia may be due to the effects of induced hypothermia (Heard 2000).

Efforts to reduce thermal loss under anesthesia usually involve placing the bird on an insulated pad, a heated circulating water mattress, or wrapping in bubble wrap (Harrison 1994). These methods have little effect because of the high insulative value of feathers. A radiant energy source placed just above anesthetized birds was the only effective technique for maintaining a constant body temperature (Phalen et al. 1996; Rembert et al. 2001). The effectiveness of radiant heat was demonstrated in a sun conure (*Aratinga solstitialis*) that died of heat stroke (body temperature of 48.1°C) during surgery under an unusually hot surgical lamp (Hofmeister & Hernandez-Divers 2005).

RECOVERY

For recovery, the anesthetized bird is positioned in lateral to slightly ventral recumbency. The bird remains intubated and respiration is assisted until it shows controlled, voluntary motion and objects to the presence of the endotracheal tube. The tube and esophageally placed monitoring sensors are removed at that time. Newly extubated birds remain sedated by the anesthetic and may become quiescent.

Many recovering birds go through a period of disorientation, wing flapping, and struggling (emergence delirium) that may result in self-inflicted trauma (Curro 1998). To avoid this, recovering birds are wrapped in a towel (unless hyperthermic) and observed closely for continued respirations. Only when the bird holds its head erect and steady is it replaced in the recovery

container. It is then regularly observed for flexion of its head and neck that may obstruct the airway. If this occurs, the bird is repositioned or removed from the recovery container and held until fully recovered. Recovery time depends on the choice of anesthetic, anesthetic duration, and extent of physiologic alteration that has occurred. A bird that is hypothermic, hypoglycemic, or that has impaired drug elimination mechanisms will take longer to recover (Heard 2000).

ANTICHOLINERGICS

Anticholinergic drugs (atropine or glycopyrrolate IM) reduce pharyngeal and tracheal secretions, but may also increase their viscosity. Consequently, they are recommended only for treatment of severe bradycardia.

INHALATION ANESTHESIA

Inhalation anesthetics offer the advantages of familiarity and ready availability of equipment for veterinarians. With an inhalation anesthetic in birds, an agent-specific vaporizer and a nonrebreathing circuit (e.g., Bain) are usually used. Anesthetic breathing systems are disinfected between uses, but must be thoroughly rinsed to remove residual toxic substances that may damage the respiratory system (Greenacre 1993).

Isoflurane has been the primary inhalant anesthetic for birds since the mid-1980s (Bednarski et al. 1985; Ludders et al. 1988b, 1989a). Others (i.e., methoxyflurane and halothane) are rarely used now because their manufacture has been discontinued (Goelz et al. 1990; Greenlees et al. 1990; Ludders et al. 1988a). The recently introduced sevoflurane is increasingly used in clinical settings. Due to its lower blood gas partition coefficient, induction and recovery of birds occur more rapidly than with isoflurane (Korbel 1998; Quandt & Greenacre 1999). Sevoflurane is less pungent than isoflurane for human beings (TerRiet et al. 2000). The pungency of volatile anesthetics may contribute to the breath holding seen in birds when an anesthetic mask is placed over their faces.

In mallard ducks, isoflurane has a minimum anesthetic concentration of 1.3% (Ludders et al. 1990). In birds generally, it causes dose-dependent reduction in spontaneous ventilation that extends to apnea at high concentrations (Ludders et al. 1990). The calculated Anesthetic Index (anesthetic concentration causing apnea/minimal anesthetic concentration) for ducks (1.65) is lower than for dogs (2.51), cats (2.40), and horses (2.33) (Ludders et al. 1990, 1995; Steffey & Howland 1977; Steffey et al. 1977). The lower Anesthetic Index for ducks indicates hypoventilation occurs at lower isoflurane concentrations in this species than in others. In Pekin ducks, isoflurane caused tachycardia and hypotension (Goelz et al. 1990). Although arrhythmias were uncommon, one duck died when ventricular bigeminy and multifocal ventricular rhythms progressed to ventricular fibrillation (Goelz et al. 1990). In other avian species, arrhythmias, cardiac irritability, and premature ventricular contractions have also been observed (Aguilar 1996; Greenlees et al. 1990; Jaensch et al. 1999; Langlois et al. 2003; Ludders et al. 1988a, 1989a; Matthews et al. 1991; Naganobu & Hagio 2000; Straub et al. 2003). Once waterfowl have stabilized under isoflurane anesthesia, cardiopulmonary variables should be carefully monitored (Table 29.3).

Induction

Inhalant anesthetics are often administered through a mask for induction. Commercially available cat or dog masks are used for small ducks and geese. Shorebirds may require custom masks fashioned from tubing or syringe cases to accommodate their long bills. The mask must include the nares at the base of the upper bill. The mask aperture can be altered with a piece of surgical glove stretched over the opening, taped around the edges and with a slit cut into the center. The apnea and bradycardia that occur when an induction mask is placed over a bird's beak and face are commonly attributed to a "dive response," but more likely are owing to a stress response caused by stimulation of trigeminal nerve receptors (Butler 1988; Jones et al. 1988; Woakes 1988). Preoxygenating ducks with 100% oxygen for several minutes reduced this response in dabbling ducks, but not in diving ducks (Furilla & Jones 1986).

The isoflurane vaporizer is set to 3–4% for induction. Although it is recommended the concentration be slowly increased to prevent breath holding, this author has not found this to be effective. In ducks and geese, the oxygen flow rate is 1–2 L/min to allow relatively rapid changes in anesthetic concentration as vaporizer setting is altered. A system for scavenging or venting waste anesthetic gases is used for safety (Altman 1992; Mason et al. 1998). Alternatively, for portable anesthetic machines, a canister filled with activated charcoal is used. However, not all cartridge brands work equally well (Smith & Bolon 2004). The charcoal canister is always laid on its side to avoid blocking the bottom vents, causing unwanted back-pressure on the nonrebreathing circuit. If apnea is prolonged during induction, respiration is encouraged by lifting the bird at the base of the wings, then gently pressing its body down on the table. Inflation and deflation of the reservoir bag is used to monitor breathing and ventilation, assuming the mask is snugly fitted against the face of the bird. Anesthetic depth is judged by pulling out a wing or a foot and releasing it. A conscious bird will withdraw either into the folded position. When the bird is assessed as unconscious, oxygen flow is turned to zero. It is preferable to turn the oxygen flow on and off (stopping flow of anesthetic through the vaporizer) rather than turning the vaporizer down and then back up again (during which time isoflurane vapor continues to flow through the dead space and into the room).

Intubation

Except for very brief procedures, all birds are intubated and ventilated. Waterfowl and shorebirds generally have long necks, allowing for a long endotracheal tube. Since the syrinx is inside the thoracic inlet, the length of the neck is used to measure the maximum endotracheal tube length.

Some male waterfowl have a bulbous expansion of the trachea, and some geese and swans have tracheal loops that lie in the caudal cervical area or within the thorax (McLelland 1989b). The avian trachea is 2.7 times as long and 1.29 times as wide as the trachea of a similarly sized mammal (McLelland 1989a). Consequently, the anatomical dead space is about 4.5 times that of a mammal (McLelland 1989a). The increased dead space is compensated for by a low respiratory frequency, about one-third that of mammals. This results in minute tracheal ventilation of about 1.5–1.9 times that of mammals (McLelland 1989a). However, respiration is depressed under general anesthesia, causing a larger percentage of minute ventilation to be devoted to dead space.

Birds have complete endotracheal rings and cuffless endotracheal tubes are preferred to prevent trauma. However, careful use of cuffed endotracheal tubes has been suggested to obtain a good seal (Curro 1998). Overinflation of a cuffed endotracheal tube may cause a longitudinal rupture of the tracheal rings that is not obvious for 5–7 days after intubation, until healing of the lesion and fibrotic narrowing of the tracheal lumen occur (Ludders 1998). A Cole endotracheal tube is appropriate for very small birds or chicks and ducklings, to prevent passing the tube too far into the trachea. The appropriate diameter of endotracheal tube must be chosen for the species of bird and its gender and age. An estimate of the external tracheal diameter is made by palpating the throat. In waterfowl, females may require one-half to one full size-larger endotracheal tube than males of the same species. In this author's experience, all ducks and geese can be intubated and ventilated with 2- to 4-mm (internal diameter) cuffless tubes. Because of the comparatively long necks found in most waterfowl and shorebird species, overintubation is a problem only with small species or immature birds. However, care is always taken to avoid striking the syrinx with the end of the endotracheal tube.

Except for birds with very long bills and small oral openings, intubation of waterfowl and shorebirds is relatively easy. The glottis is positioned at the base of the tongue and easily seen in most species. In some, a dorso-ventral septum (*crista ventralis*) is present just inside the glottal opening. If a tube cannot be readily passed through the glottis into the trachea, a tube with a smaller outside diameter is used.

Table 29.3. Mean cardiopulmonary values given as mean with SD (±) or range (−) for waterfowl after at least 15 minutes under injectable anesthesia

A. Mean Cardiopulmonary Values Given as Mean with SD (±) or Range (−) for Waterfowl after at Least 15 Minutes under Isoflurane Anesthesia

Species	Heart Rate (beats/min)	Respiration Rate (breaths/min)	Body Temperature (°C)	Systolic Blood Pressure (mmHg)	Diastolic Blood Pressure (mmHg)	Mean Blood Pressure (mmHg)	pHa	PaO₂ (mmHg)	PaCO₂ (mmHg)	HCO₃	Reference
Canada goose (*Branta canadensis*)	115 ± 12.6	11 ± 1.6	40.0 ± 0.65	140 ± 7.2	75 ± 5.0	101 ± 2.0					Valverde et al. (1990)
Pekin duck (*Anas platyrhynchos*)	190 ± 70	10 ± 2	±			119 ± 17					Goelz et al. (1990)
Pekin duck	283 ± 23	6 ± 1	41.3 ± 0.2			103 ± 11	7.168 ± 0.050	348.1 ± 18.1	93.9 ± 11.8	29.6 ± 1.1	Ludders et al. (1990)
Pekin duck		6 (3–8)					7.33 (7.23–7.40)	369 (315–433)	42 (32–54)	19 (16–27)	Seaman et al. (1994)
Mallard duck		10	(37.2–37.5)			(95–105)	7.42	102	24		Wilson and Pettifer (2004)
Pekin duck	227 ± 42	22 ± 6	41.1 ± 0.2			121 ± 11	7.37 ± 1.05	74.4 ± 12.4	43.3 ± 3.7	23.6 ± 1.2	Rode et al. (2003)

B. Mean Cardiopulmonary Values Given as Mean with SD (±) or Range (−) for Waterfowl after at Least 15 Minutes under Injectable Anesthesia

Species	Anesthetic	Heart Rate (beats/min)	Respiration Rate (breaths/min)	Body Temperature (°C)	Systolic Blood Pressure (mmHg)	Diastolic Blood Pressure (mmHg)	Mean Blood Pressure (mmHg)	pHa	PaO₂ (mmHg)	PaCO₂ (mmHg)	HCO₃	Reference
Canvasback duck (*Aythya valisneria*)	Propofol (15 mg/kg IV induction; 0.8 mg/kg/min infusion)	239 ± 16	31 ± 5	38.7 ± 0.9	186 ± 24	164 ± 25	173 ± 24	7.34 ± 0.02	83.0 ± 8.2	40 ± 4.9		Machin and Caulkett (1999)
Pekin duck (*Anas platyrhynchos*)	Pentobarbital (160 mg/kg IV)	218 ± 32	17 ± 4	40.9 ± 0.4			124 ± 13	7.40 ± 0.04	84.4 ± 11.5	40.3 ± 2.7	23.7 ± 1.1	Rode et al. (2003)

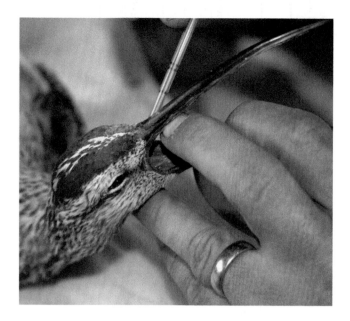

Figure 29.5. Bristle-thighed curlew (*Numenius tahitiensis*) being intubated. The left hand is used to hold the upper and lower bills apart while the right hand inserts the endotracheal tube. It is sometimes easier to intubate long-billed birds by holding the head dorsal side down, which permits the slight curve of the endotracheal tube to follow the curve of the beak (photograph courtesy of Dan Ruthrauff).

For intubation, the upper and lower bills are held agape with the fingers of one hand while inserting the endotracheal tube into the glottis with the other (Fig. 29.5). Alternatively, in large or long-billed birds, an assistant holds both bills, so the person intubating can use one hand to pull the tongue forward while passing the endotracheal tube with the other. Endotracheal tubes are usually inserted without lubrication.

Correct tube position is confirmed by direct visualization of the tube in the glottis, condensation on the inside of the tube, and chest excursions during mechanical ventilation or by the use of capnography. It is a good habit to immediately confirm proper placement by palpating the throat of the bird. If the tube is within the trachea, only one hard tubular structure, the trachea, will be felt ventral to the cervical vertebral column. If the tube was inadvertently passed into the esophagus, two hard tubular bodies will be felt, and corrective action can be immediately taken. The endotracheal tube is secured in place by tying or taping to the lower bill. Since the glottis is located on the ventral oral cavity, taping the tube to the upper bill would allow for movement of the glottis independent of the tube, which may cause inadvertent extubation.

After intubation the anesthetic system is reconnected and oxygen flow restarted to restore isoflurane flow. The vaporizer setting is reduced to maintenance. Anesthetists must ensure the bird's head and neck are

in extension to prevent kinking of the endotracheal tube. They must also be alert for gurgling sounds and exaggerated respiratory movements indicative of a blocked endotracheal tube. The use of a mechanical ventilator may reduce the likelihood of endotracheal tube blockage (Kramer 2002).

The minimal anesthetic concentration (MAC) is relatively constant (about 1.5% for isoflurane) for most species of birds. Many birds will be apneic following induction. It is prudent to use a lower vaporizer setting initially to slightly reduce anesthetic depth and to restore spontaneous ventilation. A decision to lighten anesthetic depth following induction is accompanied by attention to the anesthetic status of the patient to prevent sudden motion.

Ventilation

Most surgical procedures are performed in dorsal recumbency. This position can cause profound respiratory alteration. In conscious chickens placed in dorsal recumbency, tidal volume decreased 40–50%, although breathing frequency increased by 20–50% (King & Payne 1964). King penguins (*Aptenodynes patagonicus*) injected with tiletamine-zolazepam were immobilized about 50% longer if held in dorsal compared with ventral recumbency, and body temperatures were also significantly higher (Thil & Groscolas 2002). Respiratory compromise may be worsened in waterfowl by the inertial resistance of the relatively large pectoral muscle mass to respiratory excursions of the keel. The pressure of viscera on the abdominal air sacs also reduces their effective volume.

Inhalant anesthetics cause a dose-dependent depression of spontaneous ventilation (Ludders 1992; Ludders et al. 1988b, 1989a, 1990). Intermittent positive pressure ventilation is used in anesthetized birds, even if some spontaneous breathing is continuing, to assure adequate oxygenation of the blood (Edling et al. 2001). In geese, an average $PaCO_2$ of 53 mmHg was necessary for spontaneous respiration to occur; no respiration occurred with a $PaCO_2 \leq 40$ mmHg (Pizarro et al. 1990). Ventilation is assisted manually using the reservoir bag on the breathing system or a mechanical ventilator (Carpenter & Mason 2001; Hernandez-Divers 2001; Pettifer et al. 2002). Analysis of blood gases has showed that effective gas exchange is achieved using mechanical ventilation (Edling et al. 2001; Ludders et al. 1989a; Mitchell et al. 2001; Pettifer et al. 2002; Piiper et al. 1970).

Although a decrease in mean arterial blood pressure is observed in mammals during positive pressure ventilation, in sandhill cranes (*Grus canadensis*), pigeons (*Columba livia*), and Amazon parrots (*Amazona ventralis*), blood pressures increased or were maintained during ventilation (Ludders et al. 1989a; Pettifer et al. 2002; Wilson & Pettifer 2004). However, blood pressure decreased in positive pressure-ventilated chickens anesthetized with sevoflurane (Naganobu et al. 2003). The cardiovascular effects of positive pressure ventilation in birds are still uncertain, and have not been examined in waterfowl and shorebirds.

A spontaneously breathing bird is given at least 2 assisted breaths/min. If an anesthetized bird is apneic, the assisted ventilation rate is 8–15 breaths/min depending on size (large birds require fewer breaths than small). If pulse oximetry and capnography are used to monitor respiration, the rate is guided by the end-tidal CO_2 level and the relative hemoglobin saturation (Fig. 29.3).

OXYGEN AND ANESTHESIA

Inhalant anesthetics depress spontaneous ventilation (Ludders et al. 1988a, 1989a, 1990; Goelz et al. 1990). It is essential to avoid hypoventilation during anesthesia because birds lack the respiratory reserve capacity to compensate. Oxygen within air sacs does not diffuse into the blood to any great extent (Magnussen et al. 1976).

Using oxygen to deliver inhalant anesthetics to birds can alter respiratory variables. Respiratory rate decreased (but not significantly) as the fraction inspired oxygen increased to more than 90% (Seaman et al. 1994). Increasing oxygen concentration above 40% decreased tidal volume, a decrease that was significantly correlated with arterial CO_2 (Seaman et al. 1994). High oxygen concentrations may depress ventilation by acting on O_2-responsive chemoreceptors (Ludders et al. 1995). The use of air instead of oxygen during avian anesthesia would not depress the O_2-sensitive chemoreceptors and should have a less depressive effect on ventilation.

Air Sac Cannulation

Air flow through the lung is continuous and unidirectional. It is, therefore, possible to ventilate and to provide anesthesia through an air sac cannula (Brown & Pilny 2006; Jaensch et al. 2001; Rode et al. 2003; Whittow & Ossario 1970). A common application of this technique is in patients with tracheal obstructions (Clippinger & Bennett 1998; Graham 2004; Mama et al. 1996; Rode et al. 2003). The abdominal air sacs are generally used (Good et al. 2001). The clavicular air sac has been used, but it appears to participate less in ventilation than the thoracic and abdominal air sacs (Jaensch et al. 2002; Rode et al. 2003). Cannulation of the caudal thoracic air sac has been used to anesthetize zebra finches (*Taeneopygia guttata*) as small as 10 g (Nilson et al. 2004). The technique could easily be adapted for anesthesia of very small ducklings and shorebird chicks.

Placing an air sac cannula requires the selected site (on the lateral abdominal wall well ventral to the spine so as to avoid damage to the kidney) be prepared as with any surgical site. Feathers are taped aside and the skin is prepped. While general anesthesia makes placement easier, in conscious birds, the surgical site is infiltrated with lidocaine (≤2 mg/kg). The skin is incised with a scalpel blade. The muscle layer is penetrated with either sharp dissection by making a puncture with a blade or by blunt dissection using hemostats to work through the muscles and air sac membrane. The cannula, often an endotracheal tube, is pushed into the air sac. The tube is secured by suturing tape butterfly wings to the skin. The breathing system is then connected and the animal ventilated. Waste anesthetic gases exit through the trachea and are an exposure risk to personnel. The cannula is removed when spontaneous ventilation is reliable. Sutures or surgical glue are used to close the incision.

Ducks anesthetized with phenobarbital and breathing room air through clavicular air sac cannulas had no significant differences in arterial blood gas values compared to ducks that were tracheally intubated (Rode et al. 2003). Caudal thoracic air sac cannulation in sulfur-crested cockatoos (*Cacatua galerita*), anesthetized with isoflurane in 100% oxygen, provided adequate blood oxygenation and maintained tidal and minute volumes (Jaensch et al. 2001). However, clavicular air sac cannulation did not provide adequate ventilation or anesthetic maintenance (Jaensch et al. 2001).

PARENTERAL ANESTHESIA

Parenteral anesthesia has several advantages over inhalant anesthesia, including ease of use, rapid onset, minimal equipment, reasonable cost, and minimal contamination of the work space with toxic chemicals. Like inhalants, parenteral anesthetics produce dose-dependent cardiopulmonary depression. Few parenteral anesthetics are reversible; once injected, they cannot be adjusted, and most require renal or hepatic biotransformation to be cleared. Other potential disadvantages include species and individual differences, the need to determine body weight for accurate administration, and a relatively narrow margin of safety. In waterfowl, most parenteral anesthetics are delivered into the pectoral muscles, although the large leg muscles can be used.

Empirically derived dosages for parenteral drugs are only available for a few avian species. Alternatively, allometric scaling is used to approximate effective dosages. However, allometrically derived drug dosages in new species should be used with caution (Dorrestein 1991; Dorrestein & Van Miert 1988). Allometric scaling can be used to estimate respiratory variables in birds (Frappell et al. 2001). Monitoring of cardiopulmonary variables is essential when using parenteral anesthetics (Table 29.4).

Table 29.4. Injectable drugs used in waterfowl anesthesia

Common Name	Purpose	Primary Drug	Dosage (mg/kg)/Route	Second Drug	Dosage (mg/kg)/Route	Additional Drug	Dosage (mg/kg)/Route	Reference
Pekin duck (*Anas platyrhynchos*)	Liver biopsy	Tiletamine-zolazepam	13 IM[a]	Lidocaine	100 mg infiltrated			Carp et al. (1991)
Canada goose (*Branta canadensis*)	Sedation for radiology	Midazolam	2.0 IM					Valverde et al. (1990)
Pekin duck	Anesthesia research	Xylazine	1 IV					Ludders et al. (1989b)
Mallard duck (*Anas platyrhynchos*)	Anesthesia research	Ketamine	20 IV	Xylazine	1 IV			
		Ketamine	20 IV	Midazolam	2 IV			
		Ketamine	10 IV			Medetomidine	0.05 IV	Machin and Caulkett (1998a)
Mallard duck	Pre-anesthetic sedation	Midazolam	2 IM	Butorphanol	1 IM			Wilson & Pettifer (2004)
Mallard duck	Neuromuscular blockade	Cis-atracurium	0.25 IV					Wilson & Pettifer (2004)
Tufted duck (*Aythya fuligula*)	Surgery	Ketamine	10 IV	Midazolam	2 IV	Medetomidine	0.05 IV	Blogg et al. (1998)
						Buprenorphine	0.06 IM	
Pekin duck	Surgery	Ketamine	10 IV	Midazolam	2 IV	Medetomidine	0.05 IV	Blogg et al. (1998)
						Buprenorphine	0.06 IM	
Canvasback duck (*Aythya valisneria*)	Anesthesia research	Propofol	15 IV induction; 0.8/min IV infusion					Machin and Caulkett (1999)
Wood duck (*Aix sponsa*)	Prevent nest abandonment	Propofol	9–10 IV					Hepp and Manlove (2001)
Pekin duck	Anesthesia research	Pentobarbital	160 IV					Rode et al. (2003)
Mallard duck	Anesthesia research	Ketoprofen	5 IM					Machin and Livingston (2002)
Spectacled eider (*Somateria fischeri*)	Transmitter implantation	Ketoprofen	5.4 IM					Mulcahy et al. (2003)
King eider (*Somateria spectabilis*)	Transmitter implantation	Ketoprofen	2.2 IM					Mulcahy et al. (2003)
Common eider (*Somateria mollisima*)	Transmitter implantation	Ketoprofen	3.4 IM					Mulcahy et al. (2003)
Pekin duck	Pre-anesthetic sedation	Buprenorphine	0.05 IM					Wilberg (2005)
Canvasback duck	Transmitter implantation	Propofol	10 IV induction; 1–2 IV bolus	Bupivacaine	2 IM			Machin and Caulkett (2000)
Bar-tailed godwit (*Limosa lapponica*)	Transmitter implantation	Propofol	8–15 IV induction; 1–4 IV bolus	2:1 Bupivacaine/lidocaine	1.5–2.0 IM			Mulcahy et al. (2011)
Mallard duck	Anesthesia research	Xylazine	5 IM	Midazolam	5 IM			Machin and Caulkett (1998b)
		Midazolam	0.1 IM	Medetomidine	0.1 IM			
		Ketamine	8 IM	Medetomidine	0.1 IM			
		Ketamine	8 IM	Medetomidine	0.2 IM			
		Ketamine	8 IM	Medetomidine	0.3 IM			
		Ketamine	8 IM	Medetomidine	0.4 IM			

Species	Indication	Agent 1	Agent 2	Agent 3	Reference
Mute swan (*Cygnus olor*)	Induction	Ketamine 8 IM	Medetomidine 1 IM		Cooke(1995)
		Ketamine 8 IM	Medetomidine 2 IM		
		Ketamine 20 IM	Medetomidine 2 IM		
		Midazolam 2.5 IM	Fentanyl 0.025 IM		
		Midazolam 5 IM	Fentanyl 0.05 IM		
		Midazolam 5 IM	Sufentanil 0.025 IM		
		Midazolam 5 IM	Butorphanol 1 IM		
		Midazolam 2 IM	Ketamine 20 IM		
		Midazolam 2 IM	Methohexital 10 IM		
		Midazolam 10 IM	Alphaxalone-Alphadolone 36 IM		
		Midazolam 1 IV	Alphaxalone-Alphadolone 18 IV		
		Midazolam 1 IV	Ketamine 20 IV		
		Midazolam 1 IV	Ketamine 40 IV		
		Midazolam 2 IV	Ketamine 40 IV		
		Midazolam 5 IV	Ketamine 50 IV		
		Midazolam 1 IV	Ketamine 20 IV	Xylazine 5 IV	
		Midazolam 1 IV	Ketamine 10 IV	Xylazine 3 IV	
		Midazolam 1 IV	Ketamine 10 IV	Xylazine 1 IV	
		Midazolam 1 IV	Ketamine 10 IV	Medetomidine 0.03 IV	
		Midazolam 2 IV	Ketamine 10 IV	Medetomidine 0.05 IV	
		Alphaxalone-alphadolone 3.0–4.2 IV			
Mallard duck	Anesthesia research	Propofol 8 IV induction; 2.9 IV bolus			Müller et al. (2011)
Muscovy duck (*Calrina moschata*)	Anesthesia research	Propofol 8 IV induction; 0.85 IV infusion			Müller et al. (2011)
Hawaiian goose (*Branta sandvicensis*)	Sedation for handling	Ketamine 24 IM			Samour et al. (1984)
Mallard duck		Ketamine 20 IM			
Muscovy duck		Ketamine 20 IM			
Hawaiian goose		Alphaxalone-Alphadolone 23 IM			
Mallard duck		Alphaxalone-Alphadolone 11 IM			
Muscovy duck		Alphaxalone-Alphadolone 3 IM			
Muscovy duck		Xylazine 9 IM			
Mallard duck		Xylazine 8 IM			
Muscovy duck		Xylazine 51 IM			
Hawaiian goose		Ketamine 20 IM	Xlazine 5 IM		
		Ketamine 70 IM	Xlazine 10 IM		
		Ketamine 20 IM	Xlazine 5 IM		
Mallard duck	Analgesia research	Ketoprofen 5 IM			Machin and Livingston (2002)

[a]Additional doses of 3 mg/kg were used to extend anesthesia.

493

Tiletamine/Zolazepam

Tiletamine/zolazepam has been used both as an injectable and as an oral immobilizing drug in birds, especially larger animals (e.g., ratites, raptors, cranes, and penguins) (Howard et al. 1993; Janovsky et al. 2002; Kreeger et al. 1993; Lin & Ko 1997; Lin et al. 1997; Thil & Groscolas 2002; Van Heerden & Keefen 1991). This combination is rarely used in waterfowl because it does not provide adequate analgesia for painful procedures. In Pekin ducks (*Anas platyrhynchos*) tiletamine/zolazepam (13 mg/kg IM), with lidocaine (100 mg) infiltrated into the skin and musculature at the incision site, was used for anesthesia to surgically collect liver biopsies (Carp et al. 1991).

Ketamine

Ketamine alone is not used in waterfowl and shorebirds because of poor muscle relaxation and spontaneous movement, even at high dosages. It is often combined with other drugs to minimize these unwanted side effects. In Pekin ducks, xylazine alone (1 mg/kg IV) or combined with ketamine (20 mg/kg IV) induced hypoventilation and hypoxemia (Ludders et al. 1989b). In Pekin, mallard, and tufted ducks (*Aythya fuligula*), a combination of ketamine (10 mg/kg IV), midazolam (2 mg/kg IV), and medetomidine (0.05 mg/kg IV) was effective for anesthesia and surgery (Blogg et al. 1998; Machin & Caulkett 1998b).

Alpha 2-Adrenergic Agonists

Xylazine/ketamine combinations were commonly used for avian field anesthesia. Xylazine has largely been replaced by medetomidine. In mallards IV, but not IM, medetomidine/midazolam/ketamine produced adequate analgesia and anesthesia for a 30-minute period (Machin & Caulkett 1998a). In the same study, various combinations of medetomidine, ketamine, fentanyl, midazolam, butorphanol, methohexital, or alphaxalone-alphadolone delivered IM or intranasally were either ineffective or lethal. Medetomidine and xylazine, alone or in combination with other drugs, are used with caution. Sometimes, they fail to immobilize birds or else they produce significant cardiopulmonary side effects (Atalan et al. 2002; Pollock et al. 2001; Sandmeier 2000; Uzun et al. 2003; Varner et al. 2004). An advantage to the use of α-2 agonists alone or in combination with other drugs is their reversibility with the α-2 antagonists, atipamezole and yohimbine.

Local Anesthetics

Lidocaine and bupivacaine, both lipophilic amino-amides, are most commonly used. Their duration of effect has not been determined in birds, but in mammals, lidocaine lasts 1–2 hours and bupivacaine 4–6 hours (Lemke & Dawson 2000; Skarda 1996). Use of local anesthetics in birds has been limited by fear of toxicity. To avoid adverse side effects (i.e., depression, drowsiness, seizures, and cardiovascular collapse), the maximum dose is calculated prior to the start of the procedure (4 mg/kg lidocaine, 2 mg/kg bupivacaine) (Hocking et al. 1997; Machin 2005a). Vasoconstrictors (i.e., epinephrine) have been added to lidocaine solutions to slow systemic absorption and extend the duration of action. However, when a longer duration of action is desired, a longer-acting drug (e.g., bupivacaine) should be chosen instead. A recent pilot study reported the use of lidocaine and bupivacaine in the development of a brachial plexus nerve blockade in mallard ducks (Brenner et al. 2010).

Propofol

Propofol has found increasing popularity in waterfowl anesthesia. It can be used for induction followed by an inhalant for maintenance (Goulden 1995). Although not a widely used technique in birds, propofol can be administered by a constant rate infusion. Canvasback ducks (*Aythya valisneria*) were maintained with a constant rate infusion (0.8 mg/kg/min) following a bolus induction (15 mg/kg) (Machin & Caulkett 1999). More commonly, it is given by bolus, both to induce and to maintain anesthesia, and the frequency and size of the boluses are titrated to maintain the desired anesthetic depth. Propofol has a narrow therapeutic index. Artificial ventilation may mask overdosage because the initial sign of toxicity is hypoventilation (Machin & Caulkett 1999). With waterfowl and shorebirds, apnea should be expected in all individuals given propofol.

Alphaxolone/Alphadalone

A mixture of alphadolone acetate (3 mg/mL) and alphaxalone (9 mg/mL) has found limited use in waterfowl. This combination has been used for induction and as a sedative for handling (Cooke 1995; Machin & Caulkett 1998b; Samour et al. 1984).

VASCULAR ACCESS

The veins most commonly used for vascular access are the jugular, medial metatarsal, and basilic. For both waterfowl and shorebirds, the jugular vein is used to obtain blood samples of greater than 1 mL and can be used for placement of relatively large catheters. The jugular is the largest peripheral vein, has a fairly thick wall, and hematoma formation is uncommon. The right jugular vein is often stated to be larger than the left, but either is used.

The basilic vein crosses the medial distal humerus and, because it is visible under the skin, is a favorite phlebotomy site for the inexperienced. However, its narrow lumen, thin walls, and curving course make it difficult to obtain more than a small blood sample. In small birds, it can be pierced with a needle tip and a few blood drops collected on the skin using capillary tubes. Hematomas occur very commonly, because of its thin wall and poor technique. Their formation is prevented in several ways. First, place pressure over the needle and vein prior to withdrawing the needle, preventing blood leakage. Second, place just enough pressure to reduce blood flow, but not to empty the vessel. If the latter occurs, a hematoma forms when the pressure is lifted and blood rushes back into the vein and out the puncture. Finally, place gentle pressure over the puncture site for at least 2 minutes to allow adequate clotting.

The medial metatarsal vein courses along the medial aspect of the tarsometatarsal bone and crosses the tibiotarsal joint. The presence of scaly skin may increase the level of discomfort for the bird when this site is used. However, the vein is usually visible, the featherless skin permits good disinfection, and the tightness of the skin discourages hematoma formation. Blood is obtained using the needle-nick technique, a needle and syringe, or a butterfly catheter. The relatively small diameter of the vein minimizes the amount of blood that can be obtained, especially in small birds. However, it is useful for administration of drugs, including propofol. Although clotting at this site is usually not a problem, clotting enhancers can be used.

ANALGESIA

In waterfowl and shorebirds, any procedure that would cause pain in humans or result in tissue damage should be performed under anesthesia with consideration for analgesia (see Chapter 3). However, species differences in response to analgesics, and the relative paucity of published research in waterfowl, makes selection and dosing difficult. As with mammals, preemptive administration of analgesics is more effective in easing the pain caused by tissue damage during surgery than is postoperative analgesic administration.

Nonsteroidal Anti-Inflammatory Drugs (NSAIDs)

Flunixin meglumine, ketoprofen, meloxicam, and carprofen have all been used in waterfowl. Flunixin meglumine is not recommended because of a greater risk of adverse effects than in mammals (Clyde & Paul-Murphy 1999). These effects, noted in other bird species, include renal toxicity, regurgitation, tenesmus, and injection site necrosis (Clyde & Paul-Murphy 1999; Machin 2005a; Machin et al. 2001; Mansour et al. 1988). Nonsteroidal drugs that are not selective for cycloxygenase-2 are used with caution. In male eiders, the nonselective NSAID ketoprofen was implicated in renal toxicosis and death when given perioperatively (Mulcahy et al. 2003). Female eiders were not adversely affected. This sex-related difference was thought to be due to physiologic changes associated with male behavior on the nesting grounds. Ketoprofen (5 mg/kg IM) takes about

30 minutes from injection to the onset of analgesia (Machin & Livingston 2002).

Birds eliminate NSAIDs rapidly, but differences in elimination rates occur between species (Baert & De Backer 2003). Compared with chickens, ostriches (*Struthio camelus*), turkeys (*Meleagris gallopavo*), and pigeons (*Columba livia*), ducks (*Anas platyrhynchos*) are intermediate in elimination half-life for meloxicam (0.72 hour), a NSAID selective for cyclooxygenase-2 (Baert & De Backer 2003). Allometric scaling can be used to predict clearance of drugs, including NSAIDs, but caution should be used using this technique (Hunter et al. 2008).

Opioids

Opioids have generally been avoided in waterfowl because of fear of respiratory depression. Birds differ from mammals in their response to μ agonist opioids. This appears to be due to a preponderance of κ opioid receptors over μ (Mansour et al. 1988). Butorphanol (1 mg/kg) combined with midazolam (2 mg/kg) was used as premedication for isoflurane anesthesia in a mallard duck (Wilson & Pettifer 2004). Buprenorphine (0.05 mg/kg, IM) given to domestic ducks 1 hour before induction with isoflurane effectively reduced reaction to painful stimuli, but had strong respiratory depressant effects (Wilberg 2005). In tufted ducks buprenorphine (0.06 mg/kg IM) was given at the time of anesthetic induction to provide postsurgical analgesia (Blogg et al. 1998). Premedication with butorphanol (1 mg/kg IM) or morphine (0.1–3.0 mg/kg IV) allows a dose-dependent reduction in inhalant anesthetics in chickens (Concannon et al. 1995) and in a psittacine (Curro et al. 1994), but not turkeys (Reim & Middleton 1995). In harlequin ducks (*Histrionicus histrionicus*), preanesthetic administration of butorphanol (0.5–2.0 mg/kg IM) did not reduce isoflurane requirement for surgery (D. Mulcahy, unpubl data, 1997).

FIELD TECHNIQUES

Free-living waterfowl and shorebirds are anesthetized for a variety of reasons, including restraint. Laparoscopic sexing was a common indication (Fiala 1979; Garcelon et al. 1985; Greenwood 1983; Ketterson & Nolan 1986; Richner 1989; Risser 1971). However, unless immediate results are needed, surgical sexing has largely been supplanted by molecular techniques (Boutette et al. 2002; Griffiths 2000). An increasing number of field anesthesia and surgeries are done to collect liver biopsies for determination of cytochrome P450 1A, a hepatic enzyme induced by exposure to hydrocarbons from spilled oil (Esler et al. 2002; Golet et al. 2002; Jewett et al. 2002; Mulcahy & Esler 2010; Peterson et al. 2003; Trust et al. 2000;). Isoflurane is the anesthetic of choice for taking surgical liver biopsies from birds (Degernes et al. 2002). The cytochrome

P450 isoenzyme responsible for the limited isoflurane metabolism that occurs is different from that assayed for oil spill exposure (Kharasch & Thummel 1993).

There is a growing need for avian field anesthesia to surgically implant transmitters and data loggers (Butler & Woakes 1979; Olsen et al. 1992). Many waterfowl species, especially diving birds, do not tolerate external attachment of transmitters. Implanted transmitters are better tolerated, but signal strength is greatly attenuated. An important advance in the technique has been the addition of percutaneous antennas that solved the signal attenuation problem (Korschgen et al. 1996). Percutaneous antennas also allowed recently miniaturized satellite transmitters (PTT-100, Microwave Telemetry, Columbia, MD) to be implanted in waterfowl, especially sea ducks (Petersen et al. 1995, 1999, 2003, 2006). Coelomically implanted transmitters are placed in an abdominal air sac, but no studies have evaluated the respiratory effects of a large foreign body in this air sac.

Complicating the anesthesia required to implant transmitters into the air sacs is that the surgeries are often done in remote locations in tents, on boats, or even inside helicopters (Brown & Luebbert 2002). The opening of part of the respiratory system to the atmosphere carries its own complications. In spontaneously breathing pigeons anesthetized with isoflurane, the opening of an air sac for endoscopic splenic biopsy worsened hypoventilation, despite an increased respiratory rate (Touzot-Jourde et al. 2005). This response was possibly due to high $PaCO_2$ or to a lighter anesthetic plane following dilution with room air entering the incision. If the birds were ventilated mechanically, the ventilator did not achieve the selected inspiratory pressure due to leakage through the open air sac. In those birds, a respiratory alkalemia developed, and $PaCO_2$, HCO_3, base excess, heart rate, and mean arterial blood pressure were all significantly decreased, although PaO_2 was maintained (Touzot-Jourde et al. 2005). The incision required to implant a transmitter creates a much larger opening in the abdominal air sac than does that for an endoscopic biopsy. This suggests the cardiovascular effects during implantation are the same or worse.

When free-living birds require general anesthesia, it is rarely practical to do more than a quick physical examination prior to induction. The ability to do hematology and serum chemistries is rarely available. However, the emergence of point-of-care blood analyzers has begun to permit at least some screening of patients in the field (Stoskopf et al. 2010). Consumer-grade blood glucose analyzers have begun to be used in seabird rehabilitation (Lieske et al. 2002). The prandial status of wild avian anesthetic candidates is usually unknown, and it is advisable to hold wild birds for as short a time as possible, to limit stress. It is recommended to hold birds for about an hour before anesthesia, to prevent intra-operative draining of crop contents with subsequent aspiration.

Holding, Transportation, and Handling

Surgical facilities for field research are usually centralized and the birds are transported by truck, boat, aircraft, or by being hand-carried from the capture site. Birds are transported in soft bags, boxes, or animal carriers. Cardboard boxes are rarely suitable because of the lack of air circulation, even if holes are punched through the sides. Techniques for carrying birds are directed at protecting them from trauma, minimizing stress, and preserving the protective function of the feathers. It is preferable to transport birds individually, to prevent fighting. If more than one bird must be placed in a transport container, mixing birds of the same sex is avoided.

The size of the container should be sufficient to allow the bird to stand and turn around. Shorebirds especially prefer standing, and it may be detrimental to place them in a container that prevents them from doing so. Placing a number of birds into a larger container is not recommended; the birds generally huddle in the back of the container and will not use the extra space. If too many birds are placed into a single container, trauma or death from suffocation may result from birds piling up in a corner.

The insulation of feathers and aquatic lifestyle of waterfowl contribute to hyperthermia during dry transportation. This author has seen body temperatures as high as 43.9°C at induction in birds that survived anesthesia and surgery. A transport container must have adequate ventilation to prevent hyperthermia. Commercial cat and dog crates have grated windows, which let air circulate (Fig. 29.6). However, the grid may permit bird bills to pass through and suffer damage. This is especially important when holding long-billed shorebirds. The existing grid is covered with finer mesh netting that prevents trauma, but still allows air circulation and observation of the bird.

Prevention of feather soiling during transportation and holding is very important. Soiled feathers are a source of infection during surgery, and are less capable of maintaining a constant body temperature during anesthesia and recovery. Following release, a soiled bird has to devote more time to preening. This leads to increased energy expended, reduced feed consumption, and increased risk of predation. A towel or other absorbent material is placed on the bottom of the transport container. If the bird is permitted to rest directly on the bottom of the container, the towels are changed frequently to assure a clean and dry substrate. It is preferable to have waterfowl and shorebirds rest on netting suspended from a frame on the bottom of the container (Fig. 29.2). The mesh size should be small enough to prevent toe entanglement, but allow excreta

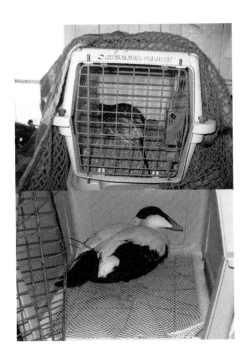

Figure 29.6. Examples of holding and recovering cages made by modifying an animal carrier by the addition of artificial turf (top) or mesh surrounding a PVC-pipe frame (bottom) to reduce fecal soiling of feathers. A turf bottom (top) is safer for a bird like the bar-tailed godwit (*Limosa lapponica*), that has a long bill and toes, to reduce the chance of entanglement. A finer mesh net should be attached to the inside of the wire-grid door and air holes to prevent damage to bills of shorebirds and ducks such as the common eider (*Somateria mollissima*), shown in the bottom picture.

to pass through. Alternatively, artificial turf is used for the substrate (Fig. 29.2).

When captured, wild birds rarely eat or drink in transport or temporary holding facilities, especially with humans nearby. Pretreatment holding times are, therefore, usually limited to 1–2 hours to reduce stress and dehydration. For most procedures, birds are returned to their holding containers for about an hour after they have recovered, then released.

The feathers are often disarranged or damaged during capture and initial handling to free the bird from nets or traps. Handling must be gently done to maintain feather integrity and waterproofing, especially for waterfowl that will be released into cold waters. If surgery is done on wild-caught water birds intended for immediate release, feathers are not be plucked because it will increase the amount of heat lost when the bird is released into cold water. It also imposes an increase in energy demand during feather replacement. Instead of plucking, the feathers are swept clear of a surgical site and held to the side with a water-soluble "liquid bandage" (e.g., Facilitator, IDEXX Pharmaceuticals, Greensboro, NC). The covering feathers are held apart to expose the down and a line of liquid bandage is

placed on them and massaged in. The liquid bandage collapses the structure of the down feathers, allowing them to be swept to the side, exposing the skin. The liquid bandage quickly becomes tacky, holding the collapsed down to the sides. The cleared surgical field is relatively small, but is sufficient to allow an incision. Since it is water soluble, the liquid bandage is quickly preened free of the feathers within hours of the bird's release. Honey has been used to in lieu of liquid bandage in field work (Cheryl Scott, personal communication). Tape (Micropore Surgical Tape®, 3M Health Care, St. Paul, Minnesota, USA) can be applied to the feathers wetted with liquid bandage to further prevent contamination of the surgical site. A transparent sterile barrier drape (Veterinary Specialty Products, Mission, Kansas, USA) with an adhesive backing will stick to the tape, and following the procedure, both tape and drape can be peeled off with minimal feather loss.

Lingering sedative effects are undesirable in field anesthesia of wild birds. Birds are released relatively quickly after recovery from anesthesia, placing them at risk of injury or predation or unable to maintain social status in a flock or a pair bond commitment. Due to these risks, analgesics that might compromise reactivity (e.g., opioids) are not used.

Field Anesthesia

Oral Drug Administration Waterfowl and other birds have been captured using bait treated with alpha-chloralose, a centrally active chloral derivative of glucose (Bailey et al. 1999; Belant & Seamans 1997, 1999; Belant et al. 1999). Other oral drugs used to capture waterfowl have not had the same level of use and experimentation (Cline & Greenwood 1972). Alpha-chloralose is a soporific and narcotic; it does not produce general anesthesia. It has been most used as an avicide to control nuisance birds. Although usually added to corn, it has also been combined (30 mg/kg) with margarine and used in tablet form to capture Canada geese (*Branta canadensis*) (Belant & Seamans 1997; Crider 1967). This approach is used for birds that habitually use a certain area. When applied to a substrate like bread, individual birds can be targeted if they can be approached and thrown the bait. However, induction is very long and recovery may take many hours. As a result, this drug is not suitable for birds that are to be quickly released after a procedure. Multiple exposures may be complicated by drug accumulation in the tissues.

Alpha-chloralose is hazardous to use, and a current Material Safety Data Sheet must be obtained from the manufacturer and consulted for the proper personal protective equipment. Legal use of alpha-chloralose in the United States requires an Investigational New Animal Drug Application (#6602) issued by the Food and Drug Administration to the Animal and Plant Health Inspection Service, U.S. Department of Agriculture. In mallard ducks, the effective dose (ED$_{50}$) is 15 mg/kg, and the lethal dose (LD$_{50}$) is 34 mg/kg, resulting in a therapeutic index (TI = LD$_{50}$/ED$_{50}$) of 2.2 (Cline & Greenwood 1972). Alpha-chloralose is much less safe in mallard ducks than chickens where ED$_{50}$ = 45 mg/kg, LD$_{50}$ = 300 mg/kg, and TI = 6.7 (Loibl et al. 1988). This difference indicates that interspecies variability in susceptibility must be carefully considered. Overdosing is a potential problem; birds that have ingested alpha-chloralose are at risk of drowning if they enter the water. Drugged birds that escape and die in wetlands are a slight risk for starting an outbreak of avian botulism in waterfowl (Goldberg et al. 2004). Care is taken to prevent secondary poisoning of nontarget species, including domestic animals (Segev et al. 2006).

Other drugs have been added to bait, but none are registered for use as veterinary drugs. Although tiletamine-zolazepam (80 mg/kg PO) caused deep sedation of common buzzards (*Buteo buteo*), this combination has not been evaluated in wild waterfowl (Janovsky et al. 2002).

Inhalation Anesthesia

Inhalation anesthesia in free-living birds is usually performed with isoflurane. The minimum equipment for administration includes a tank of oxygen, regulator and pressure tubing, flow meter, vaporizer, and breathing system (see also Chapter 6). Most people prefer the vaporizer and flow meter mounted on a stand for convenience. Concepts of portability vary, and a "mobile" anesthesia apparatus to anesthetize 150-g doves might be one that fits snugly into the back of a truck (Small et al. 2004).

Use of compressed oxygen in the field at low ambient temperatures may contribute to loss of body heat. If safely possible, oxygen cylinders are kept in a warmed environment. Exposure to very cold temperatures can shrink metal parts and seals causing gas leakage. This author has had oxygen cylinders fresh from refilling plants prove to be empty after transportation to very cold field sites. Cylinder valves transported to cold environments should be tightened more than usual and checked upon arrival at the field location. It is prudent to always have a plan for an alternative anesthetic technique (e.g., injectable drugs).

Induction of wild-caught waterfowl is done using isoflurane and a mask. The vaporizer is set at 4% with a minimum oxygen flow of 1 L/min for most ducks and small geese. Occasionally, a wild bird is sufficiently stressed to resist induction, and the vaporizer is turned to 5%. If induction resistance occurs regularly, consideration should be given to preanesthetic sedation of the birds.

Intranasal Drug Administration

Intranasal administration of sedative drugs has seldom been used in avian anesthesia. In mallard ducks, intra-nasal alphaxalone-alphadolone had no effect (Machin & Caulkett 1998a). Intranasal ketamine, midazolam, methohexital, and butorphanol alone or in combination produced light sedation at best, as did intranasal ketamine and midazolam when combined with IV propofol (Machin & Caulkett 1998a). However, intranasal delivery was not combined with isoflurane administration. Intranasal midazolam or diazepam sedated canaries (*Serinus canarius*) and ring-necked parakeets (*Psittacula krameri*) sufficiently that they tolerated dorsal recumbency, while xylazine and detomidine caused sedation (Vesal & Eskandari 2006; Vesal & Zare 2006). The effects took only 1–2 minutes to occur. Diazepam and midazolam administered intranasally to domestic pigeons (*Columba livia*) caused sedation sufficient to maintain dorsal decumbency for mean times of 47 and 23 minutes for the two drugs, respectively (Moghadam et al. 2009). Diazepam and midazolam administered intranasally to finches (*Taeneopygia guttata*) permitted dorsal recumbency to be maintained for mean times of 68 and 32 minutes, respectively (Bigham & Moghaddam 2013). Intranasal xylazine caused sedation, but it was not sufficient to permit dorsal recumbency of pigeons or finches (Bigham & Moghaddam 2013; Moghadam et al. 2009). Flumazenil and yohimbine are also successfully used via the intranasal route to reverse the alpha-agonist sedatives. The same agonists can be given IM as preanesthetic sedatives, but onset of action will not be as fast. Flumazenil should not be given IM due to the pain caused by its acidity. The rapid onset and duration of action of sedatives given intranasally to birds warrants further attention for use in reducing stress in captured wild birds intended for anesthesia and surgery.

Injectable Anesthesia

Given the difficulties of transporting inhalant anesthetics and compressed oxygen cylinders, it is not surprising that injectable anesthetics have been assessed for their usefulness in field surgeries. For the intracoelomic implantation of radio transmitters, propofol has been used as a general anesthetic, combined with bupivacaine or a 2:1 mixture of bupivacaine/lidocaine infused at the incision site (Machin & Caulkett 1999, 2000; Mulcahy et al. 2011). The propofol/bupivacaine anesthetic system eliminates shipping hazardous materials. In addition, the equipment required for propofol/bupivacaine is much less expensive, and the mass of materials required is a fraction of that required using isoflurane as an anesthetic (Fig. 29.7).

For several years, the author has used propofol and bupivacaine/lidocaine in field surgeries to implant transmitters into hundreds of birds. The medial aspect of the tibiotarsus is prepared for catheter placement by cleaning and disinfecting with nondetergent iodophor solution. A 0.508-mm (25-g), 1-cm butterfly catheter (No. 4573, Abbott Laboratories, North Chicago, IL), or

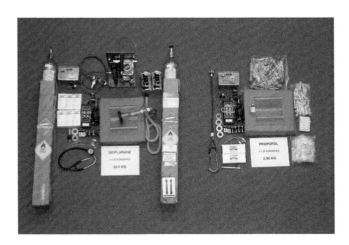

Figure 29.7. Comparison of equipment and supplies required to perform an identical number of surgeries using isoflurane (left) or propofol (right). The latter system totals about 10% of the weight of the former. The cartons containing the oxygen cylinders bear Hazardous Materials labels.

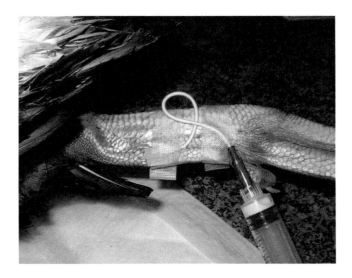

Figure 29.8. A 0.508-mm (25-gauge), 1-cm butterfly catheter placed in the tibiotarsal vein of a yellow-billed loon (*Gavia adamsii*) and connected to a syringe holding propofol. The wings of the "butterfly" have been cut off to reduce the chance of dislodging the needle.

an alternative catheter of suitable size and length for the bird, is placed in the medial metatarsal vein (Fig. 29.8). Stability of the catheter is improved by snipping the plastic butterfly wings from the needle. Other butterfly catheters and over-the-needle catheters can also be used, depending on the length of the bird's leg. Birds are induced by slow administration of propofol (20 mg/kg or to effect, depending on the temperament and level of excitement of the bird). Following induction, which occurs within seconds, the catheter and its tubing are taped in place. Following preparation of the surgical site, bupivacaine or bupivacaine/lidocaine

mixture (2 : 1 v/v) is infused at and around the incision site to a maximum of 2 mg/kg. Additional propofol is given by bolus (1–4 mg/kg) to maintain a plane of anesthesia suitable for the procedure being done. Clues to indicate the need for additional propofol are movement or tone in the legs and wings, or opening of the eye with the presence of a reflex movement of the nictitating membrane. Following induction, bar-tailed godwits and bristle-thighed curlews *Numenius tahitiensis*) were given the first additional bolus of propofol at 1–11 minutes (median 2 minutes) for godwits and at 1–10 minutes (median 3 minutes) for curlews (Mulcahy et al. 2011).

Following induction with 8 mg/kg of propofol, a continuous rate infusion (0.85 mg/kg/min) was compared to bolus administration (2.9 mg/kg) in mute swans (*Cygnus olor*) (Müller et al. 2011). In that study, bolus administration of propofol was considered to be unsatisfactory due to sudden awakening of the swans. However, that result suggests a difficulty by the researchers to detect signs of anesthetic lightening in time to administer additional propofol. The present author has used propofol administered by bolus to anesthetize tundra swans (*Cygnus columbianus*) without problems with unexpected awakenings.

Hazardous Material Shipping

Inhalant anesthetics and compressed oxygen cylinders are classified as hazardous materials for air transportation and can only be shipped as cargo, never as checked baggage (Anonymous 2006). Failure to follow regulations governing shipment of hazardous materials may result in significant legal sanctions. They must be shipped in specific packaging, with appropriate hazard labels and forms. Hazardous materials shipping agents should be consulted to assure proper packaging and labeling. Adequate time and planning must be allowed to assure the anesthetic and oxygen will arrive when needed. Additional regulations apply to moving hazardous materials on other forms of public transportation (e.g., buses, trains, and ferries) and via transportation corridors, such as tunnels and bridges. Empty oxygen cylinders are not classified as hazardous materials and may be transported on passenger aircraft. To avoid confusion and delay, empty oxygen tanks and their packaging should have all hazardous materials labels removed or covered. It is prudent to leave the valves of empty cylinders open during shipping to avoid partial repressurization due to temperature or air pressure changes, and to attach a large label stating "Empty" to the container.

Properly packaged and labeled isoflurane and other inhalant anesthetics can be shipped (as cargo) on an aircraft bearing passengers, but compressed oxygen cylinders can only be carried on purely cargo flights. In some cases, it may be possible to transport isoflurane, but not compressed oxygen, to a field site because of

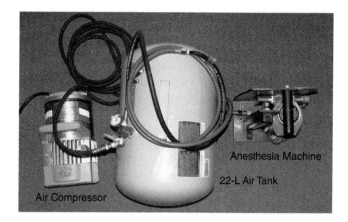

Figure 29.9. Assembly of an air-driven inhalant anesthetic system that drives a vaporizer with compressed air from a low pressure, small-volume air tank filled by an electrical air compressor.

the types of aircraft services available to the nearest staging area. If medical-grade oxygen cannot be shipped to a location, a large tank regulator can be fitted to a tank of welder's oxygen, which can often be found in remote villages and on commercial fishing boats. Alternatively, it is possible to drive an anesthetic vaporizer using compressed air. A small electric air compressor and a low pressure, 22-L portable air tank such as those used by house painters to power paint sprayers can be shipped to the field as baggage without concern for Hazardous Material shipping regulations. Most field camps have small electrical generators for recharging batteries. The air tank is filled using the air compressor and then is connected to a flow-meter and thence to the vaporizer (Fig. 29.9). The air pressure in the tank should not fall below 0.34 Mpa (50 psi), limiting this technique to short-duration procedures unless the compressor is run continuously. It is theoretically possible to fill the air tank using a hand-driven bicycle tire air pump, assuming sufficient enthusiasm for prolonged physical exertion. Specialized draw-over vaporizers, developed for military use, use ambient air, and have been adapted for use in wild animals (Lewis 2004). With any inhalant anesthetic system that uses air, it is critical to provide adequate ventilation to assure oxygenation.

Anesthesia to Prevent Nest Abandonment

Waterfowl are commonly captured while sitting on nests during laying or incubating eggs. These captures may be of short duration for the purposes of marking, measuring, or sampling. The stress of removing a sitting bird and the presence of humans when the bird is replaced on the nest causes a high rate of nest abandonment. Briefly anesthetizing gray partridges (*Perdix perdix*) and mallards being returned to the nests on which they had been captured almost eliminated nest abandonment (Rotella & Ratti 1990; Smith et al. 1980).

Despite widespread use, it is considered inappropriate and hazardous to use any inhalant anesthetic by pouring it onto cotton balls (Heard 1997). In that technique, methoxyflurane is placed on cotton in a container at the nest site; the head of the bird is then placed into the container until muscle relaxation occurs. The bird is then placed on the nest with its head tucked under its wing and the researcher quickly withdraws. The bird is closely monitored to prevent anesthesia becoming too deep because no vaporizer is used. A light anesthetic depth is sufficient because the bird only needs to be obtunded for the length of time it takes to place it on the nest and withdraw. When methoxyflurane manufacture was discontinued in the 1990s, some biologists switched to isoflurane delivered via cotton ball to birds being replaced on nests. However, the properties of isoflurane make it more hazardous than methoxyflurane to use for this purpose.

Propofol has recently been used to render birds unconscious to prevent nest abandonment (Hepp & Manlove 2001; Machin & Caulkett 2000). Propofol (10 mg/kg over 1 minute followed by additional 1–2 mg/kg boluses until induction) is delivered via a catheter in the medial metatarsal vein (Machin & Caulkett 2000).

Induction of wood ducks (*Aix sponsa*) with methoxyflurane averaged 5 minutes; although not stated, it is presumed that wood ducks given propofol IV were immediately induced (Hepp & Manlove 2001). There was no significant difference in mean time to recovery for wood ducks anesthetized with methoxyflurane (11.8 ± 1.6 minutes) compared with propofol (9.2 ± 0.8 minutes) (Hepp & Manlove 2001). The disadvantage of using propofol is that the biologist must be able to deliver it into a vein at the nest site. An advantage of propofol is that it is not classified as a hazardous material for the purpose of shipping.

Mention of trade names does not imply government endorsement.

REFERENCES

Abou-Madi N. 2001. Avian anesthesia. *The Veterinary Clinics of North America. Exotic Animal Practice* 4:147–167.

Adamson TP, Burger RE. 1986. Sodium bicarbonate infusion increases discharge frequency of intrapulmonary chemoreceptors only at high CO_2. *Respiration Physiology* 66:83–93.

Aguilar RF. 1996. Arrhythmias associated with isoflurane anesthesia in bald eagles (*Haliaeetus leucocephalus*). *Journal of Zoo and Wildlife Medicine* 26:508–516.

Altman RB. 1992. A method for reducing exposure of operating room personnel to anesthetic gas. *Journal of the Association of Avian Veterinarians* 6:99–101.

Anonymous. 2006. *IATA Dangerous Goods Regulations*. Montreal: International Air Transport Association.

Atalan G, Uzun M, Demirkan I, et al. 2002. Effect of medetomidine-butorphanol-ketamine anaesthesia and atipamezole on heart and respiratory rate and cloacal temperature of domestic pigeons. *Journal of Veterinary Medicine. A, Physiology, Pathology, Clinical Medicine* 49:281–285.

Baert K, De Backer P. 2003. Comparative pharmacokinetics of three non-steroidal anti-inflammatory drugs in five bird species. *Comparative Biochemistry and Physiology. C: Comparative Pharmacology* 134:25–33.

Bailey TA, Toosi A, Samour JH. 1999. Anaesthesia of cranes with alphaxolone-alphadolone. *The Veterinary Record* 145:84–85.

Bebout DE, Hempleman SE. 1999. Chronic hypercapnia resets CO_2 sensitivity of avian intrapulmonary chemoreceptors. *American Journal of Physiology—Regulatory Integrative and Comparative Physiology* 276:R317–R322.

Bednarski RM, Ludders JW, LeBlanc PH, et al. 1985. Isoflurane-nitrous oxide-oxygen anesthesia in an Andean condor. *Journal of the American Veterinary Medical Association* 187:1209–1210.

Belant JL, Seamans TW. 1997. Comparison of three formulations of alpha-chloralose for immobilization of Canada geese. *Journal of Wildlife Diseases* 33:606–610.

Belant JL, Seamans TW. 1999. Alpha-chloralose immobilization of rock doves in Ohio. *Journal of Wildlife Diseases* 35:239–242.

Belant JL, Tyson LA, Seamans TW. 1999. Use of alpha-chloralose by the Wildlife Services program to capture nuisance birds. *Wildlife Society Bulletin* 27:938–942.

Bigham AS, Moghaddam AKZ.2013. Finch (*Taeneopygia guttata*) sedation with intranasal administration of diazepam, midazolam or xylazine. *Journal of Veterinary Pharmacology and Therapeutics* 36:102–104.

Blogg SL, Townsend PP, Butler PJ, et al. 1998. A method of anaesthesia and post-operative care for experimental procedures in avian species. *Animal Technology: Journal of the Institute of Animal Technicians* 49:101–109.

Boedeker NC, Carpenter JW, Mason DE. 2005. Comparison of body temperatures of pigeons (*Columba livia*) anesthetized by three different anesthetic delivery systems. *Journal of Avian Medicine and Surgery* 19:1–6.

Boutette JB, Ramsay EC, Potgieter LND, et al. 2002. An improved polymerase chain reactionrestriction fragment length polymorphism assay for gender identification in birds. *Journal of Avian Medicine and Surgery* 16:198–202.

Brenner DJ, Larsen S, Dickinson PJ, et al. 2010. Development of an avian brachial plexus nerve block technique for perioperative analgesia in mallard ducks (*Anas platyrhynchos*). *Journal of Avian Medicine and Surgery* 24:24–34.

Brown C, Pilny AA. 2006. Air sac cannula placement in birds. *Lab Animal* 35:23–24.

Brown CS, Luebbert J. 2002. Arctic research: spectacled eiders, surgery, satellites, and summer solstice. *Journal of Avian Medicine and Surgery* 16:53–56.

Burger RE, Estavillo J. 1978. The alteration of CO_2 respiratory sensitivity in chickens by thoracic visceral denervation. *Respiration Physiology* 32:251–263.

Butler PJ. 1988. The exercise response and the "classical" diving response during natural submersion in birds and mammals. *Canadian Journal of Zoology* 66:29–39.

Butler PJ, Woakes AJ. 1979. Changes in heart rate and respiratory frequency during natural behaviour of ducks, with particular reference to diving. *The Journal of Experimental Biology* 79:283–300.

Carp NZ, Saputelli J, Halbherr C, et al. 1991. A technique for liver biopsy performed in Pekin ducks using anesthesia with Telazol. *Laboratory Animal Science* 41:474–475.

Carpenter JW, Mason DE. 2001. Use of a heated, artificial ventilator in exotic animal anesthesia. *Exotic DVM* 3(3):15.

Cline DR, Greenwood RJ. 1972. Effect of certain anesthetic agents on mallard ducks. *Journal of the American Veterinary Medical Association* 161:624–633.

Clippinger TL, Bennett RA. 1998. Successful treatment of a traumatic tracheal stenosis in a goose by surgical resection and anastomosis. *Journal of Avian Medicine and Surgery* 12:243–247.

Clyde VL, Paul-Murphy J. 1999. Avian analgesia. In: *Zoo & Wild Animal Medicine* (ME Fowler, RE Miller, eds.), pp. 309–314. Philadelphia: W.B. Saunders.

Concannon KT, Dodam JR, Hellyer PW. 1995. Influence of mu- and kappa-opioid agonist on isoflurane minimal anesthetic concentration in chickens. *American Journal of Veterinary Research* 56:806–811.

Cooke SW. 1995. Swan anaesthesia. *The Veterinary Record* 136:476.

Crider ED. 1967. Alpha-chloralose used to capture Canada geese. *The Journal of Wildlife Management* 31:258–264.

Curro TG. 1998. Anesthesia of pet birds. *Seminars in Avian and Exotic Pet Medicine* 7:10–21.

Curro TG, Brunson DB, Paul-Murphy J. 1994. Determination of the ED50 of isoflurane and evaluation of the isoflurane-sparing effect of butorphanol in cockatoos (*Cacatua* spp.). *Veterinary Surgery* 23:429–433.

Davenport J, O'Halloran J, Smiddy P. 2004. Plumage temperatures of dippers Cinclus cinclus on the roost and in the hand: implications for handling small passerines. *Ringing and Migration* 22:65–69.

Degernes LA, Harms CA, Golet GH, et al. 2002. Anesthesia and liver biopsy techniques for pigeon guillemots (*Cepphus columba*) suspected of exposure to crude oil in marine environments. *Journal of Avian Medicine and Surgery* 16:291–299.

Dorrestein GM. 1991. The pharmacokinetics of avian therapeutics. *The Veterinary Clinics of North America. Small Animal Practice* 21:1241–1264.

Dorrestein GM, Van Miert A. 1988. Pharmacotherapeutic aspects of medication of birds. *Journal of Veterinary Pharmacology and Therapeutics* 11:33–44.

Edling TM, Degernes LA, Flammer K, et al. 2001. Capnographic monitoring of anesthetized African grey parrots receiving intermittent positive pressure ventilation. *Journal of the American Veterinary Medical Association* 219:1714–1718.

Esler D, Bowman TD, Trust KA, et al. 2002. Harlequin duck population recovery following the "Exxon Valdez" oil spill: progress, process and constraints. *Marine Ecology Progress Series* 241:271–286.

Fedde MR, Gatz RN, Slama H, et al. 1974. Intrapulmonary CO_2 receptors in the duck. I. Stimulus specificity. *Respiration Physiology* 22:99–114.

Fiala KL. 1979. A laparotomy technique for nesting birds. *Bird-Banding* 50:366–367.

Frappell PB, Hinds DS, Boggs DF. 2001. Scaling of respiratory variables and the breathing pattern in birds: an allometric and phylogenetic approach. *Physiological and Biochemical Zoology* 74:75–89.

Furilla RA, Jones DR. 1986. The contribution of nasal receptors to the cardiac response to diving in restrained and unrestrained redhead ducks (*Aythya americana*). *The Journal of Experimental Biology* 121:227–238.

Garcelon DK, Martell MS, Redig PT, et al. 1985. Morphometric, karyotypic, and laparoscopic techniques for determining sex in bald eagles. *The Journal of Wildlife Management* 49:595–599.

Geist NB. 2000. Nasal respiratory turbinate function in birds. *Physiological and Biochemical Zoology* 73:581–589.

Gill RE Jr, Piersma T, Hufford G, et al. 2005. Crossing the ultimate ecological barrier: evidence for an 11000-Km-long nonstop flight from Alaska to New Zealand and eastern Australia by bar-tailed godwits. *Condor* 107:1–20.

Goelz MF, Hahn AW, Kelley ST. 1990. Effects of halothane and isoflurane on mean arterial blood pressure, heart rate, and respiratory rate in adult Pekin ducks. *American Journal of Veterinary Research* 51:458–460.

Goldberg DR, Samuel MD, Rocke TE, et al. 2004. Could blackbird mortality from avicide DRC-1339 contribute to avian botulism outbreaks in North Dakota? *Wildlife Society Bulletin* 32:870–880.

Golet GH, Seiser PE, McGuire AD, et al. 2002. Long-term direct and indirect effects of the "Exxon Valdez" oil spill on pigeon guillemots in Prince William Sound, Alaska. *Marine Ecology Progress Series* 241:287–304.

Good DA, Heatley JJ, Tully TN Jr, et al. 2001. Anesthesia case of the month. *Journal of the American Veterinary Medical Association* 219:1529–1531.

Goulden S. 1995. Swan anaesthesia. *The Veterinary Record* 136:448.

Graham JE. 2004. Approach to the dyspneic avian patient. *Seminars in Avian and Exotic Pet Medicine* 13:154–159.

Greenacre CB. 1993. Possible toxic disinfectant build-up in anesthetic tubing. *Journal of the Association of Avian Veterinarians* 7:104.

Greenlees KJ, Clutton RE, Larsen CT, et al. 1990. Effect of halothane, isoflurane, and pentobarbital anesthesia on myocardial irritability in chickens. *American Journal of Veterinary Research* 51:757–758.

Greenwood AG. 1983. Avian sex determination by laparoscopy. *The Veterinary Record* 112:105.

Griffiths R. 2000. Sex identification in birds. *Seminars in Avian and Exotic Pet Medicine* 9:14–26.

Gunkel C, Lafortune M. 2005. Current techniques in avian anesthesia. *Seminars in Avian and Exotic Pet Medicine* 14:263–276.

Harrison GJ. 1991. Pre-anesthetic fasting recommended. *Journal of the Association of Avian Veterinarians* 5:126.

Harrison GJ. 1994. Bubble-wrap for surgical patients. *Journal of the Association of Avian Veterinarians* 7:221.

Hawkins MG, Paul-Murphy J. 2011. Avian Analgesia. *The Veterinary Clinics of North America. Exotic Animal Practice* 14:61–80.

Heard D. 2000. Perioperative supportive care and monitoring. *The Veterinary Clinics of North America. Exotic Animal Practice* 3:587–615.

Heard DJ. 1993. Principles and techniques of anesthesia and analgesia for exotic practice. *The Veterinary Clinics of North America. Small Animal Practice* 23(6):1301–1327.

Heard DJ. 1997. Anesthesia and analgesia. In: *Avian Medicine and Surgery* (RB Altman, SL Clubb, GM Dorrestein, et al., eds.), pp. 807–827. Philadelphia: W.B. Saunders.

Hempleman SC, Bebout DE. 1994. Increased venous PCO_2 enhances dynamic responses of avian intrapulmonary chemoreceptors. *American Journal of Physiology: Regulatory Integrative and Comparative Physiology* 266:R15–R19.

Hempleman SC, Burger RE. 1984. Receptive fields of intrapulmonary chemoreceptors in the Pekin duck. *Respiration Physiology* 57:317–330.

Hempleman SC, Adamson TP, Burger RE. 1986. Sensitivity of avian intrapulmonary chemoreceptors to venous CO_2 load. *Respiration Physiology* 66:53–60.

Hempleman SC, Rodriguez TA, Bhagat YA, et al. 2000. Benzolamide, acetazolamide, and signal transduction in avian intrapulmonary chemoreceptors. *American Journal of Physiology: Regulatory Integrative and Comparative Physiology* 279:R1988–R1995.

Hempleman SC, Adamson TP, Begay RS, et al. 2003. CO_2 transduction in avian intrapulmonary chemoreceptors is critically dependent on transmembrane Na^+/H^+ exchange. *American Journal of Physiology: Regulatory Integrative and Comparative Physiology* 284:R1551–R1559.

Hepp GR, Manlove CA. 2001. A comparison of methoxyflurane and propofol to reduce nest abandonment by wood ducks. *Wildlife Society Bulletin* 29:546–550.

Hernandez-Divers SJ. 2001. New small animal ventilator. *Exotic DVM* 3:18.

Hocking PM, Gentle MJ, Bernard R, et al. 1997. Evaluation of a protocol for determining the effectiveness of pretreatment with local analgesics for reducing experimentally induced articular pain in domestic fowl. *Research in Veterinary Science* 63:263–267.

Hofmeister EH, Hernandez-Divers SJ. 2005. Anesthesia case of the month. *Journal of the American Veterinary Medical Association* 227:718–720.

Howard PE, Dein FJ, Langenberg JA, et al. 1993. Surgical removal of a tracheal foreign body from a whooping crane (*Grus americana*). *Journal of Zoo and Wildlife Medicine* 22:359–363.

Hunter RP, Mahmood I, Martinez MN. 2008. Prediction of xenobiotic clearance in avian species using mammalian or avian data: how accurate is the prediction? *Journal of Veterinary Pharmacology and Therapeutics* 31:281–284.

Jackson DC, Schmidt-Nielsen K. 1964. Countercurrent heat exchange in the respiratory passages. *Proceedings of the National Academy of Sciences of the United States of America* 51:1192–1197.

Jaensch SM, Cullen L, Raidal SR. 1999. Comparative cardiopulmonary effects of halothane and isoflurane in galahs (*Eolophus roseicapillus*). *Journal of Avian Medicine and Surgery* 13:15–22.

Jaensch SM, Cullen L, Raidal SR. 2001. Comparison of endotracheal, caudal thoacic air sac, and clavicular air sac administration of isoflurane in sulfur-crested cockatoos (*Cacatua galerita*). *Journal of Avian Medicine and Surgery* 15:170–177.

Jaensch SM, Cullen L, Raidal SR. 2002. Air sac functional anatomy of the sulfur-crested cockatoo (*Cacatua galerita*) during isoflurane anesthesia. *Journal of Avian Medicine and Surgery* 16:2–9.

Janovsky M, Ruf T, Zenker W. 2002. Oral administration of tiletamine/zolazepam for the immobilization of the Common Buzzard (*Buteo buteo*). *Journal of Raptor Research* 36:188–193.

Jewett SC, Dean TA, Woodin BR, et al. 2002. Exposure to hydrocarbons 10 years after the Exxon Valdez oil spill: evidence from cytochrome P4501A expression and biliary FACs in nearshore demersal fishes. *Marine Environmental Research* 54:21–48.

Jones DR, Furilla RA, Heieis MRA, et al. 1988. Forced and voluntary diving in ducks: cardiovascular adjustments and their control. *Canadian Journal of Zoology* 66:75–83.

Ketterson ED, Nolan VJ. 1986. Effect of laparotomy of tree sparrows and dark-eyed Juncos during winter on subsequent survival in the field. *Journal of Field Ornithology* 57:239–240.

Kharasch ED, Thummel KE. 1993. Identification of cytochrome P450 2E1 as the predominant enzyme catalyzing human liver microsomal defluorination of sevoflurane, isoflurane, and methoxyflurane. *Anesthesiology* 79:795–807.

King AS, Payne DC. 1964. Normal breathing and the effects of posture in *Gallus domesticus*. *The Journal of Physiology* 174:340–347.

Korbel R. 1998. Vergleichende untersuchungen zur inhalationsanästhesie mit isofluran (Forene®) und sevofluran (Sevorane®) bei haustauben (*Columba livia* Gmel., 1789, var. *domestica*) und vorstellung eines referenz-narkoseprotokolls für vögel. *Tierarztl Prax Augs K Klientiere Heimtiere* 26:211–223.

Korschgen CE, Kenow KP, Gendron-Fitzpatrick A, et al. 1996. Implanting intra-abdominal radiotransmitters with external whip antennas in ducks. *The Journal of Wildlife Management* 60:132–137.

Kramer MH. 2002. Managing endotracheal tube mucus plugs in small birds. *Exotic DVM* 4:9.

Kreeger TJ, Degernes LA, Kreeger JS, et al. 1993. Immobilization of raptors with tiletamine and zolazepam (Telazol). In: *Raptor Biomedicine* (PT Redig, JE Cooper, JD Remple, eds.), pp. 141–144. Minneapolis: University of Minnesota Press.

Langlois I, Harvey RC, Jones MP, et al. 2003. Cardiopulmonary and anesthetic effects of isoflurane and propofol in Hispaniolan Amazon parrots (*Amazona ventralis*). *Journal of Avian Medicine and Surgery* 17:4–10.

Lemke KA, Dawson SD. 2000. Local and regional anesthesia. *The Veterinary Clinics of North America. Small Animal Practice* 30:839–857.

Lewis JCM. 2004. Field use of isoflurane and air anesthetic equipment in wildlife. *Journal of Zoo and Wildlife Medicine* 35:303–311.

Lichtenberger M. 2004. Principles of shock and fluid therapy in special species. *Seminars in Avian and Exotic Pet Medicine* 13: 142–153.

Lichtenberger M. 2005. Determination of indirect blood pressure in the companion bird. *Seminars in Avian and Exotic Pet Medicine* 14:149–152.

Lieske CL, Ziccardi MH, Mazet JAK, et al. 2002. Evaluation of 4 handheld blood glucose monitors for use in seabird rehabilitation. *Journal of Avian Medicine and Surgery* 16:277–285.

Lin H-C, Ko JC. 1997. Anesthetic management of ratites. *Compendium on Continuing Education for the Practising Veterinarian* 19:S127–S132.

Lin H-C, Todhunter PG, Powe TA, et al. 1997. Use of xylazine, butorphanol, tiletamine-zolazepam, and isoflurane for induction and maintenance of anesthesia in ratites. *Journal of the American Veterinary Medical Association* 210:244–248.

Loibl MF, Clutton RE, Marx BD, et al. 1988. Alpha-chloralose as a capture and restraint agent of birds: therapeutic index determination in the chicken. *Journal of Wildlife Diseases* 24: 684–687.

Ludders JW. 1992. Minimal anesthetic concentration and cardiopulmonary dose-response of halothane in ducks. *Veterinary Surgery* 21:319–324.

Ludders JW. 1998. Respiratory physiology of birds: considerations for anesthetic management. *Seminars in Avian and Exotic Pet Medicine* 7:3–9.

Ludders JW. 2008. Anesthesia and analgesia in birds. In: *Anesthesia and Analgesia in Laboratory Animals* (RE Fish, MJ Brown, PJ Danneman, AZ Karas, eds.), pp. 481–500. Amsterdam: Elsevier.

Ludders JW, Mitchell GS, Schaefer SL. 1988a. Minimum anesthetic dose and cardiopulmonary dose response for halothane in chickens. *American Journal of Veterinary Research* 49: 929–932.

Ludders JW, Rode JA, Mitchell GS. 1988b. Isoflurane ED50 and cardiopulmonary dose-response during spontaneous and controlled breathing in sandhill cranes (*Grus canadensis*). *Veterinary Surgery* 13:174–175.

Ludders JW, Rode J, Mitchell GS. 1989a. Isoflurane anesthesia in sandhill cranes (*Grus canadensis*): minimal anesthetic concentration and cardiopulmonary dose-response during spontaneous and controlled breathing. *Anesthesia and Analgesia* 68: 511–516.

Ludders JW, Rode J, Mitchell GS, et al. 1989b. Effects of ketamine, xylazine, and a combination of ketamine and xylazine in Pekin ducks. *American Journal of Veterinary Research* 50:245–249.

Ludders JW, Mitchell GS, Rode J. 1990. Minimal anesthetic concentration and cardiopulmonary dose response of isoflurane in ducks. *Veterinary Surgery* 19:304–307.

Ludders JW, Seaman GC, Erb HN. 1995. Inhalant anesthetics and inspired oxygen: implications for anesthesia in birds. *Journal of the American Animal Hospital Association* 31:38–41.

Machin K. 2004. Waterfowl anesthesia. *Seminars in Avian and Exotic Pet Medicine* 13:206–212.

Machin KL. 2005a. Avian analgesia. *Seminars in Avian and Exotic Pet Medicine* 14:236–242.

Machin KL. 2005b. Controlling avian pain. *Compendium on Continuing Education for the Practising Veterinarian* 27:299–308.

Machin KL, Caulkett NA. 1998a. Investigation of injectable anesthetic agents in mallard ducks (*Anas platyrhynchos*): a descriptive study. *Journal of Avian Medicine and Surgery* 12:255–262.

Machin KL, Caulkett NA. 1998b. Cardiopulmonary effects of propofol and a medetomidine-midazolam-ketamine combination in mallard ducks. *American Journal of Veterinary Research* 59:598–602.

Machin KL, Caulkett NA. 1999. Cardiopulmonary effects of propofol infusion in canvasback ducks (*Aythya valisneria*). *Journal of Avian Medicine and Surgery* 13:167–172.

Machin KL, Caulkett NA. 2000. Evaluation of isoflurane and propofol anesthesia for intraabdominal transmitter placement in nesting female canvasback ducks. *Journal of Wildlife Diseases* 36:324–334.

Machin KL, Livingston A. 2002. Assessment of the analgesic effects of ketoprofen in ducks anesthetized with isoflurane. *American Journal of Veterinary Research* 63:821–826.

Machin KL, Tellier LA, Lair S, et al. 2001. Pharmacodynamics of flunixin and ketoprofen in mallard ducks (*Anas platyrhynchos*). *Journal of Zoo and Wildlife Medicine* 32:222–229.

Magnussen H, Wilmer H, Scheid P. 1976. Gas exchange in air sacs: contribution to respiratory gas exchange in ducks. *Respiration Physiology* 26:129–146.

Mama KR, Phillips LG, Pascoe PJ. 1996. Use of propofol for induction and maintenance of anesthesia in a barn owl (*tyto alba*) undergoing tracheal resection. *Journal of Zoo and Wildlife Medicine* 27:397–401.

Mansour A, Khachaturian H, Lewis ME, et al. 1988. Anatomy of CNS opioid receptors. *Trends in Neurosciences* 11:308–314.

Mason D, Heard D, Ritchey M, et al. 1998. Isoflurane waste gas management. *Journal of Avian Medicine and Surgery* 12:112–114.

Matthews NS, Burba DJ, Cornick JL. 1991. Premature ventricular contractions and apparent hypertension during anesthesia in an ostrich. *Journal of the American Veterinary Medical Association* 198:1959–1961.

McLelland J. 1989a. Anatomy of the lungs and air sacs. In: *Form and Function in Birds* (AS King, J McLelland, eds.), pp. 221–280. London: Academic Press.

McLelland J. 1989b. Larynx and trachea. In: *Form and Function in Birds* (J McLelland, ed.), pp. 69–103. London: Academic Press.

Midtgård U. 1980. Heat loss from the feet of mallards *Anas platyrhynchos* and arterio-venous heat exchange in the rete tibiotarsale. *Ibis* 122:354–359.

Mitchell GS, Powell FL, Hopkins SR, et al. 2001. Time domains of the hypoxic ventilatory response in awake ducks: episodic and continuous hypoxia. *Respiration Physiology* 124:117–128.

Moghadam AZ, Sadegh AB, Sharifi S, et al. 2009. Comparison of intranasal administration of diazepam, midazolam and xylazine in Pigeons: clinical evaluation. *Iranian Journal of Veterinary Science and Technology* 1:19–26.

Mueller NS. 1982. Hypothermia used instead of anesthesia for surgery on nestling passerines. *Journal of Field Ornithology* 53:60.

Mulcahy DM, Esler D. 2010. Survival of captive and free-ranging harlequin ducks (*Histrionicus histrionicus*)following surgical liver biopsy. *Journal of Wildlife Diseases* 46:1325–1329.

Mulcahy DM, Tuomi P, Larsen RS. 2003. Differential mortality of male spectacled eiders (*Somateria fischeri*) and king eiders (*Somateria spectabilis*) subsequent to anesthesia with propofol, bupivacaine, and ketoprofen. *Journal of Avian Medicine and Surgery* 17:117–123.

Mulcahy DM, Gartrell B, Gill RE Jr, et al. 2011. Coelomic implantation of satellite transmitters in the bar-tailed godwit (*Limosa lapponica*) and the bristle-thighed curlew (*Numenius tahitiensis*), using propofol, bupivacaine and lidocaine. *Journal of Zoo and Wildlife Medicine* 42:54–64.

Müller K, Holzapfel J, Brunnberg L. 2011. Total intravenous anaesthesia by boluses or by continuous rate infusion of propofol in mute swans (*Cygnus olor*). *Veterinary Anaesthesia and Analgesia* 38:286–291.

Naganobu K, Hagio M. 2000. Dose-related cardiovascular effects of isoflurane in chickens during controlled ventilation. *The Journal of Veterinary Medical Science* 62:435–437.

Naganobu K, Ise K, Miyamoto T, et al. 2003. Sevoflurane anesthesia in chickens during spontaneous and controlled ventilation. *The Veterinary Record* 152:45–48.

Nilson PC, Teramitsu I, White SA. 2004. Caudal thoracic air sac cannulation in zebra finches for isoflurane anesthesia. *Journal of Neuroscience Methods* 143:107–115.

Nye PCG, Burger RE. 1978. Chicken intrapulmonary chemoreceptors: discharge at static levels of intrapulmonary carbon dioxide and their location. *Respiration Physiology* 33:299–322.

Olsen GH, Dein FJ, Haramis GM, et al. 1992. Implanting radio transmitters in wintering canvasbacks. *The Journal of Wildlife Management* 56:325–328.

Olsen JH. 1994. Anseriformes. In: *Avian Medicine: Principles and Applications* (BW Ritchie, GJ Harrison, LR Harrison, eds.), pp. 1236–1275. Lake Worth, FL: Wingers.

Paul-Murphy J, Ludders JW. 2001. Avian analgesia. *The Veterinary Clinics of North America. Exotic Animal Practice* 4:35–45.

Petersen MR, Douglas DC, Mulcahy DM. 1995. Use of implanted satellite transmitters to locate spectacled eiders at-sea. *Condor* 97:276–278.

Petersen MR, Larned WW, Douglas DC. 1999. At-sea distribution of spectacled eiders: a 120-year-old mystery resolved. *Auk* 116:1009–1020.

Petersen MR, McCaffery BJ, Flint PL. 2003. Post-breeding distribution of long-tailed ducks *Clangula hyemalis* from the Yukon-Kuskokwim Delta, Alaska. *Wildfowl* 54:103–113.

Petersen MR, Bustnes JO, Systad GH. 2006. Breeding and moulting locations and migration patterns of the Atlantic population of Steller's eiders *Polysticta stelleri* as determined from satellite telemetry. *Journal of Avian Biology* 37:58–68.

Peterson CH, Rice SD, Short JW, et al. 2003. Long-term ecosystem response to the Exxon Valdez oil spill. *Science* 302:2082–2086.

Pettifer GR, Cornick-Seahorn J, Smith JA, et al. 2002. The comparative cardiopulmonary effects of spontaneous and controlled ventilation by using the Hallowell EMC Anesthesia WorkStation in Hispaniolan Amazon parrots (*Amazona ventralis*). *Journal of Avian Medicine and Surgery* 16:268–276.

Phalen DN, Mitchell ME, Cavazos-Martinez ML. 1996. Evaluation of three heat sources for their ability to maintain core body temperature in the anesthetized avian patient. *Journal of Avian Medicine and Surgery* 10:174–178.

Piiper J, Drees F, Scheid P. 1970. Gas exchange in the domestic fowl during spontaneous breathing and artificial ventilation. *Respiration Physiology* 9:234–245.

Pizarro J, Ludders JW, Douse MA, et al. 1990. Halothane effects on ventilatory responses to changes in intrapulmonary CO_2 in geese. *Respiration Physiology* 82:337–348.

Pollock CG, Schumacher J, Orosz SE, et al. 2001. Sedative effects of medetomidine in pigeons (*Columba livia*). *Journal of Avian Medicine and Surgery* 15:95–100.

Powell FL, Gratz RK, Scheid P. 1978. Response of intrapulmonary chemoreceptors in the duck to changes in PCO_2 and pH. *Respiration Physiology* 35:65–77.

Quandt JE, Greenacre CB. 1999. Sevoflurane anesthesia in psittacines. *Journal of Zoo and Wildlife Medicine* 30:308–309.

Redig PT. 1998. Recommendations for anesthesia in raptors with comments on trumpeter swans. *Seminars in Avian and Exotic Pet Medicine* 7:22–29.

Reim DA, Middleton CC. 1995. Use of butorphanol as an anesthetic adjunct in turkeys. *Laboratory Animal Science* 45:696–697.

Rembert MS, Smith JA, Hosgood G, et al. 2001. Comparison of traditional thermal support devices with the forced-air warmer system in anesthetized Hispaniolan Amazon parrots (*Amazona ventralis*). *Journal of Avian Medicine and Surgery* 15:187–193.

Richner H. 1989. Avian laparoscopy as a field technique for sexing birds and an assessment of its effects on wild birds. *Journal of Field Ornithology* 60:137–142.

Risser AC Jr. 1971. A technique for performing laparotomy on small birds. *Condor* 73:376–379.

Rode JA, Bartholow S, Ludders JW. 2003. Ventilation through an air sac cannula during tracheal obstruction in ducks. *Journal of the Association of Avian Veterinarians* 4:98–102.

Rosskopf WJ Jr, Woerpel RW. 1996. Practical anesthesia administration. In: *Diseases of Cage and Aviary Birds*, 3rd ed. (WJ Rosskopf Jr, RW Woerpel, eds.), pp. 664–671. Baltimore: Williams & Wilkins.

Rotella JJ, Ratti JT. 1990. Use of methoxyflurane to reduce nest abandonment of mallards. *The Journal of Wildlife Management* 54:627–628.

Samour JH, Jones DM, Knight JA. 1984. Comparative studies of the use of some injectable anaesthetic agents in birds. *The Veterinary Record* 115:6–11.

Sandmeier P. 2000. Evaluation of medetomidine for short-term immobilization of domestic pigeons (*Columba livia*) and Amazon parrots (*Amazona* species). *Journal of Avian Medicine and Surgery* 14:8–14.

Sap R, Vanwandelen RM, Hellebrekers LJ. 1993. Spontaneous respiration versus intermediate positive pressure ventilation in pigeons. *Tijdschrift Voor Diergeneeskunde* 118:402–404.

Scheid P, Slama H, Gatz RN, et al. 1974. Intrapulmonary CO_2 receptors in the duck: III. Functional localization. *Respiration Physiology* 22:123–136.

Schmidt-Nielsen K, Hainsworth FR, Murrish D. 1970. Countercurrent heat exchange in the respiratory passages: effect on water and heat balance. *Respiration Physiology* 9:263–276.

Schmitt PM, Gobel T, Trautvetter E. 1998. Evaluation of pulse oximetry as a monitoring method in avian anesthesia. *Journal of Avian Medicine and Surgery* 12:91–99.

Seaman GC, Ludders JW, Erb HN, et al. 1994. Effects of low and high fractions of inspired oxygen on ventilation in ducks anesthetized with isoflurane. *American Journal of Veterinary Research* 55:395–398.

Segev G, Yas-Natan E, Shlosberg A, et al. 2006. Alpha-chloralose poisoning in dogs and cats: a retrospective study of 33 canine and 13 feline confirmed cases. *Veterinary Journal (London, England: 1997)* 172:109–113.

Shams H, Powell FL, Hempleman SC. 1990. Effects of normobaric and hypobaric hypoxia on ventilation and arterial blood gases in ducks. *Respiration Physiology* 80:163–170.

Shoemaker JM, Hempleman SC. 2001. Avian intrapulmonary chemoreceptor discharge rate is increased by anion exchange blocker "DIDS". *Respiration Physiology* 128:195–204.

Skarda RT. 1996. Local and regional anesthetic and analgesic techniques. In: *Lumb and Jones' Veterinary Anesthesia* (JC Thurmon, WJ Tranquilli, GJ Benson, eds.), pp. 426–447. Baltimore: Williams & Wilkins.

Small MF, Baccus JT, Waggerman GL. 2004. Mobile anesthesia unit for implanting radiotransmitters in birds in the field. *Southwestern Naturalist* 49:279–282.

Smith JC, Bolon B. 2004. Comparison of three commercially available activated charcoal canisters for passive scavenging of waste isoflurane during conventional rodent anesthesia. *Contemporary Topics in Laboratory Animal Science* 42:10–15.

Smith LM, Hupp JW, Ratti JT. 1980. Reducing abandonment of nest-trapped gray partridge with methoxyflurane. *The Journal of Wildlife Management* 44:690–691.

Steffey EP, Howland D Jr. 1977. Isoflurane potency in the dog and cat. *American Journal of Veterinary Research* 38(11):1833–1836.

Steffey EP, Howland D Jr, Giri S, et al. 1977. Enflurane, halothane, and isoflurane potency in horses. *American Journal of Veterinary Research* 38:1037–1039.

Stoskopf MK, Mulcahy DM, Esler D. 2010. Evaluation of a portable automated serum chemistry analyzer for field assessment of harlequin ducks, *Histrionicus histrionicus*. *Veterinary Medicine International* 2010: Art 418596. doi: 10.4061/2010/418596.

Straub J, Forbes NA, Thielebein J, et al. 2003. The effects of isoflurane anaesthesia on some Doppler-derived cardiac parameters in the common buzzard (*Buteo buteo*). *Veterinary Journal (London, England: 1997)* 166:273–276.

TerRiet MF, DeSouza GJA, Jacobs JS, et al. 2000. Which is most pungent: isoflurane, sevoflurane or desflurane? *British Journal of Anaesthesia* 85:305–307.

Thil M-A, Groscolas R. 2002. Field immobilization of king penguins with tiletamine-zolazepam. *Journal of Field Ornithology* 73:308–317.

Touzot-Jourde G, Hernandez-Divers SJ, Trim CM. 2005. Cardiopulmonary effects of controlled versus spontaneous ventilation in pigeons anesthetized for coelioscopy. *Journal of the American Veterinary Medical Association* 227:1424–1428.

Trust KA, Esler D, Woodin BR, et al. 2000. Cytochrome P450 1A induction in sea ducks inhabiting nearshore areas of Prince William Sound, Alaska. *Marine Pollution Bulletin* 40:397–403.

Uzun M, Yildiz S, Atalan G, et al. 2003. Effects of medetomidine-ketamine combination anaesthesia on electrocardiographic findings, body temperature, and heart and respiratory rates in domestic pigeons. *Turkish Journal of Veterinary & Animal Sciences* 27:377–382.

Valverde A, Honeyman VL, Dyson DH, et al. 1990. Determination of a sedative dose and influence of midazolam on cardiopulmonary function in Canada geese. *American Journal of Veterinary Research* 51:1071–1074.

Valverde A, Bienzle D, Smith DA, et al. 1993. Intraosseous cannulation and drug administration for induction of anesthesia in chickens. *Veterinary Surgery* 22:240–244.

Van Heerden J, Keefen RH. 1991. A preliminary investigation into the immobilising potential of tiletamine/zolazepam mixture, metomidate, a metomidate and azaperone combination and medetomidine in ostriches (*Struthio camelus*). *Journal of the South African Veterinary Association* 62:114–117.

Varner J, Clifton KR, Poulos S, et al. 2004. Lack of efficacy of injectable ketamine with xylazine or diazepam for anesthesia in chickens. *Lab Animal* 33:35–39.

Vesal N, Eskandari MH. 2006. Sedative effects of midazolam and xylazine with or without ketamine and detomidine alone following intranasal administration in ring-necked parakeets. *Journal of the American Veterinary Medical Association* 228:383–388.

Vesal N, Zare P. 2006. Clinical evaluation of intranasal benzodiazepines, α_2-agonists and their antagonists in canaries. *Veterinary Anaesthesia and Analgesia* 33:143–148.

Whittow GC, Ossario N. 1970. A new technique for anesthetizing birds. *Laboratory Animal Care* 20:651–656.

Wilberg C. 2005. Untersuchungen zur inhalationsnarkose mit isofluran sowie mit buprenorphinprämedikation bei der warzenente (*Anas platyrhynchos*). PhD Dissertation. University of Munich.

Wilson D, Pettifer GR. 2004. Anesthesia case of the month. *Journal of the American Veterinary Medical Association* 225:685–688.

Woakes AJ. 1988. Metabolism in diving birds: studies in the laboratory and the field. *Canadian Journal of Zoology* 66:138–141.

Zantop D, Bowles H. 2000. Evaluating avian patients with the Parks Doppler flow monitor. *Exotic DVM* 2:44–45.

30 Birds: Miscellaneous

Darryl Heard

INTRODUCTION

The orders of birds are summarized in Table 30.1. This chapter covers the anesthesia of bird groups not specifically covered elsewhere. The anesthetic principles, regimens, and drug dosages described in the other avian chapters can, for the most part, be extrapolated to the birds of a similar size in this chapter.

ANATOMY AND PHYSIOLOGY

For those readers interested in a more detailed discussion of avian anatomy and physiology, I recommend King and McLelland (1984) and Whittow (2000). The anatomy and physiology of birds is similar across all orders and is summarized in Chapter 23. This similarity is probably due to the evolutionary constraints of flight. These include the needs to minimize weight (lightweight bone structure, rapid digestion, and assimilation of nutrients) while at the same time maximize cardiopulmonary and muscular function. The main differences between species are related to capture and prehension of food (e.g., beak shape and size), and lifestyle (aquatic, terrestrial, and arboreal). For example, in one study (Mortola & Seguin 2009), the respiration rate in aquatic birds was lower (allometric equation $14.5\ W[kg]^{-0.56}$) compared with terrestrial species ($13.4\ W^{-0.26}$).

All birds, except kiwis, have their nares at the base of the upper beak. The nares of toucans and related birds (Piciformes) are also in this position, but covered by feathers and the edge of the beak. Gannets, pelicans (Pelecaniformes), and some other diving birds have partially or fully occluded nares, and breathe through a gap in the commissure of the beak (Fig. 30.1a) (King & McLelland 1984). Many species of marine, as well as terrestrial birds from arid environments secrete salt through their nares from glands located within the head (Gerstberger & Gray 1993). The operculum in procellariiformes (albatrosses and petrels) is converted into a tube on the dorsal aspect of the bill (King & McLelland 1984).

The large beaks of hornbills (Coraciformes), toucans (Piciformes), storks (Ciconiiformes), and cranes (Gruiiformes) are lightweight, yet able to deliver powerful blows to kill small vertebrates, excavate tree cavities for nests and defend themselves (Seki et al. 2010). Unfortunately, the beaks of these animals are easily damaged if too much side to side pressure is applied. The toco toucan (*Ramphastos toco*), possesses the largest beak relative to body size of all birds. It is able to regulate heat distribution by modifying blood flow, using the bill as a transient thermal radiator (Tattersall et al. 2009) (Fig. 30.2a).

Cranes, similar to currasows and guans discussed in Chapter 29, possess long convoluted tracheas that may extend back into their sternum. This anatomy makes these species very susceptible to the adverse effects of fluid accumulation in the trachea. Pelicans possess subcutaneous air cells not connected to the respiratory system. These cells can expand during administration of nitrous oxide (Reynolds 1983).

CAPTURE AND PHYSICAL RESTRAINT

The main defensive weapon of birds is the beak, although the sharp talons of some species can also cause pain and injury (Fig. 30.1b). When restrained, birds will often orient on the handler's eyes as a place to strike. This is because the eyes are constantly moving and attract the attention of the bird. Long-necked birds, such as egrets, herons, cranes, loons, and pelicans,

Table 30.1. Classification of the class Aves

Order	Common Names	Chapter
Struthioniformes	Ostrich, rheas, cassowaries, emu, and kiwis	26
Tinamiformes	Tinamous	26
Sphenisciformes	Penguins	25
Gaviiformes	Divers (loons)	30
Podicipediformes	Grebes	30
Procellariformes	Albatrosses, petrels, shearwaters, storm petrels, and diving petrels	30
Pelecaniformes	Tropicbirds, pelicans, gannets, boobies, cormorants, darters, and frigatebirds	30
Ciconiiformes	Herons. hammerkop, storks, shoebill, ibises, and spoonbills	30
Phoenicopteriformes	Flamingos	30
Anseriformes	Screamers, ducks, geese, and swans	29
Falconiformes	Vultures, osprey, hawks, eagles, secretary bird, caracaras, and falcons	27
Galliformes	Megapodes, guans, chachalacas, currasows, pheasants, grouse, and hoatzin	28
Gruiformes	Mesites, buttonquails, plains-wanderer, cranes, limpkin, trumpeters, rails, coots, finfoots, kagu, sunbittern, seriemas, and bustards	30
Charadriiformes	Shorebirds	29
Columbiformes	Doves and pigeons	28
Psittaciformes	Parrots	24
Cuculiformes	Turacos and cuckoos	30
Strigiformes	Owls	27
Caprimulgiformes	Oilbird, frogmouths, potoos, and owlet-nightjars	30
Apodiformes	Swifts and hummingbirds	30
Coliformes	Mousebirds	30
Trogoniformes	Trogons	30
Coraciformes	Kingfishers, todies, motmots, bee-eaters, rollers, hoopoes, and hornbills	30
Piciformes	Jacamars, puffbirds, barbets, honeyguides, toucans, and woodpeckers	30
Passeriformes	Small perching birds, including crows and ravens.	30

Source: de Juana (1992).

are particularly dangerous. Consequently, protective glasses are recommended when working with these species.

Restraint is similar for most bird species. For large species, protective gloves may be worn. They, however, reduce the dexterity of the handler, and also may act as a fomite for pathogens if not properly cleaned. Towels are a useful alternative because they are more easily cleaned or discarded after use. They are perceived as a barrier by the birds and facilitate holding the wings and the legs at the same time. Covering the head and eyes will also calm many species (Fig. 30.3).

When holding any bird, regardless of size, care must be taken to prevent inhibiting respiration. The breathing pattern is similar, yet different from mammals. For a bird to inhale, the sternum must be able to move rostral and outward, along with the ribs.

Hyperthermia is common during restraint. This is exacerbated in birds adapted to cold environments. Prolonged muscle contraction including isometric, will produce heat, lactic academia, and hyperkalemia. Death may occur due to cardiac arrhythmia and muscle injury (capture myopathy or exertional rhabdomyolysis) (Burgdorf-Moisuk et al. 2012; Businga et al. 2007; Hanley et al. 2005; Marco et al. 2006; Ruder et al. 2012; Windingstad et al. 1983; Chapter 13). Physical restraint, whether it be using a towel or gloves, or tying the legs, will also potentially inhibit a bird's ability to dissipate heat. Dehydration and malnutrition exacerbate hyperthermia and muscle damage.

Conversely, care must be taken with cold-adapted species to not interfere with their adaptive thermoregulatory anatomy and physiology. For example, anesthetic drugs may alter blood flow affecting countercurrent heat exchange. Disruption of their protective feather covering with alcohol or plucking to facilitate jugular blood collection and surgery can impair their ability to return immediately to a cold or aquatic environment. Restraint devices have been designed to facilitate handling many avian species. These include body wraps and hoods with Velcro attachments (Fig. 30.3). As mentioned previously, care must be taken using these devices to ensure adequacy of breathing and thermoregulation. Many, but not all species are quieter when their eyes and ears are covered, or they are maintained in a quiet darkened environment (Fig. 30.3).

Good quality nets are essential regardless of a bird's ability to fly. Many can outrun humans and a long-handled net can be invaluable for capture. It is important to have a variety of small to large nets available.

Diurnal birds will often stay still in a dark environment and are unable to perceive red light. If a handler approaches slowly, deliberately, and directly at a bird, they may stay still long enough to allow a close approach and then a grab by hand or with a towel.

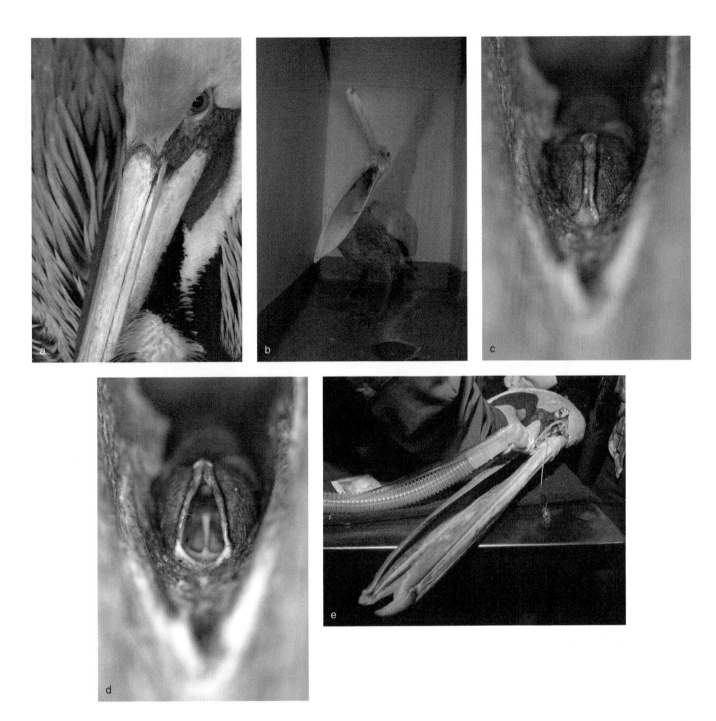

Figure 30.1. (a) The nares of brown (*Pelecanus occidentalis*) and other pelicans are partially occluded making them predominantly mouth breathers. As in most birds the nares are located at the base of the upper bill. (b) An aggressive American white pelican (*Pelecanus erythrorhynchos*) demonstrating the potential danger of the beak to handlers. Birds will orient on the human eyes to attack because they are constantly moving. The glottis is located deep within the caudal portion of the oropharynx and very mobile. (c) The closed glottis of a brown pelican (*Pelecanus occidentalis*) deep in the caudal portion of the oropharynx. (d) The open glottis of a brown pelican (*Pelecanus occidentalis*). The cartilaginous septum in the larynx can be gently displaced by the tube for endotracheal intubation. Stabilization of the glottis from outside the pouch and a good light source will facilitate intubation. (e) An intubated pelican connected to a nonrebreathing system. A circle breathing system would also be appropriate for this-size bird. The cuff of the endotracheal tube is not inflated to prevent damage to the tracheal mucosa. This bird was induced with propofol administered to effect into a catheter placed in the medial metatarsal vein.

509

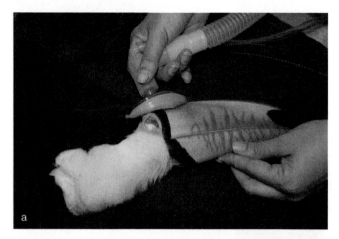

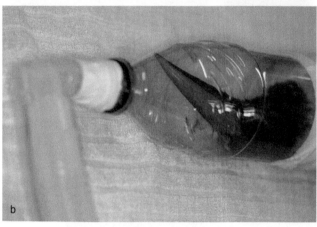

Figure 30.2. (a) Inhalant anesthetic induction of a toco toucan (*Ramphastos toco*) using a small human pediatric mask placed over the nares at the base of the bill and connected to a nonrebreathing system. (b) An aracari being induced using a mask made from a plastic bottle to accommodate the long beak.

VASCULAR ACCESS

The main sites for blood collection in all avian species are the external jugular vein, the basilic vein, and the medial saphenous vein. As the species gets smaller, the main site is the jugular vein. The right jugular vein is usually the most developed. In some individuals, however, the left is most prominent. Even when the right is prominent, the left will often be identifiable, but smaller. The basilic vein on the medial surface of the elbow can be used in large birds. It is problematic, however, because hemostasis is difficult and keeping the wing still to prevent accidental movement of the needle is hard. The medial saphenous vein is useful for collecting blood from birds restrained by a handler in the upright position. In hornbills, the jugular veins are often covered by extension of the air sacs, making accurate venipuncture difficult. This author consequently uses the medial saphenous vein for these birds.

Not all birds, especially aquatic and cold-adapted birds, have feather spaces (apterylae) over the jugular.

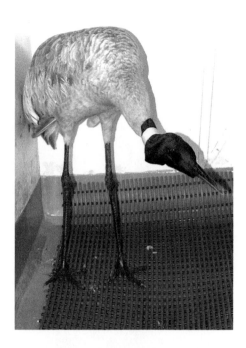

Figure 30.3. A hospitalized sandhill crane (*Grus canadensis*) demonstrating the use of purpose-made hood to keep the animal quiet. This can also be used during physical restraint and examination, or for transportation.

In birds without apterylae, the author wets the feathers over the vein with alcohol and treats the feathers as the outer skin. Wetting the feathers down will often allow the occluded jugular vein to be identified. Alternatively, it can be palpated through the feathers.

In healthy birds, 10% of the blood volume can be collected safely without any adverse effects. Since the blood volume is approximately 10% of the bodyweight (1 g = 1 mL), then 1% of the bodyweight can be collected. More athletic birds are able to tolerate greater blood loss than ground-dwelling species. Obese animals have proportionately smaller blood volumes, since fat has a relatively small blood supply.

Although not recommended in the living bird, blood can also be collected terminally or after death from the vertebral vessels, as well as the heart. To collect blood from the vertebral vessels, the needle is placed as for a CSF tap in a mammal. That is, the head is flexed ventrally and a 22- to 25-gauge needle is inserted into the space between the back of the skull and the atlas. A 1- or 3-mL syringe is then used to collect the blood. Cardiac puncture in most birds is made difficult by the complete sternum. A long needle must either be introduced in the midline from the caudal or rostral aspect of the sternum.

Depending on the size of the bird, catheters for fluid administration can be placed in either the jugular or medial saphenous veins. Keeping a catheter in the jugular vein of an awake bird is not recommended

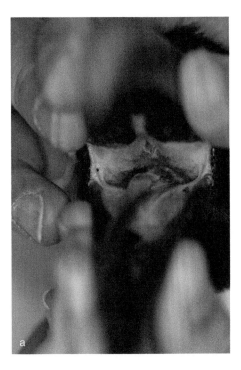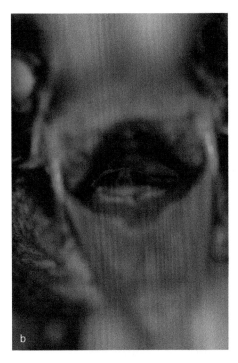

Figure 30.4. (a) The oral cavity of an aracari demonstrating the position of the glottis at the base of the thin tongue. (b) The oral cavity of a kookaburra (*Dacelo novaeguineae*) also showing the closed glottis at the base of the tongue.

because of the potential for hemorrhage if the bird struggles. Intraosseous catheters in either the proximal and distal ulna, or the proximal tibiotarsal bones are alternatives to intravenous catheterization. In very small birds, regular hypodermic needles can be used, but spinal needles are recommended in larger birds. In pelicans, the ulna is pneumatic and, therefore, intraosseous catheterization is contraindicated.

ENDOTRACHEAL INTUBATION

Despite the extreme variation in tongues of some birds, the glottal opening is always at its base (Fig. 30.1c,d and Fig. 30.4a,b). The jaws of flamingos do not open very far, inhibiting visualization of the glottis and placement of the endotracheal tube. The tube is either placed blindly by palpation or with the use of an endoscope. Some birds have septa at the glottal opening; these can be gently displaced to the side with the endotracheal tube (Fig. 30.1d). The glottis of pelecaniformes is located deep in the pouch and very mobile (Fig. 30.1b–d). Outside manipulation may be necessary to keep it still to allow intubation. A good light source is necessary for the intubation of some species. A head lamp makes glottal visualization easier in some species.

PREANESTHETIC CONSIDERATIONS

Regurgitation or vomiting in the perianesthetic period must be prepared for in many avian species. Some birds will regurgitate as a defensive mechanism when

handled (e.g., both New and Old World vultures). Fish-eating and fruit-eating birds seem particularly prone to regurgitation or reflux of stomach contents under anesthesia. Fasting is usually not an option in birds either because of the situation or the size of the bird. The smaller the bird the higher the metabolic rate and the more likely it will develop hypoglycemia. It is virtually impossible and not recommended to fast a bird to the point of no gastrointestinal contents. Water may be removed a couple hours before a procedure. When reflux is a concern, use a gauze roll placed past the glottis to prevent the liquid from entering the glottal area. The gauze is attached to tape that extends outside the bird's head so it is not forgotten at the end of the procedure.

The tracheal rings of birds are complete. Consequently, it is recommended cuffed endotracheal tubes not be used or the cuff inflated. This is because of the greater potential for tracheal mucosal damage. Trauma also occurs from the tip of endotracheal tube. The trachea of most birds narrows from the glottis. If a large tube is jammed into the trachea, mucosal damage will occur. This is exacerbated by head and neck movement during anesthesia.

ANALGESIA

Analgesia is described in detail in Chapters 6 and 24. Nonsteroidal anti-inflammatory drugs (NSAIDs) are highly variable in their effects and ability to cause injury across avian species. Great care must, therefore,

be taken in drug and dosage selection. Birds appear to respond predominantly to kappa opioid agonists, but there are some studies indicating mu opioids may produce analgesia in some species (Chapter 24). Tramadol is an alternative for use postoperatively in avian species. The judicial use of local anesthetics and blocks can also be a valuable part of a multi-modal analgesia plan.

INDUCTION/MAINTENANCE PROTOCOLS

Parenteral anesthetic regimens and response to drugs are similar across all birds and described in the other chapters. Ketamine alone is not recommended because of poor muscle relaxation. Consequently, parenteral anesthetic regimens based around this drug usually include either a benzodiazepine (diazepam and midazolam) or an alpha-2 adrenergic agonist (xylazine, detomidine, medetomidine, and dexmedetomidine). Unfortunately, birds seem to be very resistant to the effects of the latter drugs, requiring dosages much higher than in mammals of a similar size.

Propofol and alfaxolone can be used in all species of birds when vascular access is available, but they do produce dose and administration rate dependent cardiopulmonary depression. Although alfaxalone can be given intramuscularly, the large injection volume of drug required in anything, but the smallest of birds is inhumane.

All birds can be induced and maintained with an inhalant anesthetic. For some species, however, mask induction is problematic. In birds with long or large beaks, commercially available masks do not extend to cover the nares at the base of the beak. In these species, masks can be made from water bottles or a plastic bag (Fig. 30.2b). Alternatively, a small mask can be placed over the nares (Fig. 30.2a). Some species of birds do not have patent nares, but rather breathe around the side of the mouth (Fig. 30.1a). It is important to ensure the nares are patent in obligate nasal breathers when using a mask that closes the beak.

MONITORING

Mortality during anesthesia appears higher for birds than mammals. Monitoring is, therefore, very important in preventing injury and death. One person should always be dedicated to monitoring during the perianesthetic period. Clear surgical drapes facilitate visualization of respiration and auscultation of small patients during surgery. Redundancy in monitoring when possible is also important. For example, the use of both a Doppler flow detection device and an esophageal stethoscope to monitor heart rate.

Anesthetic depth is determined using basic reflexes and responses; muscle and cloacal tone, pupil size, palpebral and corneal response, toe pinch, response to surgical incision, feather plucking, heart rate, and so on. Interestingly, birds appear more likely to respond to feather plucking than a skin incision. This may be related to the clustering of nociceptors and mechanoreceptors around the feather follicles. Palpebral response is usually absent at light surgical planes of anesthesia. Sudden pilo-erection under anesthesia can be indication of cardiac arrest rather than decreased anesthetic depth.

Hypothermia is common in anesthetized birds, and temperature monitoring is essential. Unfortunately, cloacal may not accurately reflect core body temperature. Forced air warmers are preferred for maintaining normothermia in anesthetized birds.

Heart rate is monitored by palpation or placement of a Doppler flow probe on a peripheral artery (metatarsal and ulna), auscultation of the heart (stethoscope, including esophageal), pulse oximeter, or by electrocardiography. Positional maintenance of the Doppler flow probe is sometimes difficult. A soft clamp can be constructed from two tongue depressors and used to keep the probe in place over the ulna artery. Alternatively, in large birds, the flow probe can be placed in the oropharynx or esophagus and directed at the major arteries ventral to the neck vertebra. Pulse oximetry is inaccurate and unreliable in birds. Capnography can be used to monitor respiration, but is also inaccurate for reasons discussed in previous chapters.

RECOVERY CONSIDERATIONS

The recovery period is a critical period for anesthetized avian patients and a common time for mortality. This may be related to the physiologic instability associated with transitioning from anesthetized to an awake animal. For example, as a hypothermic bird becomes warmer peripheral vessels dilate and metabolic rate increases. The former may unmask hypovolemia and hypotension, leading to decreased cardiac output. Increased metabolic rate increases glucose and oxygen use exacerbating or precipitating hypoglycemia and hypoxemia, respectively.

FIELD IMMOBILIZATION (WILD CAPTURE)

Physical capture of most birds is well described by Bub et. al. (1991). The main issues when working with free-living birds is injury due to struggling, hyperthermia, and exertional rhabdomyolysis (capture myopathy) (Burgdorf-Moisuk et al. 2012; Businga et al. 2007; Hanley et al. 2005; Marco et al. 2006; Ruder et al. 2012; Windingstad et al. 1983; Chapter 13). Restraint and anesthesia time should be minimized by planning and preparation, and rapid processing. When birds are to be kept for periods of time, care must be taken to use appropriately designed crates or holding structures appropriate to the species (e.g., see Chapter 29).

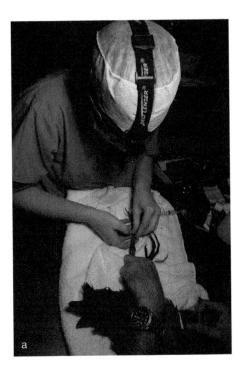
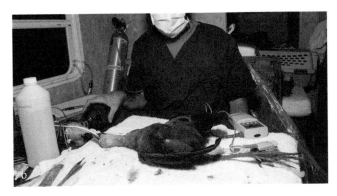

Figure 30.5.   (a) Intravenous administration of propofol into the medial metatarsal vein of a purple swamp hen (*Porhyrio porphyrio*). (b) A purple swamp hen (*Porhyrio porphyrio*) anesthetized with propofol for surgical implantation of a radiotransmitter. The mid-line surgical site was infiltrated with a combination of lidocaine and bupivacaine. Meloxicam was also administered for additional analgesia. Note the use of a flexible esophageal thermometer (white line) and esophageal stethoscope for monitoring. The bird is intubated and ventilated four to six times a minute using an Ambu bag.

Intranasal midazolam (0.5–2.0 mg/kg) administration may be a rapid way to provide sedation in wild birds (Ward et al. 2011). Propofol or alfaxalone can be used for short-term immobilization, as well as maintenance of anesthesia (Chapter 29) (Fig. 30.5a,b). Neither drug provides good analgesia, and other drugs must be added to the anesthetic regimen when painful procedures are planned. As with all avian anesthesias, respiratory support must be provided. Inhalation anesthesia can also be used for induction and maintenance. Administration of the inhalant anesthetic is preferably done using a precision vaporizer. The use of isoflurane without a vaporizer is not recommended because of the potential for anesthetic over dosage.

REFERENCES

Bub H, Hamerstrom F (trans.), Wuertz-Schaefer K (trans.). 1995. *Bird Trapping & Bird Banding*. Ithaca: Cornell University Press.

Burgdorf-Moisuk A, Wack R, Ziccardi M, Larsen RS, Hopper K. 2012. Validation of lactate measurement in American flamingo (*Phoenicopterus ruber*) plasma and correlation with duration and difficulty of capture. *Journal of Zoo and Wildlife Medicine* 43: 450–458.

Businga NK, Langenberg J, Carlson L. 2007. Successful treatment of capture myopathy in three wild greater sandhill cranes (*Grus canadensis tabida*). *Journal of Avian Medicine and Surgery* 21: 294–298.

de Juana E. 1992. Class aves (birds). In: *Handbook of Birds of the World*, Vol. 1 (J del Hoyo, A Elliott, J Sargatal, eds.), pp. 35–74. Barcelona: Lynx Edicions.

Gerstberger R, Gray DA. 1993. Fine structure, innervation, and functional control of avian salt glands. *International Review of Cytology* 144:129–216.

Hanley CS, Thomas NJ, Paul-Murphy J, Hartup BK. 2005. Exertional myopathy in whooping cranes (*Grus americana*) with prognostic guidelines. *Journal of Zoo and Wildlife Medicine* 36: 489–497.

King AS, McLelland J. 1984. *Birds. Their Structure and Function*. London, England: Bailliére Tindall.

Marco I, Mentaberre G, Ponjoan A, Bota G, Mañosa S, Lavín S. 2006. Capture myopathy in little bustards after trapping and marking. *Journal of Wildlife Diseases* 42:889–891.

Mortola JP, Seguin J. 2009. Resting breathing frequency in aquatic birds: a comparative analysis with terrestrial species. *Journal of Zoology* 279:210–218.

Reynolds WT. 1983. Unusual anesthetic complication in a pelican. *The Veterinary Record* 113:204.

Ruder MG, Noel BL, Bednarz JC, Keel MK. 2012. Exertional myopathy in pileated woodpeckers (*Dryocopus pileatus*) subsequent to capture. *Journal of Wildlife Diseases* 48:514–516.

Seki Y, Bodde SG, Meyers MA. 2010. Toucan and hornbill beaks: a comparative study. *Acta Biomaterialia* 6:331–343.

Tattersall GJ, Andrade DV, Abe AS. 2009. Heat exchange from the toucan bill reveals a controllable vascular thermal radiator. *Science* 325:468–470.

Ward JM, Gartrell BD, Conklin JR, Battley PF. 2011. Midazolam as an adjunctive therapy for capture myopathy in Bar-tailed Godwits (*Limosa lapponica baueri*) with prognostic indicators. *Journal of Wildlife Diseases* 47:925–935.

Whittow GC, ed. 2000. *Sturkie's Avian Physiology*. San Diego: Academic Press.

Windingstad RM, Hurley SS, Sileo L. 1983. Capture myopathy in a free-flying greater sandhill crane (*Grus canadensis tabida*) from Wisconsin. *Journal of Wildlife Diseases* 19:289–290.

REFERENCES

Section IV
Mammal Anesthesia

31 Monotremes (Echidnas and Platypus)

Peter Holz

INTRODUCTION

The monotremes are unique among mammals as they lay shell-covered eggs but nurse their young. There are five species: the short-beaked echidna (*Tachyglossus aculeatus*) found throughout Australia and New Guinea, three species of long-beaked echidna (*Zaglossus attenboroughi*, *Zaglossus bartoni*, and *Zaglossus bruijnii*) found in New Guinea only, and the platypus (*Ornithorhynchus anatinus*) found in Tasmania and along the east coast of mainland Australia (Van Dyke & Strahan 2008).

ECHIDNAS

Short-beaked echidnas weigh between 2 and 7 kg, while long-beaked echidnas can weigh up to 10 kg. Their dorsal surface is completely covered in spines, which are firmly attached to the skin and do not pull out the way porcupine spines do.

Capture and Physical Restraint

Echidnas have strong front feet and large pectoral muscles adapted for digging. When approached, the echidna will attempt to bury itself into the ground, rolling into a partial ball with its head tucked under its body, leaving only its spine covered dorsum exposed. Although they do not contain venom, the spines are sharp and can injure the unwary handler.

Male echidnas have spurs on their hindlegs which, until recently, were not believed to contain venom. However, new research has found that these spurs connect to a crural gland that contains proteins similar to those found in platypus venom (Koh et al. 2010). At this stage, it is unknown if the echidna "venom" is toxic to humans, and echidnas do not strike out with their spurs the way platypus do.

To dislodge the semi-buried echidna, a spade is required to dig under its body and lift it up. Alternatively, a hindfoot can sometimes be grasped. The entire echidna can then be lifted up by the foot and placed in a suitable receptacle, such as a plastic garbage can. Bags are not suitable for holding or transporting echidnas because of their spines.

If the echidna is placed on a solid surface, it will attempt to curl into a ball if approached. Again, a hand should be slid under the rear of the body and attempts made to grasp a foot. Alternatively, the entire echidna can be picked up either with a towel to protect the hands or while wearing sturdy leather gloves. If picking the echidna up by the leg, it is important to be wary of the cloaca, as stressed echidnas frequently spray urine and feces.

Anesthesia

General anesthesia is required for examination because of the echidna's tendency to roll into a ball. As the echidna usually tucks its beak quite tightly into its body it is often not possible to access the beak for mask induction. Consequently, the echidna should be placed in an induction chamber connected to an anesthetic machine and flooded with a mixture of isoflurane and oxygen. Once sufficiently sedated, the animal is removed, a mask is placed over its beak, and it is maintained with the inhalant anesthetic. Intubation is not possible because of the narrow oral cavity, inability to visualize the larynx, and presence of a keratinous pad on the dorsal surface of the base of the tongue.

Occasionally, echidnas are presented wedged into the luggage compartment of automobiles or other areas where they cannot be physically removed. Injectable agents will be required to anesthetize the echidna and extract it. A combination of xylazine (2 mg/kg IM) and ketamine (10 mg/kg IM) works well. This can be reversed with yohimbine (0.1 mg/kg IV). Alternatively, tiletamine/zolazepam (3–10 mg/kg IM), or a combination of medetomidine (0.5 mg/kg IM) and ketamine (5 mg/kg) have also been reported to be effective (Vogelnest & Woods 2008). The latter combination can be reversed with atipamezole given IM at five times the medetomidine dose. Intramuscular injections can be administered into the hindleg, proximal to the stifle.

Analgesics that have been used in echidnas include butorphanol (0.1 mg/kg IM, IV BID), buprenorphine (1 mg/kg IM, IV SID), flunixin meglumine (0.5 mg/kg SC, IM, IV SID), ketoprofen (1 mg/kg SC, IM, IV SID), and meloxicam (0.5 mg/kg SC, IV SID or 0.2 mL PO SID).

Vascular Access

On the dorsal surface of the beak, just caudal to the nostrils, lies a soft swelling that represents a venous sinus. This sinus is suitable for blood collection using a 25-gauge needle and 2- to 3-mL syringe. A heparinized winged infusion set (butterfly catheter) will reduce the likelihood of the needle coming out of the sinus if the echidna moves. Do not exert too much pressure on the syringe, as this will collapse the sinus (Johnston et al. 2006). The jugular vein can also be used, but is more difficult to access because of the echidna's short neck (Fig. 31.1).

Physiology

Normal body temperature is 28–33°C, heart rate is 80–110 beats per minute, and respiratory rate is 8–14 breaths per minute (Jackson 2003).

PLATYPUS

Capture and Physical Restraint

Platypuses weigh from 0.6 to 3.0 kg. Males possess a sharp spur on each hindleg that is connected to a venom gland located in the upper thigh region. Spurring and envenomation, although not fatal, is extremely painful (Jackson 2003). Platypuses are more aggressive and their venom more potent during the breeding season (August–October). Consequently, extra care is required when handling them during this time.

Platypuses are restrained by holding them by the tail base (Fig. 31.2). This keeps the spurs out of reach. Docile or hand-raised platypuses can be cradled in the hands. Platypuses are easily transported in bags such as pillow cases.

Anesthesia

Platypuses are anesthetized using a mask placed over the bill and induced with isoflurane and oxygen (Fig. 31.3). They are impossible to intubate because of their small gape, inability to visualize the larynx, and bulbous structure (torus linguae) at the base of the tongue (Vogelnest & Woods 2008).

Vascular Access

A vascular sinus suitable for blood collection is located running transversely along the rostral border of the bill (Fig. 31.4). A 25-gauge needle, attached to a 2- to 3-mL syringe, is inserted either side of the midline. Alternatively, a heparinized winged infusion set can be used as the needle is less likely to come out of the sinus if the platypus moves. Gentle pressure on the syringe is required to avoid collapsing the sinus. Blood can also be collected with greater difficulty from the ventral coccygeal vessels.

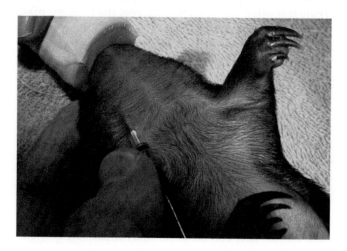

Figure 31.1. A dorsally recumbent, anesthetized echidna demonstrating the technique for blood collection from the jugular vein.

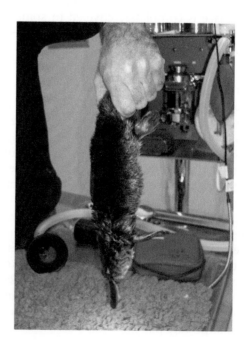

Figure 31.2. A manually restrained adult platypus demonstrating the correct position of the hand at the base of the tail to avoid the spurs in adult males.

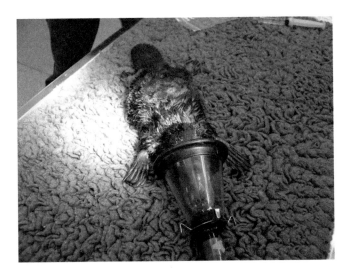

Figure 31.3. An anesthetized platypus induced and maintained with isoflurane in oxygen administered through a mask.

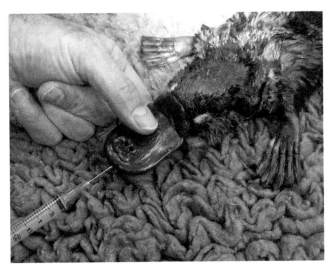

Figure 31.4. Venipuncture can be achieved in platypuses by introducing a small-gauge needle into the sinus at the edge of the bill.

Physiology

Normal body temperature is 32.5–34.5°C, heart rate is 60–150 beats per minute and respiratory rate is approximately 25 breaths per minute (Jackson 2003).

REFERENCES

Jackson S. 2003. *Australian Mammals: Biology and Captive Management*. Collingwood: CSIRO Publishing.

Johnston SD, Madden C, Nicolson V, Cowin G, Pyne M, Booth R. 2006. Venipuncture in the short-beaked echidna. *Australian Veterinary Journal* 84:66–67.

Koh JM, Haynes L, Belov K, Kuchel PW. 2010. L-to-D-peptide isomerase in male echidna venom. *Australian Journal of Zoology* 58:284–288.

Van Dyke S, Strahan R, eds. 2008. *The Mammals of Australia*, 3rd ed. Sydney: Reed New Holland.

Vogelnest L, Woods R, eds. 2008. *Medicine of Australian Mammals*. Collingwood: CSIRO Publishing.

32 Marsupials

Peter Holz

INTRODUCTION

Marsupials are a diverse group of mammals comprising approximately 330 species located predominantly in Australasia, with representatives in North and South America (Tyndale-Biscoe 2005; Van Dyke & Strahan 2008). The subclass Marsupialia is divided into seven orders: Dasyuromorphia (carnivorous marsupials), Peramelemorphia (bandicoots and bilbies), Diprotodontia (koala [*Phascolarctos cinereus*], wombats, possums, and macropods), Notoryctemorphia (marsupial moles), Didelphimorphia (opossums), Paucituberculata (shrew opossums), and Microbiotheria (monito del monte [*Dromiciops gleroides*]).

ANATOMY AND PHYSIOLOGY

The physiology of marsupials is well described by Tyndale-Biscoe (2005). Marsupials have a lower metabolic rate and a lower body temperature than eutherians. Instead of a separate anus and urogenital opening they combine the two into a single cloaca. To effectively measure a marsupial's temperature, the thermometer needs to be inserted into the dorsal part of the cloaca, leading to the rectum. Thermoregulatory ability is slow to develop, for example, kowaris (*Dasyuroides byrnii*) cannot thermoregulate until about 100 days after birth. Consequently, it is important to provide supplemental heat if young animals, particularly unfurred, are anesthetized. Marsupials combat cold by shivering. They do not have brown adipose tissue, which is used by some eutherians to generate heat. They cope with excessive heat by panting and licking. Kangaroos, in particular, will lick their forelegs to keep cool.

The majority of marsupials weigh less than 10 kg (Table 32.1) and can be manually restrained with minimal risk to the handler. Consequently, where possible, mask induction with isoflurane is the anesthetic technique of choice. Standard analgesics and anti-inflammatory agents have been used at small animal dosages with no adverse effects (Table 32.2). Venipuncture sites are listed in Table 32.3 (Fig. 32.1a–d). Reference ranges for heart rate, respiratory rate and body temperature for a variety of marsupials are given in Table 32.4.

DASYUROMORPHIA

Physical Restraint

Physical restraint is only used for minor procedures or to induce general anesthesia, as restrained animals will struggle and attempt to bite. Antechinus or dunnart bites are only mildly painful, but larger members of the group, such as the Tasmanian devil (*Sarcophilus harrisii*), can inflict severe injuries (Fig. 32.2).

Small dasyurids are gripped by the scruff of the neck or held around the body and placed in a bag (Fig. 32.3). Do not clasp them too firmly, as suffocation is possible. Larger dasyurids, such as quolls and devils, can be caught in a net or restrained by the tail and then lowered into a bag. They should not be carried long distances held only by the tail. Devils must be closely monitored while in the bag as they can chew their way out.

Smaller dasyurids, such as antechinus, dunnarts, and phascogales, should not be restrained by the tail as severe degloving injuries and tail fractures can occur. If quolls are held by the tail, care is required as some are agile enough to turn and potentially bite the handler.

Bags are a convenient way of transporting dasyurids short distances. They can range in size from a pillow case for smaller animals up to a large hessian (burlap) sack for Tasmanian devils. Animals in bags tend to relax

Zoo Animal and Wildlife Immobilization and Anesthesia, Second Edition. Edited by Gary West, Darryl Heard, and Nigel Caulkett.
© 2014 John Wiley & Sons, Inc. Published 2014 by John Wiley & Sons, Inc.

Table 32.1. Body weights of selected marsupial species (Van Dyke & Strahan, 2008)

Species	Body Weight	Species	Body Weight
Tasmanian devil	7–10 kg	Ring-tail possum	700–900 g
Eastern quoll	0.7–2.0 kg	Feathertail glider	10–15 g
Tiger quoll	1–5 kg	Sugar glider	95–160 g
Brown antechinus	20–70 g	Eastern gray kangaroo	17–85 kg
Fat-tailed dunnart	10–20 g	Western gray kangaroo	17–72 kg
Kowari	70–170 g	Red kangaroo	17–92 kg
Brush-tailed phascogale	100–300 g	Red-necked wallaby	12–24 kg
Southern brown bandicoot	0.4–1.8 kg	Swamp wallaby	10–20 kg
Bilby	0.8–2.5 kg	Tasmanian pademelon	2–12 kg
Koala	4–15 kg	Parma wallaby	3–6 kg
Common wombat	22–39 kg	Tammar wallaby	4–10 kg
Southern hairy-nosed wombat	18–36 kg	Marsupial mole	40–70 g
Brush-tail possum	1.2–4.5 kg	Virginia opossum	2.0–5.5 kg

Table 32.2. Dosages (mg/kg) of analgesics and anti-inflammatory drugs used in marsupials (Vogelnest & Woods 2008)

Drug	Dose	Species
Butorphanol	0.4 SC/IM	Macropods
	0.2 IM	Koalas
	0.4 SC/IM	Possums and gliders
Buprenorphine	0.01–0.05 SC/IM TID	Macropods
	0.01 SC/IM BID	Koalas, bandicoots and bilbies
	0.005–0.01 SC/IV BID	Possums and gliders
Fentanyl	5 µg/kg IV bolus, then 3 µg/kg/h IV infusion	Koalas
Pethidine	1 SC/IM/IV q 4–8 h	Koalas
Methadone	0.25–0.50 SC/IM q 4–6 h	Koalas
Paracetamol +/− codeine	15 PO BID-TID	Koalas
Flunixin meglumine	1 IM/IV SID 3 days	Macropods
	1 SC/IM/IV SID 1–3 days	Koalas
Carprofen	2–4 SC SID	Macropods
	4 PO SID-BID 24 h, then 2 PO SID	Koalas
	4 SC once	Possums and gliders
	2 SC BID	Bandicoots and bilbies
Meloxicam	0.2 PO/SC SID	Macropods
	0.1–0.2 PO SID	Koalas
	0.2 PO/SC followed by 0.1 PO SID for 5 days	Possums and gliders
	0.3 PO followed by 0.1 PO SID for 5 days	Bandicoots and bilbies
Tolfenamic acid	4 SC q 48 h	Macropods
	4 SC SID for 5 days	Possums and gliders

Table 32.3. Accessible veins in marsupials

Ventral coccygeal vein (artery):
Insert the needle perpendicular to the tail in the ventral midline, and advance it until the vertebrae are reached. Withdraw the needle slightly and blood should enter the hub. This vein is useful for smaller dasyurids, possums, and gliders.
Lateral coccygeal vein:
A large vein is present on both lateral aspects of the tail. Applying pressure or a tourniquet to the tail base will raise the vein. This vein is useful for macropods and opossums.
Femoral vein and artery:
Direct the needle at the pulse felt in the inguinal region. Arterial blood is often obtained and digital pressure is required to prevent hematoma formation. This vein is useful for dasyurids, bandicoots, bilbies, koalas, wombats, possums, gliders, and opossums.
Medial metatarsal (saphenous) vein:
This is a small vein running along the medial aspect of the hindleg. It is useful for small dasyurids, wombats, possums, gliders, and macropods.
Cephalic vein:
This vein is present on the dorsal surface of either foreleg. It is useful for Tasmanian devils, quolls, bandicoots, bilbies, koalas, wombats, larger possums, gliders, macropods, and opossums.
Jugular vein:
This vein is useful for dasyurids, bandicoots, bilbies, koalas, wombats, possums, gliders, and macropods, but can be difficult to access in wombats and possums due to their short necks.

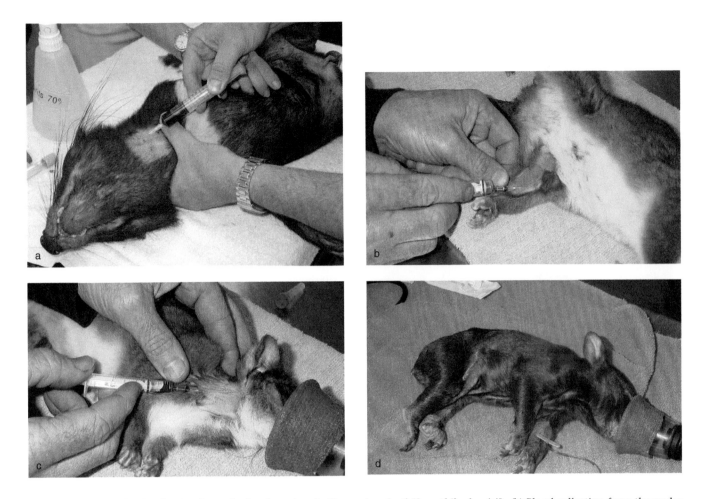

Figure 32.1. (a) Blood collection from the jugular vein of a Tasmanian devil (*Sarcophilus harrisii*). (b) Blood collection from the saphenous vein of a ringtail possum (*Pseudocheirus peregrinus*). (c) Blood collection from the jugular vein of a ringtail possum (*Pseudocheirus peregrinus*). (d) Blood collection from the cephalic vein of a juvenile common wombat (*Vombatus ursinus*).

Table 32.4. Heart rate, respiratory rate, and body temperature of selected marsupials

Species	Heart Rate/ Minute	Respiratory Rate/Minute	Temperature (°C)
Tasmanian devil	85–120	20	31–38
Bandicoot		31–37	33–34
Sugar glider	200–300	16–40	35–36
Koala	65–90	10–15	35.5–36.5
Wombat	60–120	12–30	32.0–36.5
Macropod[a]	60–150	10–30	35–36
Virginia opossum	90–160	12–24	35–36

[a]Heart rate and respiratory rate varies with the species, the rate decreases with increasing body size.

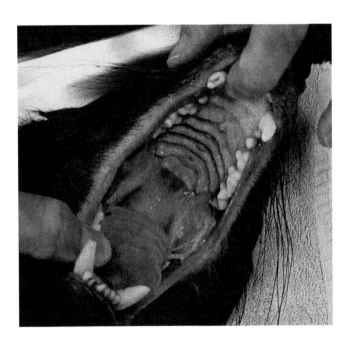

Figure 32.2. A Tasmanian devil (*Sarcophilus harrisii*) demonstrating its large gape and powerful jaws.

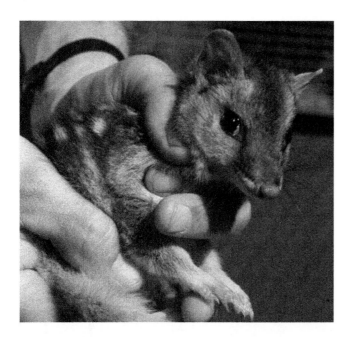

Figure 32.3. Physical restraint of an eastern quoll (*Dasyurus viverrinus*), a small carnivorous marsupial.

as outside stimuli and visual threats are removed. The chance of injury is also decreased, as they cannot lash out against solid objects. Most wild dasyurids are small enough to be caught in pit fall traps or Elliott traps baited with meat.

Anesthesia

Dasyurids are not prone to regurgitation under anesthesia, but preanesthetic fasting for 6–8 hours is recommended (Vogelnest & Woods 2008).

Inhalation anesthesia via mask induction is the method of choice. For animals in bags, anesthesia can be induced by extracting the head and placing it in the mask. It is important to grasp quolls and devils very firmly behind the head, as they will attempt to pull back out of the mask to bite the handler. Tasmanian devils and quolls have a wide gape and are easily intubated for more prolonged procedures (Fig. 32.2).

If the animal cannot be mask induced, an injectable induction is required (Table 32.5). While tiletamine/zolazepam (TZ) is a useful drug combination because of its low volume and rapid effect relaxation is variable and constant limb movement can occur in Tasmanian devils. Recoveries can also be prolonged, in excess of 6 hours in one Tasmanian devil (Holz 1992).

PERAMELEMORPHIA

Physical Restraint

Bandicoots and bilbies are nervous animals. Care is required with physical restraint as they will attempt to kick and can struggle so vigorously that spinal damage results. They have sharp teeth and will bite if provoked.

Table 32.5. Dosages (mg/kg) of tiletamine/zolazepam (TZ), xylazine/ketamine (X/K), medetomidine/ketamine (M/K), and alfaxalone for immobilization of marsupials (Vogelnest 1999; Vogelnest & Woods 2008)

	TZ	X/K	M/K	Alfaxalone
Dasyurids	7–10	4/20		2–3
Bandicoots and bilbies		10/30		
Koalas	4–10	5/15		1.5 IV / 3.0 IM
Wombats	3–8	4/20	0.125/2	3–5
Possums and gliders	4–10	6/30	0.02–0.1/1–3	5–8
Macropods	4–10	2–5/10–25	0.1/5[a]	1.5–3.0 IV / 5–8 IM
Opossums	15	5/10	0.05–0.1/2–3	

Note: Administration is by IM injection unless otherwise indicated.
[a]See Macropod section.

To restrain a bandicoot, grasp it firmly behind the neck between the first two fingers of one hand and support the rump with the palm of the other. This form of restraint should only be used for minor procedures or to transfer the bandicoot into a bag. Bilbies can be grasped by the base of the tail and then transferred to a bag.

Anesthesia

Preanesthetic fasting is not necessary. Both bandicoots and bilbies can be mask induced and maintained on isoflurane and oxygen. Because of their wide gape, visualization of the glottis and intubation is not difficult. A 2-mm uncuffed endotracheal tube can be used for bandicoots and a 3.0- or 3.5-mm tube is suitable for bilbies (Vogelnest & Woods 2008).

KOALAS (DIPROTODONTIA)

Physical Restraint

Depending on the temperament of the koala manual restraint may be sufficient for blood sampling, examination or minor treatments (Fig. 32.4). However, care is required as agitated koalas can deliver serious bites and painful scratches.

If the koala is in a tree, and within reach, it can be coaxed down using a pole with a hessian (burlap) sack or piece of material tied to the end. Waving the sack just above the koala's head will encourage it to descend. When it is close enough, a bag is placed over the koala's head, back, and rump. With the koala's body contained within the sack, the claws are disengaged from the tree and the koala should tumble into the bag. It is important to keep the bag over the koala's head and detach the animal from the top down. Otherwise it will attempt to climb back up the tree (Jackson 2003). One person can catch docile koalas. However, agitated animals need at least two people, one to cover the koala with the sack and one to detach its claws.

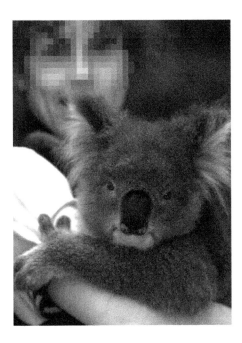

Figure 32.4. Physical restraint of a juvenile koala (*Phascolarctos cinereus*) adapted to human contact. These animals are still capable of injuring with their claws an unwary handler.

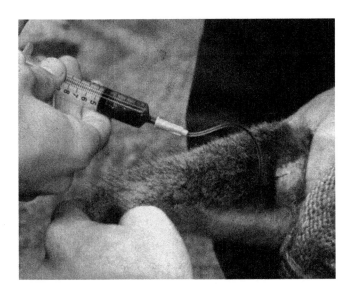

Figure 32.5. Blood collection from the cephalic vein of an awake koala restrained in a large bag.

Once in the bag, a foreleg can be extended for blood sampling (Fig. 32.5). Detailed examination and treatment should be performed under general anesthesia. When transporting the koala in the bag, it is important to hold the bag away from the body and not sling it over the shoulder, as the koala can bite and scratch through the bag.

Young hand-raised koalas can be carried on the handler's body, like a human child, with one hand supporting the rump. Make sure there is enough padding between the koala and the handler's skin, as claws will readily penetrate a shirt. Quiet adult koalas can be held with one hand on the scruff and the other supporting the rump.

Anesthesia

Preanesthetic fasting is not necessary. For inhalant induction, the koala's head is extracted from the bag and placed into the anesthetic mask. Koalas are very strong and the head must be firmly grasped as it is placed into the mask.

For prolonged procedures, koalas should be intubated. Intubation is difficult as they have a narrow oral cavity and small gape. However, if the neck is extended and a long straight-bladed laryngoscope is used, it is possible to visualize the larynx. An endotracheal tube of approximately 3- to 5-mm internal diameter can then be passed.

If the koala cannot be restrained to induce inhalation anesthesia, it will require an injectable induction (Table 32.5). Koalas high up in trees have been successfully darted with a combination of TZ (3.5 mg/kg) and medetomidine (55 µg/kg), reversed with atipamezole (2 mg IV) (Lynch & Martin 2003). Relaxation with TZ (7 mg/kg IM) alone is variable and moderate salivation can occur. Koalas take 3–4 hours to recover (Bush et al. 1990). Alfaxalone can be administered either IV or IM and provides approximately 10 minutes of anesthesia, if given by the former route. Propofol (6–8 mg/kg IV) can be used for very short procedures (Vogelnest & Woods 2008).

WOMBATS (DIPROTODONTIA)

Physical Restraint

Wild wombats are extremely strong and can be aggressive, potentially inflicting painful bites on unwary handlers. Manual restraint should not be attempted. Hand-raised wombats may permit themselves to be carried. One or both arms should be placed under the axilla, behind the forelegs, and the wombat picked up. A hand may be used to support the rump (Jackson 2003).

Anesthesia

Preanesthetic fasting is not necessary for adult wombats. Milk dependent juveniles should be fasted for at least one hour. Juvenile and hand-raised wombats can be mask induced and maintained on isoflurane. Diazepam (0.5–1.0 mg/kg IM) provides sedation for several hours. Wild adult wombats are unlikely to allow mask induction and an injectable agent will be required (Table 32.5). Despite their bulk and short legs, wombats can run as fast as a human and, given the opportunity, will rapidly dive down their burrow. As they are nocturnal, chasing wombats can be extremely hazardous due to the danger of tumbling down an unseen burrow. To catch a wild wombat, blind it by shining a powerful light at it. The handler should then approach the wombat in the dark, trap it with a net and inject it. TZ is the combination of choice as it results in rapid induction and a good level of relaxation. Recoveries can take several hours. Alfaxalone can also be used but more than 10 mL may be required to anesthetise an adult wombat.

For prolonged procedures wombats should be intubated. Intubation is difficult as they have a narrow oral cavity and small gape. However, if the neck is extended and a long straight-bladed laryngoscope is used, it is possible to visualize the larynx. Adult wombats require a 5- to 7-mm diameter endotracheal tube.

The use of long-acting neuroleptics cannot be recommended at this time. Fluphenazine decanoate (2 mg/kg IM) caused prolonged (4 weeks) sedation and inappetance in both southern (*Lasiorhinus latifrons*) and northern hairy-nosed wombats (*Lasiorhinus krefftii*) (Vogelnest & Woods 2008). The author has seen similar effects in common wombats (*Vombatus ursinus*).

POSSUMS AND GLIDERS (DIPROTODONTIA)

Physical Restraint

Many possums scratch and the larger ones will deliver painful bites. They are often presented in boxes or other containers, such as wire traps, that make restraint difficult. Bags or pillow cases are preferable. If presented in a trap, a towel should be used to cover the possum. Thick gloves can be worn, but large possums are able to bite through these and they markedly decrease sensitivity. Once under the towel, the possum is grasped firmly behind the head. Brush-tail possums (*Trichosurus spp.*), in particular, are stronger than they appear and will pull back out of a grasp that is too lax. The handler is more likely to be bitten than strangle the possum, so be firm. It is also necessary to grasp the base of the tail with the other hand. Otherwise, the possum will swing its hindlegs forward in an attempt to scratch. It can then be examined or anesthetized.

Anesthesia

Regurgitation is unlikely but 1–2 hours preanesthetic fasting has been recommended (Vogelnest & Woods 2008). If the possum is presented in a bag, the material is rolled back and the face placed in an anesthetic mask for induction.

If the animal cannot be restrained to induce inhalant anesthesia, it will require an injectable induction (see Table 32.5). Relaxation with TZ is variable and deaths occurred when it was used in squirrel gliders (*Petaurus norfolcensis*) (Holz 1992).

MACROPODS (DIPROTODONTIA)

Physical Restraint

Manual restraint is only used for minor procedures or prior to the induction of general anesthesia as macro-pods will attempt to kick the individual restraining them. Because of the size of the claw on digit four and the powerful hindlimb muscles, this can cause serious injury to the handler. Macropods will also bite and can inflict painful injuries with their teeth. Large kangaroos should never be manually restrained, as their hindlegs cannot be adequately controlled. Chemical restraint is strongly recommended.

Smaller macropods can be caught in a net. Care is required with exhibit design (Jackson 2003), since macropods will tend to run close to the fence when pursued. All poles and supporting structures must be outside the pen. The inside wall of the pen must be smooth with no protuberances. Patience and quiet are required. Many species panic easily and may collide with the fence, resulting in soft tissue trauma and cervical fractures.

Once caught in a net, the macropod can be grasped by the base of the tail and lowered into a hessian (burlap) sack or pillowcase, depending on the size of the animal. It is important not to hold the bag against the handler's body while the animal is being transported. They can still kick or bite through the bag injuring the handler.

If restraint and examination of the conscious macropod is required, small wallabies can be grasped by the tail base and held firmly behind the head. A second handler is required to restrain the hindlegs, which should be held above the hock. Otherwise, if the animal kicks out, it may break a leg. The animal can then be examined.

It is important to emphasize that animals restrained in this way, unless they are tame or hand-raised, will be extremely stressed and struggle vigorously against the restraint. It should only be used for short term procedures or as a prelude to chemical restraint.

Anesthesia

Sedation suitable for transport will occur 5–20 minutes after diazepam injection (1–2 mg/kg IM). Duration of effect is approximately 1–2 hours. Midazolam (0.3–0.4 mg/kg IM or IV) is a shorter acting alternative. If necessary, the benzodiazepines can be antagonized with flumazenil (1 mg flumazenil per 25 mg benzodiazepine). Azaperone (1–2 mg/kg IM) may also be used. Effects appear after 15–20 minutes and last for 6–8 hours (Vogelnest & Woods 2008).

For animals in bags, anesthesia is induced by extracting the macropod's head and placing the face in the mask. In this way, the handler is protected to some extent from the powerful hindlimbs, as they are contained within the bag.

If the animal cannot be restrained to induce inhalation anesthesia, it will require an injectable induction (Table 32.5). TZ inductions are swift and the low volume required makes it an ideal combination for immobilization by dart. However, recoveries can be prolonged (1–5 hours). Ketamine combined with medetomidine provides superior relaxation to TZ and, if concentrated medetomidine (10 or 20 mg/mL) is used, is also suitable for remote immobilizations. It is, however, extremely expensive. Induction times are longer than with TZ (up to 20 minutes). It is important not to stimulate the animal during induction, as this will extend the time to recumbency or result in inadequate immobilization.

The author has successfully used a combination of ketamine (5 mg/kg) and medetomidine (100 μg/kg) for immobilization of docile red (*Macropus rufus*) and western gray kangaroos (*Macropus fuliginosus*). A recent study also used this combination to immobilize Bennett's wallabies (*Macropus rufogriseus*) (Bouts et al. 2011). However, in the author's experience, this combination at this dose failed to effectively immobilize the more nervous species, such as eastern gray kangaroos (*Macropus giganteus*), or smaller macropods, such as pademelons (*Thylogale* spp.) and parma wallabies (*Macropus parma*). There are several published dosages for ketamine/medetomidine combinations in macropods (2–3 mg/kg/50–100 μg/kg, Shima 1999; 2–3 mg/kg/40–80 μg/kg, Vogelnest 1999; and 4 mg/kg/40 μg/kg, Pye & Booth 1998). However, in the author's experience, these dosages are too low to induce effective immobilization.

Recent studies have also described immobilization of Bennett's wallabies using combinations of ketamine (15 mg/kg) and xylazine (2 mg/kg), ketamine (5 mg/kg) and dexmedetomidine (0.05 mg/kg) (Bouts et al. 2010), and alfaxalone (4 mg/kg) and medetomidine (0.1 mg/kg) (Bouts et al. 2011).

Ketamine/medetomidine and ketamine/dexmedetomidine anesthesia is reversed using atipamezole (IM or SC) at five times the dose of medetomidine or dexmedetomidine. The author has successfully used this dosage IV with no adverse effects. Animals are standing, but still ataxic, approximately 10–20 minutes after reversal.

TZ (0.5–1.0 mg/kg) can be combined with either medetomidine (30–40 ug/kg) or dexmedetomidine (30–40 μg/kg) for remote injection of captive red kangaroos (Heard pers. communication). This combination allows a small injection volume (when using a concentrated solution of medetomidine), relatively rapid induction and relatively shorter recovery period after reversal (60 minutes+).

For wild macropods, the TZ combination is preferred. A recent study recommended 4.7–4.9 mg/kg for wild eastern gray kangaroos, which resulted in a mean induction time of 7–10 minutes with a recovery time of 116–130 minutes (Roberts et al. 2010).

For prolonged procedures, macropods should be intubated as they may regurgitate. Intubation is difficult as they have a narrow oral cavity and small gape. However, if the neck is extended and a long straight-bladed laryngoscope is used it is possible to visualize the larynx. An endotracheal tube can then be passed. Alternatively, the animal can be placed in dorsal recumbency and a guide catheter used to facilitate passage of the tube. Lidocaine sprayed on the glottis may assist passage of the tube.

Long-Acting Tranquilizers

Many macropod species are naturally nervous and may benefit from the use of long-acting tranquilizers when settling into new exhibits. The author has successfully used a combination of zuclopenthixol decanoate (10 mg/kg IM) and pipothiazine palmitate (10 mg/kg IM) administered to red-necked wallabies (*Macropus rufogriseus*). This dosage is much higher than that recommended for hoofstock but lower dosages proved ineffective. Duration of effect was approximately 10 days (Holz & Barnett 1996). Others have recommended using fluphenazine decanoate (2.5 mg/kg IM), the effect of which peaks by 72 hours and lasts up to 10 days, zuclopenthixol acetate (5–10 mg/kg) which has an effective duration of 72 hours, or haloperidol decanoate (4–6 mg/kg) (Vogelnest & Woods 2008). There are anecdotal reports of mortalities in bridled nail-tailed wallabies (*Onychogalea fraenata*) and agile wallabies (*Macropus agilis*) following the use of zuclopenthixol (Portas pers. comm.).

NOTORYCTEMORPHIA

Marsupial moles are rarely found in captivity. They can be held in the hand and do not attempt to bite, but resent being restrained (Jackson 2003). They can be mask induced and maintained with isoflurane.

DIDELPHIMORPHIA, PAUCITUBERCULATA AND MICROBIOTHERIA

Physical Restraint

Opossums will defend themselves by biting, but they may also feign death. It is important to remain vigilant if this happens as the opossum may suddenly become active and either bite or attempt to escape. To restrain the opossum, a towel should be placed over the animal, which can then be firmly grasped behind the head. They can also be lifted by grasping the base of the tail. However, some animals may be able to lift themselves to bite and require additional restraint around the nape of the neck.

Anesthesia

The opossum is placed in a bag for transport or mask induction with isoflurane. A plastic induction chamber, connected to an isoflurane machine, can also be used. If inhalation anesthesia is not possible, an injectable induction is required. Dosages are given in Table 32.5.

High doses of TZ or xylazine/ketamine were used in the past (Stoskopf et al. 1999), but more recent literature recommends using a combination of medetomidine (50–100 μg/kg IM) and ketamine (2–3 mg/kg IM) (Johnson-Delaney 2006), or medetomidine (70 μg/kg IM) and ketamine (10 mg/kg IM), combined with butorphanol (0.5 mg/kg SC) (Capello 2007).

REFERENCES

Bouts T, Harrison N, Berry K, Taylor P, Routh A, Gasthuys F. 2010. Comparison of three anaesthetic protocols in Bennett's wallabies (*Macropus rufogriseus*). *Veterinary Anaesthesia and Analgesia* 37:207–214.

Bouts T, Karunaratna D, Berry K, Dodds J, Gasthuys F, Routh A, Taylor P. 2011. Evaluation of medetomidine-alfaxalone and medetomidine-ketamine in semi-free ranging Bennett's wallabies (*Macropus rufogriseus*). *Journal of Zoo and Wildlife Medicine* 42:617–622.

Bush M, Graves JAM, O'Brien SJ, Wildt DE. 1990. Dissociative anaesthesia in free-ranging male koalas and selected marsupials in captivity. *Australian Veterinary Journal* 67:449–451.

Capello V. 2007. Surgical technique for neutering the female Virginia opossum. *Exotic DVM* 8(2):31–36.

Holz P. 1992. Immobilization of marsupials with tiletamine and zolazepam. *Journal of Zoo and Wildlife Medicine* 23:426–428.

Holz P, Barnett JEF. 1996. Long acting tranquillizers: their use as a management tool in the confinement of free-ranging red-necked wallabies (*Macropus rufogriseus*). *Journal of Zoo and Wildlife Medicine* 27:54–60.

Jackson S. 2003. *Australian Mammals: Biology and Captive Care.* Collingwood: CSIRO Publishing.

Johnson-Delaney CA. 2006. What every veterinarian needs to know about Virginia opossums. *Exotic DVM* 6(6):38–43.

Lynch M, Martin R. 2003. Capture of koalas (*Phascolarctos cinereus*) by remote injection of tiletamine-zolazepam (Zoletil) and medetomidine. *Wildlife Research* 30:255–258.

Pye GW, Booth RJ. 1998. Medetomidine-ketamine immobilization and atipamezole reversal of eastern grey kangaroos (*Macropus giganteus*). Proceedings American Association of Zoo Veterinarians and Proceedings American Association of Wildlife Veterinarians Joint Conference, Omaha, NE, pp. 306–309.

Roberts MW, Neaves LE, Claasens R, Herbert CA. 2010. Darting eastern grey kangaroos: a protocol for free-ranging populations. In: *Macropods: The Biology of Kangaroos, Wallabies and Rat-Kangaroos* (G Coulson, M Eldridge, eds.), pp. 325–339. Collingwood: CSIRO Publishing.

Shima A. 1999. Sedation and anesthesia in marsupials. In: *Zoo and Wild Animal Medicine: Current Therapy 4* (ME Fowler, RE Miller, eds.), pp. 333–336. Philadelphia: W.B. Saunders.

Stoskopf MK, Meyer RE, Jones M, Baumbarger DO. 1999. Field immobilization and euthanasia of American opossum. *Journal of Wildlife Diseases* 35:145–149.

Tyndale-Biscoe H. 2005. *Life of Marsupials.* Collingwood: CSIRO Publishing.

Van Dyke S, Strahan R, eds. 2008. *The Mammals of Australia*, 3rd ed. Sydney: Reed New Holland.

Vogelnest L. 1999. Chemical restraint of Australian native fauna. Wildlife in Australia. Sydney: Proceedings No. 327 of the Post-Graduate Committee in Veterinary Science, pp. 149–187.

Vogelnest L, Woods R, eds. 2008. *Medicine of Australian Mammals.* Collingwood: CSIRO Publishing.

33 Insectivores (Hedgehogs, Moles, and Tenrecs)

Darryl Heard

TAXONOMY AND BIOLOGY

The order Insectivora has traditionally been used to unite several disparate mammalian groups (i.e., hedgehogs, moles, tenrecs, shrews, and solenodons) based on size and "primitive characters" (Nowak 1999). Recent revisions based on molecular evidence has redistributed insectivores into several orders: Afrosoricida (tenrecs and golden moles, 51 species), Erinaceomorpha (hedgehogs, 24), and Soricomorpha (moles, shrews, and solenodons, 428) (Wilson & Reeder 2005). For this discussion, however, these animals are grouped together. The tree shrews appear more closely related to primates and are classified within their own order Scandentia (Wilson & Reeder 2005).

The most commonly encountered insectivores in clinical practice in Europe and North America are the West European (*Erinaceus europaeus*) and four-toed or white-bellied (*Atelerix albiventris*) hedgehogs, respectively. The biology, anatomy, and physiology of hedgehogs are well described by Reeve (1994). Their major anatomical characteristic is their spines. Each is erected by a muscle originating in the deeper layers (Reeve 1994). When threatened and unable to flee, hedgehogs usually roll into a ball using several specialized muscles. All spiny hedgehogs appear able to hibernate during adverse conditions. Hibernation is associated with polycythemia and relative hypoglycemia (Reeve 1994). The "normal" body temperature of nonhibernating European hedgehogs is 35 ± 2°C (Reeve 1994). Heart rate is approximately 200–280 bpm, declining to ≤25 bpm during hibernation.

Moles and shrews are occasionally encountered as injured wildlife. Torpor occurs in shrews, some golden moles, and tenrecs (Reeve 1994). Shrews have some of the highest metabolic rates, oxygen consumption rates, water turnover, and heart and respiration rates of any mammal (Ishii et al. 2002; Ochocinska & Taylor 2005). Although moles are adapted to low oxygen environments and can tolerate prolonged hypoxemia, it is no reason to allow this to occur during the perianesthetic period.

PHYSICAL RESTRAINT

All insectivores can bite. In addition to the trauma that may be inflicted, shrews have venom, blarina toxin, within their saliva (Kita et al. 2004).

Reeve (1994) describes several techniques for unrolling a hedgehog. Leather gloves are worn to protect from the spines, as well as bites. If you are right-handed, gently lift the hedgehog's hind end in your right palm. Use your left hand under its front, head turned away from you. Gently bounce it up and down in your hands. The hedgehog will extend its feet and unroll its snout. Without hurrying, keep bouncing it gently and allow the snout to poke between the thumb and index finger of the left hand. Place the thumb on the back of its neck using gentle, firm pressure. This prevents it from tucking its head back down. Gently gripping the rear underside of the animal with your right fingers put your right thumb in the small of its back and gently open out the animal by flexing it backwards. Alternatively, the rolled-up animal is held head down over a table. It then usually unrolls cautiously and tries to reach the surface. The back legs can then be grasped gently and the animal held by them. Alternatively, the animals are transferred directly to an inhalant anesthetic induction chamber.

Zoo Animal and Wildlife Immobilization and Anesthesia, Second Edition. Edited by Gary West, Darryl Heard, and Nigel Caulkett.
© 2014 John Wiley & Sons, Inc. Published 2014 by John Wiley & Sons, Inc.

PREANESTHETIC PREPARATION

Fasting is not recommended since most insectivores are very small, have high metabolic rates and small glucose reserves, and are prone to develop hypoglycemia. Cardiomyopathy is a relatively common postmortem finding in captive white-bellied hedgehogs (Black et al. 2011; Raymond & Garner 2000). Orbits in hedgehogs are shallow and the palpebral fissures are large. This may predispose them to proptosis during the perianesthetic period, especially if the periocular area is damaged and inflamed (Wheler et al. 2001).

House musk shrews (*Suncus murinus*), and perhaps other shew species, are very sensitive to inhalant- and parenteral anesthetic-induced emesis (Gardner & Perren 1998; Horn et al. 2012). Conversely, morphine alone appears not to produce emesis in musk shrews (Selve et al. 1994). The NK1 antagonist GR205171 (1–3 mg/kg SC) and the 5-HT3 antagonist ondansetron (3 mg/kg SC) each inhibited inhalant anesthetic induced emesis in house shrews (Gardner & Perren 1998).

PARENTERAL ANESTHESIA

Description of parenteral anesthesia in insectivores is scant—drugs and dosages are extrapolated from those used in rodents (Chapter 66). Although inhalation (isoflurane and sevoflurane) is preferred, parenteral anesthesia may be indicated for remote field work. Xylazine (3 mg/kg SC), and ketamine alone (20–30 mg/kg IM) or in combination with midazolam (1–2 mg/kg IM) will cause a hedgehog to unroll and to allow examination (Reeve 1994). Buprenorphine (0.01–0.03 mg/kg SC q 12 h) has been used by this author for analgesia (Table 33.1).

Injection Sites

For SC injections in hedgehogs, forceps are used to grasp a small fold of the spiny skin over the rump. Injection is made into the connective tissue at the base of the pleat formed with the needle parallel to the animal's body (Reeve 1994). A skin fold can also be raised by pulling upward on a spine. Alternatively, an injection is made in the flank while a gloved helper pins the animal on a table. Intramuscular injections are made in the large muscles of the thigh, not the back. This route is avoided in most other insectivores because of the potential to cause irritation and self-trauma. Intraperitoneal injection is as described for rodents. Intravenous injection is difficult or impossible in most. Potential sites include cephalic (over the forearm) and intraosseous injection into the femur, tibia, and possibly the humerus.

INHALATION ANESTHESIA

Inhalation anesthesia provides rapid induction and recovery. An induction chamber can be constructed from a plastic container with an attachment for administration of the inhalant and another for removal of waste gases. Alternatively, a mask is held over the nose or used to completely enclose a small insectivore (Fig. 33.1). Animals caught in traps are either dropped into the induction chamber, or the trap enclosed in a plastic bag for anesthetic administration.

Most insectivores are too small for endotracheal intubation. A large adult white-bellied hedgehog may be intubated with a 2 mm uncuffed endotracheal tube. Alternatively, an endotracheal tube made from an over-the-needle catheter can be used.

Table 33.1. Anesthetic and analgesic drugs used in insectivores

	Drug		Hedgehogs	Moles	Shrews	Tenrecs	Comments
Inhalant anesthetics	Isoflurane	Induction	5%	5%	5%	5%	
		Maintenance	2–5%	2–5%	2–5%	2–5%	
	Sevoflurane	Induction	7–8%	7–8%	7–8%	7–8%	
		Maintenance	3–4%	3–4%	3–4%	3–4%	
	Halothane	Induction	5%	5%	5%	5%	
		Maintenance	1–2%	1–2%	1–2%	1–2%	
Parenteral anesthetics	Ketamine		20 mg/kg IM				
	Ketamine/ midazolam						
	Ketamine/ xylazine		20–40/3–5 IP IV	50–70/2–3 IP	50–200/5–10 IP	20–40/3–5 IP IV	
	Ketamine/ medetomidine		5/0.06 IM				
	Propofol		6–8 mg/kg IV				
Opioid analgesics	Morphine						
	Meperidine						
	Buprenorphine						
	Butorphanol						
NSAIDs	Ketoprofen						
	Carprofen						
	Meloxicam		0.2–0.5 mg/kg IM PO				
	Tramadol		1–5 mg/kg PO				

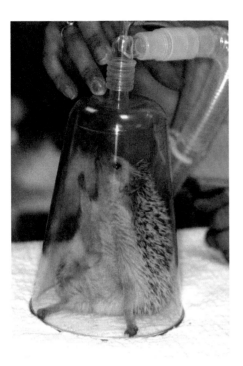

Figure 33.1. Inhalation anesthesia is preferred for anesthesia in all insectivores. This white-bellied hedgehog (*Atelerix albiventris*) is being induced with isoflurane in oxygen administered into a commercial dog mask connected to a nonrebreathing system.

MONITORING AND SUPPORTIVE CARE

Monitoring and supportive care are as for rodents (Chapter 68). The high metabolic rate, oxygen requirement and water turnover of many insectivores (especially shrews) make them very susceptible to hypothermia, hypoglycemia, hypoxemia, and dehydration. All effort should be made to minimize the duration of anesthesia. As described earlier, vascular access is very difficult or impossible to attain. Intraosseous catheterization of

the humerus, tibia or femur is a possible alternative. Monitoring should include pulse oximeter, Doppler flow detection, or ECG.

REFERENCES

Black PA, Marshall C, Seyfried AW, Bartin AM. 2011. Cardiac assessment of African hedgehogs (*Atelerix albiventris*). *Journal of Zoo and Wildlife Medicine* 42(1):49–53.

Gardner C, Perren M. 1998. Inhibition of anaesthetic-induced emesis by a NK1 or 5-HT3 receptor antagonist in the house musk shrew, *Suncus murinus*. *Neuropharmacology* 37:1643 –1644.

Horn CC, Meyers K, Pak D, Nagy A, Apfel CC, Williams BA. 2012. Post-anesthesia vomiting: impact of isoflurane and morphine on ferrets and musk shrews. *Physiology & Behavior* 25:562–568.

Ishii K, Uchino M, Kuwahara M, Tsubone H, Ebukuro S. 2002. Diurnal fluctuations of heart rate, body temperature and locomotor activity in the house musk shrew (*Suncus murinus*). *Experimental Animals* 51:57–62.

Kita M, Nakamura Y, Okumura Y, Ohdachi SD, Oba Y, Yoshikuni M, Kido H, Uemura D. 2004. Blarina toxin, a mammalian lethal venom from the short-tailed shrew Blarina brevicauda: isolation and characterization. *Proceedings of the National Academy of Sciences of the United States of America* 101:7542–7547.

Nowak RM. 1999. *Walker's Mammals of the World*, Vol. 1, 6th ed. Baltimore: The Johns Hopkins University Press.

Ochocinska D, Taylor JR. 2005. Living at the physiological limits: field and maximum metabolic rates of the common shrew (*Sorex araneus*). *Physiological and Biochemical Zoology* 78: 808–818.

Raymond JT, Garner MM. 2000. Cardiomyopathy in captive African hedgehogs (*Atelerix albiventris*). *Journal of Veterinary Diagnostic Investigation* 12(5):468–472.

Reeve N. 1994. *Hedgehogs*. London: T & AD Poyser Ltd.

Selve N, Friderichs E, Reimann W, Reinartz S. 1994. Absence of emetic effects of morphine and loperamide in *Suncus murinus*. *European Journal of Pharmacology* 256:287–293.

Wheler CL, Grahn BH, Pocknell AM. 2001. Unilateral proptosis and orbital cellulitis in eight African hedgehogs (*Atelerix albiventris*). *Journal of Zoo and Wildlife Medicine* 32(2):236–241.

Wilson DE, Reeder DM, eds. 2005. *Mammal Species of the World. A Taxanomic and Geographic Reference*, Vol. 1, 3rd ed. Baltimore: The Johns Hopkins University Press.

34 Edentata (Xenartha)

Gary West, Tracy Carter, and Jim Shaw

INTRODUCTION

Edentata are immobilized to facilitate diagnostic procedures and treatment of medical conditions in zoological institutions (Ferrigno et al. 2003). These species have also been immobilized for a variety of captive and field research projects (Carter 1983; Deem & Fiorello 2002; Herrick et al. 2002; Shaw et al. 1987). Although several studies have been done describing immobilization of these species, very little scientific data exists on anesthesia and monitoring of this order (Table 34.1).

PREANESTHETIC PREPARATIONS

The Edentata encompass animals with a wide range of body sizes and unique anatomical features (Divers 1986; Gillespie 2003; Wallach & Boever 1983). Body weights of edentates are often underestimated prior to immobilization (Deem & Fiorello 2002). Edentates are often characterized as heterothermic or incompletely homeothermic with wide ranges in normal body temperatures. For instance, sloths have a normal body temperature range of 24–40°C. Body temperatures in edentates may be influenced by ambient temperatures. Captures should be avoided during cold or inclement weather conditions (Deem & Fiorello 2002). The capture of free-ranging edentates during cold weather may prolong their recovery and contribute to postimmobilization mortality. Fasting smaller species of edentates for 4–6 hours is appropriate, and large species (giant anteater, giant armadillo, and sloths) should be fasted for 12–24 hours.

Preparation for the capture of free-ranging giant armadillos is labor intensive. The location of an active giant armadillo burrow must be made before capture can be attempted (Carter 1983). Giant armadillos will create new burrows nightly, unless they are rearing young (Carter & Encarnacao 1983). Occupied burrows are located using domestic dogs, or by observation of recent digging activity at a burrow entrance. Large traps constructed of reinforced metal are set at the entrance of occupied giant armadillo burrows. As the armadillos exit their burrows, they enter the trap. The armadillo is confined in the trap by closing a metal door. The metal door is often propped open with a small wooden stick and the armadillo bumps the stick and the door closes. Capture teams must wait near the trap site and immediately immobilize the animals after they are caught, since giant armadillos often destroy the traps and injure themselves if they are left in the traps for prolonged periods of time (see Fig. 34.1).

PHYSICAL RESTRAINT

Most armadillos can be manually restrained by grabbing the animal by the sides (Fig. 34.2 and Fig. 34.3, restraint). Gloves are often used to avoid claw or biting injuries. *Euphractus*, the six-banded armadillo, will readily bite handlers. Wild giant armadillos are typically captured in traps as previously mentioned, and caution should be used with this species, as they are powerful and can inflict serious trauma to handlers before being fully immobilized. Sloths can be manually restrained with gloves or nets. Two-toed sloths can move very quickly when harassed, and will bite. Restrained sloths are capable of using their powerful forelimbs for pulling themselves closer to a restrainer's hand and inflict serious bite injuries using their large, sharp, caniform incisors. Individual sloths can be restrained for exams, blood collections, or induction of anesthesia by holding in dorsal recumbency with forelimbs extended laterally over a flat surface at a distance

Zoo Animal and Wildlife Immobilization and Anesthesia, Second Edition. Edited by Gary West, Darryl Heard, and Nigel Caulkett.
© 2014 John Wiley & Sons, Inc. Published 2014 by John Wiley & Sons, Inc.

Table 34.1. Normal adult body weights of select Edentate species

Giant armadillo, *Priodontes maximus*	40–60 kg
Six-banded armadillo, Euphractus sexcinctus	3–6.5 kg
Three-banded armadillo, *Tolypeutes* spp.	1–2.0 kg
Long-nosed armadillo, *Dasypus* spp.	3–10 kg
Fairy armadillo, *Chlamyphorus* spp.	100 g
Giant anteater, *Mymecophaga tridactyla*	18–50 kg
Lesser anteater, *Tamandua* spp.	2–8 kg
Silky anteater, *Cyclopes didactylus*	0.4–0.8 kg
Two-toed sloth, *Choloepus* spp.	4–9 kg
Three-toed sloth, *Bradypus* spp.	3–5 kg

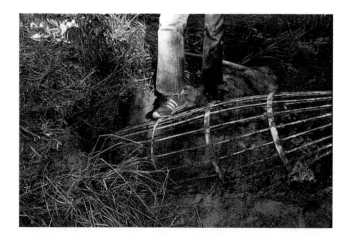

Figure 34.1. Reinforced metal trap placed at the entry to a giant armadillo (*Priodontes maximus*) burrow.

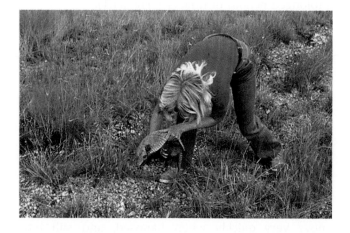

Figure 34.2. Manual capture of a six-banded armadillo (*Euphractus sexcintus*).

where the sloth cannot reach and bite. A second handler can help restrict hindlimb movements.

Lesser anteaters can be restrained with gloved hands, or held by the tail for injections. In one study, animals were restrained with their head and forelimbs in a bag while held by the tail for hand injections of immobilizing agents (Fournier-Chambrillion et al. 1997). Lesser

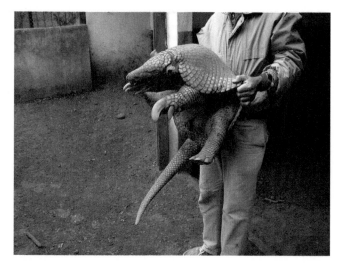

Figure 34.3. Manual restraint of captive giant armadillo (photo by Bob Klemm at Compleo Ecológico Municipal at Saenz Peña, Argentina).

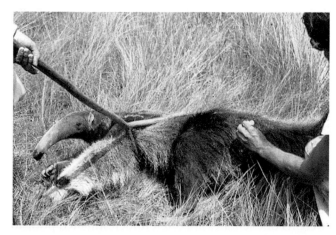

Figure 34.4. Free-ranging giant anteater (*Myrmecophaga tridactyla*) being restrained with wooden forked stick and hand injected with immobilization drugs.

anteaters have powerful claws that must be avoided. Giant anteaters have very powerful front limbs, with prominent claws, and are difficult to restrain manually. Wild giant anteaters can be pinned to the ground with forked wooden sticks, and immobilizing drugs are then administered by hand (Shaw et al. 1987); see Figure 34.4. Nets should not be used for anteater capture as their lips and mouths may be easily abraded (Wallach & Boever 1983).

INDUCTION

All edentates can be effectively immobilized with cyclohexamine (ketamine or tiletamine) drugs in combination with benzodiazepienes or alpha-2 agonists. Such combinations include ketamine-midazolam, tiletamine-zolazepam, ketamine-xylazine, or ketamine-medetomidine. In smaller species of edentates, manual restraint and induction with inhalants is preferred. All armadillo species, except the giant armadillo, can be manually restrained for mask or chamber induction with inhalants. Isoflurane or sevoflurane are very effective induction agents in these species. But anesthetic induction with inhalants can be prolonged due to breath holding of most edentates. Wild armadillos have been induced with isoflurane-soaked cotton balls (Deem & Fiorello 2002). Caution must be used with this method of administration, as isoflurane can be vaporized to very high concentrations at normal atmospheric pressures (up to 33%), and inhalant overdose could easily occur.

A variety of injectable immobilizing agents has been used effectively in armadillo species, and may be used in field conditions. These include: tiletamine-zolazepam, ketamine-midazolam, ketamine, ketamine-xylazine, or ketamine-medetomidine. Ketamine-medetomidine appeared to be a superior option in field conditions, due to the ability to reverse the medetomidine component (Fournier-Chambrillion et al. 2000). Tiletamine-zolazepam will cause good muscle relaxation, but prolonged recoveries are a problem in free-ranging species. Intraperitoneal or intravenous pentobarbital has also been used experimentally in armadillos, but does not have the margin of safety of other immobilizing combinations. Droperidol and fentanyl (Innovar-vet®) in combination have also been used effectively in armadillos, but this combination is no longer commercially available in the United States (Thurmon et al. 1996). Giant armadillos are most easily caught in burrow traps, and are successfully immobilized with ketamine and xylazine given intramuscularly (see Fig. 34.5). Drugs should be administered with 16- or 18-gauge, 1.5-in needles. Giant armadillos immobilized with ketamine-xylazine are not routinely given alpha antagonists, but the use of the alpha-2 antagonist, atipamezole at 0.1 mg/kg IM, may help shorten recoveries (Table 34.2).

Sloth species can often be approached and hand injected for immobilization while they are perching or resting. As the drugs take effect, the sloth can be supported with gloved hands to avoid biting injuries. A sedated sloth that is incapable of holding onto a support branch but capable of biting can be manipulated into a restraint box or container until maximum effect of induction drugs is reached. Sloths may also be manually restrained and induced by facemask using an anesthetic inhalant, such as sevoflurane. But sloths may hold their breath for prolonged periods, making mask inductions difficult. A variety of injectable immobilizing drug combinations has been used in sloths (Gilmore et al. 2000; Hanley, et al. 2008; Vogel et al. 1998). Ketamine-medetomine IM was found to be the best for field conditions due to its reversibility (Vogel et al. 1998). Tiletamine-zolazepam IM is a safe and effective immobilizing drug in captive situations, but recoveries are prolonged. A combination of ketamine-midazolam is also a good choice for induction. Animals may need to be confined during recovery before allowing them to climb again.

Anteater species have been immobilized with a ketamine-xylazine (Shaw et al. 1987) combination. Xylazine does not seem to cause regurgitation as reported in other species (Fournier-Chambrillion et al. 1997). In one study of lesser anteaters, increased ketamine doses seemed to increase relaxation, but also caused severe bradycardia. (Fournier-Chambrillion et al. 1997). Giant anteaters can be induced with ketamine and alpha-2 agonist combinations with good recovery after reversal of the alpha agonist. Ketamine-medetomidine will adequately immobilize captive

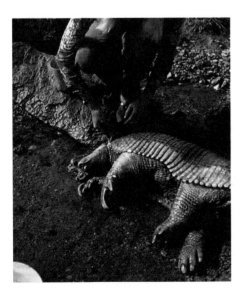

Figure 34.5. Immobilized giant armadillo (*Priodontes maximus*) having ear tag applied (photo by Bob Klemm, Compleo Ecológico Municipal, Saenz Peña, Argentina).

Table 34.2. Doses for anesthetic induction agents in Edentata

Armadillos	
Tiletamine/zolazepam	2–8 m/kg IM
Ketamine + midazolam	5 mg/kg (K) + 0.2 mg/kg (Mi) IM
Ketamine	10–15 mg/kg IM
Ketamine + xylazine	5 mg/kg (K) + 1 mg/kg (X) IM
Ketamine + medetomidine	5 m/kg (K) + 0.02–0.07 mg/kg (M) IM
Sloths	
Ketamine + medetomidine	3 mg/kg (k) + 0.04 mg/kg (M)
Tiletamine/zolazepam	2–6 mg/kg IM
Ketamine + midazolam	5–10 mg/kg + 0.2 mg/kg IM
Anteaters	
Ketamine + midazolam	5–10 mg/kg (k) + 0.2 mg/kg (Mi)
Ketamine + xylazine	5–10 mg/kg (K) + 0.5–1.5 mg/kg (x) IM
Ketamine + medetomidine	2–4 mg/kg (k) + 0.02–0.04 (M)

anteaters. In captive situations, blow darts can be used to administer immobilizing drugs. Giant anteaters can be darted in leg musculature. However, in free-ranging giant anteaters, darting episodes caused severe agitation, longer induction, and incomplete immobilization. The preferred field capture method is to approach the animal from a downwind location, restrain them with a forked stick, and quickly administer the immobilizing agent by hand injection in a hind limb, which resulted in more reliable immobilization (see Fig. 34.4). Etorphine, in combination with diazepam and atropine, may be an effective immobilizing combination for giant anteaters (Gillespie 2003; Gillespie & Adams 1985). No cardiac or respiratory depression was noted, but details were not given on how these parameters were monitored (Gillespie 2003; Gillespie & Adams 1985). The advantage of the combination would be rapid recovery after opioid antagonist administration. Salivation may be controlled by anticholinergics, but blood pressure monitoring is essential if anticholinergics are given in conjunction with alpha agonists (Sinclair 2003; Wallach & Boever 1983).

MAINTENANCE

After immobilization, edentates are typically maintained in lateral recumbency. In a captive situation, anesthesia is maintained with inhalants, and the alpha agonist drugs can be antagonized. Alpha agonists are antagonized because they cause severe bradycardia, bradyarrythmias, decreased myocardial contractility, and likely cause decreased cardiac output (Sinclair 2003). Armadillo and sloth species are easily intubated with the aid of a laryngoscope, whereas anteater species are not routinely intubated. Anteaters have very small mouths, and appropriate-sized endotracheal tubes cannot be advanced orally (Gillespie 2003; Gillespie & Adams 1985). Giant anteaters may accommodate a 10- to 14-mm endotracheal tube, and tracheotomy supplies should be available for emergency situations. Armadillos can hold their breath and seem to tolerate hypoxemia better than other mammalian species (Thurmon et al. 1996).

Often the front claws of giant anteaters are bandaged during anesthesia to prevent claw injuries to handlers. However, if the animal is adequately immobilized and monitored, this should not be necessary. In the field, immobilized edentates will have their eyes covered with a blindfold to protect them from direct sunlight.

SUPPORT

Blood pressure can be monitored in edentates with indirect methods, since intravenous and intra-arterial access sites are challenging to locate in edentates. Catheterization may require a venous cut down procedure

(Gillespie 2003; Gillespie & Adams 1985). Intravenous access sites include the femoral and cephalic veins in all edentates. Sloths also have cubital veins and vertebral veins that can be used for blood collection (Divers 1986; Wallace & Oppenheim 1996). Anteaters and armadillos also have jugular or ventral tail veins. Jugular cut down procedures have been used to administer intravenous fluids in giant anteaters, although thick skin and large salivary glands make this a challenging task (Gillespie 2003; Gillespie & Adams 1985). Cardiocentesis has been advocated for armadillos or sloths, but could have severe complications and cannot be recommended (Divers 1986). Intraosseus or intraperitoneal fluid administration may also be appropriate in emergency situations.

It has been reported that armadillos will spontaneously recover from ventricular fibrillation with no treatment (Thurmon et al. 1996). Armadillos can also tolerate longer periods of apnea and hypoxemia than most mammals (Thurmon et al. 1996). Heart rates (HRs) for immobilized armadillos range from 120 to 220 beats per minute and respiratory rates (RRs) from 60 to 80 breaths per minute. Body temperatures in armadillos may range from 30 to 35°C. Cardiac output studies have been done in three-toed sloths using a dye solution technique, and these data were similar to domestic species (Gilmore et al. 2000). EKG evaluation in the three-toed sloth has been completed (Silva et al. 2005). Sloths have extreme lability in their blood pressure, and stress can have a great influence on these values. (Gilmore et al. 2000). Pulse oximetry has been used in the sloth and may be influenced by hypothermia, hypotension, and pigmentation of tissues. Sloths immobilized with ketamine/alpha-2 agonists or tiletamine/zolazepam exhibited hypoxemia based on pulse oximetry readings (Vogel et al. 1998). But blood gas values were not collected in these sloths to confirm these readings (Vogel et al. 1998). The normal HR for sloths is 45–60 bpm, and RR 10–80. Anteaters may have HR of 110–160 bpm and RR of 10–30 bpm normally.

Capnography can be used in edentates and the readings are more accurate in intubated animals. The difficulty in locating arteries can make blood gas analysis challenging, but blood gases should be monitored when possible.

RECOVERY AND COMPLICATIONS

Severe cardiovascular abnormalities can occur when alpha-adrenergic agonist agents are used for immobilization (Sinclair 2003). Alpha-adrenergic drugs can be antagonized with atipamezole, both as a treatment for negative cardiovascular effects and to hasten recoveries. Antagonism of benzodiazepines with the use of flumazenil may reduce recovery times. However, the short duration of flumazenil antagonism (60 minutes) makes its use impractical, since. The duration of benzodiazepine effects can be up to 4 hours. Captured, free-ranging animals may require treatment of dart or injection sites to prevent screwworm infestation (Deem & Fiorello 2002). Postrecovery excitement and self-trauma can occur if the animals are confined after recovery. Animals may pace excessively and injure claws and feet by pawing at shift doors.

Isoflurane administered by cotton balls was associated with postcapture mortality in armadillos (Deem & Fiorello 2002). The authors suggest that liver failure may have been caused by isoflurane, although when properly administered, isoflurane is the least likely inhalant to cause liver damage (Steffey 1996). In addition, anesthetic-induced hepatic damage would not cause liver failure for several days after anesthetic administration. The administration of isoflurane by cotton ball may have caused severe anesthetic overdose and cardiovascular failure, with resulting liver congestion. Vaporization of isoflurane in room air could reach 33% concentrations and cause inhalant gas overdose.

Hypothermia in field situations is possible and difficult to treat in remote locations. Trauma from capture in traps can occur as animals may rub their face or head on the traps. Claw trauma can occur from animals trying to escape enclosures after being darted.

Intubation of anteaters would require tracheotomy and close monitoring as they heal. Tracheostomy was described in a cadaver specimen of the giant anteater (*Myrmecophaga tridactyla*). The authors stated that the procedure was possible but difficult due to the large submaxillary salivary glands and deep location of the larynx beneath neck musculature (Brainard et al. 2008). Additionally, the position of the larynx can enter the thoracic cavity, and full extension of the neck must be performed to access the larynx. Handling wild nine-banded armadillos in the Southeastern United States could expose human handlers to *Mycobacterium leprae* or *Sporothrix schenkeii* (Kaplan et al. 1982; Truman 2005; Wenker et al. 1998).

Respiratory arrest was suspected in a giant anteater immobilized with ketamine and xylazine (Strom 2003). The animal began to breathe after the administration of doxapram hydrochloride. Ketamine will cause apnea in certain individuals. Doxapram will stimulate respiratory centers in the central nervous system and increase ventilation, but will not be effective during respiratory arrest.

REFERENCES

Brainard BM, Newton A, Hinshaw KC, et al. 2008. Tracheostomy in the giant anteater (*Myrmecophaga tridactyla*). *Journal of Zoo and Wildlife Medicine* 39(4):655–658.

Carter TS. 1983. The burrows of giant armadillos, *Priodontes maximus* (Edentata: Dasypodidae). *Saugetierkundliche Mitteilungen* 31:47–53.

Carter TS, Encarnacao C. 1983. Characteristics and use of burrows by four species of armadillos in Brazil. *Journal of Mammalogy* 64(1):103–108.

Deem SL, Fiorello CV. 2002. Capture and immobilization of free-ranging edentates. In: *Zoological Restraint and Anesthesia* (D Heard, ed.), Document No. B0135.1202. Ithaca: International Veterinary Information Service. http://www.IVIS.org (accessed January 23, 2014).

Divers BJ. 1986. Edentates. In: *Zoo and Wild Animal Medicine* (ME Fowler, ed.), pp. 621–630. Philadelphia: WB Saunders.

Ferrigno CRA, Fedullo DL, Kyan V, et al. 2003. Treatment of radius, ulna, and humerus fractures with the aid of a bone morphogenetic protein in a giant anteater (*Myrmecophaga tridactyla*). *Veterinary and Comparative Orthopaedics and Traumatology* 16:196–199.

Fournier-Chambrillion C, Fournier P, et al. 1997. Immobilization of wild collared anteaters with ketamine and xylazine-hydrochloride. *Journal of Wildlife Diseases* 33(4):795–800.

Fournier-Chambrillion C, Vogel I, Fournier P, et al. 2000. Immobilization of free-ranging nine-banded and great long-nosed armadillos with three anesthetic combinations. *Journal of Wildlife Diseases* 36(1):131–140.

Gillespie D 2003. Xenarthra: Edentata (anteaters, armadillos, sloths). In: *Zoo and Wild Animal Medicine*, 5th ed. (ME Fowler, RE Miller, eds.), pp. 304–310. Philadelphia: W.B. Saunders.

Gillespie D, Adams C. 1985. Anatomy, husbandry, and anesthesia of the giant anteater (*Myrmecophaga tridactyla*). American Association of Zoo Veterinarians Annual Proceedings. 35–36.

Gilmore DP, Da-Costa CP, Duarte DPF. 2000. An update on the physiology of two- and three-toed sloths. *Brazilian Journal of Medical and Biological Research* 33:129–146.

Hanley CS, Siudak-Campfield J, Paul-Murphy J, et al. 2008. Immobilization of free-ranging Hoffmann's two-toed and brown-throated three-toed sloths using ketamine and medetomidine: a comparison of physiologic parameters. *Journal of Wildlife Diseases* 44(4):938–945.

Herrick JR, Campbell MK, Swanson WF. 2002. Electroejaculation and semen analysis in the La Plata three-banded armadillo (*Tolypeutes matacus*). *Zoo Biology* 21:481–487.

Kaplan W, Broderson JR, Pacific JN. 1982. Spontaneous systemic sporotrichosis in nine-banded armadillos (*Dasypus novemcintus*). *Sabouraudia* 20(4):289–294.

Shaw JH, Machado-Neto J, Carter TS. 1987. Behavior of free-living giant anteaters (*Myrmecophaga tridactyla*). *Biotropica* 19: 255–259.

Silva EM, Duarte DPF, da Costa CP. 2005. Electrocardiographic studies of the three-toed sloth, *Bradypus variegatus*. *Brazilian Journal of Medical and Biological Research* 38:1885–1888.

Sinclair MD. 2003. A review of the physiological effects of alpha2-agonists related to the clinical use of medetomidine in small animal practice. *Canadian Veterinary Journal* 44(11):885–897.

Steffey E. 1996. Inhalants. In: *Lumb and Jones, Veterinary Anesthesia* (J Thurmon, W Tranquili, GJ Benson, eds.), pp. 785–806. Philadelphia: John Wiley & Sons.

Strom H. 2003. Can you intubate an anteater? *Dansk Veterinaertidsskrift* 86(12):19–21.

Thurmon JC, Tranquili WJ, Benson GJ. 1996. *Lumb & Jones' Veterinary Anesthesia*, p. 690. Baltimore: William and Wilkins.

Truman R. 2005. Leprosy in wild armadillos. *Leprosy Review* 76(3): 198–208.

Vogel I, Thoisy B, Vie J. 1998. Comparison of injectable anesthetic combinations in free-ranging two-toed sloths in French Guiana. *Journal of Wildlife Diseases* 34(3):555–566.

Wallace C, Oppenheim YC. 1996. Hematology and serum chemistry profiles of captive Hoffman's two-toed sloths (*Choloepus hoffmanni*). *Journal of Zoo and Wildlife Medicine* 27(3):339–346.

Wallach JD, Boever WJ. 1983. Edentates. In: *Diseases of Exotic Animals*, pp. 612–629. Philadelphia: W.B. Saunders.

Wenker CJ, Kaufman L, Bacciarini LN, Robert N. 1998. Sporotrichosis in a nine-banded armadillo (*Dasypus novemcinctus*). *Journal of Zoo and Wildlife Medicine* 29(4):474–478.

35 Tubulidentata and Pholidota

Jennifer N. Langan

INTRODUCTION

Data on captive husbandry, medicine, and anesthesia of both aardvarks and pangolins in captivity are very limited. They are infrequently kept in zoos and are not favored as exhibit specimens because of their inactivity and nocturnal propensities. Some specimens of aardvarks have lived up to 20 years in zoological institutions, but the life span of captive pangolins has been significantly less.

TUBULIDENTATA

The aardvark (*Orycteropus afer*) is the only living representative of the order Tubulidentata. Their natural habitat is confined to Africa, south of the Sahara Desert. They have solid bodies, a long snout, and powerful legs. They have long spadelike toenails that are used to dig burrows, find food, and defend themselves. Aardvarks range in weight from 50 to 70 kg. The animal's thick skin is covered with bristly hair. Aardvarks have a long extensible tongue used to collect termites and ants in the wild. Their teeth lack enamel and are continuously growing; this predisposes them to malocclusion and dental disease. Their cheek teeth are composed of numerous hexagonal prisms of dentin surrounding a tubular pulp cavity. This pattern of growth gives the order its name, Tubulidentata (tubule-toothed). The dental formula for aardvarks is I 0/0, C 0/0, P 2/2, M 3/3 (Fig. 35.1). They are primarily nocturnal and sleep most of the day in underground burrows (Nowak 1991).

Aardvarks can be conditioned to allow physical examination and minor clinical procedures (skin scrapes and conjunctival swabs) without chemical restraint, but sedation is usually required for noxious or invasive procedures, such as venipuncture. Aard-

varks are extremely strong animals with an incredibly powerful kick. Manual restraint of adult aardvarks is not recommended. Neonates and juveniles can be physically restrained for procedures, but should be sedated once they are greater than 10 kg to prevent injury to the animal and the handler.

Chemical restraint for aardvarks is generally required for most medical procedures. A variety of anesthetic agents have been used successfully in aardvarks. A combination of ketamine and medetomidine intramuscularly is currently one of the most widely used anesthetic protocols (Table 35.1) (Langan 2003; Stetter 2003). This combination provides rapid, smooth inductions, and at least 30 minutes of anesthesia. In the author's experience, hand injection has not yielded consistent drug delivery because of the explosive reaction of the aardvark upon needle insertion. Contrastingly, remote drug delivery using CO_2-propelled darts has provided excellent results. However, owing to the aardvark's extremely tough skin, several modifications to dart removal have been needed. Pliers are used to pull out intramuscular darts, and pressure is applied around the area of needle insertion to prevent subcutaneous air accumulation during dart withdrawal. When invasive or painful procedures are necessary, supplementation with gas anesthesia is recommended. At the completion of the procedure, atipamezole is given intramuscularly to antagonize the effects of medetomidine and speed recovery. Recoveries are substantially smoother if the reversal is given at least 30 minutes after induction when medetomidine and ketamine are used in combination. Other successful drug combinations have included the following: tiletamine and zolazepam, ketamine, and detomidine (Vodicka 2004), ketamine and xylazine (Nel et al. 2000), ketamine and midazolam (Nel et al. 2000), ketamine and droperidol in combination

Zoo Animal and Wildlife Immobilization and Anesthesia, Second Edition. Edited by Gary West, Darryl Heard, and Nigel Caulkett.
© 2014 John Wiley & Sons, Inc. Published 2014 by John Wiley & Sons, Inc.

with fentanyl (Dieterich 1986), and etorphine with acepromazine (Stetter 2003) (Table 35.1).

Inhalant anesthetics reported in aardvarks include both halothane and isoflurane (Langan 2003; Nel et al. 2000; Stetter 2003). Animals can be maintained with gas anesthesia using either a mask or endotracheal intubation. Precautions should be taken to prevent nasal edema caused by tightly fitting face masks or gauze used to secure the endotracheal tube. Medical problems seen in aardvarks in captivity, such as conjunctivitis, postoperative wound dehiscence, and decubital ulcers can be treated by maintaining animals on a face mask using isoflurane.

Dental disease is by far the most common medical problem reported in captive aardvarks. Tooth root abscesses typically present as painful firm swellings. Buccostomies are often required to access teeth that need to be extracted because of the small size of the oral opening (Fig. 35.2 and Fig. 35.3). Curettage to remove surrounding infected bone can lead to significant hemorrhage associated with dental infections. Endotracheal intubation in these cases is especially important to protect the animal's airway. The long and narrow oral cavity of the aardvark can make intubation challenging. Blind intubation with a size 10-mm endotracheal tube for adult aardvarks has been very reliable for the author. Following induction, the animal is placed in sternal or lateral recumbency, and the animal's head and neck are maximally extended. Gentle traction is used to pull the

tongue cranially out of the oral cavity (Fig. 35.4), at which point the endotracheal tube is advanced over the base of the tongue. While holding one's ear to the proximal open end of the tube, the tip of the endotracheal tube is slowly moved into the larynx to the position at which maximal audible respiratory sounds and expiration are noted. Frequently, the tube is inadvertently advanced past this point and introduced into the cranial esophagus instead of the trachea. This happens most frequently when the animal is still swallowing. Supple-

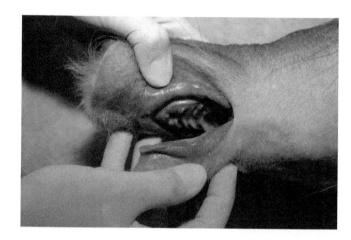

Figure 35.2.   Lateral view of the extent to which the oral cavity can be opened in the aardvark.

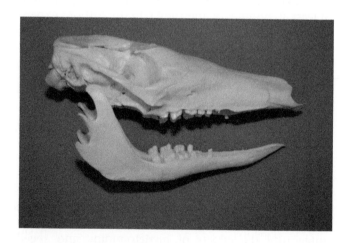

Figure 35.1.   Normal dentition of the aardvark. Dental formula I 0/0, C 0/0, P 2/2, M 3/3.

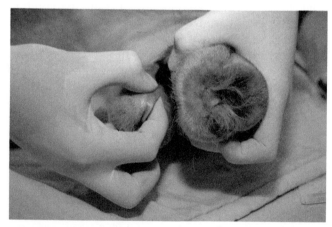

Figure 35.3.   Anterior view of the narrow oral opening of the aardvark which makes endotracheal intubation and oral examination challenging.

Table 35.1.   Chemical restraint agents used for aardvarks

Immobilization Drug	Dose	Antagonist	Dose	Reference
Tiletamine/zolazepam	4–5 mg/kg	Flumazenil	0.01 mg/kg	Langan (2003)
Ketamine/medetomidine	3 and 0.03–0.07 mg/kg	Atipamezole	0.15–0.4 mg/kg	Langan (2003)
Ketamine/detomidine	4–8 and 0.09–0.18 mg/kg	Atipamezole	0.05–0.09 mg/kg	Vodicka (2004)
Ketamine/midazolam	15–20 and 0.28–0.68 mg/kg			Nel et al. (2000)
Ketamine/xylazine	14 and 0.94 mg/kg	Atipamezole	0.3 mg/kg	Nel et al. (2000)
Ketamine/diazepam	11 and 0.26 mg/kg			Goldman (1986)

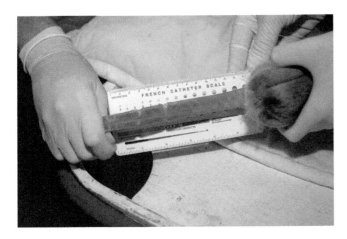

Figure 35.4. Withdrawing the aardvark's long tongue out of the mouth provides the needed space within the oral cavity and larynx to intubate the animal with an endotracheal tube.

menting with isoflurane via a mask until the animal no longer swallows makes intubation much simpler. While auscultating and watching the chest cavity, the tube is gently advanced into the trachea during inspiration. Rotation of the tube during advancement facilitates placement of the endotracheal tube. Alternatively, a long slender-bladed laryngoscope or flexible endoscope may be helpful to facilitate intubation; but these typically are not necessary in the author's experience. The tongue should be manually returned to the oral cavity after the animal is intubated to prevent lingual edema. In one instance, an animal was unable to retract its edematous tongue and subsequently stepped on it, causing a severe laceration during recovery. The animal later required amputation of the distal third of its tongue. Because of the very small oral opening and depth of the cavity, dental examination with a laryngoscope blade prior to intubation is essential. Once the endotracheal tube is in place, there is insufficient space to do a thorough dental and oral examination.

It is the author's experience that many aardvarks pace excessively once they recover from anesthesia, causing excessive wear and bleeding of the toenails during the first 24–72 hours following immobilization. Oral diazepam given once a day at 10 mg/aardvark in the late afternoon has prevented excessive pacing behavior during their nocturnal activity.

Occasionally, females are extremely restless and do not allow their infants to nurse sufficiently or injure them inadvertently because of excessive activity in the nest box. In these cases, low doses of oral diazepam (0.25–0.45 mg/kg SID-BID) have alleviated this behavior and allowed successful rearing of the calf by the dam. The female is weaned off diazepam after 3–4 weeks, once the infant is sufficiently ambulatory and is more efficient at nursing.

Data from aardvarks that have been anesthetized between 1999 and 2006 at Brookfield Zoo have included

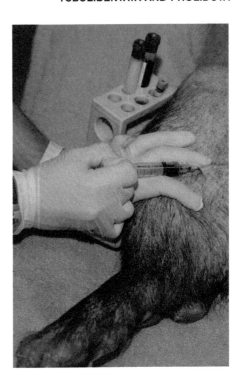

Figure 35.5. Venipuncture from the medial saphenous vein in an aardvark.

heart rates ranging from 60 to 95 beats per minute, respiratory rates between 12 and 18 breaths per minute, and temperatures of 95 to 100°F.

Anesthetic monitoring using auscultation, pulse oximetry, ECG, and temperature is as in other mammals. Blood collection and intravenous catheterization can be best accomplished from the medial saphenous vein (Fig. 35.5), but is also possible using the cephalic, ventral tail, or facial vein. Frequently, peripheral vessels appear to contract during venipuncture attempts, yielding very little blood despite large vessel diameter and good blood pressure. Large-bore (18-gauge) needles and slow manual syringe collection appear to yield the best results. The aardvark's skin is extremely thick and tough, often necessitating a modified cut-down procedure for catheter placement. The location of catheter placement is selected and appropriately prepared by clipping the fur and disinfecting the skin. The skin over the vessel is pulled lateral to the vein, and a scalpel blade is used to make a small stab incision through the skin. The skin is then allowed to return to its normal position over the vessel, at which point the intravenous catheter can be routinely placed.

Infrequent monitoring of blood pressure has been attempted using a cuff distal hind limb and proximal tail with varying results. Arterial blood samples for blood gas analysis are easily obtained from the femoral or auricular artery. Arterial catheterization for continuous direct blood pressure monitoring would also likely be possible from the auricular artery. Field techniques used to capture free-ranging aardvarks include the use of nets and funnel traps set at burrow entrances. All animals require immobilization to be handled and examined (Nel et al. 2000).

PHOLIDOTA

Animals belonging to the order pholidota include one genus (*Manus*) and seven species, and are often referred to as scaly anteaters. The white-bellied tree pangolin (*Manus tricuspis*), long-tailed tree pangolin (*Manus tetradactyla*), giant pangolin (*Manus gigantean*), and Cape pangolin (*Manus. teminckii*) are African, whereas Asia is inhabited by the Indian (*Manus crassicaudata*), Chinese (*Manus pentadactyla*), and Malayan pangolins (*Manus javanica*). Some are arboreal and have strong prehensile tails, whereas others live in burrows. Pangolins attain a weight of 4–27 kg, with males being larger than females. They feed primarily on ants and termites at night, which they mechanically digest in a crop-like stomach modified for the grinding process (Wilson 1994). Pangolins have stout powerful clawed limbs used for digging and long, ribbon-like tongues. The musculature of the tongue is remarkable and has attachments reaching along the xiphoid all the way to the pelvis. It retracts into a sheath in the chest cavity when at rest. Pangolins have very well-adapted salivary glands that extend posteriorly, nearly to the shoulder. The glands produce sticky secretions that facilitate the collection of their insect prey. Pangolins completely lack teeth, and the lower jaw is a small blade-like bone. The most obvious feature of pangolins is their scaly epidermal armor. The dorsal surface of their elongate body is covered in continuously growing, overlapping scales. Confronted with a threat, pangolins curl into a tight ball to protect their soft underparts and spray urine and noxious anal gland secretions (Nowak 1991).

Large pangolins must be handled with caution because their surprising strength and sharp body coverings can injure personnel. Smaller specimens may be safely restrained with leather gloves. The normal pangolin behavior upon handling is to curl into a protective ball. Forced manual attempts to uncoil a pangolin can result in injury to the animals, and chemical restraint is typically advised to permit examination and specimen collection. Captive animals can be accustomed to handling and may become quite tractable, which facilitates routine veterinary procedures (Heath & Vanderlip 1988; L. Greer, pers. comm.).

Historically, ketamine has been used for sedating *M. pentadactyla* (Heath 1986) and *M. tetradacyla* (Robinson 1983), with doses of approximately 16–25 mg/kg, administered IM in the hind limbs. Uncoiling is possible at the higher dose; however, some muscle tone persists and salivation occurs. The duration of effective restraint is relatively short (10–20 minutes) (Robinson 1983). More recently, chamber or mask induction and maintenance with isoflurane has replaced injectable

anesthesia with excellent results (L. Greer, pers. comm., 2006).

Resting heart rates have been reported to range from 80 to 86 beats per minute, and respiratory rates varied from 14 to 53 breaths per minute (Heath & Vanderlip 1988).

Literature on clinical medicine of pangolins is sparse. The most common reported disease concerns are related to gastrointestinal ailments. Captive pangolins have the propensity to ingest bedding materials (wood shavings and saw dust), which have resulted in gastric impactions and death (Griner 1983; Heath & Vanderlip 1988). Inappropriate diet, parasitism, and malnutrition are commonly reported problems in the literature (Heath & Vanderlip 1988; Kuehn 1986; Robinson 2003). One source reports that pangolins appear to be highly susceptible to *Cryptococcus* spp. when they were housed in mixed-species exhibits (Wilson 1994).

Conventional peripheral vessels are difficult to access. Blood sampling can be accomplished under chemical restraint from a ventral surface of the tail by clipping a portion of a scale to gain access to the skin (Heath 1986; Heath & Vanderlip 1988).

REFERENCES

Dieterich RA. 1986. Tubulidentata. In: *Zoo and Wild Animal Medicine*, 2nd ed. (ME Fowler, ed.), pp. 595–597. Philadelphia: W.B. Saunders.

Goldman CA. 1986. A review of the management of the aardvark (*Orycteropus afer*) in captivity. *International Zoo Yearbook* 24/25: 286–294.

Griner LA. 1983. *Pathology of Zoo Animals, San Diego*. San Diego: Zoological Society of San Diego.

Heath ME. 1986. Hematological parameters of four Chinese pangolins (*Manis pentadacytla*). *Zoo Biology* 5:387–390.

Heath ME, Vanderlip SE. 1988. Biology, husbandry, and veterinary care of captive Chinese pangolins (*Manis pantadacytla*). *Zoo Biology* 7:293–313.

Kuehn G. 1986. Pholidota. In: *Zoo and Wild Animal Medicine*, 2nd ed. (ME Fowler, ed.), pp. 618–620. Philadelphia: W.B. Saunders.

Langan J. 2003. Managing dental disease in aardvarks (*Orycteropus afer*). Proceedings of the American Association of Zoo Veterinarians, pp. 93–95.

Nel PJ, Taylor A, Meltzer DGA, et al. 2000. Capture and immobilization of aardvark (*Orycteropus afer*) using different drug combinations. *Journal of the South African Veterinary Association* 71: 58–63.

Nowak RM. 1991. *Walker's Mammals of the World*, Vol. 11. Baltimore: Johns Hopkins University Press.

Robinson PT. 1983. The use of ketamine in restraint of a black-bellied pangolin (*Manis tetradactyla*). *Journal of Zoo Animal Medicine* 14:19–23.

Robinson PT. 2003. Pholidota. In: *Zoo and Wild Animal Medicine*, 5th ed. (ME Fowler, ER Miller, eds.), pp. 407–410. Philadelphia: W.B. Saunders.

Stetter MD. 2003. Tubulidentata. In: *Zoo and Wild Animal Medicine*, 5th ed. (ME Fowler, ER Miller, eds.), pp. 538–541. Philadelphia: W.B. Saunders.

Vodicka R. 2004. Chemical immobilization in captive aardvark (*Orycteropus afer*). *Journal of Zoo and Wildlife Medicine* 35: 544–545.

Wilson AE. 1994. Husbandry of pangolins (*Manis* spp.). *International Zoo Yearbook* 33:248–251.

36 Chiropterans (Bats)

Darryl Heard

INTRODUCTION

After rodents, bats are the most diverse and widely distributed mammal group (Wilson & Reeder 2005). They are also the most abundant and form the biggest mammalian aggregations known (Nowak 1999). The order Chiroptera contains 18 recent families and ≥1116 bat species (Wilson & Reeder 2005). It is divided into suborders Microchiroptera and Megachiroptera. The latter comprises just one family, the Pteropodidae, with 42 genera and ≥186 species.

Bats inhabit most of the temperate and tropical areas of the world, except for some remote oceanic islands and beyond the tree growth line in the colder parts of either hemisphere. The Megachiroptera are confined to the tropical and subtropical regions of the Old World, east to Australia, and the Caroline and Cook Islands.

PHYSIOLOGY AND ANATOMY

"Chiroptera" is derived from the Greek *cheir* (hand) and *pteron* (wing). Skeletal adaptations for flight include a keeled sternum and elongated second to fifth metacarpals that form long rigid spokes for wing membrane. The thumb (digit one) is an agile grasping tool, and the only digit with a functional claw. The thoracic vertebrae are interconnected to form a rigid column that supports the flight muscles.

Compared with other mammals, the acetabular opening is rotated and shifted dorsally, and the legs are rotated 180° around their long axis so the knees face the rear. Since they usually perch inverted, their legs are adapted for pulling rather than pushing. At rest, the entire bodyweight is suspended from the toes. Most have a locking mechanism that keeps the claws in a flexed position without muscular contraction (Fig. 36.1). Consequently, bats must be "unhooked" from a perch rather than pulled; excessive force will injure toes and in juveniles may cause epiphyseal fractures. The hind limb claws are compressed into hooked blades that will lacerate skin during restraint of larger bats.

The maximal aerobic capacities are the same as similar-sized birds. The minimal metabolic requirement in level flight is 1.5 greater than the maximal aerobic capacity of a similar-sized nonflying mammal. Consequently, bats at rest are not likely to manifest overt clinical signs until respiratory dysfunction is well advanced.

Active bats are homeotherms, maintaining their body temperature between 35 and 39°C. They utilize a large amount of energy to compensate for heat loss due to a high body surface area to metabolically active tissue ratio. Additionally, large lungs and naked flight membranes result in heat loss from a surface area six times larger, and a thermal conductance 1.5–4 times greater, than wingless animals. Some bats compensate for this with heterothermy; temperate bats and tropical Vespertilionids and Molossids have a variable ability to lower body temperature and go into torpor (diurnal lethargy) or hibernation. This is based not only on temperature, but also food availability and reproductive condition. Lowered body temperature and metabolic rate in hibernating or torpid animals is assumed to reduce anesthetic requirement, and alter drug uptake and elimination.

Bats consume large quantities of food relative to their body size. Gastrointestinal transit is also very rapid, possibly to minimize bodyweight for flight. Vomiting is, therefore, unlikely unless animals are anesthetized immediately after feeding. Bats usually feed at night when they are most active. Consequently,

Zoo Animal and Wildlife Immobilization and Anesthesia, Second Edition. Edited by Gary West, Darryl Heard, and Nigel Caulkett.
© 2014 John Wiley & Sons, Inc. Published 2014 by John Wiley & Sons, Inc.

blood glucose and tissue glycogen levels are lowest at dusk before the animals begin feeding (Widmaier & Kunz 1993).

ZOONOTIC DISEASES

Bats populations are known reservoirs for several infectious agents of significance to humans and other

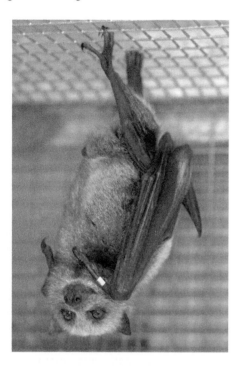

Figure 36.1.   Most bats possess a locking mechanism in the toes that allows them to hang without effort. Pulling downward causes the claws to turn inward. To remove bats from a perch the claws must be unhooked to prevent injury. Golden-mantled flying fox (*Pteropus pumilus*).

animals (e.g., Lyssaviruses, Henipaviruses, and *Leptospira* spp) (Calisher et al. 2006; Constantine 1970; Rupprecht et al. 2001). It is recommended that all personnel working with bats should be vaccinated against rabies and other lyssaviruses (Rupprecht et al. 2001). Care is taken to minimize contact with blood, saliva, and other secretions or emissions that may contain infectious organisms. Although the teeth of many Microchiropterans are very small, they can still penetrate human skin. Furthermore, saliva contact with skin is also a possible source of infection. It is recommended bats be anesthetized for procedures requiring close contact to reduce biting and transmission of secretions.

PHYSICAL RESTRAINT

Techniques used for capturing free-living bats are described by Kunz and Kurta (1988). All restrained bats are capable of delivering a defensive bite. Most have jaws that are shortened giving them a powerful bite. Neonatal bats possess needle-like, caudally directed milk teeth for gripping the nipple. The thumbs and associated claws of large bats will scratch an unprotected handler and are used to pull fingers in for a bite.

Bats are restrained with leather gloves (Fig. 36.2a,b). Alternatively, a towel is used to cover the head and confine the limbs. In small bats, nets can be used for initial capture, but are cumbersome in larger animals. However, they should always be available in case of an escape. The duration of manual restraint is minimized to reduce stress and prevent hyperthermia. Prolonged restraint induces marked elevations in cortisol and glucose (Widmaier & Kunz 1993). Carrying cages must be sufficiently tall to prevent the head of the bat from touching the floor.

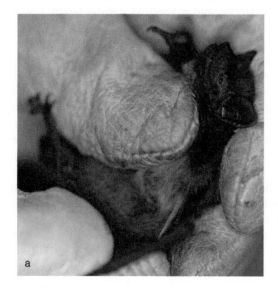
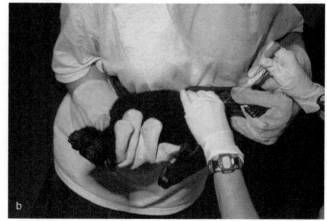

Figure 36.2.   (a) Leather gloves are recommended for handling even small bats, such as this evening bat, from bites. (b) Physical restraint of a large flying fox (*Pteropus vampyrus*) for sample collection. Note the use of long-sleeved gloves to protect the holder from scratches, and the hold around the neck and feet.

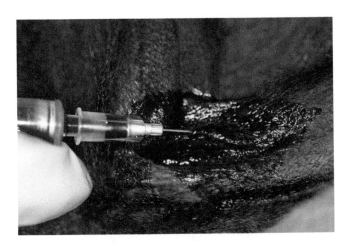

Figure 36.3. Venepuncture of the right median vein in an anesthetized large flying fox (*Pteropus vampyrus*). Note the positioning of the elbow in a right angle to facilitate access to the vessels on the ventral aspect of the distal humerus.

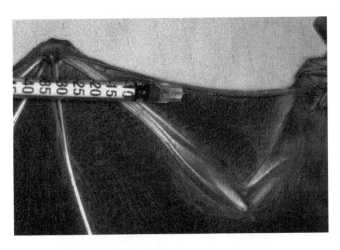

Figure 36.4. Venepuncture of the cephalic vein in an anesthetized Egyptian fruit bat (*Rousettus aegyptiacus*).

Wimsatt et al. (2005) describes the use of a restraint device made of polyvinyl chloride tubing in big brown bats (*Eptesicus fuscus*). An attachment at one end is used to administer inhalant anesthesia.

BLOOD COLLECTION AND HANDLING

The blood volume of active bats is approximately 9.0–11.0 mL/100 g. Blood is collected in bats ≥ 100 g from the median artery or vein on the medial aspect of the distal humerus with a 25-gauge needle and 1- or 3-mL syringe (Fig. 36.3). If the collector is right handed, the right wing of the supine bat is extended until the elbow joint forms a 90° angle. The left hand of the collector is then used to rotate the biceps muscle laterally while compressing the median veins to cause their distension. The right hand is supported on the table surface and the needle and syringe rest across the proximal radius as the needle enters the vessel. Once blood is identified in the needle hub, continued flow must be "finessed" with gentle alteration in suction, rotation of the needle, and patience. There are usually two or more veins and an artery in close contact at the insertion site. Although arterial blood can be used for sampling, care must be taken to ensure adequate hemostasis. Large hematomas are common, even with venous puncture, and in small bats may result in death. Since collection time may be prolonged, heparinization of the syringe is recommended when a plasma sample is appropriate (Heard et al. 2006a). However, if collection lasts >2 minutes and is traumatic, the anticoagulant effect of the heparin will be overcome by thromboplastin released from tissue. Further excessive pressures will result in hemolysis.

In small bats, blood samples are collected from the cephalic vein along the leading edge of the patagium

(Fig. 36.4). A 25-gauge needle is used to make a hole in the vessel and blood is collected into a microhematocrit tube from the incision site. Alternatively, a 1/2-mL insulin syringe with attached 27-gauge needle is used. This technique is also used to collect blood from the interfemoral (Fig. 36.5a,b) and saphenous vessels. In very small bats, the uropatagial vessels can be dilated with the application of a warm pack (Wimsatt et al. 2005).

The external jugular veins are large in Microchiropterans and may in some species be used for collection. Cranial vena caval collection has also been successful in some large bat species. The internal and external jugular veins of Megachiropterans are small and of similar size.

Bat blood is easily altered by inappropriate collection, handling, and storage. Even moderate hemolysis during sample collection will cause pseudo-hyperkalemia, hyponatremia, hypochoremia, and elevated aspartate transaminases (Day et al. 2001). Hyperkalemia in otherwise healthy animals is usually an indication of sample collection error. If the plasma remains in contact with the red cells for ≥6 hours, there will be an elevation in phosphorus and decreases in chloride and glucose concentrations (Day et al. 2001). Heparinized blood samples allow centrifugation immediately after collection and the plasma to be removed from the blood cells and frozen until analysis (Day et al. 2001; Heard et al. 2006).

PARENTERAL ANESTHESIA

Inhalation anesthesia is preferred in bats. There are circumstances, however, where it is either not available or appropriate to the situation (i.e., anesthesia of free-living animals in remote locations). Parenteral anesthetic regimens are summarized in Table 36.1.

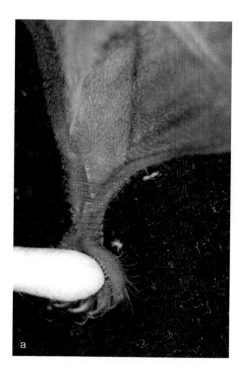

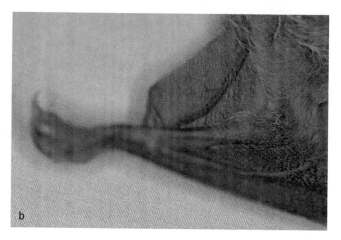

Figure 36.5.   (a) The interfemoral vein in the uropatagium of a microchiropterans, a Mexican free-tail bat (*Tadarida brasiliensis*). This vessel can be used for small volume blood collection. (b) The interfemoral vein in the uropatagium of an Egyptian fruit bat (*Rousettus aegyptiacus*).

Injection Sites

When possible, intramuscular injection in the flight muscles is avoided. However, in large aggressive bats, it is easier to press them into sternal recumbency and administer drugs in the large triceps or thigh muscles. The sternum is relatively narrow, and pectoral muscle injection may result in the needle passing between the ribs if the bat moves.

Intravenous injection sites are the same as those used for blood collection: cephalic (Fig. 36.4), median, and femoral or saphenous. Small-gauge catheters are placed temporarily in the cephalic and median veins. Awake bats usually do not tolerate catheters. Intraosseous catheterization of the radius is an alternative route for administration of fluids. This route can be used in even the smallest bats.

Microchiropterans

Although there are several examples of "big" little bats, most Microchiropterans are <50 g. Small body size is usually associated with a higher anesthetic dosage required for a given level of analgesia or anesthesia. Most reported studies of parenteral anesthetics in Microchiropterans investigate their effects on wing membrane capillary function; no mention is made of anesthetic effect (Harris et al. 1971; Longnecker & Harris 1972; Longnecker et al. 1974).

Megachiropterans

In variable flying foxes (*Pteropus hypomelanus*), ketamine alone (30–37.5 mg/kg IM) produced short-term

chemical restraint, but poor muscle relaxation and struggling during recovery (Heard et al. 1996). In the same species, xylazine (2 mg/kg IM)/ketamine (10 mg/kg IM) and medetomidine: ketamine (50 μg/kg: 5 mg/kg IM) combinations produce short-term immobilization (30 minutes), with good muscle relaxation and quiet recovery (Heard et al. 1996, 2006b). Similar dosages have been used in free-living variable flying foxes, both IM and IV (Epstein et al. 2011; Sohayati et al. 2008).

During induction with medetomidine/ketamine, the palpebral response was lost first, followed by clinch and bite response (Heard et al. 2006b). These responses returned in the reverse order during recovery. It is recommended xylazine or medetomidine not be reversed, except in an emergency, because the adverse effects of ketamine (wing flapping and struggling with associated hyperthermia) will be unmasked during recovery. In other bat species, the dosages/kg are increased as the size of the animal decreases.

Tiletamine/zolazepam (20–40 mg/kg) produces immobilization, but prolonged recovery. However, it has been used to immobilize free-living animals suspected of being rabid or trapped in barbwire (Vogelnest 1999). The drug combination is sprayed into the open mouth, preventing contact with people until anesthetized.

Propofol (8–10 mg/kg IV) provides 5–15 minutes of anesthesia in animals in which a vessel can be accessed for injection. Propofol may be diluted 1 : 4 with saline to facilitate administration (A. Olsson, pers. comm.).

Table 36.1. Anesthetic and analgesic drugs used in megachiropteran and microchiropteran bats

Drug	Route	Dosage Megachiroptera	Dosage Microchiroptera	Comments
Parenteral				
Ketamine	IM	40–50 mg/kg	≥100 mg/kg	Not recommended because of poor muscle relaxation, and prolonged recovery with wing flapping.
Xylazine/ketamine	IM	Combine equal volumes xylazine (20 mg/mL) and ketamine (100 mg/mL); 0.4 mL/kg		Variable flying fox (*Pteropus hypomelanus*) (Heard et al. 1996). Australian flying foxes (*Pteropus* spp.) (A. Olsson, pers. comm.)
Xylazine/ketamine	IV	Xylazine 1 mg + ketamine 5 mg in 0.1 mL		Free-living variable flying foxes. Provided safe short-term immobilization for collection of biological samples (Sohayati et al. 2008).
Medetomidine	IV	0.03 mg/kg		Free-living variable flying foxes (Epstein et al. 2011).
Medetomidine/ketamine	IM	Combine equal volumes medetomidine (1 mg/mL) with ketamine (100 mL/kg); 0.5 mL/kg		Captive variable flying foxes (Heard et al. 2006a).
Medetomidine/ketamine	IV	0.05/5.0 and 0.025/2.5 mg/kg		Free-living variable flying foxes (Epstein et al. 2011).
Tiletamine/zolazepam	PO	40 mg/kg		For immobilization of large bats when physical restraint is dangerous (i.e., suspect rabid bats or animals caught in barbwire). Drug combination is squirted into mouth of animal (Vogelnest 1999). Recovery is prolonged—not recommended for routine anesthesia/immobilization.
Propofol	IV	6–8 mg/kg	8–10 mg/kg	Dilute 1 : 4 with saline to obtain injection volume in small bats. (A. Olsson, pers. comm.).
Inhalation				
Halothane	Inhalation	Induction 4–5%, maintenance 1–1.5%		
Isoflurane	Inhalation	Induction 5%, maintenance 2.5%		
Sevoflurane	Inhalation	Induction 6–7%, maintenance 3–4%		Expensive
Analgesics				
Butorphanol	SC, IM	0.4 mg/kg q 4 h	2 mg/kg q 4 h	
Buprenorphine	SC, IM	0.03 mg/kg q 6–12 h	0.05–0.1 mg/kg q 6–12 h	
Morphine	SC, IM	0.5–1.0 mg/kg q 4–6 h	2–5 mg/kg q 4 h	
Carprofen	SC, IM, PO	1–4 mg/kg q 24 h (q 12 h PO)	3–5 mg/kg q 12 h	
Meloxicam	SC, IM, PO	0.1–0.3 mg/kg q 12 h	1–2 mg/kg q 12 h	
Tramadol	PO	0.5–2.0 mg/kg q 24 h		

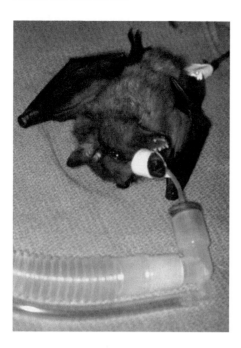

Figure 36.6. Medium to large bats, as in this Wahlberg's epauletted fruit bat (*Epomorphorus wahlbergi*) can be intubated with commercially available endotracheal tubes (≥2 mm ID). The trachea is relatively short and the endotracheal tube should be premeasured before placement.

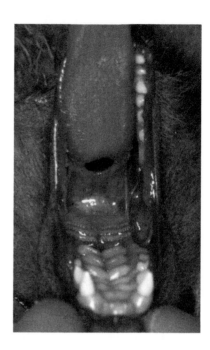

Figure 36.7. The oral cavity of a dorsally recumbent Wahlberg's epauletted fruit bat (*Epomorphorus wahlbergi*) before endotracheal intubation. The tongue is pulled dorsally. The epiglottis lies just beyond the opening in the soft palate.

Rapid injection is associated with marked cardiopulmonary depression and possibly apnea; endotracheal tubes, laryngoscope, and a mechanism for providing assisted ventilation must be available.

INHALATION ANESTHESIA

Inhalation anesthesia is very safe and effective in both captive and free-living bats (Wimsatt et al. 2005). An efficient respiratory system (Canals et al. 2005) makes induction and recovery times comparable with those of birds. Isoflurane (5% by mask, then maintenance 2–2.5%) provides rapid (1–2 minutes) induction and recovery, as well as rapid response to changes in vaporizer setting. For prolonged anesthesia, bats are attached to a nonrebreathing system with either an endotracheal tube or a mask (Fig. 36.6). Portable, lightweight inhalant anesthetic systems developed for avian anesthesia (Chapter 25) are ideal for field immobilization.

Endotracheal Intubation

Bats ≥150 g are intubated with a ≥2-mm internal diameter endotracheal tube. For intubation, the author prefers to place the bat in dorsal recumbency to visualize the glottis (Fig. 36.7). The mouth is opened using gauze placed around the upper and lower jaws and the tongue pulled forward and to the side. A laryngoscope with a small straight pediatric blade is used for illumination. Topical anesthetic applied to the glottal opening decreases reflex coughing.

Monitoring

Cardiovascular Heart rates range from 100 beats/min (bpm) in large Megachiropterans at rest to 1000 in the smallest. Heart rates are influenced by restraint, anesthesia, environmental temperature, and size. The rate of the 5- to 10-g *Myotis lucifugus* ranges from around 350 bpm at thermoneutrality (33–38°C) to as low as 6 bpm during hibernation (rectal 6°C) (Kallen 1977). Although the electrocardiogram is typically mammalian, its configuration in Microchiropterans varies with rate, and there are species differences. In some Vespertilionids, at high rates, the T and R waves fuse, and the P wave is difficult to identify. Active and dormant bats may develop a functional bradycardia interrupted by transitory compensatory tachycardias. At low body temperatures, supraventricular arrhythmias and second-degree heart block are common, but reverse with warming. However, bats appear resistant to hypothermia-associated ventricular fibrillation (Kallen 1977). Heart rate and rhythm and peripheral blood flow are assessed with a Doppler flow probe secured over the tibial artery behind the knee or the pedal artery on the palmar surface of the feet.

Respiratory Hemoglobin saturation and heart rate are monitored with a pulse oximeter probe placed on the tongue, foot, or median artery, or with a rectal reflectance probe. Arterial blood samples can be collected from the ulnar artery on the medial surface of the humerus.

Body Temperature The thermoneutral zone is for setting environmental temperatures for captive bats. This is the ambient temperature range in which a resting, fasting animal consumes the least amount of oxygen. Within this range, an animal can maintain a constant body temperature without additional energy cost. For large flying foxes (500–1000 g), the thermoneutral zone lies between 24 and 35°C, whereas for a lightweight bat, such as *Saccopteryx bilineata* (7 gm), it is restricted to 30–35°C.

Bats die quickly if the ambient temperature is above body temperature, particularly if the humidity is high. Their only means of lowering body temperature are evaporative cooling and the creation of convection currents by air movement. Flying foxes roost in large trees, often in full sun. As the ambient temperature rises, they initially start fanning the air with bent wings. If the ambient temperature approaches body temperature, they wet their fur with saliva and urine and pant, but they cannot sweat. Microchiropterans and smaller Megachiropterans avoid intense heat through their choice of diurnal roosts. Caves, crevices, and hollow trees are ideal, thermally stable environments with temperatures in or near the thermoneutral zone. Because the bats only fly out at night, they never run the risk of overheating. Since most bats roost in sites with localized climates, preferred roost humidity is likely to be greater than 30%, and may approach 100%. Humidity is an important influence on the elasticity of the patagium, and very dry conditions will be associated with dry membranes.

A temperature probe is placed in either the rectum or esophagus; the latter is preferred because it reflects core body temperature. Rectal temperatures in healthy animals may be as low as 35°C.

Metabolic Hypoglycemia is very likely to occur in the perianesthetic period, particularly in very small, anorectic animals (Widmaier & Kunz 1993). Blood glucose levels should be maintained above 80 mg/dL.

Supportive Care

To prevent hypothermia, the wings are folded to the body, and the animal is placed on a circulating water blanket. When possible, the bat is wrapped in either a blanket or bubble-wrap. Alternatively, a commercial forced air warmer developed for human surgery is used. Electric and chemical heating pads, as well as heated water bottles, are avoided because they will cause severe burns to the wing membranes. The wing membrane is also very susceptible to ischemic damage from bandaging and taping.

Intravenous over-the-needle catheters can be placed in anesthetized bats in the cephalic (Fig. 36.8), ulnar, and saphenous veins. The catheter needs to be removed before recovery or the animal will chew it out. Catheters are secured with glue or tape.

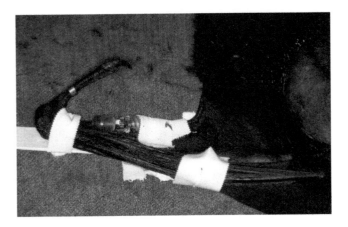

Figure 36.8. Cephalic vein catheterization in an anesthetized large flying fox (*Pteropus vampyrus*). Most bats are intolerant of catheters when awake. Care is taken to not compress the patagium (wing membrane) within constrictive bandages.

Recovery

For recovery, bats are wrapped in a towel and left in a quiet cage to prevent struggling and wing flapping; the animals are usually sufficiently recovered when they able to crawl out. Alternatively, once gripping returns the bat is suspended from its perch.

REFERENCES

Calisher CH, Childs JE, Field HE, Holmes KV, Schountz T. 2006. Bats: important reservoir hosts of emerging viruses. *Clinical Microbiology Reviews* 19:531–545.

Canals M, Atala C, Olivares R, Guajardo F, Figueroa DP, Sabat P, Rosenmann M. 2005. Functional and structural optimization of the respiratory system of the bat *Tadarida brasiliensis* (Chiroptera, Mollossidae): does airway geometry matter? *Journal of Experimental Biology* 208:3987–3995.

Constantine DG. 1970. Bats in relation to the health, welfare, and economy of man. In: *Biology of Bats* (WA Wimsatt, ed.), pp. 319–449. New York: Academic Press.

Day RL, Heard DJ, LeBlanc D. 2001. The effect of the time at which plasma separation occurs on biochemical values in small island flying foxes (*Pteropus hypomelanus*). *Journal of Zoo and Wildlife Medicine* 32:206–208.

Epstein JH, Zambriski JA, Rostal MK, Heard DJ, Daszak P. 2011. Comparison of intravenous medetomidine and medetomidine/ketamine for immobilization of free-ranging variable flying foxes (*Pteropus hypomelanus*). *PLoS ONE* 6(10):e25361. doi: 10.1371/journal.pone.0025361.

Harris PD, Hodoval LF, Longnecker DE. 1971. Quantitative analysis of microvascular diameters during pentobarbital and thiopental anesthesia in the bat. *Anesthesiology* 35:337–342.

Heard DJ, Beale C, Owens J. 1996. Ketamine and ketamine: xylazine ED₅₀ for short-term immobilization of the island flying fox (*Pteropus hypomelanus*). *Journal of Zoo and Wildlife Medicine* 27:44–48.

Heard DJ, Ruiz MR, Harr KE. 2006a. Comparison of serum and plasma for blood biochemical value determination in variable flying foxes (*Pteropus hypomelanus*). *Journal of Zoo and Wildlife Medicine* 37:245–248.

Heard DJ, Towles J, LeBlanc D. 2006b. Evaluation of medetomidine/ketamine for short-term immobilization of variable flying foxes (*Pteropus hypomelanus*). *Journal of Wildlife Diseases* 42:437–441.

Kallen FC. 1977. The cardiovascular systems of bats: structure and function. In: *Biology of Bats*, Vol. III (WA Wimsatt, ed.), pp. 289–483. New York: Academic Press.

Kunz TH, Kurta A. 1988. Capture methods and holding devices. In: *Ecological and Behavioral Methods for the Study of Bats* (TH Kunz, ed.), pp. 1–29. Washington, DC: Smithsonian Institution Press.

Longnecker DE, Harris PD. 1972. Dilatation of small arteries and veins in the bat during halothane anesthesia. *Anesthesiology* 37:423–429.

Longnecker DE, Miller FN, Harris PD. 1974. Small artery and vein response to ketamine HCl in the bat wing. *Anesthesia and Analgesia* 53:64–68.

Nowak RM. 1999. *Walker's Mammals of the World*, Vol. 1, 6th ed. Baltimore: The Johns Hopkins University Press.

Rupprecht CE, Stohr K, Meredith C. 2001. Rabies. In: *Infectious Diseases of Wild Mammals*, 3rd ed. (ES Williams, IK Barker, eds.), pp. 3–36. Ames: Iowa State Press.

Sohayati AR, Zaini CM, Hassan L, Epstein J, Siti Suri A, Daszak P, Sharifah SH. 2008. Ketamine and xylazine combinations for short-term immobilization of wild variable flying foxes (*Pteropus hypomelanus*). *Journal of Zoo and Wildlife Medicine* 39(4): 674–676.

Vogelnest L 1999. Chemical restraint of Australian native fauna. In: *Wildlife in Australia: Healthcare and Management*, Proceedings 327, pp. 149–188. Postgraduate Foundation in Veterinary Science, The University of Sydney.

Widmaier EP, Kunz TH. 1993. Basal, diurnal, and stress-induced levels of glucose and glucocorticoids in captive bats. *The Journal of Experimental Zoology* 265:533–540.

Wilson DE, Reeder DM, eds. 2005. *Mammal Species of the World. A Taxanomic and Geographic Reference*, Vol. 1, 3rd ed. Baltimore: The Johns Hopkins University Press.

Wimsatt J, O'Shea TJ, Ellison LE, Pearce RD, Price VR. 2005. Anesthesia and blood sampling of wild big brown bats (Eptesicus fuscus) with an assessment of impacts on survival. *Journal of Wildlife Diseases* 41:87–95.

37 Prosimians

Cathy V. Williams and Randall E. Junge

INTRODUCTION

The group of primates referred to as prosimians or strepsirhine primates include lemurs, lorises, pottos, and bush babies. All lemurs are endemic to the island of Madagascar. Under current classification, there are five families and over 90 separate species of lemurs recognized (Mittermeier et al. 2010), although taxonomic groupings continue to change as more information on their genetics becomes available. Lorises, pottos, and bush babies are small bodied, nocturnal primates. Lorises are native to Southeast Asia and India while pottos and galagos are endemic to Africa (Nowak 1999; Rowe 1996).

When using anesthetic agents in prosimians, it is important to remember that there is very little controlled data on the pharmacokinetics of any drug class in these species. The information contained in this chapter is predominately derived from the authors' personal experiences and the few published reports that mention use of a particular drug without apparent side effects. Thus, the doses provided here may not be the most pharmacologically appropriate, and there is no guarantee the drugs are entirely safe even though problems have not been documented. It is important to use all drugs conservatively in this group and to monitor animals' physiologic and behavioral responses carefully to minimize complications.

Prosimians are a very diverse group of primates and physiological responses to a particular drug may vary by species. It is unknown if prosimians respond to anesthetic agents similar to other primates but, in most instances, studies performed in anthropoid primates are the best resource from which to derive information when extrapolating drug doses. The reader is referred to chapters in this book discussing anesthesia in monkeys, gibbons, and great apes, and to other selected references for more extensive information on the pharmacologic action of anesthetic agents particular to higher primates (Horne 2001; Popilskis & Kohn 1997).

SPECIAL PHYSIOLOGY

Prosimian primates exhibit considerable anatomical and physiological variation (Mittermeier et al. 2010; Rowe 1996; Sussman 1999). Size ranges from 30g for the smallest mouse lemur (*Microcebus myoxinus*) to more than 8kg for some members of the Indridae family: diademed sifakas (*Propithecus diadema*) and indri (*Indri indri*). Table 37.1 gives approximate adult weight ranges for a variety of prosimian species. Prosimians have a low basal metabolic rate compared to other primates (Ross 1992). Several behaviors exhibited by lemurs, such as basking and huddling, are related to energy conservation and thermal regulation. Dwarf lemurs (*Cheirogaleus sp.*) and mouse lemur (*Microcebus sp.*) are unique among primates in that they hibernate or undergo periods of torpor, an adaptation which allows them to conserve energy during periods of reduced food and water availability (Hladik et al. 1980; Schmid et al. 2000; Schülke & Ostner 2007).

The body temperature of lemurs and bush babies generally ranges between 97 and 99°F, however dwarf and mouse lemurs undergoing torpor may have temperatures significantly below 90°F (Dausmann et al. 2005; Schmid et al. 2000). Core body temperatures of fat-tailed dwarf lemurs track ambient temperatures for hours or days a time during deep torpor (Dausmann et al. 2005). The rectal temperature of lorises is slightly lower than that of lemurs and bush babies and ranges between 95 and 97°F at normal room temperatures (Müller et al. 1985; Whittow et al. 1977).

Zoo Animal and Wildlife Immobilization and Anesthesia, Second Edition. Edited by Gary West, Darryl Heard, and Nigel Caulkett.
© 2014 John Wiley & Sons, Inc. Published 2014 by John Wiley & Sons, Inc.

Table 37.1. Body weight ranges for various prosimian species

Scientific Name	Common Name	Adult Weight (kg)
Avahi	Woolly lemur	1.0–1.5
Cheirogaleus medius	Fat-tailed dwarf lemur	0.16–0.25
Daubentonia	Aye-aye	2.5–3.0
Eulemur coronatus	Crowned lemur	1.5–2.0
Eulemur fulvus	Brown lemur	2.0–2.7
Eulemur macaco	Black lemur	2.0–2.5
Eulemur mongoz	Mongoose lemur	1.4–1.6
Galago moholi	Southern lesser bush baby	0.15–0.25
Hapalemur griseus	Eastern lesser bamboo lemur	0.75–2.50
Indri indri	Indri	6.00–7.25
Lemur catta	Ring-tailed lemur	2.0–3.0
Lepilemur	Sportive lemur	0.5–1.0
Loris tardigradis	Slender loris	0.15–0.25
Microcebus murinus	Mouse lemur	0.06–0.09
Mirza spp.	Giant mouse lemur	0.028–0.320
Nycticebus pygmaeus	Pygmy loris	0.35–0.45
Nycticebus coucang	Slow loris	0.80–1.30
Otolemur crassicaudatus	Thick-tailed greater bush baby	0.70–0.85
Perodicticus potto	Potto	0.85–1.60
Propithecus coquereli.	Coquerel's sifaka	3.3–4.5
Varecia sp.	Ruffed lemur	3.0–3.8

Prosimians have no active mechanism for cooling, such as sweating or panting, and temperature regulation is accomplished primarily by limiting activity, seeking cool locations during hot weather, and licking hands to generate evaporative cooling. Therefore, capture and handling during warm weather should be done either early in the morning while outdoor ambient temperatures are cool or indoors in temperature-controlled environments.

The amount of time necessary to withhold food prior to anesthesia varies by species due to differing rates of gastric emptying. While all prosimians have simple stomachs, the size and conformation of the cecum and large bowel varies depending on the dietary profile of the species. Campbell et al. (2004) measured gastric emptying times in four species of lemurs. Gastric emptying times ranged from 3 to 4 hours in the ruffed lemur (*Varecia variegata*), a frugivorous species, and up to 24 hours in eastern lesser bamboo lemurs (*Hapalemur griseus*) and Coquerel's sifaka (*Propithecus coquereli*), both species that are highly folivorous. The brown lemur (*Eulemur sp.*), a generalist feeder, had gastric emptying times of 8 hours. Thus, while withholding food for 8 hours is sufficient for the majority of lemur species, longer periods of fasting are likely necessary for highly folivorous species.

RESTRAINT

Physical restraint of small prosimians weighing < 1 kg is relatively simple. Animals are restrained by grasping initially over the back of the neck and around the mandible with a gloved hand to control the head while using a second hand to control the lower abdomen and back legs.

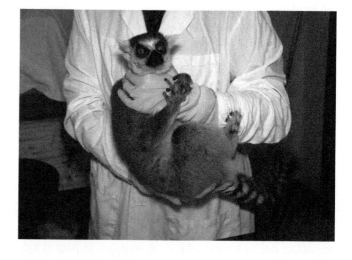

Figure 37.1. Single handler technique for manual restraint of lemurs weighing 1–4 kg.

For animals weighing between 1 and 4 kg, the animal is first netted in its enclosure or out of a transport kennel. The head is initially controlled by placing one hand around the back of the neck with fingers extending under the jaw to secure the animal. The second hand is then placed under the neck and mandible to prevent serious bites. The animal is allowed to grasp the handler's arm with front and back limbs. Limited exams and minor treatments, such as the administration of subcutaneous fluids or SC or IM injections, can be performed with animals in this position (Fig. 37.1). When manually restraining lemurs, it is recommended that the handler wear arm guards to protect against scratches when animals grasp the handler's forearm. If more control is needed, a second handler is employed to restrain the hind limbs and

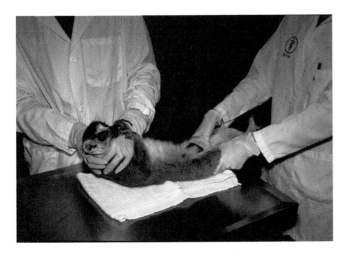

Figure 37.2. Two-handler technique for manual restraint of lemurs for physical examination or collection of blood and urine.

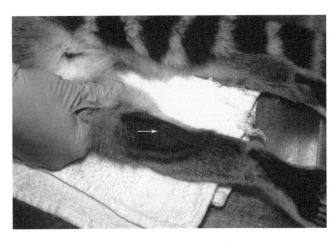

Figure 37.3. Route of the external saphenous vein on the caudal aspect of the tibia and positioning for occlusion of the proximal venous return in a ring-tailed lemur.

extend the hind legs while the animal is positioned on its back (Fig. 37.2). It is important that the person restraining the hind legs grasp the thighs above the stifles to prevent injury to the knee joint. Although it is possible for experienced handlers to physically restrain lemurs weighing more than 5 kg, the larger species are usually anesthetized for procedures.

Squeeze cages can also be used to restrain medium- to large-size lemurs for the administration of IM injections. Animals should be squeezed slowly to avoid undue stress.

VASCULAR ACCESS SITES

Several standard sites are accessible in prosimians; however, the preferred site depends on the species, the size of the animal, and whether it is under manual or chemical restraint. Blood can be collected from the cephalic, external saphenous, and jugular veins, and from the femoral artery or vein. Peripheral veins, such as the cephalic and external saphenous, tend to collapse easily, making withdrawal of more than minimal amounts of blood difficult from these sites. The authors prefer the region of the femoral triangle site in the inguinal region for blood collection requiring more than 1 mL of blood. With the animal in dorsal recumbency, the pulse of the femoral artery is palpable in the femoral triangle. The femoral vein lies immediately adjacent and medial to the femoral artery. In most cases, the close approximation of the vessels means that the artery is sampled nearly as often as the vein. The main disadvantage with using this site for blood collection is the increased risk of hematoma formation if the artery is sampled and inadequate attention paid to ensuring proper hemostasis after needle withdrawal. This is particularly true in animals that are manually restrained as blood pressure can be substantially higher

than in animals under chemical restraint. In extreme cases, lemurs have died from exsanguination secondary to inadequate hemostasis following blood collection from the femoral artery.

For indwelling catheter placement in lemurs, the external saphenous vein is most accessible; however, the cephalic and jugular veins can be used in larger species. When placing a catheter in the external saphenous vein, position the animal in ventral recumbency with the hind legs extended behind the animal. After shaving and preparing the skin of the caudal aspect of the tibia, an assistant grasps the caudal thigh of the hind leg and places his/her thumb horizontally across the mid- to lower thigh, thus closing off the proximal return of the external saphenous vein. The route of the external saphenous vein is visible along the posterior aspect of the tibia (Fig. 37.3).

ENDOTRACHEAL INTUBATION

Endotracheal intubation is relatively straightforward in most prosimians but can be challenging in select species. In lemurs, the epiglottis is long and points dorsally, completely obscuring visualization of the glottis. With the animal in sternal recumbency, the tongue is grasped and pulled forward to visualize the epiglottis. A small blade laryngoscope is useful to aid visualization and move the epiglottis ventrally to expose the glottis. When inserting the endotracheal tube, direct the tube toward the ventral aspect of the glottis.

Some lemurs, in particular aye-aye (*Daubentonia madagascariensis*) and ring-tailed lemurs (*Lemur catta*), are more challenging to intubate. The heavy musculature of the jaws in aye-aye prevents the mouth from opening widely and the long upper and lower incisors obscure visualization of the caudal oral and pharyngeal cavities. In ring-tailed lemurs, the opening of the vocal folds is narrow compared with other species. Intubation is most easily performed in both aye-ayes and ring-tailed lemurs by first inserting an 8–Fr plastic urinary catheter into the trachea as a guide, then passing the endotracheal tube over the catheter into the trachea. Once the endotracheal tube is in place, the guide catheter is removed.

Prosimians, like other primates, have a short trachea. Care must be taken to avoid inserting the endotracheal tube too far and thus intubating a mainstem bronchus. Measuring the length of the endotracheal tube relative to the animal prior to intubation is advised. Once the tube is in place, auscult both sides of the chest for air sounds and monitor end-tidal CO_2 by capnography whenever possible. Cuffed endotracheal tubes ranging in size from 3.0 to 4.5 mm are suitable for animals weighing between 1.5 and 5 kg, while 2.5-mm uncuffed Murphy tubes can be used for individuals ranging in size between 750 g and 1.5 kg. For animals weighing less than 1 kg, infant feeding catheters or urinary catheters can be used as endotracheal tubes (Morris et al. 1997).

PRE-ANESTHETIC CONSIDERATIONS

As with any animal, disease or abnormalities that alter metabolic pathways or gas exchange affect the safety of anesthesia in prosimian primates. It is important to do a thorough preanesthetic evaluation when possible

prior to using anesthetic agents. The ease of manual restraint in prosimians makes it possible to perform limited exams and even draw blood without chemical immobilization in many cases. However, if preanesthetic evaluations are not possible, careful selection of agents, using the minimum dosage necessary to accomplish the procedure, improves safety.

When developing a preoperative regime, it is important to consider the analgesic potential of drugs under consideration. Analgesia is most effective when provided preemptively and the administration of analgesics preoperatively decreases the amount of drugs needed to manage pain postoperatively and may lessen the amount of anesthetic needed by blunting pain perception during the procedure.

It is not always possible to give preanesthetic medications, but when possible, their administration provides a smoother induction, a more stable plane of anesthesia, and decreases the amount of other drugs needed to produce general anesthesia. Non-steroidal anti-inflammatory drugs (NSAIDs), benzodiazepines, alpha-2 agonists, and opiods, have all been used in prosimians successfully. Each can be combined with other drugs to take advantage of the synergistic effects of using drugs that have differing mechanisms of action. Dosages of anesthetic agents commonly used in prosimians are given in Table 37.2, and doses of analgesic drugs are given in Table 37.3.

Table 37.2.   Drugs commonly used for sedation and anesthesia in prosimian primates

Agent	Dosage (mg/kg)	Route	Duration	Reversal[a]
Diazepam	0.5–2.5	IV	30 minutes	Flumazenil
Midazolam	0.1–0.3	IM, IV	30 minutes	Flumazenil
Butorphanol	0.1–0.4	IM, IV, SC	3–4 hours	Naloxone
Dexmedetomidine	0.02	IM	30–60 minutes	Atipamazole
Ketamine	5–15	IM, IV	30 minutes	None
Tiletamine/zolazepam	3–5	IM		None/flumazenil
Propofol	3–6	IV	10–15 minutes	None
Fentanyl	0.001–0.03/h	IV CRI[b]		Naloxone

[a]Doses for reversal agents: atipamizole (0.2 mg/kg IM); naloxone (0.02 mg/kg IM); flumazenil (0.02 mg/kg IV).
[b]Constant rate infusion.

Table 37.3.   Doses of analgesic drugs used in prosimian primates

Agent	Dosage (mg/kg)	Frequency	Route
NSAIDS			
Acetaminophen	10–15	q 8–12 h	PO
Aspirin (Acetylsalicylic acid)	10–20	q 8–12 h	PO
Ibuprofen	10	q 8–12 h	PO
Ketoprofen	2 first dose then 1	Once q 24 h	PO, SC, IM, IV
Flunixin meglumine	0.25–0.50	q 24 h	SC, IM, IV
Meloxicam	≤0.2 first dose then ≤0.1	Once q 24 h	PO, SC, IV
OPIOIDS			
Butorphanol	0.1–0.4	q 3–4 h	SC, IM, IV
Buprenorphine	0.01–0.02	q 8–12 h	SC, IM, IV
Tramadol	1–4	q 12 h	PO

NONSTEROIDAL ANTI-INFLAMMATORY DRUGS (NSAIDS)

NSAIDs have no inherent sedative qualities; however, their analgesic effects make their use beneficial perioperatively as well as for the management of acute and chronic pain not associated with surgery. NSAIDs used in prosimians without obvious side effects include acetaminophen, aspirin, ibuprofen, ketoprofen, meloxicam, and flunixin meglumine (Table 37.3). As a class cyclooxygenase, inhibitory NSAIDs may be associated with adverse gastrointestinal side effects and renal toxicity. All animals receiving NSAIDs should be closely monitored for signs of gastric ulceration or bleeding and remain well hydrated during treatment. Because of potential side effects on renal and platelet function, the use of NSAID's preoperatively is controversial. (Crandell et al. 2004; Lemke et al. 2002; Lobetti & Joubert 2000). Careful patient and drug selection is important if this class of drugs is used preemptively.

BENZODIAZIPINES

Benzodiazepines are beneficial premedication agents due to their antianxiety, sedative, and muscle relaxant effects, and for antiseizure activity. Diazepam and midazolam have similar pharmacological actions; however, midazolam has advantages over diazepam in that it can be given IM whereas diazepam in incompletely absorbed when given IM. When used alone in lemurs, midazolam provides minimal or no detectable sedation, but when used in conjunction with other medications has a synergistic effect. When midazolam is combined with ketamine for induction, muscle relaxation is improved and the likelihood of seizures is reduced. The authors frequently use midazolam in combination with dexmedetomine prior to induction with gas anesthesia. The combination produces a moderate level of sedation, increasing the ease of handling during mask induction.

OPIOIDS

Information on the physiologic response of prosimians to opioids is limited. Butorphanol has been shown to cause profound respiratory depression in primates. This is largely due to the fact that in primates, butorphanol's effect on the mu receptor is one of a strong agonist rather than the weak agonist or antagonistic effect seen in domestic species (Butelman et al. 1995). Whether butorphanol has the same respiratory depressant effects in lemurs or other prosimians is unclear. Studies in ring-tailed lemurs (*Lemur catta*) using butorphanol at 0.3 mg/kg IM in combination with medetomidine and ketamine, or medetomidine and midazolam to provide complete anesthesia resulted in only mild decreases in

respiratory rates relative to animals receiving no butorphanol. Oxygen-hemoglobin saturation, end-tidal CO_2, and $PaCO_2$ values were not affected suggesting oxygenation was not compromised. Butorphanol is used by the authors both for short-term analgesia and as a premedication prior to inhalation anesthesia in lemurs; however, until more data is available on receptor activity in this group of primates, it is recommended that respiratory parameters be monitored.

The authors routinely use buprenorphine and tramadol for relief of moderate pain postoperatively with good results. Buprenorphine is often combined with an NSAID to provide stronger analgesia for moderate to severe pain. Although there are no references for the use of morphine in prosimians, it is reasonable to expect that it can be employed safely if used judiciously and animals are appropriately monitored.

ALPHA-2 AGONISTS

Alpha-2 agonists are very useful in prosimians both for their sedative and analgesic qualities and as a means of decreasing the amount of other anesthetic agents needed. The alpha-2 agonist, medetomidine, is one of the few agents studied in lemurs. Medetomidine administered IM to ring-tailed lemurs under isoflurane had no effect on heart rate, blood pressure, or oxygen-hemoglobin saturation (Williams et al. 2003). In contrast, bradycardia occurs in many domestic animals as a compensatory response to rapid and intense vasoconstriction resulting in significant hypertension (Cullen 1996; Paddleford & Harvey 1999). Dexmedetomidine combined with midazolam is used at the Duke Lemur Center for premedication prior to inhalation anesthesia. The use of dexmedetomidine preoperatively decreases the amount of inhalant anesthesia needed and reduces the degree of hypotension seen when isoflurane or sevoflurane are used alone.

INDUCTION AGENTS

Ketamine is a widely used anesthetic agent in primates for chemical restraint. The effect of ketamine on prosimians, however, is variable. There are both species and individual differences in the degree and duration of immobilization, the character of recovery, and the frequency of side effects. When used alone, ketamine provides unpredictable levels of immobilization, poor muscle relaxation, and frequently, vomiting on recovery. In the authors' experience, seizures may occur in ruffed and black lemurs at doses of 5–10 mg/kg IM. Side effects of ketamine are diminished and the quality of anesthesia improved when it is combined with either midazolam and/or dexmedetomidine; however, the duration of effective immobilization remains short at only 10–15 minutes.

Telazol®, a combination of tiletamine and zolazepam, is frequently used in lemurs, particularly for field immobilizations. Benefits of using Telazol include a wide margin of safety, good muscle relaxation, and smooth recoveries. The main disadvantages include prolonged recovery times in the range of 2–6 hours and a short shelf life of the reconstituted drug. In a clinical setting, reversible injectable combinations allow better control over recovery time and depth of anesthesia.

In a study in ring-tailed lemurs, combining medetomidine with either ketamine and butorphanol, or midazolam and butorphanol produced heavy sedation to complete immobilization lasting from 20 to 60 minutes (Williams et al. 2003). Both combinations can be used for induction prior to gas anesthesia or as complete injectable regimes. The combinations produce minimal cardiorespiratory effects, and the level of analgesia is sufficient to perform minor surgical procedures. Members of the *Eulemur* genus (brown and black lemurs) tend to require higher doses of the drug combinations than ring-tailed lemurs, ruffed lemurs, and Coquerel's sifaka (*Propithecus coquereli*) to produce equal effects. When mild to moderate sedation is desired for premedication or to increase the ease of handling during manual restraint, administering dexmedetomidine in combination with midazolam is effective. Table 37.4 lists several useful combinations.

Propofol is an injectable alkylphenol that acts similarly to the ultra-short acting barbiturate, thiopental. Propofol can be used for induction to provide short duration immobilization for diagnostic procedures or as a constant rate infusion to achieve a light plane of anesthesia for longer periods (Short & Bufalari 1999). Because the compound must be administered intravenously its use in prosimians, it is most feasible in animals receiving premedication in advance of induction. Propofol decreases cardiac contractility and is a potent vasodilator, which can result in hypotension. It is also a respiratory depressant. Administering propofol slowly and to effect minimizes the occurrence of cardiopulmonary effects. The quality of induction and the rapid rate of metabolism, and hence recovery, make the use of propofol advantageous in some circumstances.

INHALATION ANESTHESIA

Both isoflurane and sevoflurane work well in prosimians and are safe in most species; however, respiratory arrest has been reported in giant mouse lemurs (*Mirza* spp.) induced with isoflurane and inhalation agents should be used with extreme caution in this species until more information is available. Both isoflurane and sevoflurane are potent vasodilators, and hypotension is frequently observed in prosimians anesthetized with these agents. It is important to monitor blood pressure in animals under inhalant anesthesia and be prepared to administer IV fluids or other supportive measures as necessary to maintain adequate blood pressure. Information is not available regarding the mean alveolar concentration (MAC) of either agent in prosimians; however, it is the authors' impression that MAC may vary by species. Aye-ayes, in particular, seem acutely sensitive to inhalant anesthetics and require lower concentrations relative to other lemur species to achieve a surgical plane of anesthesia. Hypotension unresponsive to fluid administration alone is a frequent complication of inhalant anesthetic use in lemurs. Until more information is available, it is advisable to intensively monitor cardiopulmonary function and be prepared to support blood pressure if needed.

Prosimians can be induced with gas anesthetics via facemask or in an induction chamber. Administering premedication markedly improves the quality of mask induction. Sevoflurane offers advantages over isoflurane for mask or chamber induction as it is nonirritating to airways. Animals induced by mask with sevoflurane are more compliant than those induced with isoflurane and appear less stressed during the initial phases of induction. Induction rates are faster with sevoflurane compared with isoflurane due to very low blood and tissue solubility of sevoflurane. The cardiopulmonary effects of sevoflurane are similar to isoflurane (Clark 1999).

MONITORING

All anesthetic agents have the potential to adversely affect the major organ systems of the body. Body tem-

Table 37.4. Useful combination regimes for prosimian primates[a]

Drug Combination	Dosage[a] (mg/kg)	Duration of Effect (minute)	Level of Sedation
Dexmedetomidine/	0.02	30–40	Light to moderate sedation
Midazolam	0.2		
Dexmedetomidine/Ketamine	0.02	10–20	Heavy sedation to
	3–5		complete immobilization
Butorphanol/	0.3–0.4	15–30	Complete immobilization
Dexmedetomidine/	0.02		
Ketamine	3–5		
Butorphanol/	0.3–0.4	20–50	Complete immobilization
Dexmedetomidine/	0.02		
Midazolam	0.2–0.3		

[a]All drugs are given IM.

perature, heart rate and rhythm, respiratory rate, and capillary refill time can be monitored in even the smallest lemur or loris. With experience and the proper equipment, monitoring cardiac electrical activity (ECG) and obtaining reliable readings for oxygen-hemoglobin saturation (pulse oximetry), end-tidal CO_2 (capnography), and blood pressure (oscillotometry) can be accomplished in patients weighing more than 1.0 kg. Monitoring should start in the preoperative phase and continue until the animal is in sternal recumbency or until safety precludes further measurements.

Lemurs are highly prone to developing hypothermia under anesthesia due to their lean body confirmation and high surface area to body mass ratio. Heat loss is further compounded by shaving and using skin cleansing solutions during aseptic preparation of the surgical site. Opening a body cavity during surgery further enhances the loss of body heat. Hypothermia decreases liver and renal blood flow and slows the elimination of anesthetic agents, prolonging recovery (Sessler 2000). It is important to monitor temperature regularly during anesthetic procedures. Heat loss can be minimized by insulating animals from cold surfaces using warm water-circulating blankets, warm air blankets, placing hot-water bottles under the drapes; and minimizing exposure by covering body areas outside of the surgical field. Additional precautions include prewarming surgical skin preparation solutions and fluids used for intravenous support or lavage. (Haskins 2007)

Blood pressure can be measured directly by arterial catheterization or indirectly using either Doppler sphygmomanometry or automated oscillotonometry. In the majority of instances, the authors find that automated oscillotonometry units made for small companion animals are easy to use and provide reliable readings in animals over 1.5 kg. The cuff is placed on the hind leg just above the tarsal joint. Additional sites for cuff placement in lemurs include the base of the tail and the upper forearm close to the axilla. It is important to maintain the mean arterial pressure (MAP) above 60 mmHg to ensure adequate tissue blood flow.

Pulse oximetry can be challenging in prosimian primates. Their tongues are short and thin and probes tend to slip off easily. Several lemur species have heavy pigmentation of the tongue, mucous membranes of the oral cavity, and skin of the hands and feet, making readings inconsistent and difficult to obtain. In lightly pigmented animals, reliable readings can generally be obtained by placing a fingertip probe on the cheek wall, tongue, or first digit of the fore or hind limbs. In heavily pigmented lemurs, rectal readings using a rectal probe provide reliable readings. To ensure proper placement of the rectal probe, place the animal in dorsal recumbency and direct the probe signal toward the dorsal wall of the rectum. Manual evacuation of feces in the rectum avoids trapping feces between the probe and rectal mucosa, which interferes with signal transduction.

The use of capnography in prosimians is similar to that in other small animals. Capnography provides important information on cardiac function and pulmonary perfusion. For more information on the use of capnography and interpretation of end-tidal CO_2 measurements, the reader is referred to articles describing their use in veterinary patients (Grosenbaugh 1998; Marshall 2004).

Arterial blood gas analysis is the most reliable method of assessing pulmonary function. The development of relatively inexpensive hand-held analyzers makes measuring blood gases possible and practical, even in field settings. In prosimians, arterial blood samples are easiest to obtain from the femoral artery.

RECOVERY

The quality and speed of recovery depends on the agent used, the general health of the animal, and the success of maintaining physiological processes within optimal ranges through the use of monitoring and appropriate supportive care. Reversible agents allow smooth and controlled recovery from anesthesia. Providing supplemental heat during recovery is beneficial for animals in which body temperatures drop during anesthetic procedures. Animals should be recovered in a quiet, confined space and prevented from attempting to climb or jump until well coordinated.

REMOTE IMMOBILIZATION AND FIELD TECHNIQUES

Remote immobilization of lemurs is routinely performed in the field; however, the safety of the procedure is related to the skill of the darter, the type of darting equipment used, and the extent to which animals are monitored during immobilization. Lemurs present a difficult target, particularly when high up in a tree. Lemurs are small animals with lean body conformation and safe sites for dart placement are limited. The caudal thigh muscles provide the safest location to dart lemurs. Because of lemurs' small size and minimal muscle mass, low impact delivery devices such as blow guns are the least traumatic and provide the greatest margin of safety when darting. The lower impact pressure of darts delivered by blow gun may result in incomplete delivery of anesthetic in some instances, however, resulting in the need to use more than one dart for successful immobilization. While complete drug delivery is more likely to occur when using CO_2-powered remote injection devices, it is important that the discharge power be adjusted downward as much as possible to minimize tissue injury associated with high pressure dart impact. Dissociative anesthetics are the most frequently used class of drugs for field immobilizations in lemurs. Telazol is widely used and provides rapid induction and a wide margin of safety though muscle relaxation may not be adequate for some procedures, such as taking dental impressions. A main disadvantage of Telazol is a long recovery time, in the range of 4–6 hours. Published doses for Telazol used in lemurs in the field vary from 10 to 20 mg/kg (Dutton et al. 2003; Glander et al. 1992; Junge & Louis 2005, Larsen et al. 2011). Larsen et al. (2011) reported that young ring-tailed lemurs (2–4.9 years of age) required both higher initial doses and higher total doses of Telazol for successful immobilization than mature lemurs (≥5 years of age) in the field. The authors commented that young animals in the study were smaller and leaner than mature animals, making dart placement more challenging and resulting in incomplete injections.

Initial doses of Telazol provide 30–40 minutes of immobilization. If longer periods of immobilization are needed, supplemental doses of either Telazol or alpha-2 agonists, with or without the addition of butorphanol, can be given via hand syringe. In one study, depth of anesthesia and muscle relaxation improved following the administration of medetomidine (0.04 mg/kg) IM or medetomidine (0.04 mg/kg) + butorphanol (0.2 mg/kg) IM 20 minutes after initial induction with Telazol (Larsen et al. 2011). The authors noted that the time to recovery in mature lemurs was correlated with total Telazol dose. The ability to reverse both medetomidine and butorphanol may result in quicker recoveries for animals needing supplementation than if additional doses of Telazol are given.

Ketamine at doses of 17–50 mg/kg (Garell & Meyers 1995; Glander et al. 1992; Richard et al. 1991) has been used for field immobilizations in lemurs, but the results are generally inferior to those produced with Telazol. Ketamine immobilizations are typically plagued by poor muscle relaxation, unpredictable levels of restraint, and rocky recoveries. Vomiting on recovery is common.

REFERENCES

Butelman ER, Winger G, Zernig G, et al. 1995. Buthorphanol: characterization of agonist and antagonist effects in rhesus monkeys. *The Journal of Pharmacology and Experimental Therapeutics* 272:845–853.

Campbell JL, Williams CV, Eiseman JH. 2004. Characterizing gastrointestinal transit time using barium impregnated polyethylene spheres (BIPS). *American Journal of Primatology* 64:309–321.

Clark KW. 1999. Desflurane and sevoflurane. *The Veterinary Clinics of North America. Small Animal Practice* 29:793–811.

Crandell DE, Mathews KA, Dyson D. 2004. The effect of meloxicam and carprofen on renal function when administered to healthy dogs prior to anesthesia and painful stimulation. *American Journal of Veterinary Research* 65:1384–1390.

Cullen LK. 1996. Medetomidine sedation in dogs and cats: a review of its pharmacology, antagonism and dose. *The British Veterinary Journal* 152:519–535.

Dausmann KH, Glos J, Ganshorn JU, et al. 2005. Hibernation in the tropics: lessons from a primate. *Journal of Comparative Physiology. B, Biochemical, Systemic, and Environmental Physiology* 175:147–155.

Dutton CJ, Junge RE, Louis EE. 2003. Biomedical evaluation of free-ranging ring-tailed lemurs (*Lemur catta*) in Tsimanampetsotsa Strict Nature Reserve, Madagascar. *Journal of Zoo and Wildlife Medicine* 34:16–24.

Garell DM, Meyers DM. 1995. Hematology and serum chemistry values for free-ranging golden crowned sifaka (*Propithecus tattersalli*). *Journal of Zoo and Wildlife Medicine* 26(3):382–386.

Glander KE, Wright PC, Daniels PS, et al. 1992. Morphometrics and testicle size of rain forest lemur species from southeastern Madagascar. *Journal of Human Evolution* 22:1–17.

Grosenbaugh DA. 1998. Using end-tidal carbon dioxide to monitor patients. *Veterinary Medicine* 93:67–74.

Haskins SC. 2007. Monitoring anesthetized patients. In: *Lumb and Jones' Veterinary Anesthesia and Analgesia*, 3rd ed. (WJ Tranquilli, JC Thurmon, KA Grimm, eds.), pp. 533–558. Ames: Blackwell Publishing.

Hladik P, Charles-Dominique P, Petter JJ. 1980. Feeding strategies of five nocturnal prosimians in the dry forest of the west coast of Madagascar. In: *Nocturnal Malagasy Primates: Ecology, Physiology, and Behavior* (P Charles-Dominique, HM Cooper, A Hladik, et al., eds.), pp. 41–73. New York: Academic Press.

Horne WA. 2001. Primate anesthesia. *The Veterinary Clinics of North America. Exotic Animal Practice* 4:239–266.

Junge RE, Louis EE. 2005. Preliminary biomedical evaluation of wild ruffed lemurs. *American Journal of Primatology* 66:85–94.

Larsen RS, Moresco A, Sauther ML, et al. 2011. Field anesthesia of wild ring-tailed lemurs (*Lemur catta*) using tiletamine-zolazepam, medetomidine, and butorphanol. *Journal of Zoo and Wildlife Medicine* 42:75–87.

Lemke KA, Runyon CL, Horney BS. 2002. Effects on preoperative administration of ketoprofen on whole blood platelet aggregation, buccal mucosal bleeding time, and hematologic indices in dogs undergoing elective ovariohysterectomy. *Journal of the American Veterinary Medical Association* 220:1818–1822.

Lobetti RG, Joubert KE. 2000. Effect of administration of nonsteroidal anti-inflammatory drugs before surgery on renal function in clinically normal dogs. *American Journal of Veterinary Research* 61:1501–1507.

Marshall M. 2004. Capnography in dogs. *Compendium on Continuing Education for the Practicing Veterinarian* 26:761–778.

Mittermeier RA, Louis EE, Richardson M, et al. 2010. *Lemurs of Madagascar*, 3rd ed. Washington, DC: Conservation International.

Morris TH, Jackson RK, Acker WR, et al. 1997. An illustrated guide to endotracheal intubation in small non-human primates. *Laboratory Animals* 31:157–162.

Müller EF, Nieschalk U, Meier B. 1985. Thermoregulation in the slender loris (*Loris tardigradus*). *Folia Primatologica* 44:216–226.

Nowak RM. 1999. *Walker's Mammals of the World*, 6th ed. Baltimore: Johns Hopkins University Press.

Paddleford RR, Harvey RC. 1999. Alpha₂ agonists and antagonists. *The Veterinary Clinics of North America. Small Animal Practice* 29:737–745.

Popilskis SJ, Kohn DF. 1997. Anesthesia and analgesia in nonhuman primates. In: *Anesthesia and Analgesia in Laboratory Animals* (DF Kohn, SK Wixson, WJ White, et al., eds.), pp. 233–255. New York: Academic Press.

Richard AF, Rakotomanga P, Schwartz M. 1991. Demography of *Propithecus verreauxi* at Beza Mahafaly, Madagascar: sex ratio, survival, and fertility, 1984–1988. *American Journal of Physical Anthropology* 84:307–322.

Ross C. 1992. Basal metabolic rate, body weight and diet in primates: an evolution of the evidence. *Folia Primatologica* 58:7–23.

Rowe N. 1996. *The Pictorial Guide to Living Primates*. New York: Pagonias Press.

Schmid J, Ruf T, Heldmaier G. 2000. Metabolism and temperature regulation during daily torpor in the smallest primate, the pygmy mouse lemur (*Microcebus myoxinus*) in Madagascar.

Journal of Comparative Physiology. B, Biochemical, Systemic, and Environmental Physiology 170:59–68.

Schülke O, Ostner J. 2007. Physiological ecology of cheirogaleid primates: variation in hibernation and torpor. *Acta Ethologica* 10:13–21.

Sessler DI. 2000. Perioperative heat balance. *Anesthesiology* 92:578–596.

Short CE, Bufalari A. 1999. Propofol anesthesia. *The Veterinary Clinics of North America. Small Animal Practice* 29:747–779.

Sussman RW. 1999. *Primate Ecology and Social Structure. Vol 1: Lorises, Lemurs, and Tarsiers.* Needham Heights: Pearson Custom Publishing.

Whittow GC, Scammell CA, Manuel JK, et al. 1977. Temperature regulation in a hypometabolic primate, the slow loris (*Nycticebus coucang*). *Archives internationales de physiologie et de biochimie* 85:139–151.

Williams CV, Glenn KM, Levine JF, et al. 2003. Comparison of the efficacy and cardiorespiratory effects of medetomidine-based anesthetic protocols in ring-tailed lemurs (*Lemur catta*). *Journal of Zoo and Wildlife Medicine* 34:163–170.

38 Monkeys and Gibbons

Rolf-Arne Ølberg and Melissa Sinclair

INTRODUCTION

Primates are found in the wild, research facilities, zoos, and kept as pets. Anesthesia is an integral part of veterinary work with nonhuman primates. It is used to relive stress, pain, or discomfort, as well as to ensure safe handling when performing medical examinations, treatments, and research.

TAXONOMY AND BIOLOGY

Monkeys belong to the suborder Haplorhini (higher primates) which, excluding great apes and humans, contains five families and over 200 species (Table 38.1). The Tarsiidae, Cercopithecidae, and Hylobatidae families are Old World primates from Africa or Asia, while the Callitrichidae and Cebidae are New World primates from the neotropics.

Tarsiers are small nocturnal insectivorous species; they can turn their head 360° and some can leap as far as 5–6m between trees. Callitrichids (marmosets and tamarins) are small, diurnal, and live in family groups. They have good eyesight and hearing, and are usually active and agile. Their thumbs are not apposable and they have claw-like nails on all digits except the thumbs. Cebids (Cebidae) vary in weight, from 1 to 15kg, and many have prehensile tails. Most are good jumpers and runners. The *Cercopithecidae* all have longer hind limbs than forelimbs, none have prehensile tails, and they range in weight from 1 to 55kg. The upper canines are elongate, while the lower are curved slightly inward and backward. Hylobatidae include gibbons and siamangs. They all lack a tail, have a slender body, relatively long arms, and prominent canine teeth. For an extensive description of the various species, the reader is referred to *Walker's Mammals of the World* (Nowak 1999).

PHYSIOLOGY

Primates have a large surface-area-to-body mass ratio; consequently, rapid body heat loss commonly occurs during anesthesia. This is compounded by drug suppression of hypothalamic thermoregulation and impairment of shivering. Heat loss is most pronounced in small species. Normal rectal temperature for rhesus macaques is listed as 36.7–38.9°C (Bourne 1975).

There are few reports of normal reference ranges for cardiovascular and respiratory values in primates. Values obtained while the primate is physically restrained are likely not representative of "normal" resting values. Unsedated rhesus macaques restrained in chairs had the following mean values: mean arterial pressure 113mmHg, heart rate 174, cardiac output of 1.31L/min, stroke volume 7.5mL, blood volume 73 to 77mL/kg, respiratory tidal volume of 12.5mL/kg, respiratory minute volume 479mL/kg, and a respiratory rate of 39/min (Bourne 1975). For cynomolgus macaques, also restrained in chairs, the mean arterial pressure is reported to be 87mmHg, and the heart rate 227 beats/min (Morita 1995). Generally, heart rates are approximately 100–200 beats/min (bpm) for animals ≥1kg, and 200–300bpm for primates ≤1kg (Bourne 1975; Haruo 1995; Johnson-Delaney 1994). For most species, the respiratory rate is 20–50 breaths/min. These physiological reference ranges are altered by anesthesia and restraint (Bush et al. 1977; Liu & DeLauter 1977).

Some hematology and serum biochemistry values might be altered by serial anesthesia, and should be

Zoo Animal and Wildlife Immobilization and Anesthesia, Second Edition. Edited by Gary West, Darryl Heard, and Nigel Caulkett.
© 2014 John Wiley & Sons, Inc. Published 2014 by John Wiley & Sons, Inc.

Table 38.1. Taxonomy of monkeys including approximate adult body weights

Scientific Name	Common Name	ABW (kg)
Family: Tarsiidae		
Tarsius/5 species	Tarsiers	0.08–0.17
Family: Callitrichidae		
Callimico/1 species	Goeldi's monkey	0.4–0.9
Saguinus/12 species	Tamarins	0.2–0.9
Callithrix/17 species	Marmosets	0.2–0.5
Cebuella/1 species	Pygmy marmoset	0.08–0.15
Family: Cebidae		
Lagothrix/2 species	Woolly monkey	5–11
Ateles/6 species	Spider monkeys	6–8
Brachyteles/1 species	Woolly spider monkey	7–10
Alouatta/9 species	Howler monkeys	4–12
Pithecia/5 species	Sakis	0.7–1.7
Cacajao/2 species	Uakaris	2.7–3.5
Callicebus/13 species	Titi monkeys	0.5–2.0
Aotus/10 species	Night monkeys	0.6–1.0
Cebus/6 species	Capuchins	1.1–4.3
Saimiri/5 species	Squirrel monkeys	0.7–1.1
Family: Cercopethicidae		
Erythrocebus/1 species	Patas monkey	7–13
Chlorocebus/4 species	Savannah guenons	2–9
Cercopithecus/20 species	Guenons	2–12
Miopithecus/1 species	Talapoin	0.7–1.2
Cercocebus/3 species	Mangabeys	3–20
Lophocebus/1 species	Black mangabeys	4–11
Macaca/20 species	Macaques	2–18
Papio/5 species	Baboons	14–41
Mandrillus/2 species	Mandrills	12–25
Theropithecus/1 species	Gelada baboon	13–20
Nasalis/1 species	Proboscis monkey	7–22
Simias/1 species	Pig-tailed langur	7
Pygathrix/1 species	Douc langur	
Rhinopithecus/4 species	Snub-nosed langurs	
Presbytis/8 species	Langurs	5–8
Semnopithecus/1 species	Hanuman langur	5–24
Trachypithecus/9 species	Brown-ridges langurs	4–14
Colobus/5 species	Black-white colobus	5–15
Piliocolobus/5 species	Red colobus	5–12
Procolobus/1 species	Olive colobus	3–5

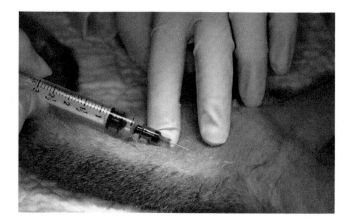

Figure 38.1. Blood collection from the femoral vein of a squirrel monkey. The vein is located in the femoral triangle, medial to the artery. It is important to provide good hemostasis; a small primate can become hypovolemic and die from blood loss into a large hematoma.

taken into account if animals are anesthetized many days in a row (Lugo-Roman et al. 2010).

HUMAN SAFETY

Most primates when restrained or confined deliver a nasty bite that may transmit several zoonotic pathogens. Herpes B virus is endemic and nonpathogenic in macaques, but can be fatal in humans (Hummeler et al. 1959; Ott-Joslin 1993). Therefore, a primary aim when handling primates is prevention of traumatic injury and transmission of zoonoses to humans.

VASCULAR ACCESS

Common vascular access sites are the femoral and the saphenous (popliteal) veins. The femoral vein is entered just distal to the inguinal canal. With the animal on its back and its legs abducted, the pulsing femoral artery is palpated. The femoral vein lies caudal to the artery and just under the skin in the triangle formed by the abdominal, sartorius, and pectineus muscles (Fig. 38.1). The saphenous (popliteal) vein is located superficially on the caudal aspect of the lower leg. It is suitable for catheter placement in most primates, including callitrichids. Less common vascular access sites include the jugular and the cephalic veins. In monkeys with tails, the lateral coccygeal veins can also be used. They are palpable on the dorsolateral surface of the base of the tail.

PHYSICAL RESTRAINT

There are a variety of physical restraint techniques in primates that are safe, both for the handler and the primate. These include nets, squeeze cages, and head-lock devices. However, any restraint is stressful to the animal, and its duration must be minimized (Bush et al. 1977). Physical restraint also increases the possibility of human bites, and contact with secretions infected with zoonotic pathogens.

Hoop nets are useful for catching smaller species (≤4 kg). The animal is physically secured within the net by pinning it to the ground or closing off the entrance by twirling the net. The animal is then moved directly to a transport cage or induction box, injected with an anesthetic drug, or administered inhalant anesthetic through the net using a mask placed over the nose and mouth.

Manual restraint is excellent for small species like tamarins and marmosets. These species are caught in a hoop net and then secured by locking the head with thumb and index finger, the upper body with the other three fingers and the hind legs with the other hand.

This restraint technique is suitable for minor procedures such as inspection of wounds, to facilitate injection of drugs, and blood sampling. Leather gloves or a towel will reduce the risk of bite wounds.

Squeeze cages are indicated for animals too dangerous to handle by hand. Once in a squeeze cage, the animal is compressed for intramuscular (IM) injection of a parenteral anesthetic. A properly compressed primate will not be able to move allowing accurate injection.

PSYCHOLOGICAL RESTRAINT (TAMING)

Taming and training methods are used for "psychologically restraining" animals. This is a common method used for domestic animals, such as horses and dogs, but it can also be used on nondomestic animals to facilitate, for example, hand injection of drugs. Through positive reinforcement, many primates will accept an IM injection or even extend an arm out of the cage for blood collection (Phillippi-Falkenstein & Clarke 1992) or IV injection.

ENDOTHRACHEAL INTUBATION

Endothracheal intubation is readily achieved in most species with the aid of a laryngoscope and a suitable endothracheal tube. Intubation can be achieved with the primate positioned in dorsal recumbency on a table with the head flexed slightly backwards (Fig. 38.2a,b). Alternatively, the animal is placed in a sitting position and an assistant flexes the head backwards. The tongue is gently pulled outwards to visualize the glottis with a laryngoscope. The use of topical local anesthetic on the glottis will reduce laryngospasm and bucking after intubation. Lidocaine 2% can be diluted to 10 mg/mL or lower to ensure dosing of local anesthetic does not exceed 4 mg/kg.

Primates have a relatively short trachea, with the bifurcation located close to the neck. It is easy to introduce an endotracheal tube too far, intubating a main bronchus and ventilating only one lung (Horne 2001). To prevent this, the endotracheal tube length is pre-measured to the base of the neck, before placement. Once the tube is in position, the animal is ventilated and both the left and right thorax auscultated. If the tube is located in one bronchus, there will be no respiratory sound on the opposite side. In addition, if a pulse oximeter is used desatruration may be noted with one lung intubation. For species smaller than a squirrel monkey, an endotracheal tube can be made from a urinary catheter or infant feeding tube. For species the size of a squirrel monkey, an uncuffed 2.0- to 2.5-mm tube can be used. For most other species between 1 and 20 kg, a cuffed tube ranging in size from 3 to 5 mm is usually appropriate (Horne 2001).

PREANESTHETIC CONSIDERATIONS

Observing the animal prior to the anesthetic procedure will provide useful information about its health status. Social interaction, lethargy, diarrhea, vomiting, anorexia, body condition, and the presence of wounds can often be evaluated this way.

If possible, it is recommended to withhold food from primates for at least 12 hours prior to the anesthetic procedure. For smaller primates (≤1 kg), it is recommended food be withheld for only 6–8 hours prior to the procedure. These animals often have a higher metabolic rate and are more likely to develop hypoglycemia.

SEDATION AND GENERAL ANESTHESIA

There are several options for administering drugs to primates. Drugs can be administered orally, parenterally, or by inhalation of anesthetic gases.

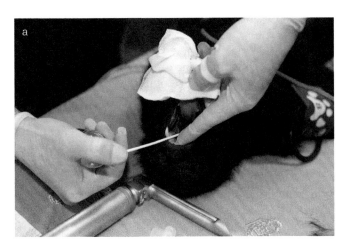
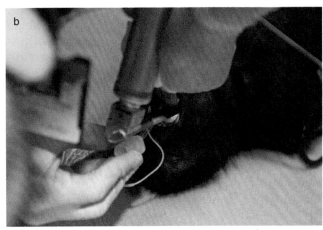

Figure 38.2. (a and b) Endotracheal intubation in primates, as in this spider monkey, is facilitated by placing the animal in dorsal recumbency, extending the head and neck, using a laryngoscope and applying topical anesthetic to the glottis to reduce laryngospasm.

Oral Administration of Drugs

Drugs can be administered orally by squirting the sedative or anesthetic dose into the mouth, or mixing it in liquid or solid treats (Knottenbelt & Knottenbelt 1990; Martin et al. 1972; Miller et al. 2000; Ølberg 2004; Pulley et al. 2004; Winterborn et al. 2008). Ingestion of the full drug dose by the animal is a voluntary action, and depends primarily on palatability. It can also be influenced by person presenting the food and even if the food has been altered in any way. Another challenge with this route of administration is unpredictable absorption. There is a difference in bioavailability and absorption time of drug dose depending on how much is absorbed through the oral mucosa compared with the intestinal mucosa. If the drug is swallowed, first pass metabolism may have a significant effect on lowering the effective drug concentration (Paine et al. 1996; Thummel et al. 1996). Despite the positive aspect of a voluntary oral drug administration to sedate or anesthetize primates, there are no reports of using this as a consistent, safe, and reliable method.

Parenteral Anesthesia

Hand injection requires physical or psychological restraint. For larger species, the use of a projectile dart to deliver drugs is common practice, and darts typically are used for immobilizing primates in the wild (Burroughs 1993; Sapolsky & Share 1998) (Chapter 12). Darting is fast and effective, but has significant disadvantages, including stress, pain, and even trauma on injection. Primates have relatively small target areas for darting, and these can be difficult to hit, especially on a moving animal. Targets usually used for injection are the muscles in the hip and thigh area, or, in rare instances, the triceps or shoulder area of larger primates.

Several review articles describe parenteral anesthesia of primates (Beck 1972; Cohen & Bree 1978; Horne 2001; Martin et al. 1972; Sainsbury et al. 1989). Most recommendations include a dissociative anesthetic alone, or in combination with an α_2-adrenoceptor agonist or benzodiazepine. It is common to combine two or more drugs to achieve immobilization of primates (Horne 2001; Jalanka 1989). This is done to minimize volume, increase potency, achieve a stable safe plane of anesthesia with adequate muscle relaxation and analgesia, improve recovery quality and time, and minimize side effects.

Alphaxolone/alphadolone, methohexitone, thiamylal, droperidol, acepromazine, butophanol, and propofol have been used, but are not included in this review. (For more information on these anesthetic agents see Bowden et al. 1974; Box & Ellis 1973; Connolly & Quimby 1978; Fowler et al. 2001; Kalema-Zikusoka et al. 2003; Marsboom et al. 1963; Porter 1982; Reed & Staple 1976; Sainsbury et al. 1989.). The drugs and combinations most commonly used for primate anesthesia are reviewed later.

Ketamine Ketamine has been used alone in a wide variety of primates, and most reports describe it as safe and reliable (Martin et al. 1972; Vercruysse & Mortelmans 1978). The duration of effect is relatively short (depending on dosage), mainly due to rapid redistribution from the central compartment and efficient metabolism in the liver. Ketamine causes reliable immobilization, and maintains stable cardiopulmonary function while maintaining the laryngeal reflex.

Effective intramuscular dosages vary from 5 to 12 mg/kg for chemical restraint, and up to 10–30 mg/kg for surgical anesthesia (Beck & Dresner 1972; Colillas 1978; Ochsner 1977). Some authors give a general recommendation of dosages from 5 to 40 mg/kg IM (Cohen & Bree 1978). A significant advantage of ketamine is its high therapeutic index. It has been given experimentally to five squirrel monkeys at dosages of 250 mg/kg without any deaths (Greenstein 1975). It can be administered safely several days in a row for repeated anesthesia (Bree et al. 1967).

However, there are several disadvantages to using ketamine alone, such as poor muscle relaxation, spontaneous movement, and hypersalivation. When high dosages of ketamine are used alone, the recovery period is prolonged and rough (Banknieder et al. 1978; Sun et al. 2003). A severe and common side effect of ketamine alone in humans is emergence delirium (Reich & Silvay 1989), which occurs in approximately 5–30% of cases (White et al. 1982). This state is associated with visual, auditory, proprioceptive, and confusional illusions (Stoelting 1999). The same effects are likely the cause of poor recoveries with ketamine alone in monkey and gibbon species. There are no antagonists to ketamine.

The side effects and dosage of ketamine can markedly be reduced by adding sedative agents, such as α_2-agonists or benzodiazepines (Levanen et al. 1995; Lilburn et al. 1978). In addition, both the α_2-agonists and the benzodiazepines are reversible. Using these anesthetic drugs in combination with ketamine at lowered doses will likely reduce side effects and enhance safety of the procedure.

Ketamine/Benzodiazepine Immobilization of olive baboons with ketamine (10 mg/kg, IM) and diazepam (0.20–0.36 mg/kg, IM) was safe and efficient (Woolfson et al. 1980). This combination was preferred for procedures requiring good muscle relaxation compared with ketamine alone (10 mg/kg, IM).

The combination of ketamine (10 mg/kg, IM) and midazolam (1 mg/kg, IM) in common marmosets and black-tufted marmosets resulted in rapid immobilization and good muscle relaxation, with a duration of 30–45 minutes (Furtado et al. 2010).

Ketamine/α_2-Adrenoceptor Agonist The addition of an alpha-2 adrenoceptor agonist (alpha-2 agonist) to ketamine has several beneficial effects. It increases muscle relaxation and analgesia and decreases the hypersalivation and required dose of ketamine. It also adds the possibility of reversing the effects of the α_2-agonist with an α_2-adrenoceptor antagonist. A disadvantage of the $\alpha2$-agonists is their dose-dependent cardiovascular depressant effects. Many dosage variations have been tried in different species of primates in order to investigate the effects and give recommendations.

The combination of ketamine (5.25 mg/kg, IM) with xylazine (0.45 mg/kg, IM) enhanced analgesia, anesthesia, and muscle relaxation in rhesus macaques, compared with ketamine alone (Banknieder et al. 1978). Animals remained anesthetized for 44 minutes (range 23–63 minutes). However, an important observation with this combination is that anesthetic emergence was fast. Animals were alert and standing only a few minutes after the anesthetic period. The presence of the pedal reflex preceded the end of the anesthetic immobilization by only 2–3 minutes. This duration likely coincides with ketamine redistribution, and the quick recovery is probably due to the arousability noted with α_2-agonists. Hence, the veterinarian needs to monitor depth closely and be aware of the procedure time with these combinations.

In rhesus macaques, the minimum effective IM dosages were 2.5 mg/kg of ketamine with 0.25 mg/kg xylazine (Naccarato & Hunter 1979). These investigators found a wide safety margin with this combination, although xylazine markedly reduced the thermoregulatory abilities of the animals. The IM dosages of 5 mg/kg ketamine and 0.5 mg/kg xylazine produced safe immobilization for 30 minutes, while increasing the dosage of xylazine to 1 and 2 mg/kg prolonged immobilization time to 60 and 80 minutes, respectively. Similar results were obtained with ketamine (5 mg/kg, IM) and xylazine (1 mg/kg, IM) in Japanese macaques (Hayama et al. 1989). Yellow baboons receiving ketamine (11 mg/kg, IM) and xylazine (0.5 mg/kg, IM) were easily intubated, and anesthesia lasted from 90 to 125 minutes (White & Cummings 1979). Other recommendations for wild savanna baboons are ketamine (10–15 mg/kg, IM) combined with xylazine (1 mg/kg, IM) (Sapolsky & Share 1998).

Medetomidine is a more selective, potent and specific α_2-agonist than xylazine (Chapter 2). Medetomidine alone is not sufficient to immobilize rhesus macaques even at intravenous dosages as high as 0.2 mg/kg (Capuano et al. 1999). Intravenous dosages of 0.05, 0.10, 0.15, and 0.2 mg/kg of medetomidine produced similar and significant bradycardia, hypotension, loss of thermoregulation, decrease in respiratory rate, and inconsistent sedation. But the advantages of medetomidine with ketamine are similar to xylazine, such as enhanced analgesia, anesthesia, and muscle relaxation.

Ketamine/medetomidine has been used in several primate species (Horne et al. 1998; Jalanka 1989; Vie et al. 1998).

Resus macaques (*Macaca mulatta*) anesthetized with ketamine (2 mg/kg, IM) and medetomidine (0.075 mg/kg, IM) had a heart rate of 135 5 minutes after injection, declining to 115 25 minutes after injection. Mean arterial pressures were 70 and 65 mmHg respectively (Settle et al. 2010).

In cynomolgus macaques, there was little difference in the level of sedation, anesthesia time, and recovery time between ketamine alone (10 mg/kg, IM) or a combination of ketamine (2 mg/kg, IM) and medetomidine (0.05 mg/kg, IM). However, due to some unexpected quick recoveries, the investigators felt that this combination was unreliable and recommended caution in using it at the earlier dosages (Young et al. 1999). In the same species, a dosage of ketamine (3 mg/kg, IM) and medetomidine (0.15 mg/kg, IM) provided good muscle relaxation when compared with ketamine (10 mg/kg, IM) alone (Lee et al. 2010). Another study in capuchin monkeys demonstrated that ketamine (4 mg/kg, IM) combined with medetomidine (0.15 mg/kg, IM) provided rapid induction of anesthesia sufficient for handling, while ketamine (2 mg/kg, IM) and medetomidine (0.2 mg/kg, IM) was not sufficient for handling (Theriault et al. 2008). In this study, the evaluation of the lower dose of ketamine was based on only one capuchin monkey, and the monkeys were reversed shortly after induction.

Japanese macaques given ketamine (5 mg/kg, IM) and medetomidine (0.05 mg/kg, IM) had a mean induction time of 4 minutes and anesthetic duration of 65 minutes, with excellent muscle relaxation (Ølberg 2004). After induction they had an initial heart rate of 100 bpm that slowly decreased to 60 bpm during anesthesia. The mean arterial pressure also decreased slowly from approximately 110 mmHg after induction, to 70 mmHg at the end. The respiratory rates were 40 breaths per minute throughout anesthesia. Hypoxemia ($PaO_2 < 60$ mmHg) was evident in the Japanese macaques after induction on room air. A normal SPO_2 and PaO_2 were measured when the monkeys were given supplemental oxygen through a face mask (4 L/min).

At lower dosages, the negative cardiopulmonary effects of α_2-agonists are reported to be minor and not clinically noticeable (Capuano et al. 1999; Dyck et al. 1993; Horne et al. 1997), suggesting that low dose medetomidine might be favorable; however, further investigations are warranted to confirm.

In golden-headed lion tamarins (*Leontopithecus chrysomelas*), a combination of dexmedetomidine (0.01 mg/kg, IM) with ketamine (5 mg/kg, IM) produced anesthesia with good muscle relaxation for 45 minutes with minor cardiovascular effects and arterial oxygen saturation over 94% in room air (Selmi et al. 2004a). The same dosage of dexmedetomidine and higher ketamine (10 mg/kg, IM) had a similar effect but longer duration and a slight decrease in mean arterial pressure. In the same species, medetomidine (0.02 mg/kg, IM) with ketamine (10 mg/kg, IM) had a similar effect and was evaluated as safe and reliable in this species (Selmi et al. 2004b). A lower dosage of dexmedetomidine (0.005 mg/kg, IM) with ketamine (10 mg/kg, IM) had poor muscle relaxation and anesthetic quality compared with the higher dexmedetomidine dose.

Based on these reports and clinical experience, ketamine ≤2 mg/kg may not be sufficient even in combination with medetomidine. In the protocols using a relatively low dosage of ketamine (2 mg/kg), the corresponding dose of medetomidine is relatively high (0.05–0.15 mg/kg). In the authors' opinion, higher dose of ketamine (>2 mg/kg, IM) and lower dose of medetomidine is preferable for cardiorespiratory stability, as well as anesthesia quality and time.

It is difficult to give minimum dose recommendations for the combination of ketamine and medetomidine. For most species, the author would recommend a ketamine dose of 5–8 mg/kg combined with a low dose medetomidine of 0.02–0.04 mg/kg for induction or short duration anesthesia.

Tiletamine/Zolazepam   Tiletamine/zolazepam has been widely used in primates (Bree 1972; Bree et al. 1972; Gray et al. 1974; Horne 2001; Schobert 1987).

Wild black spider monkeys were anesthetized with dosages ranging from 11.6 to 18 mg/kg (Karesh et al. 1998), with the higher dosage resulting in more reliable and stable planes of anesthesia. Induction times were 2–4 minutes, with immobilization lasting from 80 to 150 minutes. Adult, free-living red howler monkeys were anesthetized with 22.5 mg/kg, IM, and juveniles received 30.5 mg/kg, IM. With these dosages, the induction period was 1–6 minutes, and immobilization varied from 40 to 300 minutes, with no apparent adverse effects (Agoramoorthy & Rudran 1994).

Other researchers also describe the use of tiletamine/zolazepam for field anesthesia in various species with a good overall effect (Glander et al. 1991; Sleeman et al. 2000). In cynomolgus macaques and vervet monkeys tiletamine/zolazepam (5–10 mg/kg, IM) was adequate for ophthalmologic surgery. These dosages produced a rapid onset and 30–50 minutes of surgical anesthesia, excellent muscle relaxation, absence of ocular movement, and a gradual emergence with no adverse effects (Kaufman & Hahnenberger 1975).

In rhesus monkeys, this combination induced little or no impairment of thermoregulation (Holmes & Hunter 1980).

Tiletamine/zolazepam has a high therapeutic index, as reflected by the variety of published dosage recommendations. There are likely species differences, but the dosages probably reflect the different subjective opinions of investigators, and no dose titration studies are available. Recommended dosages for capture of free-living animals are high compared with those used in captive animals. A major advantage of this combi-

nation is high potency, which allows a small drug volume.

There are no reversal agents for tiletamine; and prolonged recovery periods are common. Hence, the investigator may have to spend time monitoring the recovery of immobilized wild animals that cannot be abandoned in a sedated state.

Tiletamine/Zolazepam/Medetomidine   Tiletamine/zolazepam (0.8–2.3 mg/kg, IM) with medetomidine (0.02–0.06 mg/kg, IM) have been used in Bornean orangutans, Bornean gibbons, and long-tailed and pigtailed macaques (Fahlman et al. 2006). This combination results in rapid smooth induction within 1–7 minutes, good muscle relaxation, and anesthesia, although the data suggest hypotension and hypoxemia in some of the animals. For the gibbons and macaques, respiratory rates were 20–56 breaths per minute, heart rate ranged from 68 to 160 beats per minute and SpO2 ranged from 88% to 99%. A major advantage observed by the investigators were that induction in wild orangutans with this combination resulted in a gradual descent from the trees, compared with rapid loss of consciousness and falling from the trees with tiletamine/zolazepam alone.

Medetomidine/Midazolam   The combination of medetomidine and midazolam has been tried in Japanese macaques as an alternative to using dissociative anesthetics (Kimura et al. 2007). It was found that a dose of medetomidine (0.06 mg/kg, IM) with midazolam (0.3 mg/kg, IM) gave reliable immobilization within 13–19 minutes, with profound sedation and moderate muscle relaxation. The animals were given atipamezole 30 minutes after medetomidine/midazolam injection and completely recovered within 12 minutes. This drug combination might be useful for minor short procedures, although cardiovascular and pulmonary effects were not evaluated.

Benzodiazepines   The main clinical effects of benzodiazepines are sedation, anxiolysis, anticonvulsive actions, spinal cord-mediated skeletal muscle relaxation, and anterograde amnesia (Ashton 1994). Benzodiazepines have few side effects and a high therapeutic index (Du Plooy et al. 1998). However, these drugs may cause mild respiratory depression, which may become significant when benzodiazepines are combined with other sedative or anesthetic agents (Gerak et al. 1998). When used in combination, they significantly decrease the minimum alveolar concentration (MAC) of inhalational agents, or dose of injectable, if used in combination with inhalational or injectable anesthetics in people (Melvin et al. 1982). With clinical doses, they have minimal effects on heart rate, blood pressure, cardiac output, and contractility, and blood pressure in veterinary species (Thurmon et al. 1996). There are numerous benzodiazepine drugs on the market. They all have similar pharmacologic profiles, but vary in potency and duration of effect, related to their affinity for the benzodiazepine receptor and their pharmacokinetic properties (Stoelting 1999).

Flumazenil is a competitive benzodiazepine antagonist, and antagonizes the sedative and amnesic qualities of benzodiazepines (Stoelting 1999). Minimal information exists on the use of these drugs specifically in primates.

Inhalation Anesthesia

Inhalation anesthesia may be used alone or to maintain anesthesia after induction with injectable agents. The most commonly used inhalants, isoflurane, and sevoflurane, have a MAC in primates of 1.2% and 2%, respectively. The MAC of halothane in primates is approximately 0.9% (Soma et al. 1988). Small primates (i.e., tamarins and marmosets) can be manually restrained in a net and induced with an inhalant anesthetic through a facemask or in an induction chamber (Fig. 38.3). A clear advantage of inhalant anesthetics is reversibility and that oxygen is used as carrier gas. This normally ensures adequate partial pressure of oxygen in the arterial blood during anesthesia. As in other species, inhalants are expected to cause dose-related cardiovascular and respiratory depression in primate species (Thurmon et al. 1996).

MONITORING

A preanesthetic physical examination with full laboratory evaluation (CBC and biochemistry panel) is typically not possible without major sedation or general anesthesia. Once the animal can be restrained adequately or is induced, heart rate, respiratory rate, capillary refill time, mucous membrane color, peripheral pulse, and airway should be assessed. If available, pulse

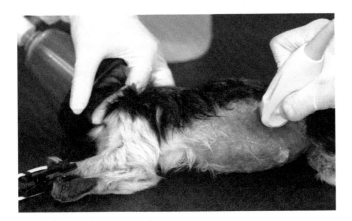

Figure 38.3. Small primates, such as this cotton-top marmoset, can be manually restrained and masked induced with an inhalant anesthetic.

oximetry and indirect blood pressure will provide additional information on circulation and oxygenation. End-tidal CO_2 measurements will give valuable information about ventilation. An accurate body weight, rectal temperature, hematocrit, serum total protein, urea, and creatinine should also be obtained. Careful monitoring of cardiovascular and respiratory function, as well as reflexes, will give information of the anesthetic depth. Also, keeping track of time and record keeping is an important part of the monitoring procedure.

ANALGESIA

Opioid agonists are powerful analgesic agents, but one should exercise care when using them in primates due to their strong ventilatory depressant effects.

Opioids are mainly used for analgesia, and the μ receptor agonists are the ones producing the strongest effect, with regard to both supraspinal and spinal analgesia (Atcheson & Lambert 1994). Analgesia, sedation, and respiratory depression increase with increased plasma concentrations.

In rhesus monkeys, fentanyl IV produced respiratory depression and analgesia at dosages as low as 2 μg/kg, and apnea was seen consistently at 60 μg/kg (Nussmeier et al. 1991). There may be large differences in dosage requirements among different species, due to variations in concentration and distribution of opioid binding sites (Robson et al. 1985). This difference may be marked when compared with unrelated species, such as dogs, which do not develop apnea even at 3000 μg/kg IV (Arndt et al. 1984; Bailey et al. 1987).

Butorphanol is an example of an agonist-antagonist opioid. However, it has significant respiratory depressant effects in primates (Liguori et al. 1996), compared with the minimal respiratory depressant effects seen in other animals, such as dogs and cats. Minute ventilation in rhesus monkeys is reduced 60–75% by butorphanol (0.1–0.3 mg/kg IM).

Buprenophine, another opioid agonist–antagonist, has much less respiratory depressant effect in primates (Liguori et al. 1996). It is approximately 30 times more potent analgesic than morphine and the duration of action of at least 8 hours in humans (Stoelting 1999). A study in rhesus monkeys suggests that buprenophine has a wide margin of safety in clinical use (Kishioka et al. 2000). It has been used for postoperative analgesia in a siamang monkey at a dose of 5 μg/kg IM (Weiland et al. 2007).

Naloxone, naltrexone, and nalbuphine are μ opioid receptor antagonists, and effectively displace the agonists from the receptor-binding sites, reversing the effects (Stoelting 1999).

Ketamine and medetomidine have strong analgesic properties, and are often used in the anesthetic protocol.

COMPLICATIONS

Catching the animal and administering anesthetic agents for sedation or induction are two critical parts of primate anesthesia. There is a possibility of causing a traumatic injury when using projectile darts. Furthermore, there is a possibility that the primate will fall down if sitting in a tree or on a shelf once it becomes sedated. Nets can be used to catch the sedated primate before it hits the ground. Once induction of anesthesia is achieved, complications are often related to the health state of the animal, drugs used, and the delivered dose of each drug. Hypothermia is common and body temperature should be monitored throughout the procedure.

Hypoxemia may occur due to hypoventilation, pulmonary shunting, or ventilation-perfusion mismatch. The use of a pulse oximeter will help evaluate oxygen saturation throughout the procedure. Supplemental oxygen should be administered through a face mask or an endotracheal tube. Commonly used anesthetic agents, such as ketamine (5 mg/kg, IM) and medetomidine (0.05 mg/kg, IM), may cause mild to severe hypoxemia if the animals are breathing room air shortly after induction (Ølberg 2004). The use of reversible anes-

thetic agents adds safety to the procedure. A laryngoscope and a suitable endotracheal tube should always be available during anesthesia, as well as equipment necessary to give IV fluid.

RECOVERY

Recovery is performed in a quiet, confined space that prevents climbing and allows constant monitoring. A towel or other insulating material minimizes heat loss to the floor. The primate should not be reunited with its group until it is fully recovered.

FIELD IMMOBILIZATION (WILD CAPTURE)

Anesthesia of free-living primates comprises numerous challenges compared to controlled captive environments. One should carefully consider factors including environment, temperature, humidity, use of darts or traps, species, social groups, and potential for zoonotic diseases (Sapolsky & Share 1998).

It is possible to use traps (Aguiar et al. 2007), as well as remote darting equipment depending on the species and situation. With darting, one must consider the risk

Table 38.2. Recommended drugs and drug combinations for immobilization of monkeys and gibbons

Drug	Dosage (mg/kg)	Reversal Agent	Comments
Ketamine	10–30	None	Fast induction, high therapeutic index. Often hypersalivation, spontaneous movements, and rigidity. Not recommended to use as sole agent.
Ketamine/medetomidine	5–8/0.02–0.05	None for ketamine Atipamezole for medetomidine	Commonly used combination in many primate species for induction or short-term anesthesia. Fast induction and anesthesia for 30–45 minutes with good muscle relaxation. Be aware that recovery can be very fast. The low dosage 0.02 mg/kg medetomidine with ketamine has only been evaluated in golden-headed lion tamarins but probably works well for other species. A low dose medetomidine is preferred for cardiorespiratory stability.
Ketamine/xylazine	5/0.5–1	None for ketamine Yohimbine or atipamezole for xylazine	Approximately 30 minutes of immobilization with good muscle relaxation. Be aware that recovery can be very fast.
Ketamine/midazolam	10/1	None for ketamine Flumazenil for midazolam	Rapid immobilization, good muscle relaxation for 30–45 minutes in marmosets.
Ketamine/diazepam	10/0.2–0.4	None for ketamine Flumazenil for diazepam	Good muscle relaxation and described as safe and efficient in olive baboons.
Tiletamine-zolazepam	5–10	None for tiletamine Flumazenil for zolazepam	Commonly used for many species. High therapeutic index and large variation in dosage recommendations. Good muscle relaxation and anesthesia time of 30–50 minutes. Can be prolonged recoveries.
Tiletamine-zolazepam/ medetomidine	1–3/0.02–0.06	None for tiletamine Flumazenil for zolazepam Atipamezole for medetomidine	Rapid induction in macaques and gibbons, with a smooth induction. Good muscle relaxation. Data suggest some hypotension and hypoxemia with the highest dosages.
Medetomidine/midazolam	0.03–0.06/0.3	Atipamezole for medetomidine Flumazenil for midazolam	Reliable immobilization in Japanese macaques. Induction within 13–19 minutes. Totally reversible. Cardiovascular and pulmonary effects not evaluated.

that the animal will fall down from high trees during induction or get lost after darting. Other considerations are hyperthermia/hypothermia and aspiration of regurgitated food material. A small dart volume and fast induction times are favorable when darting free-ranging primates. Recommended drug combinations are tiletamine/zolazepam (Karesh et al. 1998), tiletamine/zolazepam/medetomidine (Fahlman et al. 2006), or ketamine/medetomidine (Vie et al. 1998). Remote areas may restrict the amount of equipment available, and one may not have oxygen supplementation during anesthesia. One should also keep the primate in a cage until fully recovered before release back into the wild.

SUGGESTED PROTOCOLS

Animals weighing less than or equal to 4 kg are manually restrained and anesthetized with isoflurane through a facemask or in an induction box. If inhalation anesthesia is not available, then 0.02–0.05 mg/kg of medetomidine and 5–8 mg/kg of ketamine is given IM.

Animals weighing greater than 4 kg are anesthetized with 5–8 mg/kg of ketamine and 0.02–0.05 mg/kg of medetomidine IM, by use of remote darting equipment (Table 38.2). Most primates will sleep with this combination for approximately 30–45 minutes, but be aware that they may awake suddenly. It is recommended to spray the epiglottis with lidocaine spray and intubate anesthetized primates, as well as giving them supplemental oxygen. Inhalation anesthesia with isoflurane is excellent for maintenance once induction is achieved. The primate should be kept in a separate cage without possibility to climb until fully recovered, before returned to the enclosure and other members of the group.

REFERENCES

Agoramoorthy G, Rudran R. 1994. Field application of Telazol (tiletamine hydrochloride and zolazepam hydrochloride) to immobilize wild red howler monkeys (Alouatta seniculus) in Venezuela. Journal of Wildlife Diseases 30:417–420.

Aguiar LM, Ludwig G, Svoboda WK, Teixeira GM, Hilst CL, Shiozawa MM, Malanski LS, Mello AM, Navarro IT, Passos FC. 2007. Use of traps to capture black and gold howlers (Alouatta caraya) on the islands of the Upper Parana River, southern Brazil. American Journal of Primatology 69:241–247.

Arndt J, Mikat M, Parasher C. 1984. Fentanyl's analgesic, respiratory, and cardiovascular actions in relation to dose and plasma concentration in unanesthetized dogs. Anesthesiology 61:355–361.

Ashton H. 1994. Guidelines for the rational use of benzodiazepines. When and what to use. Drugs 48:25–40.

Atcheson R, Lambert DG. 1994. Update on opioid receptors. British Journal of Anaesthesia 73:132–134.

Bailey PL, Port JD, McJames S, Reinersman L, Stanley TH. 1987. Is fentanyl an anesthetic in the dog? Anesthesia and Analgesia 66:542–548.

Banknieder AR, Phillips JM, Jackson KT, Vinal SI Jr. 1978. Comparison of ketmine with the combination of ketamine and xylazine for effective anesthesia in the rhesus monkey (Macaca mulatta). Laboratory Animal Science 28:742–745.

Beck CC. 1972. Chemical restraint of exotic species. Journal of Zoo and Wildlife Medicine 3:3–66.

Beck CC, Dresner AJ. 1972. Vetalar (ketamine HCl) a cataleptoid anesthetic agent for primate species. Veterinary Medicine 67:1082–1084.

Bourne GH. 1975. The Rhesus Monkey. London: Academic Press.

Bowden DM, Holm R, Morgan MK. 1974. General anesthesia for surgery in the infant pigtail monkey (Macaca nemestrina). Laboratory Animal Science 24:675–678.

Box PG, Ellis KR. 1973. Use of CT1341 anaesthetic ("saffan") in monkeys. Laboratory Animals 7:161–170.

Bree MM. 1972. Dissociative anesthesia in Macaca mulatta. Clinical evaluation of CI 744. Journal of Medical Primatology 1:256–260.

Bree MM, Feller I, Corssen G. 1967. Safety and tolerance of repeated anesthesia with CI 581 (ketamine) in monkeys. Anesthesia and Analgesia 46:596–600.

Bree MM, Cohen BJ, Rowe SE. 1972. Dissociative anesthesia in dogs and primates: clinical evaluation of CI 744. Laboratory Animal Science 22:878–881.

Burroughs REJ. 1993. The Capture and Care Manual. Pretoria: South African Veterinary Foundation.

Bush M, Custer R, Smeller J, Bush L. 1977. Physiologic measures of nonhuman primates during physical restraint and chemical immobilization. Journal of the American Veterinary Medical Association 171:866–869.

Capuano SV, Lerche NW, Valverde CR. 1999. Cardiovascular, respiratory, thermoregulatory, sedative, and analgesic effects of intravenous administration of medetomidine in rhesus macaques (Macaca mulatta). Laboratory Animal Science 49:537–544.

Cohen BJ, Bree MM. 1978. Chemical and physical restraint of nonhuman primates. Journal of Medical Primatology 7:193–201.

Colillas OJ. 1978. Repeated sedation of the howler monkey with ketamine hydrochloride. Laboratory Animal Science 28:101.

Connolly R, Quimby FW. 1978. Acepromazine-ketamine anesthesia in the rhesus monkey (Macaca mulatta). Laboratory Animal Science 28:72–74.

Du Plooy WJ, Schutte PJ, Still J, Hay L, Kahler CP. 1998. Stability of cardiodynamic and some blood parameters in the baboon following intravenous anaesthesia with ketamine and diazepam. Journal of the South African Veterinary Association 69:18–21.

Dyck JB, Maze M, Haack C, Vuorilehto L, Shafer SL. 1993. The pharmacokinetics and hemodynamic effects of intravenous and intramuscular dexmedetomidine hydrochloride in adult human volunteers. Anesthesiology 78:813–820.

Fahlman A, Bosi EJ, Nyman G. 2006. Reversible anesthesia of Southeast Asian primates with medetomidine, zolazepam and tiletamine. Journal of Zoo and Wildlife Medicine 37:558–561.

Fowler KA, Huerkamp MJ, Pullium JK, Subramanian T. 2001. Anesthetic protocol: propofol use in rhesus macaques (Macaca mulatta) during magnetic resonance imaging with stereotactic head frame application. Brain Research. Brain Research Protocols 7:87–93.

Furtado MM, Nunes ALV, Intelizano TR, Teixeira RHF, Cortopassi SRG. 2010. Comparison of racemic ketamine versus (S+) ketamine when combined with midazolam for anesthesia of Callithrix jaccus and Callithrix penicillata. Journal of Zoo and Wildlife Medicine 41:389–394.

Gerak LR, Brandt MR, France CP. 1998. Studies on benzodiazepines and opioids administered alone and in combination in rhesus monkeys: ventilation and drug discrimination. Psychopharmacology 137:164–174.

Glander KE, Fedigan LM, Fedigan L, Chapman C. 1991. Field methods for capture and measurement of three monkey species in Costa Rica. *Folia Primatologica; International Journal of Primatology* 57:70–82.

Gray CW, Bush M, Beck CC. 1974. Clinical experience using CI-744 in chemical restraint and anesthesia of exotic specimens. *Journal of Zoo and Wildlife Medicine* 5:12–21.

Greenstein ET. 1975. Ketamine HCl, a dissociative anesthetic for squirrel monkeys. *Laboratory Animal Science* 25:774–777.

Haruo M. 1995. Ventricular wall thickness and blood pressure values in normal cynomolgus monkeys. *The Journal of Veterinary Medical Science/The Japanese Society of Veterinary Science* 57:1045–1048.

Hayama S, Terazawa F, Suzuki M, Nigi H, Orima H, Tagawa M. 1989. Immobilization with a single dose of ketamine hydrochloride and a combination of xylazine hydrochloride-ketamine hydrochloride and antagonism by yohimbine hydrochloride in the Japanese monkey (*Macaca fuscata*). *Primates; Journal of Primatology* 30:75–79.

Holmes KR, Hunter WS. 1980. Thermoregulation in Telazol (CI-744)-anesthetized rhesus monkey (*Macaca mulatta*). *The American Journal of Physiology* 239:241–247.

Horne WA. 2001. Primate anesthesia. *The Veterinary Clinics of North America. Exotic Animal Practice* 4:239–266.

Horne WA, Norton TM, Loomis MR. 1997. Cardiopulmonary effects of medetomidine-ketamine-isoflurane anesthesia in the gorilla (*Gorilla gorilla*) and chimpanzee (*Pan troglodytes*). Proceedings: American Association of Zoo Veterinarians, p. 140.

Horne WA, Wolfe BA, Norton TM, Loomis MR. 1998. Comparison of the cardiopulmonary effects of medetomidine-ketamine and medetomidine-telazol induction on isoflurane maintenance anesthesia in the chimpanzee (*Pan troglodytes*). Proceedings: American Association of Zoo Veterinarians, p. 22.

Hummeler K, Davidson WL, Henle W, Laboccetta AC, Ruch HG. 1959. Encephalomyelitis due to infection with *Herpesvirus simiae* (herpes B virus); a report of two fatal, laboratory-acquired cases. *The New England Journal of Medicine* 261:64–68.

Jalanka H. 1989. The use of medetomidine, medetomidine-ketamine combinations and atipamezole at Helsinki Zoo: a review of 240 cases. *Acta Veterinaria Scandinavica* 85:193.

Johnson-Delaney C. 1994. Primates. *The Veterinary Clinics of North America. Small Animal Practice* 24:121.

Kalema-Zikusoka G, Horne WA, Levine J, Loomis MR. 2003. Comparison of the cardiorespiratory effects of medetomidine-butorphanol-ketamine and medetomidine-butorphanol-midazolam in patas monkeys (*Erythrocebus patas*). *Journal of Zoo and Wildlife Medicine* 34:47–52.

Karesh WB, Wallace RB, Painter RL, Rumiz D, Braselton WE, Dierenfeld ES, Puche H. 1998. Immobilization and health assessment of free-ranging black spider monkeys (*Ateles paniscus chamek*). *American Journal of Primatology* 44:107–123.

Kaufman PL, Hahnenberger R. 1975. CI-744 anesthesia for ophthalmological examination and surgery in monkeys. *Investigative Ophthalmology* 14:788–791.

Kimura T, Koike T, Matsunaga T, Sazi T, Hiroe T, Kubota M. 2007. Evaluation of a medetomidine-midazolam combination for immobilizing and sedating Japanese monkeys (*Macaca fuscata*). *Journal of the American Association for Laboratory Animal Science* 46:33–38.

Kishioka S, Paronis CA, Lewis JW, Woods JH. 2000. Buprenophine and methoclocinnamox: agonist and antagonist affects on respiratory function in rhesus monkeys. *European Journal of Pharmacology* 391:289–297.

Knottenbelt MK, Knottenbelt DC. 1990. Use of an oral sedative for immobilisation of a chimpanzee (*Pan troglodytes*). *The Veterinary Record* 126:404.

Lee VK, Flynt KS, Haag LM, Taylor DK. 2010. Comparison of the effects of ketamine, ketamine-medetomidine, and ketamine-midazolam on physiologic parameters and anesthesia-induced stress in rhesus (*Macaca mulatta*) and cynomolgus (*Macaca fas-

cicularis*) macaques. *Journal of the American Association for Laboratory Animal Science* 49:57–63.

Levanen J, Makela ML, Scheinin H. 1995. Dexmedetomidine premedication attenuates ketamine-induced cardiostimulatory effects and postanesthetic delirium. *Anesthesiology* 82:1117–1125.

Liguori A, Morse WH, Bergman J. 1996. Respiratory effects of opioid full and partial agonists in rhesus monkeys. *The Journal of Pharmacology and Experimental Therapeutics* 277:462–472.

Lilburn JK, Dundee JW, Nair SG, Fee JP, Johnston HM. 1978. Ketamine sequelae. Evaluation of the ability of various premedicants to attenuate its psychic actions. *Anaesthesia* 33:307–311.

Liu C, DeLauter R. 1977. Pulmonary functions in concious and anesthetized rhesus macaques. *American Journal of Veterinary Research* 38:1843–1848.

Lugo-Roman LA, Rico PJ, Sturdivant R, Burks R, Settle TL. 2010. Effects of serial anesthesia using ketamine or ketamine/medetomidine on hematology and serum biochemistry values in rhesus macaques (*Macaca mulatta*). *Journal of Medical Primatology* 39:41–49.

Marsboom R, Mortelmans J, Vercruysse J. 1963. Neuroleptanalgesia in monkeys. *The Veterinary Record* 75:132–133.

Martin DP, Darrow CC 2nd, Valerio DA, Leiseca SA. 1972. Methods of anesthesia in nonhuman primates. *Laboratory Animal Science* 22:837–843.

Melvin MA, Johnson BH, Quasha AL, Eger EI. 1982. Induction of anesthesia with midazolam decreases halothane MAC in humans. *Anesthesiology* 57:238–241.

Miller M, Weber M, Mangold B, Neiffer D. 2000. Use of oral Detomidine and ketamine for anesthetic induction in nonhuman primates. Proceedings: American Association of Zoo Veterinarians and International Aassociation for Aquatic Animal Medicine Joint Conference, pp. 179–180.

Morita H. 1995. Ventricular wall thickness and blood pressure values in normal cynomolgus monkeys. *The Journal of Veterinary Medical Science/The Japanese Society of Veterinary Science* 57:1045–1048.

Naccarato EF, Hunter WS. 1979. Anaesthetic effects of various ratios of ketamine and xylazine in rhesus monkeys (*Macacca mulatta*). *Laboratory Animals* 13:317–319.

Nowak RM. 1999. *Walker's Primates of the World*. Baltimore: Johns Hopkins University Press.

Nussmeier NA, Benthuysen JL, Steffey EP, Anderson JH, Carstens EE, Eisele JH, Stanley TH. 1991. Cardiovascular, respiratory, and analgesic effects of fentanyl in unanesthetized rhesus monkeys. *Anesthesia and Analgesia* 72:221–226.

Ochsner AJ. 1977. Cardiovascular and respiratory responses to ketamine hydrochloride in the rhesus monkey (*Macaca mulatta*). *Laboratory Animal Science* 27:69–71.

Ott-Joslin LE. 1993. Zoonotic diseases of nonhuman primates. In: *Zoo and Wild Animal Medicine: Current Therapy 3* (MF Fowler, ed.), pp. 358–373. Philadelphia: W.B. Saunders.

Ølberg R-A. 2004. Sedation of non-human primates using oral and injectable regimes. University of Guelph, University of Guelph.

Paine MF, Shen DD, Kunze KL, Perkins JD, Marsh CL, McVicar JP, Barr DM, Gilles BS, Thummel KE. 1996. First-pass metabolism of midazolam by the human intestine. *Clinical Pharmacology and Therapeutics* 60:14–24.

Phillippi-Falkenstein K, Clarke M. 1992. Procedure for training corral-living rhesus monkeys for fecal and blood-sample collection. *Laboratory Animal Science* 42:83–85.

Porter WP. 1982. Hematologic and other effects of ketamine and ketamine-acepromazine in rhesus monkeys (*Macaca mulatta*). *Laboratory Animal Science* 32:373–375.

Pulley ACS, Roberts JA, Lerche NW. 2004. Four preanesthetic oral sedation protocols for rhesus macaques (*Macaca mulatta*). *Journal of Zoo and Wildlife Medicine* 35:497–502.

Reed M, Staple PH. 1976. Improved technique for anaesthesia of *Macaca speciosa* with methohexitone sodium. *Laboratory Animals* 10:65–67.

Reich DL, Silvay G. 1989. Ketamine: an update on the first twenty-five years of clinical experience. *Canadian Journal of Anaesthesia* 36:186–197.

Robson L, Gillan M, Kosterlitz HW. 1985. Species differences in the concentrations and distributions of opioid binding sites. *European Journal of Pharmacology* 112:65–71.

Sainsbury AW, Eaton BD, Cooper JE. 1989. Restraint and anaesthesia of primates. *The Veterinary Record* 125:640–643.

Sapolsky RM, Share LJ. 1998. Darting terrestrial primates in the wild: a primer. *American Journal of Primatology* 44:155–167.

Schobert E. 1987. Telezol use in wild and exotic animals. *Veterinary Medicine* 33:1080–1088.

Selmi AL, Mendes GM, Boere V, Cozer LAS, Filho ES, Silva CA. 2004a. Assessment of dexmedetomidine/ketamine anesthesia in golden-headed lion tamarins (Leontopithecus chrysomelas). *Veterinary Anaesthesia and Analgesia* 31:138–145.

Selmi AL, Mendez GM, Figueiredo JP, Barbudo-Selmi GR, Lins B. 2004b. Comparison of medetomidine-ketamine and dexmedetomidine-ketamine anesthesia in golden-headed lion tamarins. *The Canadian Veterinary Journal* 45:481–485.

Settle TL, Rico PJ, Lugo-Roman LA. 2010. The effect of daily repeated sedation using ketamine or ketamine combined with medetomidine on physiology and anesthetic characteristics in rhesus macaques. *Journal of Medical Primatology* 39:50–57.

Sleeman JM, Cameron K, Mudakikwa AB, Nizeyi JB, Anderson S, Cooper JE, Richardson HM, Macfie EJ, Hastings B, Foster JW. 2000. Field anesthesia of free-living mountain gorillas (Gorilla gorilla beringei) from the Virunga Volcano region, Central Africa. *Journal of Zoo and Wildlife Medicine* 31:9–14.

Soma L, Tierny W, Satoh N. 1988. Sevoflurane anesthesia in the monkey: the effects of multiples of MAC. *Hiroshima Journal of Anesthesia* 24:566–573.

Stoelting RK. 1999. *Pharmacology & Physiology in Anesthetic Practice*, 3rd ed. Philadelphia: Lippincott Williams & Wilkins.

Sun FJ, Wright DE, Pinson DM. 2003. Comparison of ketamine versus combination of ketamine and medetomidine in injectable anesthetic protocols: chemical immobilization in macaques and tissue reaction in rats. *Contemporary Topics in Laboratory Animal Science* 42:32–37.

Theriault BR, Reed DA, Niekrasz MA. 2008. Reversible medetomidine/ketamine anesthesia in captive capuchin monkeys (Cebus paella). *Journal of Medical Primatology* 37:74–81.

Thummel KE, O'Shea D, Paine MF, Shen DD, Kunze KL, Perkins JD, Wilkinson GR. 1996. Oral first-pass elimination of midazolam involves both gastrointestinal and hepatic CYP3A-mediated metabolism. *Clinical Pharmacology and Therapeutics* 59:491–502.

Thurmon JC, Tranquilli WJ, Benson GJ. 1996. *Lumb & Jones' Veterinary anesthesia*, 3rd ed., pp. 241–242. Philadelphia: Lippincott Williams & Wilkins.

Vercruysse J, Mortelmans J. 1978. The chemical restraint of apes and monkeys by means of phencyclidine or ketamine. *Acta Zoologica et Pathologica Antverpiensia* 70:211–220.

Vie JC, De Thoisy B, Fournier P, Fournier-Chambrillon C, Genty C, Keravec J. 1998. Anesthesia of wild red howler monkeys (*Alouatta seniculus*) with medetomidine/ketamine and reversal by atipamezole. *American Journal of Primatology* 45:399–410.

Weiland L, Vlaminck L, Tavernier P, Gasthuys F. 2007. Anesthesia of a siamang monkey (*Hylobates syndactylus*) for the surgical correction of a hand injury. *The Veterinary Record* 161:234–236.

White GL, Cummings JF. 1979. A comparison of ketamine and ketamine-xylazine in the baboon. *Veterinary Medicine, Small Animal Clinician* 74:392–396.

White PF, Way WL, Trevor AJ. 1982. Ketamine: its pharmacology and therapeutic uses. *Anesthesiology* 56:119–136.

Winterborn AN, Bates WA, Feng C, Wyatt JD. 2008. The efficacy of orally dosed ketamine and ketamine/medetomidine compared with intramuscular ketamine in rhesus macaques (*Macaca mulatta*) and the effects of dosing route on haematological stress markers. *Journal of Medical Primatology* 37:116–127.

Woolfson MW, Foran JA, Freedman HM, Moore PA, Shulman LB, Schnitman PA. 1980. Immobilization of baboons (*Papio anubis*) using ketamine and diazepam. *Laboratory Animal Science* 30:902–904.

Young SS, Schilling AM, Skeans S, Ritacco G. 1999. Short duration anaesthesia with medetomidine and ketamine in cynomolgus monkeys. *Laboratory Animals* 33:162–168.

39 Great Apes

Shannon Cerveny and Jonathan Sleeman

INTRODUCTION

Anesthesia of great apes is often necessary to conduct diagnostic analysis, provide therapeutics, facilitate surgical procedures, and enable transport and translocation for conservation purposes. Anesthesia of great apes can be challenging due to their relatively large size, physical strength, agility, and intelligence. In particular, great apes can be very sensitive to changes in their normal environment. Even very subtle perturbations can cause apes to become excited or aggressive, such that anesthetic induction can be very distressing to both animal and anesthesiologist. However, there are sizeable populations of great apes in zoological collections and research institutions due to their endangered status and use as animal models for human diseases, respectively. Consequently, anesthesia is frequently performed on these species, which has resulted in the development of a body of knowledge. However, captive apes often suffer from medical conditions such as cardiomyopathy that can complicate anesthetic events. Recent studies have focused on orally administered, transmucosally absorbed, anesthetic agents as alternative, less stressful methods of premedication and anesthetic induction. Finally, there is increasing conservation management of *insitu* great ape populations, which has resulted in the development of field anesthesia techniques for free-living great apes for the purposes of translocation, reintroduction into the wild, and clinical interventions.

TAXONOMY, BIOLOGY, AND ANATOMICAL CONSIDERATIONS

Great apes include the bonobo (*Pan paniscus*), four subspecies of chimpanzees (*Pan troglodytes*), two species of

gorillas (*Gorilla gorilla* and *Gorilla beringei*), each with two subspecies, and two subspecies of orangutans (*Pongo pygmaeus*). They are all tropical Old World species, and all are considered endangered.

Bonobos are the smallest of the great apes, with an adult weight range of 25–45 kg. Chimpanzees usually weigh 40–90 kg, orangutans weigh 40–189 kg, and gorillas are the largest with an adult weight range of 70–340 kg. Males are larger than females for all species. All are social animals with complex social structures and behaviors, except for orangutans, which are solitary. Great apes have a close taxonomic relationship with humans. Consequently, there are many anatomical similarities, and human anesthetic equipment, such as facemasks, is often used in preference to veterinary equipment. In addition, there is a high potential for pathogen exchange between humans and great apes, necessitating appropriate disease preventive measures.

Their large size, agility and physical strength, as well as large teeth and strong jaws, create the potential for human injury during anesthetic procedures. For this reason, physical restraint and sedation of apes is generally not practical, and most procedures require the animal to be at least stage III of anesthesia. Human safety is of paramount importance during any anesthetic event involving great apes, and it is important to have an experienced, well-trained team of individuals. Due to the zoonotic disease concerns mentioned earlier, all persons in close proximity to apes must wear personal protective equipment, such as facemasks and latex gloves. It would also be prudent to establish escape and bite-wound protocols, as well as have access to a "bite-wound kit" for first aid treatment of persons who may be bitten.

Unique respiratory anatomical features of great apes include laryngeal air sacs, which are present in all

Zoo Animal and Wildlife Immobilization and Anesthesia, Second Edition. Edited by Gary West, Darryl Heard, and Nigel Caulkett.

species, but are most extensive in gorillas and orangutans (Lawson et al. 2006; Nishimura et al. 2007; Raven 1950). In addition, great apes have relatively short tracheas, and care must be taken to ensure that a primary bronchus is not inadvertently intubated (Loomis 2003). Excessive caudal pharyngeal tissue, thick tongues, and long flaccid soft palates may create challenges for airway maintenance during anesthesia (Kenny et al. 2003). Captive apes are also prone to obesity, which may further complicate access to the airway.

Some Old World nonhuman primates in estrus will develop large genital tumescence. This swelling of the sexual skin can be quite prominent in chimpanzees, and is very vascular and friable. Care must be taken to avoid darting this area as severe hemorrhage may result (Fowler 1995).

Venous access can be accomplished at several sites. The femoral vein at the femoral triangle is readily available. In addition, the saphenous vein on the posterior surface of the lower leg and the cephalic vein are usually visible, especially in larger animals. Intravenous (IV) catheters are typically placed in the cephalic or saphenous vein. IV access is important for administration of fluids, and to provide a rapid route of anesthetic drug supplementation or emergency drug administration should the need arise (Fig. 39.1).

PREANESTHETIC CONSIDERATIONS

As with any species, a preanesthetic assessment is vital. However, this can be challenging in great apes and significant diseases may go unrecognized. Furthermore, estimated body weights are often inaccurate, with one study reporting that even experienced personnel overestimated the weights of chimpanzees by as much as 28% (Adams et al. 2003).

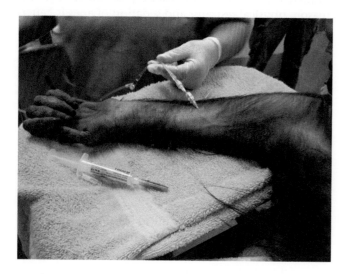

Figure 39.1. Intravenous catheter placed in the cephalic vein of a Bornean orangutan (courtesy Gary West).

Great apes should be fasted and water withheld for 12–24 hours prior to anesthesia. However, this is often a clue that a procedure is imminent and will result in increased agitation, vocalization, and aggression. Consequently, it is important to keep the environment as stress-free and close to the normal routine as possible to avoid this distress. In addition, some individuals will practice pica or coprophagy as a result of fasting(Loomis 2003). Furthermore, apes can remember and recognize individual persons, and the presence of the veterinarian will often induce a violent response.

PREANESTHETICS/SEDATIVES

Due to the stress of remote delivery injection of anesthetic agents, recent studies have focused on oral delivery and/or transmucosal absorption of preanesthetic and anesthetic agents. The techniques described can have variable and unpredictable results, but are a useful alternative method of delivery to consider. Despite the introduction of liquid or food material into the oral cavity immediately before anesthetic induction, potentially increasing the risk of aspiration, such complications have not been reported. Use of metoclopramide (0.4 mg/kg) orally to prevent emesis prior to orally administered anesthetic induction agents has been described (Miller et al. 2000).

Benzodiazepines

Benzodiazepines have minimal effects on cardiopulmonary function and are considered safe to use in primates (Horne 2001). Diazepam can be given orally as a preanesthetic agent and may provide some degree of sedation prior to anesthetic induction. Raphael et al. (2001) reported administering 5 mg diazepam orally to juvenile gorillas 2 hours prior to anesthetic induction with ketamine by hand injection. In addition, Miller et al. (2000) described the use of diazepam for its sedative effect at 0.2 mg/kg given orally 90–120 minutes prior to anesthetic induction. Premedication with midazolam (0.7–1.2 mg/kg PO) delivered in orange juice has been described in chimpanzees and orangutans (Hess et al. 2010). Effects ranged from slight to marked sedation.

Opioids

Transmucosal fentanyl formulations approved for human use have also been used in great apes. Hunter et al. (2004) trained animals to accept, after an overnight fast, a placebo candy lollipop and to suck on it slowly. After 4–6 weeks of training, the apes were then offered the fentanyl lollipop at an intended dose of 10–15 μg/kg. Orangutans and gorillas accepted the treated lollipops and displayed signs of adequate sedation in 30–45 minutes, and responded minimally to darting. However, the chimpanzees acceptance of the fentanyl lollipops was suboptimal and visible sedation was not appreciated. The authors suggested a greater fentanyl concentration in the treated lollipop may be necessary to achieve sedation in chimpanzees. The resulting plasma concentrations of fentanyl in animals accepting treated lollipops supported transmucosal absorption. Success of this technique was dependent on an effective training program, cooperation of the keeper staff, and adequate housing facilities.

Neuroleptic Agents

For anxiolytic effects, the neuroleptic drug zuclopenthixol at dosages of 0.1–0.36 mg/kg by mouth twice daily was used in gorillas undergoing a prolonged journey (Vogelnest 1998). These animals were calm, traveled well, and maintained good appetites during their transportation.

Opioid/Neuroleptic Combinations

The administration of oral droperidol at a dose of 1.25 mg for a juvenile chimpanzee and 2.5 mg for adult chimpanzees 45 minutes prior to transmucosalcarfentanil administration at 2.0 μg/kg provided an effective premedication regimen that produced profound sedation prior to the IM delivery of tiletamine-zolazepam for anesthetic induction (Kearns et al. 2000). Carfentanil was administered by enticing the animal to the front of the cage and expelling the drug from a 0.5-mL syringe directly onto the oral mucosa. This combination produced smooth induction and heavy sedation or light anesthesia approximately 25 minutes after carfentanil administration (Kearns et al. 2000). At that time, naltrexone and tiletamine-zolazepam were combined into one intramuscular injection for anesthetic induction. Naltrexone was administered at 100 times the carfentanil dose in milligrams. The primary side effect noted was respiratory depression, but was adequately managed by administration of the narcotic antagonist at the time of anesthetic induction with tiletamine-zolazepam. However, the authors also recommended providing supplemental oxygen as well as preparing a naltrexone dart in advance as a precaution. In addition, a side-effect of facial pruritus was noted in some individuals.

Kearns et al. (2000) noted that during initial carfentanil dosing trials, direct application of carfentanil onto the oral mucosa produced the deepest level of sedation, followed by offering the drug in foods that contact the mucosa, such as marshmallow crème. When the drug was administered in fruit, only stage 2 or 3 of sedation was reached, which was attributed to the poor gastric absorption of narcotics compared withmucosal absorption.

Alpha-2 Agonists

Medetomidine transmucosally administered at 50–100 μg/kg in marshmallow crème prior to immobilization with ketamine by injection resulted in variable effects (Kearns et al. 1998). Some animals that had not had previous immobilization experience were noticeably sedated, whereas other more experienced chimpanzees showed little or no sedation.

Naples et al. (2010) compared chimpanzees receiving oral medetomidine at 0.1 mg/kg in marshmallow crème or applesauce prior to immobilization with tiletamine-zolazepam at 3 mg/kg IM by remote injection, with animals that were immobilized with medetomidine at 0.05 mg/kg and tiletamine-zolazepam at 3 mg/kg both given IM by remote injection. Although there was not a significant difference between the two groups in the time between tiletamine-zolazepam administration and a degree of sedation considered safe for human contact, animals receiving oral medetomidine exhibited less excitatory behavior and agitation associated with darting than animals that did not receive medetomidine as a premedication.

INDUCTION AGENTS

Intramuscular induction agents can be given by hand injection or remote delivery into a large muscle mass, such as the shoulder or thigh. Immobilization by darting can be very stressful for great apes. Urinary cortisol consistent with a stress response has been demonstrated in chimpanzees following ketamine administration by remote injection (Anestis et al. 2006). Animals scoring highly in the "mellow" behavioral component exhibited a higher peak cortisol and change in cortisol overall, contrary to what the authors predicted. The authors speculated that this behavioral type is an adaptive response, in which animals'do not react to neutral situations, such as group member approaches, but will respond to perceived real threats, such as darting. Urinary cortisol was also demonstrated to be significantly higher in chimpanzees following remote injection with tiletamine-zolazepam, than other stressful events including restriction to an indoor enclosure due to a hurricane, and changes in group composition (Anestis 2009).

Operant conditioning to train individuals to present a muscle mass for hand injection of anesthetic agents may limit the stress experienced by the animal, but is not always possible. Otherwise, the agents are usually delivered in lightweight darts propelled by remote delivery systems, such as blow pipes or muzzle velocity adjustable dart guns. The least traumatic remote delivery system should be used to prevent injury. A pole syringe can also be used to administer supplemental drugs in a sedated animal. All attempts should be made to dart the animal without warning as once alerted the individual, or group, will become agitated and mobile, making darting very difficult. Protective clothing, including face shields may be necessary, as chimpanzees have a propensity to spit water, throw fecal matter and other material with surprising accuracy, as well as returning darts with some force. In addition, apes have surprisingly long limbs and will grab at loose clothing, glasses, and even the dart gun. Ideally, potent drugs that require a small volume for injection should be used, as apes can remove a dart very quickly prior to full injection of the drug.

Darting individuals housed in a social group can be particularly challenging, and isolation of the targeted individual from the group prior to anesthesia may not be possible, or could be very stressful. Once alerted to the event the whole group may act aggressively toward humans in close proximity, which can be very intimidating. However, it is important to have a mechanism to isolate and retrieve the anesthetized individual, especially in the event of an anesthetic emergency. Appropriate facilities that allow shifting of animals, and securing areas or rooms, is very helpful. Removal of enclosure furniture and bedding prior to darting may be beneficial as apes can be very adept at hiding, or adopting body positions, to avoid the dart.

Injectable induction agents and dosages commonly used alone or in combination are listed in Table 39.1. The protocols described in this section pertain to captive great apes unless otherwise noted.

Ketamine Hydrochloride

Ketamine hydrochloride alone has been used successfully in chimpanzees with smooth and rapid induction (3–5 minutes) using standard IM dosages in Table 39.1 (April et al. 1982). Adequate muscle relaxation, good analgesia and minimal cardiopulmonary changes were reported. Recovery occurred 40–60 minutes after injection with signs of awareness at 20–30 minutes, and the majority of individuals were calm with minimal anxiety

and natural movements. Ketamine was also used as an induction agent in gorillas with some animals receiving a premedication of diazepam (Raphael et al. 2001). Ketamine is irreversible, has a short duration of action with sudden unexpected recoveries, and tolerance develops with repeated use (April et al. 1982; Lewis 1993). Conversely, incremental doses of ketamine to prolong anesthesia can result in an extended recovery time of several hours. Ketamine does maintain laryngeal reflexes to some extent, but this does not obviate the need for careful airway management. It can also induce hypersalivation, which can be prevented or controlled using an anticholinergic agent. Another disadvantage of ketamine when used alone is the large volume required. A concentrated 200 mg/mL solution may aid delivery in larger animals.

Ketamine and Alpha-2 Agonists

The disadvantages of ketamine resulted in the development of protocols combining ketamine with alpha-2 agonists. April et al. (1982) reported the use of a combination of ketamine (15–20 mg/kg) and xylazine (1 mg/kg) in chimpanzees delivered IM that resulted in similar induction time compared withketamine alone, but with a greater depth of anesthesia characterized by greater muscle relaxation and analgesia, as well as cardiopulmonary stability, and longer but uneventful recoveries.

When medetomidine is delivered in combination with ketamine, the total ketamine dose can be reduced to at least one-fifth of the ketamine dose if it is used as the solo agent (Horne 2001). Lewis (1993), Horne et al. (1997), and Adams et al. (2003) have investigated the use of IM delivery of ketamine in combination with

Table 39.1. Range of dosages of injectable anesthetic induction and reversal agents used in wild and captive great apes

Drug	Chimpanzee	Gorilla	Orangutan	References
Induction agents				
Ketamine	15–20	6–14		April et al. (1982); Raphael et al. (2001); Sleeman et al. (2000)
Ketamine/xylazine	15–20/1		5–7/1–1.4	Andau et al. (1994); April et al. (1982); Kilbourn et al. (1997, 2003)
Ketamine/ medetomidine	2–3/0.02–0.04	2/0.03–0.04	3/0.02–0.03	Hess et al. (2010); Horne et al. (1997, 1998)
Ketamine/midazolam	2.5/0.25	9/0.05	1–2/0.03	D'Agostino et al. (2007); Hendrix (2006); Liang et al. (2005)
Tiletamine-zolazepam	2–6	2–6	2–6.9	Andau et al. (1994); Fowler (1995); Kilbourn et al. (2003); Loomis (2003); Cerveny et al. (2012); Sleeman et al. (2000); Vogelnest (1998)
Tiletamine-zolazepam/ medetomidine	1.25–3/0.03–0.05		0.8–2.3/0.02–0.06	Fahlman et al. (1999, 2006); Horne et al. (1998); Naples et al. (2010)
Reversal agents: all species				
Atipamezole	0.1–0.25			Loomis (2003)
Yohimbine	0.125–0.25			Loomis (2003)
Flumazenil	0.02–0.1 (IV)			Loomis (2003)
Naloxone	0.02 (IM/IV)			Loomis (2003)

Note: Dosages listed as mg/kg for intramuscular (IM) injection unless stated.

medetomidine by remote injection. This combination provided a rapid and safe method of anesthetic induction, with complete immobilization achieved within 3–15 minutes for both chimpanzees and gorillas (Horne et al. 1997). Horne et al. (1997) reported that it was very important for the animal to be left undisturbed for the initial 10 minutes after administration as attempts to manipulate or move it prior to this time resulted in rapid arousal. Cardiovascular effects appeared to be minimal; the only noteworthy change was a modest increase in blood pressure soon after induction (Horne et al. 1997). However, IV administration of medetomidine may induce a transient bradycardia (Horne 2001). Reversal with atipamezole given IM, at five times the dose of medetomidine, was smooth and complete in chimpanzees but with variable recovery times (Adams et al. 2003). However, Horne et al. (1997) reported full recovery within 10–13 minutes in chimpanzees and gorillas following atipamezole administration with either a full dose given IM, or a partial dose administered IV with the remainder given IM. This combination also provided a smooth transition to inhalation anesthesia. Recoveries can be quite sudden, even without use of the reversal agent (J. Sleeman, unpubl. data, 1997–200), which could create a dangerous situation for the unprepared anesthesiologist. Ketamine (100 mg) and medetomidine (1 mg) delivered IM have also been used to immobilize a bonobo (Halbwax et al. 2009).

Orally administered detomidine (0.32 mg/kg) and ketamine (9.6 mg/kg) have been investigated as anesthetic induction agents in gorillas (Miller et al. 2000). Some animals received diazepam (0.2 mg/kg PO) and metoclopramide (0.4 mg/kg PO) 90–120 minutes prior to delivery of other agents. The drugs were administered by keeper staff using husbandry training techniques. Lateral recumbency was achieved at 17 minutes in one animal that received a full dose of oral detomidineand ketamine, but supplemental tiletamine-zolazepam was administered (0.94 mg/kg) by remote injection. For the other animals that received partial doses, the first signs of sedation were seen around 15 minutes, and tiletamine-zolazepam was required to achieve lateral recumbency. In all cases, the gorillas had only mild responses to darting and were subjectively judged to be less stressed than darting alone based on decreased screaming, charging, and other stress behaviors.

Napthylmedetomidine use has been investigated in chimpanzees and orangutans (Hess et al. 2010). Animals were premedicated with midazolam (0.7–1.2 mg/kg PO) and immobilized with ketamine (3 mg/kg IM) and hyaluronidase (150 M. U.) and either medetomidine (0.02–0.03 mg/kg) or napthylmedetomidine (0.05–0.07 mg/kg IM). Immobilization with napthylmedetomidine was less complete and shorter in duration than that with medetomidine, and was incompletely antagonized by

atipamezole. However, although cardiorespiratory parameters were not statistically evaluated, animals receiving medetomidine had lower heart rates after treatment than animals receiving napthylmedetomidine. In addition, napthylmedetomidine provided antiaggressive effects in the postoperative period.

Tiletamine-Zolazepam and Tiletamine-Zolazepam Combinations

Tiletamine, a cyclohexamine, and zolazepam, a benzodiazepine has been used widely in primates in a 1:1 combination (Telazol™) (Table 39.1). In addition, tiletamine-zolazepam has been used in combination with medetomidine for chimpanzees, (Horne et al. 1998) and free-ranging orangutans (Fahlman et al. 1999, 2006; see Field Anesthesia section). In all these studies, tiletamine-zolazepam alone, or in combination with medetomidine, produced smooth rapid induction within 1–15 minutes and with stable cardiopulmonary parameters, although significantly lower blood pressures were observed in chimpanzees induced with tiletamine-zolazepam/medetomidine and maintained with isoflurane, compared with animals anesthetized with ketamine/medetomidine and isoflurane (Horne et al. 1998). Furthermore, recoveries from tiletamine-zolazepam/medetomidine anesthesia in chimpanzees were prolonged (1–5 hours) and were characterized by signs of extreme drowsiness, dizziness, ataxia, and adverse gastrointestinal effects, such as vomiting. Flumazenil (0.025 mg/kg IV) transiently increased alertness in chimpanzees but did not significantly enhance the speed or quality of recovery (Horne et al. 1998). A similar effect after administration of flumazenil to gorillas has been noted (Sleeman et al. 2000).

Tiletamine-zolazepam delivered orally at a dosage of 16 mg/kg, administered in about 30 mL of a cola beverage was used to successfully immobilize a chimpanzee (Knottenbelt & Knottenbelt 1990). Lateral recumbency was achieved within 7 minutes with no response to external stimuli. Cardiopulmonary function was considered stable, and both pharyngeal and laryngeal reflexes were present. The chimpanzee began to respond to external stimuli after 40 minutes, and recovery was uneventful.

Fowler (1995) noted that the recovery time for tiletamine-zolazepam alone is dose dependent and recommended the use of low doses for quick procedures. The authors have observed excessive prolonged recovery times in silverback western lowland gorillas immobilized with tiletamine-zolazepamand maintained with inhalation agents (Cerveny et al. 2012, J. Sleeman, unpubl. data). In one case, an initial dose of 4.36 mg/kg given intramuscularly was only partially received and two supplemental doses of 2.02 mg/kg (estimate 30% was received) and 2.45 mg/kg were given. Time from cessation of administration of inhalation agents until voluntary movement of the animal was 13.5

hours. Other gorillas supplemented with ketamine following tiletamine-zolazepam delivery did not experience profoundly prolonged recoveries, and the authors recommend ketamine supplementation if necessary.

Carfentanil

Preliminary trials with orally delivered, transmucosally absorbed carfentanil citrate alone at dosages of 2–4 μg/kg in chimpanzees provided nearly complete or complete immobilization after 22 minutes, but were accompanied by severe respiratory depression, including one case of respiratory arrest and death (Kearns et al. 1999). Consequently, administration of transmucosalcarfentanil alone for immobilization of chimpanzees is not recommended.

Other Combinations

Ketamine/midazolam combinations have also been reported in a chimpanzee (2.5/0.25 mg/kg IM; D'Agostino et al. 2007) and in gorillas (9/0.05 mg/kg IM; Liang et al. 2005). Loomis (2003) also lists various other combinations in great apes, including ketamine/xylazine/tiletamine-zolazepam (1/0.25/1.25 mg/kg), as well as ketamine/medetomidine/butorphanol (2–3 mg/kg/20–30 μg/kg/0.2–0.4 mg/kg) and ketamine/butorphanol/midazolam (3/0.4/0.3 mg/kg), although no details were given. Hanley et al. (2006) also reported the use of a combination of ketamine (5.66 mg/kg) and tiletamine-zolazepam (3.4 mg/kg) delivered IM to induce anesthesia in an orangutan.

Use of adjuncts such as atropine sulfate at 2–5 mg IM for juvenile chimpanzees (April et al. 1982), 0.04 mg/kg IM for gorillas (Raphael et al. 2001), 0.01 mg/kg IM for an orangutan (Hendrix 2006), and glycopyrrolate at 0.01 mg/kg (Greenberg et al. 1999) IM also for an orangutan have been reported, presumably to control hypersalivation and/or bradycardia.

ANESTHETIC MAINTENANCE

Endotracheal Intubation

Maintenance of the airway and provision of oxygen is an important aspect of anesthesia in great ape species. At a minimum, flow-by oxygen should be provided. For prolonged procedures, intubation and maintenance of anesthesia using inhalation agents delivered in oxygen is recommended. For most of the induction agents mentioned earlier, the plane of anesthesia may not be adequate to allow intubation, and it may be necessary to deliver inhalation agents to the animal using a tightly fitting human facemask prior to intubation. Great apes are best intubated in dorsal recumbency with the head extended off the edge of the table which will help to extend the neck. Pulling the tongue forward may help to visualize the larynx. The base of the tongue should then be depressed using a Macin-

tosh laryngoscope blade. Great apes are prone to hypersalivation and laryngospasm, especially when ketamine is given at high doses as the sole anesthetic agent (Horne 2001). Applying small amounts of lidocaine to the glottis several minutes before intubation will help to prevent this (Adams et al. 2003; Horne 2001). A mucosal atomization device can be used for lidocaine application. Great apes require cuffed Murphy tubes ranging in size from 6–12 mm. As mentioned, the short tracheas predispose to intubation of a primary bronchus; thus, once the tube is in place both sides of the chest should be auscultated and monitored for air sounds.

Laryngeal Mask Airway

The laryngeal mask airway (LMA) is an alternative to endotracheal intubation that creates a seal around the larynx with an inflatable cuff (Brain 1983). LMA use has been reported in pediatric chimpanzees (Johnson et al. 2010), and one adult (Vilani et al. 2000). Cerveny et al. (2012) found the LMA to be an effective device for airway control in western lowland gorillas (Fig. 39.2). Gorillas were immobilized with IM tiletamine-zolazepam, and anesthesia was maintained with sevoflurane delivery via either LMA or endotracheal tube. Arterial oxygen was significantly greater in the animals in which LMAs were placed 15 and 45 minutes after placement of the device. The authors speculate that this was due to intubation of a bronchus in the animals in which an endotracheal tube was placed. The LMA is easy to insert and can be used during spontaneous and intermittent positive pressure ventilation. In humans, lower anesthetic requirements have been reported for tolerance of placement, compared withendotracheal tubes (Brimacombe 1995). However, the LMA does not protect against aspiration and should not be used in animals that have not been fasted.

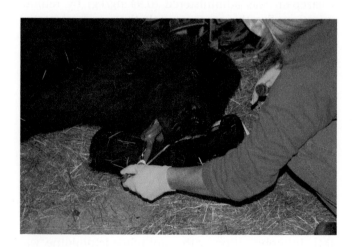

Figure 39.2. Removal of a laryngeal mask airway during anesthetic recovery of a western lowland gorilla.

Inhalatory Agents

Isoflurane is commonly used to prolong and maintain anesthesia in great apes (Adams et al. 2003; Cook & Clarke 1985; Hendrix 2006; Horne et al. 1997, 1998; Liang et al. 2005); however, it has potent vasodilatory properties that can cause severe hypotension (Horne 2001). In addition, as most animals will have received an anesthetic induction agent, the minimum alveolar concentration (MAC) of isoflurane must be reduced accordingly. For example, chimpanzees and gorillas induced with medetomidine and ketamine required masking with 2–3% isoflurane in 100% oxygen to permit intubation followed by 0.5–1.5% isoflurane for anesthetic maintenance using a nonrebreathing circuit (Horne et al. 1997). Blood pressures were elevated immediately following induction but steadily decreased and remained within normal limits after the first 15 minutes, as did heart rate, respiratory rate, hemoglobin saturation (SpO_2), and end-tidal CO_2. Animals induced with medetomidine and Telazol required a lower MAC and could be maintained at a mean level of 0.8% isoflurane in 100% oxygen (Horne et al. 1998). In addition, the latter anesthetic induction combination appeared to potentiate the vasodilatory effects of isoflurane, placing the animals at risk for hypotension, requiring close monitoring of blood pressure.

Sevoflurane is less noxious than isoflurane and can be useful for facemask delivery of an inhalant agent but is more expensive. Like isoflurane, sevoflurane had minimal effects on cardiac output at typical anesthetic concentrations (1.2 times MAC) in domestic dogs (Bernard et al. 1990). In humans, sevoflurane does not appear to sensitize the myocardium to catecholamines, a situation that may induce arrhythmias (Navarro et al. 1994). Cerveny et al. (2012) reported use of sevoflurane for anesthetic maintenance of western lowland gorillas.

Intravenous Anesthesia

Injectable agents have also been used to maintain anesthesia in great apes. Fentanyl (10 μg/kg), midazolam (0.4 mg/kg), and vecuronium (0.1 mg/kg) were delivered IV as part of a balanced anesthesia for a juvenile orangutan undergoing heart surgery. Ketamine infusion (50 μg/kg/min) and low dose isoflurane between 0.2% and 1%, in a 1:1 air:oxygen mixture were used to maintain anesthesia in this patient (Greenberg et al. 1999). Historically, supplemental doses of ketamine have been used to prolong anesthesia, but this can result in a prolonged recovery (Lewis 1993).

Hendrix (2006) reported the use of thiopental (2.1 mg/kg IV) to allow intubation after anesthetic induction with IM ketamine (1 mg/kg) and midazolam (0.03 mg/kg) in an orangutan undergoing laparoscopic tubal ligation. After intubation, the animal was maintained on 1.5–2.25% isoflurane delivered in 100% oxygen at 1.5 L per minute via a rebreathing system.

Intermittent positive pressure ventilation at a rate of 10–20 breaths per minute, 800-mL tidal volume, and a peak inspiratory pressure of 20-cm water was used to overcome the respiratory compromise induced by the head down (Trendelenburg) position and abdominal insufflation. Hypertension (highest mean arterial blood pressure was 158 mmHg) was also noted and was thought to also be due to the insufflation or use of ketamine. Increasing the inhalant concentration improved the animal's relaxation and resolved the hypertension.

Use of propofol to maintain anesthesia has been reported in an orangutan at 50 mg/kg (total dose) IV in a drip, although this did not provide sufficient sedation (Kenny et al. 2003). Propofol has also been administered to an orangutan at 0.19 mg/kg/min IV in combination with intermittent supplemental boluses of ketamine (Hanley et al. 2006), as well as a gorilla (dose not reported; Raphael et al. 2001).

ANALGESIA

Although there is little pharmacological data available for great ape species, provision of analgesia is an important aspect of the anesthesia protocol for any procedure involving painful stimuli. Opioids and nonsteroidal anti-inflammatory drugs (NSAIDs) are often administered alone, or in combination to provide multi-modal analgesia. Human drugs and drug dosages are often used. Pollock et al. (2008) describe continuous IV administration of morphine and diazepam to an orangutan to facilitate postoperative management of intra-pelvic abscess removal and to provide analgesia. Perioperative buprenorphine (0.005 mg/kg IM) was administered during an appendectomy in a chimpanzee (D'Agostino et al. 2007). During recovery, the chimpanzee was given butorphanol (0.01 mg/kg IM). When the animal was alert and able to accept food, the chimpanzee was offered acetaminophen (300 mg PO 3 times a day). Respiratory depression with opioid use has been reported in humans (Taylor et al. 2005), as well as other nonhuman primates (Carpenter 1998; Liguori et al. 1996), so caution is warranted when administering these drugs to great apes. Administration of opioid antagonists may ameliorate these effects.

Synthetic opioids are frequently administered in painful conditions in human medicine and may prove useful for great apes. One of the authors has administered tramadol at 1 mg/kg PO BID to a silverback western lowland gorilla (S. Cerveny et al., unpubl. data). This appeared to have a mild sedative effect.

Peri-operative diclofenac was given to a bonobo (75 mg IM) during removal of a retained placenta. In addition, one of the authors has administered ibuprofen to western lowland gorillas (200–800 mg PO 2–3 times a day), and chimpanzees (400 mg PO twice a day), and ketoprofen (2 mg/kg IM) to a western lowland

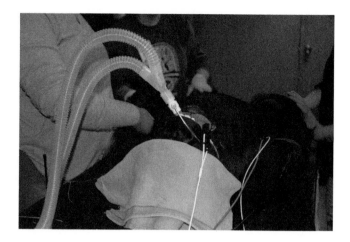

Figure 39.3. Gorilla under anesthesia with monitoring equipment. Note pulse oximeter probe placement, use of side-stream capnography, and blood pressure cuff on the upper forelimb.

gorilla without any adverse effects (S. Cerveny et al., unpubl. data). NSAIDs should be administered with caution if dehydration or renal disease is suspected.

MONITORING

Careful and close anesthetic monitoring is warranted for great apes, whenever possible. A pulse oximeter probe can be placed on the tongue to monitor SpO_2 (Fig. 39.3). End-tidal CO_2 (capnography) can be obtained from an endotracheal tube or LMA.

A cuff can be placed on a limb for indirect oscillometric blood pressure measurement. Significant increases in blood pressure with increasing age have been reported in chimpanzees, necessitating closer monitoring in older individuals to detect possible hypertension (Eichberg & Shade 1987).

Cardiac electrical activity (ECG) can be monitored with leads in standard placement. ECGs were evaluated in three chimpanzees receiving a premedication of 30 mg diazepam and anesthetized with ketamine and xylazine (Erickson & Olsen 1985). Values were similar to previous studies of unanesthetized chimpanzees, although QT and PR intervals were slightly longer due to a lower heart rate in anesthetized chimpanzees. A retrospective study of ECGs from chimpanzees anesthetized with Telazol found ventricular premature contractions (VPCs) to be the most commonly detected arrhythmia (Doane et al. 2006). Other arrhythmias included: atrial premature contractions, second-degree AV block, right bundle branch block, trigeminy, and accelerated idioventricular rhythm. A significantly higher incidence of arrhythmias was found in males, animals with structural heart disease, and animals between 20 and 39 years as compared with those younger than 20 or older than 39.

Frequent analysis of arterial blood gases can also be very useful. Hendrix (2006) reports the use of the dorsal

pedal artery as a site for direct blood pressure measurement and blood-gas sampling in an orangutan. Arterial blood gas can also be sampled from the tibial or femoral arteries. Published cardiopulmonary parameters for great apes under various anesthetic regimens are summarized in Table 39.2. Hendrix (2006) also reports arterial blood-gas and end-tidal CO_2 values for an orangutan undergoing a laparoscopic procedure. Naples et al. (2010) reported arterial blood gas, end-tidal CO_2, and indirect blood pressure values in chimpanzees anesthetized with medetomidine and tiletamine-zolazepam.

ANESTHETIC RECOVERY

Injectable reversal agents and dosages commonly used are listed in Table 39.1. As noted previously, once reversed, recovery can be quite sudden. Consequently, except for emergency situations, these agents should only be administered once the animal is safely secured. The immobilized animal should be allowed to recover in isolation to prevent attack from other members of the group. If the procedure has lasted for only a few hours, then return to the group should be uneventful. If an animal must be separated for longer periods, then behavioral problems may ensue with reintroduction (Fowler 1995).

COMPLICATIONS

A retrospective study of anesthetized great apes in the United Kingdom and Ireland found a 30-fold risk of peri-anesthetic mortality in animals over 30 years of age when compared with animals between 10 and 30 years (Masters et al. 2007). Animals that were preanesthetically assessed as sick were associated with a 26-times greater risk. Overall, perianesthetic mortality risk was 1.35% when cases of euthanasia were excluded from the data, with 80% of deaths occurring in the postanesthetic period.

Cardiovascular diseases are a significant cause of morbidity in captive great apes. Fibrosing cardiomyopathy and aortic dissection are particularly common in older male gorillas (Kenny et al. 1994; Schulman et al. 1995). Unexpected death due to cardiovascular causes was reported in 13 chimpanzees at a captive facility, with systemic hypertension reported in two of the animals (Lammey et al. 2008). Cardiac dysrhythmia was speculated as the cause of death, as all of the animals had exhibited antemortem cardiac arrhythmias. Other cardiac conditions include, for example, idiopathic cardiomyopathy (Seiler et al. 2009), congestive heart failure, and coronary atherosclerosis (Loomis 2003). All of these conditions could complicate anesthesia or result in anesthetic death. Older apes, as well as animals with a history of cardiovascular disease, should be carefully evaluated prior to anesthesia, and carefully monitored during the procedure. Consulta-

Table 39.2. Range of physiologic parameters reported in great apes under various anesthetic regimens

Physiologic Parameter	Chimpanzee	Gorilla	Orangutan	References
Heart rate (beats/min)	60–200	44–144	64–114	Fahlman et al. (2006); Horne (2001); Horne et al. (1997, 1998); Naples et al. (2010); Sleeman et al. (2000)
Respiratory rate (breaths/min)	20–60	14–41	24–120	Fahlman et al. (2006); Horne (2001); Horne et al. (1997, 1998); Naples et al. (2010); Sleeman et al. (2000)
Rectal body temperature (°C)	36.5–37	35.4–40.0	34.7–38.6	Fahlman et al. (2006); Naples et al. (2010); Sleeman et al. (2000)
Systolic arterial blood pressure (mmHg)	72–194	125–154	71–148	Eichberg and Shade (1987); Fahlman et al. (2006); Horne et al. (1997); Naples et al. (2010)
Diastolic arterial blood pressure (mmHg)	40–121	75–87		Eichberg and Shade (1987); Horne et al. (1997); Naples et al. (2010)
Mean arterial blood pressure (mmHg)	50–215	73–121		Horne et al. (1997, 1998); Naples et al. (2010)

tion with human anesthesiologists experienced with these medical conditions in human patients may be beneficial.

In a retrospective study of 226 great ape chemical restraint procedures at the San Diego Zoo, difficulty with airway maintenance was the primary reported problem (Robinson & Lambert 1986). Excessive salivation and upper airway obstruction caused by pharyngeal tissue were reported. Laryngeal air sac infections due to bacteria or yeast have been described frequently in great ape species (Hastings 1991; Hill et al. 2001; Lawson et al. 2006). Laryngeal air sacculitis could complicate general anesthesia due to the risk for fatal pneumonia from the aspiration of purulent material. Apes with air sacculitis should be intubated with cuffed endotracheal tubes, and the condition should be treated prior to any elective anesthesia.

Fatal acute respiratory distress syndrome due to negative pressure pulmonary edema was reported in an orangutan under Telazol-induced anesthesia (Kenny et al. 2003). The authors speculated that an acute upper airway obstruction was the precipitating factor. During early anesthetic induction, this orangutan was noted to be slumped forward, with the head flexed toward the chest. The propensity of orangutans for laryngospasm during anesthesia as well as the pharyngeal anatomy of this species may predispose these animals to this syndrome during anesthesia. Obesity and respiratory disease could also create further complications for respiratory function during anesthesia. Kenny et al. (2003) recommended that orangutans should be properly positioned with a patent airway during anesthetic induction, as well as the use of thick-walled, armored, or reenforced endotracheal tubes with a stylet to facilitate rapid intubation.

FIELD ANESTHESIA

There is increasing conservation management of *insitu* great ape populations, which has resulted in the devel-

opment of field anesthesia techniques for free-living great apes for the purposes of translocation, reintroduction into the wild, and clinical interventions. Anesthesia of great apes under field conditions is inherently riskier for the animals and humans conducting the procedure due to more variables and less control over the animal.

Sleeman et al. (2000) summarized the field anesthesia of 24 free-living human-habituated mountain gorillas (*Gorilla beringei beringei*) using either ketamine (dosage 7 mg/kg) or tiletamine-zolazepam (dose range 90–325 mg) delivered by remote injection. Anesthesia was mostly performed to facilitate medical treatment. Induction time for both agents was approximately 5 minutes, and recovery was significantly shorter for ketamine (mean = 42 minutes) compared with tiletamine-zolazepam (mean = 75 minutes). The authors concluded that anesthesia could be safely performed, even among a large group of gorillas, although the procedures frequently required the entire day. Success of the procedures was dependent on the assistance of local field staff, who had extensive knowledge of gorilla behavior as well as the landscape. Other key factors included darting the animals without warning; keeping the other gorillas away from the anesthetized animal by creating a visual barrier; remaining with the gorilla until it was fully recovered and able to rejoin its group; and reassuring the patient during recovery by grooming the animal and mimicking gorilla vocalizations. Neither drug appeared to produce novel physiologic effects, although some gorillas had low SpO$_2$ values (range = 86–88%). The authors reported that the relatively high altitude at which the procedures were performed may have contributed to the apparent hypoxemia, and consequently recommended providing supplemental oxygen (Fig. 39.4).

Habitat destruction and fragmentation results in scattered and isolated populations of orangutans, and translocation of isolated individuals to protected habitat is an important, albeit somewhat controversial,

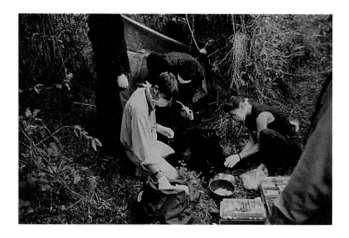

Figure 39.4. Field anesthesia of a mountain gorilla (*Gorilla gorilla beringei*). It is important to wear personal protective equipment such as facemasks and latex gloves to prevent possible pathogen exchange. Note the visual barrier to keep the other gorillas away from the anesthetized animal (photo © Jonathan Sleeman).

conservation strategy (Andau et al. 1994; Kilbourn et al. 1997, 2003). The use of various anesthetic protocols to assist with orangutan translocations have been described, including tiletamine-zolazepam (3–6.9 mg/kg; Andau et al. 1994; Kilbourn et al. 1997, 2003), combined ketamine (5–7 mg/kg), and xylazine (1–1.4 mg/kg) (Andau et al. 1994; Kilbourn et al. 1997, 2003), as well as medetomidine (0.018–0.025 mg/kg) combined with tiletamine-zolazepam (0.8–2.3 mg/kg) (Fahlman et al. 1999, 2006). Kilbourn et al. (1997) recommended tiletamine-zolazepam due to shorter induction times and smaller dart volume. However, Andau et al. (1994) advised the use of ketamine/xylazine, where rapid recovery is desired due to the availability of the xylazine reversal agent, yohimbine hydrochloride. The induction time for both tiletamine-zolazepam and ketamine/xylazine was 4.38 minutes; however, if additional doses were required then induction time increased to 15.67 minutes (Andau et al. 1994). Recovery times were around 42 minutes for ketamine/xylazine and slightly longer for tiletamine-zolazepam.

In typical translocation operations, the orangutan was darted approximately 15 meters up a tree. Both Telinject and Distinject™ systems were used along with 1- or 3-mL plastic or metal darts with 19- to 20-mm needles with retaining collars. The animals were allowed to fall naturally to the ground (the tangle of vines providing natural cushioning), or nets were used to catch the animal. Andau et al. (1994) reported no mechanical injuries from the capture, handling, and transport of animals, although the authors cautioned against darting animals at a height of over 30 m. Two fatalities were recorded. One was due to hyperthermia as a result of an immobilized animal remaining high in the nest

fully exposed to the sun, and the other was a nursing infant that accidentally received the dart intended for its mother. The authors concluded that both Telazol and ketamine/xylazine provided satisfactory immobilization to facilitate the capture and translocation of orangutans, although the need to provide additional doses of drug in several animals suggested that a somewhat higher initial dose may be appropriate.

Medetomidine/Telazol combination delivered intramuscularly to semi-captive or free-ranging orangutans provided rapid smooth induction, with recumbency within 1–7 minutes (Fahlman et al. 1999, 2006). It was considered favorable for remote drug delivery to free-ranging orangutans when compared with Telazol alone due to low drug volume and more controlled descent from the trees. This combination resulted in the animals being able to grip branches during the descent down the tree, making the fall more gradual with less risk for injury. This is in contrast with Telazol alone in which the animals rapidly became immobilized and fell unconscious from the tree. Adequate anesthetic depth with good muscle relaxation was also reported. Heart and respiratory rates and hemoglobin oxygen saturation remained stable, although occasional SPO_2 measurements were below 90% and significant declines in systolic blood pressure (below 80 mmHg in some cases) and body temperature were recorded. The authors recommended using IV fluids and oxygen supplementation to prevent these side effects. One orangutan developed hyperthermia and apnea during translocation, but was successfully resuscitated. The authors reported that additional doses of Telazol were required during the orangutan translocations, and recommended further studies to determine optimal dosages in free-ranging orangutans. Atipamezole was administered intramuscularly at five times the dosage of medetomidine 23–54 minutes after injection of medetomidine/Telazol, or the last additional dose of Telazol. First signs of recovery from anesthesia were noted on average approximately 10 minutes (range 3–27 minutes) after reversal. The recoveries were reported to be smooth and calm.

Returning confiscated and orphaned chimpanzees to native habitat is also an increasingly considered as well as controversial conservation strategy. Tutin et al. (2001) described the successful release of 20 wild-born chimpanzees, and the use of anesthesia to facilitate this project. Capture of chimpanzees prior to release was performed by administering an anesthetic either by hand or remote injection. In addition, chimpanzees were maintained under anesthesia during the boat journey to the release site in order to minimize stress. While details of the anesthetic protocols used were not given, having an experienced team to decrease the risks of drowning as chimpanzees were often in trees overhanging a lagoon, as well as controlling aggression to humans was recommended.

REFERENCES

Adams WA, Robinson KJ, Jones RS, Sanderson S. 2003. Isoflurane to prolong medetomidine/ketamine anaesthesia in six adult female chimpanzees (*Pan troglodytes*). *Veterinary Record* 152(1): 18–20.

Andau PM, Hiong LK, Sale JB. 1994. Translocation of pocketed orangutans in Sabah. *Oryx* 28(4):263–268.

Anestis SF. 2009. Urinary cortisol responses to unusual events in captive chimpanzees (*Pan troglodytes*). *Stress (Amsterdam, Netherlands)* 12(1):49–57.

Anestis SF, Bribiescas RG, Hasselschwert DL. 2006. Age, rank, and personality effects on the cortisol sedation stress response in young chimpanzees. *Physiology and Behavior* 89(2):287–294.

April M, Tabor E, Gerety RJ. 1982. Combination of ketamine and xylazine for effective anaesthesia of juvenile chimpanzees (*Pan troglodytes*). *Laboratory Animals* 16:116–118.

Bernard JM, Wouters PF, Doursout MF, Florence B, Chelly JE, Merin RG. 1990. Effects of sevoflurane and isoflurane on cardiac and coronary dynamics in chronically instrumented dogs. *Anesthesiology* 72(4):659–662.

Brain AIJ. 1983. The laryngeal mask: a new concept in airway management. *British Journal of Anaesthesia* 55(8):801–806.

Brimacombe J. 1995. The advantages of the LMA over tracheal tube or facemask: a meta-analysis. *Canadian Journal of Anaesthesia* 42(11):1017–1023.

Carpenter NA. 1998. Anesthetic apnea in two black and white colobus monkeys (*Colobus guereza*) postulated to have resulted from butorphanol tartrate administration. Proceedings of the American Association of Zoo Veterinarians, pp. 193–195.

Cerveny SN, D'Agostino JJ, Davis MR, Payton ME. 2012. Comparison of laryngeal mask airway use with endotracheal intubation during anesthesia of western lowland gorillas (*Gorilla gorilla gorilla*). *Journal of Zoo and Wildlife Medicine* 43(4): 759–767.

Cook RA, Clarke DA. 1985. The use of isoflurane as a general anesthetic in the western lowland gorilla (*Gorilla gorilla gorilla*). *Journal of Zoo Animal Medicine* 16(4):122–124.

D'Agostino J, Isaza R, Fingland R, Hoskinson J, Ragsdale J. 2007. Acute appendicitis in a chimpanzee (*Pan troglodytes*). *Journal of Medical Primatology* 36(3):119–123.

Doane CJ, Lee DR, Sleeper MM. 2006. Electrocardiogram abnormalities in captive chimpanzees (*Pan troglodytes*). *Comparative Medicine* 56(6):512–518.

Eichberg JW, Shade RE. 1987. "Normal" blood pressure in chimpanzees. *Journal of Medical Primatology* 16(5):317–321.

Erickson HH, Olsen SC. 1985. Electrocardiogram, heart rate, and blood pressure in the chimpanzee. *Journal of Zoo Animal Medicine* 16(3):89–97.

Fahlman Å, Bosi EJ, Nyman G. 1999. Immobilization of southeast Asian primates with medetomidine, zolazepam and tiletamine, and reversal with atipamezole. Proceedings of the American Association of Zoo Veterinarians, p. 334.

Fahlman Å, Bosi EJ, Nyman G. 2006. Reversible anesthesia of southeast Asian primates with medetomidine, zolazepam and tiletamine. *Journal of Zoo and Wildlife Medicine* 37(4): 558–561.

Fowler ME. 1995. Nonhuman primates. In: *Restraint and Handling of Wild and Domestic Animals* (ME Fowler, ed.), pp. 236–246. Ames: Iowa State University Press.

Greenberg MJ, Janssen DL, Jamieson SW, Rothman A, Frankville DD, Cooper SD, Kriett JM, Adsit PK, Shima AL, Morris PJ, Sutherland-Smith M. 1999. Surgical repair of an atrial septal defect in a juvenile Sumatran orangutan (*Pongo pygmaeus sumatraensis*). *Journal of Zoo and Wildlife Medicine* 30(2):256–261.

Halbwax M, Mahamba CK, Ngalula A-M, André C. 2009. Placental retention in a bonobo (*Pan paniscus*). *Journal of Medical Primatology* 38(3):171–174.

Hanley CS, Simmons HA, Wallace RS, Clyde VL. 2006. Visceral and presumptive neural baylisascariasis in an orangutan (*Pongo pygmaeus*). *Journal of Zoo and Wildlife Medicine* 37(4):553–557.

Hastings BE. 1991. The veterinary management of a laryngeal air sac infection in a free-ranging mountain gorilla. *Journal of Medical Primatology* 20(7):361–364.

Hendrix PK. 2006. Anesthetic management of an orangutan (*Pongo abelii/pygmaeus*) undergoing laparoscopic tubal ligation. *Journal of Zoo and Wildlife Medicine* 37(4):531–534.

Hess L, Votava M, Schreiberova J, Málek J, Horáček M. 2010. Experience with a napthylmedetomidine-ketamine-hyaluronidase combination in inducing immobilization in anthropoid apes. *Journal of Medical Primatology* 39(3):151–159.

Hill LR, Lee DR, Keeling ME. 2001. Surgical technique for ambulatory management of airsacculitis in a chimpanzee (*Pan troglodytes*). *Comparative Medicine* 51(1):80–84.

Horne WA. 2001. Primate anesthesia. *Veterinary Clinics of North America. Exotic Animal Practice* 4(1):239–266.

Horne WA, Norton TM, Loomis MR. 1997. Cardiopulmonary effects of medetomidine-ketamine-isoflurane anesthesia in the gorilla (*Gorilla gorilla*) and chimpanzee (*Pan troglodytes*). Proceedings of the American Association of Zoo Veterinarians, pp. 140–142.

Horne WA, Wolfe BA, Norton TM, Loomis MR. 1998. Comparison of the cardiopulmonary effects of medetomidine-ketamine and medetomidine-Telazol™ induction on maintenance isoflurane anesthesia in the chimpanzee (*Pan troglodytes*). Proceedings of the American Association of Zoo Veterinarians, pp. 22–25.

Hunter RP, Isaza R, Carpenter JW, Koch DE. 2004. Clinical effects and plasma concentrations of fentanyl after transmucosal administration in three species of great ape. *Journal of Zoo and Wildlife Medicine* 35(2):162–166.

Johnson JA, Atkins AL, Heard DJ. 2010. Application of the laryngeal mask airway for anesthesia in three chimpanzees and one gibbon. *Journal of Zoo and Wildlife Medicine* 41(3):535–537.

Kearns KS, Afema J, Duncan A. 1998. Dosage trials using medetomidine as an oral preanesthetic agent in chimpanzees (*Pan troglodytes*). Proceedings of the American Association of Zoo Veterinarians, p. 511.

Kearns KS, Swenson B, Ramsay EC. 1999. Dosage trials with transmucosalcarfentanil citrate in non-human primates. *Zoo Biology* 18(5):397–402.

Kearns KS, Swenson B, Ramsay EC. 2000. Oral induction of anesthesia with droperidol and transmucosalcarfentanil citrate in chimpanzees (*Pan troglodytes*). *Journal of Zoo and Wildlife Medicine* 31(2):185–189.

Kenny DE, Cambre RC, Alvarado TP, Prowten AW, Allchurch AF, Marks SK, ZubaJR. 1994. Aortic dissection: an important cardiovascular disease in captive gorillas (*Gorilla gorilla gorilla*). *Journal of Zoo and Wildlife Medicine* 25(4):561–568.

Kenny DE, Knightly F, Haas B, Hergott L, Kutinsky I, Eller JL. 2003. Negative-pressure pulmonary edema complicated by acute respiratory distress syndrome in an orangutan (*Pongo pygmaeus abelii*). *Journal of Zoo and Wildlife Medicine* 34(4):394–399.

Kilbourn AM, Bosi EJ, Karesh WB, Andau M, Tambing E. 1997. Translocation of wild orangutans (*Pongo pygmaeus pygmaeus*) in Sabah, Malaysia. Proceedings of the American Association of Zoo Veterinarians, p. 301.

Kilbourn AM, Karesh WB, Wolfe ND, Bosi EJ, Cook RA, Andau M. 2003. Health evaluation of free-ranging and semi-captive orangutans (*Pongo pygmaeus pygmaeus*) in Sabah, Malaysia. *Journal of Wildlife Diseases* 39(1):73–83.

Knottenbelt MK, Knottenbelt DC. 1990. Use of an oral sedative for immobilisation of a chimpanzee (*Pan troglodytes*). *Veterinary Record* 126(16):404.

Lammey ML, Lee DR, Ely JJ, SleepervMM. 2008. Sudden cardiac death in 13 captive chimpanzees (*Pan troglodytes*). *Journal of Medical Primatology* 37(Suppl. 1):39–43.

Lawson B, Garriga R, Galdikas BMF. 2006. Airsacculitis in fourteen juvenile southern Bornean orangutans (*Pongo pygmaeus wurmbii*). *Journal of Medical Primatology* 35(3):149–154.

Lewis JCM. 1993. Medetomidine-ketamine anaesthesia in the chimpanzee (*Pan troglodytes*). *Journal of Veterinary Anaesthesia* 20(1):18–20.

Liang D, Alvarado TP, Oral D, Vargas JM, Denena MM, McCulley JP. 2005. Ophthalmic examination of the captive western lowland gorilla (*Gorilla gorilla gorilla*). *Journal of Zoo and Wildlife Medicine* 36(3):430–433.

Liguori A, Morse WH, Bergman J. 1996. Respiratory effects of opioid full and partial agonists in rhesus monkeys. *The Journal of Pharmacology and Experimental Therapeutics* 277(1):462–472.

Loomis M. 2003. Great apes. In: *Zoo and Wild Animal Medicine: Current Therapy 5* (ME Fowler, ed.), pp. 381–397. St. Louis: Elsevier Science.

Masters NJ, Burns FM, Lewis JCM. 2007. Peri-anaesthetic and anaesthetic-related mortality risks in great apes (*Hominidae*) in zoological collections in the UK and Ireland. *Veterinary Anaesthesia and Analgesia* 34(6):431–442.

Miller M, Weber M, Mangold B, Neiffer D. 2000. Use of oral detomidine and ketamine for anesthetic induction in nonhuman primates. Proceedings of the American Association of Zoo Veterinarians, pp. 179–180.

Naples LM, Langan JN, Kearns KS. 2010. Comparison of the anesthetic effects of oral transmucosal versus injectable medetomidine in combination with tiletamine-zolazepam for immobilization of chimpanzees (*Pan troglodytes*). *Journal of Zoo and Wildlife Medicine* 41(1):50–62.

Navarro R, Weiskopf RB, Moore MA, Lockhart S, Eger EI II, Koblin D, Lu G, Wilson C. 1994. Humans anesthetized with sevoflurane or isoflurane have similar arrhythmic response to epinephrine. *Anesthesiology* 80(3):545–549.

Nishimura T, Mikami A, Suzuki J, Matsuzawa T. 2007. Development of the laryngeal air sac in chimpanzees. *International Journal of Primatology* 28(2):483–492.

Pollock PJ, Doyle R, Tobin E, Davison K, Bainbridge J. 2008. Repeat laparotomy for the treatment of septic peritonitis in a Bornean orangutan (*Pongo pygmaeus pygmaeus*). *Journal of Zoo and Wildlife Medicine* 39(3):476–479.

Raphael BL, James S, Calle PP, Clippingerv TL, Cookv RA. 2001. The use of ketamine as a primary immobilizing agent in gorillas (*Gorilla gorilla*). Proceedings of the American Association of Zoo Veterinarians, pp. 169–170.

Raven HC. 1950. Regional anatomy of the gorilla. In: *The Anatomy of the Gorilla, Raven Memorial Volume* (WK Gregory, ed.), pp. 23–24. New York: Columbia University Press.

Robinson PT, Lambert D. 1986. A review of 226 chemical restraint procedures in great apes at the San Diego Zoo. Proceedings of the American Association of Zoo Veterinarians, p. 183.

Schulman FY, Farb A, Virmani R, Montali RJ. 1995. Fibrosing cardiomyopathy in captive western lowland gorillas (*Gorilla gorilla gorilla*) in the United States: a retrospective study. *Journal of Zoo and Wildlife Medicine* 26(1):43–51.

Seiler BM, Dick EJ Jr, Guardado-Mendoza R, Vandeberg JL, Williams JT, Mubiru JN, Hubbard GB. 2009. Spontaneous heart disease in the adult chimpanzee (*Pan troglodytes*). *Journal of Medical Primatology* 38(1):51–58.

Sleeman JM, Cameron K, Mudakikwa AB, Nizeyi J-B, Anderson S, Cooper JE, Richardson HM, Macfie EJ, HastingsB, Foster JW. 2000. Field anesthesia of free-ranging mountain gorillas (*Gorilla gorilla beringei*) from the Virunga Volcano region, central Africa. *Journal of Zoo and Wildlife Medicine* 31(1):9–14.

Taylor S, Kirton OC, Staff I, Kozol RA. 2005. Postoperative day one: a high risk period for respiratory events. *American Journal of Surgery* 190(5):752–756.

Tutin CEG, Ancrenaz M, Paredes J, Vacher-Vallas M, Vidal C, Goossens B, Bruford MW, Jamart A. 2001. Conservation biology framework for the release of wild-born orphaned chimpanzees into the Conkouati Reserve, Congo. *Conservation Biology* 15(5):1247–1257.

Vilani RGD'OC, Vilani PD'OC, Pachaly JR, Mangini PR, Machado GV, Susko I. 2000. Inhalatory anesthesia with laryngeal mask in a chimpanzee. *Archives of Veterinary Science* 5(1):17–21.

Vogelnest L. 1998. Transport of ten western lowland gorillas (*Gorilla gorilla gorilla*) from the Netherlands to Australia, and their subsequent anaesthesia and health assessment. Proceedings of the American Association of Zoo Veterinarians, pp. 30–32.

40 Canids

R. Scott Larsen and Terry J. Kreeger

INTRODUCTION

The 36 species of nondomestic canids currently recognized by the World Conservation Union Canid Specialist Group (Sillero-Zubiri et al. 2004) are listed in Table 40.1.

SPECIES-SPECIFIC PHYSIOLOGY AND UNIQUE ANATOMIC FEATURES

The anatomy and physiology of nondomestic canids are similar to those of domestic dogs and do not warrant extensive review. The panting mechanism is important in evaporative cooling and thermoregulation. Lateral nasal glands supply moisture needed for evaporation and heat is dissipated as the animal breathes in through the nose and out through the mouth (Kennedy-Stoskopf 2003). This panting mechanism may be compromised during anesthesia, so careful attention to body temperature is warranted, especially if the mouth is held closed. Body temperature may become markedly elevated during restraint, so other methods must be used to prevent severe persistent hyperthermia if the animal cannot pant.

Cardiac parameters are generally presumed to be similar to those for comparably sized domestic dog; there are a few studies documenting cardiac values in nondomestic canid species (Estrada et al. 2009; Guglielmini et al. 2006). In a study evaluating maned wolves, several have had low-grade systolic murmurs due to mitral insufficiency (Estrada et al. 2009). There was increased contact with the sternum as maned wolves aged, and many animals >6 years old had mitral thickening.

A few canids go through seasonal torpor or hibernation. Raccoon dogs hibernate during the coldest winter periods. At these times, they have increased fat deposits and lower basal metabolic rates, as well as lower cortisol, thyroid, and insulin levels (Asikainen et al. 2004), all of which may influence the species' response to anesthetic drugs.

PHYSICAL RESTRAINT

Canids are strong, fast, and agile. Their teeth are large and sharp, their jaw muscles are strong, and most canids can bite through heavy leather gloves. Gloves may be worn to handle canids, not to protect the handler from bite injuries but to protect against scratches from the nails. However, gloves may restrict hand agility and decrease grip control, so some handlers prefer not to use gloves.

Many noninvasive procedures can be performed without anesthesia in smaller species such as foxes (Brash 2003). Canids can be caught and temporarily restrained in large fishing nets, but substantial proficiency is needed to safely restrain large canids this way. Once in the net, animals can be pinned behind the head using a soft broom, forked stick, net, or catch pole. Canids should be pinned while injections are made (Kreeger 1992). A towel or cloth should be placed over the eyes to decrease visual stimulation, calm the animal, decrease stress, and speed induction for chemical sedation/immobilization.

Small-to-medium-sized canids can be grabbed from behind and held by the scruff (Brash 2003) or by grabbing around the neck, with the fingers closing underneath the jaws. If grabbing around the neck, care should be taken not to damage the trachea. At the same time that the neck is grabbed, the body is pushed firmly and gently against the ground by the handler or an assistant. Once in hand, a muzzle can be applied using

Zoo Animal and Wildlife Immobilization and Anesthesia, Second Edition. Edited by Gary West, Darryl Heard, and Nigel Caulkett.
© 2014 John Wiley & Sons, Inc. Published 2014 by John Wiley & Sons, Inc.

Table 40.1.   Taxonomic and biologic information for canids

| Genus | Species | Common Name | Adult Body Wt (kg) | | | Longevity (year) |
			Female	Male	Combined	Captive (Wild)
Alopex	*lagopus*	Arctic fox	2.4–4.8	2.7–5.4		11
Atelocynus	*microtis*	Short-eared dog			9–10	9–11
Canis	*adustus*	Side-striped jackal	7–10	7–12		10–12
	aureus	Golden jackal	6.5–7.8	7.6–9.8		14
	latrans	Coyote	7.7–15	7.8–15		21 (16)
	lupus	Gray wolf			23–60[a]	16 (13)
	lupus dingo	Dingo	8–17	7–22		13 (7–8)
	mesomelas	Black-backed jackal	6–10	6–12		(10–12)
	rufus	Red wolf	20–30	22–34		(13)
	simiensis	Ethiopian wolf	11–14	14–19		(12)
Cerdocyon	*thous*	Crab-eating fox			4.5–8.5	(9.2)
Chrysocyon	*brachyurus*	Maned wolf			21–30	16
Cuon	*alpinus*	Dhole	10–13	15–20		16 (7–8)
Lycaon	*pictus*	African hunting dog	19–27	25–35		(11)
Nyctereutes	*procyonoides*	Raccoon dog	3–13	3–12		13
Otocyon	*megalotis*	Bat-eared fox	3.2–5.4	3.4–4.9		13
Pseudalopex	*culpaeus*	Culpeo (Andean fox)	4–10	3.4–14		(11)
	fulvipes	Darwin's fox	1.8–3.7	1.9–4.0		(7)
	griseus	Chilla	2.5–5	3.1–4.9		5
	gymnocercus	Pampas fox	3.0–5.7	4.0–8.0		14
	sechurae	Sechuran fox			2.6–4.2	
	vetulus	Hoary fox	3.0–3.6	2.5–4.0		8
Speothos	*venaticus*	Bush dog			5–8	13
Urocyon	*cinereoargenteus*	Gray fox	2.0–3.9	3.4–5.5		14–15
	littoralis	Island gray fox	1.3–2.4	1.4–2.5		(10)
Vulpes	*bengalensis*	Indian fox	>1.8	2.7–3.2		6–8
	cana	Blanford's fox	0.8–1.5	0.8–1.4		6 (4–5)
	chama	Cape fox	2.0–4.0	2.0–4.2		
	corsac	Corsac fox	1.9–2.4	1.6–3.2		9
	ferrilata	Tibetan sand fox	3.0–4.1	3.8–4.6		
	macrotis	Kit fox	1.6–2.2	1.7–2.7		
	pallida	Pale fox			2.0–3.6	3
	rueppelli	Sand fox	1.1–1.8	1.1–2.3		6 (7)
	velox	Swift fox	1.6–2.3	2.0–2.5		(8)
	vulpes	Red fox	3.6–6.5	4.4–7.6		(9)
	zerda	Fennec fox	1.0–1.9	1.3–1.7		13–14

[a]Data from Kreeger & Arnemo 2007; all other data from compiled information in Sillero-Zubiri et al. 2004.

a small rope, gauze bandage, or tape. Caution must be used with muzzles because they impair the animal's ability to pant (see earlier). If an animal appears overheated or distressed, the muzzle may need to be removed.

Appropriately sized squeeze chutes can be used for any canid, but care should be taken that the animal cannot get its mouth or legs through the spaces in the chute. Many canids can be trained to walk into a chute.

Box traps, padded-jaw traps, or offset-jawed foothold traps are typically used. Although coyotes do not usually fight a trap for long (Kreeger 1992), other canids may fight against the trap frantically (especially when approached by humans) and may pull out of the trap and/or injure themselves. Leg fractures may occur when steel-jawed traps are used to capture red foxes, but are not common (White et al. 1990). Box traps may be used on naïve fox populations, but are ineffective

on many red foxes. Leg snares may be useful for this species (Jessup 1982). Small leg snares will also capture coyotes and other canids. Leg snares are more likely to result in compromise of blood supply and edema of the paw, but are less likely than jawed traps to cause crushing, contusion, lacerations, or fractures. In colder climates, snares may result in frostbite-type lesions and should not be used. Always check for trap injuries when such means of capture are employed. A restraint pole and double leather gloves can be used to remove animals from traps (Jessup 1982).

Animals in traps are sometimes administered oral medication through "tranquilizer tabs" (Balser 1965). The device is attached to the jaw of the trap and the tablet is ingested when the animal bites at the trap, resulting in sedation. Such sedation may decrease the chance of the animal injuring itself, but is insufficient for handling (Jessup 1982). This technique was originally described in coyotes using high doses of powder-form diazepam (48–96 mg/kg) wrapped in semirotten cloth; ataxia often lasted 18–36 hours and sedation could last days (Balser 1965). Some deaths were reported using this technique, but it is unknown what effect the drug has had on mortality as compared with other factors (Balser 1965). Modifications to these "tranquilizer tabs" have since been made. One device includes a balloon with 3 mL of petroleum jelly, covered by two layers of gauze (Jessup 1982). If the trap may get wet, the tabs can be sealed by dipping them repeatedly in a melted mixture of 25% refined beeswax and 25% paraffin wax (Balser 1965). Tablets of diazepam (6–7 mg/kg), midazolam (3–4 mg/kg), or acepromazine (5 mg/kg) have also been used. Acepromazine interferes with thermoregulation, so this drug should not be used if trapping is conducted at high ambient temperatures or if the traps are infrequently checked. When using tablets, doses are relatively high because of the likely loss of drug during chewing (Jessup 1982). More recently, propiomazine has been used, to good effect, in gray wolves (Sahr & Knowlton 2000). Gray wolves in traps with propiomazine had less trap-associated trauma on their legs than those that received no tranquilizers; no mortality was associated with use of this drug, even when doses of 1000 mg were consumed by wolf pups or smaller nontarget species (Sahr & Knowlton 2000).

VASCULAR ACCESS

Arterial and venous access sites are comparable with those of domestic dogs. Medetomidine often causes vasoconstriction and may predispose to vasospasm, so vascular access may be more difficult with the use of this drug. Xylazine exerts similar changes, although vasodilation may follow the initial period of vasoconstriction. Venipuncture and catheterization should be done as soon as possible if medetomidine is used, preferably within the first 15–20 minutes post induction, because vasospasm makes these procedures more difficult later during the immobilization. Typical sites for phlebotomy are the jugular, cephalic (brachial), and lateral saphenous veins. Venous catheters are typically placed in the cephalic or saphenous veins. For blood gas analysis, arterial samples are readily obtained from the femoral artery (Larsen et al. 2002).

INTUBATION

Intubation of the anesthetized canid is not always essential, but should be performed during prolonged procedures (especially if inhalant anesthetics are used), if animals are hypoxemic, or if they are hypoventilating. Intubation is as described for domestic dogs. Endotracheal sizes increase in proportion to the size of the animals: 3–4 mm for adult fennec foxes, 5–6 mm for adult red foxes (Bertelsen & Villadsen 2009), 9–10 mm

for adult red wolves (Sladky et al. 2000), and 10–12 mm for adult gray wolves.

PREANESTHETIC CONSIDERATIONS

Anticipation and avoidance of potential complications are key points in preparation for canid anesthesia. Respiratory depression is a common complication for immobilized canids and can be induced by alpha-two adrenoceptor agonists or opioids. Respiratory depression often manifests as hypoxemia and hypercapnia. Hypoxemia can be addressed by providing supplemental oxygen in the nares or through an endotracheal tube. Hypopnea and hypercapnia may be corrected through intubation and assisted ventilation. Opioids and alpha-two agonists may be antagonized, but the animal may not remain anesthetized and effects from residual dissociative agents may occur. A respiratory stimulant, such as doxapram, may increase respiratory rate and ventilation, at least transiently.

Prolonged exertion may result in hyperthermia, which needs to be treated quickly. Heavily furred animals can also become hyperthermic when under a warm sun, even with cold ambient temperatures. Most canids dissipate heat through panting, which is often compromised during immobilization. Hyperthermia should be suspected if rectal temperature is >40°C and treatment is mandatory if the temperature is >41°C. Hyperthermic animals should be moved out of direct sunlight. Cooling measures may be warranted such as spraying the body with water, packing with ice packs, application of isopropyl alcohol to proximal legs and ears, cold water enemas, and administration of cool IV fluids. Be careful to remove these cooling methods as body temperature declines to prevent hypothermia.

Hypothermia occasionally occurs under cold conditions, prolonged immobilizations, or in animals with hair loss or debilitated body condition. Warm water containers, warm blankets, heat pads, heat lamps, and hand warmers can be used to increased body temperature. Recovery will be slowed if the animal remains below normal body temperature.

Severe sustained hypertension may be seen with concurrent use of dissociative agents and alpha-two adrenoceptor agonists. Ketamine-medetomidine-induced hypertension can be particularly severe, but this can also be seen with ketamine-xylazine, or with alpha-two agonists in the absence of a dissociative agent (Kreeger et al. 1986; Larsen et al. 2002; Sladky et al. 2000). Blood pressure typically declines over time and is less severe in calm animals. Anticholinergics should be used sparingly and judiciously to avoid exacerbating hypertension.

Vomiting may occur and can result in aspiration of stomach contents. To prevent this problem, captive animals should be fasted 12–24 hours prior to immobilization, but this is not an option for free-ranging animals. Water can be withheld up to 12 hours in advance, but 2 hours is typically sufficient. Vomiting upon recovery is typically less hazardous than at induction because the animal has control of its glottis and is less likely to aspirate. If an animal vomits when anesthetized, it should be placed in sternal recumbency with the neck extended and the nose pointed down.

Seizures may occur with the use of dissociative anesthetics, although they may be seen with less frequency as lower doses of dissociatives are used and as benzodiazepines are more commonly used as part of immobilization combinations. If the animal only experiences one or two short seizures, treatment is not necessary, but if more seizures occur, or if seizures are sustained, diazepam or midazolam should be administered IV or IM. Remember to administer diazepam over 10–20 seconds IV to prevent cardiac arrest from the propylene glycol.

Wounds are common and should be treated with appropriate medical care. All anesthetized canids should be checked for wounds from traps, needles, and conspecifics. Removal of hair should be minimized if the coat is needed for thermoregulation.

Gastrointestinal dilatation (bloat) may sometimes occur in larger canids, particularly in animals that have recently eaten (and especially if the food ingested was rotten). Although rare, gastrointestinal dilatation and volvulus may also occur. Care should be taken to avoid unnecessary rolling of animals, particularly onto their backs.

There is much discussion in the literature regarding the stress of capture and immobilization of African wild dogs, with speculation that handling-induced stress contributed to mortality in this species through elevated corticosteroids and recrudescence of latent viruses. The evidence for this is scant and analysis of the pertinent data suggests that handling does not increase the likelihood of disease in this species (de Villiers et al. 1995).

CHEMICAL RESTRAINT AND ANESTHESIA

Monitoring and Supportive Care

Approach the recumbent animal quietly and cautiously. The ear seems to be one of the more sensitive parts of the canid body to stimulation, so attempting to elicit an ear twitch with a stick or pole can be a good way of assessing anesthetic depth. If an ear twitch is still present 10–15 minutes after agent administration, supplemental drugs may be warranted. Keep in mind, however, that some animals will maintain an ear twitch despite being otherwise adequately immobilized, so supplement judiciously. Jaw tone should always be assessed and is highly predictive of an animal's depth. Deeply sedated or anesthetized animals do not have appreciable jaw tone. Animals with some degree of residual jaw tone may not be adequately anesthetized

and are more prone to become reactive and cause injury from teeth.

The animal should be placed in lateral recumbency with the head and neck extended to provide a clear airway. Respiratory rate and depth are the most important parameters to monitor. These should be checked immediately and monitored throughout the procedure. Body temperature should also be checked and the animal should be kept out of direct sunlight, if possible, to avoid hyperthermia. Efforts to cool the animal should be instituted if rectal temperature exceeds 40°C.

Once respiration and body temperature are evaluated, heart rate and rhythm should be checked. Any necessary ophthalmic exam should be performed early in the procedure so that lubrication can be applied to the cornea and the eyes can be covered. Muzzling the animal and hobbling the legs may be necessary if the animal is only sedated or lightly anesthetized.

Monitoring the Respiratory and Cardiovascular Systems Regular monitoring should be performed, with respiratory rate and depth assessed constantly. Heart rate, heart rhythm, and body temperature should be regularly evaluated every few minutes. Portable monitors that gauge blood pressure, peripheral oxygen saturation, end-tidal carbon dioxide, and electrocardiogram (ECG) profile are quite helpful in better monitoring each patient. These portable devices can be expensive and are not always essential for procedures (especially field immobilizations), but they tend to work well in canids of all different sizes and may contribute substantially to good anesthetic management. Their use would be more important for prolonged procedures, clinical settings, and high-risk animals.

Recovery Considerations The immobilized animal should not be left unattended until it has recovered, unless it is in captivity or held such that it can be kept away from other animals and hazards. Monitoring should intensify when hazards such as water and precipices are in the immediate area. For these reasons, immobilization combinations that can be antagonized are ideal. Yohimbine may be given IV to rapidly antagonize xylazine; similarly naloxone or naltrexone may be given IV to antagonize butorphanol. Some authors advocate IV atipamezole, but this may put undue strain on the cardiovascular system due to the drug's potent and specific nature. Atipamezole IM appears to result in acceptably swift recovery times. Once antagonists are administered, the animal should be left undisturbed in a shaded quiet area; if moved after antagonists are administered, the animal may become agitated and tend to stand and run before having fully recovered.

Dissociative Agents

The dissociative anesthetic, ketamine, is a mainstay of canid anesthesia. Tiletamine is also used commonly, but this drug is only available in combination with zolazepam (in Telazol®) and recoveries are typically long with this drug combination. Phencyclidine was commonly used many years ago (Seal & Erickson 1969), but is no longer available. Ketamine has been used alone to immobilize African hunting dogs, gray wolves, coyotes, red foxes, gray foxes, and kit foxes (Ebedes & Grobler 1979; Jessup 1982; Kreeger & Seal 1986a). Induction times are rapid (3–6 minutes), but immobilization times are short (18–22 minutes) relative to recovery times (50–90 minutes) (Kreeger & Seal 1986a). Typically only light anesthesia is achieved, but heart rate and respiratory rate are stable (Ebedes & Grobler 1979). Increasing doses do not decrease induction times or substantially increase immobilization times, but recoveries are longer (Jessup 1982).

If used alone, dissociative agents induce rough inductions and recoveries, hyperthermia, skeletal muscle hypertonicity, muscle spasms, uncontrolled head movements, ptyalism, and convulsions (Jessup 1982; Kreeger 1992), so they are typically combined with alpha-two agonists, benzodiazepines, and/or opioids. Dissociatives cannot be antagonized, although yohimbine was tried in gray wolves (Kreeger & Seal 1986a). Wolves that received yohimbine had their heads up more quickly, but took longer to stand, than those receiving a placebo (Kreeger & Seal 1986a). If ketamine is given with other agents that can be antagonized, the antagonists should not be administered until most of the dissociative has been metabolized. Early reversal may result in convulsions, tremors, hyperthermia, or rough recoveries due to residual ketamine. A 45-minute wait generally appears adequate. Waiting times seem less critical with the use of Telazol because zolazepam ameliorates the effects of the dissociative.

Alpha-Two Adrenergic Agonists

Alpha-two adrenoceptor agonists, including xylazine and medetomidine, are potent, reversible sedatives that are commonly used to smooth induction and recovery when either ketamine or tiletamine-zolazepam is used. Alone these agents can heavily sedate canids to the point of relatively safe handling, but these animals may also be aroused with stimulation and are capable of directed attack. For these reasons, it is usually preferable to combine an alpha-two agonist with at least one other drug.

Xylazine Xylazine has been used alone in wolves, coyotes, red foxes, gray foxes, and kit foxes (Jessup 1982; Philo 1978). Doses need to be higher for excited animals because they have higher sympathetic tone that can override the adrenergic agonist. Use of xylazine alone is best for short procedures requiring only moderate handling (Kreeger et al. 1988); for longer, or more stimulatory procedures, additional drugs are warranted. Initial effects occur in 2–3 minutes, animals are

sternal in 4–10 minutes, and maximal effect is in 15 minutes (Philo 1978). Induction is no quicker with higher doses, but respiration is more depressed and there is a greater chance of apnea (Philo 1978). Animals can be approached and safely handled if there are no loud noises and contact with the animal is not abrupt (Kreeger et al. 1988). Vomiting may occur shortly after xylazine administration (Jessup 1982; Philo 1978). Low heart rates may occur; historically, this has been counteracted by use of the anticholinergic drug, atropine (Philo 1978), but low heart rates do not necessarily need to be treated if cardiac output and perfusion are good. Xylazine sedation typically lasts 30–60 minutes, but complete recovery takes 2–3 hours without reversal (Kreeger et al. 1988; Philo 1978). Yohimbine is usually used for reversal, but tolazoline and atipamezole are other options. Recovery typically occurs 4–6 minutes after IV administration of yohimbine (Kreeger et al. 1988).

Medetomidine Medetomidine is more potent and specific than xylazine. Like xylazine, high doses of medetomidine alone can effect complete immobilization in relatively calm canids. Complete immobilization was achieved in farmed Arctic foxes using 0.1 mg/kg (Jalanka 1990). Similarly, calm, habituated gray wolves have been induced with 0.05 mg/kg. Medetomidine has even been effective in field settings with coyotes (0.12 mg/kg) and red foxes (0.14 mg/kg), although it should be noted that only noninvasive and minimally stimulating procedures could be accomplished using medetomidine alone (Baldwin et al. 2008). At high doses of medetomidine, there is better muscle relaxation and less chance of spontaneous recovery, but mucous membranes may be cyanotic, oxygenation may be poor (as low as 74%), and respiration may be impaired (Kreeger et al. 1996). Second-degree atrioventricular heart blocks are common with the use of medetomidine and occur with increased frequency at higher doses. Atropine has been administered to relieve bradycardia; although the anticholinergic drug may double the heart rate, oxygen saturation does not necessarily improve. Without administration of reversal agents, immobilization with medetomidine lasts about 60 minutes (Kreeger et al. 1996). Recoveries are quick (2–5 minutes) with the administration of atipamezole (0.25 mg/kg, IV) and are slower if yohimbine (0.2 mg/kg, IV) is used (Kreeger et al. 1996). Although some sources advocate IV administration of atipamezole, we do not. IV atipamezole appears to effect extremely rapid changes in cardiovascular parameters, with potentially deleterious consequences; such changes are not as rapid with IM atipamezole or IV yohimbine (Ambrisko & Hikasa 2003).

Phenothiazine Derivatives

The phenothiazine derivative, acepromazine, is a tranquilizer that is occasionally used alone to calm canids that are trapped (5 mg/kg; McKenzie 1993). Since aceopromazine interferes with thermoregulation, it should not be used if ambient temperatures are high or if traps are not checked frequently. Aceopromazine is not effective alone as an immobilizing agent, but has occasionally been used successfully for South American canids in combination with ketamine (Pessutti et al. 2001).

Opioids

Some opioids can be useful in combination with other drugs for sedation, immobilization, and anesthesia. Butorphanol is used most often as it is inexpensive, has relatively mild respiratory effects, and is readily absorbed via intramuscular injection. Fentanyl and morphine have also been used. By itself, butorphanol has produced "apathetic sedation" in wolves (Kreeger 1992). Anesthesia can be achieved when butorphanol is combined with an alpha-two agonist, but these combinations work best on calm, captive animals and are not potent enough to anesthetize free-ranging or otherwise highly excited canids (Kreeger 1992).

Ultrapotent opioids (etorphine, carfentanil, sufentanil) have been used historically in large canids, but the human and animal hazards of these drugs, along with the availability of safer options, make it less likely that they would be used for canids today (Kreeger & Seal 1990).

Benzodiazepines

Benzodiazepines, such as diazepam, midazolam, and zolazepam, are useful sedatives for facilitating muscle relaxation and preventing convulsions, particularly in combination with dissociative agents. They are also helpful in treating animals experiencing seizures or convulsions. Both diazepam and midazolam have been used with ketamine; zolazepam is combined with tiletamine in Telazol. Benzodiazepines are reversible with flumazenil; however, flumazenil is relatively expensive and in many situations, benzodiazepine reversal is probably not necessary. Benzodiazepines have minimal adverse cardiorespiratory effects and residual sedation is the most commonly observed occurrence post immobilization. Flumazenil administration may be warranted in animals that are going through cardiorespiratory decompensation or when animals are to be immediately released into the wild after immobilization.

Ketamine-Xylazine Ketamine-xylazine combinations were the standard protocols used for many canid species for several years. Small canids generally need higher doses of ketamine than large canids, but doses for xylazine tended to remain constant for different body weights. Some have advocated administration of xylazine 10 minutes prior to administration of ketamine (Cornely 1979), but this is often impractical in the field setting and it is our experience that temporal

separation of the drugs is not needed. Lower doses of ketamine with higher doses of xylazine result in quicker recoveries by taking advantage of the reversibility of the alpha-two agonist while minimizing the amount of ketamine that persists; quicker recoveries often occur even without reversal (Kreeger & Seal 1986b). In coyotes, if the dose of ketamine is decreased from 4 to 2 mg/kg, the recovery time is shortened from 2–3 to <1 hour (Kreeger & Seal 1986b).

Induction with ketamine-xylazine is variable, occurring in 2–20 minutes; faster inductions occur when using relatively high doses of ketamine and relatively low doses of xylazine. Working times are typically 20–40 minutes, and complete recovery occurs in 1–2 hours (Cornely 1979; Kreeger & Seal 1986b). Heart rate may be either slowed or elevated; tachycardia is seen with high doses of ketamine; bradycardia is seen with high doses of xylazine (Kreeger & Seal 1986b). Premature ventricular contractions (PVCs) may occasionally occur, but do not typically cause clinical problems (Kreeger & Seal 1986b). It is less common to see PVC arrhythmias if atropine is administered (Fuller & Kuehn 1983), but it is more common to see hypertension and mean arterial blood pressures may be over 170 mmHg (Kreeger & Seal 1986b). Since atropine will exacerbate this hypertension without improving oxygenation, the use of an anticholinergic drug is usually contraindicated. Oxygenation is typically stable, but may be lower than desired (83–94%; Osofsky et al. 1996). Blood pressure values tend to normalize after antagonists are administered (Kreeger et al. 1986). Respiratory rate is often elevated when ketamine-xylazine is used (Sladky et al. 2000). Canids immobilized with ketamine-xylazine have poor thermoregulatory ability and hyperthermia is also frequently observed (Fuller & Kuehn 1983), although temperatures tend to decrease over the course of the immobilization (Fuglei et al. 2002; Sladky et al. 2000).

The xylazine component can be antagonized with yohimbine (0.1–0.2 mg/kg) or tolazoline (8 mg/kg) (Kreeger et al. 1986, 1990b), but antagonists should not be administered until 45 minutes after the last injection of ketamine; otherwise, tachycardia, severe hypotension (<30 mmHg), mouth gaping, face scratching, twitching, and hyperreflexia may occur (Kreeger & Seal 1986b). With yohimbine, arousal occurs in 1–8 minutes, sternal recumbency in 5–6 minutes, and uncoordinated ambulation in 10–25 minutes (Kreeger & Seal 1986b). Doses of yohimbine higher than 0.2 mg/kg do not improve or hasten reversal, but instead cause ataxia, hyperreflexion, tachycardia, and hypersalivation (Kreeger et al. 1990b). Yohimbine may be given IV, IM, or a percentage by both routes (Osofsky et al. 1996).

Some immobilization-associated deaths have been reported with ketamine-xylazine, but the reasons for these deaths were not clear (Fuller & Kuehn 1983).

Ketamine-Medetomidine In the past decade, many clinicians have switched from using ketamine-xylazine to ketamine-medetomidine. Much is similar about the two protocols; however, medetomidine is more potent and specific than xylazine so lower doses of ketamine are effective and reversal is quicker and more complete. For canids, some authors have recommended ketamine (2.5–3 mg/kg) and medetomidine (0.06–0.1 mg/kg), to insure complete immobilization and operator safety (Jalanka & Röken 1990); however, in our experience, slightly higher doses of ketamine (4–6 mg/kg) can be safely combined with lower doses of medetomidine (0.02–0.04 mg/kg) to provide effective immobilization with fewer adverse cardiopulmonary effects.

Animals are typically ataxic in 1–5 minutes, recumbent in 5–10 minutes, and induced in 10–15 minutes. Inductions may be much faster in captive animals that are accustomed to handling than in less acclimated individuals (Fuglei et al. 2002; Jalanka 1990). Animals should be kept as calm as possible during induction. Vomiting occasionally occurs (Arnemo et al. 1993; Fuglei et al. 2002; Holz et al. 1994), particularly if animals have not been fasted. Animals acclimated to handling and people may have stable body temperatures, but hyperthermia is common and temperatures tend to decrease over time (Arnemo et al. 1993; Jalanka 1990; Sladky et al. 2000). Decline in body temperature may be substantial in raccoon dogs that are anesthetized during the winter when they hibernate; this decrease may critically affect their metabolism so special care to body temperature should be paid in this species (Arnemo et al. 1993).

Heart rate may increase or decrease over time in canids (Aguirre et al. 2000; Arnemo et al. 1993; Fuglei et al. 2002; Sladky et al. 2000). Heart rate is increased by atropine administration (Holz et al. 1994), but use of this drug is not typically warranted for the reasons described with ketamine-xylazine. Oxygenation is typically stable, but may be somewhat low. Arctic fox pups anesthetized with ketamine-medetomidine had SpO2 values of 78–95% (Aguirre et al. 2000), while mean values were 92–94% in red wolves (Sladky et al. 2000). Respiratory rate tends to increase over time (Aguirre et al. 2000; Jalanka 1990; Sladky et al. 2000). Raccoon dogs anesthetized with ketamine (5 mg/kg) and medetomidine (0.1 mg/kg) exhibited intermittent apnea and tachypnea, but breathing became more regular as time went on (Arnemo et al. 1993). These respiratory effects may have been due to the relatively high dose of medetomidine that was used.

Some authors have cited excess salivation as a reason for use of atropine in immobilization protocols (Holz et al. 1994). It is true that animals salivate less if an anticholinergic is administered; however, we have not appreciated hypersalivation to be a clinically important problem.

Ketamine-medetomidine immobilization typically lasts approximately 60 minutes after initial injection, although individual animals may rouse more quickly (Jalanka 1990) and some animals do not regain corneal or pedal reflexes until >120 minutes (Arnemo et al. 1993). Recovery is usually rapid, with animals standing 5–20 minutes post antagonist and fully recovered 10–35 minutes post antagonist (Aguirre et al. 2000; Arnemo et al. 1993; Jalanka 1990). Without antagonist agents, complete recovery occurs in about 3 hours (Arnemo et al. 1993). Medetomidine is typically antagonized with atipamezole (5 mg/mg medetomidine 5:1). For most species, high doses of atipamezole are contraindicated; foxes given 0.25 mg/kg atipamezole were reported to be nervous, overalert, and developed muscle fasiculations (Jalanka 1990). However, it is important to note that raccoon dogs were not effectively antagonized when given 5:1 atipamezole:medetomidine and 10:1 was needed instead (Arnemo et al. 1993). Although this dose is higher than for any other canid, it did not cause raccoon dogs to be excited or overly alert (Arnemo et al. 1993). Antagonism may be quicker with IV administration of atipamezole than with IM delivery, but the difference is a matter of 2–5 minutes. In blue foxes, IV atipamezole caused a 200% increase in heart rate 1.5 minutes post administration (Jalanka 1990). Given the rapid and dramatic changes in blood pressure and cardiovascular output that occurs when atipamezole is given IV, this route of administration poses unnecessary risks and should not be performed. Theoretically, yohimbine may also be used to antagonize medetomidine, but even in domestic dogs, there is sparse literature about dosing.

Unexplained mortalities have been seen with use of ketamine-medetomidine. Of 20 Arctic foxes anesthetized with ketamine (3 mg/kg)-medetomidine (0.5 mg/kg) for implantation of heart-rate transmitters, two died 30–35 minutes into surgery (Fuglei et al. 2002). The cause of death was not explained so surgical factors cannot be discounted.

Xylazine-Butorphanol Butorphanol (0.4 mg/kg) has been combined with xylazine (2 mg/kg) to immobilize gray wolves (Kreeger et al. 1989). Animals were induced in 12 minutes; bradycardia, respiratory depression, and normotension were observed. Immobilization was rapidly antagonized with yohimbine and naloxone. After antagonists were administered, heart rate and respiratory rate rapidly increased (Kreeger et al. 1989).

Medetomidine-Butorphanol Butorphanol has also been combined with medetomidine in canids; this drug combination can be fully antagonized, with few side effects, but requires minimal visual and auditory stimulation to be effective. Medetomidine (0.04 mg/kg) with butorphanol (0.4 mg/kg) was successfully used to immobilize 23 of 24 red wolves (Larsen et al. 2002).

Induction times were 5–15 minutes. Some wolves received supplemental diazepam (0.2 mg/kg, IV) at induction, others received ketamine (1 mg/kg, IV) 30 minutes post induction, and others received no additional anesthetics. A few red wolves experienced bradycardia (<40 beats/min); heart rate and blood pressure increased when ketamine was given. Second-degree heart block and sinus arrhythmia were observed, but there were no other cardiac arrhythmias. Initial blood pressure values were high (98–194 mmHg), but decreased over time. Oxygenation was initially poor in a few animals, but improved over time and was generally good ($SpO_2 > 93\%$). Effects of the medetomidine-butorphanol lasted 30–40 minutes; longer recumbency times were achieved with addition of diazepam or ketamine. Antagonism with atipamezole (0.2 mg/kg)-naloxone (0.02 mg/kg) effected quick recovery times, with animals fully recovered in about 7 minutes. Flumazenil (0.04 mg/kg) was also administered to wolves that had received diazepam. When low doses of glycopyrrolate were added, there appeared to be a threshold effect on heart rate and blood pressure. At low doses (0.0025–0.005 mg/kg), heart rate and blood pressure did not change, but at higher doses (0.0075–0.0175 mg/kg), acute tachycardia and severe sustained hypertension occurred (Larsen et al. 2001).

Xylazine-Fentanyl Similar to xylazine-butorphanol, xylazine (1 mg/kg)-fentanyl (0.1 mg/kg) has been used successfully to immobilize canids, African wild dogs, in particular (de Villiers et al. 1995; Hattingh et al. 1995). This combination can be antagonized with yohimbine (0.125 mg/kg) and naloxone (1.2 mg/animal). Animals were ataxic in 1.5–3 minutes and recumbent in 5–7.5 minutes (Hattingh et al. 1995). If approached too soon, animals would respond to touch by getting up and running with ataxia. With any alpha-two agonist-opioid combination, canids should be left as undisturbed as possible until 10 minutes post darting. Immobilization with xylazine-fentanyl typically lasts 45–60 minutes. During this time, canids are normoxemic, but hypercapnic ([pCO_2] = 64 mmHg) and acidemic (pH = 7.18–7.28). Supplementation with small doses of xylazine-fentanyl can extend the immobilization by 45–60 minutes. Once antagonists are administered (IV), complete antagonism occurs within 1–2 minutes (Hattingh et al. 1995). Detomidine-fentanyl has been used in African wild dogs in a similar manner (Hattingh et al. 1995).

Ketamine-Medetomidine-Butorphanol These three drugs have been combined together to take advantage of the properties of each agent while minimizing side effects. This combination was compared with ketamine-xylazine, ketamine-medetomidine, and ketamine-medetomidine-acepromazine in red wolves (Sladky et al. 2000). While all combinations were effective,

hypertension was not as severe in the ketamine-medetomidine-butorphanol group and recoveries were faster and smoother. In some animals, mild hypoxemia ($SaO_2 = 87–90\%$) was observed early in the procedures, but improved over time (Sladky et al. 2000). Although respiration rate was lower in this group, hypercapnia was not observed.

A recent study reported minimal hypertension with mild cardiac changes (first- and second-degree atrioventricular blocks, sinus arrhythmia, and depressed left ventricular systolic function) using a combination of ketamine (2 mg/kg)-medetomidine (0.03 mg/kg)-butorphanol (0.2 mg/kg)-acepromazine (0.02 mg/kg)-isoflurane (1–2%) in gray wolves (Valerio et al. 2005). However, this report did not measure blood pressure or assess arrhythmias until 35 minutes post injection, and recovery times were not reported, so it is difficult to compare these results with other investigations (Guglielmini et al. 2006; Valerio et al. 2005).

Ketamine-Midazolam This combination has been reported in red foxes, with induction times of 4–6 minutes and head-up times of 14–23 minutes. Compared with other drug regimens, inductions were longer and there were more spontaneous recoveries (Kreeger et al. 1990b). Ketamine-midazolam has not been a combination that been extensively investigated for wild canids, probably because of the availability of Telazol, a relatively inexpensive, high concentration dissociative-benozodiazepine alternative.

Tiletamine-Zolazepam Tiletamine-zolazepam (Telazol) has been used in a wide variety of species and may be the preferred agent for helicopter captures or escape situations where accurate dosing may be compromised and quick induction is essential. Induction in gray wolves was no shorter using 10 versus 5 mg/kg (5–8 minutes), but arousal time was twice as long with the higher dose (Kreeger et al. 1990a). For helicopter captures, doses over 10 mg/kg may need to be used in order for wolves to be adequately induced (Ballard et al. 1991). Telazol has also been effectively combined with xylazine in wolves (Kreeger et al. 1995).

High stepping was often the first drug response observed, followed by disoriented gait, loss of use of hind legs, licking lips, loss of use of forelegs, loss of head and neck movement, nystagmus, and loss of tongue movement (Ballard et al. 1991). In maned wolves anesthetized with 3 mg/kg tiletamine-zolazepam, many had compulsive licking, excessive salivation, muscle twitching, or muscle tremors (Furtado et al. 2006). In other canids, extreme salivation may occur and mild seizures are not uncommon (Ballard et al. 1991; van Heerden et al. 1991). Within reason, differences in Telazol doses do not seem to have a substantial effect on heart rate, respiratory rate, blood pressure, or temperature. Working times are typically 60–90 minutes at these doses and recovery time is highly variable (25–300 minutes) (Ballard et al. 1991). Complete recovery times have been reported to be as long as 5–6 hours with 5 mg/kg Telazol and some wolves have very rough recoveries with ataxia, paddling, falling backward, and severe mutilation (Kreeger et al. 1990a). When supplementing canids induced with Telazol, it is generally recommended to administer ketamine, rather than additional Telazol, if only injectable anesthetics are given. Supplemental ketamine has produced substantially shorter arousal times (30–45 minutes post injection) than equivalent doses of Telazol (80–130 minutes post injection) (Kreeger et al. 1990a).

Tiletamine-Zolazepam-Medetomidine Recovery qualities may be much improved with lower doses of Telazol combined with medetomidine. When tiletamine-zolazepam (2 mg/kg) was administered to red foxes in combination with medetomidine (0.04 mg/kg), the anesthetic quality and recovery times (6 minutes) were similar to procedures performed using ketamine-medetomidine (Bertelsen & Villadsen 2009). Other cardiorespiratory changes also appear to be similar to ketamine-medetomidine as an initial tachycardia gradually decreased during anesthesia, an initial moderate hypertension decreased over time, and an initially low respiratory rate gradually increased to normal. Telazol-medetomidine has also been used with success in dingoes (Vogelnest 1999).

Medetomidine-Midazolam Medetomidine (0.06 mg/kg)-midazolam (0.5 or 1 mg/kg) has been used successfully in red foxes (Shilo et al. 2010) with faster induction times in animals given 1 mg/kg midazolam than those given 0.5 mg/kg midazolam (Table 40.2). Recovery times were similar between the two doses and were approximately 10 minutes post-atipamezole-administration. In that study, blood pressure values were suggestive of mild hypertension and were similar between animals given ketamine-medetomidine and those given medetomidine and 0.5 mg/kg midazolam; interestingly, foxes given medetomidine and 1 mg/kg midazolam had higher blood pressure values than animals given ketamine-medetomidine.

Medetomidine-midazolam has been similarly effective in golden-backed jackals (King et al. 2008). In that study, recovery times were slightly longer than with ketamine-medetomidine, but were also smoother. It is notable that medetomidine doses were particularly high (0.09 ± 0.02 mg/kg), but bradycardia was not observed and hypertension was not severe.

Medetomidine-Midazolam-Butorphanol Medetomidine-midazolam-butorphanol has been used in red foxes, but with lower doses of medetomidine (0.04 mg/kg) and midazolam (0.3 mg/kg) than with medetomidine-midazolam and no butorphanol (Bertelsen & Villadsen 2009). Induction times with this protocol were slower (9 minutes) compared with combinations that included ketamine (3–4 minutes) or Telazol (4 minutes); similarly, recovery times were longer post atipamezole (10 minutes) than with combinations that included a cyclohexamine (6 minutes). More important to note is that inductions and recoveries with medetomidine-midazolam-butorphanol were more variable, with some animals becoming rousable before atipamezole was administered and others still sedate long after atipamezole administration (Bertelsen & Villadsen 2009). Medetomidine-midazolam-butorphanol has also been used with success in free-ranging African wild dogs (Fleming et al. 2006).

Drug Choice

As with any group of animals, drugs used for immobilization of canids will vary by the species and situation, as well as the preferences and experience of personnel.

For small canids, induction and maintenance with isoflurane or sevoflurane (Crawshaw et al. 2007) is an easy way of quickly providing anesthesia from which animals can rapidly recover. Animals can either be manually restrained and induced via face cone or induced via chamber. Mask induction can be accomplished with animals up to the size of red wolves and coyotes, if there are trained personnel capable of good manual restraint. Chamber induction can occur in purpose-built plastic induction chambers or by placing a plastic bag around a transport kennel. When using these devices, the patient must be closely monitored to insure that the animal does not have complications or become overanesthetized. Animals can become overheated in induction chambers, so these devices should not be used if temperatures cannot be controlled. Some people prefer to use clear bags when placing plastic bags around kennels, so that the animals can be observed throughout induction. By using isoflurane induction, there is increased risk of exposure of personnel to inhalant anesthetics.

Isoflurane can also be used for maintenance of anesthesia. Animals may be maintained with a face mask over the mouth or through an endotracheal tube after intubation. There will be less environmental release of isoflurane if an endotracheal tube is used. Intubation is recommended for animals with complications or for any prolonged immobilization procedure. Sevoflurane can probably be used with equal efficacy and safety, but there is less experience with this drug as it has been more expensive and requires a vaporizer with different calibration settings.

Injectable anesthetic drugs may also be used safely and are particularly appropriate for larger canids and for remote anesthetic delivery. Recommended doses from the literature are to be listed later. Although there have been many anesthetic combinations

Table 40.2. Injectable immobilization drug dosages for canids

Alopex lagopus (Arctic fox)
    Ketamine (2.5 mg/kg)-medetomidine (0.05 mg/kg); atipamezole (0.25 mg/kg) (Aguirre et al. 2000; Jalanka 1990)
    Medetomidine (0.025–0.1 mg/kg) (Jalanka 1990)
    Telazol® (10 mg/kg) (Kreeger & Arnemo 2007)
Atelocynus microtis
    Telazol (10 mg/kg) (Kreeger & Arnemo 2007)
Canis audustus, Canis aureus, Canis mesomelas (jackals)
    Medetomidine (0.09 mg/kg)-midazolam (0.5 mg/kg); atipamezole (0.45 mg/kg) (King et al. 2008)
    Ketamine (2 mg/kg)-medetomidine (0.11 mg/kg); atipamezole (0.55 mg/kg) (King et al. 2008)
    Ketamine (5–8 mg/kg)-xylazine (0.5 mg/kg) (McKenzie & Burroughs 1993)
    Telazol (3–4 mg/kg, 6–8 mg/kg if not enclosed) (McKenzie & Burroughs 1993)
Canis latrans (coyote)
    Medetomidine (0.06–0.12 mg/kg); atipamezole (0.6 mg/kg) (Baldwin et al. 2008; Miller et al. 2009)
    Ketamine (4 mg/kg)-xylazine (2 mg/kg); yohimbine (0.15 mg/kg) (Kreeger & Seal 1986b)
    Telazol (10–11 mg/kg) (Gray et al. 1974; Kreeger & Arnemo 2007).
Canis lupus (gray wolf)
    Ketamine (3–4 mg/kg)-medetomidine (0.06–0.08 mg/kg); atipamezole (0.3–0.4 mg/kg IM) (Holz et al. 1994; Kreeger & Arnemo 2007).
    Medetomidine (0.05 mg/kg); atipamezole (0.25 mg/kg IM) (Kreeger et al. 1996)
    Xylazine (2 mg/kg)-butorphanol (0.4 mg/kg); yohimbine (0.125 mg/kg IV)-naloxone (0.05 mg/kg IV) (Kreeger et al. 1989).
    Ketamine (4–10 mg/kg)-xylazine (1–3 mg/kg); yohimbine (0.15 mg/kg IV), (Kreeger 1992; Kreeger et al. 1987)
    Xylazine (2 mg/kg captive, 3–4 mg/kg wild); yohimbine (0.15 mg/kg IV) (Kreeger et al. 1988; Philo 1978)
    Telazol (10 mg/kg)-xylazine (1.5 mg/kg) (Kreeger & Arnemo 2007)
    Telazol (3–10 mg/kg, 10–13 mg/kg for helicopter captures) (Ballard et al. 1991; Boever 1977; Kreeger et al. 1987)
Canis lupus dingo (dingo)
    Telazol (1–2 mg/kg)-medetomidine (0.04 mg/kg) (Vogelnest 1999)
    Ketamine (7.5 mg/kg)-xylazine (1 mg/kg) (Wentges 1975)
    Telazol (7–10 mg/kg) (Vogelnest 1999)
Canis rufus (red wolf)
    Medetomidine (0.04 mg/kg)-butorphanol (0.4 mg/kg), supplement with diazepam 0.2 mg/kg IV) or ketamine (1 mg/kg IV);
      atipamezole (0.2 mg/kg)-naloxone (0.02 mg/kg) ± flumazenil (0.02 mg/kg) (Larsen et al. 2001)
    Ketamine (2 mg/kg)-medetomidine (0.02 mg/kg)-butorphanol (0.2 mg/kg); atipamezole (0.2 mg/kg) (Sladky et al. 2000)
    Ketamine (2 mg/kg)-medetomidine (0.04 mg/kg); atipamezole (0.2 mg/kg) (Sladky et al. 2000)
    Ketamine (8–10 mg/kg)-xylazine (2 mg/kg); yohimbine (0.1 mg/kg) (Kreeger & Arnemo 2007; Sladky et al. 2000)
    Telazol (10 mg/kg) (Kreeger & Arnemo 2007)
Canis simiensis (Ethiopian wolf)
    Telazol (2–7 mg/kg) (Sillero-Zubiri 1996)
Cerdocyon thous (crab-eating fox)
    Ketamine (10 mg/kg)-xylazine (0.5–1 mg/kg) (Pessutti et al. 2001)
    Telazol (10 mg/kg) (Kreeger & Arnemo 2007)
Chrysocyon brachyurus (maned wolf)
    Ketamine (2.5 mg/kg)-medetomidine (0.08 mg/kg); atipamezole (0.4 mg/kg) (Kreeger & Arnemo 2007)
    Telazol (1.2–5 mg/kg), supplement with ketamine (25–50 mg) or isoflurane (Deem & Emmons 2005; Estrada et al. 2009; Norton
      1990)
    Ketamine (6–9 mg/kg)-xylazine (0.5–2 mg/kg); yohimbine (0.1–0.2 mg/kg) (Norton 1990; Pessutti et al. 2001)
Cuon alpinus (dhole)
    Telazol (10 mg/kg) (Kreeger 1992)
Lycaon pictus (African wild dog)
    Ketamine (3–5 mg/kg)-medetomidine (0.05–0.1 mg/kg); atipamezole (0.15 mg/kg) (Cirone et al. 2004; van Heerden 1993)
    Medetomidine (0.045 mg/kg)-butorphanol (0.24 mg/kg)-midazolam (0.3 mg/kg); atipamezole (3 mg)- naltrexone (10 mg)-flumazenil
      (0.2 mg) (Fleming et al. 2006)
    Xylazine (0.7–1.1 mg/kg)-fentanyl (0.1 mg/kg); yohimbine (0.125 mg/kg)-nalxone (0.04 mg/kg), supplement with xylazine (10 mg)-
      fentanyl (0.5 mg) (de Villiers et al. 1995; van Heerden 1993)
    Ketamine (1.6 mg/kg)-xylazine (2.2 mg/kg); yohimibine (0.2 mg/kg IV/IM) (Osofsky et al. 1996)
    Telazol (1–4 mg/kg, ild African wild dogs are more sensitive than captive ones) (Hattingh et al. 1995; van Heerden 1993)
Nyctereutes procyonoides (raccoon dog)
    Ketamine (5 mg/kg)-medetomidine (0.1 mg/kg); atipamezole (1 mg/kg) (Arnemo et al. 1993)
    Telazol (7 mg/kg) (Gray et al. 1974)
Otocyon megalotis (bat-eared fox)
    Ketamine (5–8 mg/kg)-xylazine (0.5 mg/kg) (McKenzie & Burroughs 1993)
    Telazol (5 mg/kg) (McKenzie & Burroughs 1993)
Pseudalopex culpaeus (South American fox)
    Telazol (10 mg/kg) (Kreeger 1992)
Pseudalopex vetulus (hoary fox)
    Ketamine (3–5 mg/kg)-xylazine (0.6–0.8 mg/kg) (Pessutti et al. 2001)
Speothos venaticus (bush dog)
    Telazol (10 mg/kg) (Pessutti et al. 2001)

Table 40.2. *(Continued)*

Urocyon cineoereoargenteus (gray fox)
  Ketamine (11–15 mg/kg)-xylazine (2–3 mg/kg) (Jessup 1982)
  Telazol (9 mg/kg) (Gray et al. 1974)
Vulpes chama (Cape fox)
  Ketamine-xylazine (5–8 and 0.5 mg/kg) (McKenzie & Burroughs 1993)
  Telazol (5 mg/kg) (McKenzie & Burroughs 1993)
Vulpes macrotis (kit fox)
  Telazol (10 mg/kg) (Kreeger & Arnemo 2007)
Vulpes pallida (pale fox)
  Telazol (10 mg/kg) (Kreeger 1992)
Vulpes velox (swift fox)
  Ketamine (10 mg/kg)-xylazine (1 mg/kg); yohimbine (0.125 mg/kg) (Telesco & Sovada 2002)
  Telazol (10 mg/kg) (Kreeger & Arnemo 2007).
Vulpes vulpes (red fox)
  Ketamine (2–4 mg/kg)-medetomidine (0.04–0.07 mg/kg); atipamezole (0.20–0.35 mg/kg) (Bertelsen & Villadsen 2009; Shilo et al. 2010)
  Medetomidine (0.14 mg/kg); atipamezole (0.80 mg/kg) (Baldwin et al. 2008)
  Medetomidine (0.04 mg/kg)-midazolam(0.3 mg/kg)-butorphanol(0.1 mg/kg); atiapmezole (0.15 mg/kg) (Bertelsen & Villadsen 2009)
  Medetomidine (0.07 mg/kg)-midazolam(0.8 mg/kg); atipamezole (0.35 mg/kg) (Shilo et al. 2010)
  Ketamine (4 mg/kg)-medetomidine (0.02 mg/kg)-butorphanol (0.04 mg/kg), reversed with atipamezole (0.1 mg/kg) (Brash 2003)
  Ketamine (25–30 mg/kg)-midazolam (0.6 mg/kg) (Kreeger & Arnemo 2007; Kreeger et al. 1990b)
  Ketamine (20–23 mg/kg)-xylazine (1–1.2 mg/kg); yohimbine (0.15 mg/kg) (Brash 2003; Kreeger et al. 1990b)
  Telazol (2 mg/kg)-medetomidine (0.04 mg/kg); atipamezole (0.2 mg/kg) (Bertelsen & Villadsen 2009)
  Telazol (4–10 mg/kg) (Boever 1977; Brash 2003; Kreeger et al. 1990b)
Vulpes zerda (fennec fox)
  Telazol (10 mg/kg) (Kreeger & Arnemo 2007)

Note: Drugs or drug combinations are listed in order in which they are recommended

recommended in the literature (see previous section), the following list only incorporates those that we recommend. These recommendations are based on literature reports, current drug availability, and personal experience.

For most routine procedures, on young healthy animals in a controlled environment, we recommend medetomidine-butorphanol. This combination provides profound sedation and 45–60 minutes of working time for many canids. Induction times with medetomidine-butorphanol are typically 5–15 minutes; it is not a highly potent combination, so this is not an appropriate combination for situations where the animals are uncontained, such as darting from a helicopter. One of the authors prefers to use medetomidine-butorphanol for short procedures in medium-to-large *Canis* spp. (wolves, red wolves, and coyotes) particularly in situations where the animal is to be released immediately back into the wild (RSL). Medetomidine-butorphanol induces profound sedation, and procedures such as phlebotomy, radio collar attachment, measurements, and skin biopsies can be performed. However, this combination should not be used for more invasive procedures as there is no general anesthetic incorporated. It should be noted that there will be a subset of the population that will not be adequately immobilized with this combination. For these animals, another agent, such as ketamine, diazepam, or midazolam, may be needed. If ketamine is used, atipamezole-naloxone should not be administered for 30–45 minutes, but there is still rapid, smooth recovery.

In a less controlled situation, such as emergency captures or helicopter darting, Telazol, ketamine-medetomidine, or ketamine-xylazine may be more appropriate since there is a lower volume of drug and induction is more rapid. Induction with medetomidine-butorphanol is often 10–15 minutes, whereas induction with Telazol is typically <5 minutes.

In animals that are ill or aged, particularly if cardiac or respiratory disease is suspected, it is probably not advisable to use medetomidine or other alpha-two agonists. Although these agents can be rapidly antagonized, their effects on blood pressure, heart rate, and respiration make them unnecessarily risky in high-risk patients. For compromised patients, inhalant induction may be the safest option. However, clinical judgment must be used to determine if the stress of handling will be detrimental to the animal's condition. Injectable combinations such as ketamine-midazolam, ketamine-midazolam-butorphanol, or Telazol can also be used.

Field Immobilization Considerations (Wild Capture)

Most canids are fast, elusive, and cunning, making them challenging to successfully immobilize in the wild. Some are also nocturnal. Free-ranging canids are typically trapped before drugs are administered (Kreeger 1992), although field-darting occurs in some cases. Jackals have extremely fast reaction times to sound and can move out of the path of slow-moving darts (McKenzie & Burroughs 1993).

Injectable anesthetic drugs are most commonly administered intramuscularly by hand injection, pole syringe, or dart. Hand injection during physical restraint should be performed in smaller species to avoid errant needle placement and unnecessary tissue trauma. Larger canids can be safely darted with a blowpipe or dart gun.

Gray wolves can be relatively safely pursued and darted from helicopters because they are large and inhabit areas with open country. For this type of a procedure, a pilot and a shooter are typically needed. Rapid projectile dart rifles are needed to insure accurate dart placement. Complications of helicopter darting may include pneumothorax secondary to inadvertent thoracic dart placement (Kreeger et al. 1995) or exhaustion. Coyotes have also been effectively captured in this manner (Baer et al. 1978), and with helicopter-launched net guns, although the impact of the net may cause mortality using this latter technique (Gese et al. 1987).

African wild dogs can be darted from a vehicle at a range of 15–30 m (van Heerden 1993) and should be darted in the upper hind leg. Wild dogs can also be captured by using a helicopter to chase a pack into a funnel-shaped boma. Jackals have occasionally been darted from vehicles to which they have been habituated, but trapping is a much more practical method of capturing these animals (McKenzie & Burroughs 1993). Small animals such as foxes will not normally approach to within darting distances. These animals have small muscle masses and damage to vital organs is very possible, even with light darts (McKenzie & Burroughs 1993). Bat-eared foxes may retreat into burrows if darted; they also have a bushy coat that makes accurate dart placement difficult, so darting is not recommended (McKenzie & Burroughs 1993). In some cases, capture collars (Wildlink Capture Collar, Advanced Telemetry Systems, Isanti, Minnesota 55040, USA) have been used to facilitate immobilization through the automated injection of drugs using a remote signal (Federoff 2001).

POSTANESTHETIC CHALLENGES

Many canids are pack animals. Reintroduction after prolonged separation (>12 hours) may result in extensive fighting, so animals should be kept with the pack as much as possible. Even if it is necessary to perform frequent immobilizations on an individual, it is generally preferable to perform procedures as quick as possible and return the animal to the pack each time, rather than separating the animal and then attempting reintroduction (Kreeger 1992).

REFERENCES

Aguirre A, Alonso A, Principe B, et al. 2000. Field anesthesia of wild Arctic fox (*Alopex lagopus*) cubs in the Swedish Lapland using medetomidine-ketamine-atipamezole. *Journal of Zoo and Wildlife Medicine* 31:244–246.

Ambrisko TD, Hikasa Y. 2003. The antagonistic effects of atipamezole and yohimbine on stress-related neurohomoral and metabolic responses induced by medetomidine in dogs. *Canadian Journal of Veterinary Research* 67:64–67.

Arnemo JM, Moe R, Smith AJ. 1993. Immobilization of captive raccoon dogs with medetomidine-ketamine and remobilization with atipamezole. *Journal of Zoo and Wildlife Medicine* 24:102–108.

Asikainen J, Mustonen A-M, Hyvarinen H, et al. 2004. Seasonal physiology of the wild raccoon dog (*Nyctereutes procyonoides*). *Zoological Science* 21:385–391.

Baer CH, Severson RE, Linhart SB. 1978. Live capture of coyotes from a helicopter with ketamine hydrochloride. *The Journal of Wildlife Management* 42:452–455.

Baldwin JR, Winstead JB, Hyden-Wing D, et al. 2008. Field sedation of coyotes, red foxes, and raccoons with medetomidine and atipamezole. *The Journal of Wildlife Management* 72:1267–1271.

Ballard WB, Ayres LA, Roney KE, et al. 1991. Immobilization of gray wolves (*Canis lupus*) with a combination of tiletamine hydrochloride and zolazepam hydrochloride. *The Journal of Wildlife Management* 55:71–74.

Balser DS. 1965. Tranquilizer tabs for capturing wild carnivores. *The Journal of Wildlife Management* 29:438–442.

Bertelsen MF, Villadsen L. 2009. A comparison of the efficacy and cardiorespiratory effects of four medetomidine-based anaesthetic protocols in the red fox (*Vulpes vulpes*). *Veterinary Anaesthesia and Analgesia* 36:328–333.

Boever WJ. 1977. Use of Telazol (CI-744) for chemical restraint and anesthesia in wild and exotic carnivores. *Veterinary Medicine, Small Animal Clinician* 72:1722–1725.

Brash MGI. 2003. Foxes. In: *BSAVA Management of Wildlife Casualties* (E Mullineaux, R Best, JE Cooper, eds.), pp. 154–165. Gloucester: British Small Animal Veterinary Association.

Cirone F, Gabriella E, Marco C, et al. 2004. Immunogenicity of an inactivated oil-emulsion canine distemper vaccine in African wild dogs. *Journal of Wildlife Diseases* 40:343–346.

Cornely JE. 1979. Anesthesia of coyotes with ketamine hydrochloride and xylazine. *The Journal of Wildlife Management* 43:577–579.

Crawshaw GJ, Mills KJ, Mosley C, Patterson BR. 2007. Field implantation of intraperitoneal radio transmitters in Eastern Wolf (*Canis lycaon*) pups using inhalation anesthesia with sevoflurane. *Journal of Wildlife Diseases* 43:711–718.

de Villiers MS, Meltzer DGA, Van Heerden J, et al. 1995. Handling induced stress and mortalities in African wild dogs (*Lycaon pictus*). *Proceedings of the Royal Society of London. Series B. Biological Sciences* 262:215–220.

Deem SL, Emmons LH. 2005. Exposure of free-ranging maned wolves (*Chyrsocyon brachyurus*) to infectious and parasitic disease agents in the Noel Kempff Mercado National Park, Bolivia. *Journal of Zoo and Wildlife Medicine* 36:192–197.

Ebedes G, Grobler M. 1979. The restraint of the Cape Hunting dog *Lycaon pictus* with phencyclidine hydrochloride and ketamine hydrochloride. *Journal of the South African Veterinary Association* 50:113–114.

Estrada AH, Gerlach TJ, Schmidt MK, et al. 2009. Cardiac evaluation of clinically healthy captive maned wolves (*Chryocyon brachyurus*). *Journal of Zoo and Wildlife Medicine* 40(3):478–486.

Federoff NE. 2001. Antibody response to rabies vaccination in captive and free-ranging wolves (*Canis lupus*). *Journal of Zoo and Wildlife Medicine* 32:127–129.

Fleming GJ, Citino SB, Bush M. 2006. Reversible anesthetic combination using medetomidine-butorphanol-midazolam in in-situ African wild dogs (*Lycaeon pictus*). Proceedings of the American Association of Zoo Veterinarians, pp. 214–215.

Fuglei E, Mercer JB, Arnemo JM. 2002. Surgical implantation of radio transmitters in Arctic foxes (*Alopex lagopus*) on Svalbard, Norway. *Journal of Zoo and Wildlife Medicine* 33: 342–349.

Fuller TK, Kuehn DW. 1983. Immobilization of wolves using ketamine in combination with xylazine or promazine. *Journal of Wildlife Diseases* 19:69–72.

Furtado MM, Kashivakura CK, Fero C, et al. 2006. Immobilization of free-ranging maned wolf (*Chrysocyon brachyurus*) with tiletamine and zolazepa in central Brazil. *Journal of Zoo and Wildlife Medicine* 37:68–70.

Gese EM, Rongstad OJ, Mytton WR. 1987. Manual and net-gun capture of coyotes from helicopters. *Wildlife Society Bulletin* 15:444–445.

Gray CW, Bush M, Beck CC. 1974. Clinical experience using C–744 in chemical restraint and anesthesia of exotic specimens. *Journal of Zoo Animal Medicine* 5:12–21.

Guglielmini C, Rocconi F, Brugnola L, et al. 2006. Echocardiographic and Doppler echocardiographic findings in 11 wolves (*Canis lupus*). *The Veterinary Record* 158:125–129.

Hattingh J, Raath JP, Knox CM, et al. 1995. Anesthesia of free ranging wild dogs (*Lycaon pictus*) with fentanyl and xylazine. Proceedings of the American Association of Zoo Veterinarians, pp. 287–289.

Holz P, Holz RM, Barnett JEF. 1994. Effects of atropine on medetomidine/ketamine immobilization in the gray wolf (*Canis lupus*). *Journal of Zoo and Wildlife Medicine* 25: 209–213.

Jalanka HH. 1990. Medetomidine- and medetomidine-ketamine induced immobilization in blue foxes (*Alopex lagopus*) and its reversal by atipamezole. *Acta Veterinaria Scandinavica* 31:63–71.

Jalanka HH, Röken BO. 1990. The use of medetomidine, medetomidine-ketamine combinations, and atipamezole in nondomestic mammals: a review. *Journal of Zoo and Wildlife Medicine* 21:249–282.

Jessup DA. 1982. Restraint and chemical immobilization of carnivores and furbearers. In: *Chemical Immobilization of North American Wildlife* (L Nielsen, J Haigh, MF Fowler, eds.), pp. 227–244. Madison: Wisconsin Humane Society.

Kennedy-Stoskopf S. 2003. Canidae. In: *Zoo & Wild Animal Medicine*, 5th ed. (ME Fowler, RE Miller, eds.), pp. 482–491. St. Louis: Elsevier Science.

King R, Lapid R, Epstein A, et al. 2008. Field anesthesia of golden jackals (*Canis aureus*) with the use of medetomidine-ketamine or medetomidine-midazolam with atipamezole reversal. *Journal of Zoo and Wildlife Medicine* 39:576–581.

Kreeger TJ. 1992. A review of chemical immobilization of wild canids. Proceedings of the American Association of Zoo Veterinarians, pp. 271–283.

Kreeger TJ, Arnemo JM. 2007. *Handbook of Wildlife Chemical Immobilization*, 3rd ed. Laramie: TJ Kreeger.

Kreeger TJ, Seal US. 1986a. Failure of yohimbine hydrochloride to antagonize ketamine hydrochloride immobilization in gray wolves. *Journal of Wildlife Diseases* 22:600–603.

Kreeger TJ, Seal US. 1986b. Immobilization of coyotes with xylazine–hydrochloride-ketamine hydrochloride and antagonism by yohimbine-hydrochloride. *Journal of Wildlife Diseases* 22:604–606.

Kreeger TJ, Seal US. 1990. Immobilization of gray wolves (*Canis lupus*) with sufentanil citrate. *Journal of Wildlife Diseases* 26: 561–563.

Kreeger TJ, Seal US, Faggella AM. 1986. Xylazine hydrochloride-ketamine hydrochloride immobilization of wolves and its antagonism by tolazoline hydrochloride. *Journal of Wildlife Diseases* 22:397–402.

Kreeger TJ, Fagella AM, Seal US, et al. 1987. Cardiovascular and behavioral responses of gray wolves to ketamine-xylazine immobilization and antagonism by yohimbine. *Journal of Wildlife Diseases* 23:463–470.

Kreeger TJ, Seal US, Callahan M, et al. 1988. Use of xylazine sedation with yohimbine antagonism in captive gray wolves. *Journal of Wildlife Diseases* 24:688–690.

Kreeger TJ, Mandsager RE, Seal US, et al. 1989. Physiological response of gray wolves to butorphanol-xylazine immobilization and antagonism by naloxone and yohimbine. *Journal of Wildlife Diseases* 25:89–94.

Kreeger TJ, Seal US, Callahan M, et al. 1990a. Physiological and behavioral responses of gray wolves to immobilization with Tiletamine and zolazepam (Telazol). *Journal of Wildlife Diseases* 26:190–194.

Kreeger TJ, Seal US, Tester JR. 1990b. Chemical immobilization of red foxes. *Journal of Wildlife Diseases* 26:95–98.

Kreeger TJ, Hunter DL, Johnson MR. 1995. Immobilization protocol for free-ranging gray wolves (*Canis lupus*) translocated to Yellowstone National Park and central Idaho. Proceedings of the American Association of Zoo Veterinarians, p. 466.

Kreeger TJ, Callahan M, Beckel M. 1996. Use of medetomidine for chemical restraint of captive gray wolves (*Canis lupus*). *Journal of Zoo and Wildlife Medicine* 27:807–812.

Larsen RS, Loomis MR, Kelly B, et al. 2001. Immobilization of red wolves (*Canis rufus*) using medetomidine and butorphanol. Proceedings of the American Association of Zoo Veterinarians, pp. 171–175.

Larsen RS, Loomis MR, Kelly B, et al. 2002. Cardiorespiratory effects of medetomidine-butorphanol, medetomidine-butorphanol-diazepam, and medetomidine-butorphanol-ketamine in captive red wolves (*Canis rufus*). *Journal of Zoo and Wildlife Medicine* 33:101–107.

McKenzie AA. 1993. *The Capture and Care Manual: Capture, Care, Accommodation and Transportation of Wild African Animals*, pp. 161–164. Menlo Park: Wildlife Decision Support Services.

McKenzie AA, Burroughs REJ. 1993. Chemical capture of carnivores. In: *The Capture and Care Manual: Capture, Care, Accomodation and Transportation of Wild African Animals* (AA McKenzie, ed.), pp. 224–254. Menlo Park: Wildlife Decision Support Services.

Miller DL, Schrecengost J, Merrill A, et al. 2009. Hematology, parasitology, and serology of free-ranging coyotes (*Canis latrans*) from South Carolina. *Journal of Wildlife Diseases* 45: 863–869.

Norton TM. 1990. Medical management of maned wolves (*Chyrsocyon brachurus*). Proceedings of the American Association of Zoo Veterinarians, pp. 67–70.

Osofsky SA, McNutt JW, Hirsch KJ. 1996. Immobilization of free-ranging African wild dogs (*Lycaon pictus*) using a ketamine/xylazine/atropine combination. *Journal of Zoo and Wildlife Medicine* 27:528–532.

Pessutti C, Bodini Santiago ME, Fernandes Oilveira LT. 2001. Order carnivora, family Canidae (dogs, foxes, maned wolves). In: *Biology, Medicine, and Surgery of South American Wild Animals* (ME Fowler, ZS Cubas, eds.), pp. 279–290. Ames: Iowa State University Press.

Philo LM. 1978. Evaluation of xylazine for chemical restraint of captive arctic wolves. *Journal of the American Veterinary Medical Association* 173:1163–1166.

Sahr DP, Knowlton FF. 2000. Evaluation of tranquilizer trap devices (TTDs) for foothold traps used to capture gray wolves. *Wildlife Society Bulletin* 28:597–605.

Seal US, Erickson AW. 1969. Immobilization of carnivora and other mammals with phencyclidine and promazine. *Federation Proceedings* 28:1410–1419.

Shilo Y, Lapid R, King R, et al. 2010. Immobilization of red fox (*Vulpes vulpes*) with medetomidine-ketamine or medetomidine-midazolam and antagonism with atipamezole. *Journal of Zoo and Wildlife Medicine* 41:28–34.

Sillero-Zubiri C. 1996. Field immobilization of Ethiopian wolves (*Canis simensis*). *Journal of Wildlife Diseases* 32:147–151.

Sillero-Zubiri C, Hoffmann M, Macdonald DW, eds. 2004. *Canids: Foxes, Wolves, Jackals and Dogs. Status Survey and Conservation Action Plan.* Cambridge: IUCN/SSC Canid Specialist Group.

Sladky KK, Kelly BT, Loomis MR, et al. 2000. Cardiorespiratory effects of four alpha-two adrenoceptor agonist-ketamine combinations in captive red wolves. *Journal of the American Veterinary Medical Association* 217:1366–1371.

Telesco RL, Sovada MA. 2002. Immobilization of swift foxes with ketamine hydrochloride-xylazine hydrochloride. *Journal of Wildlife Diseases* 38:764–768.

Valerio F, Brugnola L, Rocconi F, et al. 2005. Evaluation of the cardiovascular effects of an anaesthetic protocol for immobilization and anesthesia in grey wolves (*Canis lupus* L, 1758). *Veterinary Research Communications* 29:315–318.

van Heerden J. 1993. Chemical capture of the wild dog. In: *The Capture and Care Manual: Capture, Care, Accommodation and Transportation of Wild African Animals* (AA McKenzie, ed.), pp. 251–254. Menlo Park: Wildlife Decision Support Services.

van Heerden J, Burroughs REJ, Dauth J, et al. 1991. Immobilization of wild dogs (*Lycaon pictus*) with a tiletamine hydrochloride/zolazepam hydrochloride combination and subsequent evaluation of collected blood chemistry parameters. *Journal of Wildlife Diseases* 27:225–229.

Vogelnest L. 1999. Chemical restraint of Australian native fauna. Wildlife in Australia. Healthcare Management Proceedings, 327, pp. 149–188.

Wentges H. 1975. Medicine administration by blowpipe. *The Veterinary Record* 97:281.

White PJ, Seal US, Tester JR. 1990. Pathological responses of red foxes to foothold traps. *The Journal of Wildlife Management* 54:147–160.

41 Ursids (Bears)

Nigel Caulkett and Åsa Fahlman

SPECIES-SPECIFIC PHYSIOLOGY

In the wild, free-ranging bears are often subject to physical restraint via snares or traps prior to anesthesia. Physical restraint can result in stress, hemoconcentration, or injury (Cattet et al. 2003a). In Scandinavia, free-ranging brown bears (*Ursus arctos*) are only captured by helicopter darting, whereupon hyperthermia, hypoxemia, and lactic acidemia are commonly recorded during anesthesia (Fahlman et al. 2011). A careful physical examination should be performed as part of any capture to identify capture-related injuries. Bears are monogastrics, as such, they are prone to vomiting on induction, or regurgitation during anesthesia. It is best to avoid anesthetizing bears that have recently eaten. This is not always possible in management situations, but may be an option in research situations, and should be adhered to with captive animals. Despite previous fasting, vomiting is a common adverse effect during induction of captive sun bears (*Helarctos malayanus*) with medetomidine-zolazepam-tiletamine (MZT) (Onuma 2003). On the contrary, vomiting has not been observed in free-ranging brown bears (thus not fasted) anesthetized with the same drug combination (Fahlman et al. 2011).

Human safety must always be considered during capture and anesthesia of bears. It is important to know the behavior of the target species. With free-ranging bears, it is also important to consider other bears in the vicinity; these animals can pose a threat to the anesthetized bear or to the capture personnel.

Physical Capture and Restraint

In forested areas without large clear cuts, aerial capture is generally not a safe option. Physical capture techniques are often employed in these situations. The two most common methods, in North America, are culvert traps and snares. Following physical capture, the animal may be anesthetized without the risk of losing it in a forest environment. Bears captured in culvert traps may experience hemoconcentration (Cattet et al. 2003a). Brown bears captured with snares demonstrated a stress leukogram, hemoconcentration, and muscle damage, evidenced by elevations in serum muscle enzymes (Cattet et al. 2003a). Snared bears often exhibit increased serum myoglobin and pathological lesions indicative of capture myopathy have been observed (Cattet et al. 2005, 2008). Fractures and soft tissue injuries may also be encountered in snared animals. If used, snares should be checked frequently, to minimize time spent in the snare, and snared animals should be closely examined to identify and treat snare-related injuries.

CHEMICAL RESTRAINT AND ANESTHESIA

Vascular Access

Venous blood can be sampled from the jugular or medial saphenous vein. IV catheters may be placed in the jugular or cephalic vein. The femoral pulse can easily be palpated in the groin for collection of arterial blood samples for blood gas analysis. A pulsating flow confirms insertion of the needle into the femoral artery. Firm pressure must be applied to the arterial sample site for a minimum of 2 minutes post sampling to avoid development of a hematoma (Fig. 41.1).

Intubation

Intubation of bears is not difficult if the bear is in a sufficiently deep plane of anesthesia. The oral and pharyngeal anatomy is similar to that of a canid. Intubation is easiest with the bear positioned in sternal recumbency. A long laryngoscope and a light source

Zoo Animal and Wildlife Immobilization and Anesthesia, Second Edition. Edited by Gary West, Darryl Heard, and Nigel Caulkett.
© 2014 John Wiley & Sons, Inc. Published 2014 by John Wiley & Sons, Inc.

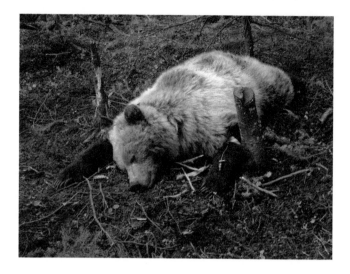

Figure 41.1. Grizzly bear, with IV catheter placed in the cephalic vein.

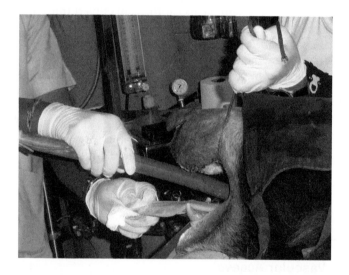

Figure 41.2. Intubation of a sloth bear at the Bannerghatta Bear Rescue Center. International Animal Rescue; Wildlife SOS India.

will facilitate visualization of the glottis prior to intubation. Endotracheal tube size is dependent on size of the bear. We typically carry size 8–14 tubes (internal diameter in millimeters) for black bears and 8–18 tubes for brown bears (Fig. 41.2).

Preanesthetic Concerns

There are two major methods to facilitate capture of wild bears. Bears can be pursued and darted from a helicopter in open areas, such as tundra, alpine meadows, frozen lakes, marshland, or on large clear cuts in the forest. Management situations may dictate that a free-ranging animal is darted by a ground based capture team. These situations can be risky as there is a possibility that the capture team will lose track of the

animal during the induction period. Trained dogs should be available to track the bear if it is lost out of sight after darting.

Aerial capture techniques are best suited for capture of polar bears (*Ursus maritimus*) and brown bears. It is important to assess the terrain for any hazards prior to pursuit. If the bear is in unsuitable terrain, the helicopter can fly at a distance to slowly drive the bear to an area where darting can take place. The dart is delivered at close range (4–6 m). The time of intensive helicopter pursuit, when the helicopter approaches the bear for the actual darting, is usually less than 30 seconds. If a darted bear during the induction period moves toward risky terrain, such as open water, a second dart might be needed to rapidly induce recumbency. In Scandinavia, helicopter darting of family groups including radio-marked mother and dependent offspring (yearlings or 2-year-old cubs, no cubs of a year are being darted) are conducted. Up to four brown bears are captured at once. The cubs are darted one after the other, with the mother being darted last. After successful darting of the first cub, it is being observed from the helicopter at a high altitude throughout the induction period until recumbency, before darting of the next family member. When a darted cub starts to slow down, as the drugs starts to have an effect, the other family members usually leave it and are then not followed by the helicopter for a while. It is often 10–20 minutes between the intensive pursuits for darting of different family members (Fahlman et al. 2011).

The major complications encountered with helicopter darting of bears are hyperthermia and acidosis (Cattet et al. 2003a; Fahlman et al. 2011). The risk of these complications can be minimized by keeping pursuit and induction times as short as possible. Other factors that can influence the degree of exertion during the induction include pursuit intensity (distance and elevation gained), the type of terrain, snow depth, and the ambient temperature.

Drug Delivery

Drug delivery systems must be reliable and accurate. Systems that have low impact energy and deliver drugs at a low velocity are generally preferable. Captive bears may be injected with a pole syringe or blow dart. Volume limitations with blow darts necessitate the use of potent drug combinations for large bears. Potent drugs may be incorporated into a sticky bait, to facilitate capture in zoological settings.

It is advisable to dart free-ranging bears from a safe distance. Dart rifles will facilitate drug delivery in these situations. Many bear species will demonstrate seasonal variation in fat distribution. Black bears and brown bears will deposit a thick layer of fat over the rump in fall, and the shoulder or neck is the preferred location for dart placement. In spring, these animals can be darted in the hindquarters. Polar bears may have a thick layer of fat at any time of the year and the shoulder or neck should be targeted.

MONITORING ANESTHESIA AND SUPPORTIVE CARE

Anesthetic Depth

Depth of anesthesia should be closely monitored as some drug combinations have proven to be unreliable in bears. Sudden recoveries have been encountered with xylazine-ketamine and medetomidine-ketamine (Cattet et al. 1999b; Jalanka & Roeken 1990). These combinations are best avoided in most situations. Factors that increase the risk of sudden arousal include loud noise, particularly distress vocalization of cubs (Jalanka & Roeken 1990). Other factors that can induce arousal include movement of the bear, that is, changing the body position or location of the anesthetized animal, or painful stimuli, such as tooth extraction. Local anesthesia should be considered whenever possible to decrease pain-related stimulation during painful procedures.

Techniques for monitoring depth of anesthesia will depend on the agent used. Zolazepam-tiletamine (Telazol®, Zoletil® [ZT]) will produce reliable anesthesia with predictable signs of recovery. Lightening of anesthesia is evidenced by spontaneous blinking, increased jaw tone, chewing, and paw movement. As the depth of anesthesia further decreases, animals will demonstrate head movement. Animals anesthetized with ZT alone with significant head movement generally require a "top-up" of tiletamine-zolazepam or ketamine, unless they are to be left to recover. Top-up doses of tiletamine-zolazepam can significantly prolong recovery and should only be used if >30 minutes of additional anesthetic time is required. Ketamine is a better choice if 5–20 minutes of additional time is needed.

In xylazine-ketamine or medetomidine-ketamine anesthetized bears, head lifting or limb movement signals that the bear is extremely light and should not be approached or manipulated. Increased intensity of the palpebral reflex or nystagmus are early indicators that the bear is light.

With both xylazine-zolazepam-tiletamine (XZT) or MZT, head lifting should be absent before the bear is approached. The palpebral reflex can be used to determine depth of anesthesia. Lightly anesthetized bears will begin to breathe deeply, and may sigh. They may start to lick, and will develop a spontaneous palpebral and an increased jaw tone. Head lifting or paw movement should be a sign to be extremely cautious, as the bear may soon rouse.

Pulmonary Function

Hypoxemia can occur in bears during anesthesia with different drug protocols, as demonstrated by arterial blood gas studies in brown bears, black bears, and polar bears (Caulkett & Cattet 1997; Caulkett et al. 1999; Fahlman et al. 2011). Both free-ranging and captive brown bears anesthetized with MZT developed hypoxemia, despite lower drug doses used in the captive bears (Fahlman et al. 2011).

Oxygenation can be monitored with a pulse oximeter with the probe placed on the tongue. Pulse oximetry readings may be difficult to achieve in bears lightly anesthetized with ZT, as they tend to chew. A hemoglobin saturation below 95% is indicative of hypoxemia, which can generally be treated with supplemental inspired oxygen. It is important to note that pulse oximetry may not reliably indicate hypoxemia or normoxemia. Inconsistent pulse oximetry values have been reported in polar bears anesthetized with ZT and in brown bears anesthetized with MZT (Cattet et al. 1999a; Fahlman et al. 2010). Since pulse oximeters tend to overestimate saturation at lower ranges of partial pressure of arterial oxygen (PaO_2), hypoxemia can be missed if arterial oxygenation is evaluated only by pulse oximetry (Fig. 41.3).

Portable equipment available to facilitate oxygen delivery include oxygen cylinders and oxygen concentrators. An ambulance-type regulator and aluminum D-cylinder is lightweight, portable, and sturdy. Portable battery driven oxygen concentrators are small, lightweight, and easy to operate. They produce oxygen on site and thus less logistic is necessary compared to when using oxygen cylinders (see Chapter 5 on Oxygen Therapy). A nasal catheter is a simple method to provide supplemental inspired oxygen. Oxygen flow can be adjusted to maintain a saturation of 95–98% with the minimum required oxygen flow. Low flow rates of intranasal oxygen effectively treats hypoxemia in brown bears anesthetized with MZT (Fahlman et al. 2009, 2010). In relation to the body weight of the bears, the following flow rates are recommended: 0.5 L/min to bears up to 25 kg, 1 L/min to bears from 25–100 kg,

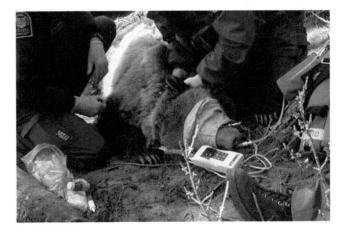

Figure 41.3. Grizzly bear receiving supplemental inspired oxygen.

2 L/min to bears from 100–200 kg, and 3 L/min to bears from 200–250 kg.

Intranasal oxygen administered by pulsed delivery from a portable oxygen concentrator (EverGo™ Portable Oxygen Concentrator, Respironics®) effectively treats hypoxemia in anesthetized brown bears (Fahlman et al. 2012). This concentrator weighs 4.5 kg and it delivers oxygen in a pulsed flow with pulse volumes from 12–70 mL up to a maximum capacity of 1.05 L/min. With pulse dose technology, the negative pressure of the patient's inspiration triggers oxygen delivery. Thus oxygen is provided during the inspiratory phase, which is the crucial time for participation of gas exchange in the lungs. The arterial oxygenation in brown bears improved significantly from mean $\pm$ SD (range) pre-O_2 PaO_2 values of 73 ± 11 (49–93) to 134 ± 29 (90–185) mmHg during supplementation (Fahlman et al. 2012).

Monitoring the Cardiovascular System

The cardiovascular system should be closely monitored. Polar bears, black bears, and brown bears anesthetized with ZT commonly have heart rates of 70–90 beats/min. Heart rate is slightly lower with XZT and MZT, 50–70 beats/min. Bradycardia is common with medetomidine-ketamine, and heart rates of 30–40 beats/min are not uncommon in polar bears. The femoral artery is the best location to palpate a pulse, but the brachial artery can also be used.

Blood pressure can be measured directly from the femoral artery. Oscillometric monitors can be useful in smaller bears. The cuff width should be approximately 0.4 times the limb circumference. Mean arterial pressure (MAP) in polar bears anesthetized with ZT was approximately 150 mmHg (Caulkett et al. 1999). Polar bears anesthetized with MZT are hypertensive (MAP > 200 mmHg) (Caulkett et al. 1999). Black bears are also hypertensive with this combination (Caulkett & Cattet 1997).

Thermoregulation

Rectal temperature should be closely monitored. Rectal temperature tends to decrease over time with ZT, whereas it tends to increase with XZT and MZT. In hot ambient temperatures, after intense physical activity, and in stressed animals, body temperature can increase to dangerous levels (>41°C). Treatment of hyperthermia may include cooling the animal with snow or water, fanning, intravenous drip, cold water enema, and intranasal oxygen.

Supportive Care

The eyes should always be lubricated, and caution must be exercised to avoid corneal abrasions or ulceration. A blindfold should be placed to protect the eyes and decrease visual stimuli.

Bears can be positioned in sternal or lateral recumbency, but can also be positioned in dorsal recumbency with few adverse effects.

When possible, anesthesia should be reversed in free-ranging animals. This is particularly important for sows with cubs, and in areas where high concentrations of bears are present.

Translocation of bears in cargo nets, by helicopter, can result in mortality (Cattet et al. 1999a). Slinging in a cargo net can induce hypertension and hypoxemia (Cattet et al. 1999a). Ideally, these bears should be transported or weighed with their head and neck extended and their body extended (Cattet et al. 1999a). We have used a stretcher-type sling or a "wooden board" to facilitate this positioning. If bears are to be relocated in culvert traps, they should be awake before transport (Fig. 41.4a,b).

PHARMACOLOGICAL CONSIDERATIONS

The following section deals with drug combinations that can be used to anesthetize bears. Mean doses of these combinations can be found in Table 41.1.

Xylazine-Ketamine

This combination may be suitable for short procedures in small bears, but the risk of sudden arousal limits its utility in larger, more aggressive bears. Xylazine can be antagonized with atipamezole or yohimbine, but since a high dose of ketamine is required, adverse effects of the ketamine (rigidity, convulsions, hyperthermia) are unmasked (Ramsay et al. 1985).

Medetomidine-Ketamine

The major advantages of medetomidine-ketamine over xylazine-ketamine are that small volumes are required. Since a low dose of ketamine is used, reversal of the effects of medetomidine with atipamezole is less likely to induce rigidity or convulsions due to ketamine residual effects. Medetomidine-ketamine may be useful for small bears, but should not be used in larger potentially aggressive bears. Sudden recoveries have occurred in brown bears (Jalanka & Roeken 1990), and polar bears (Cattet et al. 1999b). This combination should only be used by experienced personnel, for short procedures, and depth of anesthesia should be closely monitored.

Zolazepam-Tiletamine (Telazol, Zoletil)

This drug combination produces reliable anesthesia in bears. Recovery is usually slow, smooth, and predictable. ZT produces minimal adverse effects on the respiratory or cardiovascular systems; therefore, it has a high margin of safety (Caulkett et al. 1999). The major disadvantages of ZT are lack of analgesia (Caulkett et al. 1999) and lack of reversability (Cattet et al. 1999b; Caulkett et al. 1999). Recovery can be prolonged,

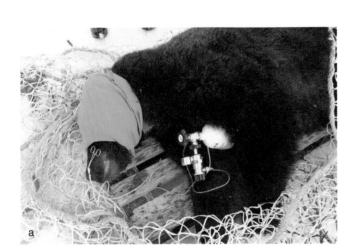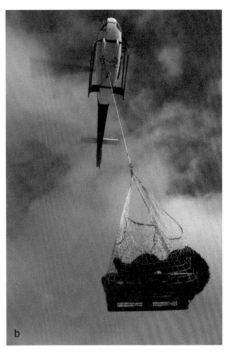

Figure 41.4. (a and b) Intranasal oxygen supplementation from an oxygen cylinder, and positioning on a palate during translocation of a brown bear.

Table 41.1. Recommended mean doses (mg/kg) of immobilizing agents used to facilitate capture of free-ranging American black bears, brown bears, and polar bears

Drug Combination	Black Bear	Brown Bear	Polar Bear
Xylazine/ketamine	2/4	NR	NR
Medetomidine/ketamine	0.04/1.5	NR	NR
Medetomidine/zolazepam-tiletamine	0.05/2	Free ranging 0.08/4.1 Captive 0.03/2.2	0.06/2.2
Xylazine/zolazepam-tiletamine	2/3	2.5/3.8	2/3
Zolazepam-tiletamine	7	8	8

NR, not recommended in this species.

particularly in large bears, and if repeated doses are administered.

Medetomidine-Zolazepam-Tiletamine (MZT)

This combination can be delivered in small volumes, which increases its utility in large polar bears or brown bears. MZT provides better analgesia than ZT alone (Caulkett et al. 1999). The major advantage of this combination is that it is readily and rapidly reversible with atipamezole, administered IM at three to five times the medetomidine dose. The major disadvantages of MZT are hypertension and hypoxemia (Caulkett & Cattet 1997; Caulkett et al. 1999; Fahlman et al. 2011). Hypoxemia can be offset by the provision of supplemental oxygen (Fahlman et al. 2010). MZT has been used in black bears (Caulkett & Cattet 1997), polar

bears (Cattet et al. 1999b), and brown bears (Arnemo et al. 2001; Fahlman et al. 2011).

Xylazine-Zolazepam-Tiletamine (XZT)

XZT has many of the same characteristics as MZT (Cattet et al. 2003b, 2003c). It provides analgesia and can be delivered at approximately half the volume of ZT alone. XZT produces hypertension and hypoxemia (Cattet et al. 2003b). Hypoxemia is generally not severe and responds well to supplemental inspired oxygen. XZT will produce effective immobilization. It is important to note that quality of anesthesia is different from ZT alone, and head lifting or limb movement may immediately precede arousal. This combination is potentially reversible with yohimbine or atipamezole, whereas tolazoline appears to be ineffective. Our current experience is that although recovery is not as rapid as with medetomidine-ketamine or MZT, it is still faster than with ZT alone. The longer recovery is probably a result of the higher ZT requirement with this mixture, compared with MZT. We generally use 0.1–0.2 mg/kg of yohimbine or 0.1 mg/kg of atipamezole to antagonize the xylazine component of this mixture.

Oral and Intranasal Drug Administration

Oral or intranasal drug administration may be preferable in captive bears, when injection is not desired. Carfentanil has been used orally in captive bears (Mama et al. 2000; Mortenson & Bechert 2001; Ramsay et al. 1995). The drug can be mixed in honey. The sticky base will coat the mouth and allow for sublingual absorption. In black bears, oral carfentanil produced effective immobilization that was accompanied by rigidity and muscle tremors (Ramsay et al. 1995). Diazepam was administered at a dose of 25 mg IV to treat these tremors (Ramsay et al. 1995). Bears immobilized with oral carfentanil were hypoxemic; this was readily treated with supplemental inspired oxygen (Ramsay et al. 1995).

Volatile Anesthesia

Volatile anesthesia may be required for invasive or prolonged procedures. The bear is induced with one of the earlier injectable drug combinations, intubated, and maintained on volatile anesthesia delivered via an appropriately sized circuit. Bears under 150 kg body weight may be maintained on a small animal circle system. A large animal machine should be used for heavier animals. Isoflurane is a good choice for maintenance of anesthesia. Isoflurane-induced vasodilation tends to offset the hypertension that can result from administration of potent alpha-2 agonists. The major side effects of isoflurane are hypotension and respiratory depression. It is advisable to monitor blood pressure and end tidal or arterial CO_2 in bears anesthetized with isoflurane (Fig. 41.5).

Recovery from isoflurane is generally smooth. Alpha-2 agonist drugs should be antagonized at the termination of surgery to hasten recovery.

SPECIES-SPECIFIC CONCERNS

Polar Bear (*U. maritimus*)

Polar bears can have substantial fat deposits throughout the year. The shoulder and neck are the best sites for drug delivery. Male polar bears can be large and heavy. Potent drug combinations are required to keep drug volume and dart size to a minimum. Polar bears should be positioned carefully to avoid excessive pressure on limbs that could result in compartment syndrome. In summer, polar bears enter a hypometabolic state. At this time of the year, animals are fasting and body temperature is decreased (34–35°C). Immobilizing

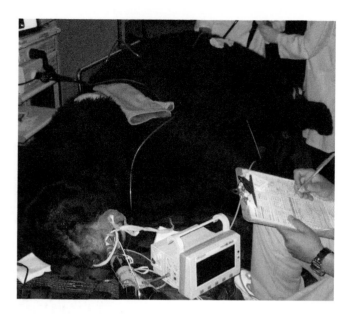

Figure 41.5. Maintenance of anesthesia with isoflurane in a black bear.

drug requirements may also be decreased at this time of the year. In areas where large numbers of polar bears congregate, reversible anesthetic protocols should be considered. This will decrease the risk of predation from other bears. Reversible protocols should also be considered for mother bears with cubs.

Zolazepam-tiletamine (Table 41.1) will produce reliable immobilization, but can also result in prolonged recoveries. Volume requirements are high, which will necessitate the use of large darts, and this can result in excessive tissue trauma.

Xylazine-zolazepam-tiletamine (Table 41.1) can be delivered at approximately half the volume of ZT alone. Although potentially reversible with yohimbine or atipamezole, reversal of this mixture is not reliable. This is probably due to residual ZT sedation. Animals immobilized with this mixture will benefit from supplemental inspired oxygen.

Medetomidine-zolazepam-tiletamine (Table 41.1) will produce reliable immobilization. This combination will produce rapid onset of immobilization; it can be delivered in a small volume and it is readily reversible with atipamezole, administered at five times the medetomidine dose. Animals will benefit from supplemental inspired oxygen (Caulkett et al. 1999).

Brown Bear (*U. arctos*)

A variety of techniques can be used to anesthetize brown bears. Drug combinations should be reliable and potent. Reversible combinations are desirable in certain situations, particularly in free-ranging sows with cubs. Brown bears enter a hypometabolic state in the winter. Drug requirements are decreased at this time (Evans et al. 2010).

Zolazepam-tiletamine (Table 41.1) is routinely used for management of brown bears in North America. ZT will not only produce reliable immobilization but can also result in prolonged recoveries. High volume requirements necessitate the use of large darts, which can produce excessive tissue trauma.

Xylazine-zolazepam-tiletamine (Table 41.1) is potentially reversible with yohimbine or atipamezole. Reversal of this mixture is not reliable. This is probably due to residual effects of ZT. Animals immobilized with this mixture will benefit from supplemental inspired oxygen.

Medetomidine-zolazepam-tiletamine (Table 41.1) will induce a rapid onset of immobilization and it can be delivered in a small volume. It is readily reversible with atipamezole, administered at five times the medetomidine dose. MZT is the drug combination of choice used for immobilization of brown bears in Scandinavia (Arnemo et al. 2001; Fahlman et al. 2011). Doses and physiological evaluation of capture and MZT anesthesia in brown bears have been described in detail (Fahlman et al. 2011).

Low doses of MZT + ketamine (MZTK) can be used for anesthesia of free-ranging brown bears during hibernation in the wild (Evans et al. 2010). Two to 4-year-old bears were darted in their dens with medetomidine at 0.02–0.6 mg/kg, ZT at 0.9–2.8 mg/kg, and ketamine at 1.1–3.0 mg/kg. Hypoxemia was corrected with intranasal oxygen therapy. One bear that was darted with the higher dose of MZTK developed apnea and was intubated followed by manual ventilation with a bag valve mask.

Oral carfentanil has been used at a dose of 8 µg/kg in a captive brown bear. This dose-induced deep sedation, sufficient for intubation to maintain anesthesia on isoflurane and oxygen. The bear also received 0.02 mg/kg of atropine IM. Naltrexone was administered at a dose of 0.42 mg/kg split IM and IV to speed recovery (Mama et al. 2000).

American Black Bears (*U. americanus*)

These bears have a more placid nature than brown bears; dose requirements are lower with ZT. A variety of drugging techniques can be used. Black bears are frequently immobilized for management purposes in North America. The bear may be snared or captured in a culvert trap prior to drug administration. Physical capture of the bear will facilitate drug administration and limit mobility on induction. Free-ranging bears are often treed prior to drug administration. This will also facilitate drug administration and decrease mobility on induction. Ideally, a coniferous tree should be picked, as the boughs will help to break the bear's fall on induction. Air filled bags or mattresses can be placed at the base of the tree to soften the landing. Bears that remain in the tree, after induction, may need to be placed in a sling and lowered with ropes.

Zolazepam-tiletamine (Table 41.1) will produce reliable immobilization and can be delivered at a relatively low volume in most bears.

Xylazine-zolazepam-tiletamine (Table 41.1) is a useful combination in black bears. The dose we have used is similar to a brown bear or polar bear dose. The dose could possibly be lowered. Further work is needed to determine an appropriate dose for this species.

Medetomidine-zolazepam-tiletamine (Table 41.1) will induce a rapid onset of immobilization; it can be delivered in a small volume and it is readily reversible with atipamezole, administered at five times the medetomidine dose. Animals will benefit from supplemental inspired oxygen (Fahlman et al. 2010).

Xylazine-ketamine (Table 41.1) can be used, cautiously, in black bears. It is important to monitor the bear closely for signs of arousal. Rapid nystagmus and brisk tongue withdrawal are signs of light anesthesia. An IV top up of xylazine-ketamine at one-third of the original dose may be considered, or procedures may be terminated.

Oral carfentanil has been used in captive black bears. A dose of 6.8–18 µg/kg was administered in honey. Bears demonstrated muscle rigidity that was readily treated with diazepam (10–25 mg IV). Bears also developed hypoxemia that resolved with 5 L/min of supplemental oxygen (Ramsay et al. 1995).

Sloth Bear (*Melurus ursinus*), Sun Bear (*Ursus malayanus*), Asiatic Black Bear (*Ursus thibetanus*), Spectacled Bear (*Tremarctos ornatus*), and Giant Panda (*Ailuropda melanoleucia*)

These species are grouped at the end of the section because there is a paucity of information in the literature about anesthesia of these animals. It is very probable that XZT, MZT, or oral carfentanil will be as effective in these species as in other bear species. ZT has been used in sun bears at a dose of 4.0–5.5 mg/kg, in sloth bears at a dose of 5.5–6.6 mg/kg, in Asiatic black bears at a dose of 2.8–4.4 mg/kg, and in spectacled bears at a dose of 3.2–11.1 mg/kg (Schobert 1987). Sloth bears have been anesthetized with 1.4–2.4 mg/kg of xylazine, combined with 5.8–9.7 mg/kg of ketamine (Page 1986). Sun bears have been anesthetized with 60–80 µg/kg of medetomidine + 2–3 mg/kg of ketamine (Jalanka & Roeken 1990). Giant pandas have been anesthetized with a variety of drug combinations. Ketamine at a dose of 4.8 mg/kg in combination with xylazine at 0.43 mg/kg has been described as a suitable protocol for healthy pandas (Kreeger et al. 2002). Alternatively, 5.8 mg/kg of ZT can be used (Kreeger et al. 2002).

REFERENCES

Arnemo JM, Brunberg S, Ahlqvist P, et al. 2001. Reversible immobilization and anesthesia of free-ranging brown bears (*Ursus arctos*) with medetomidine-tiletamine-zolazepam and atipamezole: a review of 575 captures. Proceedings of the Annual Meeting of the American Association of Zoo Veterinarians, pp. 234–236.

Cattet M, Stenhouse G, Bollinger T. 2008. Exertional myopathy in a grizzly bear (*Ursus arctos*) captured by leghold snare. *Journal of Wildlife Diseases* 44:973–978.

Cattet MRL, Caulkett NA, Streib KA, Torske KE, Ramsay MA. 1999a. Cardiopulmonary response of anesthetized polar bears to suspension by net and sling. *Journal of Wildlife Diseases* 35:548–556.

Cattet MRL, Caulkett NA, Polischuk SC, Ramsay MA. 1999b. Anesthesia of polar bears with zolazepam-tiletamine, medetomidine-ketamine, and medetomidine-zolazepam-tiletamine. *Journal of Zoo and Wildlife Medicine* 30:354–360.

Cattet MRL, Christison K, Caulkett NA, Stenhouse GB. 2003a. Physiologic responses of grizzly bears to different methods of capture. *Journal of Wildlife Diseases* 39:649–654.

Cattet MRL, Caulkett NA, Lunn NJ. 2003b. Anesthesia of polar bears using xylazine-zolazepam-tiletamine or zolazepam-tiletamine. *Journal of Wildlife Diseases* 39(3):655–664.

Cattet MRL, Caulkett NA, Stenhouse GB. 2003c. Anesthesia of grizzly bears using xylazine-zolazepam-tiletamine or zolazepam-tiletamine. *Ursus* 14:88–93.

Cattet MRL, Caulkett NA, Boulanger JG, Duval J, Cranston J, Stenhouse GB. September/ 2005. Long-term health effects of capture and handling of grizzly bears in West-Central Alberta: Implications for Animal Welfare and Good Science. Proceedings of The International Bear Association Annual Meeting, September 2005, Riva Del Garde.

Caulkett NA, Cattet MRL. 1997. Physiological effects of medetomidine-zolazepam-tiletamine immobilization in black bears (*Ursus americanus*). *Journal of Wildlife Diseases* 33: 618–622.

Caulkett NA, Cattet MRL, Caulkett JM, Polischuk SC. 1999. Comparative physiological effects of Telazol, medetomidine-ketamine, and medetomidine-Telazol in polar bears (*Ursus maritimus*). *Journal of Zoo and Wildlife Medicine* 30:504–509.

Evans A, Madslien K, Fahlman Å, Brunberg S, Støen O-G, Frøbert O, Swenson JE, Arnemo JM. 2010. Capture and anesthesia of free-ranging brown bears during hibernation. Abstract. Proceedings of the American Association of Zoo Veterinarians/ American Association of Wildlife Veterinarians Joint Conference, South Padre Island, Texas, USA, pp. 24–29.

Fahlman Å, Arnemo JM, Pringle J. 2009. Blue blood in brown bears (*Urus arctos*): effects of intranasal oxygen therapy on hypoxemia during anesthesia. Proceedings of the American Association of Zoo Veterinarians/American Association of Wildlife veterinarians Joint Conference, Tulsa, Oklahoma, USA, p. 96.

Fahlman Å, Pringle J, Arnemo JM, et al. 2010. Treatment of hypoxemia during anesthesia of brown bears (*Ursus arctos*). *Journal of Zoo and Wildlife Medicine* 41:161–164.

Fahlman Å, Arnemo JM, Swenson JE, et al. 2011. Physiologic evaluation of capture and anesthesia with medetomidine-zolazepam-tiletamine in brown bears (*Ursus arctos*). *Journal of Zoo and Wildlife Medicine* 42:1–11.

Fahlman Å, Caulkett N, Arnemo JM, et al. 2012. Efficacy of a portable oxygen concentrator with pulsed delivery for treatment of hypoxemia during anesthesia of wildlife. *Journal of Zoo and Wildlife Medicine* 43:67–76.

Jalanka HH, Roeken BO. 1990. The use of medetomidine, medetomidine-ketamine combinations, and atipamezole in nondomestic mammals: a review. *Journal of Zoo and Wildlife Medicine* 21:259–282.

Kreeger TJ, Arnemo JM, Raath JP. 2002. *Handbook of Wildlife Chemical Immobilization*. Fort Collins: Wildlife Pharmaceuticals Inc. 236.

Mama KR, Steffey EP, Withrow SJ. 2000. Use of orally administered carfentanil prior to isoflurane-induced anesthesia in a Kodiak brown bear. *Journal of the American Veterinary Medical Association* 217:546–549.

Mortenson J, Bechert U. 2001. Carfentanil citrate used as an oral anesthetic agent for brown bears (*Ursus arctos*). *Journal of Zoo and Wildlife Medicine* 32:217–221.

Onuma M. 2003. Immobilization of sun bears (*Malayanus helarctos*) with medetomidine-zolazepam-tiletamine. *Journal of Zoo and Wildlife Medicine* 34:202–205.

Page CD. 1986. Sloth bear immobilization with a ketamine-xylazine combination: reversal with yohimbine. *Journal of the American Veterinary Medical Association* 189:1050–1051.

Ramsay EC, Sleeman JM, Clyde VL. 1995. Immobilization of black bears (*Ursus americanus*) with orally administered carfentanil citrate. *Journal of Wildlife Diseases* 31:391–393.

Ramsay MA, Stirling I, Knutsen LØ, Broughton E. 1985. Use of yohimbine hydrochloride to reverse immobilization of polar bears by ketamine hydrochloride and xylazine hydrochloride. *Journal of Wildlife Diseases* 21:396–400.

Schobert E. 1987. Telazol use in wild and exotic animals. *Veterinary Medicine* 82:1080–1088.

42 Procyonids and Mustelids

George V. Kollias and Noha Abou-Madi

INTRODUCTION

Chemical restraint and anesthesia techniques and protocols applicable to captive mammals in the families Mustelidae and Procyonidae are similar in many respects to the techniques used for domestic dogs and cats. Chemical restraint and anesthesia of free-ranging members of these families present challenges not dissimilar to those encountered for mammals in other families and genera, including the capture techniques employed and stress associated with capture and restraint. The metabolic impact of physical restraint and general anesthesia on animals is often underestimated. As an example, ferrets manually restrained showed significant increase in their plasma concentration of cortisol and andrenocorticotropic hormone (ACTH) and a decrease in alpha-melanocyte stimulating hormone (MSH), while isoflurane anesthesia resulted in significant increase in plasma MSH directly after induction (Schoemaker et al. 2003). Applying the basic principles of restraint and anesthesia are essential to insuring a successful outcome. Specialized equipment and supplies (small endotracheal tubes, special face masks, small intravenous and intraosseous catheters, and cannulas) should be on hand at the outset of the procedure. Additionally, emergency drug doses should be calculated and drawn up in labeled syringes or vials prior to beginning the anesthetic procedures. Attempting to calculate, draw up, and administer emergency drugs for a 50g (1.8oz) ermine can be problematic at the time of an anesthetic emergency. Drug dosages used are extrapolated from the dog or cat unless specific doses are available for species such as the ferret (Carpenter & Marion 2013).

BIOLOGY

Mustelidae

Mustelids are members of the order Carnivora, which contains six additional families. There are 67 species of mutelids in 27 genera that include the wolverine, fisher, nearctic otter, sea otter, polecat, marten, ferret, badger, tayra, grison, and skunk. Mustelids are distributed in all continents except Antarctica and Australia. The otters have the widest distribution, being found in North, Central, and South America as well as in Africa, Europe, and Asia. Mustelid habitats range from Arctic tundra to tropical rainforest and they are terrestrial, arboreal, fossorial, and found on the open seas, as with the sea otter. Many are small (<1kg or 2.2lbs), while some are relatively large (45kg or 99lbs) when compared to members of other mammalian families. The smallest, the weasel, rarely exceeds 19cm (7.5in) in length. The giant river otter is the longest mustelid reaching a length of up to 190cm (6.2ft). Most are carnivorous (otter and fisher) but some are omnivorous (skunk). All have five toes on each foot with nonretractable claws. Sexual dimorphism is marked in most mustelids but is less apparent in badgers, otters, and skunks. Male skull size may range 5–25% longer than that of females. Mustelids process prominent sharp canines, cutting carnassials, heavy premolars, and powerful jaws that are capable of crushing thick bones. The dental formula varies within and between subfamilies. As examples, the European common weasel has the dental formula of I 3/3, C 1/1, P 3/3, M 1/2 = 36, whereas the dental formula of the wolverine is I 3/3, C 1/1, P 4/4, M 1/2 = 36. Mustelids lack both a clavicle and an appendix. The otters, like other

Zoo Animal and Wildlife Immobilization and Anesthesia, Second Edition. Edited by Gary West, Darryl Heard, and Nigel Caulkett.
© 2014 John Wiley & Sons, Inc. Published 2014 by John Wiley & Sons, Inc.

aquatic carnivores, have a multilobulated (reniculated) kidney (Baitchman & Kollias 2000). The renal lobules are firmly compressed against each other, forming a somewhat solid kidney. Musk is present in most species and produced by modified sebaceous glands present and stored in perianal sacs. The composition of musk varies between species and is used for demarcation of territory often for generations. In the case of skunks, musk is used for defense purposes. The reproductive biology of mustelids also varies between species, with males and females of most species living separately the majority of the year. Mustelids are induced ovulators and require vigorous copulation for ovulation. Males have a baculum (os penis) and females an os clitoris. Delayed implantation, up to 10 months, is exhibited in 16/67 mustelid species. The mediators of delayed implantation are largely unknown and may include environmental factors such as photoperiod. Delayed implantation can occur in semidormancy.

Procyonidae

The Procyonidae are small- to medium-sized, long-bodied, and long-tailed mammals in the order Carnivora. There are 16 New World species including the raccoon, white-nosed coati, kinkajou, and so on. New World procyonids inhabit temperate, tropical, and neotropical regions. Procyonids are generally omnivores but are known to be opportunistic carnivores. The dental formula is I 3/3, C 1/1, P 4/4, M2/2 = 40. An exception to this formula is the kinkajou which has P3/3. The molars of all procyonids are large and well adapted to crushing. There is some interspecies variation in dentition which relates to food preferences. Subsequently procyonids have highly specialized gastrointestinal systems with all members of the family lacking a cecum. The feet of procyonids have five toes and they walk partly or wholly on the soles of their feet (plantigrade). Claws are nonretractable, except the ringtails which have semiretractable claws on their front feet. All procyonids have agile front feet which make them excellent climbers. Excepting the coati, procyonids are generally nocturnal or crepuscular. Females usually breed in the spring of their first year and males from their second year on. The small procyonids live 10–15 years in captivity. The authors are aware of a male kinkajou that lived until 32 years of age in a zoo. In the wild, it is unusual for procyonids to exceed 7 years of age.

CHEMICAL RESTRAINT, IMMOBILIZATION, AND ANESTHESIA

Delivery of injectable agents to procyonids and mustelids, as with other wild mammals, often requires physical restraint and specialized supplies and equipment (see Chapters 8 and 12). Squeeze cages or boxes and transfer boxes (Fig. 42.1 and Fig. 42.2) greatly facilitate delivery of injectable drugs and help to minimize stress

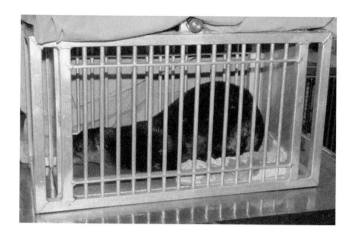

Figure 42.1. Large procyonids and mustelids are restrained in squeeze cages to facilitate intramuscular injection of parenteral anesthetic drugs.

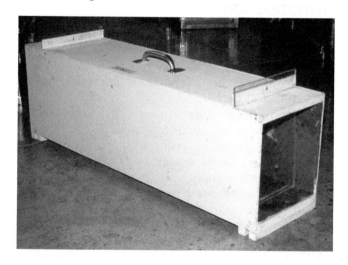

Figure 42.2. A transport cage for a Nearctic river otter (*L. canadensis*). Note the solid wood sides to reduce visual stimulation and prevent damage to the teeth and feet that can occur when confined to a wire cage. A clear door allows inspection of the animal during transport.

while maximizing the quality of induction, immobilization, and recovery of procyonids and mustelids. As an example, when recently captured nearctic river otters (*Lontra canadensis*) are transferred from their holding cages to a small squeeze cage, injected, and the squeeze cage is then covered with a drape or towel and minimal environmental noise occurs, the otters are consistently immobilized in 10–12 minutes and remained so for 35–45 minutes. If this protocol is not consistently adhered to otters never reach an acceptable level of immobilization, complications such as hyperthermia occur due to excessive movement, and recovery is unacceptable due to hyperkinesis vocalization and disorientation (Kollias 1999). Numerous general and specific single drugs or drug combinations have been reported for chemical restraint, immobilization, and anesthesia of procyonids (Table 42.1 and Table 42.2) and mustelids (Table 42.3 and Table 42.4).

Table 42.1. General Procyonidae chemical restraint agent doses (IM)

Agent(s) and Dose(s)	Reversal Agent	Comments
Ketamine (10–30 mg/kg)[a]	None	High end of dose range used for smaller animals
Ketamine (10 mg/kg) + diazepam (0.5 mg/kg)[a]		Minimal respiratory depression
Ketamine (10 mg/kg) + midazolam (0.25–0.5 mg/kg)[a]		Minimal respiratory depression
Ketamine (10 mg/kg) + xylazine (1–2 mg/kg)[b]		Good muscle relaxation
Ketamine (2.0–5.0 mg/kg) + medetomidine (0.025–0.05 kg)[c]	Antipamezole (0.1 mg/kg) Ketamine: none	
Ketamine (5–15 mg/kg) + xylazine (1–2 mg/kg) + atropine (0.04 mg/kg)[d]		Induction: 3–5 minutes Anesthesia: 15–20 minutes Recovery: 60–90 minutes
Tiletamine/zolazepam (10–25 mg/kg)[a]	Tiletamine: none Zolazepam: flumazenil	Chemical capture and minor surgery
Tiletamine/zolazepam (3–5 mg/kg)[e]	Tiletamine: none Zolazepam: flumazenil	

[a]Labate et al. (2001).
[b]Nielsen (1999).
[c]Jalanka and Roeken (1990).
[d]Mehren (1986).
[e]Denver (1999).

Table 42.2. Specific Procyonidae chemical restraint agent doses (IM)

Adult Weight Range (kg)	Agents and Doses (mg/kg)	Reversal Agent (mg/kg)	Comments
Coatimundi (*Nausa* spp.)			
3–6	Ketamine + xylazine[a]	None reported	
3–13	Medetomidine(0.051–0.064) + ketamine (2.5–7.7) + butorphanol(0.34–0.36)[b]	atipamezole (0.25) (1/2 SC; 1/2 IM)	Prolonged recovery in some cases with higher ketamine doses
Olingo (*Bassaricyon gabbii*)			
0.9–1.5	Tiletamine/zolazepam (5)[a]		Supplement with ketamine (5)
Raccoon (*Procyon lotor*)			
2–12	Ketamine (20) + xylazine (4)[c]	Yohimbine (0.15)	
	Tiletamine/zolazepam (12)[c]		Alternatives
	Ketamine (20) + acepromazine (0.1)		
	Tiletamine/zolazepam (3) + xylazine (2)[d]		60 minutes handling time; 120 minutes to full recovery
Kinkajou (*Potus flavas*)			
1.4–4.6	Ketamine (5.5) + medetomidine (0.1)[e]	Atipamezole (0.5)	Wild/free-ranging kinkajous
	Ketamine (25)[d]		Alternative choice
	Tiletamine/zolazepam (10)[d]		Alternative choice
Ringtail (*Bassariscus astutus*)			
0.8–1.3	Tiletamine/zolazepam (10)[a]		
	Ketamine (10) + acepromazine (0.2)[f]		Alternative choice

[a]Seal and Kreeger (1987).
[b]Georoff et al. (2004).
[c]Kreeger et al. (2002).
[d]Belant (2004).
[e]Fournier et al. (1998).
[f]Jessup (1982).

Table 42.3. General mustelid chemical restraint agent doses (IM)

Agents and Doses (mg/kg)	Reversal Agent (mg/kg)	Comments
Ketamine (10) + xylazine (1–2)[a]	Xylazine: yohimbine (0.125) or antipamezole (0.02–0.06)	
Ketamine (10–15)[a]	None	
Tiletamine/zolazepam (3–6)[a]	None	
Ketamine (10–40)[b]	None	Immobilization
Ketamine (20) + xylazine (2)[b]	Xylazine: same as above	Immobilization
Tiletamine/zolazepam (1.5–10)[b]	None	Higher end of dosage range may produce prolonged recovery
Ketamine (22) + diazepam (0.4)[b]	None given	
Tiletamine/zolazepam (2.2–22)[c]	Zolazepam: flumazenil (0.05–0.10)	Reported for numerous species of mustelids

[a]Fowler (2008).
[b]Pimentel et al. (2001).
[c]Fernandez-Moran (1999).

Table 42.4. Specific mustelid chemical restraint agent doses (IM)

Adult Weight Range (kg)	Agents and Doses (mg/kg)	Reversal Agent (mg/kg)	Comments
Badger, European (*Meles meles*)			
5.5–12.5	Ketamine (20)[a]	None	Recovery considered prolonged; 0h = 170 beats/min
0 = 9.3	Ketamine (15) + midazolam (0.4)[a]	None given	Few advantages over ketamine alone; 0h = 150 beats/min
	Ketamine (10) + midazolam (1.0)[a]	None given	Few advantages over ketamine alone; 0h = 160 beats/min
	Ketamine (5) + medetomidine (0.808)[a]	Medetomidine: atipamezole (0.80)	Best quality of maintenance; lower mean HR than other agents used (0 = 100 beats/min); 0 arterial blood pressure = 150mmHg was higher than other agents used; early reversal with antipamezole may cause excitement
	Ketamine (5–10) + medetomidine (0.05–0.10)[b]	Medetomidine: atipamezole (0.25–0.50)	Preferred combination
	Tiletamine/zolazepam (2.5) + medetomidine (0.04)[b]	Medetomidine: Atipamezole (0.20)	Alternative combination
10–16	Tiletamine + zolazepam (10)[c]		Supplement with ketamine (5mg/kg)
	Ketamine (15) + acepromazine (0.4)[c]		
	Ketamine (16) xylazine (6)[c]		
n = 93	Medetomidine (0.02) + ketamine (0.04) + butorphanol (0.08)[d]	None given	Induction slower than ketamine, but quality of induction similar (range = 3–22 minutes 0 = 6 minutes); paler mucous membranes than ketamine alone; recovery 37–39 minutes; sudden arousal or recovery occurred in 14/93 (15%) of the badgers using these combinations and was statistically linked to increasing rectal temperature
5.5–12.5	Medetomidine (0.02) + ketamine (0.04) + butorphanol (0.06)[d]	None given	
	Medetomidine (0.02) + ketamine (0.06) + butorphanol (0.04)[d]	None given	
Badger, Chinese ferret (*Melogale moschata*)			
1–3	Tiletamine/zolazepam (5)[c]		
Badger, hog (*Arctonyx collaris*)			
7–14	Tiletamine/zolazepam (4.4)[c]		Supplement with ketamine (5 mg/kg)
Badger, honey (ratel) (*Mellivora capensis*)			
7–13	Tiletamine/zolazepam (2.2)[e]		Supplement with ketamine (2.2mg/kg)
	Ketamine (6) + xylazine (0.5)[e]		Supplement with ketamine (2.2mg/kg)
Badger, American (*Taxidea taxus*)			
4–12	Tiletamine/zolazepam (4.4)[f]		Supplement with ketamine (4.4mg/kg)
	Ketamine (15) + xylazine (1)[f]		Alternative choice
Ermine (*Mustela erminea*)			
0.05–0.365	Ketamine (5) + medetomidine (0.0001 mg/gm) (0.1)[c]	Atipamezole (0.0005 mg/gm) (0.5); 1/2 IV + 1/2 IM	Supplement with ketamine (2.5)
	Tiletamine/zolazepam (0.011–0.022 mg/gm) (11–22)[b]		
Black-footed ferret (*Mustela nigripes*)			
0.7–1.5	Ketamine (3) + medetomidine (0.075)[b]	Medetomidine: atipamezole (0.375); 1/2 IV + 1/2 IM	
Ferret (*Mustela putorius*)			
	Ketamine (35) + diazepam (0.2)		

Dose	Drug	Antagonist	Comments
0.6–1.2	Ketamine (25) + xylazine (2)[c]		Supplement with ketamine (12)
	Ketamine (25) + acepromazine (1.1)[c]		
	Tiletamine/zolazepam (15)[c]	Medetomidine: Atipamezole (0.50)	Recovery may be prolonged
	Ketamine (5) + medetomidine (0.1)		
	Ketamine (10–30) + xylazine (1–2) or diazepam (1–2) or acepromazine (0.05–0.30)[b]		Anesthesia; poor analgesia
	Ketamine (25–35) + diazepam (2–3)[g]	Medetomidine:	Anesthesia; monitor blood pressure and ventilation
	Medetomidine (0.08) + butorphanol (0.1)[g]		
	Ketamine (5) + medetomidine (0.08)[h]	Atipamezole (0.40)	Induction for inhalation anesthesia
	Ketamine (5) + medetomidine (0.08) + butorphanol (0.1)[h]	Medetomidine: antipamezole (0.40) + butorphanol: naleoxone (0.01–0.04)	Induction for inhalation anesthesia
	Ketamine (5–10) + midazolam (0.25–0.50)[h]		Induction for inhalation anesthesia
	Propofol (5–8 IV)[i]	None	Anesthesia induction
	Diazepam (0.5–3.0 SC or IM)[i]		Premedication
	Butorphanol (0.1–0.5 SC, IM, IV)[i]	Naloxone (0.01–0.04)	Premedication analgesia
	Buprenorphine (0.01–0.03 SC, IM, IV)[i]	Naloxone (0.01–0.04)	Premedication analgesia
	Oxymorphone (0.05–0.2 SC, IM, IV)[i]	Naloxone (0.01–0.04)	Premedication analgesia
	Morphine (0.2–2.0 SC, IM)[i]	Naloxone (0.01–0.04)	Premedication analgesia
	Meperidine (5–10 SC, IM)[i]	Naloxone (0.01–0.04)	Premedication analgesia
	Atropine (0.02–0.05)[i]	None	Premedication to maintain heart rate and decrease secretions
	Glycopyrrolate (0.01)[i]	None	Premedication to maintain heart rate and decrease secretions
	Acepromazine (0.1) + butorphanol (0.2) + glycopyrrolate (0.01)[i]	Butorphanol: naloxone (0.01–0.04)	Premedication—moderate to deep sedation
	Midazolam (0.5) + oxymorphone (0.1) + glycopyrrolate (0.01)[i]	Oxymorphone: naloxone (0.01–0.04)	Premedication—moderate to deep sedation
	Acepromazine (0.05) + butorphanol (0.1) + ketamine (10)[i]	Burtorphanol: naloxone (0.01–0.04)	Premedication—moderate to deep sedation
Ferret, European or polecat (M. putorius)			
Male (n = 11) 0.84–1.04	Ketamine (10) + medetomidine (0.20)[j]	Medetomidine: atipamezole (1.0 IM) injected 28.1–54.0 minutes after ket/med injection; standing in 1.5–9.4 minutes; ambulatory in 10.0–25.7 minutes	Free-ranging polecats; captured for clinical examination; blood collection and placement of intra-abdominal radio transmitters; induction smooth and rapid (0.7–3.9 minutes); degree of anesthesia and muscle relaxation satisfactory in most individuals; all animals exhibited decreased heart rate and respiratory rate, and temperature; hypothermia was significant and was controlled/prevented by placing animals on a warmed plastic table (37°C).
Female (n = 1) 0.64			
Fisher (Martes pennanti)			
2.6–5.5	Tiletamine/zolazepam (11)[k]	None used	Wild caught/trapped
	Ketamine (30) + xylazine (3)[k]	Xylazine: antipamezole (0.02–0.06 1/2 IM, 1/2 SC) after 45 minutes immobilization	Wild caught/trapped; high dose range
4.7–5.8 (males)	Ketamine (3.2–4.2) + medetomidine (0.062–0.078)[l]	None given	Recently wild caught; 0 induction time = 4.6 minutes 0 down time = 142 minutes; 0 alert time = 147 minutes; 0 recovery time = 200 minutes; mild bradycardia and hypertension; calm recovery; temp = 38–40°C
2.3–2.9 (females)	Ketamine (3.3–3.9) + medetomidine (0.063–0.077)[l]	None given	
4.7–5.8 (males)	Ketamine (16.9–20.5)	None	
	Ketamine (17.0–21.4)	None	

(Continued)

611

Table 42.4. (Continued)

Adult Weight Range (kg)	Agents and Doses (mg/kg)	Reversal Agent (mg/kg)	Comments
2.6–5.5	Ketamine (20) + medetomidine (0.040)[c]	Medetomidine: atipamezole (0.02)	Supplement with ketamine (10)
	Ketamine (20) + acepromazine (0.10)[c]	None	
Marten (Martes americanus)			
0.5–1.5	Ketamine (10) + medetomidine (0.2)[c]	Medetomidine: atipamezole (1; 1/2 IM, 1/2 SC)	Prone to hyperthermia; supplement with ketamine (5)IM if indicated
	Ketamine (18) + xylazine (1.6)[c]	Xylazine: antipamezole (0.02–0.06) or yohimbine (0.2–0.5) IM	
Mink, American (Mustela vison)			
1.13–1.81 0 = 1.51 (males or females)	Ketamine (22.1–24.8) + 0 = 23.2[m]	None	Ranch raised and bred adults ($n = 22$); time to immobilization (lateral recumbency with no purposeful movements) = 2–4 minutes; time to anesthesia (no movement in response to [unspecified] pain) = 5–10 minutes; time to recovery (period from initial injection until mink could stand unaided) = 60 minutes; muscle relaxation improved over 60 minutes period of immobilization
0.8–1.1	Tiletamine/zolazepam (15)[c]	None specified	Supplement with Ketamine IM (15) if appropriate
	Ketamine (5) + medetomidine (0.1)[c]	Atipamezole (5), 1/2 IM, 1/2 SC	Alternative
	Ketamine (40) + xylazine (1)	Xylazine: as above for Marten	Alternative
Mink, European (Mustela lutreola)			
Males ($n = 6$) 0.77–1.03, Females ($n = 8$) 0.42–0.54	Ketamine (10) + medetomidine (0.20)[j]	Medetomidine: Atipamezone (1.0) IM injected 28.1–54.0 minutes after ket/med injection; standing in 1.5–9.4 minutes; ambulatory in 10–25.7 minutes	Free-ranging mink captured for clinical examination, blood collection and placement of intra-abdominal radio transmitters. Induction smooth and rapid (0.7–3.9 minutes); degree of anesthesia and muscle relaxation satisfactory in most individuals; all animals exhibited decreased heart rate and respiratory rate, and rectal temperature. Hypotermia was significant and was controlled/prevented by placing animals on a warmed plastic table (37°C)

Species / Weight	Agent (mg/kg)	Reversal agent (mg/kg)	Comments
Otter Nearctic (American River) (*Lontra canadensis*)			
Males 2.90–9.30; 0 = 5.64	Ketamine (15) + midazolam (0.3) or diazepam (0.5) (male and female > 4.5 kg)[n]	None used	Wild-caught otters immobilized 1–5 days post capture. Conditions of immobilization: restrained in portable squeeze cage, which was covered with a drape to block light and injected IM. Room lights out and no sound stimulation. Induction reached (lateral decumbency and no response to touch) in 10–12 minutes. Immobilization time: 30–45 minutes. Procedures (physical examination, wound care, bandaging, and blood collection) sometimes required administration of one additional 20–30 mg dose of ketamine HCl IV or isoflurane (0.5–1%) via face mask. This provided an additional 20 minute working time. If procedures extended beyond this 20 minute time frame, the otters were intubated, maintained on isoflurane (0.5–1.5%), and given intermittent positive pressure ventilation every 15 seconds if they were hypoventilating. Monitoring included HR (range = 120–264 beats/min; mean = 166), RR (range = 12–56/minutes; mean = 30/minutes) and rectal temperature (range = 99.80–104.7°F; mean = 101.8°F). Otters were recovered in their holding cage (room temp = 60°F) which was padded with towels and the front draped with a sheet to decrease light and sound stimulation. Complete recovery times (normal ambulation and mentation) ranged from 30 to 90 minutes. Hyperthermia may be an issue if otters become hyperactive during recovery. If this occurs, sedation and other corrective measure may be necessary (midazolam IM, placing a fan directed through the cage cars, decreasing ambient temperature). No mortalities, and few complications, occurred using this protocol in over 250 immobilizations and anesthetic episodes.
Females 3.6–8.0; 0 = 5.50	Ketamine (20) + midazolam (0.30) or diazepam (0.5) (male and female < 4.5 kg)[n]	None used	
Otter, Asian small clawed (*Aonyx cinerea*)			
Males and females combined (free ranging; in some geographic locations (males may be 17% heavier than females);	Ketamine (10) + midazolam (0.25)[o]	None given	Highly recommended
	Ketamine (2.5) + medetomidine (0.025)[o]	Medetomidine: atipamezole (0.125)	Avoid in hypothermic otters. May need higher doses (Ket 3.5 + Med 0.035mg/kg) but respiratory depression more likely
	Tiletamine/zolazepam (4–8)[o]	Zolazepam: flumazenil (0.08) IM	Recovery may be prolonged without flumazenil
Males and females combined (captive) 5.7–13	Ketamine (10)	None	Expect muscle rigidity and variable duration
	Ketamine (10) + diazepam (0.5–1.0)[o]	None given	Prolonged recovery compared with ketamine + midazolam
	Ketamine (5–10) + xylazine (1–2)[o]	Xylazine: yohimbine (0.125)	Variable effects from heavy sedation to immobilization. May get respiratory depression.
1–5	Azaperone (0.1) + fentanyl (0.1–0.2)[o]	Fentanyl: naloxone (0.04)	Not recommended. Reports of fatal complications.
	Ketamine (15–18) + midazolam (0.75–1.0)[b]	Medetomidine: atipamezole (0.50–0.60) IM	
	Ketamine (4–5) + medetomidine (0.10–0.12)[b]	Zolazepam: flumazenil (0.08) IM	Respiratory depression may occur. Avoid in cold environments—hypothermia.
	Tiletamine/zolazepam (6–9)[o]		
Otter, clawless (*Aonyx capensis*)			
10–12	Titeltamine/zolazepam (5)[c]	None given	Supplement with ketamine 2.5 mg/kg IM
	Ketamine (8) + xylazine (1)[c]	Xylazine: yohimbine (0.125 IV)	

(Continued)

Table 42.4. *(Continued)*

Adult Weight Range (kg)	Agents and Doses (mg/kg)	Reversal Agent (mg/kg)	Comments
Otter, sea (*Enhydra lutris*)			
Males 22–45 Females 15–32	Butorphanol (0.5) or oxymorphone (0.3)[b]	Naloxone (0.04) IV or IM	Sedation to immobilization
	Diazepam (0.5) + oxymorphone (0.3)[b]	None used	Sedation for intubation and subsequent inhalation anesthesia
	Fentanyl (0.1 ± 0.003) + diazepam $n = 294$ (0.1 ± 0.006)[p,q]	None used	Wild otters involved in oil spill rehabilitation; lighter sedation and shorter acting than when either acepromazine or azaperone was added.
	Fentanyl (0.1 ± 0.02) + azaperone (0.5 ± 0.02) + diazepam $n = 61$ (0.1 ± 0.01)[o,p]	None used	Deeper sedation than fentanyl/diazepam and duration up to 2.5 hours
	Fentanyl (0.1 ± 0.006) + acepromazine (0.14 ± 0.01) + diazepam $n = 32$ (0.2 ± 0.01)[p,q]	None used	A higher mortality rate occurred in this group compared with the others but could not be directly linked to the drug combination.
Males $n = 230$ 0 = 25.6 Females $n = 367$ 0 = 21.1	Meperidine + diazepam (13 ± 0.5) For surgical procedures fentanyl (0.33) + diazepam (0.11)[r]	None used Fentanyl: naltrexone administered at two times the total fentanyl dose (1/2 IV, 1/2 IM)	Free-ranging otters ($n = 597$) immobilized for collection of biological samples and for surgical instrumentation; smooth induction with minimal need for supplemental anesthesia during procedures lasting 30–40 minutes. Only one anesthesia related mortality (0.2% 0; reversal with naltrexone occurred in 1–3 minutes. No opioid recycling was observed.
	For nonsurgical biological sample collection procedures Fentanyl (0.22) + diazepam (0.07)[r]	Same as above	
Otter (European) Eurasian (*Lutra lutra*)			
3–14	Ketamine (18) + diazepam (0.4)[r] Ketamine (15) + diazepam (0.5)[b,s] Ketamine (5) + medetomidine (0.05)[b]	None given None given Medetomidine: atipamezole (0.25) IM	May cause respiratory depression Avoid using in cold environments—hypothermia
$n = 38$ Males and females Range (males and females) = 3–8.7 0 = 5.3	Ketamine (4.3–5.9) 0 = 5.1 + medetomidine (0.043–0.059) 0 = 0.051 (82 immobilizations in 38 animals)[b]	Medetomidine: atipamezole (0.22–0.30) five times IM medetomidine dose given 30–40 minutes post induction. Animals were able to move and respond to external stimuli in <5 minutes. Mild ataxia noted in a few animals 5 hours post atipamezole.	Recently captured free ranging otters. 0 initial effects in 3 minutes · induction time = 5.5 minutes. 0h = 95 beats/min. 0 resp rate = 32 beats/min. Relative O_2 saturation = 93%. 0 recal temp = 38.4°C (range 31.9–40.9), bradycardia (<70 beats/min) occurred in four animals (5%) and was successfully treated with atropine (0.02 mg/kg IV or IM). Apnea (<2 minutes) occurred in three animals (3.6%). Treated with O_2 via face mask until O_2 saturation >80%. Avoid use in wet or hypothermic otters.
Otter, spotted necked (*Lutra maculicollis*)			
Average 4	Titletamine/zolazepam (5)[e]	None given	Free ranging otters supplement with ketamine (5 mg/kg)
	Ketamine (5–8) + xylazine (0.5–1.0)[e]	None given	Alternative drugs
Skunk, hog nosed (*Conepatus leuconotus*)			
2.3–4.5	Tiletamine/zolazepam (10)[f]	None given	Supplement with ketamine (10)
	Ketamine (15) + acepromazine (0.2)[f]	None given	Alternative drugs
Skunk, hooded (*Mephitis macroura*)			
0.7–2.5	As above	As above	As above
Skunk, striped (*Mephitis mephitis*)			

2–3	Tiletamine/zolazepam (10)[a]	None given	Field immobilization of free ranging skunks. Supplement with 10 mg/kg ketamine
Kits 0.8–1.9 0 = 1.2 (n = 78)	Ketamine (36.3–62.0)[m] 0 = 52.4	None	Field immobilization: scent gland removal; immobilization time = 1–3 minutes; surgical anesthesia = 10–15 minutes; recovery = 60–90 minutes. One mortality due to aspiration.
Kits 0.5–1.8 0 = 1.0 (n = 43)	Ketamine (32.9–69.0)[m] 0 = 36.8	None	Field immobilization: scent gland removal; immobilization time = 2–4 minutes; surgical anesthesia = 5–10 minutes; recovery = 45–74 minutes
Kits 0.6–2.5 0 = 1.1	Ketamine (39.2–107.7)[m] 0 = 7.3	None	Field immobilization: scent gland removal; immobilization = 1–4 minutes; surgical anesthesia = 35–90 minutes; recovery = 60–120 minutes. Better muscle relaxation than above two groups.
Tayra (*Eira barbata*) 4–6	Ketamine (15) + acepromazine (0.2)[b]	None	None
Weasel, long tailed (*Mustela frenata*)	Tiletamine/zolazepam (3.3)[b]	None given	Captive
85–200	See above (Ermine)	See above	See above
Wolverine (*Gulo gulo*)	Ketamine (20) + acepromazine (0.2)[b]	None	
	Ketamine (5–8) + medetomidine (0.1–0.15)	Medetomidine: atipamezole (0.5–0.45)	
7–32	Ketamine (7) + medetomidine (0.3)[c]	Medetomidine: atipamezole (1.5, 1/2 IV, 1/2 IM)	If not immobilized in 15 minutes, repeat full dose (decrease dose by 1/2 in captive wolverines)
	Ketamine (20) + acepromazine (0.2)[c]	None	Alternative drugs
	Etorphine (0.1) + xylazine (1)[c]	Etorphine: diprenorphine (0.2 mg/kg); xylazine: yohimbine (0.15 mg/kg)	

[a]Thornton et al. (2005).
[b]Fernandez-Moran et al. (2001).
[c]Kreeger et al. (2002).
[d]McLaren et al. (2005a, 2005b).
[e]McKenzie and Burroughs (1993).
[f]Jessup 1982; Schwantje et al. (1998).
[g]Carpenter and Marion (2013).
[h]Evans and Springsteen (1998); Wolfensohn and Lloyd (1998).
[i]Cantwell (2001).
[j]Fournier-Chambrillon et al. (2003).
[k]Mitcheltree et al. (1999).
[l]Dzialak et al. (2002).
[m]Ramsden et al. (1976).
[n]Kollias (1999).
[o]Petrini et al. (2001); Spellman (1999).
[p]Haulena and Heath (2001).
[q]Sawyer and Williams (1996).
[r]Monson et al. (2001).
[s]Kulken (1988).
[t]Seal and Kreeger (1987).
[u]Larivière and Messier (1996).

In the authors' experiences, the doses listed are guidelines for use and often require modification when applied to specific individuals or collections of animals and whether they are used for captive, recently captured, or free-ranging procyonids or mustelids.

INHALATION ANESTHESIA

Generally, induction of inhalation anesthesia is facilitated by prior administration of injectable agents recommended in Table 42.1, Table 42.2, Table 42.3, and Table 42.4, and in standard veterinary anesthesia texts for domestic dogs and cats (Muir & Hubbell 2007; Seymour & Gleed 1999). The polecat and ferret are mustelid species for which a number of injectable and inhalation anesthesia protocols have been published (Table 42.3 and Table 42.4; Cantwell 2001; Evans & Springsteen 1998; Gaynor et al. 1997; Imai et al. 1999; MacPhail et al. 2004; Vastenburg et al. 2004). Isoflurane and sevoflurane have been shown to be safe and efficacious and are agents of choice in both procyonids and mustelids (Denver 2000; Gaynor et al. 1997; Schumacher 1996). Following administration of preanesthetic agents or parenteral drugs, some animals may still require restraint. They can be held in a towel or with gloves and provided the inhalant agent via face mask or induction chamber. Once the animal loses its righting reflex, it is masked until it is intubated or maintained on a face mask. With intubation or face mask maintenance, inhalants should be administered using a non-rebreathing circuit (Ayre's T-piece or Bain system). Oxygen flow should be two to three times the minute ventilation (approximately 200–350 mL/kg/min) (Cantwell 2001). Anesthesia monitoring, thermoregulation, and cardiopulmonary support, resuscitation, and recovery for these species are as discussed in Chapters 3–5 and 9.

REFERENCES

Baitchman EJ, Kollias GV. 2000. Clinical anatomy of the North American river otter (*Lontra canadensis*). *Journal of Zoo and Wildlife Medicine* 33(4):473–483.

Belant JL. 2004. Field immobilization of raccoons (*Procyon lotor*) with Telazol and Xylazine. *Journal of Wildlife Diseases* 40(4):787–791.

Cantwell S. 2001. Ferret, rabbit, and rodent anesthesia. *The Veterinary Clinics of North America. Exotic Animal Practice. Analgesia and Anesthesia* 4(1):169–191.

Carpenter JW, Marion CJ. 2013. *Exotic Animal Formulary*, pp. 561–594. St. Louis: Elsevier Saunders.

Denver M. 1999. Procyonidae and Viverridae. In: *Zoo and Wild Animal Medicine* (Fowler ME, Miller RE, eds.), pp. 516–523. Philadelphia: W.B. Saunders.

Denver M. 2000. Procyonidae and Viveridae. In: *Zoo and Wild Animal Medicine* (ME Fowler, RE Miller, eds.), pp. 516–523. Philadelphia: W.B. Saunders Press.

Dzialak MR, Serfass TL, Durland L, Shumway DL, Hedge LM, Blakenship TL. 2002. Chemical restraint of fishers (*Martes pennanti*) with ketamine and medetomidine-ketamine. *Journal of Zoo and Wildlife Medicine* 33(1):45–51.

Evans AT, Springsteen KK. 1998. Anesthesia of ferrets. *Seminars in Avian and Exotic Pet Medicine* 7:48–52.

Fernandez-Moran J. 1999. Mustelidae. In: *Zoo and Wild Animal Medicine* (ME Fowler, RE Miller, eds.), pp. 505–516. Philadelphia: W.B. Saunders.

Fernandez-Moran J, Perez E, Sanmartin M, Saavedra D, Manteca-Vilandra X. 2001. Reversible immobilization of Eurasia otters with a combination of ketamine and medetomidine. *Journal of Wildlife Diseases* 37(3):561–565.

Fournier P, Fournier-Chambrillon C, Vie J-C. 1998. Immobilization of wild kinkajous (*Potos flavus*) with medetomidine-ketimine and reversal by atipamezole. *Journal of Zoo and Wildlife Medicine* 29:190–194.

Fournier-Chambrillon C, Chusseau J-P, Dupuch J, Maizeret C, Fournier P. 2003. Immobilization of free-ranging European mink (*Mustela lutreola*) and polecat (*Mustela putorius*) with medetomidine-ketamine and reversal by atipamezole. *Journal of Wildlife Diseases* 39(2):393–399.

Fowler ME, ed. 2008. *Restraint and Handling of Wild and Domestic Animals*, 3rd ed., pp. 280–283. Ames: Wiley-Blackwell.

Gaynor JS, Wimsatt J, Mallinckrodt C, Biggins D. 1997. A comparison of sevoflurane and isoflurane for short-term anesthesia in polecats (*Mustela eversmanni*). *Journal of Zoo and Wildlife Medicine* 28(3):274–279.

Georoff TA, Boon DA, Hammond EE, Ferrell ST, Radcliffe RW. 2004. Preliminary results of medetomidine-ketamine-butorphanol for anesthetic management of captive white-nosed coati (*Nasua narica*). Proceedings of the American Association of Zoo Veterenarians, pp. 388–391.

Haulena M, Heath RB. 2001. Marine mammal anesthesia. In: *Handbook of Marine Mammal Medicine*, 2nd ed. (LA Dierauf, FMD Gulland, eds.), pp. 655–688. Boca Raton: CRC Press.

Imai A, Steffey EP, Farver TB, Ilkiw JE. 1999. Assessment of isoflurane-induced anesthesia in ferrets and rats. *American Journal of Veterinary Research* 60(12):1577–1578.

Jalanka HH, Roeken BO. 1990. The use of medetomidine, medetomidine-ketamine combinations, and atipamezole in non-domestic mammals: a review. *Journal of Zoo and Wildlife Medicine* 21:259–282.

Jessup DA. 1982. Restraint and chemical immobilization of carnivores and furbearers. In: *Chemical Immobilization of North American Wildlife* (L Nielsen, JC Haigh, ME Fowler, eds.), pp. 227–244. Milwaukee: Wisconsin Human Society, Inc.

Kollias GV. 1999. Health assessment, medical management, and prerelease conditioning of translocated North American river otters. In: *Zoo and Wild Animal Medicine* (Fowler, ME, Miller RE, eds.), pp. 443–448. Philadelphia: W.B. Saunders.

Kreeger JJ, Arnemo JM, Raath JP. 2002. *Handbook of Wildlife Chemical Immobilization*, International Edition, p. 412. Fort Collins: Wildlife Pharmaceuticals, Inc.

Kulken T. 1988. Anaesthesia in the European otter (*Lutra lutra*). *Veterinary Record* 123:59.

Labate AS, Nunes ALV, Gomes M, Passerino ASM. 2001. Order Carnivora, Family Procyonidae (raccoons, kinkajous). In: *Biology, Medicine, and Surgery of South American Wild Animals* (ME Fowler, ZS Cubas, eds.), pp. 317–322. Ames: Iowa State University Press.

Larivière SL, Messier F. 1996. Immobilization of striped skunks with Telazol®. *Wildlife Society Bulletin* 24:713–716.

MacPhail CM, Monnet E, Gaynor JS, Perini A. 2004. Effect of sevoflurane on hemodynamic and cardiac energetic parameters in ferrets. *American Journal of Veterinary Research* 65(5): 653–658.

McKenzie AA, Burroughs REJ. 1993. Chemical capture of carnivores. In: *The Capture and Care Manual* (AA McKenzie, ed.), pp.

224–243. Pretoria: Wildlife Decision Support Services and the South African Veterinary Foundation.

McLaren GW, Thornton PD, Newman C, Buesching CD, Baker SE, Mathews F, MacDonald DW. 2005a. The use of ketamine-medetomidine-butorphanol combinations for field anesthesia in wild European badgers (*Meles meles*). *Veterinary Anaesthesia and Analgesia* 32:367–372.

McLaren GW, Thornton PD, Newman C, Buesching CD, Baker SE, Mathews F, MacDonald DW. 2005b. High rectal temperature indicates a high risk of unexpected recovery in anaesthetized badgers. *Veterinary Anaesthesia and Analgesia* 32:48–52.

Mehren KG. 1986. Procyonidae. In: *Zoo and Wild Animal Medicine* (ME Fowler, ed.), pp. 816–820. Philadelphia: W.B. Saunders Press.

Mitcheltree DH, Serfass TL, Tzilkowski WM, Peper RL, Whary MT, Brooks RP. 1999. Physiological responses of fishers to immobilization with ketamine-xylazine or Telazol®. *Wildlife Society Bulletin* 27:582–591.

Monson DH, McCormick C, Ballachey BE. 2001. Chemical anesthesia of Northern sea otters (*Enhydra lutris*): results of past field studies. *Journal of Zoo and Wildlife Medicine* 32(2):181–189.

Muir WW, Hubbell JAE. 2007. *Handbook of Veterinary Anesthesia*, 4th ed., p. 656. St. Louis: Mosby.

Nielsen L. 1999. *Chemical Immobilization of Wild and Exotic Animals*. Ames: Iowa State University Press.

Petrini K, Spelman L, Reed-Smith J. 2001. Health care. In: *North American River Otter Lontra (Lutra) Canadensis Husbandry Notebook*, 2nd ed. (J Reed-Smith, ed.), pp. 165, 177–178. Grand Rapids: John Ball Zoological Gardens (Pub).

Pimentel TL, Reis ML, Passerino AS. 2001. Order Carnivora, Family Mustelidae. In: *Biology, Medicine and Surgery of South American Wild Animals* (ME Fowler, ed.), pp. 323–331. Ames: Iowa State University Press.

Ramsden RO, Coppin PE, Johnson DH. 1976. Clinical observations on the use of ketamine hydrochloride in wild carnivores. *Journal of Wildlife Diseases* 12:221–225.

Sawyer DC, Williams TD. 1996. Chemical restraint and anesthesia of sea otters affected by the oil spill in Prince William Sound, Alaska. *Journal of the American Veterinary Medical Association* 208(11):1831–1834.

Schoemaker NJ, Mol JA, Lumeij JT, Thijssen JHH, Rijnberk A. 2003. Effects of anesthesia and manual restraint on the plasma concentrations of pituitary and adenocortical hormones in ferrets. *The Veterinary Record* 152:591–595.

Schumacher J. 1996. Anesthesia of wild, exotic, and laboratory animals. In: *Lumb and Jones Veterinary Anesthesia*, 3rd ed. (JC Thurman, WJ Tranquilli, GJ Benson, eds.), pp. 297–329. Baltimore: Williams and Wilkins.

Schwantje HM, Weir R, McAdie M. 1998. Capture and immobilization of mustelids in British Columbia. Proceedings of the Joint Conference of the American Association of Zoo Veterinarians and the American Association of Wildlife Veterinarians, p. 450.

Seal US, Kreeger TJ. 1987. Chemical immobilization of furbearers. In: *Wild Furbearer Management and Conservation in North America* (M Novak, JA Baker, ME Obbard, B Malloch, eds.), pp. 191–215. Toronto: Ontario Ministry of Natural Resources.

Seymour C, Gleed R. 1999. *British Small Animal Veterinary Association Manual of Small Animal Anesthesia and Analgesia*, p. 324. London: Blackwell Publishers.

Spellman L. 1999. North American river otter anesthesia. In: *Zoo and Wild Animal Medicine* (ME Fowler, RE Miller, eds.), pp. 436–443. Philadelphia: W.B. Saunders.

Thornton PD, Newman C, Johnson PJ, Buesching CD, Baker SE, Slater D, Dominic-Johnson DP, MacDonald DW. 2005. Preliminary comparison of four anesthetic techniques in badgers (*Meles meles*). *Veterinary Anaesthesia and Analgesia* 32:40–47.

Vastenburg MH, Boroffka SA, Schoemaker NJ. 2004. Echocardiographic measurements in clinically healthy ferrets. *Veterinary Radiology and Ultrasound* 43(3):228–232.

Wolfensohn SE, Lloyd MH. 1998. *A Handbook of Laboratory Animal Management and Welfare*, 2nd ed., p. 237. Oxford: Blackwell Science Ltd.

43 Viverrids

Anneke Moresco and R. Scott Larsen

INTRODUCTION

Viverrids are small- to medium-sized carnivores and their natural habitat spans Southwestern Europe, Southern Asia, the East Indies, and Africa, including Madagascar. The phylogeny is challenging as there is a fair bit of convergence in this taxon (Gaubert & Veron 2003). Therefore, as new molecular techniques become available, the taxonomic classification of the Viverridae continues to change. This chapter follows the taxonomy detailed by the Integrated Taxonomic Information System (ITIS). Within the Viverridae family, there are now 4 subfamilies and 35 species listed. Latin names, common names, weight ranges, and longevities are given in Table 43.1. The International Union for Conservation of Nature (IUCN) lists the genus *Prionodon* in its own family Prionodontidae. The Euplerinae and Nandininae are now listed as distinct families (Eupleridae and Nandinidae, respectively) rather than within the Viverridae. The family Eupleridae contains the genera Cryptoprocta, Eupleres, and Fossa, formerly classified in the Viverridae (IUCN 2011).

The fossil record for Viverridae is the oldest among the families classified in the order Carnivora. Phylogenetically, they are classified as part of the Feliformia group and are more closely related to felids than to canids (Veron & Heard 2000).

Most viverrid species are nocturnal or crepuscular, making observations difficult. Therefore, the ecology of many species in this group is poorly understood. With the advent of smaller devices, more radiocollaring studies are being done, thus providing more data on their behavior and diet (Grassman et al. 2005). The natural social structure is typically solitary (Kingdon 2003); however, in captivity, they can be housed in pairs or small groups. This needs to be taken into account during induction and recovery, since brief separation and reintroduction will be necessary.

SPECIES SPECIFIC PHYSIOLOGY

As their taxonomic classification indicates, most viverrids are carnivorous and a high percentage of their diet (70%) consists of meat (Ray & Sunquist 2001). Binturongs (*Arctictis binturong*) and many civet species are more omnivorous, with up to 40% of their diet consisting of fruit. However, for many species, details about their diets in the wild remain unknown.

Viverrids are skilled climbers with strong, sharp, retractile or semiretractile claws, and tend to be arboreal. A few are primarily terrestrial (e.g., oriental civets) and will dig burrows, use burrows dug by other animals, or seek shelter within human-built structures (Nowak 2005). One should remember their raking power when physically restraining and handling these animals (Rettig & Divers 1986). In addition to personnel safety, nails are an important consideration when choosing a net to catch and restrain as they can injure themselves or may tear the net trying to escape.

The binturong is unique among viverrids in that it has a truly prehensile tail. It is a very thick (up to 15 cm diameter at the base) and strong appendage that can be used with great dexterity, which should be kept in mind when handling binturongs, even when they are sedated.

Mammals that consume exclusively vertebrate diets tend to have higher metabolic rates than those that also consume fruit and invertebrates (McNab 1995). The binturong, the largest of the viverrids, has a slightly lower body temperature (37–38°C) than similarly sized dogs and tends to maintain normal body temperature during anesthesia (Moresco & Larsen 2003; Mudappa

Zoo Animal and Wildlife Immobilization and Anesthesia, Second Edition. Edited by Gary West, Darryl Heard, and Nigel Caulkett.
© 2014 John Wiley & Sons, Inc. Published 2014 by John Wiley & Sons, Inc.

Table 43.1. Latin names, common names, body weights, and longevity of viverrid species

Latin Name	Common Names	Weight	Reference
Hemigalinae			
Chrotogale owstoni	Owston's palm civet	2.5–4.0 kg	King (2002; Kingdon (2003)
Cynogale bennettii	Sunda otter civet	3–5 kg	Nowak (2005)
Diplogale hosei	Hose's palm civet	Wt unk	Nowak (2005)
Hemigalus derbyanus	Banded palm civet	1.75–3.0 kg	Nowak (2005)
Paradoxurinae			
Arctictis binturong	Binturong, Asian bear cat	14 kg, in captivity up to 30 kg	Moresco & Larsen (2003); Nowak (2005) A. Moresco, pers. obs.
Arctogalidia trivirgata	Small-toothed, three-striped civet	2.0–2.5 kg	Nowak (2005)
Macrogalidia musschenbroekii	Sulawesi palm civet	3.8–4.5 kg	Nowak (2005)
Paguma larvata	Masked palm civet	3.6–5 kg	Nowak (2005)
Paradoxurus hermaphroditus	Asian palm civet, common palm civet, musang, toddy cat		
Paradoxurus jerdoni	Jerdon's palm civet, musang, toddy cat, brown palm civet	1.2–3.5 kg	Mudappa and Chellam (2001)
Paradoxurus zeylonensis	Golden palm civet		
Prionodontinae			
Prionodon linsang	Banded linsang	0.6–1.2 kg	Nowak (2005)
Prionodon pardicolor	Spotted linsang	7–20 kg	Kingdon (2003)
Viverrinae			
Civettictis civetta (V. civetta)	African civet	7–20 kg	(Kingdon 2003)
Genetta abyssinica	Ethiopian or Abyssinian genet	1.3–2 kg	Kingdon (2003)
Genetta angolensis	Angola or Miombo genet	1.3–2 kg	Kingdon (2003)
Genetta genetta	Small spotted- or common genet	1.3–2.25 kg	Haltenorth and Diller (1984)
Genetta johnstoni	Johnston's genet	1–3 kg	Kingdon (2003)
Genetta maculata	Rusty spotted genet	1.2–3.1 kg	Haltenorth and Diller (1984)
Genetta servalina	Servaline genet	1–2 kg	Kingdon (2003)
Genetta thierryi	Hausa genet	1.3–1.5 kg	Kingdon (2003)
Genetta tigrina	Large-spotted- or rusty-spotted genet	1.2–3.1 kg	Kingdon (2003)
Genetta victoriae	Giant genet	2.5–3.5 kg	Kingdon (2003)
Genetta cristata	Crested servaline genet		
Genetta piscivora	Aquatic genet	1.2–2.5 kg	Kingdon (2003)
Poiana richardsoni	African linsang or oyan	0.5–0.7 kg	Kingdon (2003)
Viverra civettina	Malabar civet	5–11 kg	Nowak (2005)
Viverra megaspila	Large spotted civet	5–11 kg	Nowak (2005)
Viverra tangalunga	Malay civet	Male: 2.45–4.3 kg; female: 3.62–3.95 kg	Colón (2002)
Viverra zibetha	Large Indian civet	5–11 kg	King (2002); Nowak (2005)
Viverricula indica	Lesser oriental civet, rasse	2–4 kg	Nowak (2005)

& Chellam 2001). The smaller viverrids have a larger surface-to-volume ratio, making them more susceptible to heat loss during anesthesia.

In the wild, the fanaloka (*Fossa fossana*) and the falanouc (*Eupleres goudotii*) can lay down fat reserves in preparation for winter. Fat may make up a significant percentage of their body weight and is laid down especially in the tail (Garbutt 1999). Therefore, the tail is not recommended as a site for intramuscular anesthetic injection in viverrids because absorption can be inconsistent (Moresco, unpublished data, 2002).

PHYSICAL RESTRAINT

In most cases, it is difficult to safely handle viverrids for examination and sample collection solely using physical restraint techniques. Typically, the goal is to choose the restraint technique that will be the least stressful and will allow the most reliable drug delivery. Recently transported animals are best left to acclimate before restraint is attempted; restraint (physical or chemical) should not be attempted if ambient temperature is above 32.2°C (90°F) (Fowler 1986).

Nets

Advantages: Net capture can be low stress if performed by well trained staff; transfer out of the net may not be necessary to administer drugs because these can be delivered through the mesh. Nets can be used to capture animals in a tree or in a den in their exhibit. With appropriately sized nets and trained personnel, nets can be used even for binturongs, the largest of the viverrids. Animals can be transferred to a kennel after injection of anesthetics and kept quiet and dark to minimize stimulation. This is particularly important when using alpha-two agonists for chemical restraint, as catecholamines released due to stress or excitement can overwhelm the sedative effect of alpha-two adrenergic agonists. If left in the net while the injectable anesthetics take effect, the animal's eyes should be covered and noise should be minimized.

Disadvantages: There is the potential for claws or teeth getting caught in mesh. Nets are not typically useful in free-ranging situations.

Trap/Kennel/Squeeze Cage

Advantages: Squeeze cages or small kennels can be low stress if the animals have been habituated to enter them voluntarily (operant conditioning). These have been used successfully in animals as small as Owston's palm civet (Streicher 2001). Transfer for drug delivery is usually not necessary because drugs can be delivered through the mesh (via pole syringe, blow pipe, or low-power dart gun if trap is not a squeeze cage). If the animal is small enough, it can be transferred to a chamber for induction with inhalant anesthesia or the entire cage can be covered with a plastic bag and inhalant anesthetics can be administered. In the field, box traps are typically used to capture small- to medium-sized carnivores (Colón 2002; Mudappa & Chellam 2001). Trap success improves if traps are located near areas such as latrines where signs of activity have been recorded. Traps should be baited, but left locked open for several days before setting the trap to close, to habituate the animals (Mudappa & Chellam 2001). Many viverrids have nocturnal habits, so traps should be set at night and checked frequently to minimize the amount of time the animals spend inside. Checks can be less frequent if traps are equipped with devices that signal when they are triggered. Animals should spend minimal time in the traps because this can increase stress and thereby affect the quality of anesthesia, as well as increase the likelihood of self injury.

Disadvantages: When trapping animals in the wild, keep in mind the presence of potential predators that may attack and kill the trapped animal. Trap-related injuries may include self-mutilation, nose trauma, or traumatized digits and limbs. Free-ranging animals will not be habituated to squeeze cages and kennels and will be stressful; in the captive setting, it can also be stressful if the animals are not habituated (see advantages).

Handling Bag

Advantages: Animals can be transferred from a trap to a handling (burlap) bag prior to injection; this facilitates hand injection and decreases visual stimulation. Appropriate gloves (e.g., Kevlar®) should be used when handling the bag containing an animal.

Disadvantages: Any additional manipulation of the animal can increase the stress to the animal as well as the risk of escape or injury to the animal or personnel.

CHEMICAL RESTRAINT AND ANESTHESIA
Vascular Access
In many viverrids, the skin is thick, the hair is coarse, and subcutaneous tissue is abundant (especially in obese captive animals), all of which makes visualization of veins difficult.

Jugular Vein The preferred site for phlebotomy is the jugular vein due to its accessibility and the possibility of obtaining relatively large amounts of blood. The neck of viverrids tends to be cylindrical, rather than cone shaped. In binturongs, the jugular vein appears to be small relative to body size and is located more lateral than in dogs and cats, similar to ferrets. In overweight animals, it is difficult to palpate or visualize the jugular vein unless the head of the animal is held slightly below the body by briefly extending the head and neck beyond the edge of the examination table (the head should remain supported). This technique can put some additional pressure on the lungs, and it is important to evaluate the cardiorespiratory status of the animal before using it. Arterial oxygen saturation can be monitored with a pulse oximeter. If using an anesthetic combination that includes medetomidine, veins are best visualized and accessed within 20 minutes after drug administration (Moresco & Larsen 2003).

Cephalic Vein The cephalic vein is a valuable site for catheterization. In binturongs, the cephalic vein courses medially and it is often large enough to place a 20-gauge 3/4-in or 1-in IV catheter. This vein is visible after clipping hair and/or moistening with isopropyl alcohol.

Femoral Vein Frequently, the femoral vein is not visible, but can be found adjacent to the easily palpable femoral artery. It is not recommended as the primary site of venipuncture because the artery can be inadvertently punctured, which may lead to formation of a large hematoma. If the femoral artery is punctured, direct pressure should be applied for several minutes to minimize hematoma formation. If accessing the femoral vein, attempt to isolate the vein between two fingers and insert the needle perpendicular to the skin and vessel. Use a small gauge needle (23–25 gauge) to minimize vascular trauma. Some viverrids have large fat deposits in the hind leg, which may make it difficult to access the femoral artery and vein.

Saphenous Vein In binturongs, the saphenous vein can be accessed on the distolateral aspect of the hind leg over the tarsus, similar to its location in dogs. It can vary considerably in size between individuals.

Tail Vein In some viverrids, the tail vein can be accessed for small amounts of blood; however, it is not useful for drug administration. This vein can neither be seen nor palpated. The needle is inserted medially on the ventral aspect of the tail, perpendicular to the long axis; the needle is "walked" cranially, similar to the technique used in cattle. In binturongs, success is most likely when inserting the needle about 10 cm caudal to the tail base.

ENDOTRACHEAL INTUBATION

Endotracheal intubation of viverrids is not described in the literature, but it is generally straightforward because the mouth can be opened wide. In binturongs, the glottis is usually easily visualized and endotracheal tube insertion is similar to cats. In contrast to felids, there is minimal laryngospasm, so topical lidocaine is generally not needed. Due to the small size of the animals, it is important not to overinflate the cuff to avoid pressure necrosis. Since many viverrids are small in size, small internal diameter endotracheal tubes are needed, making it more likely that a small amount of saliva, blood, or foreign material can obstruct the tube. If intubation is not performed, nasal insufflation may be used for oxygen supplementation.

Preanesthetic Considerations

Preanesthetic considerations are similar to other small mammals. Similar to other members of the order Carnivora, viverrids have simple stomachs and relatively short gastrointestinal tracts; in some species, the cecum is absent or vestigial (Crapo et al. 2002; Mitchell 1905). In general, hind gut fermentation does not seem to be significant despite the large amount of fruit consumed by some species (Mitchell 1905). They have correspondingly short gastrointestinal transit times and preanesthetic fasting periods of 24 hours are typically appropriate; water can be withheld for 4–8 hours.

Induction/Maintenance Protocols

Anesthetic induction is often achieved with injectable drugs. The most commonly used combinations include a dissociative agent (ketamine or tiletamine) and either an alpha-two adrenergic agonist (medetomidine or xylazine) or a benzodiazepine (diazepam or midazolam). Sometimes, an opioid (butorphanol) is added to further reduce the needed doses of other drugs.

The dissociative agent phencyclidine was successfully used in combination with promazine (a phenothiazine) in a large number of viverrids: *A. binturong*, *Arctogalidia trivirgata*, *Cryptoprocta ferox*, *Genetta genetta*, *Hemigalus derbyanus*, *Nandinia binotata*, *Paradoxurus hermaphroditus*, *Paguma larvata*, *Prionodon linsang*, *Viverra civetta*, *Viverricula indica*, and *Viverra zibetha* (Seal & Ericksson 1969). Although phencyclidine is no longer available in the United States, ketamine and tiletamine are other dissociative agents that are commonly used in viverrids. If dissociative agents are used alone, high muscle tone, persistent movement, rough inductions, and rough recoveries may occur (Seal & Ericksson 1969). These effects have been documented with phencyclidine use in viverrids and with the use of other dissociatives in other carnivore species. Therefore, the use of dissociative agents by themselves is not recommended. Instead, it is recommended to use a dissociative in combination with a sedative to improve muscle relaxation (see Table 43.2).

Table 43.2. Anesthetic drug combinations used in viverrids

Drug Combination (dose)	Species	Comment	Reference
Ketamine (10–15 mg/kg) Xylazine (1–2 mg/kg) Ketamine (3–8 mg/kg) Medetomidine (0.02–.06 mg/kg) Butorphanol (0.2–0.5 mg/kg)	(1) Viverrids (2) *Paradoxurus jerdoni* *Arctictis binturong*	(2) Induction: 3–15 minutes. Recovery: 49–138 minutes. Lower ketamine and higher medetomidine doses provide shorter recovery	(1) Denver (2003) (2) Mudappa and Chellam (2001) Moresco and Larsen (2003) Klaphake et al. (2005)
Ketamine (10 mg/kg) Diazepam (0.5 mg/kg)	Viverrids		Denver (2003)
Ketamine (10 mg/kg) Midazolam (0.25–0.50 mg/kg)	Viverrids		Denver (2003)
Tiletamine/zolazepam (1) 3–5 mg/kg (2) 5 mg/kg (3) 15 mg/kg	(1) Viverrids (2) *Viverra tangalunga* (3) Madagascar carnivores	(2) Induction: 15–20 minutes. Need redosing if excited, silence during induction. Recovery: 60–120 minutes. More docile in trap than *Arctictis binturong* or *Paguma larvata*	(1) Denver (2003) (2) Colón (2002) and Colon, pers. comm. (3) Louis, pers. comm.
Ketamine (17 mg/kg) Acepromazine (0.73 mg/kg) Atropine (0.04 mg/kg)	*Chrotogale owstoni*	Induction: 9 minutes, No vomiting, ↓ in body temp. Only HR and temp were monitored.	King (2002)
Ketamine (17.9 mg/kg) Acepromazine (0.77 mg/kg) Atropine (0.04 mg/kg)	*Viverra zibetha*	Induction: 11 minutes, No vomiting, Only HR and were temp monitored	King (2002)

The combination of ketamine-medetomidine-butorphanol has been successfully used for anesthetizing binturongs. Doses ranged from 2 to 8 mg/kg ketamine, 0.02 to 0.06 mg/kg medetomidine, and 0.2 to 0.5 mg/kg butorphanol; lower doses of ketamine were used with higher doses of medetomidine (Klaphake et al. 2005; Moresco & Larsen 2003). This combination worked well in binturongs, with good inductions, stable cardiopulmonary values, and fast, reversible recoveries. Ketamine-medetomidine-butorphanol has been used in African palm civets at similar dosages. Although ketamine-medetomidine-butorphanol is recommended as an anesthetic protocol in viverrids, there may be other combinations that offer more consistent inductions while retaining reversibility.

Ketamine (6 mg/kg) has been used in combination with a relatively high dose of xylazine (10 mg/kg) in the common genet (Palomares 1993). This combination used much lower doses than that reported for ketamine alone (66 mg/kg) (Maddock 1989). However, the actual doses used by Maddock varied widely, and 4 of 10 animals needed supplemental doses. In brown palm civets, 15 mg/kg of ketamine and 1.5 mg/kg of xylazine achieved greater induction success (Mudappa & Chellam 2001), see Table 43.2. Metoclopramide may be used during ketamine-medetomidine immobilization to counter vomiting associated with medetomidine administration (Moresco, unpublished data, 2002).

Acepromazine has also been used in combination with ketamine in viverrids (Fuller et al. 1990; Maddock 1989); however, acepromazine has a long duration of action and is nonreversible. One study in Owston's palm civets (*Chrotogale owstoni*) and large Indian civets (*V. zibetha*) used ketamine-acepromazine-atropine as a combination mixed in the bottle prior to administration (King 2002). Acepromazine was chosen to decrease the risk of vomiting, as had been reported with the use of xylazine (Mudappa & Chellam 2001; Streicher 2001). Inductions were relatively quick (~7–9 minutes) and no vomiting was observed; however, temperatures decreased substantially in spite of measures taken. No other adverse effects were noted; however, only temperature, heart rate, and recovery were evaluated. The main disadvantage of this combination is that acepromazine has a long duration of action, and that none of the drugs used are reversible.

Tiletamine-zolazepam has been recommended for several different species of viverrids, including *N. binotata*, *C. civetta*, *H. derbyanus*, *Viverri. indica*, *F. fossa*, *Pag. larvata*, *V. zibetha*, and *Par. hermaphroditus*. Dosages used for these species range from 4 to 9 mg/kg (Kreeger 1999). Smaller species often require higher dosages, up to 12 mg/kg (McKenzie & Burroughs 1993).

Isoflurane can be administered via face mask as an induction agent to small species or young animals. For small- to medium-sized animals, chamber induction can also be readily performed if adequate equipment is available.

Body Weights
See Table 43.1.

Monitoring
Ideally, heart rate, respiratory rate, temperature, blood pressure, oxygenation, ventilation (CO_2), and electrocardiogram (ECG) should be monitored during an anesthetic procedure. It is not always possible to monitor all these parameters. However, minimum monitoring equipment in captive as well as field settings should include a stethoscope for monitoring heart rate, cardiac rhythm, respiration rate, and lung field quality, as well as a thermometer for measuring temperature. Cardiac and respiratory function as well as mucous membrane color should be evaluated as soon as the animal is unconscious to assess physiologic stability before continuing with the procedure. Temperature should be taken frequently because the small species of viverrids are at increased risk for rapid loss of heat. A pulse oximeter can provide trends in oxygenation over the course of anesthesia. End tidal CO_2 (ETCO2) measurements are useful to determine if the animal is properly intubated as well as to monitor ventilation. However, if the animal is small, some capnographs may have difficulty providing accurate readings.

Blood pressure can be profoundly affected by the initial excitement of capture and also by the drugs chosen. Combinations of ketamine with medetomidine have been reported to cause hypertension in canids and ursids (Caulkett et al. 1999; Larsen et al. 2002; Sladky et al. 2000). Since changes in blood pressure are difficult to assess clinically, a means of monitoring blood pressure contributes to the ability to improve the quality of the anesthesia. In animals that are subject to regular physical examinations, recording ECGs provides a baseline for that individual; additionally, in the case of viverrids, baseline ECGs would provide valuable data for the taxon as there are no such normal values published.

Recovery Considerations
The main consideration during an anesthetic event is safety for the animal and personnel. In cases where the animal needs to go back to a group or to fend for itself in the wild, it is important that animals are fully conscious and have good motor coordination.

During recovery, the animal should be in a quiet place and isolated from other animals, but where it can be observed as it recovers. The antagonists (if any) may be given after transport to the recovery area to ensure that the patient does not start to recover prior to it being contained. Animals should be monitored continuously until they have been extubated and they can lift their head. After extubation, visual monitoring can be done at short intervals until the animal is standing, then at longer intervals until it is fully recovered. Although animals recovered in a quiet place may appear to take longer to recover than when stimulated, stimulating them into activity before the anesthetics have been fully metabolized results in activity that is uncoordinated and leads to unnecessary stress or injury.

Recovery should take place in a kennel, cage, or area from which the animal does not need to be moved once awake. Even for binturongs, the largest viverrid, a kennel can be used if the door can be opened with minimal risk to personnel. Food and water should not be provided until the animal is fully recovered.

Field Immobilization Considerations (Wild Capture)

Darting: When darting free-ranging animals, the period of time between the administration of drugs and recumbency is particularly dangerous because the animal is still ambulatory but has lost some motor coordination. If anesthesia is administered via dart, and the animal is not contained, they will attempt to escape. Many viverrids will climb trees, increasing the chance of escape or fall. It is important to make sure that the darting does not occur near water because sedated animals can easily drown if they fall into a pond, lake, or stream.

Monitoring: Similar to anesthesia in captive animals, safety of free-ranging animals and personnel should be key. Close monitoring of the patient allows for early detection of problems. There are now monitors that can provide heart rate, respiration rate, temperature, blood pressure, oxygenation, ETCO2, and ECG in one machine, weighing less than 5 kg. With monitors this small, close monitoring of anesthetized patients is no longer restricted to a clinic. Because free-ranging animals cannot be fasted, the possibility of regurgitation should be considered and additional precautions to address regurgitation should be taken. In the field, age and health status of the animals are usually not known ahead of time so problems can arise once the animal is anesthetized; emergency drugs should be on hand and dosages should be calculated prior to induction.

Recovery: Release of the animal should only happen once the animal is fully recovered. Timing of the release should be such that the animal will still have enough time to find a safe area for sleeping. Release of diurnal animals should occur well before sunset. Conversely, release of nocturnal and crepuscular animals should be timed according to their behavior.

Postanesthetic Complications

Postanesthetic complications can occur due to the presence of undetected disease. Animals that have otherwise masked disease conditions decompensate due to the effects of anesthesia and may be affected by heart

failure, renal disease, or hepatic disease. Not only may these conditions contribute to physiologic problems but they may also change how anesthetic agents are metabolized.

Other things to consider are group dynamics when returning an animal to the group with which it is housed. Group dynamics can be altered by separation and reintroduction, with increased fighting occurring during reintroduction. This is less likely in viverrids that are housed in pairs. If returning to the wild, animals should always be returned to the same place they were captured. Releases should also happen only after complete recovery has occurred. Complications from premature release can include injury sustained from falling, drowning, or being predated. Animals should be held until the next day if they have not fully recovered in time for an appropriate release.

REFERENCES

Caulkett NA, Cattet MRL, Caulkett JM, Polischuk SC. 1999. Comparative physiologic effects of Telazol (R), medetomidine-ketamine, and medetomodine-Telazol(R) in captive polar bears (*Ursus maritimus*). *Journal of Zoo and Wildlife Medicine* 30: 504–509.

Colón CP. 2002. Ranging behaviour and activity of the Malay civet (*Viverra tangalunga*) in a logged and an unlogged forest in Danum Valley, East Malaysia. *Journal of Zoology (London)* 257: 473–485.

Crapo C, Moresco A, Hurley S, Hanner T, Kadzere C. 2002. Anatomical measurements of the digestive tract and nutrient digestibility in the Asian Bear Cat (*Arctictis binturong*). *Journal of Dairy Science* 85:251.

Denver M. 2003. Procyonidae and Viverridae. In: *Zoo and Wild Animal Medicine* (ME Fowler, RE Miller, eds.), pp. 516–523. St. Louis: Saunders.

Fowler ME. 1986. Restraint. In: *Zoo and Wild Animal Medicine* (ME Fowler, ed.), pp. 37–50. Philadelphia: W.B. Saunders Company.

Fuller TK, Biknevicius AR, Kat PW. 1990. Movements and behavior of large spotted genets (*Genetta maculata Gray 1830*) near Elementeita, Kenya (Mammalia, viverridae). *Tropical Zoology* 3:13–19.

Garbutt N. 1999. *Mammals of Madagascar*. Sussex: Pica Press.

Gaubert P, Veron G. 2003. Exhaustive sample set among Viverridae reveals the sister-group of felids: the linsangs as a case of extreme morphological convergence within Feliformia. *Proceedings of the Royal Society of London. Series B. Biological Sciences* 270:2523–2530.

Grassman LI, Tewes ME, Silvy NJ. 2005. Ranging, habitat use and activity patterns of binturong *Arctictis binturong* and yellow-throated marten *Martes flavigula* in Northcentral Thailand. *Wildlife Biology* 11:49–57.

Haltenorth T, Diller H. 1984. *A Field Guide to the Mammals of Africa, including Madagascar*. London: Collins.

IUCN. 2011. IUCN Red List of Threatened Species. Version 2011.1. http://www.iucnredlist.org (accessed October 27, 2011).

King L. 2002. Physiological responses of Owston's palm civets and large Indian civets to immobilization with a combination of ketamine HCl, acepromazine and atropine sulphate. *Small Carnivore Conservation* 27:13–16.

Kingdon J. 2003. *The Kingdon Field Guide to African Mammals*. London: Christopher Helm.

Klaphake E, Shoieb A, Ramsay EC, Schumacher J, Craig L. 2005. Renal adenocarcinoma, hepatocellular carcinoma, and pancreatic islet cell carcinoma in a binturong (*Arctictis binturong*). *Journal of Zoo and Wildlife Medicine* 36:127–130.

Kreeger TJ. 1999. *Handbook of Wildlife Chemical Immobilization*. Ft. Collins: Wildlife Pharmaceuticals Inc.

Larsen RS, Loomis MR, Kelly BT, Sladky KK, Stoskopf MK, Horne WA. 2002. Cardiorespiratory effects of medetomidine-butorphanol, medetomidine-butorphanol-diazepam, and medetomidine-butorphanol-ketamine in captive red wolves (*Canis rufus*). *Journal of Zoo and Wildlife Medicine* 33:101–107.

McKenzie AA, Burroughs REJ. 1993. Chemical capture of carnivores. In: *The Capture and Care Manual* (AA McKenzie, ed.), pp. 226–238. Pretoria: Wildlife Decision Support Services cc and The South African Veterinary Foundation.

McNab BK. 1995. Energy expenditure and conservation in frugivorous and mixed-diet carnivorans. *Journal of Mammalogy* 76:206–222.

Maddock AH. 1989. Anesthesia of four species of viverridae with ketamine. *South African Journal of Wildlife Research* 19:80–84.

Mitchell PC. 1905. On the intestinal tract of mammals. *Transactions of the Zoological Society of London* 17:437–531.

Moresco A, Larsen RS. 2003. Medetomidine-ketamine-butorphanol anesthetic combinations in binturongs (*Arctictis binturong*). *Journal of Zoo and Wildlife Medicine* 34:346–351.

Mudappa D, Chellam R. 2001. Capture and immobilization of wild brown palm civets in Western Ghats. *Journal of Wildlife Diseases* 37:383–386.

Nowak RM. 2005. *Walker's Carnivores of the World*. Baltimore and London: Johns Hopkins University Press.

Palomares F. 1993. Immobilization of common genets, *Genetta genetta*, with a combination of ketamine and xylazine. *Journal of Wildlife Diseases* 29:174–176.

Ray JC, Sunquist ME. 2001. Trophic relations in a community of African rainforest carnivores. *Oecologia* 127(3):395.

Rettig T, Divers B. 1986. Viverridae. In: *Zoo and Wild Animal Medicine* (ME Fowler, ed.), pp. 822–828. Philadelphia: W.B. Saunders Company.

Seal US, Ericksson AW. 1969. Immobilization of carnivora and other mammals with phencylcidine and promazine. *Federation Proceedings* 28:1410–1419.

Sladky KK, Kelly BT, Loomis MR, Stoskopf MK, Horne WA. 2000. Cardiorespiratory effects of four alpha2-adrenoceptor agonist-ketamine combinations. *Journal of the American Veterinary Medical Association* 217:1366–1371.

Streicher U. 2001. The use of xylazine and ketamine in Owston's palm civets, *Chrotogale owstoni*. *Small Carnivore Conservation* 24:18–19.

Veron G, Heard S. 2000. Molecular systematics of the Asiatic viverridae (carnivora) inferred from mitochondrial cytochrome *b* sequence analysis. *Journal of Zoological Systematics and Evolutionary Research* 38:209–217.

WEBLIOGRAPHY

http://www.isis.org/Pages/findanimals.aspx, accesses on March 4, 2013

http://www.IUCN.org, accessed on March 4, 2013

http://www.ITIS.gov , accessed on March 4, 2013

44 Hyenidae

Nina Hahn, John M. Parker, Gregory Timmel, Mary L. Weldele, and Wm. Kirk Suedmeyer

INTRODUCTION

A breeding colony of spotted hyenas (*Crocuta crocuta*) was established at the University of California, Berkeley (UCB) in 1985 with wild cubs collected in Kenya. The spotted hyena was selected for research because of unique morphological and behavioral characteristics. Female spotted hyenas are larger than, and dominant to, males. They lack an external vagina, and instead have a hypertrophied, penis-like clitoris through which they urinate, copulate, and give birth. This makes them a useful research model in which to study the general mechanisms of sexual differentiation, and the differential development of morphology and behavior.

Colony management has included annual physical exams, which are always performed on anesthetized animals. Hyenas are also anesthetized for longer-term procedures including dentistry, diagnostic imaging, and surgery. They are also routinely immobilized to collect blood and measurements essential to research. Nearly 2000 anesthetic procedures have been performed in the over-20 years that the UCB colony has been existent, and no mortality has resulted from anesthesia. Unique characteristics of hyena anesthesia are outlined in the following chapter.

TAXONOMY AND BIOLOGY RELATED TO ANESTHESIA AND HANDLING

Hyenas resemble large canids, but because they belong to the suborder Feloidae (with cats and mongooses), they are more closely related to domestic cats (*Felis (sylvestris) catus*) than dogs (*Canis familiaris*). Reports of hyena anatomy and physiology indicate similarities to cats as well as dogs in terms of retinal anatomy (Calde-

rone et al. 2003) and susceptibility to pathogens (East et al. 2004; Ferroglio et al. 2003; Hahn et al. 2003; Harrison et al. 2004; Troyer et al. 2005). Hyenas, however, are more cat-like in several ways including dentition as well as physiological responses to xylazine and ketamine (see discussion later).

It is therefore appropriate that veterinarians utilize physical anesthetic techniques suitable for large dogs, yet rely on domestic cat references for drug choices and dosages.

VASCULAR ACCESS AND SAMPLE COLLECTION SITES

Fore- and hind-limb veins are both readily accessible for catheterization (Fig. 44.1 and Fig. 44.2). The venous anatomy as it pertains to catheterization of the fore limb is comparable with that of the domestic cat (Fig. 44.1). Catheterization of the cephalic vein can be performed with the relative ease of that of a large dog. However, care should always be taken when positioning the catheter to avoid the extensive branching and anastamoses of the superficial fore-limb vessels (Fig. 44.1).

The jugular, cephalic, and saphenous veins are accessible for blood collection and cannulation. Sublingual vessels are prominent and can provide quick vascular access for electrolyte and blood gas analysis during anesthetic procedures. Arterial pulses can be palpated midline on dorsal metacarpi; however, arterial cannulation has not been attempted by these authors. Cerebral spinal fluid can best be collected by cisternal puncture. The occipital protuberance, spinous process of axis, and wings of the atlas can palpated in an intubated hyena despite the thick neck muscles.

Zoo Animal and Wildlife Immobilization and Anesthesia, Second Edition. Edited by Gary West, Darryl Heard, and Nigel Caulkett.
© 2014 John Wiley & Sons, Inc. Published 2014 by John Wiley & Sons, Inc.

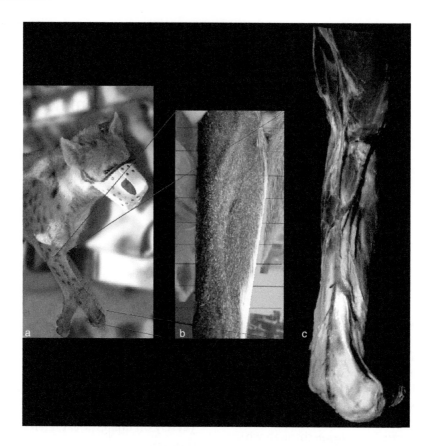

Figure 44.1. Three photographs of the spotted hyena forelimb. (a) A hyena in left lateral recumbency. Note the right antebrachium for panel (b) orientation. (b) An *in situ* cranial–medial view from the level of midelbow to proximal carpus. Note the prominent superficial veins (visualization aided by manual occlusion). (c) The venous anatomy *in situ*. Only the skin and superficial fascia have been removed. In both panels (b) and (c), extensive anastomoses and bifurcations can be observed.

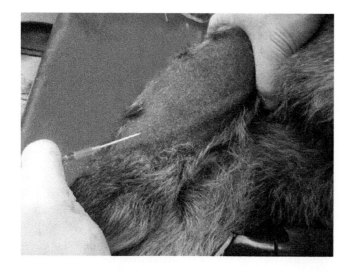

Figure 44.2. Catheter placement in the saphenous vein of a hyena.

RESTRAINT

Chemical restraint (anesthesia) is always necessary prior to performing any procedures on adult hyenas. Cubs less than 1 month of age can be manually restrained for examination and minor procedures such as blood collection and vaccinations. Hyena cubs 2–6 months of age may be placed in a "squeeze-back" cage for hand injection with anesthetics as will be described later.

FIELD TECHNIQUES

The anesthetic procedures described for anesthesia in captive hyenas (see Captive Hyena Immobilization and Anesthesia) are also used in the field (Berger et al. 1992; Place et al. 2002). The most commonly used agent for immobilization in the field, however, is a combination of tiletamine hydrochloride and zolazepam hydrochloride (Telazol®, A.H. Robbins, Richmond, VA), given at an estimated dose of 6.5 mg/kg (K. Holekamp, pers. comm., 2005; Van Horn et al. 2004). For field use in hyenas, Telazol (500-mg vial) is reconstituted with 2.5 mL of diluent instead of the label-recommended 5 mL. The resulting solution provides 86.2 mg/mL of each, tiletamine and zolazepam (combined 172.4 mg/mL of Telazol). Adult hyenas receive 1.8–2.0 mL, sub-adults 1.4–1.6 mL, and cubs ~1 mL of this solution. The actual dose used is probably <6.5 mg/kg, and 5 mg/kg of Telazol is recommended for captive hyenas. Hyenas can be darted with either a blow pipe or a CO_2-powered rifle. The blow pipe is only useful at distances of 1–5 m and only practical for animals that are very comfortable around the vehicle. It is always preferable to use the CO^2 rifle since it is silent and allows the dart to hit the animal with a smaller, less traumatic impact. Hyenas are darted in the early morning hours. They are allowed to recover in the shade and are attended until able to walk. The Telazol dose for field use has also been reported as 2.5 mg/kg (Harrison et al. 2004; Holekamp & Sisk 2003), but this is likely an error.

BODY WEIGHTS AND BLOOD VALUES

Adult colony-born female hyenas weigh 50 kg on average (range 49.5–90 kg). Adult males weigh slightly less than females, averaging 47.6 kg (range 44.5–54.5 kg). Serum chemistry, blood gas analysis, and complete blood count are similar to both cats and dogs (Table 44.1 and Table 44.2). Clot formation is frequently encountered in specimens treated with ethylenediaminetetraacetic acid (EDTA) and therefore heparin is the preferred anticoagulant.

Table 44.1. Serum chemistry ranges for captive adult spotted hyenas under KXA anesthesia

Serum Chemistry	Range	Units
Alk phos	14–136	U/L
ALT	65–162	U/L
AST	76–142	U/L
CK	149–419	U/L
GGT	1–7	U/L
Albumin	2.2–2.8	g/dL
Total protein	6.1–7.7	g/dL
Globulin	3.6–5.2	g/dL
Total bilirubin	0–0.2	mg/dL
Direct bilirubin	0–0.1	mg/dL
BUN	14–30	mg/dL
Creatinine	1.1–1.8	mg/dL
Cholesterol	165–300	mg/dL
Glucose	80–153	mg/dL
Calcium	9–10.9	mg/dL
Phosphorus	3.2–6.5	mg/dL
Chloride	106–118	mEq/L
Potassium	4.2–4.9	mEq/L
Sodium	140–149	mEq/L
A/G ratio	0.4–0.7	
B/C ratio	8.6–23.3	
Indirect bilirubin	0–0.1	mg/dL
NA/K ratio	29–35	
Anion gap	14–24	mEq/L
TCO_2	13–25	mEq/L

Notes: All parameters represent a 95% confidence interval of 210 samples collected from 103 animals over a 7-year period. All samples were treated with either heparin or EDTA. All analysis provided by IDEXX Laboratories Inc.

ALT, Alanine transaminase; AST, aspartate aminotransferase; CK, *creatine kinase*; GGT, gamma-*glutamyl transferase*; BUN, blood urea nitrogen; A/G, albumin to globulin; A/C, albumin to creatinine; NA/K, sodium to potassium.

CAPTIVE HYENA IMMOBILIZATION AND ANESTHESIA

The anesthetic regime established 20 years ago at UCB remains the protocol of choice for captive hyenas. It consists of 4–6 mg/kg ketamine, 1 mg/kg xylazine, and 0.045 mg/kg atropine (KXA). The ketamine dose has been incorrectly reported as 10 mg/kg (Berger et al. 1992; Hahn et al. 2003). Hyenas 9 months of age and older are anesthetized using a reusable, air-charged dart/blow gun system prior to handling. Telinject and Daninject systems have both been used successfully at UCB.

Prior to darting, it is usually best to isolate the hyena in a small enclosure. Hyenas are fasted overnight prior to anesthesia. Xylazine appears to be an emetic in hyenas, as in cats (Plumb 2005), and they frequently vomit after successful darting.

The hind quarters are the preferred anatomic site for dart placement. The excitement preceding darting often induces pronounced side-to-side whipping of the hyena's neck. This precludes the neck/shoulder region from being the preferred target site. Hyenas appear to undergo segmental anesthesia following KXA inoculation delivered into hind quarters; loss of function is first evident in the caudal region (lumbrosacral region, pelvic limbs, and tail).

Mature hyenas are anesthetized with KXA utilizing 3 mL darts and drug preparations of 100 mg/mL ketamine, 100 mg/mL xylazine, and 15 mg/mL atropine. Dart preparation time can be safely performed by first

Table 44.2. Complete blood count ranges for captive adult spotted hyenas under KXA anesthesia

Blood Value	Range	Units
WBC	7200–23,200	Thous./μL
RBC	4.74–8.73	Million/μL
HCT	23–46.5	%
MCV	43–65	fl
MCH	14.4–22.5	pg
MCHC	32.3–35.4	g/dL
Neutrophils	42–85	%
Lymphocytes	5–48	%
Monocytes	0–7	%
Eosinophils	1–14	%
Basophils	0–3	%
Abs. neutrophils	3942–16,353	/μL
Abs. lymphocytes	512–7708	/μL
Abs. monocytes	0–1068	/μL
Abs. eosinophils	98–2440	/μL
Abs. basophils	0–504	/μL

Notes: All parameters represent a 95% confidence interval of 210 samples collected from <100 animals over 7-year period. All samples were treated with either heparin or EDTA. All analysis provided by IDEXX.

WBC, white blood cell; RBC, red blood cell; HCT, hematocrit; MCV, mean corpuscular volume; MCH, mean corpuscular hemoglobin; MCHC, mean corpuscular hemoglobin concentration.

adding calculated doses of xylazine and atropine based on previous weights to the dart syringe, then adding ketamine to fill the remaining 3 mL volume (2.2–2.4 mL). Heavier hyenas will therefore receive a lower dose and will often need supplemental doses of ketamine (1–2 mg/kg) for full sedation. In contrast, low weight animals often require supplemental sedatives to counter the side effects associated with ketamine, such as rigidity and twitching. Intraveneous diazepam (0.1–0.5 mg/kg) is commonly used for this purpose. When supplementing KXA anesthesia, diazepam causes a transient respiratory depression evident by prolonged periods of apnea. Subadult animals may not require the amount of ketamine needed to fill the dart to capacity. Less concentrated preparations of xylazine (20 mg/mL) and atropine (0.54 mg/mL) should be used for small cubs. Hyena cubs can be either hand or squeeze-cage restrained and drugs can be delivered via hand injection. Additionally, cubs generally require approximately 80% of the weight-calculated adult ketamine and xylazine doses. The previously stated adult dose of atropine, however, is used for cubs.

Hyenas must be muzzled upon immobilization, and when applicable, remained muzzled for duration of procedure when maintained on injected anesthetics. The bite response is not as readily abolished by ketamine anesthesia, as it is with dogs, cats, and primates. Jaw tone should be cautiously and properly assessed prior to endotracheal intubation.

Yohimbine (0.11 mg/kg), up to a maximum dose of 6 mg, is administered intramuscularly to reverse the xylazine at the conclusion of the procedure, at least 20 minutes after the last injection of ketamine. The time delay and route of administration decrease the likelihood of negative reaction due to the presence of ketamine.

Telazol (5 mg/kg) has been used successfully to anesthetize "ketamine reactors" (see discussion later) but was associated with a rough, prolonged recovery in the captive colony and therefore is not recommended.

ANESTHETIC MAINTENANCE

For long-term and major surgeries, hyenas are catheterized, intubated, and maintained on isoflurane anesthesia (1–2%) after darting with KXA, as described earlier. Yohimbine given after isoflurane stabilization may help prevent xylazine-induced adverse effects such as bradycardia, respiratory depression respiratory, and loss of thermoregulation, as will be described later.

Intubation of the hyena can be performed using a size 11–12 endotracheal tube with the relative ease of a large dog. The hyena is best intubated while in sternal recumbency. The larynx is easily visualized through the mouth using a large-bladed laryngoscope. Unlike cats, laryngeal spasm during intubation has not been observed.

ANALGESIA

Analgesia is always provided following major surgeries and dental procedures. Buprenorphine (0.01 mg/kg SQ or IM) is administered at the time of intubation and repeated following the end of surgery. If additional analgesia is indicated, 10 mg/kg etodolac (Etogesic®) is administered orally once daily in food. No ill effects have been observed in any hyena receiving etodolac, including one hyena given 9 mg/kg daily for 1 month. Meloxicam (0.2 mg/kg SQ) has been used for endodontic procedures. It is given once at the completion of the procedure.

COMPLICATIONS

Xylazine frequently induces emesis, pronounced bradycardia, and loss of thermoregulation in hyenas. Atropine is included to reduce salivation typical of ketamine and offset bradycardia associated with xylazine administration. Aspiration of regurgitate was noted on necropsy in one geriatric animal (21 years old) with biliary carcinoma following immobilization with KXA, but aspiration following KXA administration has never been a clinical problem in hyenas. As a precaution, however, hyenas are always fasted prior to immobilization.

Hyenas' eyes remain open after ketamine administration, as do cat eyes (Plumb 2005), and should always be treated with ophthalmic lubricant (e.g., Lacri-lube®). Prolonged apnea is noted infrequently following bolus diazepam and ketamine/diazepam administration as occurs in cats.

Hyperthermia in response to KXA administration has been observed. Care is taken to avoid darting during hot weather, but hyperthermia has been noted on days when ambient temperature is not a contributing factor. Hyperthermia has been attributed to agitation and increased activity prior to darting; however, this may be a response to ketamine as has been observed in cats (Plumb 2005). Xylazine causes loss of thermoregulation in many animal species (Plumb 2005) and this may also contribute to hyperthermia in anesthetized hyenas.

Very rarely, respiratory depression after KXA administration is noted. Reversal of the xylazine with yohimbine will correct this. Heart rates as low as 48 beats/minute are often observed, but as clinical outcome for these animals is no different from animals with higher heart rates, this has been attributed to the effects of xylazine and considered normal. Systolic heart murmurs have been occasionally identified during physical exam under KXA anesthesia. Follow-up cardiac ultrasound examinations identified a decrease in ventricular myocardial contractility in the three animals examined. This was attributed to the xylazine component of the anesthetic combination and not considered clinically significant.

There are two types of adverse reaction to KXA anesthesia that have been observed. Some hyenas display tonic-clonic-like movements and extensor rigidity after KXA administration. This response is not uncommon in male hyenas. Male hyenas weigh on average less than female hyenas and therefore may receive the high end of the 4- to 6-mg/kg ketamine range when following the UCB KXA protocol. The adverse ketamine reaction observed in these hyenas may be due to the ensuing relatively high ketamine to xylazine ratio. This reaction may be similar to what has been described in captive macaque monkeys (*Macaca mulatta*), which undergo frequent exposure to ketamine anesthesia. In macaques, ketamine causes varying degrees of muscle rigidity in susceptible individuals. These animals may have a tonic-clonic or psychotomimetic response to the administration of ketamine (UC Davis Veterinary School, Clinical Medical Primatology lecture notes). Cats also demonstrate "myoclonic jerking and/or tonic/clonic convulsions" (package insert of Ketaset®) with ketamine administration.

Two male hyenas (brothers with the same parents but from different litters) developed generalized seizures after KXA administration. They both had been anesthetized with KXA numerous times. Both of these animals developed generalized seizures when anesthetized with KXA in their fourth year. Prior to having seizures, neither of these two animals demonstrated the tonic-clonic movements as described earlier. Hyenas at the UCB colony are routinely immobilized for research purposes seven times the first year, four times the second year, twice the third year, and yearly thereafter. Seizures have been reported to occur in 20% of cats anesthetized with therapeutic doses of ketamine (Plumb 2005). Ketamine is known to be epileptogenic (Plumb 2005), and there may be individual susceptibility to the effects of ketamine in hyenas, but the mechanism of both the seizure activity and tonic-clonic movements are purely speculative.

Diazepam (0.5–1 mg/kg IV to effect) will eliminate seizures as well as tonic-clonic muscle activity in hyenas. Diazepam should always be kept close at hand when anesthetizing hyenas.

RECOVERY

Hyenas are placed in a straw-bedded, enclosed cage for postsurgical recovery. Animals are allowed to fully recover from anesthesia prior to being reintroduced to cage mates. After short-term procedures using xylazine reversal, this can generally be within 1–2 hours of anesthesia. In longer term or major surgical procedures when xylazine reversal is not used, or if opioid analgesics are used, hyenas are allowed overnight recovery prior to reintroduction to cage mates. After laparotomy hyenas are kept separate from cage mates for up to 2 weeks.

DISEASE ISSUES (AFFECTING ANESTHESIA)

Acute and peracute pain has dramatic effects on dosage requirements and induction time. Beyond this, there are no known disease issues that affect anesthesia in hyenas.

FIELD IMMOBILIZATION OF THE BROWN HYENA (*HYAENA BRUNNEA*) IN NAMIBIA

Wm. Kirk Suedmeyer

Few references for field immobilization techniques of the brown hyena are reported in the literature. An understanding of the natural history and habits facilitates successful capture. Health assessment, placement of tracking devices, evaluation of reproductive status, and morphometric measurements are only accomplished by immobilization (Fig. 44.3).

The brown hyena is a nocturnal, cautious, silent, and solitary forager (Estes 1992; Mills 2003; Nowak 1991). However, large carcasses will attract several hyenas. As opposed to the spotted hyena (*C. crocuta*), brown hyenas generally feed singly, rather than as groups, even on larger carcasses; individuals will wait patiently in the distance until a conspecific finishes. In most instances, black-backed jackals (*Canis mesomelas*) will arrive at the site first; vocalization and activity of larger groups of jackals may attract hyenas to the location. Jackals will commonly telegraph a hyenas approach by nervously looking in the direction of the approaching animal. In some areas, hyenas disperse jackals from the site, whereas in other locations, jackals antagonize hyenas from the carcass. Use of camouflage, a low profile silhouette, and absolute stillness are paramount to success. The field marksman should be in

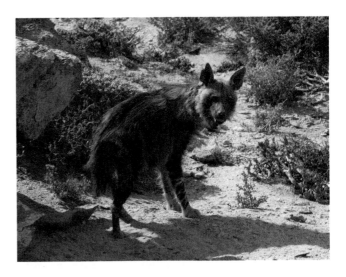

Figure 44.3. A GPS collared brown hyena (*Hyaena brunnea*) inadvertently disturbed from its daytime den. Brown hyenas are rarely observed during daylight hours.

place prior to sunset as brown hyenas are very aware of movement and changes in the environment. Utilization of enhanced lighting in the form of infrared technology facilitates darting during moonless nights. Dart placement is key to efficient immobilization. Commercially available remote delivery systems work well. A well-aimed dart placed in the shoulder or neck affords consistent success. Patience is necessary to predict the stance of the hyena while feeding. Carcasses should be placed in a position that encourages the hyena to present a lateral profile. Use of a centrally located, secured carcass with a peripheral, spoke-wheeled scent trail improves chances for success. The strength of hyenas should not be underestimated. Adult hyenas have been observed carrying entire carcasses of freshly killed Cape fur seal pups (*Arctocephalus pusillus*) (Wiesel 2010), removing springbok (*Antidorcas marsupialis*), and large carrion away from dart sites. Carcasses must be secured with 1–2 m posts driven deeply into the ground. Hyenas will carry carcasses to more secure locations if they can.

A combination of 3–4 mg/kg of ketamine hydrochloride with 0.035–0.045 mg/kg of medetomidine hydrochloride provides effect within 3 minutes and recumbency within 7 minutes on average. It is advisable to use either telemetry darts, and/or allow several minutes before attempting to locate the immobilized animal as brown hyenas are prone to running for extended distances if startled. The initial response is a sudden gallop from the dart site, followed by circling back to the general area as the drugs take effect. In most instances, the hyena can be located less than 50 yards from the initial site. On occasion, an anesthetized hyena may require 30–40 mg of supplemental ketamine hydrochloride given intramuscularly to facilitate complete recumbency. This combination provides good muscle relaxation, stable heart rate and rhythm (although bradycardia is commonly encountered; heart rates average 40–60 beats/min), slight to moderate pytalism, and 40–50 minutes of stable anesthesia. Rectal body temperatures with this combination average 1000°F.

Atropine sulfate should not be utilized to control pytalism, as it counters the alpha adrenergic effects on peripheral vasoconstriction and can lead to complications. Initial hypoxia (<75% pulse oximetry) is routinely observed but improves over time. In most instances, brown hyenas achieve pulse oximetry readings of >90% after 20–30 minutes of anesthesia. Supplemental oxygen should be provided if available. Application of a bland ophthalmic ointment protects the eyes during times of blowing sand. Covering the eyes and placing plugs in the ear canal also lessens ocular and aural stimulation, which, in turn, provides consistent recumbency (Fig. 44.4). Reversal is achieved with atipamezole hydrochloride at five times the milligram dose of medetomidine induction. Atipamezole

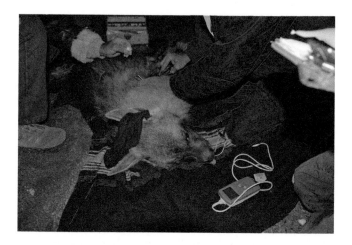

Figure 44.4. A brown hyena (*Hyaena brunnea*) anesthetized with ketamine HCl and medetomidine HCl in Namibia. Note the aural plugs, pulse oximetry, and substrate barrier.

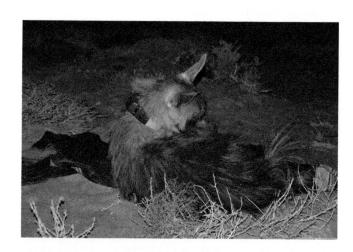

Figure 44.5. A brown hyena (*Hyaena brunnea*) shortly after reversal with atipamezole. Note the position of the head and cervical spine just prior to standing.

given intramuscularly produces smooth, reliable recovery within 5–10 minutes. Blepharospasm, followed by purposeful movement of the head and cervical spine, is a prelude to rapid recovery to standing within minutes (Fig. 44.5).

In general, the hyena stands then canters away with mild ataxia, which rapidly resolves to normal ambulation within an additional 3–5 minutes. It is advisable to remotely monitor the response to full recovery as black-backed jackals can antagonize and injure the hyena unless it is fully recovered (Fig. 44.6).

Use of ketamine/medetomidine produces, safe, reliable, and predictable results of the brown hyena in field situations and may be a suitable combination for captive anesthetic approaches.

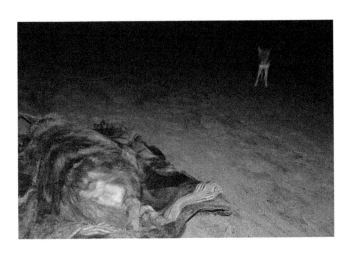

Figure 44.6. An anesthetized brown hyena (*Hyaena brunnea*) immediately after reversal with atipamezole. Note the encroachment by a black-backed jackal (*Canis mesomelas*), which can injure recumbent hyenas.

REFERENCES

Berger DMP, Frank LG, Glickman SE. 1992. Unraveling ancient mysteries: biology, behavior and captive management of the spotted hyena (*Crocuta crocuta*). Proceedings of the Joint Meeting of the American Association of Zoo Veterinarians/American Association of Wildlife Veterinarians.

Calderone JB, Reese BE, Jacobs GH. 2003. Topography of photoreceptors and retinal ganglion cells in the spotted hyena (*Crocuta crocuta*). *Brain, Behavior and Evolution* 62(4):182–192.

East ML, Moestl K, Benetka V, Pitra C, Honer OP, Wachter B, Hofer H. 2004. Coronavirus infection of spotted hyenas in the Serengeti ecosystem. *Veterinary Microbiology* 102(1–2):1–9.

Estes RD. 1992. *The Behavior Guide to African Mammals*, pp. 323–348. Los Angeles: University of California Press.

Ferroglio E, Wambwa E, Castiello M, Trisciuoglio A, Prouteau A, Pradere E, Ndungu S, De Meneghi D. 2003. Antibodies to *Neospora caninum* in wild animals from Kenya, East Africa. *Veterinary Parasitology* 118(1–2):43–49.

Hahn NE, Jenne KJ, Diggs HE. 2003. Dermatophytosis in three colony-born spotted hyenas. *Journal of the American Veterinary Medical Association* 223(12):1809–1811.

Harrison TM, Mazet JK, Holekamp KE, Dubovi E, Engh AL, Nelson K, Van Horn RC, Munson L. 2004. Antibodies to canine and feline viruses in spotted hyenas (*Crocuta crocuta*) in the Masai Mara National Reserve. *Journal of Wildlife Diseases* 40(1):1–10.

Holekamp KE, Sisk CL. 2003. Effects of dispersal status on pituitary and gonadal function in the male spotted hyena. *Hormones and Behavior* 44(5):385–394.

Mills MGL. 2003. *Kalahari Hyenas*, pp. 5–22, 33–48, 55–78, 112–200. Caldwell: Blackburn Press.

Nowak RM. 1991. *Walker's Mammals of the World*, Vol. II, 5th ed., pp. 1177–1184. Baltimore: John Hopkins University Press.

Place NJ, Weldele ML, Wahaj SA. 2002. Ultrasonic measurements of second and third trimester fetuses to predict gestational age and date of parturition in captive and wild spotted hyenas *Crocuta crocuta*. *Theriogenology* 58(5):1047–1055.

Plumb DC. 2005. *Veterinary Drug Handbook*, 5th ed. Ames: Blackwell Publishing.

Troyer JL, Pecon-Slattery J, Roelke ME, Johnson W, VandeWoude S, Vazquez-Salat N, Brown M, Frank L, Woodroffe R, Winterbach C, Winterbach H, Hemson G, Bush M, Alexander KA, Revilla E, O'Brien SJ. 2005. Seroprevalence and genomic divergence of circulating strains of feline immunodeficiency virus among *Felidae* and *Hyaenidae* species. *Journal of Virology* 79(13):8282–8294.

Van Horn RC, Engh AL, Scribner KT, Funk SM, Holekamp KE. 2004. Behavioural structuring of relatedness in the spotted hyena (*Crocuta crocuta*) suggests direct fitness benefits of clan-level cooperation. *Molecular Ecology* 13(2):449–458.

Wiesel I. 2010. Killing of cape fur seal (*Arctocephalus pusillus pusillus*) pups by brown hyenas (*ParaHyaena brunnea*) at mainland breeding colonies along the coastal Namib desert. *Acta Ethologica* 13:93–100.

45 Felids

Edward C. Ramsay

INTRODUCTION AND TAXONOMY

There are 38 species in the family Felidae and general agreement surrounding the taxonomy of the large felids, cheetah, and clouded leopard (Nowak 2005). The genus *Panthera* contains all the large cats: lions (*Panthera leo*), tigers (*Panthera tigris*), leopards (*Panthera pardus*), snow leopards (*Panthera uncia*), and jaguars (*Panthera onca*). The cheetah, *Acinonyx jubatus*, and the clouded leopard, *Neofelis nebulosa*, are the sole member of each respective genus. There is considerable controversy over the taxonomy of the smaller felids, but most small felids have been grouped, by some, in the genus *Felis*. *Felis* species range in size from the black-footed cat, *Felis nigripes* (body weight of 1.5–2.75 kg) to the cougar, *Felis concolor* (body weight of 36–103 kg). The large felids range in size from leopards (28–90 kg) to tigers (100–306 kg) (Nowak 2005).

Regardless of size or taxonomy, all adult members of the family Felidae require chemical restraint for performing a thorough physical examination and gathering samples. While some species and individuals can be trained to allow obtaining blood or other biological samples while awake (Fig. 45.1), chemical immobilization is the norm. Relatively little research has been done on small felids, but there are many reports on immobilization of the larger felids, particularly tigers, lions, leopards, and cheetahs. Additionally, the majority of the immobilization literature is based on studies of captive cats. As a result, the information in this chapter is heavily biased toward information on captive, large felids.

ANATOMY RELATED TO IMMOBILIZATION AND ANESTHESIA

The anatomy of nondomestic felids is very similar to domestic cat anatomy, such that virtually all routine clinical procedures and techniques can be based on those used in domestic cats. Once immobilized, blood is most easily obtained from the jugular veins or the medial sapheneous veins distal to the knee. These vessels are easily visualized after the overlying fur is clipped. These veins are also useful for intravenous injection and placement of intravenous catheters. Tail veins, located dorso-laterally at "10:00 and 2:00" on the tail, can be used to obtain blood samples or for administration of supplemental immobilization drugs. They can be difficult to visualize, even with the fur clipped. The femoral veins can also be used for blood collection, especially in animals where the hair cannot be clipped, but this vessel is not easily visualized and somewhat difficult to catheterize. The cephalic vein is accessible for blood collection and drug administration in some species, but it is difficult to visualize in large felids, even after clipping the hair. Dorsal pedal arteries or femoral arteries are most commonly used to obtain arterial blood samples.

PHYSICAL RESTRAINT

Some individuals of small felid species and young larger species (<10 kg) can be netted for injection by hand, but the safety of this method depends on the attitude of the individual cat, the skill of the netter, and the setup of the enclosure or room. It is preferable to transfer the animal to a small cage or squeeze cage for injection. Squeeze cages are useful for physical restraint of all felids, but even these cages do not allow much more than hand injection of drugs. As with any squeeze cage, the operator should not attempt to squeeze the cat until it is completely immobilized, as the possibility for injuring the animal increases as greater pressure is exerted. Ideally, a squeeze cage should be used to bring

Zoo Animal and Wildlife Immobilization and Anesthesia, Second Edition. Edited by Gary West, Darryl Heard, and Nigel Caulkett.
© 2014 John Wiley & Sons, Inc. Published 2014 by John Wiley & Sons, Inc.

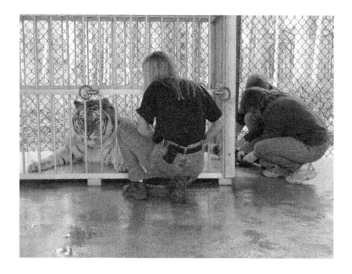

Figure 45.1. Voluntary blood draw in a tiger. This tiger is trained to get into a small cage and lie down. The tail of the animal is pulled through the bars or a small opening in the cage and the veterinary technician is able to take a blood sample from the tail vein. The trainer is located at the front of the animal and rewards verbally and with food.

the animal into close enough proximity to permit safe hand injection.

TRANQUILIZATION OR PREMEDICATION

Benzodiazepines
Diazepam and midazolam are the two benzodiazepines most commonly used for tranquilization of nondomestic felids. Both drugs are also used to treat seizures and may be selected for use in cats prone to seizures while immobilized.

Diazepam is variably absorbed when given intramuscularly and thus should be given either orally or intravenously. Oral diazepam can be used as premedication, administered 1–3 hours before immobilization. Repeated dosing of diazepam has been reported to cause idiopathic hepatic toxicity in domestic cats (Center et al. 1996). This problem has not been observed in nondomestic cats, but most clinicians use oral diazepam for short periods (the day before and/or the day of immobilization) in nondomestic felids. Oral diazepam dosages of 0.15–0.46 mg/kg (20–60 mg/adult tiger or lion) have been used for premedication with good effect in large cats. Intravenous doses are typically 0.08–0.15 mg/kg (10–20 mg/adult tiger or lion).

Midazolam has largely replaced diazepam in clinical practice because of its more predictable intramuscular absorption. Although only available in the United States as an injectable agent, the injectable preparation can be given orally as a premedication or added to other agents in a dart. Typical dosages for premedication for a tiger are 0.08–0.14 mg/kg (15 mg/adult tiger or lion), PO or IM. A similar dosage is used during

induction protocols (Curro et al. 2004). In people, midazolam has amnesic properties and whether this is true in nondomestic felids is not known. If it does have some amnesic properties, this would be an added benefit of using midazolam in immobilization combinations.

OTHER TRANQUILIZATION AGENTS
Relatively few other tranquilizing agents are used in nondomestic felids. A trial of two long-acting tranquilizers, perphenazine enanthate and zuclopenthixol acetate, used separately and together, in cheetahs showed perphenazine enanthate (3.0-mg/kg deep IM) significantly reduced the cats' behavior for days 1–6 post injection (PI) (Huber et al. 2001). Perphenazine enanthate treated cheetahs returned to normal behavior patterns by day 14 PI. Zuclopenthixol acetate at 0.6 mg/kg produced profound adverse effects (inappetance, ataxia, extrapyramidal effects), and the authors felt it "should not be used in cheetahs" (Huber et al. 2001).

INDUCTION AND CHEMICAL IMMOBILIZATION
Safety
All nondomestic felids are capable of harming, potentially mortally, those working with the cat. Every cat should, following administration of immobilizing drugs, remain restrained, either in a cage, squeeze cage, or box, until it is ascertained that the animal is sufficiently obtunded. In the author's practice, cats are assessed for depth of anesthesia by monitoring an ear twitch reflex. Using a stick or similar item (pole syringe, rake handle, etc.), the hair inside the ears is brushed and ear movement noted. No cat that moves its ear following stimulation should be handled. Wait and/or administer supplemental drugs if the anticipated induction time has passed. Additionally, supplemental ketamine should always be carried with an immobilized nondomestic cat wherever it is outside of a cage or exhibit. If an animal begins to move or awaken, an immediate injection of 1- to 3-mg/kg ketamine, IM or IV, should be administered.

Ketamine Hydrochloride
Ketamine HCl is the most common immobilization agent used in nondomestic felids and has proven itself safe and effective in a wide variety of species (Table 45.1 and Table 45.2) (Armstrong et al. 1996; Deem et al. 1998; Grassman et al. 2004; Jalanka & Roeken 1990; Kolata 2002; McKenzie & Burroughs 1993; Tomizawa et al. 1997). In smaller species or small individuals, ketamine can be used alone for chemical immobilization. In larger species, complete and satisfactory immobilization with ketamine alone may not be possible due to the adverse effects seen with greater dosages, such

Table 45.1. Dosages for immobilization agents used in large nondomestic felids (*Panthera* spp.) and cheetahs (*Acinonyx jubatus*)

Species	Agents	Dosages (Reversal Agents and Dosages)	Reference
Cheetah			
	Ketamine + medetomidine	2.5 mg/kg + 50–70 μg/kg (atipamezole 0.3 mg/kg [25% IV/75% SC])	Klein and Stover (1993)
		1.57 mg/kg + 31 μg/kg (atipamezole 0.15 mg/kg)	Deem et al. (1998)
	Tiletamine-zolazepam	1.6–3.6 mg/kg (light anesthesia)	Smeller and Bush (1997)
		4.0 mg/kg	Schumacher et al. (2003)
		3.0–4.0 mg/kg	McKenzie and Burroughs (1993)*
		4.8–7.8 mg/kg	Taylor et al. (1998)
		2.0–3.0 mg/kg	Meltzer (1999)
	Tiletamine-zolazepam 50 mg/mL + ketamine 80 mg/mL + xylazine 20 mg/mL	0.023 mL/kg (yohimbine 0.1–0.2 mg/kg)	Lewandowski et al. (2002)
	Medetomidine + butorphanol + midazolam	35 μg/kg + 0.02 mg/kg + 0.15 mg/kg (atipamezole + flumazenil + naltrexone 0.18 mg/kg + 6 μg/kg + 0.25 mg/kg)	Lafortune et al. (2005)
	Saffan® [9-mg/mL alphaxolone and 3-mg/mL alphadolone]	5.0 mL IV	Meltzer (1999)
Jaguar (*Panthera onca*)			
	Ketamine + medetomidine	4.4 mg/kg + 40 μg/kg (atipamezole 0.1 mg/kg)	Burgos-Rodriguez et al. (2004)[a]
	Ketamine + medetomidine	2.5 mg/kg + 60–80 μg/kg (atipamezole 0.12–0.24 mg/kg)	Jalanka and Roeken (1990)
Leopard (*Panthera pardus*)			
	Ketamine + xylazine	5.0 mg/kg + 1.4 mg/kg Supplemental ketamine: 50–70 mg/adult	Belsare and Athreya (2010)*
		8.0–10.0 mg/kg + 1.0 mg/kg	McKenzie and Burroughs (1993)*
		7.0–8.0 mg/kg + 3.0–4.0 mg/kg	McKenzie and Burroughs (1993)*
Amur subspecies (*Panthera p. orientalis*)			
	Ketamine + xylazine	6.6 mg/kg + 0.66 mg/kg (yohimbine 0.04–0.13 mg/kg) Supplemental drug: ketamine 1.1 mg/kg	Quigley et al. (2001)*
	Ketamine + medetomidine	2.5–3.0 mg/kg + 60–80 μg/kg (atipamezole 0.12–0.24 mg/kg)	Jalanka and Roeken (1990)
Leopard, snow (*Panthera uncia*)			
	Ketamine + medetomidine	2.5–3.0 mg/kg + 60–80 μg/kg (atipamezole 0.29 mg/kg)	Jalanka (1989)
Lion, African (*Panthera leo*)			
	Ketamine + medetomidine	1.9–5.7 mg/kg + 48–58 μg/kg (Atipamezole 0.19–0.23 mg/kg)	Tomizawa et al. (1997)
		2.0–3.0 mg/kg + 60–80 μg/kg (atipamezole 0.12–0.24 mg/kg)	Jalanka and Roeken (1990)
		2.5 mg/kg + 30 μg/kg (atipamezole 0.29 mg/kg)	Jalanka and Roeken (1990)
		2.0–3.0 mg/kg + 20–30 μg/kg (atipamezole 0.1–0.15 mg/kg)	McCain et al. (2009)
	Ketamine + xylazine	7.0–8.0 mg/kg + 3.0–4.0 mg/kg	McKenzie and Burroughs (1993)*
		10 mg/kg + 1.0 mg/kg (yohimbine 0.1 mg/kg IV)	Epstein et al. (2002); Ofri et al. (1998)
	Tiletamine-zolazepam	4.0–6.0 mg/kg	McKenzie and Burroughs (1993)*
		3.8 mg/kg	Bush et al. (1978)
	Tiletamine-zolazepam + medetomidine	1.0 mg/kg + 15 μg/kg (atipamezole: no dose given)	Roken (1997)
		0.6 mg/kg + 25 μg/kg (atipamezole: no dose given)	
		Repeat tiletamine/zolazepam dosage at 45 minutes	Roken (1997)
Tiger (*Panthera tigris*)			
	Ketamine + xylazine + midazolam	9.7 mg/kg + 0.49 mg/kg + 0.1 mg/kg (yohimbine 0.11 mg/kg)	Curro et al. (2004)
	Ketamine + xylazine	4.0–6.0 mg/kg + 0.4 mg/kg (yohimbine 0.05 mg/kg) Supplementation: ketamine 1.0 mg/kg or Diazepam 0.01–0.05 mg/kg IV (slowly) or Midazolam 0.01 mg/kg IV	Armstrong et al. (1996)

(Continued)

637

Table 45.1.   *(Continued)*

Species	Agents	Dosages (Reversal Agents and Dosages)	Reference
	Ketamine + medetomidine	200 mg + 3.0 mg (per adult tiger) (atipamezole 15 mg (per tiger))	Miller et al. (2003)
For South Chinese subspecies (*Panthera t. amoyensis*)			
	Ketamine + xylazine	7.7 mg/kg for males or 11.9 mg/kg for females + 0.4 mg/kg (yohimbine 0.05 mg/kg)	Armstrong et al. (1996)
Sumatran subspecies (*Panthera t. sumatrae*)			
	Ketamine + medetomidine	3.0 mg/kg + 18 μg/kg (atipamezole 0.06 mg/kg [50% IV/50% IM])	Forsyth et al. (1999)[a]
	Ketamine + xylazine	4.0–6.0 mg/kg; ≤0.2 mg xylazine/kg	Armstrong et al. (1996)
Amur subspecies (*Panthera t. altaica*)			
	Ketamine + medetomidine	2.5 mg/kg + 80–100 μg/kg (atipamezole 0.12–0.24 mg/kg)	Jalanka (1989)
		2.5 mg/kg + 30 μg/kg	Jalanka (1989)
	Ketamine + medetomidine + midazolam	2.5 mg/kg + 46 μg/kg + 0.1 mg/kg (atipamezole 0.23 mg/kg)	Curro et al. (2004)
	Ketamine + xylazine	10.8 mg/kg + 0.8 mg/kg	Goodrich et al. (2001)*
		6.6 mg/kg + 0.66 mg/kg (yohimbine 0.04–0.13 mg/kg)	
		Supplemental ketamine: 1.1 mg/kg	Quigley et al. (2001)*
	Tiletamine-zolazepam + medetomidine	0.8 mg/kg + 20 μg/kg (Atipamezole: no dose given)	Roken (1997)

Note: Mean dosages reported, when available. All agents administered IM, unless otherwise indicated.
[a]Only one animal immobilized.
*Dosages for immobilization of wild felids.

as seizures (Taylor et al. 1998). For these animals, ketamine is typically combined with an alpha-2 adrenergic agonist, benzodiazepine, and/or an opioid.

Ketamine inductions are usually smooth and rapid but can be stormy if an inadequate initial dose is given, either due to poor dart placement or to partial dart discharge. Felids immobilized with ketamine alone, and with some ketamine combinations, will keep their eyes open, retain palpebral reflexes, and have poor muscle relaxation. Maintaining a low amount of environmental stimulation (i.e., darkening the room, decreasing noise) during induction, immobilization, and recovery, regardless of the agent or combination of agents given, will benefit the patient. Supplemental doses of ketamine (Table 45.2) can be given IM or IV to animals immobilized with ketamine alone and with most immobilization drug combinations (Curro et al. 2004; Epstein et al. 2002). There is no reversal agent for the effects of ketamine; however, ketamine immobilizations, in dosages typically used in felids, are generally short (20–45 minutes). Felids recovering from ketamine alone may be stormy, that is, display ataxia, falling, and hallucination-like behavior.

In the United States, ketamine is commercially available in a 100-mg/mL concentration. At this concentration, large volumes (>5 mL) may be required to immobilize a very large cat, such as a Siberian tiger. More concentrated ketamine (200 mg/mL) can be compounded, and many practitioners prefer this concentration as it permits smaller injection volumes. Limited availability in the United States and issues with crystals forming in the vials, causing concern about actual concentration of preparation, have caused the author to rely on the 100 mg/mL product.

Ketamine plus an alpha-2 adrenergic agonist is the most commonly used drug combination for nondomestic felid immobilization (Table 45.1 and Table 45.2). A great advantage to the addition of an alpha-2 adrenergic agonist is their effects can be reversed with an alpha-2 antagonist (see discussion later), greatly shortening recovery times and improving the safety of the immobilization. While protocols vary, the author and others prefer to initially inject the cat with an alpha-2 agent, possibly in combination with or following premedication with midazolam. Once the animal is sedated, then ketamine is administered (Armstrong et al. 1996; Curro et al. 2004). The alpha-2 agents do not appear to cause intense irritation when injected, such as occurs with ketamine injections, and once the cat is sedated, it will frequently not respond to injection of the ketamine.

Ketamine/medetomidine combinations in felids are probably the most widely used induction "cocktails" in the past decade. A variety of dosages have been reported, with ketamine dosages ranging from 1 to 6 mg/kg and medetomidine dosages of 20–60 μg/kg (Table 45.1 and Table 45.2). The dosage of each tends to change inversely, that is, as dosages of medetomidine are increased, dosages of ketamine are decreased. Sumatran tigers may be more susceptible to effects of medetomi-

Table 45.2. Dosages for immobilization agents used in small nondomestic felids (*Felis* spp. and *Neofelis nebulosa*)

Species	Agents	Dosages (Reversal Agents and Dosages)	Reference
Bobcat (*Felis rufus*)			
	Ketamine + xylazine	13.3 mg/kg + 1.2 mg/kg	Beltrán and Tewes (1995)*
Cougar, mountain lion, puma, or panther (*Felis concolor*)			
	Ketamine/medetomidine	2.2 mg/kg + 43 μg/kg (atipamezole 0.25 mg/kg (50% IM/50% SC)	Schumacher et al. (1999)
	Ketamine + xylazine	4.7–15.8 mg/kg + 0.8–2.6 mg/kg (target dosages: 11 mg/kg + 1.8 mg/kg)	Logan et al. (1986)*
		8.4 mg/kg + 1.8 mg/kg	Schumacher et al. (1999)
	Tiletamine-zolazepam + ketamine	0.6–2.5 mg/kg + 4.0–15.5 mg/kg	Taylor et al. (1998)*
Clouded leopard (*N. nebulosa*)			
	Ketamine + xylazine	19.3 mg/kg + 1.6 mg/kg	Grassman et al. (2004)*
	Tiletamine-zolazepam	10.1 mg/kg	Grassman et al. 2004*
Golden cat (*Felis temmincki*)			
	Ketamine + medetomidine	3.0–4.0 mg/kg + 80–100 μg/kg (atipamezole 0.12–0.24 mg/kg)	Jalanka and Roeken (1990)
	Ketamine + xylazine	29.6 mg/kg + 2.1 mg/kg	Grassman et al. (2004)*
Marbled cat (*Felis marmorata*)			
	Ketamine + xylazine	24.9 mg/kg + 1.7 mg/kg	Grassman et al. (2004)*
Leopard cat (*Felis bengalensis*)			
	Ketamine + xylazine	27.4 mg/kg + 1.9 mg/kg	Grassman et al. (2004)*
	Tiletamine-zolazepam	11.6 mg/kg	Grassman et al. (2004)*
		10.0 mg/kg	Rabinowitz (1990)*
		4.0–5.0 mg/kg	McKenzie and Burroughs (1993)*
Lynx (*Felis lynx* and *Felis canadensis*)			
	Ketamine + medetomidine	5.0 mg/kg + 80–200 μg/kg (atipamizole 0.16–0.4 mg/kg)	Arnemo et al. (1999)*
	Ketamine + xylazine	4.6 mg/kg + 4.0 mg/kg	Ferraras et al. (1994)*
		6.8 mg/kg + 0.4 mg/kg (yohimbine 0.1 mg/kg SC)	Greer et al. (2003)*
	Tiletamine-zolazepam	5.0 mg/kg	Poole et al. (1993)*
	Tiletamine-zolazepam + medetomidine	0.5 mg/kg + 50 μg/kg (Atipamezole: no dose given)	Roken (1997)
Ocelot (*Felis pardalis*)			
	Ketamine + xylazine	14.7 mg/kg + 1.1 mg/kg	Beltrán and Tewes (1995)*
	Tiletamine/zolazepam	5.5 mg/kg	Shindle and Tewes (2000)*
Pallas cats (*Felis manul*)			
	Ketamine + medetomidine + butorphanol	2.0–2.5 mg/kg + 40 μg/kg + 0.15 mg/kg (atipamizole 0.2 mg/kg)	Ketz-Riley et al. (2003)
Serval (*Felis serval*)			
	Ketamine + medetomidine + butorphanol	1.0 mg/kg + 47 μg/kg + 0.2 mg/kg (atipamezole 0.24 μg/kg (50% IV/50%)	Langan et al. (2000)

Note: Mean dosages reported, when available, and all drugs administered IM, unless otherwise indicated
*Dosages for immobilization of wild felids.

dine than others (Table 45.1) (Forsyth et al. 1999). Ketamine/medetomidine inductions and recoveries tend to be more rapid than those in cats immobilized with ketamine/xylazine (Curro et al. 2004; Schumacher et al. 1999). Midazolam or butorphanol can be added to ketamine/medetomidine combinations to smooth inductions and recoveries, and prolonged sedative effects (Curro et al. 2004; Ketz-Riley et al. 2003; Langan et al. 2000).

Ketamine/medetomidine inductions are rapid (3–11 minutes) when the drugs are given together, and cats typically become deeply sedated. Vomiting during induction and transient apnea immediately following induction are the two most commonly observed adverse effects (Curro et al. 2004). Occasionally, decreased

respiratory rates persist during immobilization, especially at greater medetomidine dosages. Medetomidine effects can be reversed with atipamizole (see discussion later).

Medetomidine is a racemic mixture of dextro- and levo-medetomidine, with both enantiomers present in equal proportions. It was previously commercially available in the United States as Dormitor®, a 1-mg/mL product, but this has recently been withdrawn from the US market. More concentrated medetomidine preparations (10–40 mg/mL) remain available from compounding pharmacies in North America. Dexmedetomidine (Dexdormitor®, Pfizer, Inc., New York, NY) contains only the active dextro-enantiomer of the medetomidine and is now marketed in the United States for use in dogs and cats. It is available as a 0.5-mg/mL solution, making the volume of Dexdormitor used in immobilization cocktails the same volume as that previously used for Dormitor. Recent work in cheetahs and the author's experience indicate that one can directly substitute the volume of Dexdormitor for the volume of Dormitor previously used in immobilization combinations (Gunkel & Lafortune 2007).

Ketamine/xylazine combinations have been used to immobilize a wide range of captive and wild felids for many years. Because xylazine is the oldest alpha-2 sedative, a considerable body of information has been accumulated on its use in nondomestic felids (Table 45.1 and Table 45.2) (Beltrán & Tewes 1995; Ferraras et al. 1994; Greer et al. 2003; Sabapara 1995). Similar to ketamine/medetomidine combinations, dosages for each agent vary widely, with very large ketamine dosages (up to >20 mg/kg) used effectively in wild, small cat species (Grassman et al. 2004). Because of xylazine's profound cardiovascular effects, it has largely been replaced in immobilization combinations with medetomidine or dexmedetomidine.

Some species-specific dosage sensitivities have been noted with the ketamine/xylazine combinations. Captive Sumatran tigers (*Panthera tigris sumatrae*) appear to have a profound sensitivity to xylazine at dosages greater than 0.2 mg/kg, when given in combination with ketamine. At greater xylazine dosages, a number of Sumatran tigers show profound respiratory depression (Armstrong et al. 1996). South Chinese tigers (*Panthera tigris amoyensis*) show a gender difference in their susceptibility to ketamine, with females requiring considerably greater dosages than males, when ketamine is administered with xylazine (Table 45.1) (Armstrong et al. 1996). A similar phenomenon has been observed in wild bobcats, with females requiring 50% more ketamine per kilogram than males (Beltrán & Tewes 1995). Seizures have been reported in several species immobilized with ketamine/xylazine combinations and seem most common in tigers (Armstrong et al. 1996; Ferraras et al. 1994; Grassman et al. 2004; Quigley et al. 2001; Seal et al. 1987). Vomiting is also commonly observed in cats receiving combinations containing xylazine (Armstrong et al. 1996).

Ketamine and detomidine combinations have been used rarely in nondomestic felids. Orally delivered detomidine in combination with ketamine has been used as premedication in domestic cats, servals, and lions (Grove & Ramsay 2000; Ramsay et al. 1999). Large dosages, 0.5 mg/kg, combined with ketamine (6.7–11.4 mg/kg) squirted into the cats' mouths, reliably produced sedation and sternal or lateral recumbency in domestic cats and servals. This combination was less reliable in producing recumbency in the lions evaluated. Oral detomidine alone (0.5 mg/kg) routinely produced sternal, but not lateral, recumbency when used as a premedication in tigers (Ramsay et al. 1999). The

most common adverse effects of orally delivered detomidine or detomidine/ketamine were vomiting, salivation, and sinus bradycardia.

Ketamine and diazepam combinations have been used for immobilization of a few nondomestic felids (Epstein et al. 2002; Ofri et al. 1998; Sabapara 1995; Taylor et al. 1998). Large dosages of ketamine (20 mg/kg) were required initially, before lions could be supplemented with additional ketamine (5 mg/kg) IV and diazepam (0.5 mg/kg) IV (Ofri et al. 1998). The large injection volumes required, coupled with the variable absorption of the diazepam, generally prevent people from using this combination.

Tiletamine/Zolazepam

The combination of tiletamine, a dissociative agent, and zolazepam, a benzodiazepine, has also been used in a wide variety of felid species (Bush et al. 1978; Grassman et al. 2004; McKenzie & Burroughs 1993; Meltzer 1999; Schumacher et al. 2003; Smeller & Bush 1997). As an investigational drug, this combination was called CI744. In North America, this combination is marketed as Telazol® (Fort Dodge Animal Health, Fort Dodge, IA) and in other areas of the world as Zoletil® (Virbac Laboratories, Carros, France). For convenience, all three of these products will be referred to as Telazol in this chapter.

Telazol is marketed as a powder and is intended to be reconstituted with sterile water to produce 50-mg tiletamine and 50-mg zolazepam/mL; in routine usage, its concentration is typically identified as 100 mg/mL. This preparation is fairly potent, when compared with 100-mg/mL ketamine, and allows for small injection volumes. As a result, Telazol has been favored by some field researchers (Grassman et al. 2004; McKenzie & Burroughs 1993; Rabinowitz 1990). Telazol can also be reconstituted with less water or with another agent(s) to produce a more potent preparation. For example, the reconstitution of a bottle of Telazol with 400-mg (4.0 mL) ketamine and 100-mg (1.0 mL) xylazine is a preparation which has been used for cheetah immobilization (Lewandowski et al. 2002).

Telazol can be used alone or in combination with alpha-2 adrenergic agonists. When used alone, Telazol has a slightly faster induction time than ketamine alone and a longer duration of effect. Immobilizations with Telazol typically result in better muscle relaxation than those where only ketamine is used, but recoveries can be prolonged and stormier than ketamine recoveries.

For many years, it has been a common practice to avoid Telazol in tigers, as early reports of adverse effects (neurological signs, behavior changes, death) developed into the dogma that Telazol is contraindicated in tigers (Armstrong et al. 1996; Wack 2003). A recent reexamination of the literature regarding use of Telazol in tigers suggests that, while adverse effects may occur, the scientific literature does not support its contraindication in tigers (Kreeger & Armstrong 2010).

Telazol/medetomidine combinations have been used in a number of felids species, but recent reports on their use are rare (Deem et al. 1998; Roken 1997). Telazol combined with ketamine and xylazine or only ketamine for felid immobilization has also been reported (Lewandowski et al. 2002; Taylor et al. 1998). The latter combination was the preferred drug combination for field immobilization of Florida panthers (Taylor et al. 1998).

A FULLY REVERSIBLE INJECTABLE COMBINATION

A medetomidine-butorphanol-midazolam combination has been studied and found useful for short procedures (<40 minutes) in cheetahs (Lafortune et al. 2005). Sudden early arousals were observed in that study. The prime advantage of this combination is that each component has a reversal agent, and thus immobilization can be fully reversed. This could be an advantage for fieldwork, where quick recoveries times speed the release of an immobilized cat. Additionally, such a combination could be more easily used in range countries where dissociative agents may be difficult to obtain or import (D. Armstrong, pers. comm., 2009).

INTRAVENOUS INDUCTIONS

Few awake nondomestic felids will allow intravenous injections, and cheetahs appear to be the only species where this approach has been routinely used (Meltzer 1999). South African veterinarians and managers have developed a restraint cage that allows intravenous induction of cheetahs using Saffan®, a combination of two steroidal anesthetic agents: alphaxolone and alphadolone. This preparation produces rapid immobilization and sufficient relaxation to permit electroejaculation (Meltzer 1999). Saffan was not available in North America and appears not to be manufactured anymore. A new product Alfaxan® (Jurox Pty. Ltd., Rutherford, NSW, Australia), containing only alphaxalone, has recently become available in Canada.

SUPPLEMENTATION OF INJECTABLE AGENTS

Ketamine and midazolam are the two injectable drugs most commonly used to supplement or extend immobilization in the author's practice. Ketamine, at doses of approximately 1 or 2–3 mg/kg, can be given IV or IM, respectively, to extend immobilization for brief periods. Similar doses can be given during inhalation anesthesia, should decreased blood pressure or respiratory depression occur and it is desirable not to decrease the amount of the inhalant agent. Midazolam at doses of 0.08–0.14 mg/kg (15 mg/adult tiger or lion) IM or IV can also be used for prolonging immobilization, but its effects are not as profound as those of ketamine. Although administering additional Telazol has been recommended in one report (Roken 1997), the author avoids administering supplemental Telazol or giving additional alpha-2 agonists during immobilization.

Propofol has also been used to complete induction or prolong immobilization in a number of nondomestic cats induced with other agents (Burgos-Rodriguez et al. 2004; Epstein et al. 2002; Galloway et al. 2002). Most commonly, cats had been induced with ketamine and medetomidine, and propofol (1–2 mg/kg IV) was administered to facilitate endotracheal intubation or provide additional relaxation for a short procedure, such as a bandage change. Potential disadvantages of using propofol in large felids are apnea, cardiovascular effects, and the risk of rapid, full recovery of a dangerous animal.

INHALATION AGENTS

Isoflurane in oxygen is commonly used for inhalation anesthesia in nondomestic felids. Isoflurane can also be used for chamber anesthetic induction of small cats, in either a specially built induction chamber or by encasing a carrier or small cage in a plastic bag. Typically, 5% isoflurane with high oxygen flow rates are used for chamber inductions, and some cats take a considerable amount of time to become safe to handle. Following the cat's removal from the chamber, anesthesia can be continued with isoflurane administered via face mask or endotracheal tube.

For any long procedures, endotracheal intubation and maintenance on isoflurane in oxygen are preferred to repeated supplementation of injectable agents. The muzzle of cats is relatively short and the larynx is found at the base of the tongue, allowing for easy endotracheal intubation of most felids. Intubation rarely requires numbing of the larynx. In small felids, traditional small animal endotracheal tubes can be used. Adult lions' and tigers' tracheas are large in diameter and typically require large animal/equine endotracheal tubes (interior diameters of 18–24 mm). Intubation is greatly assisted by the use of a long laryngoscope blade and a rigid stylet, placed within the tube. Large animal endotracheal tubes are designed for animals with longer necks, so care must be taken to prevent endobroncheal intubation.

ANTAGONIST OR REVERSAL AGENTS

Benzodiazepine Antagonists

Flumazenil is the only benzodiazepine antagonist widely used in zoological medicine. It can be used to reverse the effects of diazepam or midazolam, such as when rapid reversal in the field is desired. In captive settings, however, many clinicians prefer not to reverse the benzodiazepines and retain their calming effects to "smooth" recoveries. Flumazenil can also be used to speed recovery of an animal immobilized with Telazol. One study of flumazenil (31 μg/kg IM) and sarmazenil (0.1 mg/kg IM), another benzodiazepine antagonist, in cheetahs showed administration of each decreased recovery times, and improved (smoothed) recoveries (Walzer & Huber 2002).

Alpha-2 Adrenergic Antagonists

Yohimbine and atipamizole (Antisedon®, Pfizer, Inc., New York, NY) are used to reverse the effects of xylazine and medetomidine (or dexmedetomidine), respectively. A number of yohimbine dosages have been used, but most are in the range of 0.1–0.125 mg/kg. An even wider range of atipamizole, dosages have been reported, but all are based on the amount of medetomidine administered. Typically, atipamizole is administered at two to five times the medetomidine dosage, with the lower end of that range more commonly reported from Europe, and the upper limit of that range being that recommended by the US manufacturer. Following long procedures or anesthesias (>2 hours), some clinicians will not administer an alpha-2 antagonist or will administer only a portion of the dosages discussed earlier.

Many routes of administration have also been used, including combinations of IV and IM or SC (Deem et al. 1998; Jalanka & Roeken 1990; Klein & Stover 1993; Lafortune et al. 2005; Lewandowski et al. 2002; Schumacher et al. 1999). In the author's practice, IM or SC administration of yohimbine and atipamizole is preferred. Occasionally, during ketamine-medetomidine-isoflurane immobilization/anesthesia of a lion or tiger, hypotension or hyperkalemia can occur. If this happens, the clinician may elect to give a portion of the atipamizole reversal dose. Typically 2.5- to 5.0-mg atipamizole is administered, either IV or IM. This should be done only when the animal is intubated and well controlled under inhalant anesthesia.

MONITORING

Routine monitoring of felid chemical restraint should include serial body temperature, pulse, and respiration measurements, and continuous hemoglobin saturation monitoring via pulse oximetry (Fig. 45.2). Long procedures or cool weather can result in a dramatic decrease in body temperature, and regular measurement of body temperature is especially required in these situations. Measuring body temperature just before allowing the animal to recover, or before immobilization drugs are reversed, is also important to allow for remedial efforts for a hypothermic animal. Hypothermia is a major reason for prolonged recoveries.

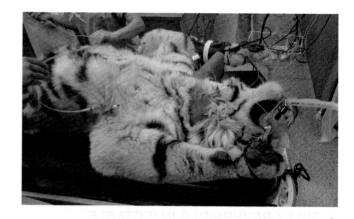

Figure 45.2. A tiger with an endotracheal tube in place and instrumented for monitoring during anesthesia. A catheter is in the left jugular vein, a pulse oximetry probe is placed on the tongue, and ECG leads are attached to the cat.

For short procedures, animals are not typically intubated, but if respiratory rates are very low (<6 breaths/min) or if hemoglobin saturation remains low (<85%), endotracheal intubation and ventilation may be required. It should be pointed out that pulse oximeters are calibrated for use in humans and, as a result, absolute accuracy of any given saturation value cannot be guaranteed. Pulse oximetry is useful, however, for monitoring trends and providing information about oxygenation, especially if hypoventilation or ventilation–perfusion mismatching are present.

Routine monitoring for surgical anesthesia includes the measurements stated earlier, serial blood pressure measurements, and continuous electrocardiography (ECG) and end-tidal CO_2 monitoring. Noninvasive oscillometric blood pressure (NIBP) measuring is routinely done, but values can be difficult to obtain on some cats. Use of human arm or thigh cuffs, placed around the foreleg just above the carpus, attached to an automated pressure monitor is the method commonly used in our practice. A study comparing direct blood pressure measurement, obtained via an arterial catheter, with NIBP with cuffs placed around the foreleg, above the elbow, showed that the latter method accurately reflected the systolic (SAP) and diastolic (DAP) pressures, but overestimated the mean arterial pressures (MAPs) (Howard et al. 2006). That same study also compared direct arterial pressure measurements to those obtained via NIBP with the cuff placed around the base of the tail. The tail cuff NIBP measurements also accurately reflected the SAP, but underestimated the MAP and DAP. The authors concluded that NIBP with cuffs placed at either site could reasonably be used to monitor blood pressure in anesthetized lions (Howard et al. 2006).

Progressive hyperkalemia has been observed in 20% of anesthetized tigers (Gunkel & Lafortune 2007); however, the condition remains poorly described and mainly anecdotal. The pathophysiology of hyperkalemia in healthy large felids under general anesthesia is not known and several mechanisms may be responsible. Alpha-2 adrenoceptor agonists, such as xylazine, medetomidine, and dexmedetomidine may play a role in increasing the serum potassium concentration. A significant increase in plasma potassium during anesthesia with xylazine and ketamine has been reported in tigers (Seal et al. 1987) and dogs (Taluker & Hikasa 2009); however, in both reports, the potassium concentration did not exceed 5.5 mmol/L. In dogs and cats, medetomidine induces hyperglycemia and hypoinsulinemia (Burton et al. 1997; Kanda & Hikasa 2008a, 2008b; Taluker & Hikasa 2009). Hypoinsulinemia may play a role in increasing serum potassium concentration during sedation with these drugs. Hyperkalemia-induced cardiac arrhythmias and ECG changes depend on the concentration of potassium in the extracellular fluid. ECG changes can include bardycardia, increase in T-wave amplitude, ST segment depression, widening of P and QRS waves, and loss of P-waves (Carroll 2008). Although ECG monitoring is recommended as an indirect mean for monitoring plasma potassium, a study on hyperkalemic domestic cats and dogs showed that 59% of the ECGs were normal or revealed abnormalities not previously described in conjunction with hyperkalemia (Tag & Day 2008). Therefore, ECG examination as a sole technique for monitoring the plasma concentration of potassium cannot be recommended. Gunkel and Lafortune (Gunkel & Lafortune 2007) recommended monitoring plasma electrolytes and blood gases every 15–30 minutes during general anesthesia of large cats. Certainly, if the anesthesia extends longer than 1 hour, routine monitoring of electrolytes and glucose seems prudent.

In a pilot study in the author's practice, plasma potassium concentration increased consistently during general anesthesia in four large captive felids (three tigers and one liger). ECG changes (bradycardia, spiked T-waves, and wide QRS complexes) were observed in three of these animals and cardiac arrest occurred in two animals. Plasma or serum glucose also rose concomitantly with the increase in circulating potassium in all these cats. A more extensive study on the pathophysiology of hyperkalemia in large felids during general anesthesia is currently underway (R. Seddighi and S. Reilly, pers. comm., 2010).

LOCAL AND REGIONAL ANESTHESIA

There are very few reports on regional anesthesia in nondomestic cats. It is assumed that most anesthetic blocks used in domestic cats can be adapted and applied to nondomestic felids. A transverse abdominis plane block has been used for abdominal surgery in a Canadian lynx (*Lynx canadensis*) (Schroeder et al. 2010). Briefly, diluted bupivacaine (0.125%) was injected, with the assistance of ultrasonography, between the facial planes of the internal oblique and transversus abdominis muscles, bilaterally. An estimated 6.25-mg bupivacaine was administered on each side, and the block affected the spinal nerves of T-10 to L1, but analgesia extended as far cranial as T-7 (Schroeder et al. 2010).

Lumbosacral epidermal analgesia has been employed in lions and tigers undergoing ovario-hysterectomy or other procedures (Gunkel & Lafortune 2007; McCain et al. 2009). In the author's practice, 10 mL (equivalent to 0.06–0.12 mg/kg) of morphine sulfate without preservative is aseptically placed in the epidural space of the caudal lumbar spinal region, immediately prior to surgery. No side effects of this block could be identified post surgery, although one cat which received >11 mL of the epidural morphine and also received a parenteral opioid postsurgery exhibited dysphoria, which responded to treatment with an opioid antagonist. Use of larger doses of morphine (0.1–0.3 mg/kg) and bupivacaine (0.3 mg/kg, not exceeding 6.0–9.0 mL total) for epidural analgesia in nondomestic felids has been used by others (Gunkel & Lafortune 2007).

ANALGESIA

Very few analgesic agents are approved for use in domestic felids, and some commonly used human products, such as acetaminophen, can be toxic to cats. These facts, coupled with the feline ability to mask or hide pain, has made selection of analgesics and evaluating their efficacy in nondomestic felids challenging.

A number of nonsteroidal anti-inflammatory drugs (NSAIDs) and analgesics have been reported in single case reports, case series, or proceedings abstracts. These include gabapentin (3.7 mg/kg PO q 24 hours long term) for arthritic and presumed intervertebral disc disease in a lion (Adkesson 2006), etodolac (5 mg/kg PO q 48 hours for five doses, then q 72 hours) in a tiger (Ball et al. 2001), buprenorphine (0.015 mg/kg IM after surgery, then 0.005 mg/kg IM q 8 hours for three doses) in a tiger undergoing abdominal surgery (Hart et al. 2000), butorphanol (0.1–0.2 mg/kg SC) for analgesia following surgeries in lions and tigers (Conrad et al. 2002; Kolata 2002), and meloxicam (0.1–0.2 mg/kg PO or SC, 0.1 mg/kg q 24 hours for 5 days for short-term pain, and then continuing 0.1 mg/kg q 48–72 hours for long-term pain relief) in several nondomestic felids (Whiteside & Black 2004).

Injectable meloxicam (Metacam®, Boehringer Ingelheim Vetmedica, Inc., St. Joseph, MO) is the only NSAID approved for use in domestic cats in the United States at this time and is approved only for short-term use. Recently, a warning was issued against its long-term use in domestic cats. Our experience indicates that adequate analgesia may be achieved in nondomestic felids with lower meloxicam doses and longer dosing intervals than those previously used in domestic cats

Table 45.3. Dosages for analgesic and NSAIDs used in nondomestic felids

Agent	Perioperative/Short-Term Treatment	Long-Term Treatment
Buprenorphine	0.01–0.02 mg/kg SC, b.i.d., or q.i.d.	May also be given IM or orally (transmucosally)
Butorphanol	0.1–0.4 mg/kg SC	0.4–1.0 mg/kg PO q 4–8 h
Tramadol	1.0–4.0 mg/kg PO b.i.d.	0.8–1.5 mg/kg PO b.i.d.
Meloxicam	0.1–0.3 mg/kg SC	Day 1: 0.1–0.2 mg/kg PO once
		Days 2–4: 0.05–0.1 mg/kg q 24 h
		Days 5 on: 0.025 mg/kg q 48–72 h
Piroxicam	0.3 mg/kg PO q 24 h for 4 days	Days 1–4: 0.3 mg/kg PO q 24 h
		Days 5 on: 0.3 mg/kg PO q 48 h

(Table 45.3) and nondomestic felids have been maintained on meloxicam for months without adverse clinical signs. Postmortem examination of the kidneys from a large series of nondomestic felids found renal papillary necrosis (RPN) was significantly associated with meloxicam treatment, but not all felids receiving meloxicam developed RPN (Newkirk et al. 2011). Piroxicam, another NSAID more commonly used in oncology, is also useful for treating chronic pain in some nondomestic felids. Domestic cats treated with piroxicam show a number of adverse effects, but these have not been observed in the author's practice.

Tramadol, a drug with opioid-like effects, is used for analgesia in domestic cats and has proved to be an effective oral analgesic in a number of nondomestic felid species. It can be used long term and very few, if any, adverse effects have been encountered. It can also be used safely in geriatric cats with renal disease or gastrointestinal problems.

For perioperative or short-term pain relief, meloxicam and tramadol are used in our practice (Table 45.3). Oral tramadol is given the night before surgery, the evening following surgery, and for 3–4 days post surgery. Meloxicam is administered SC during surgery and orally for 2–4 days thereafter. For very painful procedures, buprenorphine can be used intraoperatively, instead of postrecovery tramadol. The author has also used butorphanol 0.03–0.04 mg/kg SC (4.0- to 5.0-mg total dose) in subadult and adult lions and tigers following castration with satisfactory short-term effects. Butorphanol should be redosed at 2-hour intervals to maintain postoperative analgesia.

In domestic cats, fentanyl transdermal patches offer a method of providing long-term postsurgery analgesia, without the need to continually redose an animal. These patches require good contact between the patch and skin, and protection of the patch to prevent removal. In nondomestic felids, these requirements preclude the use of fentanyl patches in most individuals. Delivery of fentanyl, or other analgesic, via subcutaneously implanted osmotic pumps is a potential alternative method for delivery of pain relief drugs. Modeling of osmotic pump fentanyl delivery in domestic cats showed that the cats treated with pumps had shorter lag times to therapeutic serum concentrations

and faster fentanyl elimination following pump removal, as compared with cats treated with transdermal fentanyl patches (Sykes et al. 2009). The latter might be especially useful should an animal show adverse drug effects.

Large nondomestic felids appear to be more prone to osteoarthritis than has been recognized in domestic cats, and osteoarthritis can be a cause of chronic pain (Kolmstetter et al. 2000). Meloxicam, piroxicam, tramadol, and gabapentin are used in our practice for treatment of chronic pain in nondomestic felids. Meloxicam or piroxicam can be used alone, or either can be used in combination with either tramadol or gabapentin. In nondomestic felids with chronic pain, combined meloxicam and tramadol therapy is typically attempted before trying other agents or combinations.

ACKNOWLEDGMENTS

The author would like to thank Dr. Seddighi, Dr. Reilly, and Dr. Steeil for the critical review of this manuscript.

REFERENCES

Adkesson MJ. 2006. The role of gabapentin as an analgesic: potential applications in zoological medicine. Annual Conference of the AmAssoc Zoo Vet, 2006, pp. 270–272.

Armstrong DL, Miller RE, Byers O, et al. 1996. International cooperation with range country efforts to conserve tigers (*Panthera tigris*) and the veterinarian's role. Annual Conference of the American Association of Zoo Veterinarians, pp. 532–541.

Arnemo JM, Linnell JDC, Wedul SJ, et al. 1999. Use of intraperitoneal radio-transmitters in lynx *Lynx lynx* kittens: anaesthesia, surgery, and behavior. *Wildlife Biology* 5:245–250.

Ball RL, Weiner L, Richner A. 2001. Etodolac as an adjunct to managing osteoarthritis in captive Bengal tigers (*Panthera tigris bengalis*). Joint Conference of the AAZV, AAWV, AARAV, NAZWV, & AZA/NAG, pp. 137–139.

Belsare A, Athreya V. 2010. Use of xylazine hydrochloride-ketamine hydrochloride for immobilization of wild leopards (*Panthera pardus fusca*) in emergency situations. *Journal of Zoo and Wildlife Medicine* 41:331–333.

Beltrán J, Tewes ME. 1995. Immobilization of ocelots and bobcats with ketamine hydrochloride and xylazine hydrochloride. *Journal of Wildlife Diseases* 31:43–48.

Burgos-Rodriguez AG, Backues KA, Zollinger T, et al. 2004. Mid-metacarpal amputation in a jaguar. Joint Conference of the AAZV, AAWV, & WDA, pp. 365–367.

Burton SA, Lemke KA, Ilhe SL, et al. 1997. Effects of medetomidine on serum insulin and plasma glucose concentrations in clinically normal dogs. *American Journal of Veterinary Research* 58:1440–1442.

Bush M, Custer R, Smeller J, et al. 1978. The acid-base status of lions, *Panther leo*, immobilized with four drug combinations. *Journal of Wildlife Diseases* 14:102–109.

Carroll GL. 2008. *Small Animal Anesthesia and Analgesia*. Ames: Blackwell Publishers.

Center M, Elston TH, Rowlind PH, et al. 1996. Fulminant hepatic failure associated with oral administration of diazepam in 11 cats. *Journal of the American Veterinary Medical Association* 209:618–624.

Conrad J, Wendelburg K, Santinelli S, Park A. 2002. Deleterious effects on onychectomy (declawing) in exotic felids and a reparative surgical technique: a preliminary report. Annual Conference of the American Association of Zoo Veterinarians, pp. 16–20.

Curro TG, Okeson MS, Zimmerman D, et al. 2004. Xylazine-midazolam-ketamine versus medetomidine-midazolam-ketamine anesthesia in captive Siberian tigers (*Panthera tigris altaica*). *Journal of Zoo and Wildlife Medicine* 35:320–327.

Deem SL, Ko JC, Citino SB. 1998. Anesthetic and cardiorespiratory effects of tiletamine-zolazepam-medetomidine in cheetahs. *Journal of the American Veterinary Medical Association* 213:1022–1026.

Epstein A, White R, Horowitz IH, et al. 2002. Effects of propofol as an anaesthetic agent in adult lions (*Panthera leo*): a comparison with two established protocols. *Research in Veterinary Science* 72:137–140.

Ferraras P, Aldama JJ, Beltrán JF, et al. 1994. Immobilization of the endangered Iberian lynx with xylazine- and ketamine-hydrochloride. *Journal of Wildlife Diseases* 30:65–68.

Forsyth SF, Machon RG, Walsh VP. 1999. Anaesthesia of a Sumatran tiger on eight occasions with ketamine, medetomidine and isoflurane. *New Zealand Veterinary Journal* 47:105–108.

Galloway DS, Coke RL, Rochat MC. 2002. Spinal compression due to atlantal vertebral malformation in two African lions (*Panthera leo*). *Journal of Zoo and Wildlife Medicine* 33:249–255.

Goodrich JM, Kerley LL, Schleyer BO, et al. 2001. Capture and chemical anesthesia of Amur (Siberian) tigers. *Wildlife Society Bulletin* 29:533–542.

Grassman LI, Austin SC, Tewes ME, et al. 2004. Comparative immobilization of wild felids in Thailand. *Journal of Wildlife Diseases* 40:575–578.

Greer LL, Troutman M, McCracken MD, et al. 2003. Adult-onset hypothyroidism in a lynx (*Lynx canadensis*). *Journal of Zoo and Wildlife Medicine* 34:287–291.

Grove DM, Ramsay EC. 2000. Sedative and physiologic effects of orally administered α2-adrenoceptor agonists and ketamine in cats. *Journal of the American Veterinary Medical Association* 217:467–468.

Gunkel C, Lafortune M. 2007. Felids. In: *Zoo and Wildlife Immobilization and Anesthesia* (G West, D Heard, N Caulkett, eds.), pp. 443–459. Ames: Blackwell Publishing.

Hart SH, Pye G, Bennett RA. 2000. Subtotal colectomy in a tiger (*Panthera tigris*). Joint Conference of the AAZV & IAAAM, 2000, pp. 78–79.

Howard L, Bashaw M, Lamberski N, et al. 2006. Evaluation of two anatomical locations for the measurement of indirect blood pressure in anesthetized African lions (*Panthera leo*). Annual Conference of the American Association of Zoo Veterinarians, p. 253.

Huber C, Walzer C, Slotta-Bachmayr L. 2001. Evaluation of long-term sedation in cheetah (*Acinonyx jubatus)* with perphenazine enanthate and zuclopenthixol acetate. *Journal of Zoo and Wildlife Medicine* 32:329–335.

Jalanka H. 1989. Medetomidine- and ketamine-induced immobilization of snow leopards (*Panthera uncia*): doses, evaluation, and reversal by atipamizole. *Journal of Zoo and Wildlife Medicine* 20:154–162.

Jalanka HH, Roeken BO. 1990. The use of medetomidine, medetomidine-ketamine combinations, and atipamizole in nondomestic mammals: a review. *Journal of Zoo and Wildlife Medicine* 21:259–282.

Kanda T, Hikasa Y. 2008a. Effects of medetomidine or midazolam alone or in combination on the metabolic and neurohormonal responses in healthy cats. *Canadian Journal of Veterinary Research* 72:332–339.

Kanda T, Hikasa Y. 2008b. Neurohormonal and metabolic effects of medetomidine compared with xylazine in healthy cats. *Canadian Journal of Veterinary Research* 72:278–286.

Ketz-Riley CJ, Ritchey JW, Hoover JP, et al. 2003. Immunodeficiency associated with multiple infections in captive Pallas cats (*Ototcolobus manul*). *Journal of Zoo and Wildlife Medicine* 34:239–245.

Klein L, Stover J. 1993. Medetomidine-ketamine-isoflurane anesthesia in captive cheetah (*Acinonyx jubatus*) and antagonism with atipamizole. Annual Conference of the American Association of Zoo Veterinarians, p. 130.

Kolata RJ. 2002. Laparoscopic ovariohysterectomy and hysterectomy in African lions (*Panthera leo*) using Ultracision® Harmonic Scalpel®. *Journal of Zoo and Wildlife Medicine* 33:280–282.

Kolmstetter C, Munson L, Ramsay EC. 2000. Degenerative spinal disease in large felids. *Journal of Zoo and Wildlife Medicine* 31:15–19.

Kreeger TJ, Armstrong DL. 2010. Tigers and Telazol®: the unintended evolution of caution to contradiction. *Journal of Wildlife Management* 74:1183–1185.

Lafortune M, Gunkel C, Valverde A, et al. 2005. Reversible anesthetic combination using medetomidine-butorphanol-midazolam (MBMZ) n cheetahs (*Acinonyx jubatus*). Joint Conference of the AAZV, AAWV, & AZA/NAG, p. 270.

Langan JN, Schumacher J, Pollock C, et al. 2000. Cardiopulmonary and anesthetic effects of medetomidine-ketamine-butorphanol and antagonism with atipamizole in servals (*Felis serval*). *Journal of Zoo and Wildlife Medicine* 31:329–334.

Lewandowski AH, Bonar CJ, Evans SE. 2002. Tiletamine-zolazepam, ketamine, xylazine anesthesia of captive cheetah (*Acinonyx jubatus*). *Journal of Zoo and Wildlife Medicine* 33:332–336.

Logan KA, Thorne ET, Irwin LL, et al. 1986. Immobilizing wild mountain lions (*Felis concolor*) with ketamine hydrochloride and xylazine hydrochloride. *Journal of Wildlife Diseases* 22:97–103.

McCain S, Ramsay E, Allender M, et al. 2009. Pyometra in captive large felids: a review of eleven cases. *Journal of Zoo and Wildlife Medicine* 40:147–151.

McKenzie AA, Burroughs REJ. 1993. Chemical capture of carnivores. In: *The Capture and Care Manual Capture, Care, Accommodation and Transportation of Wild African Animals* (AA McKenzie, ed.), pp. 223–244. Pretoria: South African Veterinary Foundation.

Meltzer DGA. 1999. Medical management of a cheetah breeding facility in South Africa. In: *Zoo and Wild Animal Medicine: Current Therapy IV* (ME Fowler, RE Miller, eds.), pp. 415–417. Philadelphia: W.B. Saunders.

Miller M, Weber M, Neiffer D, et al. 2003. Anesthetic induction of captive tigers (*Panthera tigris*) using a medetomidine-ketamine combination. *Journal of Zoo and Wildlife Medicine* 34:307–308.

Newkirk KM, Newman SJ, White LA, et al. 2011. Renal lesions of non-domestic felids. *Veterinary Pathology* 48:698–705.

Nowak RM. 2005. *Walker's Carnivores of the World*, pp. 229–272. Baltimore: The Johns Hopkins University Press.

Ofri R, Horowitz I, Jacobson S, et al. 1998. The effects of anesthesia and gender on intraocular pressure in lions (*Panthera leo*). *Journal of Zoo and Wildlife Medicine* 29:307–310.

Poole KG, Mowat G, Slough BG. 1993. Chemical immobilization of lynx. *Wildlife Society Bulletin* 21:136–140.

Quigley KS, Armstrong DL, Miquelle DG, et al. 2001. Health evaluation of wild Siberian tigers (*Panthera tigris altaica*) and Amur leopards (*Panthera pardus orientalis*) in the Russian far east. Joint Conference of the AAZV, AAWV, & NAZW, pp. 179–182.

Rabinowitz A. 1990. Notes on the behavior and movements of leopard cats, *Felis bengalensis*, in a dry tropical forest mosaic in Thailand. *Biotropica* 22:397–403.

Ramsay EC, Grove D, Miller M, et al. 1999. Immobilization of felids using oral detomidine and ketamine. Annual Conference of the American Association of Zoo Veterinarians, pp. 47–48.

Roken BO. 1997. A potent anesthetic combination with low concentrated medetomidine in zoo animal. Annual Conference of the American Association of Zoo Veterinarians, pp. 134–136.

Sabapara RH. 1995. Chemical restraint and sedation of leopards (*Panthera pardus*). *The Indian Veterinary Journal* 72:655–657.

Schroeder CA, Schroeder KM, Johnson RA. 2010. Transversus abdominis plane block for exploratory laparotomy in a Canadian lynx (*Lynx canadensis*). *Journal of Zoo and Wildlife Medicine* 41:338–341.

Schumacher J, Erdtmann J, Pollock C, et al. 1999. Comparative cardiopulmonary and anesthetic effects of ketamine-medetomidine and ketamine xylazine in cougars (*Felis concolor*). Annual Conference of the American Association of Zoo Veterinarians, pp. 45–46.

Schumacher J, Snyder P, Citino SB, et al. 2003. Radiographic and electrocardiographic evaluation of cardiac morphology and function in captive cheetahs (*Acinonyx jubatus*). *Journal of Zoo and Wildlife Medicine* 34:357–363.

Seal US, Armstrong DL, Simmons LG. 1987. Yohimbine hydrochloride reversal of ketamine hydrochloride and xylazine hydrochloride immobilization of Bengal tigers and effects on hematology and serum chemistries. *Journal of Wildlife Diseases* 23:296–300.

Shindle DV, Tewes ME. 2000. Immobilization of wild ocelots with tiletamine and zolazepam in Southern Texas. *Journal of Wildlife Diseases* 36:546–550.

Smeller J, Bush M. 1997. A physiological study of immobilized cheetah. *Journal of Zoo Animal Medicine* 7:5–7.

Sykes JM, Cox S, Ramsay EC. 2009. Evaluation of an osmotic pump for fentanyl administration in cats as a model for non-domestic felids. *American Journal of Veterinary Research* 70:950–955.

Tag TL, Day TK. 2008. Electrocardiographic assessment of hyperkalemia in dogs and cats. *Journal of Veterinary Emergency and Critical Care* 18:61–67.

Taluker MH, Hikasa Y. 2009. Diuretic effects of medetomidine compared with xylazine in healthy dogs. *Canadian Journal of Veterinary Research* 73:224–236.

Taylor SK, Land ED, Roelke-Parker ME, et al. 1998. Anesthesia of free-ranging Florida panthers (*Puma concolor coryi*), 1981–1998. Joint Conference of the AAZV & AAWV, pp. 26–29.

Tomizawa N, Tsujimoto T, Itoh K, et al. 1997. Chemical restraint of African lions (*Panthera leo*) with medetomidine-ketamine. *The Journal of Veterinary Medical Science* 59:307–310.

Wack RF. 2003. Felidae. In: *Zoo and Wildlife Medicine*, 5th ed. (ME Fowler, RE Miller, eds.), pp. 491–501. St. Louis: WB Saunders.

Walzer C, Huber C. 2002. Partial antagonism of tiletamine-zolazepam anesthesia in cheetah. *Journal of Wildlife Diseases* 38:468–472.

Whiteside DP, Black SR. 2004. The use of meloxicam in exotic felids at the Calgary Zoo. Joint Conference of the American Association Zoo Veterinarians, American Association of Wildlife Veterinarians, Wildlife Disease Association Joint Conference, pp. 346–349.

46 Phocid Seals

Michael Lynch and Kate Bodley

INTRODUCTION

Seals, sea lions, fur seals, and walruses make up a distinctive group of mammals: the order Pinnipedia. Most members of this group can be divided into two families: the Otariidae (eared seals) contains 14 species and the Phocidae (true seals) contains 18 species (Riedman 1990).

Phocid and otariid seals share many adaptive features that enable them to occupy both aquatic and terrestrial environments. However, there are significant anatomical, physiological, and behavioral variations between these groups and between species within each group. Some of these variations must be taken into account during the planning and management of immobilization and anesthesia procedures.

ANATOMY AND PHYSIOLOGY

Phocid seal species have numerous anatomical and physiological adaptations that must be considered as part of their anesthetic management. The maintenance of a core body temperature within a narrow range is essential for the survival of endothermic mammals. This is particularly challenging for species that move between terrestrial and aquatic environments, as water conducts heat 25 times more efficiently than air (Nadel 1984). To maintain a constant core body temperature, semiaquatic species generally need to reduce heat loss when in the water, and often, heat stress when on land. Phocid seals rely on a thick layer of blubber to insulate the body core (Harrison & King 1980). In addition to behavioral means of thermoregulation, heat is conserved or off-loaded by altering the blood flow through arteriovenous anastomoses in the trunk and flippers

(Bryden & Molyneux 1978; Mauck et al. 2003). Anesthesia removes the seal's ability to employ behavioral means of thermoregulation and may also interfere with physiological mechanisms. Therefore, a consideration of likely changes in the animal's body temperature during immobilization procedures and planned responses to their potential hypo or hyperthermia is necessary.

Phocid seals also have adaptations that relate to their ability to dive. In some species such as leopard and Weddell seals, there is very little cartilaginous support of the trachea, allowing its dorso-ventral collapse while diving (Boyd 1975; Gray et al. 2006; Kooyman 1989). Phocids also have a flexible rib cage, enabling the thorax to compress, and the smaller pulmonary airways are supported by muscle rather than cartilage (Ridgway 1972; Welsch et al. 1989). During anesthesia, relaxation of pharyngeal and palatine tissues, of the musculature of the rib cage, and of the pulmonary airways may contribute to airway obstruction. This means that phocid seals, particularly large individuals, are susceptible to ventilation–perfusion mismatch. In addition, these anatomical adaptations of the respiratory system can increase the difficulty of providing adequate ventilation to anesthetized animals when employing intermittent positive pressure ventilation (Pang et al. 2006).

Physiological adaptations that aid diving in pinnipeds include a series of cardiovascular changes that are collectively known as the dive response. The dive response is most pronounced during prolonged dives and most profoundly elicited in deep diving phocid species (Kooyman 1981). The dive response is characterized by a profound bradycardia, peripheral vasoconstriction, and the shunting of blood to essential and

Zoo Animal and Wildlife Immobilization and Anesthesia, Second Edition. Edited by Gary West, Darryl Heard, and Nigel Caulkett.
© 2014 John Wiley & Sons, Inc. Published 2014 by John Wiley & Sons, Inc.

hypoxia-sensitive tissues such as the heart and brain (Scheffer 1990). The pinniped dive response is primarily controlled by central mechanisms influencing respiratory drive. Input from pulmonary stretch receptors, arterial chemo- and baroreceptors, and trigeminal receptors result in a vagally mediated bradycardia (Angell James et al. 1981). The activity of the sympathetic nervous system also increases, resulting in splenic contraction, peripheral vasoconstriction, and constriction of the muscular vena cava sphincter. Consequently, there is an increased hematocrit and pooling of blood within the hepatic sinus during diving (Thornton et al. 2001).

Profound bradycardia and periods of prolonged apnea are sometimes observed in anesthetized seals and have been suggested to be a result of an inappropriate elicitation of the dive response (Gales & Burton 1988). It is not unreasonable to suggest that the dive response could be elicited by anesthetic agents, as they generally depress central respiratory and cardiovascular centers, and may induce periods of apnea. Anesthesia may be considered as providing two of the triggers, central and peripheral, for elicitation of a dive response. However, cardiac arrest and cessation of breathing may be elicited by hypoxia in any mammal. Therefore, a conclusion of a dive response episode in an anesthetized seal may only be made if the animal's ventilation is being appropriately monitored by pulse oximetry and capnography. Careful monitoring of the physiological status of anesthetized phocid seals, including the use of capnography, allows continuous assessment of respiratory function and reduces the risk of development of hypercapnea and hypoxemia.

CAPTURE AND PHYSICAL RESTRAINT

When planning an immobilization procedure, the objectives must be clearly defined. Setting objectives clarifies whether animal restraint is needed at all, and, if restraint is necessary, what degree of immobilization is required. For all animal restraint procedures, the method of immobilization must take into account the animal's size, its demeanor, and its proximity to water. In addition, the skill level of handlers is a very important consideration.

It is possible to herd many phocid seals into trailers or transport crates using baffle boards and funneling arrangements, and this technique finds most application in the captive environment. Crates used to transport seals should be able to be opened at either end, be well ventilated, and of a width and height that does not allow the animal to turn around and become trapped. In the field, baffle boards may be suitable for herding animals to desired locations. Baffle boards are most useful when managing species that are relatively tolerant of human disturbance, such as Weddell and southern elephant seals.

Procedures of short duration that are minimally invasive may be most simply and safely achieved using physical restraint methods. Skilled and confident handlers are essential when manually restraining seals. Phocid seals up to ~100 kg can be caught using a hoop net and then manually restrained. Young pups may be captured by simply grasping the individual in front of the hind flippers and holding. Once caught in a hoop net, the animal can be restrained within the net by grasping its neck just behind the skull, and pushing it down to the ground while straddling the body. This allows a second operator to perform brief procedures such as collection of blood or delivery of anesthetic agents by face mask or injection. Small seals (<30 kg) can be removed from the net by grasping in front of the tail flippers and then restrained by straddling the body and pinning the animal's neck and head.

Larger phocid seals such as crab eater, leopard, and southern elephant seals can be physically restrained using a head bag (Harcourt et al 2010; McMahon et al. 2000; Stirling 1966). Once the head bag is in position, the animal can be manually restrained: one person straddling its shoulders and another its hindquarters (Fig. 46.1). A third handler can then perform minor procedures, such as blood collection and flipper tagging.

More elusive species may be difficult to approach on land. Harbor seals can be caught in narrow water canals using fine drift nets. Entangled animals are then hauled into a boat. Ringed seals have been captured at breathing holes in sea ice using nets (Kelly 1996). Seals that are surfacing to breathe will trigger the fall of a weight that causes the net to extend.

One advantage of physical restraint is that the animal can be immediately released on completion of the procedure without residual drug effects that might

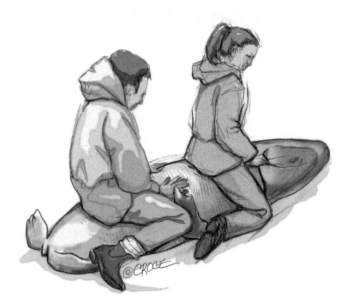

Figure 46.1. A head bag may be used to facilitate physical restraint of larger phocid seals. Once the head bag is in position, the animal can be manually restrained: one person straddles its shoulders and another its hindquarters (illustration by Beth Croce).

PHOCID SEALS **649**

impair its behavior. Physical restraint may be used to facilitate accurate delivery of chemical immobilization agents after the animal is caught. Southern elephant seals that received anesthetic agents intravenously after physical restraint had shorter induction and recovery times and less variable responses than those that were given the same agents by intramuscular injection (Slip & Woods 1996). Alternatively, animals may be sedated via intramuscular injection of chemical agents prior to physical restraint for intravenous access (Woods et al. 1994b).

The disadvantages of physical restraint include the increased risk for the handlers (i.e., bite wounds), increased animal stress, and the difficulty of monitoring the animal's physiological state adequately. Excessively vigorous restraint may compromise the animal's breathing via occlusion of the airway or constriction of the thoracic wall. This may of particular importance in phocid seals due to their tracheal and rib cage anatomy. Prolonged physical restraint in warm ambient temperatures may also cause hyperthermia.

VASCULAR ACCESS

The extradural intravertebral vein is most frequently used for intravenous access in phocid seals. The vein is located dorsal to the spinal cord, in the epidural sinus (Fig. 46.2). The animal is restrained in sternal recumbency and the vein is located by determining the dorsal midline in the lower lumbar region. The spinous processes of lumbar vertebrae 3–4 are located by palpation, and the needle is inserted perpendicularly between these processes until blood is observed in the needle hub. A 20-gauge, 25 mm (1 in.) needle has been recommended for harbor seal pups, an 18-gauge, 76 mm (3 in.) spinal needle has been recommended for harbor

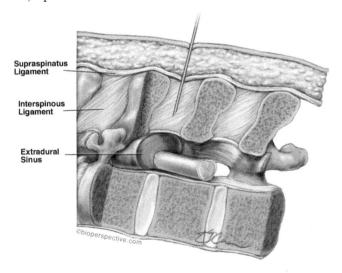

Figure 46.2. A schematic diagram of a sagittal section of the lower lumbar region of a phocid seal demonstrating the perpendicular placement of a needle to enter the extradural sinus (illustration by Beth Croce).

seal adults, and an 18-gauge, 90 mm (3.5 –in.) spinal needle has been recommended for southern elephant seal adults (Haulena & Heath 2001; McMahon et al. 2000). If extradural intravertebral venipuncture is performed without adequate skin preparation, there is potential for introduction of pathogens directly into a major vessel. Care must be taken when attempting intravenous access in a restrained seal: if the animal struggles, there is potential for vessel trauma. Inadvertent bone marrow contamination of blood samples has been reported during extradural intravertebral vein access in northern elephant seal pups (Goldstein et al. 1998).

The plantar interdigital veins of the hind flippers have also been used for intravenous access in phocid seals. A needle is inserted at the origin of the interdigital webbing, 10°–20° to the skin surface directly over the second digit or medial to the fourth digit (Gulland et al. 2001). Firm pressure must be applied to this site post venipuncture to prevent hematoma formation.

ENDOTRACHEAL INTUBATION

Intubation is strongly recommended in phocid seals to maintain the airway and provide the ability to ventilate the animal. Therefore, personnel performing chemical immobilization procedures should have the skills and capacity to intubate and ventilate animals. Intubation is required to ensure reliable maintenance of the airway during anesthesia. However, intubation may be difficult, particularly in larger animals, due to the presence of spongy peripharyngeal tissues and a flaccid soft palate that prevent visualization of the laryngeal opening. In some species such as Weddell seals, the laryngeal orifice is narrow (Hammond & Elsner 1977). This may result in difficulty of insertion of an endotracheal tube of a size suitable for the lumen of the trachea.

In larger phocid seals, intubation is most easily accomplished by manually palpating the laryngeal opening and then passing the tube. Laryngoscopes may be used for smaller species (up to around 100 kg), but often do not displace enough pharyngeal tissue to visualize the glottis opening. A spatula of 5- to 8-cm width will aid this process (Haulena & Heath 2001).

Manipulation of the glottis in apneic phocid seals will often stimulate respiration. However, apnea was associated with endotracheal tube placement in 24 of 31 previously breathing, lightly anesthetized southern elephant seals (Woods et al. 1996b). In most seals, the apnea was resolved by tube removal alone.

For assisted ventilation, intubated large seals require oxygen demand valves capable of delivering high flow rates. A modified Robert–Shaw demand and resuscitation valve (Ohmeda Pty Ltd), capable of delivering an oxygen flow of 140 L/min, has been used by the authors to ventilate phocid seals up to 300 kg body weight. Devices capable of delivering 300 L/min are used to ventilate large terrestrial mammals and would be capable of ventilating the largest phocid seals (Horne et al. 2001).

PREANESTHETIC CONSIDERATIONS

Immobilization Location

There are many features in the captive environment that can be modified to achieve safe and effective chemical immobilization of phocid seals. For example, trained behaviors may allow venipuncture and administration of intravenous sedatives or anesthetics with minimal restraint. Facilities that allow rapid and safe animal restraint, restriction of access to water, and control of environmental factors, such as temperature and animal interactions, will simplify immobilization procedures and improve handler and animal safety.

Assessment of Physiological Status

An assessment of the current physiological status of an animal should be made prior to any immobilization procedure. Most captive animals will have a known medical history; many will have a previous anesthetic history and their current disease status can be readily assessed. It is often possible to weigh captive animals prior to immobilization and assess this in relation to their annual cycle of weight fluctuation. In free-living animals, preanesthetic assessment is usually limited to characteristics that can be easily observed (such as body condition), combined with an assessment of the likely physiological status of the animal.

Weight fluctuations in phocid seals are generally the result of deposition or utilization of blubber, and lean body mass varies much less dramatically. Blubber is less metabolically active than most other tissues; therefore, it is important that doses of anesthetic agents are used without total body mass being the sole guide to their calculation. A significant inverse relationship between body condition and duration of anesthesia has been demonstrated in southern elephant seals given a single intravenous dose of a combined 1:1 mixture of tiletamine and zolazepam (Field et al. 2002). The authors suggest that lipophilic drugs move out of the blood stream and into blubber more rapidly in fatter animals, and therefore duration of anesthesia is shorter than in thinner animals given the same dose (in mg/kg) of drug. However, there may be prolonged drug effects in fatter animals due to gradual passage from saturated sites (e.g., fat), where the drug is inactive, back into the plasma. The time to complete recovery (as opposed to the duration of effective chemical immobilization) might therefore be expected to be longer in fatter animals.

Delivery of Anesthetic Agents

The method of delivery of chemical immobilizing agents requires careful consideration in the planning stages of a procedure. In general, manually restraining animals prior to delivery of anesthetic agents is not ideal, as they will be in a heightened state of excitement. However, the delivery of agents by remote means carries its own set of complicating factors, and the final decision about how to administer agents will depend on the demeanor of the species concerned, the individual's size, and whether or not the procedure is on free-ranging or captive animals. Immobilizing drugs may be safely administered by hand injection without full manual restraint in relatively tractable species such as Weddell seals (Phelan & Green 1992). Using a needle attached to extension tubing facilitates the ease of this technique (Ryding 1982). In addition, head bagging the seal prior to injection can provide for greater operator safety.

Remote injection of immobilizing agents by dart allows drugs to be delivered while minimizing animal disturbance and reduces the risk of the animal handler being bitten. Drug delivery by dart is useful for large and potentially dangerous species or for species that become agitated or flee when approached by humans. For free-ranging animals that are likely to flee, an assessment needs to be made of the likelihood that the individual will be stimulated to enter the water following darting. In most instances, this requires either stealthy approach to within the animal's flight distance or firing of darts from outside the flight distance. In most cases, flight distance will be altered depending on whether the approaching human is standing or crawling. Darting hauled out animals from a boat also often allows a much closer approach than if on land. Once the animal is chemically restrained, anesthesia can then be induced or maintained using intravenous administration of chemical agents or inhalant anesthesia.

One of the factors contributing to variability of response to any chemical immobilization agent is the site where the drug is deposited. Response to drug administration is less predictable following delivery by remote delivery systems such as darting than following accurate deposition of drug in an optimal site (e.g., into the extradural vein or directly into the lumbar musculature).

There are a number of advantages of using the inhalant anesthetics in phocid seals. Inhalation anesthesia techniques enable precise control of the animal's depth and give the anesthetist control over the animal's airway. Inhalant anesthesia is being used more frequently for field anesthesia of phocids because of the development of portable units that can be used for both large pinnipeds (Geschke & Chilvers 2009) and under a wide variety of climatic conditions (Bodley et al. 2005; Gales et al. 2005).

INDUCTION AND MAINTENANCE PROTOCOLS

Table 46.1 reviews drug regimens used in phocid seals.

Table 46.1. Some chemical immobilizing agents used in phocid seals 1990–2010

Species	Agent	Dose Rate	Route	Comments	Reference
Halichoerus grypus (gray seal)	Tiletamine and zolazepam	1 mg/kg	IM	Some animals became apneic, requiring ventilation. Tremors noted.	Baker et al. (1990)
	Tiletamine and zolazepam	0.5 mg/kg	IM	Additional doses given to maintain sedation; palpebral reflex maintained	Lawson et al. (1996)
	Medetomidine	50–100 μg/kg	IM	Note: adverse effects noted by other authors following use of medetomidine. Effects dependent on dose rate.	Barnett (1998)
Hydrurga leptonyx (leopard seal)	Ketamine, xylazine	2.2–5.9 mg/kg	IM	Muscle tremors, apnea, bradycardia, mortalities	Mitchell and Burton (1991)
	Tiletamine and zolazepam	2 mg/kg	IM	Apnea, bradycardia, mortalities	Mitchell and Burton (1991)
	Xylazine	0.8–2.8 mg/kg	IM	Variable plane of anesthesia with lower dose	Mitchell and Burton (1991)
	Midazolam, pethidine	0.18–0.27 mg/kg	IM	Unpredictable immobilization, poor airway maintenance.	Higgins et al. (2002)
	Tiletamine and zolazepam	1.0–1.5 mg/kg	IM	1.2–1.4 mg/kg IM gave most reliable response.	Higgins et al. (2002)
	Tiletamine and zolazepam	0.5–1.5 mg/kg	IM	Supplemented with midazolam (IV or IM) or ketamine (IV or IM) as required.	Vogelnest et al. (2009)
	Tiletamine and zolazepam	0.8–1.0 mg/kg	IM		
Leptonychotes weddellii (Weddell seal)	Ketamine, halothane	0.15–0.25 mg/kg	IM	Plane of anesthesia varied with dosage, mortalities	Hurford et al. (1996)
		1–4%	IH		
	Tiletamine and zolazepam	0.3–1.1 mg/kg	IM	Dose rate for midazolam based on estimated body mass only	Phelan and Green (1992)
	Midazolam, isoflurane	0.3–0.5 mg/kg	IM		Bodley et al. (2005)
		2.5–5%	IH		
	Ketamine, midazolam	1.6–2.4 mg/kg	IM	Dose rate per kilogram (animals were weighed). Induction dose administered IM and additional doses given IV if required. Five animals were treated using intravenous flumazenil +/– doxapram	Mellish et al. (2010)
		0.08–0.12 mg/kg	IV		
	Ketamine, diazepam	2.0 mg/kg	IM	Dose rate per kilogram (animals were weighed). Described as "mild sedative."	Harcourt et al. (2010)
		0.01 mg/kg			
Lobodon carcinophagus (crab-eater seal)	Ketamine, diazepam	2.9–7.7 mg/kg	IM	Some mortalities.	Shaughnessy (1991)
	Midazolam, pethidine	0.15–0.4 mg/kg	IM	Reversed using naloxone and flumazenil.	Tahmindjis et al. (2003)
		1–3 mg/kg			
	Midazolam, isoflurane	0.26–0.85 mg/kg	IM	Purpose-built gas anesthetic machine for field use.	Gales et al. (2005)
		1–5%	IH		
Mirounga angustirostris (northern elephant seal)	Medetomidine, ketamine	70–140 μg/kg	IM	Bradycardia, prolonged recovery, poor reversibility, variable plane of anesthesia	Haulena and Heath (2001)
		2.5 mg/kg	IM		
	Tiletamine and zolazepam	0.8 mg/kg	IV	Atropine given routinely (0.02 mg/kg IV) at the time of induction. IV zoletil provides 15-minute anesthesia at a level sufficient for intubation. Can then supplement with isoflurane as required.	Dailey et al. (2002); M. Haulena personal communication
Mirounga leonina (southern elephant seal)	Ketamine, diazepam	2.3–3.9 mg/kg	IM	Apnea, poor muscle relaxation	Woods et al. (1994a)
		0.02–0.35 mg/kg	IM		
	Ketamine, diazepam	4.4–8.6 mg/kg	IM	Apnea	Slip and Woods (1996)
		0.04–0.13 mg/kg			
	Ketamine, xylazine	2.1–11.4 mg/kg	IM	Prolonged apnea	Mitchell and Burton (1991)
		0.2–0.5 mg/kg			

(Continued)

651

Table 46.1. (Continued)

Species	Agent	Dose Rate	Route	Comments	Reference
	Ketamine, xylazine	2.1–3.1 mg/kg	IM	Apnea, tremors	Woods et al. (1994a)
		0.2–0.5 mg/kg	IM		
	Ketamine, xylazine	2.5–3.4 mg/kg	IM	Apnea, responsive to doxapram 2 mg/kg	Woods et al. (1996b)
		0.5–0.6 mg/kg	IM		
	Medetomidine	13–27 μg/kg	IM	Vomiting, hyperthermia, bradycardia	Woods et al. (1996a)
	Medetomidine, ketamine	12–27 μg/kg	IM	Hyperthermia, variable plane of anesthesia, poor reversibility, bradycardia	Woods et al. (1996a)
		1.4–2.2 mg/kg	IM		
	Midazolam, pethidine	0.02–0.07 mg/kg	IM	Deeper sedation with higher doses of pethidine (2.7–6.7 mg/kg), faster recovery after naloxone or naltrexone	Woods et al. (1994b)
		1.2–6.7 mg/kg	IM		
	Midazolam, pethidine, thiopentone	0.02–0.07 mg/kg	IM	Good immobilization allowing intubation of 5-minute duration after thiopentone	Woods et al. (1994b)
		2.7–6.7 mg/kg	IM		
		2.2–5.9 mg/kg	IV		
	Midazolam, pethidine, ketamine	0.02–0.07 mg/kg	IM	Incremental doses of ketamine to maintain immobilization for 1 hour	Woods et al. (1994b)
		2.7–6.7 mg/kg	IM		
		4.4–10 mg/kg	IV		
	Ketamine, midazolam	2.1–3.7 mg/kg	IM	Deep sedation, apnea, prolonged recovery, hyperthermia, bradycardia	Woods et al. (1994a)
		0.02–0.03 mg/kg	IM		
	Tiletamine and zolazepam	1 mg/kg	IM	Some animals became apneic requiring ventilation	Baker et al. (1990)
	Tiletamine and zolazepam	1.6–2.4 mg/kg	IM	Prolonged apnea, muscle tremors, mortalities.	Mitchell and Burton (1991)
	Tiletamine and zolazepam	0.7–1.2 mg/kg	IM	Apnea, tremors, possible hallucinations, prolonged recovery	Woods et al. (1994a)
	Tiletamine and zolazepam	0.46 mg/kg	IV	Mean duration of immobilization 15.48 minutes. Immobilized such that stomach lavage and blood sampling were possible.	McMahon et al. (2000)
	Tiletamine and zolazepam, supplemental ketamine	0.5–0.7 mg/kg; 1.04 ± 0.66 mg/kg	IM	Addition of ketamine useful when initial level of sedation or duration of immobilization was unsatisfactory. Induction dose rate should be adjusted depending on stage of annual cycle (molting/breeding).	Carlini et al. (2009)
Phoca vitulina (harbor seal)	Propofol	2–6 mg/kg	IV	Optimum short-acting anesthesia at 5 mg/kg. Apnea.	Gulland et al. (1999)
	Propofol, isoflurane	3–5 mg/kg	IV	Easily intubated, apnea	Gulland et al. (1999)
		2–5%	IH		
	Butorphanol	0.4 mg/kg	IM	Decreased anxiety, relaxation sufficient for minor procedures (radiographic positioning, skin scrapes)	Tuomi et al. (2000)
	Butorphanol, diazepam	0.4 mg/kg	IM	Immobilization sufficient for deep muscle biopsy, endoscopy	Tuomi et al. (2000)
		0.2 mg/kg	IV		
	Diazepam, isoflurane	0.15–0.2 mg/kg	IV	Atropine given routinely (0.02 mg/kg IV) at the time of induction. Routine induction protocol for this species.	M. Haulena personal communication
		0.5–2.5%	IH		
	Butorphanol, isoflurane	0.2 mg/kg	IV	Atropine given routinely (0.02 mg/kg IV) at the time of induction.	M. Haulena personal communication
		1.5–5.0%	IH		
	Diazepam	1.5–2.0 mg/kg	IV	Recommended as initial dose for sedation (then supplemented as required)	Lapierre et al. (2007)

Source: Haulena M, Heath RB. 2001. Marine mammal anesthesia. In: *CRC Handbook of Marine Mammal Medicine* (LA Dierauf, FMD Gulland, eds.), pp. 655–688. Boca Raton: CRC Press.
IH, inhalational; IM, intramuscular injection; IV, intravenous injection.

Ketamine

Ketamine has been commonly used for chemical immobilization of phocid seals (Gales 1989), alone or in combination with other drugs. In phocids, ketamine has the advantage of causing minimal cardiopulmonary depression over a relatively wide dosage range. Northern elephant seals were immobilized using intramuscular doses of ketamine between 1.4 and 6.9 mg/kg (Briggs et al. 1975), and intravenous ketamine has been used successfully in young harp seals at doses between 0.5 and 7.5 mg/kg (Engelhardt 1977). Adverse effects of ketamine alone have included poor muscle relaxation and muscle tremors (Briggs et al. 1975). Therefore, it has been used most often in combination with other agents, such as benzodiazepines (e.g., diazepam or midazolam) or α_2-agonists (e.g., xylazine, detomidine, or medetomidine).

Benzodiazepines

Benzodiazepines are very useful agents for phocid seal sedation because of their muscle relaxant properties, minimal cardiovascular effects, and reversibility with specific antagonists. They are often used as a premedication, delivered remotely to aid safe physical restraint in large phocids. Prior to the introduction of midazolam, mixtures of ketamine and diazepam were commonly used to immobilize many species of phocid seals. Midazolam has some advantages over diazepam: its unique solubility characteristics (water-soluble injection but lipid soluble at body pH) result in a very rapid onset of action following injection (Plumb 1999).

Diazepam at a mean dose of 0.32 mg/kg, administered intravenously to harbor seal pups, provided sufficient sedation to facilitate blood collection and muscle biopsy; however, mild-to-severe bradycardia was noted in some individuals (Lapierre et al. 2007). The authors suggested that a lower initial dose of diazepam (0.15–0.20 mg/kg IV), supplemented as required, would be effective and would not result in undesirable cardiac effects. A combination of ketamine and diazepam, given intramuscularly, has also been used to sedate male Weddell seals (Harcourt et al. 2010).

Midazolam given at dose rates of 0.15–0.2 mg/kg by intramuscular injection will produce moderate sedation, and dose rates of 0.4–0.5 mg/kg will produce heavy sedation. The higher dose rate is useful for the larger phocid species, where physical restraint in unsedated animals can be dangerous for handlers and stressful for the animal. Weddell seals have been immobilized using a preprepared 1:1 mix of ketamine 100 mg/mL and midazolam 5 mg/mL. Ongoing maintenance was then achieved using the same ketamine and midazolam mix, delivered intravenously as needed (Mellish et al. 2010). Midazolam dosages of 0.51 ± 0.19 mg/kg have been given intramuscularly to produce a moderate level of sedation in crab-eater seals (Gales et al. 2005). This level of sedation allowed restraint for

anesthetic induction using isoflurane. In contrast, premedication of harp seals, using midazolam given intramuscularly at 0.1 or 0.2 mg/kg, did not appear to improve quality of isoflurane anesthesia or ease of intubation (Pang et al. 2006). In addition, recovery from anesthesia was prolonged in some individuals.

Alpha-2 Adrenergic Agonists

Xylazine (alone and in combination with ketamine) has been used successfully in numerous phocid seals. The use of xylazine as a sole immobilization agent has been associated with hyperthermia, bradycardia, and high rates of mortality in leopard and southern elephant seals (Mitchell & Burton 1991). A medetomidine-ketamine combination used in southern elephant seals produced similar undesirable side effects (Woods et al. 1996a). Generally, the use of α_2-agonists has resulted in undesirable cardiovascular side effects such as decreased cardiac output, bradycardia, and increased peripheral vascular resistance. Prolonged anesthetic recovery, bradycardia, and variable levels of anesthesia have been observed in harbor and northern elephant seals following administration of medetomidine (Haulena & Heath 2001). However, this drug has been routinely used by other authors to sedate harbor and gray seals, and when given in combination with ketamine, to induce anesthesia in these species (Barnett 1998). The α_2-agonists offer the advantage of being reversible using antagonists such as yohimbine and atipamezole although the use of such agents is not well established in phocids.

Tiletamine and Zolazepam

A combination of tiletamine and zolazepam in a 1:1 ratio has been used in a wide range of phocids. As a combination of two drugs presented in a fixed ratio, it does not allow for fine adjustments in the dosage of either agent to suit a particular species. In general, intravenous administration of tiletamine and zolazepam produces more predictable immobilization with fewer adverse side effects (such as prolonged apnea and muscle tremors) when compared with intramuscular administration.

Tiletamine and zolazepam have been used in southern elephant seals both intramuscularly at a dose rate of 1 mg/kg (Woods et al. 1994a) and intravenously at a rate of 0.5 mg/kg (McMahon et al. 2000). Induction doses of 0.5–0.7 mg/kg given by intramuscular injection were also effective in this species although supplemental doses of ketamine were required to maintain an adequate plane of anesthesia in some animals (Carlini et al. 2009). Harbor seals have been anesthetized using 0.8–1.2 mg/kg tiletamine and zolazepam injected intravenously under physical restraint (Lander et al. 2005), and a similar regimen has been described in northern elephant seals (Dailey et al. 2002). An intramuscular dose of 1 mg/kg was also found to be effective in immobilizing gray seals (Baker et al. 1990). Intramuscular administration of tiletamine and zolazepam to 30 Weddell seals produced variable planes of immobilization. Intramuscular administration of tiletamine and zolazepam to 30 Weddell seals produced variable planes of immobilization. Six animals displayed prolonged apnea, and three of these animals eventually died (Phelan and Green 1992). Variable responses were also obtained in leopard seals following intramuscular administration of tiletamine and zolazepam 1.2–1.4 mg/kg (Higgins et al. 2002); however, a lower dose rate (0.8–1.0 mg/kg) was found to provide reliable induction when used in another study (Vogelnest et al. 2009). In this later study, supplemental midazolam or ketamine (given IM or IV) was used to maintain anesthesia.

Opioids

Anesthetic regimens that include opioids have also been used to immobilize phocid seals. There are several advantages of using opioids: they can be reversed using naloxone or naltrexone, and they usually have relatively mild cardiovascular and respiratory side effects when used at low doses. A mixture of meperidine (pethidine) and midazolam has been used with good results in southern elephant seals, inducing a reliable deep sedation that allowed intravenous access for the administration of ketamine or thiopentone (Woods et al. 1994b). However, a meperidine and midazolam combination was considered unsatisfactory in leopard seals due to the variability in response produced, a loss of muscle tone that compromised patency of the airway and respiratory depression (Higgins et al. 2002). A combination of meperidine and midazolam has also been used to induce deep sedation and light anesthesia in crab-eater seals (Tahmindjis et al. 2003) although periods of prolonged apnea were noted. Meperidine, when given as the sole sedative agent, produced moderate restraint without respiratory depression in harbor and northern elephant seals (Joseph & Cornell 1988). Butorphanol tartrate (0.4 mg/kg IM) in harbor seals produced mild sedation and decreased anxiety during minor procedures (Tuomi et al. 2000). The addition of diazepam (0.2 mg/kg IV) allowed more invasive procedures (muscle biopsy, endoscopy) to be carried out. Potent opioids (i.e., etorphine and carfentanil) produced respiratory depression, hyperexcitability, and prolonged apnea in hooded and gray seals. Their only really advantage is small drug volume delivery (Baker & Gatesman 1985; Haigh & Stewart 1979).

Intravenous Anesthetics

Propofol (5 mg/kg IV) was evaluated in harbor seal pups, two northern elephant seal pups, and two harbor seal adults and produced short-duration general anesthesia, good muscle relaxation, and rapid recoveries (Gulland & Gage 1997; Gulland et al. 1999). The primary disadvantage of this agent is that large volumes of the commercially available preparations (10 mg/mL) are required for animals over 40 kg.

Inhalation Anesthetics

Prolonged immobilization procedures or those requiring a surgical plane of anesthesia are most safely performed using inhalant techniques. Studies in gray seals have demonstrated an efficient exchange of large volumes of gases during surface breathing, in part, because the animals have a large tidal volume (Reed et al. 1994). This suggests that diving seals can achieve rapid and efficient uptake and distribution of inhalant anesthetic agents. The use of a precision vaporizer and anesthetic circuit allows the anesthetist to accurately deliver a known, clinically useful concentration of the anesthetic agent in oxygen. Intubation of the animal completes the anesthetic circuit and gives the anesthetist control over the animal's airway. Maintenance of a clear airway is particularly significant during anesthesia of phocid seals, as many of these species have reduced cartilaginous support of the trachea and so are prone to respiratory obstruction (Hammond & Elsner 1977; Higgins et al. 2002). In addition, many phocid species have a very fleshy pharyngeal region that may contribute to respiratory obstruction when muscular tone is reduced by sedation. The most frequently used inhalant anesthetic agents in pinnipeds are isoflurane and sevoflurane.

MONITORING

The plane of sedation or anesthesia in phocid seals can be assessed by basic means such as ability to move body, head and flipper movements, jaw tone, and palpebral reflex. Table 46.2 defines levels of chemical restraint observed in leopard seals according to Higgins et al. (2002).

The assessment of physiological parameters is essential for the safe management of any chemical immobilization procedure. The animal's heart rate should be continuously monitored so that bradycardia, whether resulting from hypoxemia or presumed dive response, is quickly detected and treatment instituted immediately. It is difficult to auscultate the heart through the thoracic wall and an esophageal stethoscope should be used for this purpose. Alternatively, the heart rate is counted by the visualization of movements of the thoracic wall. Monitoring devices with electrocardiographic capacity are useful for assessment of the rate and rhythm (Lapierre et al. 2007).

Prolonged apnea is common in chemically immobilized phocid seals (Haulena & Heath 2001). However, the respiratory pattern in sleeping phocid seals is also characterized by frequent periods of apnea (Castellini et al. 1994). Since anesthetic agents often produce changes in the cardiovascular and respiratory systems, direct time comparisons between these events should be interpreted with caution. The interpretation of what

Table 46.2. Classification of stages of immobilization in phocid seals

	Definition
Stage 0	No effect
Stage 1	Negligible sedation
Stage 2	Visibly sedated but mobile
Stage 3	Sedated. Sluggish movement in response to body or head touch. Locomotion may be elicited with repeated stimulus. Hand injection possible.
Stage 4	Small movements of head or eyes. Locomotion possible but sluggish. Stage of immobilization sufficient if not adjacent to water.
Stage 5	No body movement. Muscle tone variable, dependent on drug used. Eye may follow passing objects.
Stage 6	No response to vigorous shaking of the tail, body, or head. Very little muscle tone. Sluggish palpebral response.
Stage 7	As for stage 6 but slightly deeper, with some respiratory depression and negligible muscle tone. Negligible palpebral response.
Stage 8	Deep anesthesia. Cardiac or respiratory depression. Complete loss of muscle tone. No palpebral response.

Source: With permission from Higgins DP, Rogers TL, Irvine AD, Hall-Aspland SA. 2002. Use of midazolam/pethidine and tiletamine/zolazepam combinations for the chemical restraint of Leopard seals (*Hydrurga leptonyx*). *Marine Mammal Science* 18(2):483–499.

constitutes a life-threatening duration of apnea is species dependent and related to their aerobic dive capacity (Slip & Woods 1996). The aerobic dive limit (ADL) is defined as the time beyond which an animal must rely on anaerobic metabolism to prolong the dive (Kooyman 1989). Species that are capable of deep and prolonged dives (e.g., southern elephant and Weddell seals) have a greater ADL and would be expected to tolerate longer periods of apnea under anesthesia compared with shallow diving species. Ultimately, respiratory rates and periods of apnea in anesthetized phocid seals should be interpreted in light of the other physiological variables that reflect ventilation and perfusion.

Hypoventilation is a significant problem during phocid anesthesia. It is essential that both respiratory rate and tidal volume be continuously monitored. The anesthetist must be prepared to assist ventilation if hypoventilation becomes apparent (i.e., reduced thoracic excursions during breathing, increasing end-tidal CO_2 [$ETCO_2$] values).

In addition to visualization of mucous membrane color, determination of hemoglobin saturation with pulse oximetry is a valuable aid when assessing ventilation and perfusion. Probe placement sites include the vulva, lip, and tongue (Fig. 46.3). Capnography is also an extremely useful tool in anesthetized phocid seals for assessing adequacy of ventilation. Respiratory obstruction is very likely to occur in anesthetized leopard seals and is likely the major contributor to the high mortality associated with chemical immobilization procedures in this species (Higgins et al. 2002). To obtain accurate $ETCO_2$ readings, the animal must be intubated. There are no published normal values for this variable in anesthetized phocid seals, but it is the authors' belief that assisted ventilation is indicated when $ETCO_2$ exceeds 55 mmHg. This figure is based, in part, on the authors' observations of $ETCO_2$ values during the initial period of anesthetic procedures on both otariid seals and phocid seals and, in part, on experimental studies. Parkos and Wahrenbrock (1987)

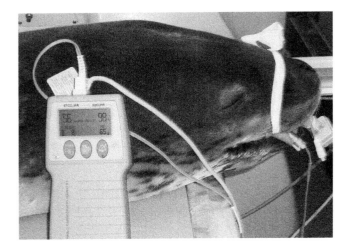

Figure 46.3. Monitoring end-tidal carbon dioxide levels and hemoglobin saturation with a capnometer and pulse oximeter, respectively, in an intubated, anesthetized leopard seal. The pulse oximeter probe is placed on the tongue, and the capnometer is attached to the end of the endotracheal tube.

found that the ventilatory response to hypercapnia in unanesthetized Weddell seals did not differ from that of terrestrial mammals. Reed et al. (1994) measured $ETCO_2$ values in freely diving gray seals and found they ranged between 28 and 35 mmHg, a range not dissimilar to that seen in terrestrial mammals.

Noninvasive blood pressure monitoring would provide additional information to aid the anesthetic management of phocid seals. However, it is generally not applicable to phocids because of their lack of readily accessible peripheral arteries.

Anesthetic agents disrupt the ability of phocid seals to thermoregulate. Seals in cold environments given vasodilatory agents may become hypothermic (Hammond & Elsner 1977), probably due to disruption of their countercurrent heat exchange mechanisms. Behavioral thermoregulation will also be affected by immobilization and may result in hyperthermia. In temperate or warmer climates, seals recovering from sedation or anesthesia should be kept wet and/or in the shade. Accurate measurement of the body temperature in larger phocid seals requires rectal temperature probes of at least 30 cm in length.

SUPPLEMENTAL DRUGS USED DURING ANESTHESIA

Doxapram

Doxapram increased the depth and frequency of respiration and stimulated breathing in apneic southern elephant seals (Woods et al. 1996b). It failed to stimulate breathing when delivered into the extradural sinus, but direct intratracheal administration (via an endotracheal tube) stimulated breathing in four of six apneic animals. The lack of efficacy of IV doxapram was probably due to low pressures and flows in this vessel during breath holding. There have been no reported studies to determine whether the doxapram administration to hypoventilating phocid seals improves respiration and/or oxygen delivery to the tissues. Doxapram (5.0 mg/kg) was a nonspecific antagonist for ketamine-diazepam sedation in southern elephant seals, but often caused shaking and hyper-responsiveness in animals, prompting a recommendation to use a lower dosage (Woods et al. 1995).

Atropine

Atropine has been used at a wide variety of dose rates in the anesthesia of phocid seals (Gales & Burton 1988; Mitchell & Burton 1991). It has been included in some anesthetic regimens in an attempt to block some of the physiologic effects of the dive response. Doses that are standard for terrestrial carnivores (0.02–0.04 mg/kg) were used in unsedated harbor seals to eliminate the reflex bradycardia that occurs during diving (Galantsev et al. 1984), and it is likely that doses of this order would be efficacious in most pinniped species. However, it would be expected that atropinization would not affect the vasoconstriction and venous pooling seen with this physiological mechanism. While atropine, historically, was often included in anesthetic drug protocols for phocid seals, a number of authors describe protocols that do not routinely include atropine, without apparent adverse effects (Bodley et al. 2005; Gales et al. 2005; McMahon et al. 2000). Increased salivation was noted following intravenous administration of diazepam to harbor seal pups (Lapierre et al. 2007) and, therefore, atropine may have a role in management of excessive salivation and upper respiratory tract secretion during anesthesia.

RECOVERY

Adequate management of the recovery of phocids following anesthestic procedures is essential. For captive animals, access to water should be denied until the individual is fully recovered. The potential for hyperthermia must be managed by wetting the animal or keeping it shaded. Conversely, individuals at risk of hypothermia can be insulated using blankets or thermal devices until they have reached a light plane of anesthesia. Timing of extubation is a key decision during recovery. Premature removal of the endotracheal tube increases the risk of respiratory obstruction, while delayed intubation increases risk to handlers. Animals that have been induced and maintained on gaseous anesthesia may recover suddenly and become startled by the close presence of the anesthetist. In the field situation, this may lead to the animal fleeing while not fully coordinated, thereby increasing its chances of injury.

Antagonists

Antagonists potentially improve safety of chemical immobilization of pinnipeds: they may be used during emergency resuscitation and to reduce recovery times.

Yohimbine and Atipamezole Yohimbine (0.5 mg/kg IM) hastened recovery from ketamine-xylazine-diazepam sedation in Weddell seals (Bornemann & Plotz 1993) and has also been used (0.06 mg/kg IV) to hasten recovery in southern elephant seals under ketamine-xylazine sedation (Woods et al. 1995). Low dose atipamazole (median dosage of 0.04 mg/kg IV) failed to arouse southern elephant seals from ketamine-medetomidine anesthesia (Woods et al. 1996a).

Flumazenil Flumazenil appears to be a useful adjunct to anesthetic management of phocid seals immobilized with benzodiazepine combinations. In crab-eater seals (250–300 kg), a combination of meperidine (1.29–2.2 mg/kg IM) and midazolam (0.29–0.37 mg/kg IM) was partially antagonized by naloxone (1.2–4 mg IV) and flumazenil (0.1–0.5) (M. Lynch, unpublished data 1997). While the time to recovery was greatly shortened, reversal of drug effects was not complete and larger doses may be indicated. Flumazenil (1 mg per 20–25 mg benzodiazepine IM) has also been used to reverse the zolazepam in southern elephant seals immobilized with tiletamine-zolazepam (Karesh et al. 1997). Mellish et al. (2010) administered flumazenil intravenously, at a dose rate of 0.002 mg/kg, to Weddell seals that had been immobilized using midazolam and ketamine; however, the authors commented that its effect was questionable.

FIELD ANESTHESIA

Free-ranging phocid seals occupy a variety of habitats, and many of these are difficult to access as well as presenting challenging environmental conditions to operate within. The grouping of sexes and age groups for each species and the physiological status of the animals may vary depending on the time of the year, as do the nature of interactions between animals and their reactions to the presence of humans. The value of the outcome gained from immobilizing an animal must always be balanced against the detrimental impacts that the intervention produces. Where possible, procedures should be conducted at times of the year when the expected impact upon animals is lowest. For example, if a procedure on a lactating female decreases the likelihood of survival of her pup, then the procedure should be delayed if possible.

A major consideration in most immobilization procedures conducted on free-ranging phocid seals is the assessment of the likelihood of the animal fleeing to the water. This is particularly important when the chemical agent is being delivered by remote injection, as sedated animals are at risk of drowning. In this situation, it is important to understand the animal's response to human interference, and carefully approach the animal to a distance where the dart can be placed as accurately as possible. Ideally, the seal should not be aware of the approach of the operator. Regardless of whether this can be achieved, the aim is that the animal remains calm to reduce the likelihood of it fleeing to the water when darted.

Optimal techniques for anesthesia, monitoring and recovery management can often be difficult to apply in a field procedure. For example, inhalant anesthetic techniques may be logistically difficult during field procedures conducted in extremely cold environments. Precision vaporizers function efficiently within a limited temperature range and must be housed in insulated containers when environmental temperatures are low (Gales et al. 2005). Effective insulation may be difficult to maintain for prolonged procedures, and the use of injectable anesthetic agents may be more practically useful in such circumstances (Mellish et al. 2010).

Optimal management of the recovery period is extremely important. As previously discussed (see Recovery section), the timing of extubation is of particular significance for phocid seals as they are prone to respiratory obstruction. It is also worthwhile to consider the potential effect of immobilization technique on physiological parameters. For example, male Weddell seals show a clear, prolonged elevation in cortisol levels in response to physical restraint (Harcourt et al. 2010). This effect may impact upon biological parameters being measured during field experiments.

ANALGESIA

Phocid seals may require analgesia during periods of illness or following trauma or surgery. Use of both opioids and nonsteroidal anti-inflammatory drugs (NSAIDs) has been reported. Nutter et al. (Nutter et al. 1998) described pharmacokinetics of single-dose butorphanol in northern elephant seals and determined that

a dose rate of $55\,\mu g/kg$ IM resulted in detectable plasma levels for up to 5 hours post injection, and produced a degree of sedation for up to 3 hours. The NSAID flunixin meglumine has been used to treat ocular inflammation in southern elephant seals (Vogelnest et al. 1996) and musculoskeletal disorders in gray and harbor seals (Barnett 1998). Anorexia has been reported in southern elephant seals treated with flunixin meglumine for more than 72 hours, possibly the result of gastric inflammation/ulceration (Barnett 1998; Vogelnest et al. 1996). The NSAIDs carprofen and meloxicam have been administered to phocid seals both orally and intramuscularly at canine dose rates without adverse effects (Barnett 1998; Lucas et al. 1999).

REFERENCES

Angell James JE, Elsner R, De Burgh Daly M. 1981. Lung inflation: effects on heart rate, respiration, and vagal afferent activity in seals. *American Journal of Physiology* 240:H190–H198.

Baker JR, Gatesman TJ. 1985. Use of carfentanil and a ketamine-xylazine mixture to immobilise wild grey seals (*Halichoerus grypus*). *The Veterinary Record* 116:208–210.

Baker JR, Fedak MA, Anderson SS, et al. 1990. Use of a tiletamine-zolazepam mixture to immobilise wild grey seals and southern elephant seals. *The Veterinary Record* 126:75–77.

Barnett J. 1998. Treatment of sick and injured marine mammals. *In Practice* 20:200–211.

Bodley K, van Polanen Petel T, Gales N. 2005. Immobilisation of free-living Weddell seals *Leptonychotes weddellii* using midazolam and isoflurane. *Polar Biology* 28:631–636.

Bornemann H, Plotz J. 1993. A field method for immobilising Weddell seals. *Wildlife Society Bulletin* 21:437–441.

Boyd RB. 1975. Gross and microscopic study of respiratory anatomy of the Antarctic Weddell seal, (*Leptonychotes weddelli*). *Journal of Morphology* 147:309–335.

Briggs GD, Henrickson RV, Le Boeuf BJ. 1975. Ketamine immobilisation of northern elephant seals. *Journal of the American Veterinary Medical Association* 167:546–548.

Bryden MM, Molyneux GS. 1978. Arteriovenous anastomoses in the skin of seals. II. The California sea lion (*Zalophus californianus*) and the northern fur seal (*Callorhinus ursinus*) (Pinnipedia: Otariidae). *The Anatomical Record* 191:253–259.

Carlini AR, Negrete J, Daneri GA, et al. 2009. Immobilization of adult male southern elephant seals (*Mirounga leonina*) during the breeding and molting periods using a tiletamine/zolazepam mixture and ketamine. *Polar Biology* 32:915–921.

Castellini MA, Milsom WK, Berger RJ, et al. 1994. Patterns of respiration and heart rate during wakefulness and sleep in elephant seal pups. *American Journal of Physiology* 266:R863–R869.

Dailey MD, Haulena M, Lawrence J. 2002. First report of a parasitic copepod (*Pennella balaenopterae*) infestation in a pinniped. *Journal of Zoo and Wildlife Medicine* 33:62–65.

Engelhardt FR. 1977. Immobilization of harp seals, *Phoca groenlandica* by intravenous injection of ketamine. *Comparative Biochemistry and Physiology* 56C:75–76.

Field IC, Bradshaw CJA, McMahon CR, et al. 2002. Effects of age, size and condition of elephant seals (*Mirounga leonina*) on their intravenous anaesthesia with tiletamine and zolazepam. *The Veterinary Record* 151:235–240.

Galantsev VP, Kovalenko SG, Popov SM. 1984. Investigation of the cholinergic mechanisms of the adaptive reactions of the heart in diving mammals. *Journal of Evolutionary Biochemistry and Physiology* 19:180–183.

Gales N, Barnes J, Chittick B, et al. 2005. Effective, field-based inhalation anesthesia for ice seals. *Marine Mammal Science* 21: 717–727.

Gales NJ. 1989. Chemical restraint and anaesthesia of pinnipeds: a review. *Marine Mammal Science* 5:228–256.

Gales NJ, Burton HR. 1988. Use of emetics and anaesthesia for dietary assessment of Weddell Seals. *Australian Wildlife Research* 15:423–433.

Geschke K, Chilvers BL. 2009. Managing big boys: a case study on remote anaesthesia and satellite tracking of adult male New Zealand sea lions (*Phocarctos hookeri*). *Wildlife Research* 36: 666–674.

Goldstein T, Johnson SP, Werner LJ, et al. 1998. Causes of erroneous white blood cell counts and differentiation in clinically healthy young northern elephant seals (*Mirounga angustirostris*). *Journal of Zoo and Wildlife Medicine* 29:408–412.

Gray R, Canfield P, Rogers T. 2006. Histology of selected tissues of the leopard seal and implications for functional adaptations to an aquatic lifestyle. *Journal of Anatomy* 209:179–199.

Gulland FMD, Gage LJ. 1997. Preliminary trials on the use of propofol for general anesthesia of phocid seals. Proceedings of the Annual Conference of the International Association of Aquatic Animal Medicine, p. 3.

Gulland FMD, Haulena M, Elliott S, et al. 1999. Anesthesia of juvenile Pacific harbor seals using propofol alone and in combination with isoflurane. *Marine Mammal Science* 15: 234–238.

Gulland FMD, Haulena M, Dierauf LA. 2001. Seals and sea lions. In: *CRC Handbook of Marine Mammal Medicine* (LA Dierauf, FMD Gulland, eds.), pp. 907–926. Boca Raton: CRC Press.

Haigh JC, Stewart REA. 1979. Narcotics in hooded seals (*Cystophora cristata*): a preliminary report. *Canadian Journal of Zoology* 57:946–949.

Hammond D, Elsner R. 1977. Anesthesia in phocid seals. *Journal of Zoo Animal Medicine* 8:7–13.

Harcourt RG, Turner E, Hall A, et al. 2010. Effects of capture stress on free-ranging, reproductively active male Weddell seals. *Journal of Comparative Physiology. A, Neuroethology, Sensory, Neural, and Behavioral Physiology* 196:147–154.

Harrison RJ, King JE. 1980. *Marine Mammals*. London: Hutchinson Publishing Group.

Haulena M, Heath RB. 2001. Marine mammal anesthesia. In: *CRC Handbook of Marine Mammal Medicine* (LA Dierauf, FMD Gulland, eds.), pp. 655–688. Boca Raton: CRC Press.

Higgins DP, Rogers TL, Irvine AD, et al. 2002. Use of midazolam/pethidine and tiletamine/zolazepam combinations for the chemical restraint of leopard seals (*Hydrurga leptonyx*). *Marine Mammal Science* 18:483–499.

Horne WA, Tchamba MN, Loomis MR. 2001. A simple method of providing intermittent positive-pressure ventilation to etorphine-immobilized elephants (*Loxodonta africana*) in the field. *Journal of Zoo and Wildlife Medicine* 32:519–522.

Joseph BE, Cornell LH. 1988. The use of meperidine hydrochloride for chemical restraint in certain cetaceans and pinnipeds. *Journal of Wildlife Diseases* 24:691–694.

Karesh WB, Cook RA, Stetter M, et al. 1997. South American pinnipeds: Immobilization, telemetry, and health evaluations. Proceedings of the Annual Meeting of the American Association of Zoo Veterinarians, Houstan, Texas, pp. 291–295.

Kelly BP. 1996. Live capture of ringed seals in ice-covered waters. *Journal of Wildlife Management* 60:678–684.

Kooyman GL. 1981. *Weddell Seal, Consumate Diver*. Cambridge: Cambridge University Press.

Kooyman GL. 1989. *Diverse Divers: Physiology and Behaviour*. Berlin: Springer-Verlag.

Lander ME, Haulena M, Gulland FMD, et al. 2005. Implantation of subcutaneous radio transmitters in the harbor seal (*Phoca vitulina*). *Marine Mammal Science* 21:154–161.

Lapierre JL, Schreer JF, Burns JM, et al. 2007. Effect of diazepam on heart and respiratory rates of harbor seal pups following intravenous injection. *Marine Mammal Science* 23:209–217.

Lucas RJ, Barnett J, Riley P. 1999. Treatment of lesions of osteomyelitis in the hind flippers of six grey seals (*Halichoerus grypus*). *The Veterinary Record* 145:547–550.

Mauck B, Bilgmann K, Jones DD, et al. 2003. Thermal windows on the trunk of hauled-out seals: hot spots for thermoregulatory evaporation? *Journal of Experimental Biology* 206:1727–1738.

McMahon CR, Burton H, McLean S, et al. 2000. Field immobilisation of southern elephant seals with intravenous tiletamine and zolazepam. *The Veterinary Record* 146:251–254.

Mellish JAE, Tuomi PA, Hindle AG, et al. 2010. Chemical immobilization of Weddell seals (*Leptonychotes weddellii*) by ketamine/midazolam combination. *Veterinary Anaesthesia and Analgesia* 37:123–131.

Mitchell PJ, Burton HR. 1991. Immobilisation of southern elephant seals and leopard seals with cyclohexamine anaesthetics and xylazine. *The Veterinary Record* 129:332–336.

Nadel ER. 1984. Energy exchanges in water. *Undersea Biomedical Research* 11:149–158.

Nutter FB, Haulena M, Bai SA. 1998. Preliminary pharmacokinetics of single-dose intramuscular butorphanol in elephant seals (*Mirounga angustirostris*). Joint Conference of the American Association of Zoo Veterinarians and the American Association of Wildlife Veterinarians, pp. 372–373.

Pang DSJ, Rondenay Y, Measures L, et al. 2006. The effects of two dosages of midazolam on short-duration anesthesia in the harp seal (*Phoca groenlandica*). *Journal of Zoo and Wildlife Medicine* 37:27–32.

Parkos CA, Wahrenbrock EA. 1987. Acute effects of hypercapnia and hypoxia on the minute ventilation in unrestrained Weddell seals. *Respiration Physiology* 67:197–207.

Phelan JR, Green K. 1992. Chemical restraint of Weddell seals (*Leptonychotes weddelli*) with a combination of tiletamine and zolazepam. *Journal of Wildlife Diseases* 28:230–235.

Plumb DC. 1999. *Plumb's Veterinary Drug Handbook*. Ames: Blackwell Publishing.

Reed JZ, Chambers C, Fedak MA, et al. 1994. Gas exchange of captive freely diving grey seals (*Halichoerus grypus*). *Journal of Experimental Biology* 191:1–18.

Ridgway SH. 1972. Homeostasis in the aquatic environment. In: *Mammals of the Sea. Biology and Medicine* (SH Ridgeway, ed.), pp. 590–748. Springfield: Charles C Thomas.

Riedman M. 1990. Evolution, classification and distribution of pinnipeds. In: *The Pinnipeds: Seals, Sea Lions and Walruses* (M Riedman, ed.), pp. 50–83. Berkeley; Los Angeles: University of California Press.

Ryding FN. 1982. Ketamine immobilisation of southern elephant seals by a remote method. *British Antarctic Survey Bulletin* 57:21–26.

Scheffer V. 1990. Adaptations for a marine existence. In: *The Pinnipeds: Seals, Sea Lions and Walruses* (M Riedman, ed.), pp. 1–49. Berkeley, Los Angeles: University of California Press.

Slip DJ, Woods R. 1996. Intramuscular and intravenous immobilization of juvenile southern elephant seal. *Journal of Wildlife Management* 60:802–807.

Stirling I. 1966. A technique for handling live seals. *Journal of Mammaology* 47:543–544.

Tahmindjis MA, Higgins DP, Lynch MJ, et al. 2003. Use of a pethidine and midazolam combination for the reversible sedation of crabeater seals (*Lobodon carcinophagus*). *Marine Mammal Science* 19:581–589.

Thornton SJ, Speilman DM, Pelc NJ, et al. 2001. Effects of forced diving on the spleen and hepatic sinus in northern elephant seal pups. *Proceedings of the National Academy of Sciences of the United States of America* 98:9413–9418.

Tuomi PA, Grey M, Christen D. 2000. Butorphanol and butorphanol/diazepam administration for analgesia and sedation of harbor seals (*Phoca vitulina*). Proceedings of the Joint Meeting of the American Association of Zoo Veterinarians and the International Association of Aquatic Animal Medicine, pp. 382–383.

Vogelnest L, Hulst F, Woods R. 1996. The veterinary management of southern elephant seals (*Mirounga leonina*) at Taronga Zoo. Proceedings of the Annual Meeting of the American Association of Zoo Veterinarians, pp. 318–325.

Vogelnest L, Edwards N, Ciaglia M, et al. 2009. Anaesthesia of leopard seals (*Hydrurga leptonyx*) on the western Antarctic peninsula. Proceedings of the Annual Meeting of the Wildlife Disease Association (Australasian Section), The Catlins, New Zealand, pp. 61–63.

Welsch U, Wagner H, Galm R, et al. 1989. Architecture and functional aspects of the distal airways of Antarctic seals with different habits, the Weddell seal (*Leptonychotes weddellii*) and the crabeater seal (*Lobodon carcinophagus*). Polar Biology 10:187–196.

Woods R, McClean S, Nicol S, et al. 1994a. A comparison of some cyclohexamine based drug combinations for chemical restraint of southern elephant seals, (*Mirounga leonina*). *The Veterinary Record* 10:412–429.

Woods R, McClean S, Nicol S, et al. 1994b. Use of midazolam, pethidine, ketamine and thiopentone for the restraint of southern elephant seals, (*Mirounga leonina*). *The Veterinary Record* 135:572–577.

Woods R, McClean S, Nicol S, et al. 1995. Antagonism of some cyclohexamine-based drug combinations used for chemical restraint of southern elephant seals (*Mirounga leonina*). *Australian Veterinary Journal* 72:165–171.

Woods R, McClean S, Nicol S, et al. 1996a. Chemical restraint of southern elephant seals, (*Mirounga leonina*); use of metomidine, ketamine and atipamazole and comparison with other cyclohexamine-based combinations. *British Veterinary Journal* 152:213–224.

Woods R, McClean S, Nicol S, et al. 1996b. Use of the respiratory stimulant doxapram in southern elephant seals (*Mirounga leonina*). *The Veterinary Record* 138:514–517.

Shaughnessy PD. 1991. Immobilization of crabeater seals *Lobodon carcinophagus*, with ketamine and diazepam. *Wildlife Research* 18:165–168.

Lawson JW, Parsons JL, Craig SJ, Eddington JD, Kimmins WC. 1996. Use of electroejaculation to collect semen samples from wild seals. *Journal of the American Veterinary Medical Association* 9(1):1615–1617.

Hurford WE, Hochachka PW, Schneider RC, et al. 1996. Splenic contraction, catecholamine release, and blood volume redistribution during diving in the Weddell seal. *Journal of Applied Physiology* 80(1):298–306.

47 Otariid Seals

Martin Haulena

INTRODUCTION

The chemical immobilization of otariid and other marine mammal species has historically been considered to be of relatively high risk and associated with high mortality (Gage 1993). Recent advances in monitoring and support, improved preanesthetic risk assessment, and the use of newer and safer immobilization agents have, however, greatly increased successful outcomes from anesthetic procedures in these species (Stringer et al. 2012).

The family Otariidae (sea lions and fur seals) within the order Pinnipedia is composed of 14 species. Otariids bear weight on all four flippers, climb, locomote quickly, and are more adept on land than phocid seals. However, their aquatic adaptations are less developed, and they generally do not dive as deep or for as long as phocids. Anatomic and physiologic adaptations for diving (i.e., large venous sinuses and a dive response) are, therefore, not as extreme (Elsner 1999; Pabst et al. 1999). Some of these differences make otariids more difficult to physically or mechanically restrain than phocids of similar mass.

CAPTURE AND PHYSICAL RESTRAINT

Many otariid species are easily trained to follow trainers and voluntarily enter different housing units or transport cages. Training of animals maintained at public display institutions is essential for enrichment, minimizing stress, and facilitating medical procedures. Animals in care for only short periods of time, as in a wildlife rehabilitation center or research facility, require the use of protective equipment by handlers. Depending on size and species, animals can be safely moved with herding boards, chutes, and mobile fencing. They can be herded into cages or transport containers for longer travel. Depending on the local topography, moving healthy adult otariids is very challenging and requires well-trained, experienced personnel.

Physical Restraint

Physical restraint is primarily limited by the animal's size and the experience of personnel. Training captive animals for a variety of behaviors minimizes the requirement for physical restraint. Towels, protective gloves, or sedative drugs may facilitate restraint of smaller individuals. Multiple personnel are required to restrain animals ≥20 kg. Mechanically or chemically assisted restraint is strongly recommended for healthy untrained animals ≥90 kg. Larger debilitated animals, such as those encountered at rehabilitation centers, may be restrained using only physical methods. The limitations of physical restraint in otariids include minimal duration of procedures, poor accessibility to various parts of the animal, lack of analgesia, risk of injury to personnel, and undue stress to the animal as a result of prolonged struggling.

Otariids are quick, agile, and strong and will use their large carnivorous teeth in defense. Controlling the head is essential. Sea lions have tremendous power in their forelimb muscles. If they gain a purchase and are able to lift their thorax off the ground, they will easily throw off a person. Care is taken to control the front flippers, raising them slightly and holding them against the side of the animal. This is particularly important in animals ≥20 kg. Animal safety concerns include ensuring airway integrity and that the head is not turned at an awkward angle or held over an edge that may collapse the trachea. Too much weight on the thorax will inhibit ventilation. Musculoskeletal problems arise from excessive restraint on the extremities.

Zoo Animal and Wildlife Immobilization and Anesthesia, Second Edition. Edited by Gary West, Darryl Heard, and Nigel Caulkett.

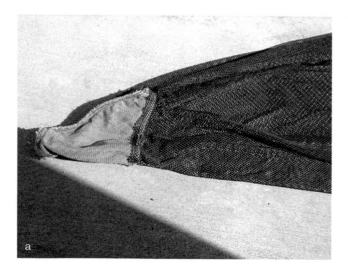 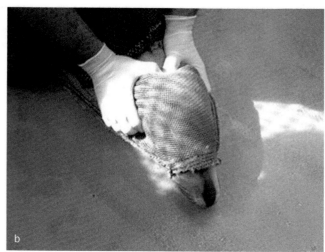

Figure 47.1.   (a and b) Nets with reinforced, small conical openings are useful for restraining small otariid seals. They can also be used for restraint for inhalant anesthesia induction with a mask. Care must be taken to prevent obstruction of the nares.

Care must be taken to avoid soft tissue injuries, including abrasions and scrapes, if restraint is on a rough substrate.

Mechanically Assisted Restraint

There are several commercially available large carnivore squeeze cages that have been used successfully in a variety of otariid species. Although many designs exist, squeeze cages that entrap the animal's neck in a vise or noose will put pressure on the trachea and should be avoided. The otariid trachea easily collapses due to incomplete tracheal rings. When using squeeze cages, it is important to closely monitor the respiratory excursions and mucous membrane color of the animal. Care is taken to avoid pinching extremities, especially as the cage begins to squeeze. Animals will bite at the bars potentially resulting in tooth fracture. The cage bars may be padded to avoid soft tissue injury and minimize dental injuries. Animals maintained in zoos or aquaria can be trained to enter a cage and be lightly squeezed for sample collection (e.g., for venipuncture). Some animals have been trained to accept delivery of an anesthetic gas through a mask without further restraint. As with physical restraint, sedative agents may decrease the degree of struggling and facilitate restraint.

Nets

There are a variety of commercially available nets custom-designed for use in otariids. Nets aid in capturing animals, can be used for restraint, and allow the administration of chemical immobilization drugs. Well-designed nets are somewhat tubular to keep the pectoral limbs against the side and prevent the animal from lifting itself up. Nets should be wide enough to easily capture the animal, but taper to a point so the head can be easily controlled. In the field, care must be

taken to monitor an animal in a net for hyperthermia and exhaustion after capture. Animals have overheated in tightly fitting nets left in the sun while other animals were being sampled or processed. Some nets have small openings at the tip that allow exposure of the nares and rostrum but are tight enough to prevent the animal from biting personnel (Fig. 47.1a,b). These openings aid in masking an animal with an inhalant anesthetic after capture.

Although most methods of mechanical restraint enhance safety for personnel, training and experience are required to ensure adequate and safe restraint. Most mechanical devices, including nets, limit access to the animal for some procedures.

VASCULAR ACCESS

Vascular access for placement of catheters for fluid and emergency drug administration is difficult in small animals, hypothermic individuals, or otariids anesthetized with certain drugs (e.g., alpha-2 agonists). Some species have readily accessible interdigital veins in the pelvic limbs. However, these are not accessible in some species (e.g., California sea lion). Other accessible veins for catheterization include the cephalic, jugular, subclavian, and vessels running along the digits of the hind flipper. Ultrasound-guided placement is recommended if available. An indwelling catheter was maintained by the author for 4 days in a juvenile California sea lion using the common jugular vein. Arterial access has also been achieved through a variety of vessels including the median artery.

ENDOTRACHEAL INTUBATION

Endotracheal intubation is strongly recommended for any prolonged procedure that requires a surgical plane of anesthesia (Sedgwick 1999; Work et al. 1993). Otariid intubation is easier than in phocids, resembling intubation of terrestrial carnivores. In general, endotracheal tubes are of similar diameter to those that would be used on terrestrial carnivores of the equivalent mass. Care is taken to ensure that endotracheal tubes do not extend past the prethoracic bifurcation of the trachea resulting in unilateral lung intubation (McGrath et al. 1981). The mouth is opened with soft nylon straps or rope. The head and neck are held straight and in a slightly hyperextended (opisthotonic) position. Ensure table edges or other equipment does not compress the trachea and interfere with passage of the endotracheal tube (Lynch et al. 1999). Gentle manipulation is used to prevent trauma to the larynx. Standard laryngoscopes facilitate visualization of the airway (Haulena et al. 2000; Heard & Beusse 1993). Very large adults can be intubated by manual palpation of the epiglottis (Heath et al. 1996). Cuffed endotracheal tubes are used to prevent aspiration. It is important not to cause tracheal injury by overinflating the cuff. Endotracheal tubes can be secured over the maxilla or mandibles using rolled gauze, rope, or tape passed caudal to the canine teeth.

PREANESTHETIC CONSIDERATIONS

Preanesthetic assessment is important for selection of the optimal method of immobilization and to decrease the incidence of adverse side effects. It is often very difficult to obtain a complete medical history for an individual animal, particularly for free-living animals or those undergoing rehabilitation. A medical history for zoo and aquarium animals may be available. However, even for these animals, the purpose of the immobilization procedure may be to gather information and samples to diagnose an unknown condition. A recent study (Stringer et al. 2012) confirmed that health status is an excellent predictor of a successful immobilization. It is important, therefore, to try to select animals that are in good body condition and of known health status for elective procedures or for field studies. In addition, it is important to have some knowledge of the common medical conditions that affect both captive and free-living animals to facilitate preprocedure planning.

Some problems are specific to species, sex, age, season, or geographic location. For example, most stranded animals entering a rehabilitation program are dehydrated, malnourished, and may have infectious disease conditions that should be stabilized prior to an anesthetic procedure. Particular attention to these potential problems will lead to better intraprocedure physiologic support. Free-living animals, particularly juveniles, may have high parasite loads. Parasitic pneumonia caused by *Parafilaroides decorus* in species such as the California sea lion (*Zalophus californianus*) (Gage

et al. 1993) may exacerbate ventilation problems encountered during an anesthetic procedure. Young animals such as northern fur seals (*Callorhinus ursinus*) may be affected by hookworm (*Uncinaria* spp.) which can cause anemia (Lyons et al. 2000). These animals are prone to hypoxemia and vascular compromise. Dehydrated juvenile and subadult California sea lions stranding during the late summer and early fall are often affected by leptospirosis, which may cause renal failure (Gulland et al. 1996). Poor renal function can significantly alter the excretion of some parenteral anesthetics. Animals with clinical leptospirosis are poor anesthetic candidates. Animals housed in zoos and aquaria may live longer than free-living animals and may be prone to developing progressive organ failure similar to domestic species.

Atropine (0.02 mg/kg IM) has been recommended 10 minutes prior to immobilization to prevent bradycardia associated with the dive reflex in anesthetized otariids (Gage 1993; Heath et al. 1996). Atropine has also been administered after injection of sedatives to control airway and oral secretion and prevent bradycardia (Spelman 2004). However, alpha-2 agonists such as medetomidine will cause bradycardia. Use of atropine with medetomidine is contraindicated in terrestrial mammals (Cullen 1996). There is currently a debate over the use of atropine in otariids, especially those anesthetized with alpha-2 agonists, with some studies indicating that the use of atropine is associated with increased mortality (Stringer et al. 2012).

INDUCTION/MAINTENANCE PROTOCOLS

Intravenous sites for injection of immobilizing agents are poorly accessible in many otariid species. This is particularly true for difficult to restrain animals and under field conditions (Work et al. 1993). Most anesthetic drugs evaluated for use have, therefore, been limited to those that can be administered IM (Bester 1988; Heard & Beusse 1993; Heath et al. 1996; Loughlin & Spraker 1989; Melin et al. 2013) and inhalant anesthetics (Heath et al. 1997; Work et al. 1993; Yamaya et al. 2006).

Intramuscular drugs are injected into the large muscle masses overlying the lower lumbar spine (Bester 1988; Loughlin & Spraker 1989), tibia, and hips (Haulena et al. 2000; Heard & Beusse 1993; Loughlin & Spraker 1989; Sepulveda et al. 1994) as well as the shoulders (Loughlin & Spraker 1989). Immobilizing IM agents have been hand injected or delivered by dart. Physical or mechanical restraint may facilitate accurate hand injection of anesthetic agents.

Inhalation anesthetics (e.g., isoflurane) appear to be the safest method for anesthetizing otariids because of the ability to titrate the level of drug to effect. The main limitation is the availability and portability of equipment to safely and reliably deliver the anesthetic in the field. In addition, delivery of a gas for a sufficient period of time to induce anesthesia may be difficult in a fractious, unrestrained animal. Most public display facilities, rehabilitation centers, and research facilities are equipped for delivery of inhalant anesthetics. A recent publication describes the use of an induction chamber for delivery of inhalant anesthesia to sea lions (Yamaya et al. 2006). The development of safe, portable gas anesthesia machines for field work has greatly increased the use of gas anesthesia in free-living species. A comprehensive animal training program, adequate physical or mechanical restraint, or the use of chemical sedative and immobilizing agents (Haulena & Gulland 2001; Haulena et al. 2000; Heard & Beusse 1993; Heath et al. 1996) facilitates the use of inhalation anesthesia.

Although chemical immobilization is the safest method of restraint for personnel and allows complete access to the entire animal, there is some risk to the animal being anesthetized. This risk is minimized by adequate preparation and preanesthetic evaluation of the patient, use of experienced anesthetists, use of safe and efficacious immobilization agents, careful monitoring, and physiologic support of the animal.

Sedation

The use of a variety of IM sedative drugs may facilitate physical or mechanical restraint and aid induction with other drugs (e.g., isoflurane) (Gales 1989). Diazepam (0.1–0.2 mg/kg PO) prior to transport aids physical restraint of some animals. More reliable sedation is achieved with midazolam in California sea lions (0.15–0.2 mg/kg IM) and fur seals (0.25–0.35 mg/kg IM) (Lynch et al. 1999). Benzodiazepines can be reversed with flumazenil (Karesh et al. 1997). Butorphanol (0.05–0.2 mg/kg IM) has been used for mild sedation and analgesia. Combination of midazolam and butorphanol results in an increased level of sedation. Medetomidine (70 μg/kg IM) is recommended for sedation of sea lions for electroencephalography because of its apparent lack of interference with brain wave patterns in contrast to a combination of medetomidine and butorphanol (0.1–0.2 mg/kg IM) (Dennison et al. 2008). Although sedation was variable, placement of multiple percutaneous leads for recordings was accomplished for greater than 30 minutes.

Chemical Immobilization

Drugs commonly used to immobilize otariids are discussed in the following section. Table 47.1 summarizes drug dosages from recent studies. Several reviews have been written and should be referred to for a complete list of pinniped immobilization methods (Gales 1989; Haulena & Heath 2001; Lynch et al. 1999; Williams et al. 1990).

Zolazepam/Tiletamine The advantages of this combination include small injection volume, low cost, and

Table 47.1. Blood gas variables from the caudal gluteal vein in 10 physically restrained California sea lions (*Zalophus californianus*)

Variable	Mean ± SD	Range
Na	149 ± 3	146–152
K	4.3 ± 0.5	3.6–5.3
TCO_2	23 ± 5	17–29
iCa (mmol/L)	1.20 ± 0.07	1.07–1.31
Hct (%)	45 ± 5	37–51
Hb (g/dL)	16 ± 2	13–17
pH	7.31 ± 0.05	7.22–7.38
PCO_2 (mmHg)	43.9 ± 4.9	38.4–53.8
PO_2 (mmHg)	74 ± 21	45–103
HCO_3 (mmol/L)	22 ± 4	16–27
BE	−4 ± 5	−11–2
SO_2 (%)	91 ± 7	77–97

dependable deep sedation and immobilization. However, some studies report significant mortality, prolonged recovery, and a narrow margin of safety (Dabin et al. 2002; Heath et al. 1996). Zolazepam/tiletamine (1.7 mg/kg IM) in California sea lions is administered 10 minutes after atropine (0.02 mg/kg IM) (Gage 1993). A slightly lower dosage (0.9–1.3 mg/kg IM) is recommended in subantarctic fur seals (*Arctocephalus tropicalis*). Additional "top-up" doses to increase anesthetic depth have been associated with increased mortality (Heath et al. 1996). However, additional ketamine has been used successfully without mortality (Karesh et al. 1997). The combination is partially reversed with flumazenil (Karesh et al. 1997).

Medetomidine/Ketamine In California sea lions, the combination of medetomidine (140 μg/kg IM) and ketamine (2.5 mg/kg IM) provides effective and safe immobilization that is reversed by atipamezole (0.2 mg/kg IM). Animals were premedicated with atropine (0.02 mg/kg IM). Disadvantages of this combination in sea lions include moderately variable anesthetic depth, large injection volume when commercially available products are used, and high cost (Haulena et al. 2000).

Medetomidine/Zolazepam/Tiletamine The combination of medetomidine (70 μg/kg IM) and zolazepam/tiletamine (1 mg/kg IM) produced reversible (atipamezole 0.2 mg/kg IM), reliable anesthesia (Haulena & Gulland 2001). Injection volume and cost were much less than for medetomidine/ketamine. Adverse effects observed during recovery included tremors, ataxia, and disorientation. These were less than with zolazepam/tiletamine alone, but occur more often than with medetomidine/ketamine. Animals were premedicated with atropine (0.02 mg/kg IM). One mortality did occur in the study. Consequently, a lower medetomidine dosage (40 μg/kg) in combination with zolazepam/tiletamine is recommended.

Medetomidine/Butorphanol/Midazolam A combination of medetomidine (10–13 μg/kg), midazolam (0.2–0.26 mg/kg), and butorphanol (0.2–0.4 mg/kg) IM was evaluated in California sea lions (Spelman 2004) maintained at a zoo. The combination is completely reversible using atipamezole (0.05–0.06 mg/kg IM), flumazenil (0.0002–0.002 mg/kg IM), and naltrexone (0.1 mg/kg IM), respectively. The combination produced safe, light anesthesia in animals that was supplemented with isoflurane for deeper planes of anesthesia. Atropine (0.02 mg/kg IM) was given immediately after injection of the immobilizing agents. This combination was further evaluated in free-ranging adult male California sea lions at a dosage of 0.03 mg/kg medetomidine, 0.15 mg/kg midazolam, and 0.1 mg/kg butorphanol, where it was found to have much superior immobilization characteristics in comparison with medetomidine/zolazepam/tiletamine and with medetomidine/midazolam (Melin et al. 2013).

Inhalant Anesthetics Inhalant anesthetics including isoflurane (Gales & Mattlin 1998; Haulena et al. 2000; Heard & Beusse 1993; Heath et al. 1996, 1997), sevoflurane, and halothane (Work et al. 1993) have all been used in otariids. The safest anesthesia with the best recovery characteristics has been obtained with isoflurane and sevoflurane. Otariids uptake anesthetic gases very rapidly and efficiently and are readily induced with a mask. Controlled studies on the efficacy of mask induction and maintenance of anesthesia with an inhalant are few for marine mammals. However, California sea lions, New Zealand fur seal (*Arctocephalus forsteri*) bulls, and adult female New Zealand sea lions (*Phocarctos hookeri*) appear to be more rapidly masked to anesthetic depths in comparison with terrestrial species (Gales & Mattlin 1998; Heath et al. 1997). The use of inhalant anesthetic agents alone appears to be a reliable and safe method of anesthesia in otariids if it is possible to accomplish restraint and masking (Fig. 47.2). Premedication and induction with intramuscular drugs facilitate masking and maintenance of anesthesia with an inhalant agent if the animals cannot be masked voluntarily or with physical restraint (Haulena & Gulland 2001; Haulena et al. 2000; Heard & Beusse 1993; Heath et al. 1996). Once anesthesia has been attained, reversible induction agents may be antagonized.

Immobilization Location

As with phocid seals, otariid immobilization success is greatly enhanced by good planning, proper equipment, experienced staff, and a well-prepared space. The ability to safely handle, restrain, and deliver anesthetic agents to the animal is essential. A surgery or procedure area that includes an accessible immobilization and recovery pen for monitoring or emergencies is recommended. The ability to control temperature, noise, and light will

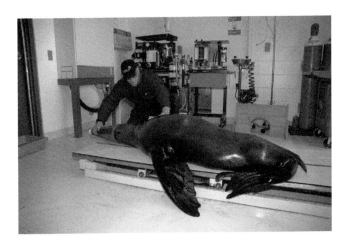

Figure 47.2. Training a Steller sea lion (*Eumetopias jubatus*) for voluntary acceptance of a mask for induction with isoflurane at the Vancouver Aquarium (photo courtesy of the University of British Columbia Marine Mammal Research Unit).

help induction and physiologic support of the patient. Immobilization of larger animals may require procedures be carried out in the animal's pen due to space and transport limitations. Adequate preprocedure planning and availability of emergency equipment are essential for a safe procedure.

MONITORING

An anesthetic plan is developed based on available history, knowledge of the species, and any available laboratory data. Monitoring physiologic variables (especially cardiopulmonary) should begin as soon as possible after induction and throughout the procedure. Most commonly used monitors can be adapted for use in the otariid (Chapter 3). Variables that are commonly measured include heart and respiratory rates, capillary perfusion, response to painful stimuli, body temperature, hemoglobin saturation (relative SpO_2), end-tidal carbon dioxide ($EtCO_2$), blood pressure, and blood gas levels. For otariids, the trends in the measured variables are more important than the point measurements.

Heart rate is one of the most important variables to monitor. It is determined by either palpation or observation of thoracic wall movement over the heart, just caudal to the axilla. Chest auscultation can be used, but thoracic noise is muffled compared with terrestrial mammals (Lynch et al. 1999). Heart rate can also be determined using electrocardiogram (ECG) leads placed externally (Heard & Beusse 1993) or attached within an esophageal probe (Haulena & Heath 2001). Pulse oximeters also generate a pulse wave that can be used to calculate heart rate. However, the pulse wave does not reflect adequacy of tissue perfusion (Chapter 3). The pulse oximeter probes can be clipped to the tongue

(Haulena et al. 2000; Heard & Beusse 1993; Heath et al. 1996, 1997), but the clips tend to slip off the short, thick tongue. Probes are placed on the nasal septum of larger animals. Reflectance probes can be placed rectally, vaginally, or along the buccal or gingival mucosa (Heath et al. 1996). Sudden or progressive bradycardia may be an early indication of initiation of the dive reflex. Some drugs, particularly the alpha-2 agonists, also cause bradycardia.

Respiratory rate is measured by observing thoracic movement, opening of the nares, or by chest auscultation. Capnography and respiratory monitors can be used to electronically calculate respiratory rate. Apnea is common in anesthetized otariids (Sedgwick 1999) and may be due to excessive anesthetic, the immobilizing drug used, or the dive reflex.

Anesthetic depth is assessed using response to various stimuli such as noise and deep pain (interdigital web pinch, ear pinch, and surgical stimulation), presence or absence of the palpebral and pupillary reflexes, respiratory rate rhythm, tidal volume, and jaw tone (Heath et al. 1996, 1997; Work et al. 1993).

Peripheral body temperature measurement does not accurately reflect core because of the thick layers of insulating blubber. Flexible temperature probes are inserted at least 10 cm into the rectum of the animal (Bester 1988; Ferreira & Bester 1999; Loughlin & Spraker 1989). Alternatively, esophageal probes inserted to the level of the heart (Heath et al. 1997) may give accurate core temperature readings.

Body temperature fluctuations resulting in either hypo- or hyperthermia can occur in anesthetized otariids. It is particularly important to monitor temperature in field conditions where control of the environment is more difficult. Temperature changes are influenced by the drugs used, species, size, geographic location, and physiologic status of the animal. For example, larger animals have a greater tendency to hyperthermia than smaller animals (Work et al. 1993). Some drugs (e.g., ketamine) may cause hyperthermia (Sepulveda et al. 1994), while others (e.g., isoflurane) cause vasodilation that promotes hypothermia (Loughlin & Spraker 1989; Work et al. 1993). Profound hyperthermia was seen in a late-term pregnant California sea lion that was anesthetized using medetomidine and ketamine. Shelter from rain, wind, and sun, while maintaining adequate ventilation, is recommended to prevent temperature irregularities. A variety of commercially available heating blankets, heated surgical tables, hot water bottles, wraps, and insulating pads can be used to prevent hypothermia (Heath et al. 1997; Sepulveda et al. 1994; Work et al. 1993). Ice or cold water applied to extremities is used to treat hyperthermia.

Mucosal membranes (oral, rectal, and vaginal) are used for monitoring color and capillary refill time as indicators of perfusion and oxygenation (Heath et al. 1997; Work et al. 1993). Capnometer probes are attached to the endotracheal tube via filter line (Haulena & Gulland 2001; Heard & Beusse 1993). Elevations or sudden decreases in $EtCO_2$ levels may indicate ventilation and perfusion problems.

Noninvasive, oscillometric blood pressure monitoring is performed by attaching cuffs to the proximal portion of the limbs or to the base of the tail. Venous blood gas samples are collected from the caudal gluteal, interdigital, or common jugular veins. Blood gas values obtained from 10 healthy California sea lions under physical restraint (Table 47.1) indicate that arterial blood is sometimes obtained from the area of the caudal gluteal vein (Haulena et al. 2001). Direct blood pressure and arterial blood gases have been collected from a variety of sites including the median artery.

Low SpO_2 values (<85%) have been reported in sea lions immobilized with zolazepam/tiletamine (Heath et al. 1996) and with medetomidine/ketamine (Haulena et al. 2000). This effect is greater in animals not intubated and provided with supplemental oxygen. Conversely, sea lion pups maintained with isoflurane in oxygen maintained higher SpO_2 values (Heath et al. 1997). This may be due to the drugs used, anesthetic depth, or to the animal's physiology. Low SpO_2 levels indicate that the anesthetist should be prepared to intubate, provide oxygen therapy, and assist ventilation.

High $EtCO_2$ (>70 mmHg) levels (Haulena & Gulland 2001; Heard & Beusse 1993) associated with acidemia (pH < 7.15) in anesthetized California sea lions support the need for assisted mechanical ventilation in some animals (Haulena et al. 2001). Some drugs are more commonly associated with hypoventilation and hypercapnia. Animals anesthetized for prolonged periods, maintained at deep anesthetic planes, and positioned in a manner that interferes with normal thoracic expansion are particularly prone to developing hypercapnia. Conversely, hyperventilation of California sea lions has resulted in alkalemia (pH > 7.5).

In anesthetized otariids, mechanical ventilation is recommended at a starting tidal volume of 15 mL/kg and a rate of 8–10 breaths/min (Haulena et al. 2001). Capnometry is essential with mechanically assisted ventilation to adjust tidal volume and rate to maintain normocapnia. Blood gas monitoring is recommended to prevent alkalosis. Venous blood gas values for California sea lions are listed in Table 47.2.

FIELD IMMOBILIZATION (WILD CAPTURE)

Many of the physical and mechanical restraint methods described earlier can be modified for use in field conditions. Immobilization of animals in the field presents significant challenges. However, portable gas anesthesia machines, battery-operated monitoring equipment, and emergency equipment are all available (Gales & Mattlin 1998). If injectable chemical immobilization is required prior to adequate physical or mechanical

Table 47.2. Parenteral and inhalant anesthetic drug dosages in otariids

Species	N	Drug(s)	Dosage	Route	Mortality	Comments	Reference
Arctocephalus australis South American fur seal	32	Tiletamine/zolazepam	1.43 mg/kg	IM dart	0%	Partial reversal with flumazenil	Karesh et al. (1997)
A. australis South American fur seal	4	Tiletamine/zolazepam, ketamine	1.43 mg/kg 0.81 mg/kg	IM	0%	Supplemental ketamine given due to insufficient sedation—partial reversal with flumazenil	Karesh et al. (1997)
A. australis South American fur seal	8	Tiletamine/zolazepam, ketamine	1.15 mg/kg 0.27 mg/kg	IM dart	0%	All administered together—partial reversal with flumazenil	Karesh et al. (1997)
A. australis South American fur seal	1	Ketamine/midazolam	1 mg/kg 0.1 mg/kg	IM dart	0%		Karesh et al. (1997)
Arctocephalus australis forsteri New Zealand fur seal	5	Isoflurane	1.2–4.0%	IH	0%		Gales and Mattlin (1998)
A. australis forsteri New Zealand fur seal	22	Midazolam	0.3–0.7 mg/kg	IM dart	0%	Light sedation and increased wariness on recapture	McKenzie et al. (2012)
A. australis forsteri New Zealand fur seal	120	Tiletamine/zolazepam	0.9–2.4 mg/kg	IM dart	na	Eighty-seven percent of darted animals were successfully captured. Ten of 16 of the animals that escaped were verified to have survived.	McKenzie et al. (2012)
Arctocephalus gazella Antarctic fur seal	172	Tiletamine/zolazepam	1.2–1.7 mg/kg	IM dart	3%	Respiratory depression	Boyd et al. (1990)
A. gazella Antarctic fur seal	30	Ketamine	6.9 ± 0.1 mg/kg	IM dart	0%	Muscle tremors	Boyd et al. (1990)
A. gazella Antarctic fur seal	23	Ketamine/diazepam		IM dart	4%		Boyd et al. (1990)
A. gazella Antarctic fur seal	45	Ketamine/xylazine	7.3 ± 0.3 mg/kg 0.6 ± 0.02 mg/kg	IM dart	7%		Boyd et al. (1990)
A. gazella Antarctic fur seal	14	Ketamine/xylazine	3.8–10.8 mg/kg 0.7–2.0 mg/kg	IM	14%	Poor sedation with ketamine ≤ 5.6 mg/kg	Bester (1988)
A. gazella Antarctic fur seal	7	Ketamine/xylazine	5.6–7.8 mg/kg 0.5–1.3 mg/kg	IM dart	0%		Ferreira and Bester (1999)
Arctocephalus phillipi Juan Fernández fur seal	12	Ketamine/diazepam	2.16–6.76 mg/kg 0.04–0.28 mg/kg	IM	17%	Decreased induction and recovery times than when used IV—variable plane of anesthesia	Sepulveda et al. (1994)
A. phillipi Juan Fernández fur seal	10	Ketamine/diazepam	2.16–6.76 mg/kg 0.04–0.28 mg/kg	IV	0%	Deeper immobilization compared with IM	Sepulveda et al. (1994)
Arctocephalus pusillus pusillus South African fur seal	27	Ketamine	4.3–7.8 mg/kg	IM dart	19%	Variable anesthesia	David et al. (1988)
A. pusillus pusillus South African fur seal	7	Ketamine/xylazine	4.2–5.2 mg/kg 0.6–0.9 mg/kg	IM dart	29%	Xylazine dosage estimated	David et al. (1988)

(Continued)

Table 47.2. (Continued)

Species	N	Drug(s)	Dosage	Route	Mortality	Comments	Reference
A. pusillus pusillus South African fur seal	5	Carfentanil/xylazine	6–18 μg/kg na	IM dart IM dart	na	Twenty percent of animals given combination with carfentanil died. Apnea, muscle convulsions, variable plane of anesthesia.	David et al. (1988)
A. pusillus pusillus South African fur seal	7	Carfentanil/xylazine/ azaperone	6–18 μg/kg na na	IM dart IM dart IM dart	na	Twenty percent of animals given combination with carfentanil died. Apnea, muscle convulsions, variable plane of anesthesia.	David et al. (1988)
A. pusillus pusillus South African fur seal	2	Carfentanil/xylazine/ azaperone/ketamine	6–18 μg/kg na na na	IM dart IM dart IM dart IM dart	na	20% of animals given combination with carfentanil died. Apnea, muscle convulsions, variable plane of anesthesia.	David et al. (1988)
A. pusillus pusillus South African fur seal	2	Carfentanil/xylazine/ ketamine	6–18 μg/kg na na	IM dart IM dart IM dart	na	Twenty percent of animals given combination with carfentanil died. Apnea, muscle convulsions, variable plane of anesthesia.	David et al. (1988)
A. pusillus pusillus South African fur seal	15	Xylazine/zaperone	0.57–2.0 mg/kg 0.57–2.0 mg/kg	IM dart IM dart	7%	Sufficient for branding, short immobilization time	David et al. (1988)
A. pusillus pusillus South African fur seal	2	Droperidol	na	IM	50%		David et al. (1988)
Arctocephalus tropicalis Subantarctic fur seal	58	Ketamine	1.9–2.8 mg/kg	IM	0%	Sufficient for tooth extraction, some tremors noted	Dabin et al. (2002)
A. tropicalis Subantarctic fur seal	32	Ketamine/xylazine	3.1–11.4 mg/kg 0.3–1.7 mg/kg	IM dart	13%	Variable anesthesia	Ferreira and Bester (1999)
A. tropicalis Subantarctic fur seal	49	Tiletamine/zolazepam	0.7–1.9 mg/kg	IM	4%	Prolonged recovery. Apnea requiring artificial respiration	Dabin et al. (2002)
Eumetopias jubatus Steller's sea lion	29	Tiletamine/zolazepam	1.8–8.1 mg/kg	IM dart	21%	Best results: 1.8–2.5 mg/kg	Loughlin and Spraker (1989)
E. jubatus Steller's (northern) sea lion	51	Tiletamine/zolazepam, isoflurane	1.6–3.3 mg/kg	IM dart IM dart IH	10%		Heath et al. (1996)
Otaria byronia South American sea lion	13	Tiletamine/zolazepam	2.75 mg/kg	IM	0%	Flumazenil 1 mg for every 20–25 mg of tiletamine and zolazepam for reversal	Karesh et al. (1997)
O. byronia South American sea lion	7	Isoflurane	na	IH	0%		Karesh et al. (1997)

668

Species / Common name	N	Agent(s)	Dose	Route	%	Comments	Reference
Phocarctos hookeri Hooker's (New Zealand) sea lion	29	Isoflurane	0.8–4.0%	IH	0%		Gales and Mattlin (1998)
P. hookeri Hooker's (New Zealand) sea lion	6	Tiletamine/zolazepam, isoflurane	1.6–2.0 mg/kg, 2–3%	IM dart, IH	0%	Adult males up to 330 kg	Geschke and Chilvers (2009)
Zalophus californianus California sea lion	4	Detomidine/ketamine, isoflurane	40–55 μg/kg, 2.0–4.3 mg/kg, 1–5% in oxygen	IM, IM, IH	0%		Heard and Beusse (1993)
Z. californianus California sea lions	60	Tiletamine/zolazepam	1.7 mg/kg	IM	0%	Apnea	Gage (1993)
Z. californianus California sea lion	115	Isoflurane	0.75–3%	IH	0%		Heath et al. (1997)
Z. californianus California sea lion	30	Halothane	0.75–5%	IH	3%		Work et al. (1993)
Z. californianus California sea lion	29	Medetomidine	70 μg/kg	IM	0%	Good sedation for ECG	Dennison et al. (2008)
Z. californianus California sea lion	12	Medetomidine/butorphanol	70 μg/kg, 0.2 mg/kg	IM, IM	0%	Butorphanol resulted in decreased quality of encephalographs due to muscle jerks	Dennison et al. (2008)
Z. californianus California sea lion	35	Medetomidine/ketamine	140 μg/kg, 2.5 mg/kg	IM, IM	0%	Variable anesthesia—reversal with atipamezole	Haulena et al. (2000)
Z. californianus California sea lion	16	Medetomidine/ketamine, isoflurane	140 μg/kg, 2.5 mg/kg, 1–5%	IM, IM, IH	0%	Reversal with atipamezole	Haulena et al. (2000)
Z. californianus California sea lion	17	Medetomidine, tiletamine/zolazepam	70 μg/kg, 1 mg/kg	IM, IM	6%	Reliable anesthesia. Reversal with atipamezole. Ataxia and disorientation during recovery in some animals	Haulena and Gulland (2001)
Z. californianus California sea lion	22	Medetomidine/tiletamine/zolazepam, isoflurane	70 μg/kg, 1 mg/kg, 1–5%	IM, IM, IH	0%	Reliable anesthesia. Reversal with atipamezole. Ataxia and disorientation during recovery in some animals	Haulena and Gulland (2001)
Z. californianus California sea lion	3	Medetomidine/midazolam/butorphanol/	30 μg/kg, 0.15 mg/kg, 0.1 mg/kg	IM, IM, IM	0%	Adult males up to 280 kg	Melin et al. (2013)
Z. californianus California sea lion	2	Medetomidine/midazolam/butorphanol/isoflurane	10–13 μg/kg, 0.2–0.26 mg/kg, 0.2–0.4 mg/kg, 0.5–2.0%	IM, IM, IM, IH	0%	Two animals anesthetized 13 times. Reversal with atipamezole, flumazenil, naltrexone	Spelman (2004)

restraint, it is essential that animals selected for capture are as far as possible from water or other hazards (Fig. 47.3 and Fig. 47.4). It is also important to choose animals that are relatively calm and have the least risk of escaping into the water or to inaccessible areas (Heath et al. 1996). This will help minimize the risk of drowning or falling from large heights.

Young animals such as pups can be herded on suitable haul-out sites into temporary pens where individual animals can then be isolated for further handling (Merrick et al. 1995). For procedures requiring immobilization, the use of portable anesthetic machines for delivery of inhalant anesthesia is preferred (Heath et al. 1997).

Large adult animals have been trapped on artificial haul outs and then funneled through chutes and into squeeze cages to facilitate sample collection and handling (Melin et al. 2013). These animals can then be

masked with inhalant anesthetics for more invasive sampling procedures.

Recently, a method of capturing free-ranging Steller sea lions (*Eumetopias jubatus*) in the water was developed using a team of divers, baited nooses attached to floats, and a surface capture team in boats (Raum-Suryan et al. 2004). This capture method requires a tremendous amount of training and planning and should only be carried out by highly experienced staff.

Delivery of immobilizing agents by dart has been used in animals undergoing rehabilitation (Haulena et al. 2000) as well as in the field (Geschke & Chilvers 2009; Heath et al. 1996; McKenzie et al. 2012). In free-living animals, delivery by dart poses some risk to animals that may escape to the water or to an inaccessible area as the anesthetic drug begins to take affect prior to complete immobilization (Heath et al. 1996). The remotely delivered use of zolazepam-tiletamine has been associated with a high degree of risk in some species such as Steller sea lions (Heath et al. 1996), while other studies report much lower risk in New Zealand fur seals and sea lions (Geschke & Chilvers 2009; McKenzie et al. 2012). Some authors report a decrease in the reliability of anesthesia when darts are employed in comparison with hand injection (Haulena et al. 2000).

More recently, the reversible combination of medetomidine, midazolam, and butorphanol (Melin et al. 2013; Spelman 2004) has been evaluated for remotely delivered use in adult female Steller sea lions (Haulena et al. 2011) (Fig. 47.2 and Fig. 47.3). Medetomidine (0.04–0.06 mg/kg), midazolam (0.20–0.22 mg/kg), and butorphanol (0.13–0.15 mg/kg) reliably and safely immobilized animals for sampling and attachment of telemetry instruments (Fig. 47.5 and Fig. 47.6a,b). The sea lions were maintained with isoflurane and reversed with atipamezole (0.25 mg/kg IM) and naltrexone (0.15 mg/kg IM). Animals that went

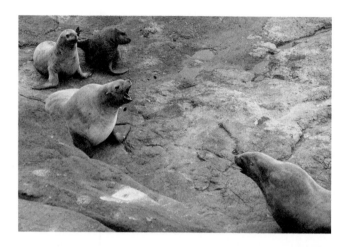

Figure 47.3. Adult female Steller sea lion reacting to nearby sea lion immediately after darting. Note darkened stabilizer. This activity was conducted pursuant to MMPA/ESA Permit No. 14326.

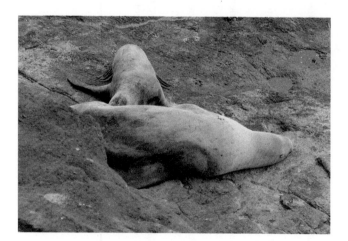

Figure 47.4. Adult female Steller sea lion settling down after darting while pup resumes nursing. This activity was conducted pursuant to MMPA/ESA Permit No. 14326.

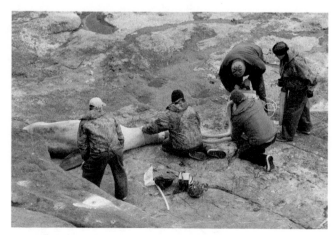

Figure 47.5. Approach to immobilized adult female Steller sea lion with portable isoflurane field machine after darting. This activity was conducted pursuant to MMPA/ESA Permit No. 14326.

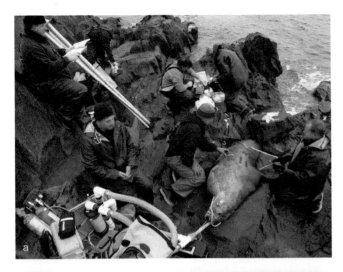

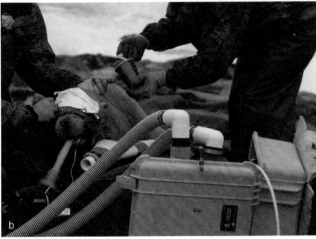

Figure 47.6. (a and b) Attachment of instruments to and biological sampling of darted adult female Steller sea lions maintained on gas anesthetic. This activity was conducted pursuant to MMPA/ESA Permit No. 14326.

into the water after darting were either darted with the reversal agents, and observed fully recovered, or monitored until they spontaneously recovered. No mortalities occurred. Advantages included a smooth induction and full recovery prior to entering the water after the procedure.

It is apparent that careful selection of individuals is very important for successful darting. Animals should be very calm and preferably sleeping. Steller sea lions darted in an undisturbed group appear to be less likely to move and enter the water after they are darted. Animals that spot darting team members after being darted are more likely to move and enter the water. Animals react more to brightly colored dart stabilizers and darkening the stabilizers with a black permanent marker is recommended. Animals also react more to darts that remain embedded, and nonbarbed and non-collared needles should be used that allow the dart to fall out as soon as possible after delivery.

ANALGESIA

There are very few studies evaluating the use of analgesics in otariids. Use and dosage of analgesic agents have been based on extrapolation from other species and personal experience. Analgesics that have been used with good clinical response in otariids include opiates, nonsteroidal anti-inflammatory drugs (NSAIDs), and alpha-2 agonists. The most commonly used opioid is butorphanol (0.05–0.2 mg/kg PO, IM, or IV q 6 h). Buprenorphine (0.01 mg/kg SC, IM, or IV BID) has been used as well as tramadol (0.5–2.0 mg/kg PO BID). NSAIDs used by the author include flunixin megulmine (1 mg/kg IM q 24 h) for up to 3 days, ketoprofen (1 mg/kg IM q 24 h) for up to 5 days, buffered acetylsalicylic acid (5 mg/kg PO q 24 h) for up to 5 days, carprofen (2–4 mg/kg PO q 24 h) for up to 14 days (Dold et al. 2004), meloxicam (0.1–0.2 mg/kg PO, SC, or IM SID), and piroxicam (0.2–0.3 mg/kg PO SID). For additional analgesia, butorphanol has been combined with an NSAID. Medetomidine (10–40 µg/kg) has also been used to provide analgesia.

ACKNOWLEDGMENTS

Sincere thanks go to the staff and volunteers of The Marine Mammal Center, the Vancouver Aquarium, the North Pacific Universities Marine Mammal Research Consortium, the National Marine Mammal Laboratory, and the University of British Columbia Marine Mammal Research Unit. Funding for research involving mechanically assisted ventilation was provided by the California Oiled Wildlife Care Network. Special thanks go to Dr. David Huff for his thoughtful review.

REFERENCES

Bester MN. 1988. Chemical restraint of Antarctic fur seals and southern elephant seals. *South African Journal of Wildlife Research* 18:57–60.

Boyd IL, Lunn NJ, Duck CD, Barton T. 1990. Response of Antarctic fur seals to immobilization with ketamine, a ketamine-diazepam or ketamine-xylazine mixture, and Zoletil. *Marine Mammal Science* 6:135–145.

Cullen LK. 1996. Medetomidine sedation in dogs and cats: a review of its pharmacology, antagonism and dose. *The British Veterinary Journal* 152:519–535.

Dabin W, Beauplet G, Guinet C. 2002. Response of wild subantarctic fur seal (*Arctocephalus tropicalis*) females to ketamine and tiletamine-zolazepam anesthesia. *Journal of Wildlife Diseases* 38:846–850.

David JHM, Hofmeyr JM, Best PB, Meyer MA, Shaughnessy PD. 1988. Chemical immobilization of free-ranging South African (Cape) fur seals. *South African Journal of Wildlife Research* 18: 154–156.

Dennison S, Haulena M, Gulland F, Greig D, Williams DC. 2008. Comparison of the use of medetomidine and medetomidine-butorphanol to facilitate electroencephalography in California sea lions (*Zalophus californianus*). Proceedings of the International Association for Aquatic Animal Medicine, pp. 275–276.

Dold C, Haulena M, Gulland FMD. 2004. Pharmacokinetics of oral carprofen in the California sea lion (*Zalophus californianus*).

Proceedings of the American Association of Zoo Veterinarians Annual Meeting, pp. 343–345.

Elsner R. 1999. Living in water: solutions to physiological problems. In: *Biology of Marine Mammals* (JE Reynolds III, SA Rommel, eds.), pp. 73–116. Washington, DC: Smithsonian Institution Press.

Ferreira SM, Bester MN. 1999. Chemical immobilization, physical restraint and stomach lavaging of fur seals at Marion Island. *South African Journal of Wildlife Research* 29:55–61.

Gage LJ. 1993. Pinniped anesthesia. In: *Zoo and Wild Animal Medicine*, 3rd ed. (ME Fowler, ed.), pp. 412–413. Philadelphia: W.B. Saunders Co.

Gage LJ, Gerber JA, Smith DM, Morgan LE. 1993. Rehabilitation and treatment of California sea lions (*Zalophus californianus*) and northern fur seals (*Callorhinus ursinus*) stranded along the central and northern California coast, 1984–1990. *Journal of Zoo and Wildlife Medicine* 24:41–47.

Gales NJ. 1989. Chemical restraint and anesthesia of pinnipeds: a review. *Marine Mammal Science* 5:228–256.

Gales NJ, Mattlin RH. 1998. Fast, safe, field-portable gas anesthesia for otariids. *Marine Mammal Science* 14:355–361.

Geschke K, Chilvers BL. 2009. Managing big boys: a case study on remote anaesthesia and satellite tracking of adult male New Zealand sea lions (*Phocarctos hookeri*). *Wildlife Research* 36: 666–674.

Gulland FMD, Koski M, Lowenstine LJ, Colagross A, Morgan L, Spraker T. 1996. Leptospirosis in California sea lions (*Zalophus californianus*) stranded along the central California coast, 1981–1994. *Journal of Wildlife Diseases* 32:572–580.

Haulena M, Gulland FMD. 2001. Use of medetomidine-zolazepam-tiletamine in California sea lions, with and without isoflurane, and reversal using atipamezole. *Journal of Wildlife Diseases* 37:566–573.

Haulena M, Heath RB. 2001. Marine mammal anesthesia. In: *CRC Handbook of Marine Mammal Medicine* (LA Dierauf, FMD Gulland, eds.), pp. 655–688. Boca Raton: CRC Press.

Haulena M, Gulland FMD, Calkins DG, Spraker TR. 2000. Immobilization of California sea lions using medetomidine plus ketamine with and without isoflurane and reversal with atipamezole. *Journal of Wildlife Diseases* 36:124–130.

Haulena M, Heath RB, Gulland F. 2001. Assisted mechanical ventilation and its affect on end-tidal carbon dioxide levels in anesthetized California sea lions. Proceedings of the American Association of Zoo Veterinarians Annual Meeting, pp. 107–108.

Haulena M, Beckmen K, Fadely BS, Lander ME, McAllister D, Melin SR, Rea L, Rehberg MJ, Snedgen G, Van Bonn W, Gelatt T. 2011. Remotely-delivered chemical immobilization of adult female Steller sea lions (*Eumetopias jubatus*) for physiological sampling and satellite telemetry attachment. Proceedings of the International Association for Aquatic Animal Medicine, p. 2011.

Heard DJ, Beusse DO. 1993. Combination detomidine, ketamine, and isoflurane anesthesia in California sea lions (*Zalophus californianus*). *Journal of Zoo and Wildlife Medicine* 24:168–170.

Heath RB, Calkins D, McAllister D, Taylor W, Spraker T. 1996. Telazol and isoflurane field anesthesia in free-ranging Steller's sea lions (*Eumetopias jubatus*). *Journal of Zoo and Wildlife Medicine* 27:35–43.

Heath RB, DeLong R, Jameson V, Bradley D, Spraker T. 1997. Isoflurane anesthesia in free ranging sea lion pups. *Journal of Wildlife Diseases* 33:206–210.

Karesh WB, Cook RA, Stetter M, Uhart MM, Hoogesteijn A, Lewis MN, Campagna C, Mailuf P, Torres A, House C, Thomas L, Braselton WE, Dierenfield ES, McNamara TS, Duignan P, Raverty S, Linn M. 1997. South American pinnipeds: immobilization, telemetry, and health evaluations. Proceedings of the American Association of Zoo Veterinarians Annual Meeting, pp. 291–295.

Loughlin TR, Spraker T. 1989. Use of Telazol to immobilize female northern sea lions (*Eumetopias jubatus*) in Alaska. *Journal of Wildlife Diseases* 25:353–358.

Lynch MJ, Tahmindjis MA, Gardner H. 1999. Immobilisation of pinniped species. *Australian Veterinary Journal* 77:181–185.

Lyons ET, Spraker TR, Olson KD, Tolliver SC, Bair HD. 2000. Prevalence of hookworms (*Uncinaria lucasi*, Stiles) in northern fur seal (*Callorhinus ursinus*, Linnaeus) pups on St. Paul Island, Alaska, USA: 1986–1999. *Comparative Parasitology* 67:218–223.

McGrath CJ, Feeney D, Crimi AJ, Ruff J. 1981. Upper airway of the California sea lion: an anesthetist's perspective. *Veterinary Medicine, Small Animal Clinician* 76:548–549.

McKenzie J, Page B, Goldsworthy SD, Hindell MA. 2012. Behavioral responses of New Zealand fur seals (*Arctophoca australis forsteri*) to darting and the effectiveness of midazolam and tiletamine-zolazepam for remote chemical immobilization. *Marine Mammal Science* 29:241–260.

Melin SR, Haulena M, Van Bonn W, Tennis MJ, Brown RF, Harris JD. 2013. Reversible immobilization of free-ranging adult male California sea lions (*Zalophus californianus*). *Marine Mammal Science* 29:E529–E536. doi: 10.1111/mms.12017.

Merrick RL, Brown R, Calkins DG, Loughlin TR. 1995. A comparison of Steller sea lion, *Eumetopias jubatus*, pup masses between rookeries with increasing and decreasing populations. *Fishery Bulletin* 93:753–758.

Pabst DA, Rommel SA, McLellan WA. 1999. The functional morphology of marine mammals. In: *Biology of Marine Mammals* (JE Reynolds III, SA Rommel, eds.), pp. 15–72. Washington, DC: Smithsonian Institution Press.

Raum-Suryan KI, Rehberg MJ, Pendleton GW, Pitcher KW, Gelatt TS. 2004. Development of dispersal, movement patterns, and haul-out use by pup and juvenile Steller sea lions (*Eumetopias jubatus*) in Alaska. *Marine Mammal Science* 20:823–850.

Sedgwick CJ. 1999. Anesthesia for small to medium sized exotic mammals, birds, and reptiles. In: *Manual of Small Animal Anesthesia* (RR Paddleford, ed.), pp. 318–356. Philadelphia: W.B. Saunders Co.

Sepulveda MS, Ochua-Acuna H, McLaughlin GS. 1994. Immobilization of Juan Fernandez fur seals, *Arctocephalus phillipi*, with ketamine hydrochloride and diazepam. *Journal of Wildlife Diseases* 30:536–540.

Spelman LH. 2004. Reversible anesthesia of captive California sea lions (*Zalophus californianus*) with medetomidine, midazolam, butorphanol, and isoflurane. *Journal of Zoo and Wildlife Medicine* 35:65–69.

Stringer EM, Van Bonn W, Chinnadurai SK, Gulland FMD. 2012. Risk factors associated with perianesthetic mortality of stranded free-ranging California sea lions (*Zalophus californianus*) undergoing rehabilitation. *Journal of Zoo and Wildlife Medicine* 43: 233–239.

Williams TD, Williams AL, Stoskopf MK. 1990. Marine mammal anesthesia. In: *CRC Handbook of Marine Mammal Medicine: Health, Disease, and Rehabilitation* (LA Dierauf, ed.), pp. 175–192. Boca Raton: CRC Press.

Work TM, DeLong RL, Spraker TR, Melin SR. 1993. Halothane anesthesia as a method of immobilizing free-ranging California sea lions (*Zalophus californianus*). *Journal of Zoo and Wildlife Medicine* 24:482–487.

Yamaya Y, Ohba S, Koie H, Watari T, Tokuriki M, Tanaka S. 2006. Isoflurane anesthesia in four sea lions (*Otaria byronia* and *Zalophus californianus*). *Veterinary Anaesthesia and Analgesia* 33: 302–306.

48 Walrus

David B. Brunson

SPECIES-SPECIFIC PHYSIOLOGY

Walruses are one of the most difficult marine animals to anesthetize. The large size, limited vascular access, and propensity for sudden physiological changes during chemical restraint have led to their reputation of high anesthetic risk. High mortality rates have been reported with both opioids and dissociative anesthetics but are most likely due to severe respiratory and circulatory compromise when the animals are anesthetized out of the water. Respiratory arrest is commonly reported during immobilization with potent opioids. Additionally, walruses have died during chemical immobilization; they have developed circulatory failure despite effective ventilatory support.

There are two subspecies of walruses; the Atlantic walrus, *Odobenus rosmarus rosmarus*, and the Pacific walrus, *O. rosmarus divergens*. A third subspecies, the Laptev sea walrus, *O. rosmarus laptevi*, has been proposed but this is not commonly recognized. The walrus is a large and powerful pinniped. The skin is typically a cinnamon-brown color which is covered by short course hair. As the animal ages, the skin becomes lighter. The name rosmarus comes from the reddened color due to cutaneous vasodilatation when warmed by the sun while the animal is out of the water. Walruses have enlarged upper canine teeth commonly referred to as tusks. The Atlantic subspecies, the males measure 300 cm and weigh 1200 kg. Females measure 250 cm and weigh 750 kg. At birth, pups are 140 cm long and weigh 50 kg. The Pacific walrus is slightly larger with males being up to 360-cm long and weighing up to 1600 kg; Pacific walrus females are 260-cm long and weigh approximately 1250 kg. Young Pacific walrus pups measure 140 cm and weigh 60 kg (Garlich-Miller & Stewart 1999).

Problems with chemical immobilization of marine mammals and, in particular, walruses have been associated with elicitation of the dive reflex. Clinical signs during chemical immobilization appear similar to this classic physiological reflex. Since walruses can submerge for extended time periods for foraging at the sea bottom, they are capable of prolonged breath holding. Additionally, the simultaneous occurrence of low heart rates with breath holding has close similarities to the classic "dive reflex." However, the ability to dive for long periods of time is not the same as the adverse reactions seen by marine mammals to anesthetic or immobilization drugs. Unlike the normal diving physiology, apnea and bradycardias during chemical immobilization are associated with high mortality. Normal dive responses are not associated with lasting metabolic derangements or cardiac failure. It appears that during chemical immobilization or general anesthesia, the physiological dive mechanisms do not function normally. A necropsy finding of a captive walrus showed disseminated myocardial fibrosis and atherosclerosis which was attributed as the cause of death. Underlying myocardial disease would increase the risk of anesthesia (Gruber et al. 2002).

The upper airway of walruses is characterized by small nostrils with large muscles to close the openings during submersion. The nasal passages are small and the nasal turbinates are such that the nasal passages lack a large meatus. This adaptation prevents water from passing through the nose into the pharynx and trachea. The oral cavity is large and characterized by a high arched hard palate. The walruses tongue is large and thick. Because the tongue lacks thin edges, standard veterinary pulse oximetry probes are not easily placed on the tongue. The lower jaw moves between the large upper canine teeth (tusks). Even in very large

Zoo Animal and Wildlife Immobilization and Anesthesia, Second Edition. Edited by Gary West, Darryl Heard, and Nigel Caulkett.
© 2014 John Wiley & Sons, Inc. Published 2014 by John Wiley & Sons, Inc.

individuals, the rostral opening to the mouth is no more than 10–12 cm in width and height. Because of the limited size of the opening, smaller walruses are difficult to manually direct an endotracheal tube into the larynx as is done in cattle.

Walruses have a unique pharyngeal pouch that can be inflated to provide buoyancy while resting on the ocean surface. Although this adaptation seems to be more highly developed in wild free-ranging walruses, it may also present a potential problem for airway management in captive raised walruses (Fay 1969). During tracheal intubation, it is important to direct the tube through the larynx and not into the pharyngeal pouch.

PHYSICAL CAPTURE AND RESTRAINT

Physical restraint of untrained wild adult walruses is impractical. Captive walruses can be conditioned to enable physical examination including oral examination and thoracic auscultation. Cargo nets are used for young animals but have limited effectiveness in animals greater than 100–150 kg of body weight.

CHEMICAL RESTRAINT AND ANESTHESIA
Vascular Access
The heavy subcutaneous fat layer and the thickness of walrus skin prevent identification and access to veins in the cervical region or the appendages. Venous access can be obtained through the dorsal extradural intravertebral vein (EIV) and the gluteal vein. Placement of a catheter into the dorsal EIV has been described (Stetter et al. 1997). The epidural IV access can be used for fluid administration, emergency drugs, and for intravenous anesthetic administration.

Needle placement for intravenous access into the epidural venous sinus is identical to placement of epidural needles or catheters via the lumbo-sacral space in other species. Palpate the wings of the ilea on each side of the spinal column and the midline of the walruses back to identify the approximate location of the last lumbar vertebra. In the author's experience, it is easiest to find these landmarks with the animal in sterna recumbency. Even in animals with normal body fat and in healthy condition, these landmarks for needle placement can be found. If an epidural catheter is being used for IV access, a tuohy needle is recommended to assist in directing the catheter cranially into the vein. The needle will be placed on the midline approximately 3–5 cm behind a line transecting the midline from the cranial aspects of each ileum. This should be approximately at the third to fourth lumbar vertebra (L3–L4). The landmarks for the proper access site are the same as those used for epidural anesthesia in the dog or cat. In adult walruses, a 16- or 17-gauge 8.9-cm-long needle is necessary to access the EIV. Advance the needle into the animal at a perpendicular angle to the skin. A

syringe can be placed on the needle and gentle aspiration used to determine entrance into the vein.

Vascular access from the flippers has been described in phocid seals but not walruses. Attempts to obtain blood samples following the landmarks described for seals would be as follows. At the level of the proximal edge of the interdigital webbing of the second and third digits, insert a 37-mm (1 1/1 in) 19-gauge needle at a 10°–20° angle until the blood is aspirated into the syringe. Blood obtained will most often be of mixed arterial and venous origin (Geraci 1978).

An alternative vascular access location is the caudal gluteal vein. A needle is inserted lateral to the sacral vertebra approximately 1/3 of the distance from the femoral trochanter to the base of the tail. In adult walruses, a 12.5-cm-long needle is necessary to reach the vessel. The needle should be held perpendicular to the skin and advanced slowly until blood can be aspirated into a syringe.

Endotracheal Intubation
Intubation of walruses is relatively easy to perform. Intubation is easier if the neck is extended to straighten the oral-laryngeal axis of the head and neck. This is facilitated by positioning the walrus in sternal recumbency. If the animal has large tusks, they can be used to prop up the head and extend the neck. Small ropes or towels placed in the mouth facilitate positioning for intubation. Because of the highly arched hard palate, using a separate rope or towel around each tusk allows better access to the oral cavity than a single one rope passed across the oral cavity. Palpation of the larynx with one hand while directing the endotracheal tube into the trachea with the other hand is recommended. Because of the small size of the oral cavity of even large walruses, it may be difficult to pass a large endotracheal tube while palpating the larynx. In these cases, the use of a small diameter stylet is recommended. The stylet must be at least twice as long as the endotracheal tube. Palpate the larynx as described earlier and pass the stylet through the larynx and into the trachea. The endotracheal tube is then fed over the stylet and into the trachea. Blind intubation is not recommended because of the difficulty in correct placement and the potential for the endotracheal tube to enter the esophagus or pharyngeal pouch.

Tracheal intubation is facilitated by muscle relaxation during immobilization and anesthetic induction. Opioids and dissociative immobilization techniques are frequently associated with extensive muscle rigidity. Small dosages of propofol (40–60 mg) via the EIV will produce muscle relaxation and facilitate endotracheal intubation.

Preanesthetic Concerns
Because of the large size and physical power of walruses, most procedures are performed with the animal

immobilized with drugs or general anesthetics. If the animal is well trained and will allow handling while awake, surgical procedures can be performed using local anesthetics. The thick skin and heavy layer of insulating fat present mechanical challenges for effective regional nerve blocks. However, infiltration of the skin can be performed to provide effective local anesthesia. Both lidocaine HCl and bupivicaine HCl are effective for blocking pain.

Opioid analgesics have been used for capture and immobilization in walruses (DeMaster et al. 1981; Gales 1989; Griffiths et al. 1993; Lynch et al. 1999). As with other marine mammals, analgesia in addition to immobilization is assumed. Of the opioids analgesics, meperidine and butorphanol have been used with benzodiazepines or alpha-2 agonists. Assessment of the analgesic effects of opioids has been limited to the responses observed during immobilization.

Drug Delivery

The walrus, like seals and sea lions, have relatively small pelvic limbs. The pelvis, femur, and tibia are short and the associated muscles are small in relations to the size of the animal. The femur of an adult 1500-kg pacific walrus is approximately ~12–14 in. in length. In addition, the upper pelvic limb is not well demarcated, resulting in injections often occurring at or below the knee joint. The muscles of the hind limbs and pelvis can be used for IM injections but are relatively smaller than the epaxial muscles.

The best sites for intramuscular injections are the large muscles of the back. The epaxial muscles are large and well developed. The areas caudal to the last rib and cranial to the pelvis on both sides of the vertebral column provide a large target area for remote drug injection. The muscles of the front limbs can also be used for IM drug administration. Caution should be used to ensure that injections do not occur into the large cervical blood vessels which are located cranial to the front legs.

During immobilization and anesthesia, injections can be made into the base of the tongue. Sublingual injections have the advantage of rapid absorption due to the high blood flow to the tissue. In emergencies, sublingual injections provide a readily available route for cardiac and respiratory support drugs. Alternatively, emergency drugs can be administered by flushing the drugs into the lungs via the endotracheal tube. A long semirigid piece of plastic tubing can be passed through the ET tube and the medications flushed into the airway. Dilution of the drugs or flushing the tubing with sterile water is recommended to ensure that the entire drug dosage has been administered. Antagonists for immobilization drugs may also be given by these routes when the end of the immobilization has been reached.

MONITORING ANESTHESIA AND SUPPORTIVE CARE

Baseline heart rate and respiratory rates should be taken prior to drug administration. Changes associated with the onset of the effects of immobilization drug can be used to determine the time to approach and to intervene.

Respiratory Function
Apnea is a common sequel to anesthetic or immobilization drugs. Ventilatory support is essential when working with these animals. End tidal gas monitoring is recommended to assess both the efficacy of ventilation and to determine the relative anesthetic concentrations in the animal. Spontaneous ventilation is likely to be inadequate and methods for assisting ventilation should be available. In contrast to the conscious animal's ability to breath hold for long time periods, apnea during immobilization and anesthesia are associated with respiratory and metabolic acidosis, arrhythmias, and poor anesthetic delivery. For this reason, controlled ventilation coupled with expired gas monitoring is important for immobilization or anesthesia. Ventilation rate is essential to monitor during all phases of handling. Adequacy of ventilation is best determined by measurement of end tidal carbon dioxide ($EtCO_2$) or by blood gas measurements. CO_2 can be monitored with battery operated side-stream style monitors with a catheter placed into the animal's airway or from an endotracheal tube in the intubated animal. Blood gases can be measured on blood samples taken from any vessel including the epidural intervertebral sinus.

Monitoring the Cardiovascular System
Captive walruses are usually immobilized with a combination of midazolam (0.1 mg/kg) and meperidine (2.2 mg/kg) (Klein et al. 2002). Atropine (0.04 mg/kg) is also recommended to prevent vagal induced bradycardia. Intramuscular injections into the hip or epaxial muscles are the recommended injections sites. A long needle (3–4 in.) is necessary to ensure effective drug injection into muscle and rapid absorption.

Heart rate during the onset of immobilization and anesthesia is usually between 80 and 100 beats/min. As anesthesia deepens, the heart rate slows to around 60 beats/min. Heart rate can be determined by observation of movement of the animal's chest wall. Once at the animal's side, auscultation of the heart with a stethoscope or use of an electrocardiograph (ECG) to determine the rate and rhythm of the heart is essential to detect early changes in cardiac function. The use of a pulse oximeter has proven difficult because of the lack of places to position the sensing probes. The author has found that a reflectance style pulse oximeter probe placed against the oral mucosa or rectum has worked intermittently.

PHARMACOLOGICAL CONSIDERATIONS

Whether immobilizing a walrus in captivity or in the wild, the attendant problems are similar. The drugs must be administered via intramuscular injection and from a distance. For this reason, drug volumes must be small and choices are restricted to alpha-2 agonists, benzodiazepines, opioids, and dissociative classes of drugs. All of these drug groups have been used successfully; however, mortalities have also been associated with all drug groups. The reversibility of alpha-2 agonists, benzodiazepines, and opioids has made them the preferred drugs.

Meperidine

Based on early studies within marine mammals, meperidine was shown to be an effective sedative and immobilization drug in a variety of species (Joseph & Cornell 1988). Meperidine was administered by hand injection to 10 walruses at a dosage of 0.23 and 0.45 mg/kg. Sedation/restraint was moderate without apparent detrimental effects. If used as an analgesic, meperidine was associated with obvious sedation (Cornell 1978). As a result of clinical experience, a higher dose of meperidine (2.2 mg/kg) is frequently used to immobilize captive walruses when combined with midazolam (0.1 mg/kg). It is recommended, because of the high incidence of bradycardia during sedation, that atropine (0.04 mg/kg) IM, SQ, or IV be included in the immobilization technique (Klein et al. 2002). A long needle (3–4 in.) is necessary for effective drug injection to ensure rapid complete absorption.

Potent Opioids +/– Alpha-2 Agonists

The use of highly potent opioid analgesics for immobilization of walruses has proven to be less than ideal. Complications include apnea, muscle spasms, rigidity, and death. Adult male Atlantic walruses on a land haul out were effectively immobilized with carfentanil with an intramuscular dose of 2.7–3.0 mg. Muscle spasms were associated with the onset of immobilization. All of the animals had extended periods of apnea; tracheal intubation was not possible due to muscle rigidity (Lanthier & Stewart 2002; Lanthier et al. 1999). The estimated effective dosage range was 4–5 µg/kg.

Many factors make accurate drug dosing difficult in field situations, the body weight can only be estimated prior to drug administration, dart placement, and vascularity of the injection site all affect the ultimate success of remote drug delivery. Pacific walruses injected with similar carfentanil dosages were not adequately immobilized despite the presence of apnea and muscle spasms.

A field study was preformed to test combinations of the alpha-2 agonist medetomidine with opioids carfentanil in adult Pacific walruses. Medetomidine was selected because of the presence of an effective antago-

nist (atipamezole) and availability of a concentrated formulation which minimized dart size and injection volume. The addition of medetomidine with carfentanil would likely decrease the opioid dose and improve muscle relaxation (Mulcahy et al. 2003). A medetomidine dose of 30 mg was combined with carfentanil doses that varied from 0.06 to 3.0 mg per animal. At the 0.06-mg carfentanil dose, immobilization was inadequate, while a dose at the 3.0 mg caused severe respiratory and circulatory depression that was judged to be life threatening. Carfentanil doses of 0.15 and 0.3 mg with 30 mg of medetomidine enabled approach and handling, but apnea occurred and immediate reversal of both drugs was administered. Due to the low numbers of animals, it was not possible to further evaluate this combination. It should be noted that the addition of medetomidine did markedly decrease the carfentanil needed for immobilization although respiratory depression was still severe. Dexmedetomidine is now available and is a purified form of medetomidine. The dosage is 1/2 of the medetomidine dose due to the elimination of the "left handed" isomer levomedetomidine. Thus it would be appropriate to use 1/2 of the milligram medetomidine dosage if using dexmedetomidine. Atipamezole is an effective and recommended reversal agent for dexmedetomidine.

Seventeen walruses were immobilized with carfentanil alone with immediate reversal with naltrexone. Carfentanil (2.4- to 2.7-mg total dose) was administered via dart to the muscular area of the rump. Sedation occurred in 7–21 minutes. Muscle twitching of the muzzle was noted with full body tremors lasting a few seconds, leading to muscle rigidity and immobilization (Tuomi et al. 2002). Naltrexone at 175- to 350-mg total dose was administered into the muscular area of the lip as soon as the walrus was safe to approach. Reversal occurred between 10 and 20 minutes after administration. One animal had a rapid reversal in approximately 5 minutes following injection. An additional dose of naltrexone (175–350 mg) was administered to each animal at the completion of the desired work time to ensure complete reversal of the carfentanil. Use of gas anesthesia provided additional anesthesia when needed (Tuomi et al. 2002).

Field immobilizations with etorphine HCl have had similar effects. Dosages between 4.0 and 15.5 mg/adult male based on estimated body weight were used in field immobilizations of Pacific walruses, with or without reversal with either diprenorphine or naloxone. A dose of 7 mg/adult male was used for the standard dose. Overall mortality rates varied but were in the range of 15–20% (Griffiths et al. 1993; Hills 1992).

Because of the rapid onset of severe respiratory depression associated with potent opioid administration in walruses, an opioid antagonist should be available. Naltrexone is recommended because the antagonism will last beyond the expected effects of opioid antagonist. A naltrexone dose of 0.1 mg/kg of the estimated body weight has been used in field immobilization situations with complete reversal occurring in less than 5 minutes. If the immobilization technique includes the use of an alpha-2 agonist such as medetomidine, atipamezole should be administered if full immediate recovery is desired. A 5:1 ratio of atipamezole to medetomidine is recommended for complete reversal.

Dissociative Anesthetics

Tiletamine and ketamine have been used to immobilize free-ranging walruses. The principal problem associated with dissociative chemical restraint is the long duration of effect and the lack of a reversal agent. Since walruses are often immobilized near water, it is imperative that conditions prevent the partially anesthetized animal from entering water.

Tiletamine and zolazepam (Telazol or Zolatil) at a dose of 1.4- to 2.2-mg/kg IM have been studied for chemical restraint of walruses. Induction time ranged from 14 to 29 minutes, and the duration of immobilization lasted from as short as 75 minutes to as long as 220 minutes. The induction and recoveries were reported to be smooth. Apnea was not reported although one of the three animals died during recovery (Griffiths et al. 1993).

Atlantic walruses have also been immobilized with a combination of Telazol and medetomidine. A total dose of Telazol and 100 mg of medetomidine (approximately 3.3 mg/kg Telazol and 17 μg/kg medetomidine) were administered by dart to two animals. The respiration rate varied between 10 and 12 breaths/min throughout the procedure. Despite oxygen supplementation via a nasal cannula, pulse oximetry showed relatively low oxygen concentration (37–79%) (Lanthier & Stewart 2002). Atipamezole was used to antagonize medetomidine. Three additional walruses (one male and two female) were injected with a total dose of 2 gm of ketamine and 90 mg of medetomidine (approximately 2.5–4.0 mg/kg of ketamine and 11–18 μg/kg of medetomidine). In each case, the respiration rate appeared to be normal (rate and depth). Immobilization occurred in 15 minutes. None of the walrus showed muscle spasms. Procedure length varied between 16 and 40 minutes. Atipamezole was injected intravenously and intramuscularly 50/50 as the antagonist (approximately 9.5–19.0 μg/kg). Recoveries were smooth and rapid (6–23 minutes) (Lanthier & Stewart 2002).

Propofol

The author has used small boluses of propofol (40–60 mg) via the EIV sinus to provide unconsciousness, muscle relaxation, and to facilitate endotracheal intubation. The use of propofol decreased the need for higher doses of the immobilization drugs and the asso-

ciated muscle relaxation appears to facilitate spontaneous ventilation. Similarly, ultrashort-acting barbiturates (thiamylal sodium) have been successfully used to produce general anesthesia in walruses. Dosages of 3.3–4.8 mg/kg with 1/2 of the calculated dose administered initially and the additional drug given to effect as needed (Walsh et al. 1990).

Volatile Anesthetics

Isoflurane has been used to maintain general anesthesia in walruses. However, because of the low blood:gas solubility of sevoflurane, both uptake and elimination will be faster and may improve the ability to reach surgical anesthesia and have shorter recovery times than with isoflurane. Since the cardiovascular and respiratory depressive effects of isoflurane and sevoflurane are similar, the lower solubility of sevoflurane would be of significant advantage in walruses. Oxygen flow rates and vaporizer settings will be similar to equine anesthesia. Oxygen should be set at >4 L/min to ensure delivery of anesthetic and oxygen for metabolic needs. Initial vaporizer settings will likely be between 3.0 and 4.5%; however, vaporizer settings should be reduced in anticipation of equilibration of the animal with the anesthetic machine. Maintenance levels of 2.0–2.5% isoflurane and 2.5–3.0 sevoflurane are expected.

ANALGESIA

Analgesic methods used in other marine mammals should be considered to decrease stress associated with painful procedures or conditions. As previously discussed, local anesthetics are effective if injected around the surgical site or on sensory nerves to a region. As with other species, total local anesthetic dosages should be kept below 4 mg/kg to avoid potential local anesthetic toxicity. Opioid analgesics have been used as a part of chemical immobilization techniques are believed to provide reduction in pain perception, modulation, and transduction. Chronic pain management has not been addressed in walruses and no recommendations can be made for the use of anti-inflammatory drugs at this time.

REFERENCES

Cornell LH. 1978. Capture, transportation, restraint and marking. In: *Zoo and Wild Animal Medicine* (ME Fowler, ed.), pp. 573–580. Philadelphia: WB. Saunders.

Cornell LH, Joseph BE. 1985. Anesthesia and tusk extraction in walrus, Abstracts. Annual Proceedings of the American Association of Zoo Veterinarians, p. 97.

DeMaster DP, Faro JB, Estes JA, Taggart J, Zabel C. 1981. Drug immobilization of walrus (*Odobenus rosmarus*). *Canadian Journal of Fisheries and Aquatic Sciences* 38:365–367.

Fay FH. 1969. Structure and function of the pharyngeal pouches of the walrus (*Odobenus Rosmarus* L.). *Extrait de Mammalia* 24(3):361–371.

Gales NJ. 1989. Chemical restraint and anesthesia of pinnipeds: a review. *Marine Mammal Science* 5:228–256.

Garlich-Miller JL, Stewart REA. 1999. Female reproductive patterns and fetal growth of Atlantic walrus (*Odobenus rosmarus rosmarus*) in Foxe Basin, Northwest Territories, Canada. *Marine Mammal Science* 15:179–191.

Geraci JR. 1978. Marine mammals. In: *Zoo and Wild Animal Medicine* (ME Fowler, ed.), pp. 523–552. Philadelphia: W.B. Saunders.

Griffiths D, Wiig Ø, Gjertz I. 1993. Immobilization of walrus with etorphine hydrochloride and Zoletil®. *Marine Mammal Science* 9:250–257.

Gruber AD, Peters M, Knieriem A, Wohlsein P. 2002. Atherosclerosis with multifocal myocardial infarction in a pacific walrus (*Odobenus Rosmarus Divergens Illiger*). *Journal of Zoo and Wildlife Medicine* 33(2):139–144.

Hills S. 1992. The effect of spatial and temporal variability on population assessment of Pacific walruses. PhD Thesis, University of Maine, Bangor, Maine, p. 217.

Joseph BE, Cornell LH. 1988. The use of meperidine hydrochloride for chemical restraint in certain cetaceans and pinnipeds. *Journal of Wildlife Diseases* 244(4):691–694.

Klein L, Calle P, Raphael B, Cook R. 2002. Anesthesia in captive pacific walrus. Report of workshop on the chemical restraint of walruses edited by Chadwick V. Jay, pp. 18–25, San Diego, U.S. Geological Survey.

Lanthier C, Stewart REA. 2002. Chemical restraint of walruses: a Canadian perspective. Report of workshop on the chemical restraint of walruses edited by Chadwick V. Jay, pp. 5–7, San Diego, U.S. Geological Survey.

Lanthier C, Stewart REA, Born EW. 1999. Reversible anesthesia of Atlantic walrus (*Odobenus rosmarus rosmarus*) with carfentanil antagonized with naltrexone. *Marine Mammal Science* 15: 241–249.

Lynch MJ, Tahmindjis MA, Gardner H. 1999. Immobilization of pinniped species. *Australian Veterinary Journal* 77:181–185.

Mulcahy DM, Tuomi PA, Garner GW, Jay CV. 2003. Immobilization of free-ranging male pacific walruses (*Odobenus Rosmarus Divergens*) with carfentanil citrate and naltrexone hydrochloride. *Marine Mammal Science* 19:846.

Stetter M, Calle PP, McClave C, Cook RA. 1997. Marine Mammal Intravenous Catheterization Techniques. Proceedings of the American Association of Zoo Veterinarians, pp. 194–196.

Tuomi P, Mulcahy D, Garner G. 2002. Immobilization of Pacific walrus (Odobenus rosmarus divergens) with carfentanil, naltrexone reversal and isoflurane anesthesia. Proceedings of the WSAVA Congress.

Walsh MT, Asper ED, Andrews B, Antrium J. 1990. Walrus biology and medicine. In: *CRC Handbook of Marine Mammal Medicine: Health, Disease, and Rehabilitation* (LA Dierauf, ed.), pp. 594–595. Boca Raton: CRC Press LLC.

49 Cetaceans

Christopher Dold and Sam Ridgway

INTRODUCTION

Cetaceans (whales, dolphins, and porpoises) are mammals whose ancestors developed on land. Around 55 million years ago, these ancestors went back to the water (Gingerich et al. 1983) and evolved anatomically, physiologically, and behaviorally for a completely aquatic existence. Most clinical experience has been with the bottlenose dolphin (*Tursiops truncatus*, *Tursiops truncatus gilli*, and *Tursiops truncatus aduncus*) since it is the species most commonly found in display, research, and rehabilitation facilities. Other odontocete species, including the killer whale (*Orcinus orca*), the beluga or white whale (*Delphinapterus leucas*), the Pacific white-sided dolphin (*Lagenorhynchus obliquidens*), and the false killer whale (*Pseudorca crassidens*), have been successfully managed in zoos and aquaria for many years. A growing amount of clinical experience with these species has led to increasingly frequent need for sedation and, in certain instances, general anesthesia.

DOLPHIN SLEEP

Bottlenose dolphins, like all cetaceans, have an apneustic style of breathing. Even when resting at the water surface, dolphins ordinarily take 1–3 breaths/min. Each breath is a deep one, rapidly filling the lung to 80 or 90% capacity (Ridgway et al. 1969). Expiratory flow rates are very rapid and empty the lung almost completely (Kooyman & Cornell 1981). Thus the effort of breathing, even at rest, appears much more pronounced than that of humans and other terrestrial mammals.

Given their need to swim and breathe air with these deep breaths, it is not surprising that many biologists and veterinarians have wondered how dolphins sleep in the water. In the early 1960s, John Lilly (1962a) suggested that bottlenose dolphins slept with one eye closed and utilized one brain hemisphere at a time. However, he produced no electroencephalograms (EEGs) to support this hypothesis. Serafetinides et al. (1970) reported the first EEG evidence of unihemispheric sleep using subcutaneous (SC) needle electrodes during a one-night recording from a pilot whale (*Globicephala scammoni*). Mukhametov et al. (1977) and Mukhametov (1984) recorded many 24-hour periods, from multiple dolphins using screw electrodes inserted through the skull in a multichannel array with a low-noise wire system that allowed some animal movement around a shallow pool. They demonstrated overwhelming evidence that the vast majority of dolphin slow waves were unihemispheric and appeared first in one hemisphere and then the other. Remarkably, each hemisphere appears to accumulate a separate sleep debt. When one hemisphere was deprived of slow wave sleep for several days, only that hemisphere showed the typical sleep rebound; the nondeprived hemisphere continued to alternate its slow wave sleep in the usual amount (Oleksenko et al. 1992). Since slow waves appeared only very rarely and then very briefly in both hemispheres simultaneously, Mukhametov (1984) and Mukhametov et al. (1977) suggested that slow waves in both hemispheres are not compatible with respiration.

Using a small implantable telemetry unit, Ridgway (2002) replicated the earlier unihemispheric EEG findings and also recorded symmetrical EEG in both hemispheres during pentothal/halothane anesthesia. There were short periods of EEG slow waves in both hemispheres during the unanesthetized state, but slow waves in both hemispheres were not seen during breaths.

Zoo Animal and Wildlife Immobilization and Anesthesia, Second Edition. Edited by Gary West, Darryl Heard, and Nigel Caulkett.
© 2014 John Wiley & Sons, Inc. Published 2014 by John Wiley & Sons, Inc.

From behavioral observations, Lilly (1962b) stated "In regard to lateralization of the sleep pattern, these animals sleep with one eye closed at a time. The eye closures are 180° out of phase; it is rare to have both eyes closed at once. The accumulated sleep in each eye runs 120–140 minutes per day. The sleep occurs in brief periods between each respiration running from 20 to 40 seconds per eye closure. A dolphin wakes up to take each breath." Extensive behavioral observations were conducted by McCormick (1969), who was able to observe bottlenose dolphins through large underwater viewing windows. He observed dolphins resting at the water surface, virtually immobile, with both eyes closed and breathing in an "automatic fashion" for periods of ≥1 hour.

McCormick (1969) also observed, unlike the bottlenose dolphin, the Dall porpoise (*Phocoenoides dalli*) swam continuously without ever stopping to rest or become immobile. Azov porpoises (*Phocoena phocoena*), in the same family as Dall porpoises, were observed to swim continuously as well (Mukhametov & Polyakova 1981). From these observations, it would be easy to conclude that Dall porpoises and Azov porpoises never sleep. Mukhametov and Polyakova (1981) fitted three of the Azov porpoises with their EEG recording equipment. The animals swam continuously around their pool. Unihemispheric slow waves alternated between the hemispheres while the porpoises continued to swim (Mukhametov & Polyakova 1981). Therefore, stopping to rest, or becoming immobile, is not an absolute requirement for sleep. Although bottlenose dolphins and the largest member of the dolphin family, the killer whale, often rest at the surface, as described by McCormick (1969), both mother and calf swim constantly for several weeks after the birth (Lyamin et al. 2005). Thus if mother and calf are sleeping, it must occur while they are continuously swimming.

HISTORY OF DOLPHIN GENERAL ANESTHESIA

The physiology of anesthesia is different from sleep, especially in cetaceans. The superficial appearances of these two physiologic states, however, gives rise to the common comparison of administering general anesthesia with inducing sleep. Although there are many differences, unconsciousness in these two different physiologic states is considered somewhat similar to humans and other land mammals. However, the phenomenon of unihemispheric sleep in cetaceans makes the comparison between sleep and anesthesia not as applicable in these species. Moreover, in all mammals, arousal from sleep by noxious stimuli has a relatively low threshold, whereas arousal from anesthesia is possible only after recovery.

The first attempt to put a dolphin "to sleep" or to give general anesthesia was made by Langworthy

(1932), who administered ether by a cone held over the blowhole. The dolphin stopped breathing and died. After a number of attempts to employ intraperitoneal barbiturate anesthesia resulted in dolphin deaths (Lilly 1962a; Nagel et al. 1964), the latter group successfully developed endotracheal intubation methods and induced anesthesia with 70% nitrous oxide (Nagel et al. 1964). Although nitrous oxide was safe, it was inadequate for major surgery. Ridgway and McCormick (1967, 1971) used halothane, and later IV thiopental, for induction and halothane for anesthesia maintenance. Other early work in dolphin anesthesia has been reviewed in French by Lecuyer (1983).

More recently, propofol has been the choice for induction followed by intubation and isoflurane maintenance (Linnehan & MacMillan 1991). When general anesthesia is achieved, dolphins do not breathe and slow waves appear on the EEG of both brain hemispheres (Howard et al. 2006; Ridgway 2002). All successful general anesthesias have required intubation and the use of a respirator. A Bird Mark 9 large animal respirator fitted with an apneustic control device has been employed to mimic the normal respiration of the animal (Nagel et al. 1964; Ridgway & McCormick 1967, 1971).

ANATOMY AND PHYSIOLOGY RELEVANT TO ANESTHESIA

Specific anatomic and physiologic adaptations of the respiratory and cardiovascular systems, although beneficial for a purely aquatic existence, pose challenges to the clinician for sedation and general anesthesia of the cetacean patient. Much of the physiological and anatomical knowledge discussed here was gained from work on bottlenose dolphins. Fortunately for the clinician, most of the adaptations are well conserved among the other odontocete species commonly encountered in zoos and aquaria.

The most obvious adaptation of the respiratory system is the blowhole, the external nasal opening of cetaceans (Fig. 49.1). It is positioned on top of the head rather than at the front of the face as it is in all other mammals. Immediately, ventral and lateral to the blowhole are right and left lateral vestibular sacs. One can readily palpate these sacs by placing a finger through the blowhole directed to the left or to the right. The right sac is larger. Paired internal nares can be seen below the nasal plug when it opens. The paired nasal cavities, separated by the nasal septum, extend from the nares ventrally along the cranial aspect of the calvarium to the naso-pharynx just above the larynx, which is beak-shaped structure frequently referred to as a "goosebeak" because of its semblance in shape (Fig. 49.1). The goosebeak is an elongation of epiglottal and cricoarytenoid cartilages supported laterally by arytenoepiglottal muscles (Green et al. 1980). It is held in

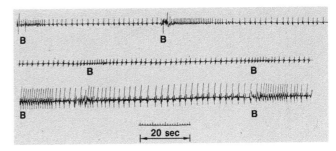

Figure 49.3. A recording of dolphin heart rhythm. Each breath is indicated by the letter B on the recording. With each breath, the heart rate increases then slows in a marked sinus rhythm of tachycardia/bradycardia. This rhythm is abolished with the induction of anesthesia.

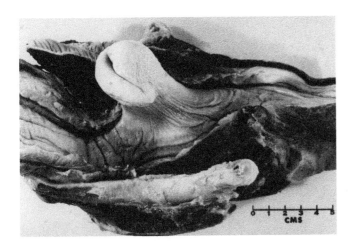

Figure 49.1. The laryngeal "goosebeak" rises from the center of the oropharynx (from Green et al. 1980, U.S. Navy photograph).

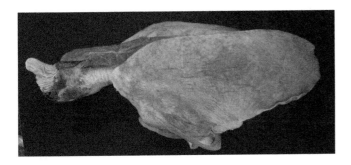

Figure 49.2. Left lateral view of excised dolphin lung, trachea, and larynx (U.S. Navy photograph).

its dorsally oriented position by the nasopharyngeal sphincter muscle along the dorsal oropharynx. Foods, usually swallowed whole, course laterally around the larynx. The larynx is not permanently affixed in this position. It can be displaced voluntarily by the animal or when swallowing large food items, and by the clinician manually when intubating the animal. The larynx leads to a short trachea (Fig. 49.3). Preceding the carina is a right-sided accessory bronchus (Green 1972), which is an important consideration when intubating these species because the separate right bronchus is required for inflation of a portion of the right lung.

Compared with terrestrial mammals, cetaceans have more extensive pulmonary support structures including complete tracheal and bronchial cartilagenous rings that extend beyond the mainstem bronchi into deep bronchioles, and plates and rings of cartilage that extend all the way to the junctions of aveoli. Smooth-muscle sphincter-like narrowings occur at the terminal bronchioles (Simpson & Gardner 1972). The lungs contain a great amount of elastic tissue. A dense elastic visceral pleura 1 mm or so in thickness covers each nonseptate, nonsegmented lung (Fig. 49.2). Since ceta-

ceans must be intubated and put on a respirator for general anesthesia, the anatomy relative to the endotracheal intubation process is especially important.

As previously mentioned, cetaceans have a specialized respiratory cycle with short, rapid exchange phases followed by long inspiratory apneustic plateaus. They take fewer and deeper breathes than their terrestrial counterparts. Bottlenose dolphins breathe an average of 2–3 times/min and have a tidal volume of 5–10 L, which may represent 80% or more of their total lung capacity (Ridgway 1972).

Anatomic adaptations of the cardiovascular system to support deep diving, long breath holds, and temperature conservation in the cold ocean include large, distensible veins, venous sinuses, venous valves in the lungs, portal triads of the liver, and a venous sphincter in the common hepatic vein at the junction of the inferior vena cava below the diaphragm. A rete mirabile, a highly developed meshwork of arteries and veins between the thoracic vertebral bodies, and periarterial venous rete represent temperature countercurrent exchange systems that allow cetaceans to peripherally vasoconstrict and still perfuse the brain with warm, oxygenated blood even under the great pressure and temperature extremes experienced at depth (McFarland et al. 1979). Finally, cetaceans have a profound respiratory sinus arrhythmia that is normal—the heart rate speeds up with each breath and slows between breaths (Fig. 49.3).

PHYSICAL RESTRAINT

Physical restraint of small cetaceans is a common practice, but requires multiple personnel. Even then it can still result in injury to both people and patient due to the substantial size and strength of most small cetaceans. It is recommended, therefore, that physical restraint be performed under the supervision of trained, experienced personnel. However, because experience

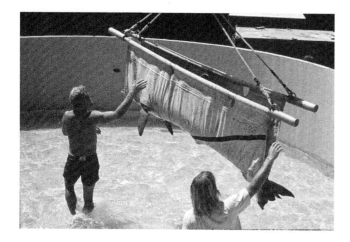

Figure 49.4. A dolphin is lifted from its pool in a fitted sling (U.S. Navy photograph).

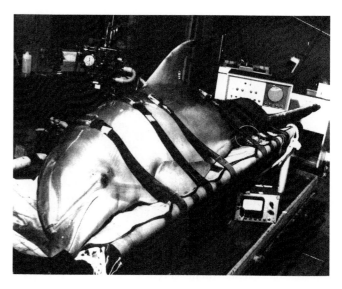

Figure 49.5. Prior to induction of anesthesia, a dolphin rests on a special table held loosely by seat belt straps (U.S. Navy photograph).

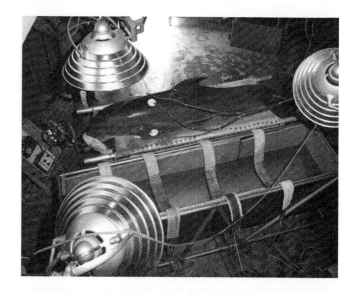

Figure 49.6. The dolphin is anesthetized and ventilated with a Bird respirator through an oral endotracheal tube. White rubber suction cups hold surface electrodes for monitoring the electrocardiogram (ECG). The suction cups provide insulation for the electrodes to allow for recording ECG while the animal is immersed. The dolphin will be supported by the warm water and padded straps in the adjacent tank during the surgical procedure. IV fluid is given through the caudal vascular bundle. Blood transfusions, if needed, may be given through the same site or via the PAVR. For long procedures, a nebulizer is placed in the line for humidification of respiratory gas (U.S. Navy photograph).

with cetacean sedation and anesthesia is still relatively limited, most, if not all, clinically relevant procedures can be, and have been, performed under physical restraint alone.

Animals requiring care can be separated from pool mates either under voluntary control or with the use of nets or stranding devices. Care must be taken when introducing a net into the water. If animals do become entangled, they must be quickly assisted to the surface so that they can breathe. Many facilities have medical pools designed to strand animals out of the water for clinical procedures without the need for nets, slings, or stretchers. Clinical procedures have been performed on dolphins and other odontocetes with animals out of the water suspended in fitted slings (Fig. 49.4), suspended in water tight boxes, or most commonly out of the water supported on a soft foam rubber pad on the ground or on large animal surgical tables. When not suspended in stretchers or slings, animals are commonly positioned onto closed-cell foam padding. Personnel are positioned on both sides of the animal; one or two people restrain the animal's tail flukes, and one or two people are positioned near the animal's head. For animals that are relaxed out of the water, simple support by only one or two people may be all that is required. For more fractious animals, multiple people may be needed to provide adequate restraint.

Due to the challenges associated with physical and chemical restraints in these animals, operant conditioning and training have resulted in many small cetaceans being conditioned to voluntarily participate in clinical procedures (blood sampling, ultrasound, radiographs, and endoscopy).

Whenever the cetacean is out of water, its skin must be kept moist for temperature control and prevention of drying. Special attention should be paid to the eyes to prevent injury or drying. During anesthesia, it is best to apply a lubricating ophthalmic ointment to prevent drying of the eyes. Special tables (Fig. 49.5) or tanks (Fig. 49.6) have been constructed to maintain the dolphin patient in proper position for monitoring and surgery.

VASCULAR ACCESS

There are several peripheral sites from which blood may be collected. The arteriovenous nature of the peripheral vasculature, however, means very few of these sites allow rapid drug or fluid administration. Consequently, central venous access is desirable and has become increasingly attainable as imaging and vascular access technologies improve. Both peripheral and central access sites are described.

Dorsal and Ventral Fluke Periarterial Vascular Rete (PAVR)

The ventral fluke PAVR is most commonly used for routine venipuncture in odontocetes species (Ridgway 1965). In dolphin collections, animals are often trained to allow venipuncture in the site under voluntary stimulus control. Blood can be collected with 19- to 23-gauge and 2- to 4-cm (3/4- to 1 1/2-in) needles, depending on animal size and species. Intravenous (IV) antibiotics and fluids can be administered into this site, but the size and microanatomy of the vessel, the accuracy of the needle stick, and the dynamic nature of the peripheral blood vessels in this species can limit the success of administration. Blood collected from this site (Fig. 49.7) is most commonly venous or an arterial–venous admixture, and rarely purely arterial.

Peduncle PAVR

This venipuncture site is located on the ventral aspect of the terminal vertebral bodies. The landmarks for injection are the ventral peduncle ridge, immediately proximal to the confluence of the right and left fluke PAVR. Venipuncture at this site is best performed with needles longer and larger than those used for fluke vessel venipuncture in the same anima: 18- to 21-gauge, 2- to 4-cm (1.5- to 2-in) needles and larger may be required. The site may be accessed from voluntary fluke presentations or in animals out of the water for exams and procedures (Fig. 49.8). The larger diameter of the artery at this site allows rapid collection of large volumes of arterial and arterial–venous admixed blood. This site has been successfully used for repeated phlebotomy to treat iron overload in bottlenose dolphins (Johnson et al. 2009). The larger vessels also make the site appropriate for IV injection. Assuming appropriate positioning, and if necessary, restraint of the flukes, the needle may be left indwelling in this site during longer procedures for constant rate infusion of fluids, as well as repeat blood samples for arterial blood gases. Arterial blood pressure has been measured at this site (Ridgway et al. 1974); however, needle placement and movement must be carefully monitored because shifts may lead to values not necessarily reflective of the patients' status.

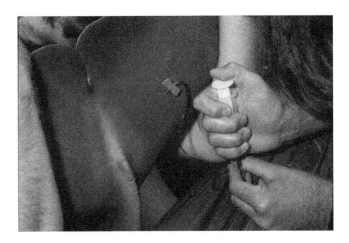

Figure 49.7. A 20 gauge butterfly needle is used to collect a blood sample from the fluke blade (U.S. Navy photograph).

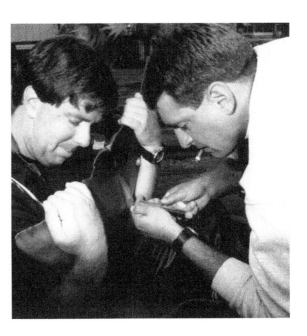

Figure 49.8. Blood is collected from the peduncle PAVR employing a 20 gauge needle and vacutainer tube. The peduncle PAVR is the best peripheral site for collecting arterial samples (U.S. Navy photograph).

Dorsal Fin PAVR

Although a challenging site for venipuncture in smaller cetaceans, this location is useful for killer whales (Fig. 49.9). For dolphins, it is usually reserved for fractious animals that will not allow access to the flukes or peduncle. It is also used as a second site for blood collection during anesthetic or sedative procedure. The dorsal fin PAVR has all of the same anatomic challenges as the fluke PAVR. When considering IV drug administration, it is important to note the blood draining from this site travels directly to a rete around animal's gonads. The authors usually access this site with needles similar to those used for fluke PAVR venipuncture.

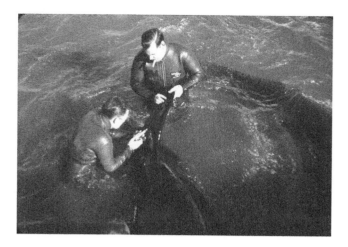

Figure 49.9. Accessing the dorsal fin PAVR is much easier in larger animals such as the killer whale (U.S. Navy photograph).

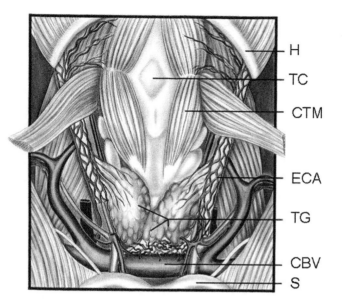

Figure 49.10. Drawing from a dissection of the ventral neck of a bottlenose dolphin. H, hyoid; TC, thyroid cartilage; CTM, cricothyroid muscle; ECA, external carotid artery; TG, thyroid gland; CBV, common brachiocephalic vein; S, sternum. Note that the ECA is covered by a meshwork of veins. Drawing by Barbara Stolen Irvine from Ridgway and Patton (1971).

Hemal Arch/Caudal Vascular Bundle

The caudal vascular bundle runs longitudinally along the ventral midline of the caudal vertebral bodies within an arch formed by the chevron bones. In an adult bottlenose dolphin, a 9-cm (3.5 in.) spinal needle is advanced transversely into the ventral intervertebral space, ventral and parallel to the lateral processes of the caudal vertebral bodies in the mid- to caudal peduncle region. The caudal vascular bundle is a low pressure, mostly venous system. This site can be catheterized (Van Bonn et al. 1996) and, when accessed, it is appropriate for IV fluid and drug administration. Given the venous rete at this site, however, rates of absorption of drugs and fluid may be more variable and delayed compared with administration into other sites.

Common Brachiocephalic Vein (CBV)

The CBV (Fig. 49.10) is not part of a PAVR. It is, therefore, an appropriate site to collect purely venous blood samples and to measure venous blood pressure. It is also large enough to allow catheterization, and indwelling catheters in this site have improved anesthesia monitoring and support capabilities in these species. Drugs and fluids given into the CBV may have more predictable and rapid absorption and effect than when injected intravenously into other peripheral sites that are part of PAVRs. Accessing the brachiocephalic vein is a challenge. In bottlenose dolphins, it lies 10- to 12-cm deep under skin, blubber, and muscle, and runs in a transverse plane. The actual site for access is large: 2- to 3-cm wide and 2-cm thick. Slight misdirection at the skin, however, can translate into significant misdirection of the long needles at the level of the vessel. The transverse orientation of the vessel also makes catheterization difficult.

The authors have had the greatest success accessing the vein using ultrasound guidance. As such, the procedure benefits from two people working together; one

person guides the probe and holds the image steady, while the other person performs venipuncture. For catheterization, we pass a 14-gauge, 16-cm needle into the vein and then feed a 60-cm polyurethane catheter through it to a depth of approximately 25 cm. For short term access (IV drugs, bolus fluids), we use a needle and no catheter. The stylet from an equine 16g, 14-cm (5.5 in) radio-opaque (Abbocath®) catheter is the sharpest, disposable needle to use. The animal is placed in lateral recumbency for the procedure. We have recent evidence that placing the animal in right lateral recumbency is more anatomically appropriate for catheterization. Right lateral recumbency, along with the natural tendency of the phlebotomist to orient the needle tip toward the floor, encourages the catheter to feed toward the heart (with left to right flow in the vessel). In left lateral recumbency, the catheter tends to feed toward the venous return from the rete (against flow). Successful catheterization, however, can also be performed with the animal in left lateral recumbency.

Hepatic Vein

Recent collaborations with interventional radiologists have enabled the development of a safe, percutaneous, transhepatic approach to the hepatic vein. Using local anesthesia and ultrasound guidance, Johnson et al. (2010) were able to reliably and repeatedly pass a 6 Fr peripherally inserted central catheter (PICC) into the hepatic vein and advance the catheter into the caudal vena cava. Catheter placement can be achieved from both the right and left sides of the animal. In addition to offering the same advantages of the brachiocephalic vein (medication and fluid administration), this site carries the added advantage of a lateral approach reducing risk of displacement. Retention times of up to 6 hours (out of water) were reported. While considered to be generally safe, the approach does carry the added risk of hepatic bleeding. The authors recommend placement of embolized Gelfoam™ during removal of the catheter (Houser et al. 2010; Johnson et al. 2010).

ENDOTRACHEAL INTUBATION

Endotracheal intubation of adult bottlenose dolphins and larger odontocete species is usually performed by an oral approach to the larynx (Fig. 49.1). This can be accomplished when the animal is either awake (in an emergency situation) or following sedation or anesthetic induction. Large animal endotracheal tubes with inflatable cuffs (size of 16- to 30-mm internal diameter) are appropriate for most adult bottlenose dolphins. Intubation usually requires multiple personnel; one person to hold the mouth open with soft rolled towels and another to pass the endotracheal tube. The oral approach to the larynx is done blind. Intubation requires manual removal of the larynx (goosebeak) from the nasopharyngeal sphincter to orient it in a rostral direction. Once the laryngeal tip is positioned rostral, two fingers can be placed into the glottis (Fig. 49.1) and the endotracheal tube guided through the glottis into the short trachea. The trachea is very short in most odontocetes (Fig. 49.2), and there is a right-sided accessory bronchus (Green 1972) that precedes the carina. Care must be taken not to advance the endotracheal tube too far and block the right bronchus.

The oral approach to intubation may not be possible in smaller odontocetes due to their small mouths and oropharynx. Intubation in these animals can be accomplished with a small tube placed through the blowhole (Fig. 49.11). This approach is more complicated than the oral due to redundant tissue and muscular folds used for vocalization and echolocation between the goosebeak and the blowhole. The tube must be inserted through either the right or left nasal cavities. This limits the size of tube that can be used. Intubation is greatly facilitated by the use of a bronchoscope for visualization of the goosebeak and a stylet to advance the endotracheal tube through the glottis. A possible adverse effect of prolonged intubation is abnormal with blowhole function when the animal is returned to the water. To our knowledge, prolonged blowhole intubation has not previously been performed.

Blowhole intubation was used in small dolphins (*Stenella styx* and *Delphinus delphis*) under experimental conditions at sea (Rieu & Gautheron 1968). Xylocaine

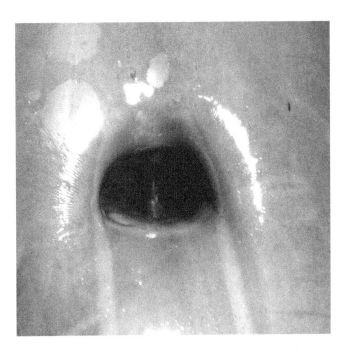

Figure 49.11. Dolphin open blowhole. Anterior is down in this photograph. The nasal septum divides the nares so that only a small tube can be inserted down one nostril through the nasal cavity to reach the glottis sitting below the opening of the distal nares (also see Fig. 49.1 and Fig. 49.2) (U.S. Navy photograph).

(2%) was injected through the tube to produce laryngeal anesthesia and analgesia.

ANESTHESIA SUPPORT AND MONITORING

Anesthesia monitoring and support is just as critical in cetaceans as in terrestrial mammals, if not more so. Since normal spontaneous ventilation, circulation, and perfusion in cetaceans are typically performed with the animals' bodyweight supported by the buoyancy forces exerted by the water column, simply removing the animals from the water for a clinical procedure may place them at a cardiopulmonary disadvantage. A collapsible thorax, gravity, and the animals' mass combine to increase respiratory effort and compress muscles and vessels. Changes in temperature and pressure may cause hyper- or hypothermia, abnormal vasoconstriction, or vasodilation with resultant blood shunts. This can happen even before any respiratory, cardiovascular, or central nervous system depressing drugs are given.

A comprehensive approach to monitoring and support should be applied to the cetacean patient and, since reported drug protocols are frequently limited to experience with only a few individual animals, the anesthetist should always be on alert for the possibility of profound and unexpected drug reactions. Applying anesthesia monitoring equipment to patients out of the water and without sedation is as important as applying it to the fully anesthetized patient, if for no other reason than it can help to build the clinician's familiarity with individual animal's normal heart and respiratory rates, core temperatures, and reflexes.

Respiratory support in sedated animals that are still spontaneously ventilating is not necessary. Many marine mammal clinicians, however, will still provide supplemental oxygen to dolphins and whales that are out of the water or sedated. For general anesthesia in dolphins, successful mechanical ventilation has been performed with use of a Bird Mark 9 respirator with an apneustic plateau modification to allow for prolonged inspiratory hold in the ventilation cycle. A respiratory rate of 2–4 breaths/min (Ridgway & McCormick 1967, 1971; Ridgway et al. 1974) is generally employed. Early experiences suggested that general anesthesia lasting longer than 4 hours without this modification resulted in reduced lung expansion and alveolar inflation, and associated respiratory acidemia, and cardiovascular depression (Ridgway & McCormick 1971). One recent report suggests that the apneustic plateau ventilatory cycle may not be necessary for shorter procedures (Reidarson 2003). Recently, one animal (*Tursiops*) maintained under isoflurane anesthesia for 2 hours by the authors and ventilated with and without the apneustic plateau pattern showed lower end-tidal CO_2 (EtCO$_2$) levels (45–50 mmHg) that more closely approximated the animal's nonanesthetized expiratory CO_2 when ventilated without the apneustic plateau pattern.

Monitoring EtCO$_2$ as an indicator of adequate ventilation and perfusion is recommended for dolphins under general anesthesia, and may be helpful even with dolphins under sedation (not intubated). For sedated animals, the sampling probe can be held in the blow stream above the blowhole. EtCO$_2$ measurements should always be checked against the patient's pCO$_2$ before determining just how representative the measured EtCO$_2$ is of true alveolar CO_2.

Blood gases can be measured as in other animals, and normal ranges appear similar to other mammals. Due to cetacean vascular anatomy, collecting a purely arterial or purely venous sample is possible, but less likely than collecting an arteriovenous admixture when sampling from peripheral sites. A truly venous sample can be collected from the brachiocephalic vein, as described earlier. In the authors experience, the best peripheral site for a purely arterial sample is the peduncle PAVR.

Heart rate can be monitored with electrocardiogram leads as in other species. The authors recommend placing the leads before the animal has received any drugs to establish baseline readings. Normal, stable animals should have a profound resting sinus arrhythmia (Fig. 49.11). Some animals that are anxious or stressed, however, will override the arrhythmia and maintain a steady, mildly tachycardic rate (100–120 beats/min). Additionally, general anesthesia results in abolition of the sinus arrhythmia (Ridgway 1972;

Ridgway et al. 1974). Published reports suggest that a heart rate of less than 60 beats/min may be a cause for concern in anesthetized dolphins (Ridgway & McCormick 1971).

Perfusion can be measured with a pulse-oximeter impedance probe placed on the tongue of anesthetized patients (Linnehan & MacMillan 1991). In sedated animals, the authors have attempted to place reflectance probes rectally and within the genital slit of some patients with little success in obtaining readings.

Mean arterial blood pressure (MAP) has been monitored and reported in bottlenose dolphins and pacific white-sided dolphins (Ridgway & McCormick 1971; Ridgway et al. 1974). These measurements were recorded from an indwelling needle within the ventral peduncle PAVR. The authors have also successfully measured central venous pressure (CVP) in several bottlenose dolphins through an indwelling IV catheter placed in the CBV. CVP can also be measured by the PICC line placed via the hepatic vein into the caudal vena cava under ultrasound guidance (Johnson et al. 2010).

Body temperature has been monitored with a flexible thermometer probe placed rectally (Fig. 49.12) to a depth of 15- to 25-cm depending on animal size (Nagel et al. 1964; Ridgway 1965; Ridgway & McCormick 1967; Ridgway et al. 1974). Clinicians should be aware that countercurrent heat exchange systems for internal gonads may interfere with thermometer readings if the probe is placed too deep or too shallow, and lead to misinterpretations of core body temperature readings (Rommel et al. 1992, 1993).

Depth of anesthesia can be determined through assessment of reflexes as in other mammals. Palpebral and corneal responses, response to manipulation of the blowhole, jaw tone, and swallow reflexes are all appropriate. Ridgway and McCormick (1967) reported that loss of swimming motion in the tail flukes may be the

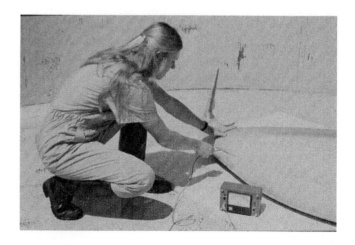

Figure 49.12. A flexible probe from an electronic thermometer is inserted 15–25 cm into the rectum, depending on the animal size, to measure temperature (U.S. Navy photograph).

most reliable indicator that a surgical plane of anesthesia has been reached. Future advances in assessing anesthetic depth may be achieved through application of entropy measuring programs and EEG monitoring, as described earlier.

FIELD TECHNIQUES AND STRATEGIES

Due to limited experience and serious potential complications associated with the use of sedatives in small cetaceans, most field work is accomplished with animals physically, rather than chemically, restrained. There appear to be no peer-reviewed publications describing data for sedation of odontocetes in a field setting. Sedation of entangled North Atlantic right whales (*Eubalaena glacialis*) has been attempted by Moore et al. (2010). Midazolam, meperidine, and butorphanol were given alone and in combination by cantilevered pole syringe and ballistic dart to two whales. The goal was to achieve a deep enough level of sedation to permit safe removal of the whales entangled in fishing gear, and still allow for the animals to protect their blowholes, ventilate, and maintain awareness and position in the water column. The authors conclude that these first attempts were conservative, and while the levels of sedation achieved were light and signs not obvious, the sedation did allow for enhanced disentanglement.

BODY WEIGHT RANGES OF SOME CETACEAN SPECIES

Body weights range with age class, sex, and species, as in other mammals. Adult weight ranges of the commonly encountered cetacean species are listed in Table 49.1. Cetaceans are relatively large, with large body mass, and therefore might require a large drug dose.

For many pharmaceuticals, a direct extrapolation of mg/kg dosing may be appropriate, however, in the specific instance of sedative and anesthetic drugs; consideration of dose scaling and basal metabolic rate must be made. In the author's experience, larger cetacean species may require smaller dosages of drug (on a mg/ kg basis) than smaller species to achieve the same level of sedation. As mentioned previously, most anesthetic and sedative drug use in cetaceans is limited to a very small sample size: in most instances, only one or a few individuals. As such, the potential for unpredictable drug reactions, even from published dosages, may exist.

ANALGESIA

If there is little published data on anesthetic drugs used in cetaceans, there is even less for analgesics. The greatest challenges to cetacean pain management are presented by the difficulty in effective assessment of pain, in measuring response to therapy, and in assessment of potential drug reactions. Several marine mammal clinicians have encountered acute, negative side effects after the use of nonsteroidal anti-inflammatory drugs in cetaceans (J. McBain, pers. comm., 2005). With that caveat, Table 49.2 lists several

Table 49.1. Common juvenile and adult weight ranges for selected species of cetaceans housed in oceanaria and aquaria

Species	Weight Range (kg)
Lagenorhynchus obliquidens	60–160
Tursiops truncatus	90–315
Orcinus orca	500–5600
Delphinapterus leucas	300–1600
Pseudorca crassidens	430–800

Table 49.2. Analgesic drugs used in cetaceans

Category	Drug Name	Species	Dosage	Route	Comments	Reference
NSAIDs	Flunixin meglamine (Banamine)	*Tursiops truncatus, Orcinus orca*	0.25–0.5 mg/ kg SID	IM	Caution with use in cetaceans as gastric ulcers are common	J. McBain, pers. comm., (2005)
	Carprofen	*T. truncatus*	0.5 mg/kg SID	PO	Gastric ulceration seen	T. Schmitt, personal comm., (2006)
	Acetaminophen	*T. truncatus, O. orca*	3–5 mg/kg SID	PO	Monitor transaminases	M. Walsh, pers. comm., (2005)
Opioids	Butorphanol	*T. truncatus, O. orca*	0.05– 0.13 mg/kg	IM	Possible excitatory response seen in one dolphin	Chittick et al. (2006)
	Tramadol	Multiple (bottlenose dolphin, common dolphin, rough tooth dolphin, spinner dolphin, spotted dolphin, and pygmy and dwarf sperm whales)	0.1–0.4 mg/ kg BID	PO	Titrate up to least effective dose. Produces good analgesia without change in appetite. Drowsiness seen at 0.73 mg/kg (can be used IM or IV as well)	C. Manire, pers. comm., (2006)

analgesic and anti-inflammatory agents that have been used in cetaceans.

ANESTHETIC AND SEDATIVE DRUGS

Drugs that have been reported or used by the authors for sedation and local or general anesthesia of several

cetacean species are presented in Table 49.2 and Table 49.3. The authors wish to caution, in most instances, that the number of animals exposed to these drugs is small and the potential for unpredictable or as yet unrevealed drug reactions is not insignificant. Also, to give perspective, we estimate that general anesthesia in cetaceans has been performed less than 100 times.

Table 49.3.   Chemical sedative and anesthetic agents used in bottlenose dolphins (*Tursiops truncatus*)

Category	Drug Name	Dosage	Route	Comments	Reference
Premedication	Atropine	0.02 mg/kg	IM		Ridgway and McCormick (1971)
Sedatives	Diazepam	0.1–0.2 mg/kg	IM		Reidarson (2003)
		0.25–1.0 mg/kg	PO	Larger doses reserved for research or for animals that may have become refractory to smaller oral doses of diazepam. Keep flumazenil available for reversal.	S. Ridgway, pers. obs.; Ridgway et al. (2006)
		0.26–0.36 mg/kg	PO		Schroeder et al. (1986)
	Midazolam	0.05–0.15 mg/kg	IM	Provides good plane of sedation lasting about 45–60 minutes. Caution when using in spp. other than *T. truncatus*	J. McBain and M. Walsh, pers. comm. (2005); S. Ridgway and C. Dold, pers. obs.
	Flumazenil	0.005 mg/kg	IM, PO, IV, sublingual	Can be given at equal volume of midazolam when midazolam is 5 mg/mL and flumazenil is 0.5 mg/mL. Usually titrate dose to effect.	J. McBain and M. Walsh, pers. comm.; S. Ridgway and C. Dold, pers. obs.
	Butorphanol	0.05–0.15 mg/kg	IM	Provides sedation adequate for bronchoscopy and other minor procedures. Possible drug reactions seen when combined with bronchodilators.	Chittick et al. (2006)
	Meperidine	0.1–2.0 mg/kg	IM	Given in combination with midazolam can produce deep level of sedation that is reversible.	Joseph and Cornell (1988); Reidarson (2003); Ridgway (1965)
	Tramadol	0.15–0.2 mg/kg	PO	Given in combination with diazepam (0.15 mg/kg) provides sedation adequate for tooth extraction.	T. Schmitt, pers. comm., (2005)
	[Naloxone]	5–10 mg/kg	IM/IV	Butorphanol and meperidine reversal	Reidarson (2003)
	[Naltrexone]	0.005 mg/kg	IM/IV	Opioid reversal	Chittick et al. (2006)
Induction agents	Ketamine	1.75 mg/kg	IM	Single case only	Reidarson (2003)
	Medetomidine	10–40 mg/kg	IM/IV	Abolishes sinus arrhythmia and causes respiratory depression, decreased CVP	Reidarson (2003); S. Ridgway and C. Dold, pers. obs.
	[Atipamezole]	50–200 mg/kg	IM/IV	Equal volume of medetomidine for reversal; medetomidine is 1 mg/mL and atapamazole is 5 mg/mL	S. Ridgway and C. Dold, pers. obs.
	Thiopental	10–15 mg/kg	IM	Requires additional inhalant anesthesia for full induction	Ridgway and McCormick (1971)
	Propofol	0.5–3.5 mg/kg	IV	Onset and duration of effect injection site dependent	Linnehan and MacMillan (1991); S. Ridgway and C. Dold, pers. obs.; W. Van Bonn, pers. comm., (2005)
Inhalational agents	Isoflurane	0.5–2.0%	IH	Higher dose for induction, lower maintenance dose	Dover et al. (1999); Linnehan and MacMillan (1991); S. Ridgway and W. Van Bonn, pers. obs., (1991–2005)
	Nitrous oxide	70%	IH	Light anesthesia	Nagel et al. (1964)

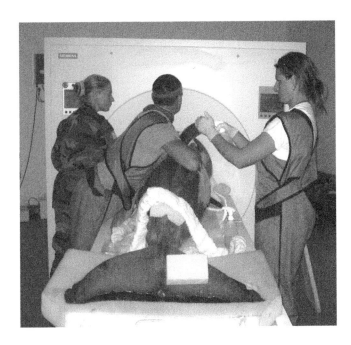

Figure 49.13. A trained dolphin remains still for a PET scan following 0.55–0.60 mg/kg of oral diazepam. The animal is kept moist with sponges and spray bottles during the 35- to 45-minute procedure (Ridgway et al. 2006) (U.S. Navy photograph).

Cetaceans have, however, been safely and, in some instances, repeatedly sedated or anesthetized with the listed drugs. Benzodiazepines and opioids are most commonly used for sedation in cetacean patients.

Benzodiazepines
Diazepam and midazolam are frequently employed for light sedation as an oral and a parenterally administered drug, respectively. Diazepam (0.55- to 0.60-mg/kg PO) has been used to help trained dolphins remain still for 35- to 45-minute functional scans such as positron emission tomography (Fig. 49.13). Diazepam (0.5-mg/kg PO) combined with tramadol (0.5-mg/kg PO) results in an enhanced sedation, as well as providing some analgesia. This combination has been used successfully for tooth extractions (with regional lidocaine) in white whales (T. Schmitt, pers. comm., 2011). Midazolam (0.05–0.1 mg/kg IM or IV) is effective and generally safe in Atlantic bottlenose dolphins (*T. truncatus*). Extreme caution, however, is indicated in species other than Atlantic bottlenose dolphins as profound sedation resulting in respiratory and cardiac depression has been witnessed in Pacific bottlenose dolphins (*T. truncatus gilli*) and Atlantic/Pacific hybrids (C. Smith, pers. comm., 2005). In the case of overdose, flumazenil may be given orally (Votey et al. 1991) or intravenously depending on the urgency (Geller et al. 1988; White et al. 1989).

Opioids
Meperidine (Demerol) is not infrequently used, but for some clinicians may be supplanted by butorphanol.

Several marine mammal clinicians are developing a growing comfort level with butorphanol (Chittick et al. 2006) as a sedative that provides analgesia, safe light sedation, and is easily reversible (Naloxone/Naltrexone).

Parenteral Anesthetics
Thiopental, pentothal, and propofol have been used for induction to general anesthesia. Reidarson (2003) reported the use of ketamine and medetomidine for the successful intubation and maintenance of anesthesia in one animal. The authors have limited experience with medetomidine, and experience with ketamine in only one patient (SR). In the author's experience, medetomidine alone produces significant respiratory and CVP depression, in addition to light sedation. The effects are reversed with atipamazole administration.

Inhalant Anesthetics
Anesthesia has been maintained with the inhalant anesthetics halothane (Ridgway 1965; Ridgway & McCormick 1967, 1971; Medway et al, 1970) and isoflurane (Dover et al. 1999; Haulena & Heath 2001; Linnehan & MacMillan 1991) in oxygen. Isoflurane is currently the inhalational anesthetic of choice (SR), although sevoflurane deserves consideration since, following induction of anesthesia with propofol, awakening from sevoflurane is faster (in people) compared with isoflurane.

RECOVERY
Perhaps greater than the challenges posed by induction and maintenance of general anesthesia in cetaceans are those encountered upon recovery. Due in part to the difficulty in observing depth of anesthesia, and also the replacement of the goosebeak as a necessary step for voluntary ventilation, great care must be taken as one attempts to recover the animal and get it breathing on its own.

LOCAL ANESTHESIA
Two percent xylocaine (Lidocaine HCl) has frequently been used for subcutaneous infiltration for surface surgical procedures. Blocking the infra-alveolar nerve, a branch of mandibular nerve, with xylocaine infiltration, has been effectively employed for dental procedures (Ridgway et al. 1975).

DISEASE ISSUES AFFECTING ANESTHESIA
Cetaceans, given their anatomy and physiology, are particularly susceptible to lung disease, and pneumonia is the most commonly diagnosed cause of severe disease in these species. Consequently, since these animals are also known to mask disease (Geraci & Sweeney 1986), a high index of suspicion should be maintained for

animals showing that evidence of disease may have some loss of normal pulmonary function and, accordingly, the potential for hypoxemia.

REFERENCES

Chittick EJ, Gearhart S, Dold C, Walsh MT, Dalton L. 2006. Preliminary findings with butorphanol sedation in cetaceans. International Association for Aquatic Animal Medicine Proceedings 37, pp. 144–145.

Dover SR, Beusse D, Walsh T, McBain JF, Ridgway S. 1999. Laparoscopic techniques for the bottlenose dolphin (*Tursiops truncatus*). International Association for Aquatic Animal Medicine Proceedings 30, pp. 128–129.

Geller E, Niv D, Nevo Y, Leykin Y, Sorkin P, Rudick V. 1988. Early clinical experience in reversing benzodiazepine sedation with flumazenil after short procedures. *Resuscitation* 16:49–56.

Geraci JR, Sweeney J. 1986. Clinical techniques. In: *Zoo and Wild Animal Medicine* (ME Fowler, ed.), pp. 771–776. Philadelphia: W.B. Saunders.

Gingerich PD, Wells NA, Russell DE, Ibrahim SM. 1983. Origin of whales in epicontinental remnant seas: new evidence from the early eocene of Pakistan. *Science* 220:403–405.

Green RF. 1972. Observations on the anatomy of cetaceans and pinnipeds. In: *Mammals of the Sea: Biology and Medicine* (SH Ridgway, ed.), pp. 247–297. Springfield: Charles C Thomas.

Green RF, Ridgway SH, Evans WE. 1980. Functional and descriptive anatomy of the bottlenosed dolphin nasolaryngeal system with special reference to the musculature associated with sound production. In: *Animal Sonar Systems* (RG Busnel, JF Fish, eds.), pp. 199–238. New York: Plenum.

Haulena M, Heath RB. 2001. Marine mammal anesthesia. In: *Marine Mammal Medicine* (LA Dierauf, FMD Gulland, eds.), pp. 655–688. Boca Raton: CRC Press.

Houser DS, Moore PW, Johnson S, Lutmerding B, Branstetter B, Ridgway SH, Trickey J, Finneran JJ, Jensen E, Hoh C. 2010. Relationship of blood flow and metabolism to acoustic processing centers of the dolphin brain. *The Journal of the Acoustical Society of America* 128(3):1460–1466.

Howard R, Finneran J, Ridgway S. 2006. Bispectral index monitoring of unihemisphere effects in dolphins. *Anesthesia and Analgesia* 103(3):626–630.

Johnson SP, Venn-Watson SK, Cassle SE, Smith CR, Jensen ED, Ridgway SH. 2009. Use of phlebotomy treatment in Atlantic bottlenose dolphins with iron overload. *Journal of the American Veterinary Medical Association* 235(2):194–200.

Johnson SP, Ferrara S, Hill LD, Jensen E, Lutmerding B, Ridgway S. 2010. Ultrasound-guided percutaneous transhepatic catheterization in the bottlenose dolphin (*Tursiops truncatus*). Proceedings of the 41st Annual Conference. International Association for Aquatic Animal Medicine, p. 38. Vancouver, Canada.

Joseph B, Cornell L. 1988. The use of meperidine hydrochloride for chemical restraint in certain cetaceans and pinnipeds. *Journal of Wildlife Diseases* 24:691–694.

Kooyman GL, Cornell LH. 1981. Flow properties of expiration and inspiration in a trained bottlenosed porpoise. *Physiological Zoology* 54:55–61.

Langworthy OR. 1932. A description of the central nervous system of the porpoise (*Tursiops truncatus*). *The Journal of Comparative Neurology* 54:437.

Lecuyer C. 1983. Respiration du dauphin applications al anesthesie de cet animal. Ecole Nationale Veterinaire De Maisons-Alfort. 53p.

Lilly J. 1962b. Cerebral dominance. In: *Interhemispheric Relations and Cerebral Dominance* (V Mountcastle, ed.), pp. 112–114. Baltimore: Johns Hopkins University Press.

Lilly JC. 1962a. *Man and Dolphin*. New York: Doubleday.

Linnehan RM, MacMillan A. 1991. Propofol/isoflurane anesthesia and debridement of a corneal ulcer in an Atlantic bottlenosed dolphin (*Tursiops truncatus*). Proceedings of the American Association of Zoo Veterinarians, pp. 290–291. Calgary, Canada.

Lyamin OI, Pryaslova J, Lance V, Siegel JM. 2005. Animal behaviour: continuous activity in cetaceans after birth. *Nature* 435:1177.

McCormick JG. 1969. Relationship of sleep, respiration, and anesthesia in the porpoise: a preliminary report. *Proceedings of the National Academy of Sciences of the United States of America* 62:697–703.

McFarland WL, Jacobs MS, Morgane PJ. 1979. Blood supply to the brain of the dolphin, *Tursiops truncatus*, with comparative observations on special aspects of the cerebrovascular supply of other vertebrates. *Neuroscience and Biobehavioral Reviews* 3(Suppl. 1):1–93.

Medway W, McCormick JG, Ridgway SH, Crump JF. 1970. Effects of prolonged halothane anesthesia on some cetaceans. *Journal of the American Veterinary Medical Association* 157:576–582.

Moore M, Walsh MT, Bailey J, Brunson D, Gulland F, Landry S, Mattila D, Mayo C, Slay C, Smith J, Rowles T. 2010. Sedation at sea of entangled North Atlantic right whales (*Eubalaena glacialis*) to enhance disentanglement. *PLoS ONE* 5(3):e9597.

Mukhametov LM. 1984. Sleep in marine mammals. *Experimental Brain Research* (Suppl. 8):227–238.

Mukhametov LM, Polyakov IG. 1981. Electroencephalographic study of sleep in sea of Azov porpoises. *Zhurnal vysshei nervnoi deiatelnosti imeni I P Pavlova* 31:333–339 (in Russian).

Mukhametov LM, Supin AY, Polyakova IG. 1977. Interhemispheric asymmetry of the electroencephalographic sleep patterns in dolphins. *Brain Research* 134:581–584.

Nagel EL, Morgane PJ, McFarland WL. 1964. Anesthesia for the bottlenose dolphin. *Science* 146:1591–1593.

Oleksenko AI, Mukhametov LM, Polyakova IG, Supin AY, Kovalzon VM. 1992. Unihemispheric sleep deprivation in bottlenose dolphins. *Journal of Sleep Research* 1:40–44.

Reidarson TH. 2003. Cetacean medicine. In: *Zoo and Wild Animal Medicine V* (M Fowler, ER Miller, eds.), pp. 442–459. Orlando: W.B. Saunders.

Ridgway SH. 1965. Medical care of marine mammals. *Journal of the American Veterinary Medical Association* 147:1077–1085.

Ridgway SH. 1972. Homeostasis in the aquatic environment. In: *Mammals of the Sea: Biology and Medicine* (SH Ridgway, ed.), pp. 590–747. Springfield: Charles C Thomas.

Ridgway SH. 2002. Asymmetry and symmetry in brain waves from dolphin left and right hemispheres: some observations after anesthesia, during quiescent hanging behavior, and during visual obstruction. *Brain, Behavior and Evolution* 60:265–274.

Ridgway SH, McCormick JG. 1967. Anesthetization of porpoises for major surgery. *Science* 158:510–512.

Ridgway SH, McCormick JG. 1971. Anesthesia of the porpoise. In: *Textbook of Veterinary Anesthesia* (LR Soma, ed.), pp. 394–403. Baltimore: Williams and Wilkins.

Ridgway SH, Patton GS. 1971. Dolphin thyroid: some anatomical and physiological findings. *Zeitschrift fur Vergleichende Physiologie* 71:129–141.

Ridgway SH, Scronce BL, Kanwisher J. 1969. Respiration and deep diving in the bottlenose porpoise. *Science* 166:1651–1654.

Ridgway SH, McCormick JG, Wever EG. 1974. Surgical approach to the dolphin's ear. *The Journal of Experimental Zoology* 188:265–276.

Ridgway SH, Green RF, Sweeney JC. 1975. Mandibular anesthesia and tooth extraction in the bottlenosed dolphin. *Journal of Wildlife Diseases* 11:415–418.

Ridgway SH, Houser D, Finneran JJ, Carder DA, Keogh M, Van Bonn W, Smith C, Scadeng M, Mattrey R, Hoh C. 2006. Functional imaging of dolphin brain metabolism and blood flow. *The Journal of Experimental Biology* 209:2902–2910.

Rieu M, Gautheron B. 1968. Preliminary observations concerning a method for introduction of a tube for anaesthesia in small delphinids. *Life Sciences* 7:1141–1146.

Rommel SA, Pabst DA, McLellan WA, Mead JG, Potter CW. 1992. Anatomical evidence for a countercurrent heat exchanger associated with dolphin testes. *The Anatomical Record* 232: 150–156.

Rommel SA, Pabst DA, McLellan WA. 1993. Functional morphology of the vascular plexuses associated with the cetacean uterus. *The Anatomical Record* 237:538–546.

Schroeder JP, Dawson WW, Cates MB. 1986. Dentistry and ophthalmology of the bottlenose and Risso's dolphin. International Association for Aquatic Animal Medicine Proceedings, 19, pp. 1–4.

Serafetinides EA, Shurley JT, Brooks RE. 1970. Electroencephalogram of the pilot whale, *Globicephala scammoni*, in wakefulness and sleep: lateralization aspects. *International Journal of Psychobiology* 2:129–133.

Simpson JG, Gardner MB. 1972. Comparative microscopic anatomy of selected marine mammals. In: *Mammals of the Sea: Biology and Medicine* (SH Ridgway, ed.), pp. 298–418. Springfield: Charles C Thomas.

Van Bonn WG, Jensen ED, Miller WG, Ridgway SH. 1996. Contemporary diagnostics and treatment of bottlenose dolphins: a case study. International Association for Aquatic Animal Medicine Proceedings, 29, pp. 40–42.

Votey SR, Bosse GM, Beyer MI, Hoffman JR. 1991. Flumazenil: a new benzodiazepine antagonist. *Annals of Emergency Medicine* 20:181–188.

White PF, Shafer A, Boyle WA, et al. 1989. Benzodiazepine antagonism does not provoke a stress response. *Anesthesiology* 70: 636–639.

50 Sirenians (Manatees and Dugongs)

Elizabeth C. Nolan and Michael T. Walsh

INTRODUCTION

Distributed throughout fresh, brackish, and marine tropical waters of North and South America and Africa, three species of manatees (Trichechidae) and one species of dugong (Dugongidae) comprise the family Sirenia (Table 50.1) (Domning & Hayek 1986; Reynolds & Odell 1991). Genetically related to elephants (Probosicidae) and hyrax (Hyracoidea), these hind gut fermenters are the sole obligate herbivores of the marine mammal world. Manatees are considered "weakly" social species, establishing no long term bonds other than mother–calf pairs and forming only temporary congregations of individuals during winter months at warm water sites or when breeding (Hartman 1979; Odell 2003; Reynolds 1981; Wells et al. 1999). Calves generally stay with their mothers for 1–2 years, and reach sexual maturity between 2 and 5 years of age (Odell 2003; U.S. Fish and Wildlife Service 2001) although this may be influenced as much by achieving biological size versus chronological age. In comparison, dugongs take approximately 9–10 years to reach sexual maturity and are often found in large herds with "amorphous" social organization, the only close identifiable social bonds being those between mother and calf (Odell 2002; Wells et al. 1999).

Due to habitat loss or degradation, human interaction problems, and natural disease in their home ranges, sirenians are currently listed under the Convention on International Trade in Endangered Species of Wild Fauna and Flora (CITES) Appendix I or II and the International Union for the Conservation of Nature (IUCN) Red List (Baillie et al. 2004; Reynolds & Odell 1991). The United States Endangered Species Act categorizes West Indian and Amazonian manatees and dugongs as endangered and the West African manatee as threatened (U.S. Fish and Wildlife Service 2001). Mortality associated with human interaction either due to hunting, watercraft interaction, or habitat loss is believed to have had significant impacts on sirenian populations, in general (Odell 2003; Reynolds & Odell 1991). Severe cold stress periods in 2010 and 2011 in Florida resulted in increased mortality for manatee populations with inadequate natural warm water refuges. Current conservation efforts for sirenians include worldwide public education campaigns, local and national legal protection, enhancement of warm water sites, and rescue and rehabilitation programs.

Medical advancements in the care of rescued sirenians have improved survivability and potential for reintroduction to the wild. The use of sedative agents was first applied in Florida manatees in the late 1980s and general anesthesia was first attempted in 1990 (Walsh et al. 1997). Anesthesia of manatees and dugongs is still an emerging field, but much has been recently learned to effectively sedate, anesthetize, and treat these species. The information presented in this chapter focuses predominately on the West Indian manatee, but likely has applications across the Sirenia family.

ANATOMY AND PHYSIOLOGY

Sirenians have a somewhat tubular body shape and a wide dorsoventrally flattened fluke that is paddle shaped in manatees and bilobed resembling a dolphin tail in dugongs. Whereas manatees tend to have more dorsoventrally flattened bodies, dugongs are more laterally compressed, particularly caudally. Sirenian skeletons are comprised of dense pachyostotic bone (Fawcett 1942a). They have relatively short but mobile pectoral flippers and lack hind limbs. Flippers of male

Zoo Animal and Wildlife Immobilization and Anesthesia, Second Edition. Edited by Gary West, Darryl Heard, and Nigel Caulkett.
© 2014 John Wiley & Sons, Inc. Published 2014 by John Wiley & Sons, Inc.

manatees are longer in length than those of females, and have more roughened epithelium medially, which likely aids in holding a female during copulation. Male manatees also tend to weigh less than females and have more lean body composition.

The skin of manatees is generally thick, tough, and sparsely haired, with the exception of the Amazonian manatee which has smooth skin (Domning & Hayek 1986; Reynolds & Odell 1991). Nill et al. (1999) found that the increased collagen network of the manatee dermis is roughly 2.5 times denser than that of terrestrial mammals. This unique skin density, along with their pachyostotic bones, helps counterbalance the positive buoyancy effects of the air-filled lungs and intralumenal gas of the gastrointestinal tract in these animals (Kipps et al. 2002; Nill et al. 1999).

Unique sirenian facial features include small eyes which close by a sphincter rather than upper and lower eyelids, a flexible upper lip and an oral disk covered with modified vibrissae for use when foraging, and nostrils with valves that close between breaths. Dentition varies between manatees and dugongs. While manatees horizontally replace their molars throughout life, dugongs do not. In addition, manatees lack functional incisors and premolars, whereas dugongs have both premolars and small tusk-like maxillary incisors (Reynolds & Odell 1991). In place of incisors, manatees have a dorsal dental pad which articulates with the lower jaw just caudal to a firm gingival ridge overlying the symphysis of the mandible. Due to manatees' relatively small mouth, laterally narrowed oral cavity, thick short tongue, and elongated soft palate, oral visualization of the glottis is very difficult. Even with maximal distension of the jaws in adult manatees, the glottis cannot usually be seen.

The manatee trachea is relatively short and bifurcates at the thoracic inlet into two separate pleural cavities or hemithorax. The specialized diaphragm of sirenians has a transverse septum separating the heart from the lungs and other organs, as well as two hemidiaphragms that horizontally extend the length of the body and divide the pleural spaces from the abdominal cavity (Rommel & Reynolds 2000). Unlike other marine mammals, manatee and dugong respiratory tracts comprise the dorsal third of their body cavity, extending from the shoulders to the pelvis and remaining dorsal to the heart (Fig. 50.1) (Rommel & Reynolds 2000). Due to this position of the lungs, IM injections are placed in the gluteal muscles to avoid injury to organs under more cranial epaxial musculature. Alternatively, IM injections can be administered in the caudal neck musculature, cranial to the shoulder. Another consideration with regards to the respiratory system of sirenians is the position of the gastrointestinal tract, which lies ventral to the thorax and can comprise 23% of an animal's weight (Reynolds & Rommel 1996). As hindgut fermenters, manatees have a distinct round cecum with

two ovoid diverticulae and an enlarged colon which aid with digestion of vegetation. In well-nourished animals, the cecum and large intestine together comprise approximately 10% of the body weight in dugongs and 14% in manatees (Marsh et al. 1977; Reynolds & Rommel 1996). The nutritional status of the animal and the amount of ingesta present in the intestinal tract can influence the respiratory capacity in the awake and sedated animal. When animals are removed from water for anesthetic procedures, pulmonary compression can occur from these internal organs and ventilatory variables must be closely monitored.

Respiratory adaptations for diving in sirenians are similar to those of other marine mammals. The terminal bronchioles of manatees are reinforced with cartilage (Pabst et al. 1999). Inspiration is closely paired with and follows forceful expiration, allowing animals to dive with replenished oxygen stores. Sirenians also have long interbreath intervals, which generally last 2–3 minutes in Florida manatees, but can extend as long as 24 minutes in "bottom resting" individuals (Reynolds 1981). In studies evaluating the response of Amazonian manatees to hypoxemia and hypercapnia in relation to respiratory drive, carbon dioxide rather than oxygen was concluded to be the "primary controller of ventilation and dive time" (Gallivan 1980). Similar to other marine mammal dive responses, dugongs and manatees develop bradycardia; however, it is generally characterized as "sluggish and modest" compared with that of cetaceans and pinnipeds (Elsner 1999; Scholander & Irving 1941).

The sirenian heart lies cranioventral to the lungs and anterior to the abdominal organs between the pectoral flippers. The heart rate can often be assessed by evaluating the skin pulse over this area when an animal is in ventrodorsal recumbency.

Unlike other marine mammals, West Indian manatee metabolic rates are 25–30% of predicted values and result in their unique warm water thermoregulatory requirements and relative cold intolerance (Irvine 1983; Worthy 2001). Amazonian manatees also have relatively low metabolic rates and limited capacity for thermogenesis (Gallivan et al. 1983). Depending on the season, Florida manatees are found in water ranging from 22°C (72°F) to over 32°C (90°F). While manatees may reside in water cooler than 21°C (70°F) during winter months, they have been observed to shiver at these temperatures and develop skin damage in temperatures ≤ 16°C (61 F). The degree of damage is dependent on length of cold water exposure, and the animal's nutritional state and size. Manatees ≤ 300 kg are physiologically less adaptable to cold stress than larger manatees; juveniles seem unable to increase their metabolic rates to compensate for cold temperatures ≤ 16°C (61°F) (Worthy 2001). For long term rehabilitation of manatees, water temperatures are generally maintained ≥24.5°C (76°F), although often raised to 27–29°C

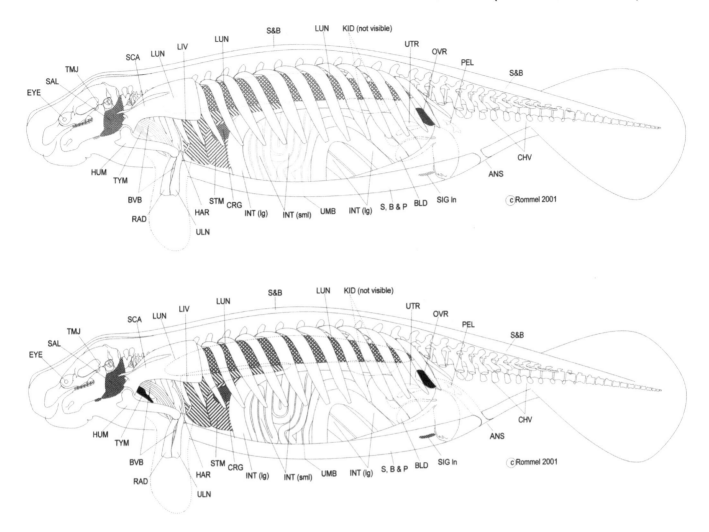

Figure 50.1. Florida manatee (*Trichechus manatus latirostris*) internal organ position. ANS, anus; BLD, urinary bladder; BVB, brachial vascular bundle; CRG, cardiac gland; CHV, chevrons; EYE, the eye; HAR, heart; HUM, humerus; INT, intestines; KID, left kidney, not visible from this vantage in the manatee; LIV, liver; LUN, lung; OVR, left ovary; PEL, pelvic vestige; RAD, radius; SAL, salivary gland; S&B, skin and blubber; SCA, scapula; SIG ln, superficial inguinal lymph node; S,B&P, skin, blubber, and panniculus muscle, cut at midline; STM, stomach; TMJ, temporomandibular joint; TYM, thymus gland; ULN, ulna; UMB, umbilical scar; UTR, uterine horn; VAG, vagina (used with permission, Dr. Sentinel Rommel).

(80–84°F) for neonates, cold stressed, or thin individuals. The recommended ambient air temperature for animals removed from the water for procedures is 22–26°C (72–79°F) (Bossart 2001). If ambient temperatures drop ≤20°C (68°F), time for out-of-water procedures is minimized to reduce exposure to cooler air. Water is often used to cool animals maintained out of water in warm ambient temperatures or in direct sunlight. In addition to thermoregulatory impacts, it has been suggested that the lower metabolic rate of sirenians has implications for drug metabolism, distribution, and elimination (Murphy 2003).

CAPTURE AND PHYSICAL RESTRAINT

To minimize injury to an animal or handlers, it is preferred that manatees are removed from the water for medical and surgical procedures. Acquisition of sick or injured wild manatees usually involves setting long nets to encircle, then "bag" an animal before pulling it onshore or into a boat. When working with nets in bodies of water, particular care is taken to avoid net entanglement of the animal(s) or personnel that lead to injury or drowning. Hoop netting has limited success with dugongs, and where regulatory and equipment constraints exist for handling this species, a "rodeo method" of capture in shallow open water has been described (Lanyon et al. 2006). Care is taken to minimize injury to animal handlers, as well as reduce dugong chase and handling time, and the potential development of fatal capture stress or myopathy (Marsh & Anderson 1983). The authors do not recommend this capture method for manatees.

In captive environments, physical restraint is accomplished using nets, dry docking with pool water drops, raising a medical pool floor above the water level, or

Table 50.1.   Family Sirenia

Genus and Species	Common Name	Length[a,b]	Mass[b]	Distribution
Dugong dugon	Dugong	Adults: 2.7 m average, up to 3.3 m Calves: 1–1.3 m	Adults: 250–300 kg average, up to 400 kg Calves: 20–35 kg	Coastal waters of Indo-Pacific
Trichechus senegalensis	West African manatee	Adults: 3–4 m	Adults: <500 kg	Coastal waters, rivers, and lakes of West-Central Africa
Trichechus inunguis	Amazonian manatee	Adults: 2.8–3 m Calves: 0.8–1 m	Adults: 450–480 kg Calves: 10–15 kg	Freshwater rivers and lakes of Amazonian basin
Trichechus manatus	West Indian manatee (two subspecies)			
Trichechus manatus manatus	Antillean manatee	Adults: 1.85–2.7 m, up to 3.5 m	Adults: max 1000 kg	West Indes, Caribbean, coastal waters and rivers of Mexico, Central America, Northeastern South America
Trichechus manatuslatirostris	Florida manatee	Adults: 2.7–4 m, average 3 m Calves: 1.2–1.4 m	Adults: 400–1775 kg, avg 400–600 kg males, max 1600 kg females Calves: 18–45 kg, average 30 kg	Coastal waters and rivers of Southeastern United States

[a]Straight length, snout to tail tip.
[b]Calf length and mass ranges at time of birth.
Sources: Converse et al. (1994); Domning and Hayek (1986); Murphy (2003); Nowak (1999); Odell (2002); Reynolds and Odell (1991); Walsh and Bossart (1999).

placing an animal within a stretcher. Whether in captivity or the wild, care is taken during any "catch-up" as these animals may actively avoid capture and restraint. The strong thrust of sirenian tails and often large body size (Table 50.1) make injury a possibility to both handlers and animals. Only trained personnel participate in the capture and restraint of sirenians.

While these animals spend their entire lives in water, they are capable of being sustained outside of the aquatic environment for a number of hours. Intermittently spraying with water throughout a procedure will help prevent skin desiccation and overheating, although their skin is much more resistant to drying than cetaceans. When "stranded" for diagnostics or therapeutics, animals are generally placed on closed or open cell foam to cushion their body mass and reduce pressure on internal organs. Animal position is adjusted with stretchers, boat sling straps (placed around the animal's body), cranes, and in smaller animals, manually. When animals are in sternal recumbency, a sheet of closed cell foam is placed over the dorsal aspect of the fluke for handlers to sit on and restrain the tail (Fig. 50.2). Handlers also position themselves on either side of the animal to prevent lateral movement. It is not uncommon for manatees to lie quietly either sternally or dorsoventrally during transport or nonpainful procedures. Care must be taken around the head and tail areas. Manatees can explosively resist restraint and are capable of touching the tips of their tails to their snouts and/or rolling quickly. Particularly fractious animals are secured to restraint boards or administered sedatives if necessary. In cases of thoracic trauma, where rib fractures exist, manatees may be sedated or strapped to

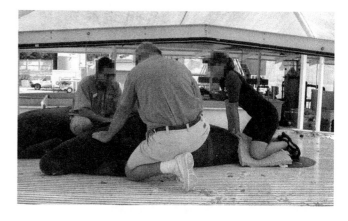

Figure 50.2.   Restraint of a Florida manatee (*Trichechus manatus latirostris*).

a board to minimize further damage to the chest during diagnostic or treatment procedures.

VASCULAR ACCESS

One of the few available vascular access sites in manatees includes a brachial vascular bundle comprised of a rete of veins and arteries in the interosseous space between the radius and ulna (Fawcett 1942b). This site is accessed from the medial or lateral sides of the pectoral flippers (Fig. 50.3a,b). A cephalic vessel has been accessed in one anesthetized Florida manatee (J. Bailey, pers. comm., 2011), and, historically, blood has been collected from the distal humeral region although this has not been investigated further. A caudal tail ventral

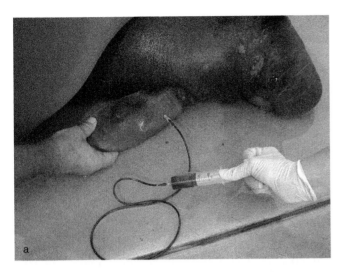

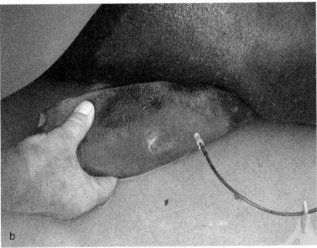

Figure 50.3. (a and b) Brachial vascular bundle venipuncture site in a Florida manatee calf (*Trichechus manatus latirostris*).

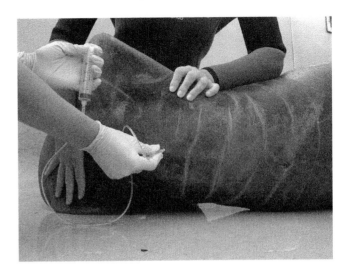

Figure 50.4. Caudal tail vascular bundle venipuncture site of the Florida manatee calf (*Trichechus manatus latirostris*).

vertebral arch vascular bundle is also available for venipuncture, particularly in younger animals where pectoral vessels are small (Fig. 50.4). Care is taken when using this caudal tail site for IV access in unanesthetized animals, since forward thrust of the fluke could injure the phlebotomist. Due to the potential danger from the fluke, this site is generally not used in awake individuals except for compromised neonates.

Spinal needles may be used to obtain IV access for drug and fluid administration in anesthetized adult manatees in the caudal tail vascular bundle. This site is accessed by elevating the tail to visualize its ventral aspect or placing the animal in lateral or dorsoventral recumbency. Tissue glue may be used to secure needles in place. Calves that are easily restrained due to size or illness are catheterized awake in the caudal tail site with 20- or 21-gauge 3.75- to 5-cm (1.5–2 in) needles. The brachial vascular bundle is difficult to catheterize due to needle placement perpendicular to the arteriovenous plexus. It is accomplished with 18-gauge 5-cm

(2 in) needles in adults and 20-gauge 3.75-cm (1.5 in) needles in juveniles (Murphy 2003). Although the pectoral flippers can be catheterized either medially or laterally, contact between the body wall and a medially placed catheter may displace it. Perivascular leakage of drugs can occur, potentially resulting in local tissue inflammation or necrosis. To reduce the likelihood of catheter displacement, venous access is best attempted after sedative administration, tracheal intubation, and/or final patient positioning for a medical or surgical procedure. During fluid administration, closely monitoring flow rates and observing vascular access sites for swelling are recommended.

ENDOTRACHEAL INTUBATION

Manatees can occasionally be intubated under midazolam or midazolam/butorphanol sedation at higher dosages, but others may require anesthetic induction with an inhalant administered by mask prior to endotracheal tube passage. Mask administration is usually done with a modified 20-L (5 gal) clear plastic water jug with the bottom removed. The edges are padded for a tighter fit over the animal's head (Walsh & Bossart 1999). A large mask allows adequate tidal volume exchange with less resistance to rapid inspiration. Even in sedated manatees, breath holding during mask induction can occur. The manatee patient may require stimulation, such as rocking side to side, to facilitate additional respirations during mask induction. Animals inadequately sedated for intubation will often respond to sound, open their eyes partially, or retract their head when stimulated.

For intubation, a manatee's trachea can be accessed, at least theoretically, from both the oral or nasal cavities. Initial attempts at oral intubation in manatees were historically unsuccessful. Given the poor visualization of the caudal pharynx and larynx due to the curved angle of the tongue, the narrow width of the buccal cavity, and the long soft palate, nasal intubation is preferred. Nasogastric tubes can be passed blindly in manatees, but dependable tracheal intubation is best accomplished with rhinoscopic assistance. Wild sirenians commonly have mild to heavy loads of nasopharyngeal trematodes, and in some cases, heavy parasitic infestations cause severe rhinitis or tracheitis and complicate intubation (Beck & Forrester 1988; Bossart 2001). In Florida manatees, it is recommended to use cuffed elongated foal endotracheal tubes (8- to14-mm internal diameter, based on the size of the animal) for intubation. Stylets may be used to assist passage of the tube into the laryngeal opening (Murphy 2003; Walsh & Bossart 1999). Due to the short length of the manatee trachea, however, intubation of a single bronchus can occur. Preplacing the endotracheal tube over the end of a bronchoscope and using the bronchoscope to guide the tube past the loose palatopharyngeal tissues into the trachea allow visual confirmation of proper positioning. An additional benefit of the bronchoscope's small diameter is that it can be gently passed into the trachea even when the glottis is closed, allowing quick and minimally traumatic intubation. Breath holding and the periodic, brief opening of the glottis in a sedated manatee can result in multiple attempts for successful intubation using other methods. Regardless of the method used to intubate manatees, bronchoscopic confirmation of endotracheal tube placement cranial to the carina is recommended. The endotracheal tube is secured to the muzzle with white waterproof tape strips secured to white tape encircling the muzzle caudal to the oral disk (Fig. 50.5). Periodic suctioning of endotracheal tubes is required to remove mucous that accumulates in the tube (Walsh & Bossart 1999). Once intubated, sirenians can be maintained

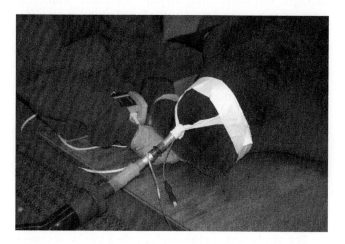

Figure 50.5.   Endotracheal tube securing on muzzle of a Florida manatee (*Trichechus manatus latirostris*).

with isoflurane levels similar to those used in domestic animals (Table 50.2).

PREANESTHETIC CONSIDERATIONS

Similar to other mammals, sirenians are physically examined and their bloodwork is evaluated prior to anesthesia to identify any health conditions that would pose risks. Florida manatees present to rescue and rehabilitation programs with a variety of injuries and illnesses secondary to both natural and human causes, as have been described in previous mortality studies (Ackerman et al. 1995; Bossart et al. 2004; O'Shea et al. 1985; U.S. Fish and Wildlife Service 2001; Walsh & Bossart 1999). Two of the more commonly seen naturally occurring conditions in Florida manatees are cold stress and brevetoxicosis. Traumatic injuries from crab trap, monofilament line entanglement, and boat strike are also common presentations to rescue and rehabilitation programs. Understanding the extent of illness or injury is critical to assessing the anesthetic risk to a manatee patient.

Prior to anesthesia, sirenians are ideally fasted for 24 hours to reduce the likelihood of regurgitation. However, these species have a slow gut transit time (4–7 days in the Florida and 5–9 days in the Amazonian manatee), so complete emptying of the gastrointestinal tract (GIT) in 24 hours does not occur (Gallivan & Best 1986; Walsh & Bossart 1999).

Respiratory rates are monitored prior to sedation and through the induction procedure. In sirenians, respirations are counted over 5 minutes to determine a rate because they are usually ≤1 breath/min. If a manatee in the water shows signs of depression or incoordination after sedatives are administered, it is removed prior to the usual 20–25 minutes before handling. In animals with pulmonary compromise, oxygen supplementation with a portable oxygen tank and Hudson or Elder demand valve is often provided during short sedative procedures or prior to administration of general anesthesia.

INDUCTION/MAINTENANCE PROTOCOLS

Reported anesthetic drugs and dosages are listed in Table 50.2. It has been suggested that the relatively low metabolic rate of sirenians may contribute to their apparent sensitivity to sedative and opioid drugs compared with terrestrial mammals (Murphy 2003) but further work has shown that manatees can be successfully sedated with similar dosages of some drugs. Diazepam and midazolam have been used extensively for both mild and preoperative sedation. Meperidine has also been used in conjunction with benzodiazepines for more fractious individuals or for procedures that may result in surgical discomfort. In captive environments, after administration of these sedatives, animals are often placed back in

Table 50.2. Analgesic, anesthetic, and reversal agents for the Florida manatee (*Trichechus manatus latirostris*)

Agent	Use	Dosage	Comments	Reference
Atipamezole	Reversal	1 mg/20 mg of xylazine IV	For xylazine reversal	Murphy (2003)
		1 mg/2 mg of detomidine IV	For detomidine reversal	Murphy (2003)
		5 mg/1 mg of detomidine IM	For detomidine reversal	
Butorphanol	Sedative, analgesic	0.01–0.025 mg/kg IV	In combination with diazepam for mild painful procedures, anesthetic induction, give butorphanol 10 minutes prior to diazepam	Murphy (2003)
		0.005–0.01 mg/kg IV	In combination with detomidine for minor surgical procedures or anesthetic induction	Murphy (2003)
		0.0086 mg/kg IM	In combination with detomidine for heavier sedation, +/− intubation	
		0.04–0.06 mg/kg IM	With midazolam 0.1 mg/kg IM for anesthesia induction or for short procedures involving fractious individuals	M.T. Walsh and A.D. Bukowski, pers. comm., 2010
		0.1 mg/kg IM	With midazolam 0.1 mg/kg IM for anesthesia induction in severely fractious individuals, results in very deep sedation, use with caution	M.T. Walsh et al., pers. comm., 2010b
Detomidine	Sedative	0.005–0.01 mg/kg IV	Moderate sedation, beware of narrow therapeutic index, cardiac and blood pressure effects not noted	Murphy (2003)
		0.025–0.005 mg/kg IV	In combination with butorphanol, excellent analgesia and muscle relaxation, beware of narrow therapeutic index	Murphy (2003)
		0.0086 mg/kg IM	In combination with butorphanol for heavier sedation, +/− intubation	
Diazepam	Sedative	0.02–0.035 mg/kg IV	For nonpainful diagnostics	Murphy (2003)
		0.01–0.025 mg/kg IV	In combination with butorphanol for mild to moderate painful procedures	Murphy (2003)
		0.066 mg/kg IM	For tranquilization, lasts 60–90 minutes	Bossart (2001)
Flumazenil	Reversal	1 mg/10–20 mg of midazolam or diazepam IV	Reversal for midazolam or diazepam	Murphy (2003)
		Equal volume as midazolam IM	Reversal for midazolam may require redosing after long procedure	Walsh and Bossart (1999)
		Equal volume as diazepam IM	Reversal for diazepam	Bossart (2001)
Isoflurane	Anesthetic	0.5–5%	Similar settings as in domestic animals	Walsh and Bossart (1999)
Ketoprofen	Analgesic	1–2 mg/kg IM	Analgesia for severe abdominal pain. Authors' note: caution in dehydrated animals, side effects not well documented in this species	R. Ball, pers. comm., 2011
Lidocaine 2%	Analgesic	Local infusion to effect	Local analgesia	
Meperidine	Sedative, analgesic	Up to 1 mg/kg IM	In combination with midazolam for more painful procedures or anesthetic induction	Walsh and Bossart (1999)
		0.5–1 mg/kg IM	Sedation/analgesia for minor surgical procedures	Bossart (2001)
Midazolam	Sedative	0.02–0.05 mg/kg IM	Mild to moderate sedation	Murphy (2003)
		0.045 mg/kg IM	Sedation for 60–90 minutes can also use in conjunction with meperidine for more painful procedures or anesthetic induction	Walsh and Bossart (1999)
		0.05–0.072 mg/kg IM	Sedation for 20–30 minutes at peak effect for endoscopy, freeze branding, or noninvasive procedures	R. Ball, pers. comm., 2011
		0.08 mg/kg IM	Anesthetic induction, intubation	Walsh and Bossart (1999)
		0.1 mg/kg IM	Anesthetic induction, in combination with butorphanol	M.T. Walsh et al., pers. comm., 2010a
Naltrexone	Reversal	1–2 mg/1 mg of butorphanol IV, IM	Reversal for butorphanol	Murphy (2003)
		Equal volume dose as meperidine IM	Reversal for meperidine	
Xylazine	Sedative	0.05–0.1 mg/kg IM	Moderate sedation, beware of narrow therapeutic index	Murphy (2003)
Xylocaine 1%	Epidural anesthetic	Dose not noted, epidural	Used in one case for vertebral fracture surgery	Bossart (2001)
Yohimbine	Reversal	1 mg/5–10 mg of xylazine IV	Reversal for xylazine	Murphy (2003)
		2–3 mg/1 mg of detomidine IV	Reversal for detomidine	Murphy (2003)
		IM at the above dosages	Reversal for xylazine, detomidine	

IM, intramuscular; IV, intravenous.

shallow water pools to allow the agent to take effect and minimize the effects of restraint overriding the sedative, in particular, the benzodiazepines. Sirenians are monitored closely with higher sedative dosages for evidence of hypoventilation or reduced ability to surface to breathe. A combination of detomidine (0.017 mg/kg IM) and butorphanol (0.017 mg/kg IM) resulted in marked respiratory depression in a 700-kg female Florida manatee (D. Neiffer and A. Stamper, pers. comm., 2006). Intravenous administration of yohimbine/naltrexone/supplemental atipamezole reversed the respiratory effects. Manatees have subsequently been sedated with lower dosages of detomidine (0.0085 mg/kg IM) and butorphanol (0.0085 mg/kg IM) without adverse side effects (D. Neiffer and A. Stamper, pers. comm., 2006). In one instance of a manatee sedated with this detomidine/butorphanol combination, an additional 0.017-mg/kg midazolam IV was administered to achieve adequate sedation for intubation.

Local infusion of 2% lidocaine at a surgical site is effective, in conjunction with sedation, for analgesia in minor procedures. Epidural administration of 1% lidocaine has been reported once in a manatee undergoing spinal surgery for a vertebral fracture (Bossart 2001). Other analgesic agents used in sirenians include nonsteroidal anti-inflammatory drugs, but care is taken to avoid gastrointestinal upset with these drugs by minimizing dosage and frequency of use. Intramuscular flunixin meglumine is not used for more than a few days in succession to avoid gastrointestinal or renal compromise. Butorphanol has also been administered for analgesia either intra or post operatively in West Indian manatees.

Sedative or analgesic drugs are administered IM or IV. Onset of drug effects after IM injection is approximately 15–20 minutes (Bossart 2001), although maximum effect may not occur until 25 minutes in some individuals. Due to the thickness of the skin and subcutaneous blubber, needles are advanced perpendicularly and forcefully to reach the deep layers of the lumbar epaxial musculature for injection of sedatives. For adult Florida manatees, 18-gauge 8.75-cm (3.5 in.) spinal needles are used to administer drugs IM, whereas 20- or 21-gauge 3.75- to 5-cm (1.5–2 in.) needles are used in calves. When administering IM injections in the caudal neck region, 18-gauge 3.75-cm (1.5 in.) or 21-gauge 5-cm (2 in.) are used on adult manatees. The individual administering the drug keeps pressure on the syringe plunger to avoid reflux of sedative back into the syringe. Digital pressure is applied to the injection site to avoid drug leakage after removal of the needle.

Mechanically assisted ventilation is preferred over manually assisted ventilation during general anesthesia to maintain adequate gas exchange and oxygenation. For shorter sedative procedures without inhalant anesthesia, oxygen supplementation is accomplished with an oxygen demand valve. When mechanically ventilat-ing a manatee, some unique anatomical and physiological traits need be considered. Mechanical ventilation does not mimic the sirenian respiratory cycle of inspiration closely following expiration. Rather, it reverses the cycle with expiration closely following inspiration. Higher respiratory rates on mechanical ventilators shorten time of lung inflation in a breath-holding species and leads to hypoventilation and hypercapnia. In the authors' experience, a slow inspiratory flow rate improves oxygenation while decreasing carbon dioxide accumulation.

In manatees, pulmonary resistance is increased from other organs when they are removed from the water. In dorsoventral recumbency, the ventilator must counter the weight and pressure of abdominal organs and ingesta on the lungs. In sternal recumbency, the ventilator must also provide enough pressure to inflate the lungs despite limited lateral mobility of the pachyostotic ribs and ventral pressure from abdominal organs. Pulmonary resistance is further increased by loss of lung function from concurrent respiratory disease (e.g., severe pyothorax, pneumothorax, or pulmonary fibrosis or adhesions secondary to thoracic trauma). In these cases, it may be difficult to alleviate hypercapnia or hypoxemia due to loss of functional tissue. In some cases, whether due to disease or patient positioning, the peak inspiratory pressure of the ventilator must be adjusted above 20 mmHg to achieve lung expansion, oxygenation, and carbon dioxide exchange. Close monitoring of physiological variables will determine the most appropriate ventilatory settings. Ventilations are initially set at 6 breaths/min (Murphy 2003). Doxapram (IV, IM) has been administered to improve respiration in sedated and anesthetized manatees although this approach should not be considered a substitute for proper ventilation management.

MONITORING

Manatees are closely monitored during sedation and anesthesia using standard techniques or modalities used in domestic animals (Chapter 3). Anesthetic depth is determined by assessing blink response, jaw tone, and resistance to limb movement. Eye position is often difficult to assess due to recession of the globe into the orbit during anesthesia.

Physiological variables of the Florida manatee are listed in Table 50.3. Heart rates are calculated by listening to the heart with a stethoscope, placing a Doppler on the skin near the heart, or observing the pulsation of the skin overlying the heart when animals are positioned in dorsoventral recumbency. Electrocardiography, either by esophageal probe or pad/needle placement of leads on skin, is used for assessment of cardiac rate and rhythm (Siegal-Willott et al. 2006). If esophageal probes are inserted orally, care is taken to prevent the probe inadvertently being advanced into

Table 50.3. Physiological parameters for the Florida manatee (*Trichechus manatus latirostris*)

Parameter	Range
Respiratory rate	Variable, average 2–4 breaths/5 min in water, 3–15 breaths/5 min out of water
Heart rate	40–60 beats/min (can be as low as 30 with diving)
Body temperature	35.5–36°C[a]
Tidal volume	2.9% of body weight[b]
Lung volume	Approximately 5% of total body weight

[a]Oral temperatures. Note that body temperatures are dependent on environmental water temperatures as well as site of thermometer placement.

[b]Based on Scholander and Irving's work, $N = 2$.

Sources: Murphy (2003); Pabst et al. (1999); Scholander and Irving (1941); Walsh and Bossart (1999).

the trachea instead of the esophagus. It may be prudent to verify placement with a bronchoscope. Placement of a pulse oximetry probe on the tongue is difficult because of the short, thick shape and reduced mobility of sirenian tongues and their firm attachment to the lower jaw (Levin & Pfeiffer 2002; Yamasaki et al. 1980). Pulse oximetry readings are occasionally collected from the nasal septum, buccal mucosa, or rostral gingival ridge of the lower jaw. Rectal reflectance pulse oximetry probes are placed in the nostril to obtain saturation readings. Gingival capillary refill time is generally ≤2 seconds in manatees.

Body temperature is measured with a rectal, oral, or nasal probe. Flexible rectal thermometers are difficult to place due to high sphincter tone and the fibrous consistency of feces obstructing advancement into the colon. Rectal temperatures may read lower than core temperatures for these reasons (Irvine 1983). Nasal passage of flexible probes is relatively easy; however, inhalation can result in spurious results due to mixture with ambient air. Oral placement of thermometers alongside the caudal buccal mucosa appears to give fairly accurate results although also lower than core body temperature. Equipment damage from the molars or accidental advancement into the trachea must be avoided.

End tidal carbon dioxide (ETCO$_2$) levels follow those of other mammals', yet no scientific study has been reported, to the authors' knowledge, to correlate results with arterial blood gases. Samples for blood gas analysis have been collected from manatees, but the arteriovenous plexus in the pectoral flipper makes interpretation difficult. Venous or mixed samples are still diagnostically valuable when the animal is used as its own control during the procedure.

RECOVERY CONSIDERATIONS

Following recovery from anesthesia, manatees are not placed in water until they are appropriately responding

to stimuli and breathing voluntarily. If possible, animals are placed in shallow water (≤1 m) so they are able to surface to breathe by pushing off the pool floor with their pectoral flippers.

The unique anatomy, physiology, and aquatic environment of sirenians make sedation and anesthesia challenging. Continued efforts to develop knowledge of sirenian anesthesia are important to advance conservation efforts and improve our ability to treat sick and injured animals.

ACKNOWLEDGMENTS

The authors would like to thank Dr. Dan Odell and Dr. Sentinel Rommel for their help in manuscript preparation, and Carol Swain for her photographic assistance. We would also like to thank the staff members of the SeaWorld Orlando Veterinary and Animal Care Departments for their photographic contributions and their help and support in the development of Florida manatee anesthesia techniques. Additional thanks to the Disney Department of Animal Health and the Seas Marine Mammal Department for their help and support with advancing our knowledge of Florida manatee anesthesia.

REFERENCES

Ackerman BB, Wright SD, Bonde RK, Odell DK, Banowetz DJ. 1995. Trends and patterns in mortality of manatees in Florida, 1974–1992. In: *Population Biology of the Florida Manatee (Information and Technology Report 1)* (TJ O'Shea, BB Ackerman, HF Percival, eds.), pp. 223–258. Washington, DC: U.S. Department of the Interior, National Biological Service.

Baillie JEM, Hilton-Taylor C, Stuart SN, eds. 2004. *2004 IUCN Red List of Threatened Species. A Global Species Assessment*, pp. 1–217. IUCN, Gland and Cambridge.

Beck C, Forrester DJ. 1988. Helminths of the Florida manatee, *Trichechus manatus latirostris*, with a discussion and summary of the parasites of sirenians. *Journal of Parasitology* 74(4): 628–637.

Bossart GD. 2001. Manatees. In: *CRC Handbook of Marine Mammal Medicine*, 2nd ed. (LA Dierauf, FMD Gulland, eds.), pp. 939–960. Boca Raton: CRC Press.

Bossart GD, Meisner RA, Rommel SA, Lightsey JD, Varela RA, Defran RH. 2004. Pathologic findings in Florida manatees (*Trichechus manatus latirostris*). *Aquatic Mammals* 30(3):434–440.

Converse LJ, Fernandes BS, MacWilliams PS, Bossart GD. 1994. Hematology, serum chemistry, and morphometric reference values for Antillean manatees (*Trichechus manatus manatus*). *Journal of Zoo and Wildlife Medicine* 25(3):423–431.

Domning DP, Hayek LAC. 1986. Interspecific and intraspecific morphological variation in manatees (Sirenia: *Trichechus*). *Marine Mammal Science* 2:87–144.

Elsner R. 1999. Living in water: solutions to physiological problems. In: *Biology of Marine Mammals* (JE Reynolds III, SA Rommel, eds.), pp. 73–116. Washington, DC: Smithsonian Institution Press.

Fawcett DW. 1942a. The amedullary bones of the Florida manatee (*Trichechus latirostris*). *The American Journal of Anatomy* 71 (2):271–309.

Fawcett DW. 1942b. A comparative study of blood-vascular bundles in the Florida manatee (*Trichechus latirostris*) and in certain cetaceans and edentates. *Journal of Morphology* 71(1): 105–133.

Gallivan GJ. 1980. Hypoxia and hypercapnia in the respiratory control of the Amazonian manatee (*Trichechus inunguis*). *Physiological Zoology* 53(3):254–261.

Gallivan GJ, Best RC. 1986. The influence of feeding and fasting on the metabolic rate and ventilation of the Amazonian manatee (*Trichechus inunguis*). *Physiological Zoology* 59(5): 552–557.

Gallivan GJ, Best RC, Kanwisher JW. 1983. Temperature regulation in the Amazonian manatee *Trichechus inunguis*. *Physiological Zoology* 56(2):255–262.

Hartman DS. 1979. *Ecology and Behavior of the Manatee (*Trichechus manatus*) in Florida*, pp. 1–153. Special publication No. 5. Pittsburgh: The American Society of Mammalogists.

Irvine AB. 1983. Manatee metabolism and its influence on distribution in Florida. *Biological Conservation* 25:315–334.

Kipps EK, McLellan WA, Rommel SA, Pabst DA. 2002. Skin density and its influence on buoyancy in the manatee (*Trichechus manatus latirostris*), harbor porpoise (*Phocoena phocoena*), and bottlenose dolphin (*Tursiops truncatus*). *Marine Mammal Science* 18(3):765–778.

Lanyon JM, Slade RW, Sneath HL, Broderick D, Kirkwood JM, Limpus D, Limpus CJ, Jessop T. 2006. A method for capturing dugongs (*Dugong dugon*) in open water. *Aquatic Mammals* 32(2): 196–201.

Levin MJ, Pfeiffer CJ. 2002. Gross and microscopic observations on the lingual structure of the Florida manatee *Trichechus manatus latirostris*. *Anatomia, Histologia, Embryologia* 31:278–285.

Marsh H, Anderson PK. 1983. Probable susceptibility of dugongs to capture stress. *Biological Conservation* 25(1):1–3.

Marsh H, Heinsohn GE, Spain AV. 1977. The stomach and duodenal diveticula of the dugong (*Dugong dugon*). In: *Functional Anatomy of Marine Mammals*, Vol. 3 (RJ Harrison, ed.), pp. 271–295. New York: Academic Press.

Murphy D. 2003. Sirenia. In: *Zoo and Wild Animal Medicine*, 5th ed. (ME Fowler, RE Miller, eds.), pp. 476–482. Saint Louis: Elsevier Science.

Nill EK, Pabst DA, Rommel SA, McLellan WA. 1999. Does the thick skin of the Florida manatee provide ballast? *American Zoologist* 39(5):114A.

Nowak RM. 1999. Order Sirenia. In: *Walker's Mammals of the World*, Vol. II, 6th ed., pp. 982–992. Baltimore: The Johns Hopkins University Press.

Odell DK. 2002. Sirenian life history. In: *Encyclopedia of Marine Mammals* (WF Perrin, B Würsig, JGM Thewissen, eds.), pp. 1086–1088. San Diego: Academic Press.

Odell DK. 2003. West Indian manatee: *Trichechus manatus*, Chapter 40. In: *Wild Mammals of North America*, 2nd ed. (GC Feldhamer, BC Thompson, JA Chapman, eds.), pp. 855–864. Baltimore: Johns Hopkins University Press.

O'Shea TJ, Beck CA, Bonde RK, Kochman HI, Odell DK. 1985. An analysis of manatee mortality patterns in Florida, 1976–81. *Journal of Wildlife Management* 49(1):1–11.

Pabst DA, Rommel SA, McLellan WA. 1999. The functional morphology of marine mammals. In: *Biology of Marine Mammals* (JE Reynolds III, SA Rommel, eds.), pp. 15–72. Washington, D.C.: Smithsonian Institution Press.

Reynolds JE III. 1981. Behavior patterns in the West Indian manatee, with emphasis on feeding and diving. *Florida Scientist* 44:233–242.

Reynolds JE III, Odell DK. 1991. *Manatees and Dugongs*, pp. 1–192. New York: Facts on File, Inc.

Reynolds JE III, Rommel SA. 1996. Structure and function of the gastrointestinal tract of the Florida manatee, *Trichechus manatus latrostris*. *Anatomical Record* 245:539–558.

Rommel SA, Reynolds JE III. 2000. Diaphragm structure and function in the Florida manatee (*Trichechus manatus latirostris*). *Anatomical Record* 259:41–51.

Scholander PF, Irving L. 1941. Experimental investigations on the respiration and diving of the Florida manatee. *Journal of Cellular and Comparative Physiology* 17(2):169–191.

Siegal-Willott J, Estrada A, Bonde R, Wong A, Estrada DJ, Harr K. 2006. Electrocardiography in two subspecies of manatee (*Trichechus manatus latirostris* and *T. m. manatus*). *Journal of Zoo and Wildlife Medicine* 37(4):447–453.

U.S. Fish and Wildlife Service. 2001. Florida manatee recovery plan, (*Trichechus manatus latirostris*), 3rd revision. U.S. Fish and Wildlife Service, Atlanta, GA, pp. 1–144.

Walsh MT, Bossart GD. 1999. Manatee medicine. In: *Zoo & Wild Animal Medicine, Current Therapy*, 4th ed. (ME Fowler, RE Miller, eds.), pp. 507–516. Philadelphia: W.B. Saunders.

Walsh MT, Webb A, Bailey J, Campbell TW. 1997. Sedation and anesthesia of the Florida manatee (*Trichechus manatus*). *IAAAM Proceedings*, 28, pp. 12–13.

Wells RS, Boness DJ, Ratheun GB. 1999. Behavior. In: *Biology of Marine Mammals* (JE Reynolds III, SA Rommel, eds.), pp. 324–422. Washington, DC: Smithsonian Institution Press.

Worthy GAJ. 2001. Nutrition and energetics. In: *CRC Handbook of Marine Mammal Medicine*, 2nd ed. (LA Dierauf, FMD Gulland, eds.), pp. 791–828. Boca Raton: CRC Press.

Yamasaki FS, Komatsu S, Kamiya T. 1980. A comparative morphological study on the tongues of manatee and dugong (Sirenia). *The Scientific Reports of the Whales Research Institute* 32:127–144.

51 Elephants

William A. Horne and Michael R. Loomis

Elephants belong to the order Proboscidae, family Elephantidae. There are two surviving genera: *Loxodonta*, the African elephant, and *Elephas*, the Asian elephant. The genus *Elephas* consists of a single species with three subspecies: *Elephas maximus indicus*, the Indian elephant; *Elephas maximus maximus*, the Sri Lankan elephant; and *Elephas maximus sumatranus*, the Sumatran elephant. A fourth subspecies, *Elephas maximus borneensis*, has recently been proposed based on genetic studies (Fernando et al. 2003).

The genus *Loxodonta* is generally considered to be divided into two species: *Loxodonta africana*, the savanna or bush elephant, and *Loxodonta cyclotis*, the forest elephant (Roca et al. 2001). A third species (or possibly a subspecies), the West African elephant, has been proposed based on recent genetic studies (Eggert et al. 2002). Table 51.1 gives geographic ranges, heights, and weights of the different elephant taxa.

As of August 2011, 606 Asian elephants and 382 African elephants were registered with the International Species Information System (ISIS). Recent estimates for numbers of free-ranging elephants are 400,000–500,000 African elephants (Blanc et al. 2007) and 35,000–50,000 Asian elephants (Focus 2005). These numbers indicate that the captive elephant population has nearly doubled in the last 15 years, and that estimates of wild elephant populations have declined by 30% (compared with Kock et al. 1993). Both captive and free-ranging elephants require sedation and anesthesia for a variety of reasons (Table 51.2). In captivity, elephants are sedated or anesthetized predominately for medical reasons (though operant conditioning has allowed many minor procedures to be performed without anesthesia or sedation). These reasons are numerous and include a range of activities from dental work on tusks to caesarian section.

Captive elephants also require long-term analgesia. In the coming decade, more than 50% of all captive elephants will be 40 years old or older; osteomyelitis in the bones of the feet has been a significant cause of morbidity, often leading to euthanasia, in elephants of this age group.

By far, however, the vast majority of anesthetic episodes occur in free-ranging populations. These episodes generally involve translocations, various types of research, disease surveillance, and tracking-collar deployment for monitoring movement and land use patterns (Fig. 51.1). Occasionally, free-ranging elephants are anesthetized for medical procedures, such as removing a snare from a foot.

GENERAL CONSIDERATIONS FOR ELEPHANT SEDATION AND ANESTHESIA

Herd and Reproductive Behavior

Social structure and reproductive behavior must be considered in planning for anesthetic procedures both in field and captive settings. Elephants are long-lived (up to 65 years in the wild, 50 years in captivity), highly social animals that live in matrilineal family groups. The family group is lead by a matriarch, who is generally the oldest and tallest female in the group. The group (Fig. 51.2, *top*) consists of the matriarch and her descendants, her sisters and their daughters and their offspring. Males are driven from the family group before reaching sexual maturity (12–15 years) and live alone or in small dynamic groups.

With age, females acquire social knowledge that benefits the entire group. For example, groups with older matriarchs have higher per capita reproductive success (McComb et al. 2001). Moreover, matriarchs retain geographical memories that define the home

Zoo Animal and Wildlife Immobilization and Anesthesia, Second Edition. Edited by Gary West, Darryl Heard, and Nigel Caulkett.

Table 51.1. Geographic distribution, height, and weight of officially recognized elephant taxa

Taxonomic Designation	Common Name	Geographic Range	Weight (kg)	Height (m)
Elephas maximus indicus	Mainland or Indian elephant	Indian Subcontinent, Southeast Asia, Peninsular Malaysia	2000–5000	2.5–3.5
Elephas maximus maximus	Sri Lankan elephant	Island of Sri Lanka	2000–5500	2.5–3.5
Elephas maximus sumatranus	Sumatran elephant	Island of Sumatra, Indonesia	2000–4000	2.5–3.2
Loxodonta africana[a]	Savanna or bush elephant	East and South Africa	4000–7000	3.0–4.0
Loxodonta cyclotis[a]	Forest elephant	Central and West Africa	2000–4500	2–3

[a]Ranges may overlap somewhat.

Table 51.2. Procedures requiring elephant sedation or anesthesia

Procedure(s)	Drug Protocol	Reference
Captive elephants: standing sedation		
Transport (juveniles)	Xylazine and ketamine	Heard et al. (1988)[a]
Abscess treatment, venipuncture, TB testing, manual ejaculation	Azaperone with local anesthetics	Ramsay (2000)[a]
Aggressive abscess debridement	Azaperone and butorphanol	Ramsay (2000)[a]
Trailer loading, cow-calf separation	Xylazine	Abou-Madi et al. 2004[c]; Ramsay (2000)[a]
Tumor excision, wound dressing, subconjunctival injection	Medetomidine	Sarma et al. (2002)[c]
Captive elephants: recumbent immobilization		
Radiographs/dental (juveniles)	Etorphine and halothane	Heard et al. (1988)[a]
Castration	Etorphine	Fowler and Hart (1973)[c]
Electroejaculation	Etorphine	Hattingh et al. (1994)[a]
Fractured tusk management/repair	Etorphine	Allen et al. (1984)[a]
	Etorphine and halothane	Stegmann (1999)[a]; Tamas and Geiser (1983)[a]
	Etorphine and isoflurane	Dunlop et al. (1994)[a]
Sole abscess	Xylazine and ketamine followed by etorphine and acepromazine	Ollivet-Courtois et al. (2003)[c]
Removal of infected phalanges	Etorphine and isoflurane	Gage et al. (1997)[c]
Umbilical herniorrhaphy (juvenile)	Xylazine, diazepam, ketamine, and isoflurane	Abou-Madi et al. (2004)[c]
Free-ranging elephants: recumbent immobilization		
Translocation (juveniles)	Etorphine and azaperone	Still et al. (1996)[a]
Laproscopic reproductive sterilization	Etorphine and azaperone	Stetter et al. (2005)[a]
Deployment of satellite and/or radio tracking collars	Etorphine	Elkan et al. (1998)[b]; Horne et al. (2001)[a]; Kock et al. (1993)[a]; Osofsky (1997)[a]; Tchamba et al. (1995)[a]
	Etorphine and acepromazine	Dangolla et al. (2004)[c]; Elkan et al. (1998)[b]
	Carfentanil	Elkan et al. (1998)[b]

Notes: All elephants were adults unless otherwise indicated.
Species of elephant sedated or anesthetized in the selected references:
[a]*Loxodonta africana,* the African savanna or bush elephant.
[b]*Loxodonta cyclotis,* the African forest elephant.
[c]*Elephas maximus,* the Asian elephant.

range and corridors of seasonal herd migration patterns. For this reason, herd matriarchs are often selected for deployment of radio/satellite tracking collars ("tagging"), which requires 30–60 minutes of field anesthesia. The ecological success of the herd is thus very dependent on the successful outcome of the anesthetic procedure. As a result, the authors are strong advocates of providing 100% oxygen, intermittent positive pressure ventilation, and cardiopulmonary monitoring (discussed later), even in very remote locations.

Females reach sexual maturity at approximately 10 years; gestation lasts 22 months. Calves are weaned at 2–3 years, and the calving interval is 4–6 years. Over her lifetime, a cow may produce seven offspring; in the field, it is not unusual to observe a cow with an infant and two older offspring. The presence of multiple offspring can complicate anesthetic procedures enormously (Fig. 51.2, *middle*). Although the oldest siblings typically follow the herd and separate from an anesthetized female when provoked by gunfire, the younger

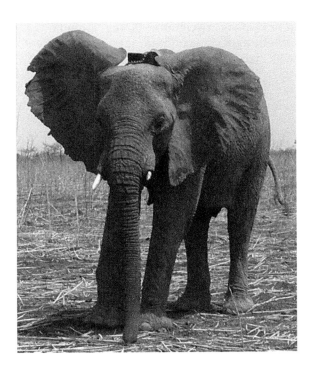

Figure 51.1. Adult free-ranging female African elephant with satellite tracking collar deployed. The transmitter can be seen dorsally between the ears. The photograph was taken 3 minutes after intravenous injection of the etorphine reversal agent, naltrexone.

ones often do not (Fig. 51.2, *bottom*). Infants weighing 100–200 lb can often be managed by physical restraint; older, more aggressive offspring may require anesthesia to protect team personnel.

Physical Restraint
Free-ranging wild elephants must be adequately anesthetized in order to ensure the safety of all those involved in an anesthetic procedure. Physical restraint is impractical and dangerous. Elephants in captivity, however, can be trained to accept some forms of handling. There are two distinct handling approaches currently in use: free contact and protected contact. The former involves direct contact between the keeper and the elephant, and often includes the use of an ankus to control the elephant. The legs are often chained for control (Fowler 1995). Negative reinforcement is sometimes employed. The elephant is essentially placed in a subservient position to the keeper.

Free contact is potentially more dangerous than protected contact for the handler. Many zoological institutions feel that protected contact is a more preferable way to manage captive elephants. The other, more acceptable approach is protected contact. Here, the keeper is separated from the elephant by a protective barrier, often with access ports to access various body parts, especially the feet or ears. The elephant, through operant conditioning, is taught to present body parts

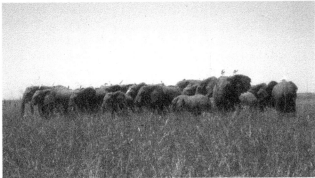
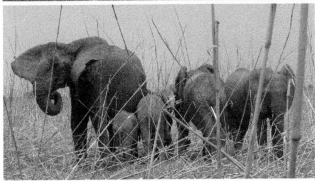
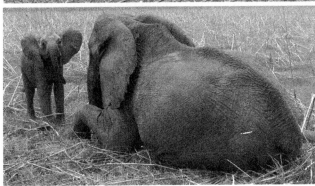

Figure 51.2. Free-ranging African elephants (*Loxodonta africana*) are highly social animals that live in matrilineal family groups. (Top) A small family group of adult females and their offspring. The activity of cattle egrets around herds is especially helpful in spotting elephants from a distance. (Middle) A single adult female may stray away from the herd and bring a number of offspring with her. (Bottom) Very young offspring are difficult to separate from their anesthetized mothers. Note the dart in the left hindquarter of the adult female. In this case, it was possible to physically restrain the infant while procedures were performed.

for inspection for minor procedures, such as foot trimming or venipuncture. The elephant is positively rewarded for performing the desired behavior, and can choose whether or not to perform the behavior (Desmond & Laule 1991).

In either approach, an elephant restraint device (ERD) may be used as an adjunct to restraint to perform more invasive procedures, such as reproductive evaluations (Fig. 51.3). An ERD should allow safe access to all four feet, trunk, tusks, ears, face, both sides, hindquarters, and back by moving parts of the ERD or the

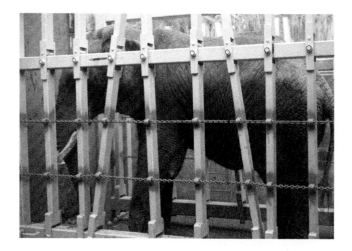

Figure 51.3. Captive elephants can be trained to stand in an elephant restraint device for minimally invasive procedures.

elephant (Schmidt 2003). Most ERDs are hydraulically operated and are large enough for an elephant to stand in comfortably for the duration of the procedure. The ERD should be constructed so that it can be quickly and easily opened in case an elephant falls down in the device.

Allometric Scaling

The energy cost of living (kJ/day) varies over a range of five orders of magnitude across species (Nagy et al. 1999). And though there is no consensus as to whether energy cost scales as the 2/3 (surface area) or 3/4 (volume) power of mass, it is widely accepted that the physiological processes that underlie metabolic scaling are the same as those that regulate uptake, distribution, and elimination of drugs. Given that the elephant is the largest of all land mammals, it is important to consider allometric scaling when calculating dosages of drugs used for anesthetic procedures. When the energy cost (kJ/d) of a variety of mammalian species is plotted against the log of their individual masses (kg), the graph that results is a straight line with a slope of approximately 0.75. This indicates that metabolic rate (MR) varies according to the following simple relationship, MR is proportional to $(Mass)^{0.75}$. This fits with the general observation that smaller mammals have higher metabolic rates than larger ones. Accordingly, this relationship can be used to extrapolate drug dosages to be used in elephants from known dosage regimens worked out for other placental mammals. (The relationship can also be applied across energy groups by introducing a taxa specific allometric constant [MR is proportioinal to $K(Mass)^{0.75}$; see Sedgwick 1993]).

The species most commonly used for comparison to elephants is the horse (Mikota and Plumb, Elephant Formulary, available at http://www.elephantcare.org/drugdex.htm, last accessed January 29, 2014). Assume, for example, that we want to give an average-sized African elephant (weighing 3000 kg) atropine as a preanesthetic agent. Though not used often in the horse, a published dosage for a 500-kg animal is approximately 0.05 mg/kg (Plumb VDH). To adjust the elephant's dose by taking the different metabolic rate into account, the following relationship applies:

$$(\text{horse dosage})(\text{horse metabolic rate}) =$$
$$(\text{elephant dosage})(\text{elephant metabolic rate}), \text{ or}$$
$$(0.05\text{ mg/kg})(500\text{ kg}^{0.75}) = (\text{elephant dosage})$$
$$(3000\text{ kg}^{0.75}).$$

Rearranging to solve for elephant dosage and solving for body mass raised to the 0.75 power,

$$\text{elephant dosage} = (0.05\text{ mg/kg})(106)/(405)$$
$$= (0.05)(0.26) = 0.013,$$

we see that the elephant dosage should be reduced by 74%. If this is a 6000-kg male elephant, a 84% reduction would be required (substitute $6000^{0.75} = 682$ into the equation above). Thus, giving the published horse dose would result in a dramatic overdose. This may explain why a 28-year-old Asian elephant developed immediate CNS signs (central excitation leading to restlessness, irritability, disorientation, and ataxia) of atropine toxicity after receiving 0.05 mg/kg atropine IV (Gross et al. 1994). The process of scaling down dosages has been applied to a variety drugs used in elephant sedation and anesthesia.

Tracheal Anatomy and Intubation

To maximize the safety of any anesthetic procedure in any species, it is very important to have access to, and control of, the patient's airway. This is especially true in the case of elephants, as etorphine, the drug used most commonly for induction and maintenance of anesthesia/immobilization, is a very potent respiratory depressant. In addition, as the animal goes down in either sternal or lateral recumbency, there is significant pressure on the diaphragm from abdominal contents. The combination of these two factors can result in severe hypoxemia and hypercapnea. Even though 70% of inhaled air is taken through the elephant's trunk, attempts of positive pressure ventilation through the nares would prove futile as most of the forced air or oxygen would escape through the mouth. Complete control of the elephant's airway requires endotracheal intubation. Elephants are relatively easy to intubate; however, success of intubation requires an understanding of the unique feature of the elephant's larynx (Fig. 51.4).

Intubation is done blindly, with the greatest success coming with hand-guided insertion of the tip of the endotracheal tube into the dorsal opening of the glottis. It is imperative that the mouth be opened wide enough

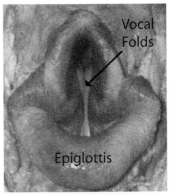

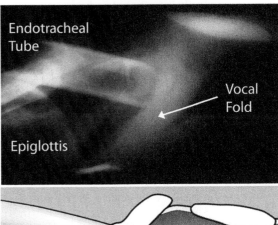

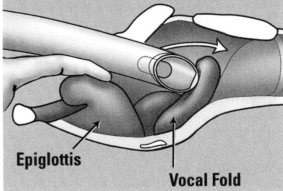

Figure 51.4. Anatomy of the elephant larynx. (Top) Elephants have a large fleshy epiglottis and extremely thick vocal folds. (Middle) The thickness of the elephant's vocal fold can be appreciated in this lateral radiograph of a dissected larynx. The curvature of the endotracheal tube makes intubation difficult. It is hard to get the end of the tube past the vocal folds. (Bottom) Intubation can be achieved by manually guiding the end of the tracheal tube to the dorsal aspect of the glottis.

to allow insertion of the arm, as elephants have large molars and a very narrow intermandibular space. The *top panel* of Figure 51.4 shows the larynx as it would be palpated when approaching from the oral cavity.

Elephants have a very large, fleshy epiglottis that is free of cartilage. It allows for a very tight seal to be formed between the trachea and the openings to the nares on the roof of the pharyngeal cavity. (The trunk and pleural adhesions that are unique to elephants are thought to have evolved for snorkeling [West 2002].) The epiglottis is very pliable and can readily be pulled

forward to allow access to the glottis. Elephants have very thick vocal folds that, at rest, largely occlude the entrance to the trachea. Difficulty in intubation, as shown radiographically in the *middle panel* of Figure 51.4, arises in part as the result of the curvature of the endotracheal tube causing its end to press up against the vocal folds. The solution to this problem is to, in coordination with breathing, manually guide the end of the tracheal tube to the dorsal aspect of the glottis where the vocal folds are much thinner and therefore more easily separated (Fig. 51.4, *lower panel*).

Physiology

Allometric scaling predicts that a 3000-kg elephant standing at rest would have a heart rate of 33 beats/min ($241 \times M^{-0.25}$), respiratory rate of 7 breaths/min ($53.5 \times M^{-0.26}$), and tidal volume of 20 L ($6.2 \times M^{1.01}$). Though there are few references to substantiate these predictions in awake elephants, the numbers are in close agreement with what has been compiled to date (Mikota 2003, at http://www.elephantcare.org, accessed January 29, 2014): heart rate, 25–30 beats/min, and respiratory rate, 4–6 breaths/min. Interestingly, the heart rate more than doubles in awake elephants lying in lateral recumbency (Honeyman et al. 1992). These physiologic variables differ somewhat in anesthetized animals, as will be discussed in later sections.

Elephants have an average rectal temperature of 36–37°C. Their packed cell volumes are comparable to other mammals (40–45%); however, elephant red blood cells are large (MCV = 130 fl vs. 50 fl for horses) and fewer in number compared with other mammals ($3–4 \times 10^6/\mu l$ vs. $8–12 \times 10^6/\mu l$). Overall the oxygen carrying capacity of elephant blood is comparable to other mammals (20–21 mL O_2/100 mL). However, elephant hemoglobin binds oxygen with somewhat higher affinity than other species [P_{50} = 23–24 mmHg vs. 23–27 mmHg for the horse, and 29–31 mmHg for the dog (Cambier et al. 2004, 2005; Dhindsa et al. 1972)].

It is also of interest to point out some physiological variables important to anesthesia that do not scale allometrically. These include mean arterial blood pressure (about 100 mmHg in all species), maximum functional capillary diameter, and fractional airway dead space (constant at about 25–30% in large species). Plasma protein concentrations vary little with size or species.

Cardiopulmonary Monitoring in Remote Locations

Regardless of procedure location, it is very important to continuously monitor the oxygenation and ventilation status, blood pressure, heart rate and rhythm, respiratory rate, and temperature of anesthetized elephants. Monitoring anesthetized animals in remote geographic locations with no electrical power can be accomplished with the use of commercially available equipment or with modifications of available equipment.

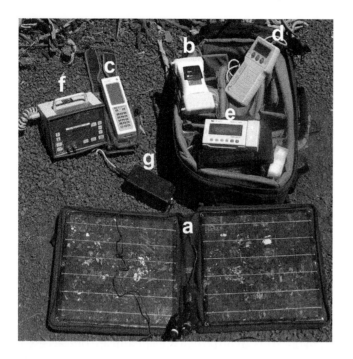

Figure 51.5. Cardiopulmonary monitoring in remote locations. A portable solar panel (a) is used to recharge batteries. Adequacy of oxygenation and ventilation can be assessed with a portable pulse oximeter (b), blood gas analyzer (c), and capnograph (d). Adequacy of cardiovascular function can be assessed with a battery-operated ECG monitor (e), and a blood pressure monitor (f) that can be charged directly from the solar panel through a voltage regulator (g).

Portable solar panels that recharge batteries can ensure adequate power to operate most equipment. Equipment for monitoring oxygenation, ventilation, cardiac rhythm and rate, blood pressure, and core temperature have been successfully used in areas without an electrical grid or electrical generators (Fig. 51.5).

Size, weight, power requirements, durability, and dependability in harsh environmental conditions should be considered when choosing monitoring equipment for field use. Of concern are power requirements and the source of the power, particularly in areas where there is no power grid or generator available. There are a number of types of rechargeable batteries on the market.

We use nickel metal hydride batteries (NiMH) in monitoring equipment in our studies (MAHA Powerx 2100 mAh, Thomas Distributing, Paris, IL). NiMH batteries have several features that make them attractive for remote use. They can be recharged 500–1000 times, have no memory, have a fairly steady discharge curve, and have a minimal negative environmental impact when disposed of. One disadvantage of NiMH batteries is that they have a self-discharge rate of 2–3% per day when not in use. AA-size NiMH batteries produce 1.2 V. Battery energy output is measured in milliamp hours (mAh), with higher mAh ratings implying greater

battery output. A battery rated at 1700 mAh will produce 1700 mA for 1 hour. Different manufacturers produce batteries with different power outputs. AA-size NiMH batteries are rated at up to 2400 mAh.

Batteries are charged using fast, smart chargers attached to portable solar panels (iPowerUS fast smart charger, iPower Corporation, El Monte, CA). A fast charger delivers the amount of current necessary to recharge the battery in 1 hour or less. In general, however, a slower charge rate will extend the overall life of the battery. To overcome the deleterious effects of rapidly charging a battery, a smart charger has a current-limiter built into it that reduces the current as the battery is charged, thereby limiting deterioration. The fast smart charger is attached to a portable solar panel (Sun Catcher Expedition solar charger, Power-Qwest, Inc., Duluth, GA) via a 12-V "cigarette lighter" type plug. The panel (Fig. 51.5a) produces 25 W of power, which is more than enough power to charge 8 AA-size NiMH batteries at a time. Monitoring equipment that uses AA- or AAA-size batteries is preferred so that a large number of different-sized rechargeable batteries are not required in the field.

There are a number of commercially available cardiopulmonary monitors that can be adapted for use in the field. Oxygenation status is assessed continuously with a pulse oximeter and intermittently by arterial blood gas determination using a portable clinical analyzer. Several brands of pulse oximeters have been successfully used and recharged in the field. An Invacare model 3402 NV (Sims BCI, Inc., Waukesha, WI) is relatively small, lightweight, and operates on 6 AA-size batteries (Fig. 51.5b). This pulse oximeter is durable and operates well on rechargeable AA-size NiMH batteries. An I-Stat portable clinical analyzer (Heska Corp., Loveland, CO) has been successfully used in the field using rechargeable 9-V NiMH batteries (Fig. 51.5c). A challenge of using the I-Stat in the field is the analyzer's normal operating temperature of 16–30°C (61–86°F), which is often exceeded in typical elephant habitat. The I-Stat can be maintained at the proper operating temperature range by placing it in a 12-V thermoelectric cooler (Coleman, Spirit Lake, IA). The thermoelectric cooler can be powered directly off the solar panel.

Ventilation status is measured continuously by capnography (end-tidal CO_2 measurement) and intermittently by arterial blood gas determination. The criteria for choosing a capnograph include availability of a waveform display, mainstream and side-stream capabilities, and power requirements. The Novametrix Tidal Wave model 615 (Novametrix Medical Systems, Inc., Wallingford, CT) meets these criteria (Fig. 51.5d). The Tidal Wave comes standard with a rechargeable computer-type battery, but can be ordered with a battery tray which holds seven AA-size batteries. This instrument is durable and operates well on rechargeable batteries. The side-stream capability allows a large-gauge needle to be placed in the lumen of a large endotracheal tube or respirator for sampling.

Cardiac rate and rhythm are monitored by use of an electrocardiograph (ECG). A compact ECG unit (Heska Vet/ECG 2000, Heska Corp., Fort Collins, CO), which operates on 3 AAA-size rechargeable NiMH batteries, is durable and dependable in the field (Fig. 51.5e).

Blood pressure can be measured using a direct arterial line or by indirect methods. Of the indirect methods, automated oscillotonometry has been successfully used in the field. We have not identified an automated blood pressure machine that runs on replaceable batteries. We have, however, modified a compact, durable instrument, Oscillomate 9300 (CAS Medical Systems, Inc., Branford, CT) for field use (Fig. 51.5f). We manufactured a voltage regulator (Fig. 51.5g), which is inserted between the internal battery of the blood pressure monitor and the solar panel. This allows the internal battery of the blood pressure monitor to be recharged directly from the solar panel.

All monitoring equipment, battery chargers, and rechargeable NiMH batteries can be transported into the field in a backpack that is designed for photographic equipment (Lowepro Supertrecker AW II, Lowepro USA, Santa Rosa, CA). All of the earlier equipment has been dependably used to monitor immobilized elephants in a variety of remote habitats in Cameroon, including forest savannah (hot and dry) and rainforest (hot and humid) locations.

IMMOBILIZATION OF FREE-RANGING ELEPHANTS

Etorphine

Etorphine is a nonselective opiate agonist that binds to μ, κ, and δ opiate receptors; consistent with the ability of the drug to activate G-proteins, its effects occur at very low fractional receptor occupancy (Perry et al. 1982). Etorphine has been used safely for elephant restraint and anesthesia for nearly 40 years (Wallach & Anderson 1968). The first in-depth report of the use of etorphine for prolonged maintenance of an elephant in lateral recumbency for a surgical procedure was published by Fowler and Hart in 1973. Etorphine was used as the sole anesthetic agent on two separate occasions for castration of a subadult Asian elephant. Several important guiding anesthetic principles emerged from this report. First, it demonstrates that by using incremental dosing or constant rate infusion of etorphine, elephants can be maintained in lateral recumbency for up to 3 hours and 40 minutes without adverse effects. Of particular importance is the fact that even in the absence of fluid administration, the elephant under study did not develop postanesthetic myopathy or nerve paralysis, conditions that are common in other large mammals subjected to prolonged recumbency.

Second, the report shows that it is possible to maintain adequate ventilation and oxygenation throughout the procedure. The authors went to great lengths to maintain a patent airway, provide a supplemental source of 100% oxygen, and maintain a surgical plane of anesthesia that did not compromise ventilation. Most importantly, they monitored for adequacy of oxygenation and ventilation by performing serial blood gas analysis.

Third, reversal of etorphine with diprenorphine was rapid and complete regardless of procedure time. The elephant stood within 8 minutes following each procedure and was immediately able to eat, drink, and urinate. The option of immediate reversal added considerably to the safety of the anesthetic procedure.

A few other points from this report are worth noting. Given that the elephant was confined, the authors were able to induce anesthesia with a relatively low intramuscular dose (5–6 mg) of etorphine. Ataxia was noticeable within 6 minutes; an additional 5–10 minutes was required for the animal to lie down on its side. Maintenance of anesthesia for 1 hour required a total of approximately 10 mg of etorphine. As is a general property of opiates in all species, etorphine had minimal effects on cardiovascular function in this study. Neither anticholinergic agents nor sympathomimetics were required to maintain hemodynamic stability. Although blood pressure was not monitored, there was no evidence of hypotension (acidosis associated with poor perfusion, tachycardia) or hypertension (pulmonary hemorrhage). The elephant had minimal postoperative complications and was considered safe for elephant rides five months after surgery.

Lessons learned from this report have for the most part been carried into the field for larger-scale immobilization projects (Horne et al. 2001; Osofsky 1997; Raath 1993; Still et al. 1996). Larger initial doses of etorphine have been recommended for free-ranging elephants, often in combination with either acepromazine or azaperone. Carfentanil (Jacobsen et al. 1988; Kreeger et al. 2002) and thiofentanyl (Kreeger et al. 2002) have been used instead of etorphine; naltrexone has been used in the place of diprenorphine as a reversal agent. Hyaluronidase has been used by some with the intent of improving uptake of the drug at intramuscular injection sites. Table 51.3 gives the doses of the

Table 51.3. Doses of opiate agonists used in elephant anesthesia

Drug	Taxa	Dose (mg/kg)
Carfentanil citrate	*Loxodonta*	0.0021
Etorphine hydrochlodide	*Loxodonta*	0.003
Thiafentanil oxalate	*Loxodonta*	0.003
Etorphine hydrochloride	*Elaphus*	0.003

Source: Kreeger (2002).

most commonly used opiate agonists used in elephant anesthesia.

Drug Delivery

Delivering anesthetic agents to free-ranging elephants can be very challenging. Terrain, equipment and infrastructure vary greatly across elephant range countries. Raath (1993) describes the use of helicopters or vehicles to approach elephants. In areas with limited infrastructure and no access to helicopters, approach on foot is necessary. Great care must be taken when approaching an elephant or a herd of elephants this way. An armed game guard and an experienced tracker should be part of the approach team. As elephants have excellent senses of smell and hearing, the approach should be from downwind and as quiet as possible. In areas where there is access to cover, the approach should be from one area of cover to the next.

Perhaps most importantly, a long-range remote delivery system (RDS) should be used. (For a thorough review of RDSs, see Kreeger et al. 2002). Both CO_2 and powder-charge rifles are available, as are polyamide and aluminum syringes. Regardless of the RDS, 50- to 65-mm needles should be used in order to ensure an intramuscular injection. The hind leg, back, and shoulder are preferred darting sites (Raath 1993). If darting in the shoulder, care must be taken to avoid darting the ear. The dart impact should be perpendicular to the target site to ensure that the drug is delivered intramuscularly.

Elephants have relatively poor eyesight. The elephant will have limited ability to see the darter at distances greater than 40 ft. It is extremely important to know the position of all of the individuals in a herd so that the approach does not place the team within the perimeter of the herd. The shot should be taken from cover if possible. Although most elephants will run away from the darter, an elephant may occasionally charge the darter. Also, elephants may initially run in random directions after a herd mate is darted; this places the approach team in jeopardy. A human cannot outrun an elephant, but can run around a tree faster than an elephant can. Finding a tree that an elephant can not easily push over, and not leaving the tree until the charging elephant is at a safe distance, is a good practice. In forests, it may be necessary to dart an elephant from a distance of 10 m or less due to the thickness of the surrounding vegetation. In such situations, it is extremely important to dart from behind cover. Once the elephant is darted, the tracker(s) should follow at a safe distance.

A "Typical" Etorphine Field Immobilization Procedure

All of our immobilization procedures have been initiated either from a vehicle (savannah regions) or on foot (forest-savannah or rainforest). What follows also applies to helicopter-assisted immobilizations, except that physiological parameters measured in these elephants often reflect significant sympathetic stimulation. Adult, free-ranging female African elephants weighing 3000–3500 kg are typically administered a single intramuscular 10–12 mg dose of etorphine delivered by dart to a region high on the hind limb. (Large males may require up to 20 mg.) At this dose, elephants show first effects in 3–5 minutes, but are capable of running at high speed over a long distance during this time. Within 10–15 minutes, the elephant will often sit down into sternal recumbency. Though some elephants will roll spontaneously into lateral recumbency, many remain in this sternal position. It is important to locate the elephant as soon as possible, as it is widely believed that elephants do not ventilate adequately while sternal. (Drug effects on breathing often cause the elephants to make a loud rumbling sound that can be heard over long distances.) While approaching the darted elephant, the remaining members of the herd, including offspring, must be frightened off with rifle fire.

An elephant found in sternal position must be rolled onto her side, which may require 6–10 people depending on the size of the elephant and the terrain. While rolling the elephant, great care should be taken to protect the airway by extending the trunk. Heart rate, pulse pressure, respiratory rate, and arterial blood gases (blood drawn from auricular artery) should be evaluated immediately. Table 51.3 lists some of the published values for physiological parameters that have been recorded under similar field conditions. The elephant should have a very strong pulse as assessed by palpating an auricular artery. The table indicates that an etorphine immobilized adult female elephant, regardless of species, typically has a heart rate of 50 beats/min and a respiratory rate of 5–7 breaths per minute. Any deviation from these values, whether higher or lower, should alert the anesthetist to the possibility of hypoxemia. This would be confirmed by arterial blood gas measurements. As is the case with most mammals, elephant hemoglobin begins to desaturate very quickly below an oxygen partial pressure of 60 mmHg (SpO_2 = 93%).

A number of elephant immobilization studies, including our own, have determined that etorphine-immobilized elephants are at-risk for developing severe hypoxemia (PaO_2 = 40–60 mmHg). Though the actual number of hypoxemic elephants we have encountered is small (approximately 1 in 10), the importance of the matriarchal female to the social structure of the herd dictates that every effort be made to provide oxygen to immobilized elephants, even in remote locations. We have developed a simple and effective respirator device to provide oxygen and intermittent positive pressure ventilation to immobilized elephants in the field (Fig. 51.6, see Horne et al. 2001). The respirator can be

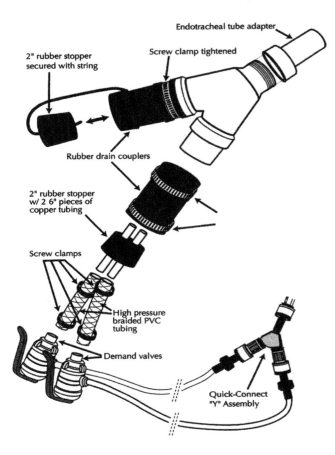

Figure 51.6.   A portable respirator can be constructed with readily available parts (for details, see Horne et al. 2001). Oxygen is delivered through two high flow (160L/min) demand valves connected to an oxygen cylinder (not shown).

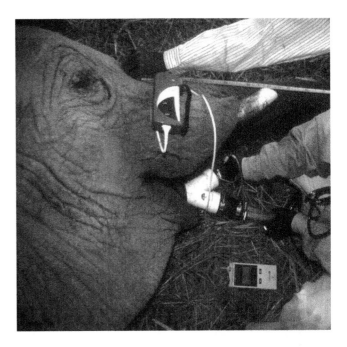

Figure 51.7.   Continuous pulmonary monitoring using a pulse oximeter and capnograph while providing intermittent positive pressure ventilation. For pulse oximetry, a large C-probe is placed on the tip of the elephant's tongue. The sidestream capnograph draws expired air through a needle inserted into the expiration port of the respirator.

driven off a single MM oxygen cylinder (aluminum cylinders weigh 45lb) which holds 3500L of oxygen, enough for at least 45 minutes of continuous use. High partial pressures of oxygen (>400mmHg) can be achieved when the oxygen is delivered in synchrony with the elephant's breathing pattern through a 35-mm endotracheal tube with an inflatable cuff.

Placement of the endotracheal tube requires a team approach. The process is easy if the elephant has been properly dosed. Higher doses of etorphine tend to cause rigidity of the muscles of the jaw, making it difficult to access the pharyngeal cavity. With one person holding the tusk and pulling dorsally, and another pulling the lower jaw ventrally (a rope is helpful), the person inserting the tube lies on the ground and reaches between the jaws with the lower arm to locate the epiglottis. In large females, this is typically a full arm's length reach. Once the epiglottis is located (see Tracheal Anatomy and Intubation), the tube is passed alongside the arm and guided into the dorsal aspect of the glottis. The arm is removed, and the endotracheal tube cuff is inflated with a large syringe. The "Y" piece of the respirator is then connected by way of a standard

endotracheal tube adapter, and oxygen is delivered through one side of the "Y" (inspiration port) by two demand valves connected in parallel. A large rubber stopper is used to plug the opposite side of the "Y" (expiration port) during inspiration and then removed during expiration. The respirator can deliver oxygen at a rate of 5L/s; delivery over 4–5 seconds (elephant inspiration time) generates an adequate 20- to 25-L tidal volume with noticeable expansion of the chest wall.

Indirect methods of cardiopulmonary monitoring work well with immobilized elephants. Heart rate and SpO_2 can be monitored continuously via pulse oximetry with a large C-probe positioned on the tip of the tongue. End-tidal CO_2 can be monitored using a sidestream capnograph drawing from a needle inserted into the endotracheal tube (Fig. 51.7). Blood pressure can be monitored oscillometrically with a small adult human cuff (12 × 30cm) positioned at the base of the tail (Fig. 51.8). As summarized in Table 51.4, three separate studies report SpO_2 values less than 93%, which is indicative of hypoxemia. Note also that end-tidal CO_2 values may under represent actual $PaCO_2$ values by up to 25%, due to the presence of physiologic dead space. Mean arterial pressures measure in the range of 80–120mmHg, indicating that the 10mg dose provides an adequate plane of anesthesia, at least for the placement of radio/satellite tracking collars.

Our experience has been that 10–12 mg of etorphine provides a full hour of immobilization without any signs of awakening; however, a typical collar deployment requires less than 45 minutes. We have not had to redose any cases in which it was clear that the drug delivery was complete with the first dart.

Pink Foam Syndrome

Opioids have been implicated as the cause of hypertension in elephants (Raath 1993), with pulmonary hemorrhage being a common sequela. The pulmonary

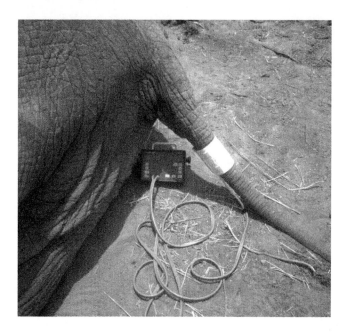

Figure 51.8. Blood pressure can be monitored continuously with a portable oscillotonometer and a small adult human cuff positioned near the base of the tail.

edema and bleeding is manifest as "pink foam" bubbling from the elephant's trunk. Surprisingly, we have not observed this effect of opioids in nearly 50 immobilizations. This is probably because the procedures we perform require that we approach elephants on foot, rather than by helicopter, as is common in South Africa where pink foam syndrome has been reported. Approach on foot causes significantly less stress to the elephant. Second, the dose of etorphine that we use may be more appropriate for our procedures compared to previous reports of documented hypertension. Hattingh et al. reported mean arterial pressures > 185 mmHg in 5000 kg bull elephants that had received only 8 mg etorphine; the pressure increased to >260 mmHg during electroejaculation. The elephants were obviously not fully anesthetized. Azaperone and acepromazine have been recommended for use in elephants because of their vasodilatory effects, and because of their potential to reduce the probability of pulmonary hypertension. We have not found them to be necessary and believe that hypertension in elephants is not a direct result of opiate administration.

Recovery

Several drugs have proven to be effective in reversing opiates in elephants, including diprenorphine, nalmefene, and naltrexone. Because of the potential for renarcotization resulting from the reversal agent wearing off too soon, we routinely reverse with naltrexone at 100 times the etorphine dose (1–1.2 g) given intravenously or 25% of the dose given intravenously and the remaining 75% given intramuscularly. First signs of recovery—movement of the trunk and ears—generally occur within two minutes, and recovery is often complete within 10 minutes. Figure 51.9 shows the first stages of

Table 51.4. Published cardiopulmonary values for etorphine-immobilized free-ranging elephants

Species (sex)	HR beats/min	MAP mm Hg	RR breaths/ min	SpO$_2$ %	PaO$_2$ mm Hg	EtCO$_2$ mm Hg	PaCO$_2$ mm Hg	Reference
Etorphine								
Loxodonta africana (♂A)	52[a]		8					Wallach and Anderson (1968)
L. africana (♀A)	50		5					Kock et al. (1993)
L. africana (♀A)	48 (34–80)[b]			87 (70–96)				Osofsky (1997)
L. africana (♂♀J)	69 (56–112)		9 (3–28)	88 (82–95)	75 (50–99)		52 (38–70)	Still et al. (1996)
L. africana (♀A)	50 (33–68)	105 (80–120)	7 (6–12)	95 (75–99) 95[c] (93–97)[c]	63 (40–77) 251[c] (97–491)[c]	47 (34–60) 47[c] (33–50)[c]	60 (45–69) 58[c] (51–67)[c]	Horne et al. (2001)
Etorphine and acepromazine								
Elephas maximus (♂♀A)	52 (40–60)		7 (4–10)					Dangolla et al. (2004)

[a]All single values are rounded averages.

[b]Values in parenthesis indicate range.

[c]Following 15 minutes of oxygen supplementation and intermittent positive pressure ventilation.

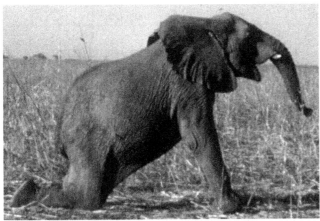

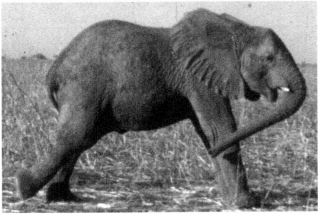

Figure 51.9. Recovery from etorphine anesthesia occurs within minutes following intravenous naltrexone administration. Elephants typically stand on their front legs first (top) and then adopt a saw-horse stance (bottom) until the drug has been completely reversed (several minutes).

a typical recovery. Elephants roll into sternal, throw their heads backward, and stand on their front legs first. They then stand on their hind legs, balance in a saw-horse position for a short time as the reversal becomes complete, and then amble off to find their herd mates. Given the promptness of recovery, it is essential that all equipment, vehicles, and personnel be a safe distance away prior to administration of the reversal agent.

CAPTIVE ELEPHANT PROCEDURES

Drug Delivery
Anesthetics and sedatives can be delivered to captive elephants by most acceptable means. Hand intramuscular or intravenous injections can be given to conditioned elephants in captivity with or without the use of an ERD. For less tractable elephants, pole syringes or a variety of RDS may be required.

Standing Sedation
Standing sedation is useful in situations where a degree of sedation is required to perform a procedure that does not require general anesthesia. Procedures performed under sedation include treatment of abscesses, tuberculin testing, trunk washes for acid fast culture, venipuncture, reproductive evaluations, manual stimulation of ejaculation, radiology, loading for transport and transport (Ramsay 2000). Sedation is often performed in conjunction with an ERD. Azaperone is preferred to α-2 agonists for reproductive procedures (Schmitt et al. 1996). But there are anecdotal reports of azaperone causing excitement in elephants. Azaperone has been reported to cause paradoxical excitement in the horse (Dodam & Waterman 1979). Xylazine/butorphanol provides a greater level of sedation than does azaperone (Ramsay 2000). Xylazine can be reversed with the intramuscular administration of yohimbine (0.5 mg per mg xylazine used), tolazoline (2 mg per mg of xylazine used) (Kock et al. 1993), or atipamizole (0.1 mg per mg xylazine used) (Kreeger et al. 2002). Table 51.5 lists drugs and dosages commonly used for standing sedation of elephants.

Etorphine Induction and General Anesthesia
A variety of anesthetic protocols have been used in captive elephants. A summary of published cardiopulmonary values obtained during these procedures are listed by protocol in Table 51.6. As mentioned earlier, the striking difference between published free-ranging and captive elephant procedures is the method of administering etorphine as an induction agent. For example, rather than a single dose of 10–12 mg etorphine IM, Dunlop et al. have reported that, in two out of three attempts, 6-mg etorphine administered by pole syringe was sufficient to allow an elephant to be positioned into sternal recumbency. An additional 2 mg of etorphine administered IV permitted positioning in lateral recumbency. In a third attempt, the elephant appeared to be apprehensive and stressed and required an additional 7 mg of etorphine and a 210-mg dose of azaperone.

Maintenance of a surgical plane of anesthesia for prolonged periods can be achieved by repeated 1- to –2-mg doses of etorphine (Allen et al. 1984; Fowler & Hart 1973) or with inhalation anesthetics (Dunlop et al. 1994; Heard et al. 1988; Stegmann 1999; Tamas & Geiser 1983). Inhalation anesthetics have also been used following induction with carfentanil (Jacobsen et al. 1988) and xylazine-ketamine (Abou-Madi et al. 2004). As with any species, recoveries from inhalation anesthetic procedures may be prolonged. Opiates should be reversed, even if it has been several hours since they were administered.

ANALGESIA

Nonsteroidal Anti-Inflammatory Agents
Although nonsteroidal anti-inflammatory agents (NSAIDs) are used extensively in elephants, very little

Table 51.5. Drugs used for standing sedation in elephants

Drug	Dosage mg/kg	Route	Species	Reference
Azaperone	0.08–0.09	IM	*Loxodonta*	Ramsay (2000)
Azaperone	0.017–0.046	IM	*Elephus*	Schmitt (1996)
Azaperone	0.060–0.150	IM	*Loxodonta*	Page (1994)
Azaperone	0.067	IM	*Loxodonta*	Raath (1993)
Haloperidol[a]	Variable with size of elephant	IM	*Loxodonta*	Raath (1993)
Butorphanol[b]	0.12	IM	*Loxodonta*	Ramsay (2000)
	0.01–0.03	IV	*Loxodonta*	Ramsay (2000)
Xylazine[c]	0.2–0.3	IM	*Loxodonta*	Ramsay (2000)
Xylazine	0.080–0.150	IM	*Elephas*	Schmidt (2003)
Xylazine	0.110–0.550	IM	*Loxodonta*	Schmidt (2003)
Medetomidine	0.005	IM	*Elephus*	Sarma et al. (2002)
Detomidine	0.0055	IM	*Elephus*	De Silva and Kuruwita (1994)
Detomidine[e] Butorphenol[e]	14.7–16.2 μg/kg	IM	*Loxodonta*	Neiffer et al. (2005)
	14.7–16.2 μg/kg	IM		
Acepromazine[d]				Kock et al. (1993)

[a]Used in conjunction with azaperone for transport of adult African elephants. See reference for dosages.
[b]Used in conjunction with xylazine.
[c]Used in conjunction with butorphanol.
[d]Total doses of: 30 mg for an adult, 10–20 mg for a juvenile-adult, and 5–10 mg for a baby-juvenile.
[e]Given simultaneously.

Table 51.6. Published cardiopulmonary values for etorphine-immobilized captive elephants[a]

Species (sex)	HR beats/min	MAP mm Hg	RR breaths/min	SpO₂ %	PaO₂ mm Hg	EtCO₂ mm Hg	PaCO₂ mm Hg	Reference
Etorphine								
Elephas maximus (♂A)	48[b] (56–76)[c,d]		8		(74–93) (85–146)[e]		(44–49)	Fowler and Hart (1973)
Loxodonta africana (♀, ♂J)	(44–100)		(7–20)		(67–73) (80–516)[f]		(29–78)	Heard et al. (1986)
L. africana (♂A)		186 263[g]						Hattingh et al. (1994)
Xylazine, ketamine, etorphine								
E. maximus (♂A)	(36–41)			(95–98)				Ollivet-Courtois et al. (2003)
Etorphine and halothane								
L. africana (♀A)	(32–42)		(5–10)					Tamas and Geiser (1983)
L. africana (♀J)	50	106	10					Heard et al. (1988)
L. africana (♀J)	61	106[h]	(4–6)		(140–277)[i]	(49–64)	(42–59)	Stegmann (1999)
Carfentanil and halothane								
E. maximus (♂A)	(47–60)[j] (110–125)[d]	(77–157)[h]	(4–12)		(40–49)[j] (249–400)[i]		(52–60)[j] (52–78)	Dunlop et al. (1985)
Etorphine and isoflurane								
L. africana (♀A)	(60–90)[j] (50–70)[d]	(120–240)[j] (110–170)	(6–8)[j] (2–5)		(45–75)[j] (100–350)[i]	(20–35)	(40–50)[j] (45–68)	Dunlop et al. (1994)
Xylazine, ketamine, and isoflurane								
E. maximus (♂ 2 mo old)	(55–60)		(10–30)	≥97	(152–558)[i]		(55–61)	Abou-Madi et al. (2004)

[a]A, adult; J, juvenile.
[b]All single values are rounded averages.
[c]Values in parenthesis indicate range.
[d]Intraoperative range.
[e]With 100% oxygen insufflation through the trunk.
[f]With 100% oxygen delivery through Hudson demand valve.
[g]During electroejaculation.
[h]Calculated [0.3(average systolic pressure − average diastolic pressure)].
[i]With 100% oxygen delivery through a semi-closed anesthetic circuit.
[j]Values with opiate alone.

714

Table 51.7. Commonly used nonsteroidal anti-inflammatory agents used in elephants[a]

Drug	Dose (mg/kg)	Method of Determination	Reference
Flunixin	1.0 every 24 hours	Empirical	Mortenson 2001
Flunixin	0.7 every 40 hours	Metabolic scaling[b]	Mortenson (2001)
Ibuprofen	0.5–4.0 every 24 hours	Empirical	Mortenson (2001)
Ibuprofen	6 mg/kg every 12 hours PO (Elaphus) 7 mg/kg every 12 hours PO (Loxodonta)	Pharmacokinetics	Bechert and Christensen (2007)
Phenylbutazone	1.0–2.0 every 24 hours	Empirical	Mortenson (2001)
Phenylbutazone	4.0 every 12 hours	Metabolic scaling[b]	Mortenson (2001)
Phenylbutazone	3 mg/kg every 48 hours PO (Elaphus) 2 mg/kg every 24 hours (Loxodonta)	Pharmacokinetics	Bechert et al. (2008)
Butorphanol	0.015 mg/kg single dose IM	Pharmacokinetics	Tana et al. (2010)
Ketoprofen	1.0–2.0 every 24–48 hours PO or IV	Pharmacokinetics	Hunter et al. (2003)

[a]Empirical doses may not be appropriate.
[b]Based on a 3200-kg elephant.

pharmacokinetic data are available. Ketoprofen was studied by Hunter et al. (2002). Dosage recommendations resulting from their study are 1–2 mg/kg every 24–48 hours, IV or PO. Table 51.7 lists NSAIDs commonly used in elephants. Care should be used in treating elephants with other NSAIDs. Extrapolation of elephant dosages from equine pharmacokinetic parameters is inappropriate (Hunter et al. 2002). Metabolic scaling dosages and treatment intervals for elephants may correlate with pharmacokinetic data (Hunter et al. 2002; Mortenson 2001).

SUMMARY

Despite their very large size, elephants can be readily anesthetized and stably maintained for hours under both free-ranging and captive conditions. Fortunately, they respond very predictably to the potent opiate agonists, etorphine and carfentanil. Whether the opiates are used alone or in combination with inhalation anesthetics, it is possible to maintain hemodynamic and respiratory stability for many hours without pharmacological intervention. Quite amazingly, a number of multiple-hour anesthetic procedures have been performed without any postanesthetic complications, such as nerve paralysis or myopathy.

As with any anesthetic procedure, it is important to monitor cardiopulmonary function and temperature continuously in elephants. Monitors developed for companion animal species are readily adapted to the elephant, even in remote locations. Of all the potential complications that might be expected during anesthesia, elephants are most at risk of developing hypoxemia. We and others have shown, however, that hypoxemia is readily corrected by simple oxygen supplementation. We recommend that, whether by continuous insufflation or by intermittent positive pressure ventilation, some means of oxygen supplementation be readily available for use when anesthetizing ele-

phants. This is especially true in field situations, where severe hypoxemia is most likely to occur.

REFERENCES

Abou-Madi N, Kollias GV, Hackett RP, Ducharme NG, Gleed RD, Moakler JP. 2004. Umbilical herniorrhaphy in a juvenile Asian elephant (*Elephas maximus*). *Journal of Zoo and Wildlife Medicine* 35(2):221–225.
Allen JL, Welsch B, Jacobsen ER, Turner TA, Tabeling H. 1984. Medical and surgical mangement of a fractured tusk in an African elephant. *Journal of the American Veterinary Medical Association* 185(11):1447–1449.
Bechert U, Christensen JM. 2007. Pharmacokinetics of orally administered ibuprophen in African and Asian elephants (*Loxodonta africana* and *Elephas maximus*). *Journal of Zoo and Wildlife Medicine* 38(2):258–268.
Bechert U, Christensen J, Nguyen C, Neelkant R, Bandas E. 2008. Pharmacokinetics of orally administered phenylbutazone in African and Asian elephants (*Loxodonta africana* and *Elephas maximus*). *Journal of Zoo and Wildlife Medicine* 39(2):188–200.
Blanc JJ, Barnes RFW, Craig GC, Dublin HT, Thouless CR, Douglas-Hamilton I, Hart JA. 2007. *African Elephant Status Report 2007: An Update from the African Elephant Database.* SSC Occasional Paper Series 33. Gland: IUCN.
Cambier C, Wierinckx M, Clerbaux T, Detry B, Liardet MP, Marville V, Frans A, Gustin P. 2004. Haemoglobin oxygen affinity and regulating factors of the blood oxygen transport in canine and feline blood. *Research in Veterinary Science* 77(1):83–88.
Cambier C, Di Passio N, Clerbaux T, Amory H, Marville V, Detry B, Frans A, Gustin P. 2005. Blood-oxygen binding in healthy Standardbred horses. *Veterinary Journal (London, England: 1997)* 169(2):251–256.
Dangolla A, Silva I, Kuruwita VY. 2004. Neuroleptanalgesia in wild Asian elephants (*Elephas maximus maximus*). *Veterinary Anaesthesia and Analgesia* 31(4):276–279.
De Silva DDN, Kuruwita VY. 1994. Sedation of wild elephants (*Elephas maximum ceylonicus*) using detomidine HCL (Domosedan) in Sri Lanka. 5th International Congress of Veterinary Anesthesia, p. 61. August 21–25.
Desmond T, Laule G. 1991. Protected contact: elephant handling. Proceedings of the 12th International Elephant Workshop, Burnet Park Zoo, Syracuse, NY, pp. 84–91.
Dhindsa DS, Sedgwick CJ, Mecalfe J. 1972. Comparative studies of the respiratory functions of mammalian blood. VIII. Asian

elephant (*Elephas maximus*) and African elephant (*Loxodonta africana africana*). *Respiration Physiology* 14:332–342.

Dodam NH, Waterman AE. 1979. Paradoxical excitement following intravenous administration of azaperone in the horse. *Equine Veterinary Journal* 11(1):33–35.

Dunlop CI, Hodgson DS, Steffey EP, Fowler ME. 1985. Observations during anesthetic management of an adult elephant. *Veterinary Surgery* 14:71–72.

Dunlop CI, Hodgson DS, Cambre RC, Kenny DE, Martin HD. 1994. Cardiopulmonary effects of three prolonged periods of isoflurane anesthesia in an adult elephant. *Journal of the American Veterinary Medical Association* 205(10):1439–1444.

Eggert LS, Rasner CA, Woodruff DS. 2002. The evolution and phylogeography of the African elephant inferred from mitochondrial DNA sequence and nuclear microsatellite markers. *Proceedings of the Royal Society of London. Series B. Biological Sciences* 269(1504):1993–2006.

Elkan PW, Planton HP, Powell JA, Haigh JA, Karesh WB. 1998. Chemical immobilization of African elephant in lowland forest, southwestern Cameroon. *Pachyderm* 25:32–37.

Fernando P, Vidya TNC, Payne J, Stuewe M, Davison G, Alfred RJ, Andau P, Bosi E, Kilbourn A, Melnick DJ. 2003. DNA analysis indicates that Asian elephants are native to Borneo and are therefore a high priority for conservation. *PLoS Biology* 1(1): 110–115.

Focus. 2005. Species spotlight: Asian elephant. Focus (World Wildlife Fund) 27/2:2.

Fowler ME. 1995. Elephants. In: *Restraint and Handling of Wild and Domestic Animals*, 2nd ed., pp. 257–269. Ames: Iowa State University Press.

Fowler ME, Hart R. 1973. Castration of an Asian elephant using etorphine anesthesia. *Journal of the American Veterinary Medical Association* 163(6):539–543.

Gage LJ, Fowler ME, Pascoe JR, Blasko D. 1997. Surgical removal of infected phalanges from an Asian elephant (*Elephas maximus*). *Journal of Zoo and Wildlife Medicine* 28(2):208–211.

Gross ME, Clifford CA, Hardy DA. 1994. Excitement in an elephant after intravenous administration of atropine. *Journal of the American Veterinary Medical Association* 205(10):1437–1438.

Hattingh J, Knox CM, Raath JP. 1994. Arterial blood pressure of the African elephant (*Loxodonta africana*) under etorphine anaesthesia and after remobilisation with diprenorphine. *The Veterinary Record* 135(19):458–459.

Heard DJ, Jacobson ER, Brock KA. 1986. Effects of oxygen supplementation on blood gas values in chemically restrained juvenile African elephants. *Journal of the American Veterinary Medical Association* 189(9):1071–1074.

Heard DJ, Kollias GV, Webb AI, Jacobson ER, Brock KA. 1988. Use of halothane to maintain anesthesia induced with etorphine in juvenile African elephants. *Journal of the American Veterinary Medical Association* 193:254–256.

Honeyman VL, Pettifer GR, Dyson DH. 1992. Arterial blood pressure and blood gas values in normal standing and laterally recumbent African (*Loxodonta africana*) and Asian (*Elephas maximus*) elephants. *Journal of Zoo and Wildlife Medicine* 23: 205–210.

Horne WA, Tchamba MN, Loomis MR. 2001. A simple method of providing intermittent positive-pressure ventilation to etorphine-immobilized elephants (*Loxodonta africana*) in the field. *Journal of Zoo and Wildlife Medicine* 32(4):519–522.

Hunter RP, Isaza R, Koch DE. 2002. Oral availability and pharmacokinetic characteristics of ketoprofen enantiomers after oral and intravenous administration in Asian elephants (*Elephas maximus*). *American Journal of Veterinary Research* 64(1):109–114.

Jacobsen ER, Kollias GV, Heard DJ, Caliguiri R. 1988. Imobilization of African elephants with carfentanil and antagonism with nalmefene and diprenorphine. *Journal of Zoo Animal Medicine* 19(1–2):1–7.

Kock RA, Morkel P, Kock MD. 1993. Current immobilization procedures used in elephants. In: *Zoo and Wild Animal Medicine, Current Therapy 3* (ME Fowler, ed.), pp. 436–441. Philadelphia: W.B. Saunders Co.

Kreeger TJ, Arnemo JM, Raath JP. 2002. *Handbook of Wildlife Chemical Immobilization*. Fort Collins: Wildlife Pharmaceuticals Inc.

McComb K, Moss C, Durant SM, Baker L, Sayialel S. 2001. Matriarchs as repositories of social knowledge in African elephants. *Science* 292(5516):491–494.

Mortenson J. 2001. Determining dosages for antibiotic and anti-inflammatory agents. In: *The Elephant's Foot: Prevention and Care of Foot Conditions in Captive Asian and African Elephants* (B Csuti, EL Sargent, US Bechert, eds.), pp. 141–144. Ames: Iowa State University Press.

Nagy KA, Girard IA, Brown TK. 1999. Energetics of free-ranging mammals, reptiles, and birds. *Annual Review of Nutrition* 19:247–277.

Neiffer D, Miller M, Weber M, Stetter M, Fontenot D, Robbins P, Pye G. 2005. Standing sedation in African elephants (*Loxodonta africana*) using detomidine-butorphenol combinations. *Journal of Zoo and Wildlife Medicine* 36(2):250–256.

Ollivet-Courtois F, Lecu A, Yates RA, Spelman LH. 2003. Treatment of a sole abscess in an Asian elephant (*Elephas maximus*) using regional digital intravenous perfusion. *Journal of Zoo and Wildlife Medicine* 34(3):292–295.

Osofsky SA. 1997. A practical anesthesia monitoring protocol for free-ranging adult African elephants (*Loxodonta africana*). *Journal of Wildlife Diseases* 33(1):72–77.

Page CD. 1994. Anesthesia and chemical restraint. In: *Medical Management of Elephants* (SK Mikota, EL Sargent, GS Ranglack, eds.), pp. 41–49. West Bloomfield: Indira Publishing House.

Perry DC, Rosenbaum JS, Kurowski M, Sadee W. 1982. [³H]Etorphine receptor binding in vivo. Small fractional occupancy elicits analgesia. *Molecular Pharmacology* 21(2):272–279.

Raath JP. 1993. Chemical capture of the African elephant, *Loxodonta africana*. In: *The Capture and Care Manual* (AA McKinzie, ed.), pp. 484–493. Pretoria: Wildlife Decision and Support Services and the South African Veterinary Foundation.

Ramsay E. 2000. Standing sedation and tranquilization in captive African elephants (*Loxodonta africana*). Proceedings of the AAZV Joint Conference, New Orleans pp. 111–113.

Roca AL, Georgiadis N, Pecon-Slattery J, Obrien SJ. 2001. Genetic evidence for two species of elephant in Africa. *Science* 293 (5534):1473–1477.

Sarma B, Pathak SC, Sarma KK. 2002. Medetomidine a novel immobilizing agent for the elephant (*Elephas maximus*). *Research in Veterinary Science* 73(3):315–317.

Schmidt MJ. 2003. Proboscidae (elephants). In: *Zoo and Wild Animal Medicine, Current Therapy 5* (ME Fowler, RE Miller, eds.), pp. 541–550. St. Louis: Saunders.

Schmitt DL, Bradford LP, Hardy DA. 1996. Azaperone for standing sedation in Asian elphants (*Elephas maximus*). Proceedings of the AAZV Annual Conference, Puerta Vallarta, Mexico, pp. 48–51.

Sedgwick CJ. 1993. Allometric scaling and emergency care: the importance of body size. In: *Zoo and Wild Animal Medicine, Current Therapy 3* (ME Fowler, ed.), pp. 34–37. Philadelphia: W.B. Saunders Co.

Stegmann GF. 1999. Etorphine-halothane anaesthesia in two five-year-old African elephants (*Loxodonta africana*). *Journal of the South African Veterinary Medical Association* 70(4):164–166.

Stetter M, Grobler D, Zuba JR, Hendrickson D, Briggs M, Castro L, Neiffer D, Terrell S, Robbins PK, Stettr K, Ament BS, Wheeler L. 2005. Laparoscopic reproductive sterilization as a method of population control in free-ranging african elephants (*Loxodonta africana*). Proceedings of the AAZV, AAWV, AZA/NAG Joint Conference, Omaha, NE, pp. 199–200.

Still J, Raath JP, Matzner L. 1996. Respiratory and circulatory parameters of African elephants (*Loxodonta africana*) anesthetized with etorphine and azaperone. *Journal of the South African Veterinary Medical Association* 67(3):123–127.

Tamas PM, Geiser DR. 1983. Etorphine analgesia supplemented by halothane anesthesia in an adult African elephant. *Journal of the American Veterinary Medical Association* 183(11):1312–1314.

Tana L, Isaza R, Koch D, Hunter R. 2010. Pharmacokinetics and intramuscular bioavailability of a single dose of butorphenol in Asian elephants (*Elephas maximus*). *Journal of Zoo and Wildlife Medicine* 41(3):418–425.

Tchamba MN, Bauer H, De Iongh HH. 1995. Application of VHF-radio and satellite telemetry techniques on elephants in northern Cameroon. *African Journal of Ecology* 33(4):335–346.

Wallach JD, Anderson JL. 1968. Oripavine (M.99) combinations and solvents for immobilization of the African elephant. *Journal of the American Veterinary Medical Association* 153(7):793–797.

West J. 2002. Why doesn't the elephant have a pleural space? *News in Physiological Sciences* 17:47–50.

52 Nondomestic Equids

Chris Walzer

INTRODUCTION AND TAXONOMY

The Equidae family encompasses the zebras, asses, and horses. These descended some 50 million years ago from the "dawn horse" (*Hyracotherium*), with the *equus* emerging in the Pleistocene, about 1.5 million years ago. The taxonomy of the nondomestic equidae is controversial; the International Species Information System (ISIS) lists eight wild species with several subspecies, three zebras and one wild ass in Africa, and three wild asses and the Przewalski's horse in Asia (Table 52.1). They are distributed solely throughout the Old World, from the deserts of Namibia across the plains of eastern Africa to the high altitude semi-deserts of central Asia. In addition to the wild equidae, feral horses and donkeys (or burros) exist on all continents except Antarctica. Generally, the present-day equids exploit the semiarid grasslands, where they play a key role in the functioning of natural grazing systems. Within their natural range, many equids are subjected to extreme weather conditions. For example, temperatures range from −45°C in the winter to 40°C in the summer, with diurnal temperature ranges in excess of 35°C at the reintroduction site for Przewalski's horses in the Dzungarian Gobi in Mongolia. The equidae utilize a great range of altitudes within their present-day distribution, 60 m b.s.l. (Danakil: Somali wild ass) and 5000 m a.s.l. (Tibet: Kiang) (Strauss 1995). For further information concerning the status and geographical distribution of the various subspecies, the reader is referred to the IUCN/SSC Equid specialist group publications (Moehlman 2002). Of particular importance in the captive and medical management of the wild equids is an understanding of their two distinct social systems (Moehlman 2002). In the equids of the arid habitats, some males defend territories—preferably near water sources, which confer mating

rights over females when they enter the territory. Asses and Grevy's zebra form loose groups, and the only long-term relationship occurs between mother and off-spring for a period of 2 years. Asses in central Asia may aggregate to loose groups in excess of several 100 individuals. The other equid species form permanent family groups, so-called harem groups. In this system, lifelong relationships between adult individuals are formed. Young males form bachelor groups. The various social systems must be considered when managing these species in general, but especially the removal of individual animals from a harem group during anesthesia must be critically evaluated.

ANATOMY AND PHYSIOLOGY

The anatomy and physiology of the wild equids is similar to that of their domesticated counterparts (Table 52.2). The mountain zebras (*Equus zebra hartmannae* and *Equus zebra zebra*) are distinguished from other zebra species by a "grid iron" pattern formed by stripes on the rump and a small dewlap on the throat (Duncan 1992). The Grevy's zebra (*Equus grevyi*) is the largest wild equid. They are easily recognizable on the one hand due to their size, and on the other due to the large ears and distinct fine stripe pattern. The plains zebras (*Equus burchelli* spp.) are one of the most abundant ungulate species in Africa. Subspecies can be distinguished by the variations in their stripe patterns. The classification and number of the subspecies is controversial. The African wild asses are sympatric throughout their range with the domestic African donkeys, and it is probable that the genomes of the wild and domestic asses are extensively mixed. Unlike the Przewalski's horse and the domestic horse, the wild asses and donkeys have the same number of chromosomes and

Zoo Animal and Wildlife Immobilization and Anesthesia, Second Edition. Edited by Gary West, Darryl Heard, and Nigel Caulkett.
© 2014 John Wiley & Sons, Inc. Published 2014 by John Wiley & Sons, Inc.

appear similar. Differences persist in leg colors, counter shading, and shoulder crosses. The Asian wild asses (*Equus onager, Equus kiang,* and *Equus hemionus*) vary little in size, but skeletal and color differences allow the various subspecies to be distinguished. The Przewalski's horse (*Equus ferus przewalskii*) is closely related to the domestic horse; though they are distinct in the number of chromosomes (Przewalski's horse $2n = 66$; domestic horse $2n = 64$) their hybrids are fertile (Ryder et al. 1978). The Przewalski's horse has an erect mane, and the proximal aspect of the tail has short guard hairs. Most Przewalski's horses have a dark stripe along the back and distinct horizontal stripping of the palmar aspects of the front legs. Latest genetic research has shown that the Przewalski's horse is most probably not the direct ancestor of the present domestic horses, but more likely a sister taxa (Wallner et al. 2003).

VASCULAR ACCESS SITES AND MONITORING

Vascular access is easily performed in the various equid species. As a routine measure, an IV catheter should be placed during all equid anesthesia procedures, as this provides constant venous access if an emergency should arise or additional drugs must be provided. The jugular veins provide an excellent venous access site for standard "over the needle" catheters. Large bore catheters should be used to provide adequate fluid flow rates. At least 14 standard wire gauge (swg) should be used (Taylor & Clarke 2007). These can be placed either with the flow or against the flow. Placing catheters against the flow (towards the head) is often easier and reduces the risk of air entrainment (Taylor & Clarke 2007). Alternative venous access sites are the distal branches of the saphenous vein and the external thoracic vein. Arterial access and catheter placement is most easily achieved in the facial and transverse facial artery. These sites can be used to determine the pulse rate, collect arterial blood samples for blood gas analysis, and direct blood pressure monitoring. The handling and storage of arterial blood samples may affect blood gas values (Klein et al. 2005).

In general, anesthesia monitoring in the wild equid species is analogous to the domestic horse. Anesthesia monitoring should be implemented as soon as the animal is fixed. Sequential rectal temperature measurements, thorax excursion to determine breaths per minute, and auscultation for heart rate are the absolute minimum in anesthesia monitoring. Relative percent oxyhemoglobin saturation measured with a battery-powered pulse oximeter (e.g., Nellcor NP-20, Nellcor Incorporated, Pleasanton, CA) is useful to determine arterial oxygenation and gives a good insight into respiratory function. Pulse oximeter probes can be affixed to the tongue, nasal septum, and the plucked ear (Fig. 52.1). Several excellent reviews have been previously published and the reader is referred to these (Saint John 1992; Taylor & Clarke 2007).

INTUBATION

Endotracheal intubation is easily achieved in the equid species. For intubation, the head is extended. When using the almost straight silicone endotracheal tubes (ET), these can be advanced directly into the trachea. When using the older curved red-rubber type ET, the

Table 52.1.   Present-day wild equids

Genus	Species	Subspecies	Common Name
Equus	*asinus*	*africanus*	Nubian wild ass
		somalicus	Somali wild ass
	onager	*khur*	Indian wild ass
		kulan	Turkmenian wild ass/kulan
		onager	Persian onager
	kiang	*holdereri*	Eastern kiang
		kiang	Western kiang
		polyodon	Southern kiang
	hemionus	*hemionus*	Mongolian wild ass
		luteus	Gobi dziggetai
	ferus	*przewalskii*	Przewalski's wild horse
	burchelli	*antiquorum*	Damara zebra
		boehmi	Grant's zebra
		burchelli	Burchel's zebra
		selousii	Selous' zebra
		chapmanni	Chapmann zebra
	grevyi		Grevy's zebra
	zebra	*hartmannae*	Hartmann's mountain zebra
		zebra	Cape mountain zebra

Table 52.2.   Biological data of the wild equids

	Birth Weight	Adult Weight	Life Expectancy	Reported Gestation Length	Nursing in Months
Przewalski's horse	45	250–375	33	330–340	6–8
Asian wild ass	25–30	200–250	29	330–360	6–9
African wild ass	20–30	250–300	24	360	4–6
Grevy's zebra	20–30	350–450	35	387–428	6–13
Plains zebra	33	350–450	29	365–375	6–10

Sources: Adapted from Strauss G. 1995. Einhufer. In: *Krankheiten der Zoo- und Wildtiere* (R Göltenboth, H-G Klös, eds.), pp. 189–200. Berlin: Blackwell Wissenschafts-Verlag; Duncan P, ed. *Zebras, Asses, and Horses: An Action Plan for the Conservation of Wild Equids*. Gland, Switzerland: UCN, 1992.

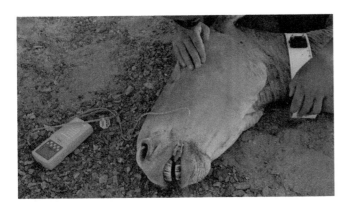

Figure 52.1. Portable pulse oximeter probe affixed to the tongue of an Asiatic wild ass.

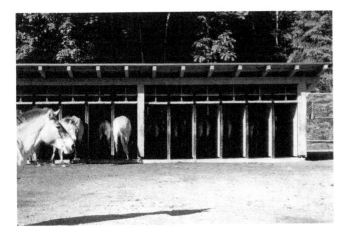

Figure 52.2. Nonchemical capture of the zoo-born horses. Individual horses are fed in large crates over a period of several weeks. These crates are subsequently closed using a cable controlled remote drop-door system.

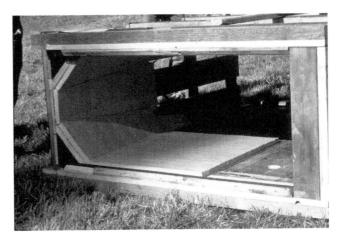

Figure 52.3. Head and neck movement in transport crates is restricted with padding in order to reduce the risk of a horse turning onto its back at take off during air transport.

ET is initially advanced with the concave curve dorsally until the soft palate is dislodged from the epiglottis and then rotated 90° and passed on down the trachea (Taylor & Clarke 2007).

NONCHEMICAL CAPTURE OF EQUIDS

Though physical restraint cannot be recommended for any wild equid, except possibly newborn foals, non-chemical capture methods have been employed in the zoo-born Przewalski's horse. In the course of the various reintroduction projects to Mongolia, specific techniques and methods have been developed in order to facilitate loading. For the first time in 2002, nonchemical capture and crating was possible for the majority of the zoo-born horses. The system was based on training each individual horse to feed in large crates over a period of several weeks. These crates are subsequently be closed using a remote system and the horses moved into the smaller transport crates (Fig. 52.2) (Walzer

et al. 2004). In 2005, a similar simplified system was also used successfully in Takhin Tal, Mongolia, to move eight horses into the west of the Gobi B Strictly Protected Area (Schönpflug and Walzer, unpubl. data, 2005).

Individual transport crates for equids are based on the IATA recommendations but have been adapted over the years for this specific airfreight transport scenario but are most probably beneficial for all equid transports (IATA 2006). Head and neck movement in the crate has been limited in order to reduce the risk of a horse turning onto its back while inside the crate at take off during air transport (Fig. 52.3). The headroom of the crates is additionally lined with high density foam mats to limit abrasions and trauma due to head—rubbing. Alternatively and for land transport, equids can be mass crated (Openshaw 1993).

CHEMICAL RESTRAINT AND CAPTURE

Oral Sedation

Varying degrees of sedation can be achieved using acepromazine as granules (Vetranquil 1%, Albrecht, Germany) or as a paste (Sedalin, Chassot, Switzerland) at a dosage of 0.5–1.5 mg/kg PO. The granules are mixed into moistened pelleted feed, and alternatively the paste is placed in apples both of which are then readily consumed by the animal. Though this is not sufficient for subsequent physical restraint, it has proven valuable as a transport and preimmobilization sedation (Wiesner 1993).

Parenteral Sedation

Various drugs, especially alpha2-agonists and acepromazine (Vetranquil 1%, Albrecht, Germany), have been used to sedate wild equids. Detomidine (Domosedan, SmithKline Beecham Animal Health) at 20–80 µg/kg IM has been used successfully in some wild equids (Morris

1992; Vitaud 1993). In contrast to the experiences gained with detomidine, these authors warn against using the alpha2 agonist medetomidine (Dormitor, SmithKline Beecham Animal Health) alone as a preanesthetic due to the occurrence of significant ataxia (Morris 1992). Similarly romifidine (Sedivet, Boehringer, Germany) has been shown to cause ataxia (Wiesner & von Hegel 1990). Acepromazine is used at a dosage of 0.15–0.25 mg/kg IM. Furthermore, Azaperone at a dosage of 200 mg has been suggested for the sedation of zebras (Burroughs 1993b). Several other drugs would potentially be useful in sedating equids but are impracticable in their use due to the large volumes necessary.

Long-Acting Neuroleptics

When long-term sedation is required, as during a transport process, this is best achieved using one of the long-acting neuroleptics (LAN). This group of drugs can be used to reduce anxiety and stress during long-distance translocation, and for reintroduction into novel enclosures and habitats. As a result of the delayed absorption of the neuroleptics, it is prudent to combine a long-acting tranquillizer with a short-acting analog (Ebedes 1992). Haloperidol belongs to the butyrophenone group of neuroleptics with a longer duration of activity. It is available in Europe as a 5-mg/mL injectable solution (Haldol, Janssen-Cilag, Vienna, Austria) that can be applied intramuscularly (IM) and IV. Furthermore, 1- and 10-mg tablet forms (Haldol, Janssen-Cilag) for oral application are also available. It is important to note that in Europe, haloperidol is also available as a decanoate ester (Haloperidol decanoate, Janssen-Cilag), an oily form that results in a long-term deposit. Haloperidol decanoate results in a prolonged sedation of up to 25 days and its effects are generally unsatisfactory due to adverse side effects, such as innappetence and central nervous system symptoms (Swan 1993). Zuclopenthixol acetate is a thioxanthene similar to the phenothiazine group of tranquillizers. Through esterification with the acetate and dissolution in a vegetable oil, absorption and duration has been extended. It is available as 50 mg/mL injectable solution (Ciatyl-Z-Accuphase, Bayer, Leverkusen, Germany). Similar to haloperidol, zuclopenthixol is also available in some countries as a decanoate ester; again, the duration is extended, but once again the effect seems inadequate

(Swan 1993). Perphenazine is a phenothiazine derivate with a piperazine side chain. It is available as a 100 mg/mL injectable solution in the enanthate ester form, dissolved in a sesame oil (Decentan Depot, Merck KgaA, Darmstadt, Germany). When compared with haloperidol and zuclopenthixol, perphenazine has a markedly prolonged duration of action that can subsist for 10 days. These neuroleptics have been used successfully in various zebra species (Swan 1993) and in the Przewalski's horse (Atkinson & Blumer 1997; Walzer et al. 2000). Extrapyramidal symptoms (EPS), a neurological side effect, causes a variety of symptoms, for example, involuntary movements, tremors, changes in breathing and heart rate, and inapetenz have been recorded as the most important side effects of LAN. The EPS can be treated with biperidine (Akineton, Knoll, South Africa) and diazepam (Valium, Roche, Switzerland). The use of long-acting neuroleptics has greatly facilitated the in-crate phase during flight (36 hours) and reloading of Przewalski's horses. This author presently recommends treatment with a combination of 0.2–0.3 mg/kg haloperidol (Haldol, Janssen-Cilag) and 150–200 mg/adult equid perphenazine (Decentan-Depot, Merck KgaA, Darmstadt, Germany). It is important to carry out this treatment at least 12–24 hours prior to transport or anticipated stressor influence (Table 52.3).

Anesthesia

Applying drugs over a greater distance requires specific remote delivery systems. For an excellent review of the various available systems, the reader is referred to Kreeger et al. (2002) and the previous chapter by Isaza in this book. The author recommends the use of a CO_2 propelled dart gun, such as the Daninject JM model (Daninject JM™, Wildlife Pharmaceuticals, Fort Collins, CO). Previous authors have warned against using high velocity gun systems (e.g., Cap-Chur® system) in zebras due to their thin skin (Burroughs 1993a). When working in the wild, this author prefers to use new 3-mL darts discharged by expanding compressed air (Daninject, Wildlife Pharmaceuticals). Old darts are not used, as these are never as accurate. By shortening the dart stabilizers to 3 cm, the effective range is 80 m under ideal conditions (Lengger et al. 2002). However, this distance is significantly reduced in the windy conditions. A sufficiently long dart needle of 55 mm is required to efficiently dart an Asian wild equid in good

Table 52.3. Suggested dosages for long-acting neuroleptics in selected wild equids

Drug	Burchell's Zebra	Hartmann's Zebra	Przewalski's Horse	Onset of Sedation	Duration
Haloperidol	0.3 mg/kg	0.28–035 mg/kg	0.2–0.3 mg/kg	5–10 minutes	8–18 hours
Zuclopenthixol	50–100 mg/adult	50–100 mg/adult	50–100 mg/adult	1 hour	3–4 days
Perphenazine	100–200 mg/adult	200 mg/adult	150–200 mg/adult	12–16 hours	10 days

Sources: Based on Swan GE. 1993. Drugs used for the immobilization, capture, and translocation of wild animals. In: *The Capture and Care Manual* (AA McKenzie, ed.), pp. 2–64. Pretoria: Wildlife Decision Support and the South African Veterinary Foundation; Walzer C, Baumgartner R, Robert N, et al. 2000. Medical aspects in Przewalski horse (*Equus przewalskii*) reintroduction in the Dzungarian Gobi, Mongolia. Proceedings of the American Association of Zoo Veterinarians, pp. 7–21.

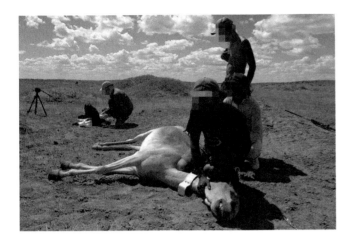

Figure 52.4. The head of a horse should be fixated at all times during an immobilization procedure. The knee is best placed laterally on the maxilla.

condition during the late summer and fall, due to significant layers of fat in the rump region. For zebras, a needle length of 25–30 mm has previously been recommended (Burroughs 1993a). In captive zebras, this is most probably too short, and the use of 55 mm should be considered. The use of wire barbs or collars on the needle to securely retain the dart in the animal is recommended in order to enable complete drug expulsion. Once an animal is successfully darted, one should attempt to keep it in sight. However, it is very important at this stage to not disturb the animal any further by chasing it or approaching before the drugs have taken full effect. Once the animal has become recumbent, an approach on foot from behind and immediate fixation of the head is recommended (Fig. 52.4). Be aware that in the first few minutes of recumbency, the animal may become aroused by voices or loud noises and attempt to rise and flee further. Anesthesia monitoring should be implemented as soon as the animal is fixed.

The agent of choice for wild equid immobilization and anesthesia is the potent opiate ethorphine. The opiates interact in the central nervous system (CNS) with stereo-specific and satuarble receptors (Kreeger et al. 2002). Various receptors have been identified. These are classified as κ, δ, σ, and μ receptors. A major advantage in the use of the opiates is the specific opiate antagonists that allow for the complete reversal of the anesthetic effects. Whereas some agents can be classed as sole antagonists (e.g., naltrexone), others have agonist–antagonist properties (e.g., diphrenorphine). The opiate ethorphine is an analog of thebaine and is in humans 500 times more potent then morphine (Jasinski et al. 1975; Kreeger et al. 2002). Ethorphine at 2.45 mg/mL is available in Europe and many other parts of the world in combination with acepromazine 10 mg/mL (Large Animal Immobilon, C-Vet Veterinary Products, Leyland, UK). Furthermore, ethorphine is

available as a mono substance at 4.9 mg/mL and 9.8 mg/mL (M99, Vericore Ltd., Dundee, Scotland). All products are supplied in a container together with the antidote diprenorphine or M5050 in the respective adequate dosages. The use of diprenorphine to antagonize etorphine in nondomestic equids may increase the likelihood of renarcotizations. In North America, due to difficulty in obtaining ethorphine, a similar, more potent opiate, carfentanil (Wildlife Pharmaceuticals) has been used extensively in equids (Allen 1992, 1994, 1997; Klein & Citino 1995). However, the effects of carfentanil cannot be equated with those of ethorphine as the procedure is markedly rougher with significant muscle contractions (Morris 1992). In the past years, several additional nonnarcotic immobilization protocols have been developed and used more or less successfully in wild equids (Matthews et al. 1995; Morris 1992; Vitaud 1993). For prolonged surgical procedures, intubation and inhalation anesthesia with isoflurane or halothane is recommended.

For wild equid anesthesia, this author presently recommends a combination of the opiate ethorphine (M99, C-Vet Veterinary Products, Lancashire, UK), the sedative alpha$_2$ agonist detomidine-HCl (Domosedan, Orion Corp. Farmos, Turku, Finland), and the mixed antagonist-agonist opioid buthorphanol (Torbugesic, Fort Dodge Animal Health, Fort Dodge, IA). Detomidine acts on the alpha$_2$-adrenergic receptors, where it inhibits the release of norephinephrine. Butorphanol is a mu-opioid receptor antagonist that alleviates the marked respiratory depression induced by the ethorphine at the μ receptor and potentiates the sedative effect at the kappa and sigma receptors. Furthermore, this combination has significantly limited the ethorphine specific pacing, which greatly reduces the distance an equid travels after darting. This is particularly important in open steppe habitats, where equids darted without the addition of butorphanol can cover several kilometers before becoming recumbent. However, the combination still allows for "walk-in" crate loading. Ethorphine is reversed with the opioid antagonist naltrexone at a rate of 20:1 (Trexonil, Wildlife Laboratories Inc., Fort Collins, CO). Naltrexone has a longer half-life than the antagonist-agonist diprenorphine (Revivon, C-Vet Veterinary Products) and eliminates in- and posttransport renarcotization. Renarcotization is an effect that occurs when using opioids. Several hours after antagonist application, the animals once again come under the influence of the opioid agonist (Kreeger et al. 2002). Especially in equids captured in the wild, this effect could be fatal as it potentially makes an individual more prone to predation and injury. However, it is important to note that due to the long half-life, a subsequent anesthesia induction with ethorphine (or any other opioid), in case of emergency, would not be possible, and an alternative method (e.g., the alpha$_2$-agonist medetomidine and ketamine) needs to be considered (Table 52.4).

Table 52.4. Selected anesthetic protocols for wild equids

Species	Drug 1	Drug 2	Additional Drugs	Antagonist	Comments	Literature
Kulan (*Equus hemionus*)	4.2-mg ethorphine	17-mg ACP	30-mg xylazine	6-mg diprenorphine + 0.125-mg/kg yohimbine	Total dose for adult	a
	0.016-mg/kg ethorphine	0.067-mg/kg ACP		0.042-mg/kg diprenorphine + 0.4-mg/kg nalorphine	n = 27 + 49	c,d
	5.4-mg ethorphine		150-mg ketamine	250-mg naltrexone	Total dose for adult n = 3 wild	i
	4.4-mg ethorphine	10-mg butorphanol	10-mg detomidine	6-mg diprenorphine	n = 17 wild	c,d
Kiang (*Equus kiang kiang*)	0.012-mg/kg ethorphine	0.05-mg/kg ACP		0.025-mg/kg diprenorphine	n = 26 + 10	c,d
Somali wild ass (*Equus onager*)	0.017 mg/kg ethorphine	0.07-mg/kg ACP		0.045-mg/kg diprenorphine	n = 14	c,d
Przewalski's horse (*Equus ferus przewalskii*)	0.008-mg/kg ethorphine	0.033-mg/kg ACP	0.033-mg/kg detomidine, 0.033-mg/kg buthorphanol	0.16-mg/kg naltrexone + 0.04-mg/kg atipamezole IV	n = 34 wild	f,i
	0.018-mg/kg ethorphine	0.075-mg/kg ACP	0.16-mg/kg xylazine	0.045-mg/kg diprenorphine IV	n = 32 + 41	c,d
	0.07- to 0.1-mg/kg medetomidine	1.8- to 2.6-mg/kg ketamine		0.17- to 0.23-mg/kg atipamezole	n = 11 from 14	b
Mountain zebra (*Equus zebra*)	0.6-mg/kg romifidine	3.3-mg/kg TZ		Tolazoline 2.5- to 3-mg/kg IV	n = 15	g
	0.35-mg/kg romifidine	1.8-mg/kg TZ		Tolazoline 2.5- to 3-mg/kg IV	n = 9	h
	4- to 6-mg ethorphine	80-mg azaperone		9.6- to 14.4-mg diprenorphine	Total dose for adult High dose for male	a
Plains zebra (*Equus burchelli*)	0.009- to 0.01-mg/kg ethorphine	0.037- to 0.044-mg/kg ACP		0.045-mg/kg diprenorphine IV	n = 53 + 69	c,d
	0.0085- to 0.01-mg/kg ethorphine	0.035- to 0.04-mg/kg ACP		0.045-mg/kg diprenorphine IV	n = 54 + 21	c,d
	5.5- to 8.3-mg/kg TZ	0.06- to 0.08-mg/kg detomidine			n = 11 long recovery	e

[a]Kreeger TJ. 1996. Individual dosages. In: *Handbook of Wildlife Chemical Immobilization* (TJ Kreeger, ed.), pp. 178–237. Laramie: International Wildlife Veterinary Services.
[b]Matthews NS, Petrini KR, Wolff PL. 1995. Anesthesia of Przewalksi's horses (*Equus przewalskii przewalskii*) with medetomidine/ketamine and antagonism with atipamezole. *Journal of Zoo and Wildlife Medicine* 2:231–236.
[c]Strauss G. 1992. Erfahrungen bei der immobilisation verschiedener Equidenarten in Tierpark Berlin-Friedrichfelde. Proceedings of the 34th International Symposium on the Diseases of Zoo and Wild Animals, pp. 163–169.
[d]Strauss G. 1999. Zur Immobilisation der Wildequiden unter Zoobedingungen. *Equus* 3:306–314.
[e]Vitaud C. 1993. Utilisation de la combinaison anesthesique tiletamine/zolazepam et detomidine chez les zebres de Grant (Equus burchelli boehmi) premiers resultats. Proceedings of the 34th International Symposium on the Diseases of Zoo and Wild Animals, pp. 277–80.
[f]Walzer C, Baumgartner R, Robert N, Suchebaatar Z, Bajalagmaa N. 2000. Medical considerations in the reintroduction of the Przewalski Horse (*Equus przewalskii*) to the Dzungurian Gobi, Mongolia. Proceedings of the European Association of Zoo and Wildlife Veterinarians (EAZWV), pp. 147–150. Paris, France.
[g]C. Walzer, unpubl. data, 2002.
[h]Wiesner H, von Hegel G. 1990. Zur Immobilisation von Wildequiden mit STH 2130 und Tiletamin/Zolazepam. *Tierärztliche Praxis* 18:151–154.
[i]Walzer C, Kaczensky P, Ganbataar O, Lengger J, Enkhsaikhan N, Lkhagvasuren D. 2006. Capture and anaesthesia of wild Mongolian equids: the Przewalski's horse (*E. ferus przewalskii*) and the Khulan (*E. hemionus*). *Mongolian Journal of Biological Sciences* 4(1):19–28.

ACP, acepromazine.

Chemical Capture of Equids in the Wild

Przewalski's Horses Due to the general lack of cover in the Gobi area wild Przewalski's horses are extremely difficult to approach in the field. During the past years, we have employed various methods to get within shooting range, such as approaching on a motorcycle and horseback or waiting at water points. Using a combination of 2.5- to 3.0-mg ethorphine, 10-mg detomidine, and 10-mg butorphanol, 14 horses have been successfully captured in the wild (and 35 procedures in the very large adaptation enclosures—20–30 ha) in Mongolia (Walzer et al. 2006). Initial effects were noticed after 3–5 minutes when the animal exhibited a stiff, high stepping gait and became ataxic. Induction to lateral recumbency occurred within 5–10 minutes. Procedures lasted on average 35 minutes. Following IV antagonist application anesthesia was smoothly reversed without any signs of excitement, and the animals were back on their feet within 2 minutes. It is important to note that the head of all equids should be fixed to the ground as long as possible following antagonist application to prevent premature uncoordinated attempts at getting up, as these could result in injury (Walzer et al. 2006) (Fig. 52.5).

Asiatic Wild Ass In Mongolia, the wild ass is extremely skittish—most probably due to poaching activities—and in some areas, flees human presence at several kilometers' distance (e.g., in Great Gobi B SPA). We have employed three distinct techniques to capture this species in the wild. In the summers of 2002 and 2005, we used a modified high pressure CO_2 dart gun (Daninject JM, Wildlife Pharmaceuticals) from a pre-placed hide, 60–80 m distant from water points. This method was especially useful in the south Gobi as the

khulan are readily approached in the area. Some water points additionally offer good cover that allows for a shooting distance of 40–55 m. If possible, it is a distinct advantage to take a position high above the animal (e.g., cliff face), as they are unwary of danger from above. As open water is lacking in large parts of the distribution range in the south Gobi, the wild ass must dig to a depth of approximately 45 cm to access ground water. At this time, it is very difficult for animal to see movements in its vicinity. Furthermore, the use of ground water increases the amount of time the animals have to remain stationary, which additionally greatly facilitates darting.

In 2003 and 2005, we also employed a chase method where the khulan was darted from a moving jeep. This method had previously been used to collar a wild Bactrian camel (*Camelus bactrianus ferus*) and is traditionally employed by wild ass poachers with 12-gauge shotguns (Blumer et al. 2002). When using the local UAZ jeeps it is important to remove the window from the passenger side and to provide seatbelts for the driver and shooter. If using the Daninject JM CO_2 dart gun, a short 4-cm barrel can be used instead of the standard barrel as this greatly facilitates movement in the jeep. Once an animal is identified, it is chased until the jeep is able to approach within approximately 10–15 m on a parallel track (see Fig. 52.6). It is then easily darted in the rump musculature using standard pressure settings. It is essential to define a chase cut off time before the procedure is started. Our experience has shown that a cut off time of 15 minutes is adequate for the Asiatic wild ass. To date, we have captured six animals with this very time-efficient method. The shortest chase time was 2 minutes and the longest 13 minutes. In all cases, induction was extremely rapid

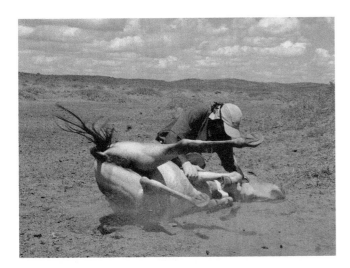

Figure 52.5. The head of all equids should be fixed to the ground as long as possible following antagonist application to prevent premature uncoordinated attempts at getting up, as these could result in injury.

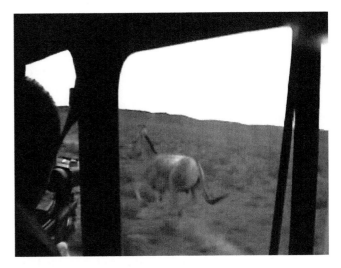

Figure 52.6. An Asiatic wild ass being darted in the rump musculature from a moving jeep (60 km/h) at a distance of approximately 10–15 m on a parallel track.

and smooth (4–8 minutes), and body temperature was below 40°C. A severe limitation to this method is that one is only able to capture males or juveniles without foals. A chase of a female with a foal would result in (permanent) separation of the young from the mare and is therefore unacceptable.

Finally, we have used a video-enabled remote controlled CO_2 gun (Walzer & Boegel 2003) at several water points in attempts to capture khulan in 2003 and 2005. To date, this method has not been successful for wild ass mainly due to the abundance of water in the areas it was employed. In the authors' view, this method has great potential in areas with small waterholes that the animals have to visit.

In all wild ass procedures, anesthesia was induced with a single 3-mL dart containing a combination of 4.4-mg ethorphine (M99, C-Vet Veterinary Products, Lancashire, UK), 10-mg Detomidine–HCl (Domosedan, Orion Corp. Farmos) and 10-mg Butorphanol (Torbugesic, Fort Dodge Animal Health). Anesthesia was initially reversed with an IV combination of 200-mg naltrexone (Trexonil Wildlife Laboratories Inc.) and the alpha$_2$-antagonist 20 mg Atipamezole (Antisedan, Orion Corp. Farmos). Reversal was rapid and generally smooth, but some signs of excitation related to radio collar placement—head shaking—were noted. Subsequently, the opioid antagonist-agonist diprenorphine (Revivon, C-Vet Veterinary Products) was used. This eliminated head shaking and provided a smoother reversal. All animals were standing and alert approximately 2 minutes following administration of the antagonists.

Zebras The chemical capture of zebras has been described previously (Burroughs 1993a). Similar to the Asiatic wild equids, zebras are very difficult to approach in the wild. The techniques employed are similar to the ones described earlier. When available, darting from a helicopter is recommended (Burroughs 1993a).

Surgical Field Anesthesia For some procedures, it can be necessary to extend and deepen the anesthesia as the chemical capture drug combinations at the doses provided, do not offer the necessary depth of anesthesia for surgical procedures as significant muscle contractions and uncontrollable movements can occur. Following recumbency, an IV catheter is placed, and an IV infusion of guaifenesin-ketamine-xylazine (1 L of 5% guaifenesin) (Myolaxin, Vétoquinol UK Ltd., Buckingham, UK), 1000 mg ketamine (Ketamidor, Richter Pharma, Wels, Austria), and 500 mg xylazine (Rompun, Bayer Austria Ges.m.b.H, Vienna, Austria) is started. Nasal oxygen at a flow rate of 10 L/min is provided. An adult Przewalski's horse received on average 733 mL of the triple drip at an average rate of 12.6 mL/min. Despite oxygen supplementation, most equids will

become hypoxemic and slightly hypercapnic throughout the procedure.

Approximately 10 minutes before the surgical procedure is finished, the IV infusion should be stopped. Subsequently, the opiate anesthesia components from the capture event are reversed with 150 mg IV naltrexone. This multidrug procedure is well adapted for surgical anesthesia in Przewalski's horses and most likely for other wild equids in a field setting. However, it is strongly recommended that adequate anesthesia monitoring is available for the early recognition of critical respiratory and metabolic problems (Walzer et al. 2009) (Fig. 52.1 and Fig. 52.7).

Figure 52.8 shows a horse post antagonism getting up.

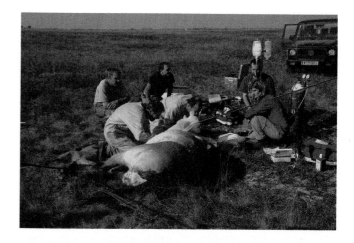

Figure 52.7. Field anesthesia and surgery setting in the Hortobágy National Park, Hungary. Following induction with etorphine-detomidine-butorphanol, surgical-depth anesthesia is maintained with a so-called triple-drip IV consisting of guaifenesin-ketamine-xylazine.

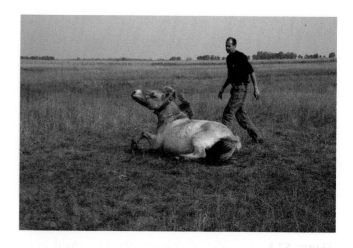

Figure 52.8. A radio-collared Przewalski's horse rising following the reversal of the opiate anesthesia components with 150-mg naltrexone.

Chemical Capture of Captive Nondomestic Equids

Carfentanil has been extensively studied as an immobilizing agent for nondomestic equids (Allen 1990, 1992, 1994, 1997; Klein & Citino 1995). Ethorphine was not available to zoo and wildlife veterinarians working in the United States for several years, so carfentanil was used as a primary immobilizing agent for nondomestic equids (Allen 1992, 1994, 1997). There are several disadvantages of using carfentanil versus ethorphine as an immobilizing agent for nondomestic equids. Oftentimes, nondomestic equids immobilized with carfentanil have to be assisted into recumbency or be given supplemental anesthetic induction agents to achieve complete immobilization (Allen 1992, 1994; Klein & Citino 1995). Supplemental anesthetic agents are given IV after the animal partially immobilized by carfentanil. Ketamine, glyceryl guaiacolate, or propofol is often used to get adequate muscle relaxation and complete immobilization (Zuba & Burns 1998). The delivery of carfentanil by dart into the muscles of the neck or shoulder will result in faster induction times and less morbidity (Allen 1992, 1994, 1997). Significant respiratory depression is commonly seen with carfentanil immobilizations (Allen 1992, 1994). This can often be successfully treated with IV administration of doxapram and the delivery of intranasal oxygen (Allen 1992, 1994, 1997). Most nondomestic equids immobilized with carfentanil alone experience a significant tachycardia, which may be due the stress of the procedure and inadequate immobilization (Allen 1992, 1994). Additionally, renarcotization may occur in nondomestic equids immobilized with carfentanil.

Renarcotization seems to be more common in the Somali wild ass (*Equus onager*) when immobilized with carfentanil alone (Allen 1997). Carfentanil, when used alone, was not adequate for the immobilization of Grevy's zebra (*Equus grevyi*) unless unacceptably high doses were used (Allen 1997).

Grevy's zebra (*Equus grevyi*) can be immobilized with carfentanil in combination with other drugs in a staged immobilization protocol (Klein & Citino 1995). First, detomidine (0.1–0.15 mg/kg) is given IM. Then approximately 20 minutes later, carfentanil (0.098 mg/kg) in combination with ketamine (2 mg/kg) is given IM. In one study, this combination was compared to medetomidine and ketamine in combination. Both study groups experienced significant hypertension with these combinations (Klein & Citino 1995). The preferred method for immobilizing captive Grevy's zebra is using ethorphine in combination with detomidine or detomidine and acepromazine (see Table 52.4).

Although carfentanil can be used to immobilize captive nondomestic equids, ethorphine is the preferred primary immobilizing agent. Diprenorphine, in most cases, will adequately antagonize the effects of ethorphine. But in one comprehensive review of renarcotization in nondomestic equids, renarcotization was relatively common in zebra and onager when using diprenorphine to antagonize ethorphine (Allen 1990). The use of naltrexone to antagonize ethorphine typically does not result in any episodes of renarcotization in nondomestic equids.

REFERENCES

Allen JL. 1990. Renarcotization following etorphine immobilization of non-domestic equidae. *Journal of Zoo and Wildlife Medicine* 21(3):292–294.

Allen JL. 1992. Immobilization of Mongolian wild horses (*Equus przewalskii przewalskii*) with carfentanil and antagonism with naltrexone. *Journal of Zoo and Wildlife Medicine* 23(4):422–425.

Allen JL. 1994. Immobilization of Hartmann's mountain zebras (*Equus zebra hartmannae*) with carfentanil and antagonism with naltrexone or nalmefene. *Journal of Zoo and Wildlife Medicine* 25(2):205–208.

Allen JL. 1997. Anesthesia of non-domestic horses with carfentanil and antagonism with naltrexone. Proceedings of the American Association of Zoo Veterinarians, p. 126.

Atkinson M, Blumer ES. 1997. The use of a long-acting neuroleptic in the Mongolian wild horse (*Equus przewalskii przewalskii*) to facilitate the establishment of a bachelor herd. Proceedings of the American Association of Zoo Veterinarians, pp. 199–200.

Blumer, ES, Namshir Z, Tuya T, Mijiddorj B, Reading RP, Mix H. 2002. Veterinary aspects of wild Bactrian camel (*Camelus bactrianus ferus*) conservation in Mongolia. In: *Ecology and Conservation of the Wild Bactrian Camel (*Camelus bactrianus ferus*)* (RP Reading, D Enkhbileg, T Galbaatar, eds.), pp. 115–122. Series in Conservation Biology. Ulaanbaatar: Mongolian Conservation Coalition.

Burroughs REJ. 1993a. Chemical capture of Burchell's zebra Equus burchelli and the mountain zebra Equus zebra. In: *The Capture and Care Manual* (AA McKenzie, ed.), pp. 627–630. Pretoria: Wildlife Decision Support and the South African Veterinary Foundation.

Burroughs REJ. 1993b. Care of Burchell's zebra and mountain zebra in captivity. In: *The Capture and Care Manual* (AA McKenzie, ed.), p. 631. Pretoria: Wildlife Decision Support and the South African Veterinary Foundation.

Duncan P. 1992. Zebras, asses, and horses an action plan for the conservation of wild equids. In: *Zebras, Asses, and Horses: An Action Plan for the Conservation of Wild Equids*. Gland: IUCN.

Ebedes H. 1992. Long acting neuroleptics in wildlife. In: *The Use of Tranquillizers in Wildlife* (H Ebedes, ed.), pp. 31–37. Pretoria: Sinoville Printers.

International Air Traffic Association (IATA). 2006. *Live Animals Regulations*, 33rd ed. Montreal, Canada: IATA.

Jasinski DR, Martin WR, Mansky PA. 1975. Progress report on studies from the clinical pharmacology section of the addiction research center, *CPDD*:121.

Klein L, Citino SB. 1995. Comparison of detomidine/carfentanil/ketamine and medetomidine/ketamine anesthesia in Grevy's zebra. Proceedings of the American Association of Zoo Veterinarians/Wildlife Disease Association/American Association of Wildlife Veterinarians, pp. 290–293.

Klein L, Bush M, Citino SB, et al. 2005. Effects of Three methods of storage on Po2, Pco2, and pH of Grevy's zebra blood (*Equus grevyi*). 2005 Proceedings of the American Association of Zoo Veterinarians, pp. 267–269.

Kreeger, JT, Arnemo JM, Raath JP. 2002. *Handbook of Wildlife Chemical Immobilization*, International ed. Fort Collins: Wildlife Pharmaceuticals.

Lengger J, Walzer C, Silinski S. 2002. A simple method of range extension in remote injection systems. Proceedings of the

European Association of Zoo and Wildlife Veterinarians (EAZWV), pp. 467–470. Heidelberg, Germany.

Matthews NS, Petrini KR, Wolff PL. 1995. Anesthesia of Przewalksi's horses (*Equus przewalskii przewalskii*) with medetomidine/ketamine and antagonism with atipamezole. *Journal of Zoo and Wildlife Medicine* 2:231–236.

Moehlman PDE. 2002. *Equids: Zebras, Asses and Horses.* Cambridge, UK: IUCN Publication Services Unit.

Morris PJ. 1992. Evaluation of potential adjuncts for equine chemical immobilization. 1992 Proceedings of the Joint Meeting American Association of Zoo Veterinarians-American Association of Wildlife Veterinarians, pp. 235–250.

Openshaw P. 1993. Transportation of antelope and zebra. In: *The Capture and Care Manual* (AA McKenzie, ed.), pp. 407–421. Pretoria: Wildlife Decision Support and the South African Veterinary Foundation.

Ryder O, Epel NC, Bernischke K. 1978. Chromosome banding studies of the equidae. *Cytogenetics and Cell Genetics* 20: 323–350.

Saint John BE. 1992. Pulse oximetry: theory, technology and clinical considerations. 1992 Proceedings of the Joint Meeting American Association of Zoo Veterinarians-American Association of Wildlife Veterinarians, pp. 223–229.

Strauss G. 1995. Einhufer. In: *Krankheiten der Zoo- und Wildtiere* (R Göltenboth, H-G Klös, eds.), pp. 189–200. Berlin: Blackwell Wissenschafts-Verlag.

Swan GE. 1993. Drugs used for the immobilization, capture, and translocation of wild animals. In: *The Capture and Care Manual* (AA McKenzie, ed.), pp. 2–64. Pretoria: Wildlife Decision Support and the South African Veterinary Foundation.

Taylor PM, Clarke KW. 2007. *Handbook of Equine Anaesthesia*, 2nd ed. Edinburgh: Saunders—Elsevier.

Vitaud C. 1993. Utilisation de la combinaison anesthesique tiletamine/zolazepam et detomidine chez les zebres de Grant (Equus burchelli boehmi) premiers resultats. Proceedings of the 35th International Symposium on Diseases of Zoo and Wild Animals, pp. 277–280.

Wallner B, Brem G, Mueller M, Achmann R. 2003. Fixed nucleotide differences on the Y chromosome indicate clear divergence between *Equus przewalskii* and *Equus caballus*. *Animal Genetics* 34:453–456.

Walzer C, Boegel R. 2003 A video-enabled, radio-controlled remote telinjection system for field applications. Proceedings of the American Association of Zoo Veterinarians, p. 228–229. October 4–10, Minneapolis, MN.

Walzer C, Baumgartner R, Robert N, Suchebaatar Z, Bajalagmaa N. 2000. Medical aspects in Przewalski horse (*Equus przewalskii*) reintroduction to the Dzungarian Gobi, Mongolia. Proceedings of the American Association of Zoo Veterinarians, pp. 7–21. New Orleans, LA.

Walzer C, Baumgartner R, Ganbataar O, Stauffer C. 2004. Boxing a wild horse for Mongolia—tips, tricks and treats. Proceedings of the European Association of Zoo- and Wildlife Veterinarians (EAZWV), pp. 153–157. Ebeltoft, Denmark.

Walzer C, Kaczensky P, Ganbataar O, Lengger J, Enkhsaikhan N, Lkhagvasuren D. 2006. Capture and anaesthesia of wild Mongolian equids—the Przewalski's horse (*E. ferrus przewalskii*) and the Khulan (*E. hemionus*). *Mongolian Journal of Biological Sciences* 4:19–28.

Walzer C, Stalder G, Petit T, Sos E, Molnar V, Brabender K, Fluch G. 2009. Surgical field anesthesia in Przewalski's horses (*Equus ferus przewalskii*) in Hortobágy national park, Hungary. Proceedings of American Association of Zoo Veterinarians/American Association of Wildlife Veterinarians, pp. 98–99.

Wiesner H. 1993. Chemical immobilization of wild equids. In: *Zoo and Wild Animal Medicine, Current Therapy 3* (ME Fowler, ed.), pp. 475–476. Philadelphia; London; Toronto: W.B. Saunders.

Wiesner H, von Hegel G. 1990. Zur Immobilisation von Wildequiden mit STH 2130 und Tiletamin/Zolazepam. *Tierarztliche Praxis* 18:151–154.

Zuba J, Burns R. 1998. The use of supplmental propofol in narcotic anesthetized non-domestic equids. Proceedings of American Association of Zoo Veterinarians/American Association of Wildlife Veterinarians, pp. 11–19.

53 Tapirs

Sonia M. Hernandez, James Bailey, and Luis R. Padilla

INTRODUCTION, TAXONOMY, AND NATURAL HISTORY

Tapirs belong to the family Tapiridae, within the order Perissodactyla, which are distinguished from the Artio-dactyla by their foot morphology and digestive system. Their closest relatives are rhinoceroses and horses. The small family of Tapiridae has only four species within the single genus *Tapirus*. There are three New World species (*Tapirus terrestris*, *Tapirus bardi*, and *Tapirus pinchaque*) and a single Old World species (*Tapirus indicus*). Tapirs are typically solitary (except mother and offspring pairs), largely nocturnal, tropical forest herbi-vores. In the wild, tapirs spend most days sleeping in dense areas and forage at night. They often inhabit aquatic habitats, spending large amounts of time in or near water (Klingel & Thenius 1990; Nowak 1991). Further, they are found to frequently urinate and def-ecate in water. These are all proposed as passive, stealth defense mechanism for survival. Despite their size, they can travel very quietly in the forest, are extremely agile, can run fast, and if threatened or protecting offspring, will charge (S. Hernandez-Diver, pers. obs., 2000).

All species, except the mountain tapir (*T. pinchaque*) are commonly exhibited in zoological institutions. To date, both captive and free-ranging individuals of all four species have been physically and chemically immobilized; however, the protocol used, and its success, varies with capture situation. Therefore, no one anesthetic protocol is recommended for all situations.

CLINICAL ANATOMY AND PHYSIOLOGY

A variety of sources have reviewed the anatomic pecu-liarities of tapirs (Janssen 2003); therefore, details pro-vided here are limited to those relevant to physical or chemical restraint. Table 53.1 summarizes the body weight and sizes for each species of Tapiridae. As with any animal of that size and weight, rough induction or recoveries can lead to severe, often untreatable, trau-matic injuries and safety concern for personnel. Unlike horses, tapirs rarely kick, but can inflict severe injury by biting, stomping, bucking, and charging. The dental formula for tapirs is $2\times$ (I-3/3, C-1/1, P-4/3, M-3/3). The upper third incisor is large, and separated from the canine by a narrow diastema which allows the manipu-lation of the tongue in the anesthetized animal. The glottis of the tapir is similar to the horse. Therefore, blind or laryngoscope-assisted intubation is possible (Fig. 53.1). Pulmonary atelectasis, ventilation-perfusion mismatch, or neuropathies associated with prolonged recumbency can complicate anesthetic procedures. The anesthetists are encouraged to review principles of large animal anesthesia when planning an immobilization procedure to minimize these risks as much as possible (Muir & Hubbell 1991; Steffey et al. 1990a,b). Supple-mental oxygen, assisted ventilation, and appropriate padding should be considered even in field captures. Tapirs, like horses, are unable to vomit; however, regur-gitation is still possible. Tapirs are hindgut fermenters, with small stomachs and large cecae and colons. Much like horses, tapirs can be at risk for gastrointestinal disease following chemical immobilization. Tapirs have a highly mobile proboscis which acts as a tactile and prehensile organ. The proboscis is a fleshy organ lacking any internal osseocartilaginous support, constructed of connective tissue and muscle (Witmer et al. 1999). This organ is highly sensitive and care should be taken not to restrict its movement during immobilization or cause it injury during anesthesia.

Zoo Animal and Wildlife Immobilization and Anesthesia, Second Edition. Edited by Gary West, Darryl Heard, and Nigel Caulkett.
© 2014 John Wiley & Sons, Inc. Published 2014 by John Wiley & Sons, Inc.

Table 53.1. Typical body weight and size for members of Tapiridae

Species	Body Weight (kg)	Body Length (cm)	Height at Shoulder (cm)
Tapirus bairdii (Baird's tapir)	150–300	198–202	Up to 120
Tapirus terrestris (lowland tapir)	250–300	180–250	77–108
Tapirus pinchaque (mountain tapir)	225–250	180	75–80
Tapirus indicus (Malayan tapir)	200–375	185–240	90–105

Physical Capture and Immobilization

Despite their large size, tapirs have had a reputation of being docile in captive environments and extremely elusive as free-ranging animals. In free-ranging situations, tapirs are adept at hiding, are extremely quiet when moving even in dense habitats, and generally stay out of sight. Reports of tapir captures for ecological studies include attracting the animal to bait stations, pitfall traps, box traps, capture pens, and using dogs for locating and chasing an individual animal (Foerster et al. 2000; Hernandez-Divers & Foerster 2001; Mangini & Velastin 2001; Mangini et al. 2001; Medici et al. 2001). All capture techniques reported were followed by chemical immobilization.

As opposed to similarly sized mammals maintained in captivity, many tapirs have traditionally been managed through "direct contact." Reports of severe biting, crushing, mutilating and possibly lethal injuries inflicted on caretakers should caution tapir handlers of the safety implications when attempting physical immobilization and the individual temperament of the animal should be taken into account. When provoked, even free-ranging tapirs can inflict fatal injuries, and at least one report exists of a tapir that killed a farmer that stabbed the animal because it was eating his crops (Haddad et al. 2005). Current standards of the Association of Zoos and Aquariums (AZA) allow for tapirs to be worked in an unprotected or protected contact setting, where caretakers enter or do not enter the same space as an animal, respectively, but the individual's temperament and institutional policies must be taken into account (AZA Tapir TAG 2013). Physical immobilization is possible with training and conditioning by using a large animal chute (Janssen 2003).

Tapirs are amenable to training using positive reinforcement techniques. Additionally, they can be "scratched down," a technique that involves using a horse brush or outdoor broom to stroke the animal's dorsum, neck, lateral, and abdominal walls (Janssen 2003). This appears to induce a pleasurable state in which the animal first sits, and then lays down in lateral recumbency. Although tapirs apparently enjoy this interaction, the level of immobilization induced

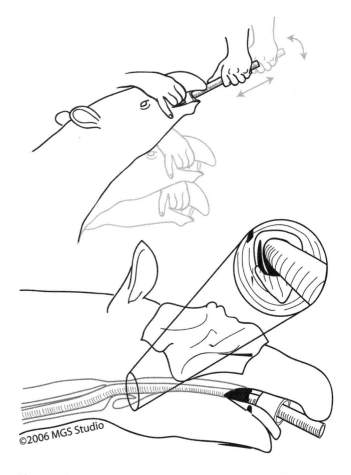

©2006 MGS Studio

Figure 53.1. How to intubate a tapir. In a fashion similar to a horse, intubation is preformed in the tapir—with ease—blindly. Optimally, the tapir's mouth is flushed with water to remove debris prior to anesthesia. In the field, the only opportunity to remove debris may be after anesthetic induction by a brief finger sweep of the buccal surfaces and examination of the oropharynx. After induction of anesthesia, the tapir is moved to lateral recumbency. The optional mouth speculum (PVC pipe segment) may be placed between the upper and lower incisors and the head extended to create a linear oral–laryngeal–pharyngeal axis. The endotracheal tube is then passed through the mouth speculum, over the base of the tongue into the pharynx. The tube may pass immediately into the larynx and trachea. More frequently, it is necessary to hold the head in extension, retract the endotracheal tube 10–15 cm, rotate the tube on its axis 45–90° and advance to the larynx once more. Multiple gentle rapid advancements and retractions, lightly tapping on the laryngeal opening will usually lead to intubation. Changing the degree of extension of the head while advancing the endotracheal tube may be of assistance. In the event blind intubation fails, a long bladed laryngoscope may be used for direct larygoscopic examination to intubation. Anticipate endotracheal tubes from 16- to 20-mm inside diameter (cuffed) will be appropriate for adult tapirs (illustration courtesy of MGS Studio).

should not be overemphasized. This technique, alone or combined with desensitization training and operant conditioning techniques, have been used for physical examination and even repeated blood collection (e.g., Kusuda et al. 2007), and can be utilized to administer injections. Positive reinforcement has also been used to move animals from one area to another, to enter crates,

Table 53.2. Criteria that should be considered when designing an anesthetic protocol for tapirs

Criteria	Free-ranging	Captive
Anesthetic onset	Rapid induction (avoid predation, trauma, and drowning)	Not as crucial, as animal is typically confined
Reversible anesthetic	Fully reversible	Not as crucial, as animal is typically confined
Anesthetic safety	Wide margin of safety (precapture body weight may not be available)	Wide margin of safety (disease is a more common indication for anesthesia in captivity)
Cost	Relatively inexpensive	Expense concerns vary
Volume	Volume should be minimized for remote delivery	Volume not as crucial, as dart distance is typically short

to present body parts for examination and to stand still for biological sample collection and intravenous catheterization.

Chemical Immobilization

The refinement in techniques using alpha-2 adrenergic agonists alone or in combination with other drugs has made them the basis of most modern, balanced anesthetic protocols used in tapirs. These drugs have largely replaced the need for ultrapotent opioids, such as etorphine or carfentanil, which had been historically associated with poor ventilation, poor oxygen saturation (Janssen 2003), hypoxemia, and personnel safety risk. The anesthetic protocol preferred may depend on whether the animal is captive or free-ranging, the facilities available, and the experience of the available personnel. Table 53.2 summarizes the major concerns in captive or free ranging scenarios.

PREANESTHETIC CONSIDERATIONS

As with any animal, individual tapirs that are calm are better candidates for anesthesia. The physiologic effects of excitement and endogenous release of catecholamines may delay or prevent anesthetic induction or muscle relaxation. In fact, the success of some anesthetic protocols utilized for free-ranging tapirs depend on the animal's degree of relaxation (Foerster et al. 2000; Hernandez-Divers & Foerster 2001). In all cases, it is important to create a quiet environment while working with these animals. If the animals cannot remain stress-free (i.e.,: transport, trauma, or disease), preanesthetic medication is highly recommended. Tapirs are often maintained in enclosures with bodies of water, and when threatened, they often retreat into the water. This must be taken into consideration when planning an anesthetic procedure. In free-ranging situations, capture protocols are designed to specifically avoid drowning by either anesthetizing animals that are contained, or are at least 200 m away from a body of water (Foerster et al. 2000; Hernandez-Divers & Foerster 2001). To maximize safety, capture techniques should be designed to minimize the probability an animal will walk or run after anesthesia has been administered. Although vomiting is generally not a consideration, fasting for 24 hours prior to anesthetic procedures is recommended. This will decrease the amount of food within the oral cavity and esophagus; minimize the probability of regurgitation, and minimize the pressure on the diaphragm related to the gastrointestinal tract distention secondary to fermentation of food material during the anesthetic period (Andersen et al. 2006). Tapirs are tropical animals; therefore, in regions with cold climate, they should be maintained in an indoor area that can be heated prior to the anesthetic period. In warmer climates, hyperthermia is a concern, and procedures should be planned for early morning or times when ambient temperatures are more favorable. In addition, methods to prevent and decrease excessive body temperatures should be available. Regardless of temperature concerns, tapirs should not be anesthetized in full sun, as their skin is sensitive to sunburn. If previous training allows, the length of the anesthetic period may be minimized by collecting samples or placing intravenous catheters ahead of time, although this must be judiciously balanced with any stress that these procedures can cause. Whenever possible, it is important to obtain a resting heart, respiratory rate, and body temperature on each individual to use as baseline for comparison during anesthetic monitoring.

PREANESTHETIC MEDICATION AND INDUCTION

Although the administration of preanesthetic medication is not always feasible in tapirs, in horses, it is considered a standard practice of care (Martinez et al. 2006; Muir & Hubbell 1991). Preanesthetic agents provide tranquilization, reduce the amount of induction and maintenance anesthetic agents required, balance the anesthetic technique to limit negative side effects, and may improve the quality of recovery. The common equine preanesthetic agents, xylazine and butorphanol, have been applied successfully in tapirs (Foerster et al. 2000; Hernandez-Divers & Foerster 2001). An estimated dosage of 0.15–0.25 mg/kg butorphanol combined with 0.3–0.5 mg/kg xylazine delivered IM produced immobilization of tapirs. Similarly, the use of a 0.06 mg/kg detomidine, an alpha-2 agonist related to xylazine, has been used in captive Baird's tapirs in combination with 0.15–0.2 mg/kg butorphanol to induce immobilization and recumbency (Pukazhenthi et al. 2011) These dosages would likely provide

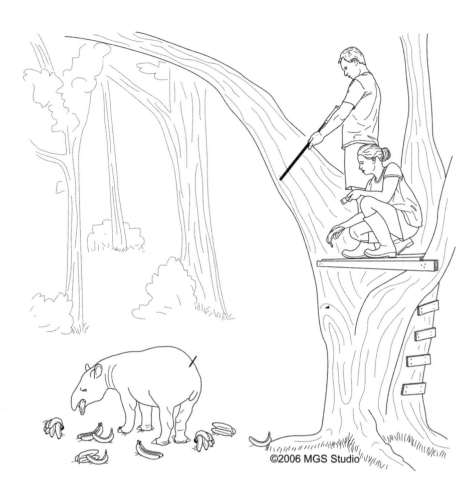

Figure 53.2. One method of immobilizing free-ranging tapirs. Bananas are placed in the center of a bait station. Additional bananas are thrown from a chosen location—such as this tree platform—into the forest and hung from nearby trees to disperse the odor of bananas for several days. Once evidence of tapir visitation is noted (tracks), captors sit at the proven bait station, starting at dusk (Foerster REF). Tapir movements are often not detected until the animal is with 20 m of the captors. Once an animal's footsteps were heard, a low power flashlight or a night-vision telescope is utilized to scan the area and confirm that the animal is a tapir. Immobilization drugs are then prepared while additional bananas are dropped every 10–20 seconds to bring the animal closer to the captors. This feeding technique distracts the tapir while the dart is being loaded and entices the tapir to move to an area for an advantageous dart shot. The tapir's reaction to thrown bananas is also used to evaluate its demeanor and level of nervousness. When the dart is loaded and the tapir is in an acceptable location for darting, a final decision is made regarding behavior and likely reaction to dart impact. A low power flashlight may be used to transiently illuminate the tapir (if night vision is unavailable) and the tapir is darted (illustration courtesy of MGS Studio).

sedation in the domestic horse, but are not likely to cause recumbency. For comparison, routine mild to moderate sedation of a horse would require xylazine 0.3–0.5 mg/kg and butorphanol 0.01–0.02 mg/kg IV. Intramuscular dosages of up to 2 mg/kg xylazine, with and without butorphanol, have been used for moderate to profound sedation of horses (Muir & Hubbell 1991). The apparent greater sensitivity of the tapir to these common equine preanesthetic agents suggests a lower dosage could be used if only mild sedation is desired. In fact, sedation (although unclear to what degree) was achieved in an ill Malayan tapir with 5-mg detomidine hydrochloride and 10-mg butorphanol administered by hand injection (Peters et al. 2012), although the animal was likely debilitated. Standing sedation, using xylazine or other alpha-2 agonist combinations, should be considered for short procedures that require little

manipulation (i.e., skin biopsy, blood collection, and portable radiography). Standing sedation using azaperone (1 mg/kg IM) has also been reported (Janssen et al. 1996).

Induction of anesthesia is typically achieved by intramuscular injections delivered by remote injection systems (free-ranging and captive), (Fig. 53.2) or by intravenous injections (captive). Despite their thick skin, a variety of peripheral vessels can be used in tapirs for administration of intravenous agents. Based on the author's experience and previous reports, the marginal auricular vein, carpal, cephalic, and saphenous veins can be used for either blood collection or short-term catheterization (Janssen 2003) (Fig. 53.3). A sedated or conditioned tapir may tolerate intravenous injection of propofol or ketamine into the saphenous, cephalic, or medial carpal vein to induce recumbency. The use of a

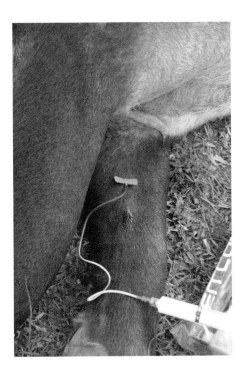

Figure 53.3. Intravenous access site in a Baird's tapir. The medial aspect of the forelimb of a tapir provides easy vascular access for short-term catheterization or administration of intravenous agents. In this image, a butterfly catheter has been placed in anesthetized tapir to provide propofol to maintain a desired plane of anesthesia (photo courtesy of Dr. Budhan S. Pukazhenthi, Smithsonian Conservation Biology Institute, Front Royal, VA).

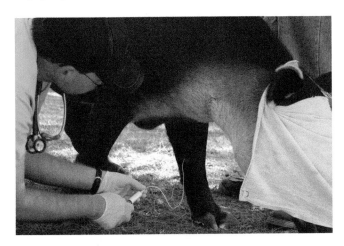

Figure 53.4. Intravenous anesthetic induction of anesthesia in a sedated Baird's tapir. An intravenous butterfly catheter has been placed in the medial aspect of the forelimb in a sedated tapir and propofol is being administered slowly to effect to induce recumbency and anesthesia (photo courtesy of Dr. Budhan S. Pukazhenthi, Smithsonian Conservation Biology Institute, Front Royal, VA).

butterfly catheter is a safe and practical way to reach the medial aspect of a forelimb for vascular access. (Fig. 53.4).

When anesthesia is induced in tapirs, they behave similarly to the horse, with some minor differences.

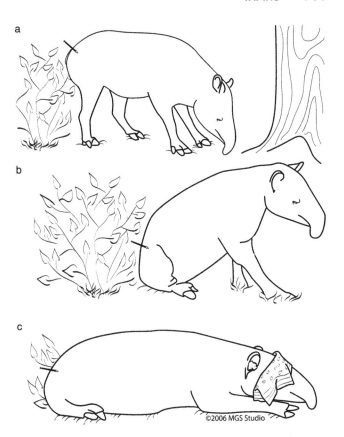

Figure 53.5. Typical induction behavior of a tapir. (a) The tapir getting drowsy; head-down with a basewide (sawhorse) stance, leaning back slightly and proboscis extended; (b) down to a sitting position with forelimbs extended; and (c) down in sternal recumbency (on its stomach), now with a blindfold applied over its eyes and gauze sponges placed in its ears (to reduce ambient sound stimulus) (illustration courtesy of MGS Studio).

Initially, they stand still, often in a saw-horse position, with limbs further apart than normal and drop their head. Tapirs may drool and loose control of their proboscis. From this position, they often sit, in a dog-like position, and then move to sternal recumbency (Fig. 53.5). In some cases, they remain standing and may need some light pressure on the hindquarters to encourage sitting. Rarely, a tapir may elevate the head from the sitting position and fall onto lateral recumbency. Table 53.3 reviews reported protocols for immobilization of free-ranging tapirs.

A wide range of drug combinations have been reported for use in captive tapirs. Table 53.4 summarizes the protocols used in captivity.

Despite their thick skin, a variety of peripheral vessels can be used in tapirs for administration of intravenous agents. Based on the author's experience and previous reports, the marginal auricular vein, carpal and medial saphenous veins can be used for both blood collection and short-term catheterization (Janssen 2003). Intravenous induction is rarely utilized, but can be accomplished in trained or sedated individuals using

Table 53.3. Summary of protocols utilized to immobilize free-ranging tapirs

Geographic Location	Species	Capture Method	Anesthetics	Comments
Costa Rica	*Tapirus bairdii*	Attracted animals to bait stations	Etorphine 1.88- and 7.7-mg acepromazine IM per animal; reversal: Diprenorphine hydrochloride at 3× the etorphine used	Administered to animals from a tree blind via a dart. The animals had been habituated to come to bait (ripe bananas) for several days and thus were relatively calm when darted (Parás et al. 1996)
Costa Rica	*Tapirus bairdii*	Attracted animals to bait stations	Total dosage for a 200- to 300-kg animal: 40–50mg of butorphanol and 100mg of xylazine in the same dart. Additional ketamine (187 ± 40.86mg/animal) or constant rate infusion of propofol (50–200µg/kg/min), administered IV. Reversal: Naltrexone 50mg IM with 1200mg of tolazoline in the same syringe IM; no sooner than 30 minutes from last administration of ketamine.	Administered to animals from a tree blind via a dart. The animals had been habituated to come to bait (ripe bananas) for several days and thus were relatively calm when darted. Animals weight estimated between 200 and 300kg. Average time to sternal recumbency: 11 minutes. Average return to standing after reversal: 12 minutes (Foerster et al. 2000; Hernandez-Divers et al. 2005).
Venezuela	*Tapirus terrestris*	Immobilized animals were captive, semi-captive, or wild tapirs	Ketamine (3.5–4mg/kg) and xylazine (2–2.2mg/kg) IM supplemented with ketamine (1.4mg/kg) IM; reversal: tolazoline 4mg/kg	Administered using darts projected by a blowpipe, or IV using syringe (Blanco Márquez & Blanco Márquez 2004).
Venezuela	*Tapirus terrestris*	Immobilized animals were captive, semi-captive, or wild tapirs	Telazol (2.5–2.8mg/kg) supplemented with ketamine (1.2–1.5mg/kg) IM; reversal: tolazoline 4mg/kg	Administered using darts projected by a blowpipe, or IV using syringe (Blanco Márquez & Blanco Márquez 2004).
Mexico	*Tapirus bairdii*		Total dosage for a 200- to 250-kg animal: 1.96-mg etorphine hydrocloride and 5.90mg of Acepromazine maleate, in the same dart; Reversal: Diprenorphine hydrochloride 5.88mg	This protocol was designed for specific environmental conditions (slopes of more than 60°) of the Sierra Madre. Induction times minimized to avoid fatalities. (I.L. Torres, pers. comm., 2006, modified from Kreeger 1997; Parás et al. 1996)
Brazil	*Tapirus terrestris*	Captured in pens or pitfalls	Butorphanol tartrate (0.15mg/kg) with medetomidine (0.03mg/kg) IM, in same dart; reversal: atipamezole (0.06mg/kg) with naltrexone (0.6mg/kg) in same syringe, IV	Adequate chemical restraint for radio collaring, and biological sampling. Average induction time: 10 minutes (Velastin et al. 2004)
Brazil	*Tapirus terrestris* and *Tapirus pinchaque*	Captured in pens or pitfalls, or immobilized by dart	Dosages were calculated using allometric scaling: ketamine (0.62 to 0.41mg/kg) and atropine (0.025 to 0.04mg/kg), and tiletamine-zolazepam (1.25 to 0.83mg/kg), and romifidine (0.05 to 0.03mg/kg) OR detomidine (0.06 to 0.04mg/kg) OR medetomidine (0.006 to 0.004mg/kg) in the same dart; reversal: atipamezole 0.06mg/kg.	Average induction time: 5 minutes. Medetomidine produced best results obtaining good muscular relaxation and more stable cardiopulmonary parameters. Authors state that the use of atropine should be at the discretion of the veterinarian in charge (Mangini & Velastin 2001; Mangini et al. 2001).

Table 53.4. Anesthetic protocols used in captive tapirs

Type of Facility	Species	Anesthetic Protocol Used	Comments
Zoological institution	*Tapirus pichanque*	Carfentanil (5.4 ug/kg), ketamine (0.26 mg/kg) and xylazine (0.13 mg/kg) IM; reversal: yohimbine (0.2 mg/kg IV) and naltrexone (100–200 mg/kg, half IV, half SC)	Six immobilizations of tapirs (1 female, 3 males; 1 juvenile male immobilized 3 times) for footwork, gastrointestinal endoscopy, and reproductive surgery (Miller-Edge & Amsel 1994).
Zoological institution	*Tapirus indicus*	Butorphanol (0.15 mg/kg) and detomidine (0.05 mg/kg) OR xylazine (0.3 mg/kg) all IM; use ketamine if needed (0.5 mg/kg IV); reversal: naloxone and yohimbine (0.2–0.3 mg/kg IV)	Nineteen immobilizations of Malayan and mountain tapirs (Janssen et al. 1996).
Zoological institution	*Tapirus bairdii*	Butorphanol (0.15–0.2 mg/kg) and detomidine (0.06 mg/kg); ketamine (1–2 mg/kg) was used to reach or maintain recumbency and light anesthesia. Boluses of propofol (0.2–2.0 mg/kg per bolus) were used to effect as needed.	Report of 11 males anesthetized for semen collection by electroejaculation in three captive institutions in Panama (Pukazhenthi et al. 2011), but one of the authors (Padilla) has also used in females with the same effects, and anesthesia was antagonized with naltrexone and yohimbine.
Zoological institution	*Tapirus bairdii*	Acepromazine (7.7 mg/animal), butorphanol (0.13–0.2 mg/kg), detomidine (0.065–0.13 mg/kg) and ketamine (2.2 mg/kg) IM; no reversal	Trim et al. (1998)
Zoological institution	*Tapirus indicus*	Etorphine 2.45 mg and acepromazine 10 mg total IM, then guaifenesin IV until intubation was possible; then isoflurane maintenance	Eighteen-month-old female; estimated to weigh 265 kg; immobilized for diagnosis and surgical management of abdominal abscess (Lambeth et al. 1998).
Zoological institution	*Tapirus indicus*	Butorphanol (80 mg IM) and Xylazine (120 mg total IM) OR detomidine (12 mg total IM); reversal: naltrexone (200 mg total IM), tolazoline (1400 mg total IM)	Estimated body weight 340 kg; repeated immobilizations of light anesthesia for diagnosis and treatment of oral squamous cell carcinoma (Miller et al. 2000).
Teaching hospital	*Tapirus terrestris*	Detomidine (0.03 mg/kg PO), 20 minutes later, carfentanil (1.85 μ/kg PO)	One animal repeatedly immobilized for wound management; variety of combinations of alpha-2 agonist/ etorphine or carfentanil were used, but eight immobilizations with detomidine/ carfentanil PO were most useful (Pollock & Ramsay 2003).

propofol or ketamine. Standing sedation, using xylazine or other alpha-2 agonist combinations, should be considered for short procedures that require little manipulation (i.e., skin biopsy, blood collection, and portable radiography). Standing sedation using azaperone (1 mg/kg IM) has also been reported (Janssen et al. 1996).

MAINTENANCE ANESTHESIA

Typically, general anesthesia is maintained in horses by inhalation anesthetics or total intravenous anesthesia (TIVA). Isoflurane, and sevoflurane and halothane are all commonly used inhalation anesthetic agents for horses (Martinez et al. 2006; Muir & Hubbell 1991). To date, isoflurane is the most common inhalant used in for maintenance of anesthesia of tapirs, but the use of sevoflurane in the future is anticipated. Mixtures of injectable anesthetic agents, such as the classic xyla-

zine, ketamine, and guaifenesin (also known as tripledrip), may be used to maintain general anesthesia for relatively short procedures in horses, but no published reports exist in tapirs (Aubin & Mama 2002). Intravenous guaifenesin in a dextrose solution has been safely used in a small number of Baird's tapirs by one of the authors (LRP) to increase relaxation, depth, and duration of anesthesia after anesthetic induction with other agents using empirical rates similar to those used in domestic horses, The effects were similar to those seen in equids, with dose and rate dependent respiratory depression. Two tapirs showed increased nasal secretions and salivation during recovery after guaifenesin usage, although a cause–effect relationship could not be established. Since guaifenesin susceptibility varies between equid species (Matthews et al. 1997), its usage in tapirs should be done with extreme caution until objective documentation of its effects has been reported. Propofol, thought not routinely used in large animals, is an acceptable TIVA method for horses. Constant rate infusions of propofol have been reported in tapirs (Hernandez-Divers & Foerster 2001), and small boluses have been used as supplements to maintain or reach deeper planes of anesthesia. Horses anesthetized with either isoflurane or propofol experience cardiopulmonary depression in a dose-dependent fashion. Propofol is more likely to lead to apnea than isoflurane (Mama et al. 1995, 1996; Reid et al. 1997).

MONITORING AND ANESTHETIC SUPPORT

Once anesthetized, tapirs can be maintained in sternal or lateral recumbency. However, sternal recumbency (Fig. 53.6) allows for better ventilation in large animals (Steffey et al. 1990a, 1990b). If lateral recumbency is necessary, proper padding and vigilance of pressure points on the recumbent side is essential, to minimize the likelihood of myositis or neuropathies, especially during prolonged anesthetic procedures. While on lateral recumbency, the "up" leg should be elevated to improve flow through major arteries, while the "down" leg should be pulled forward to minimize physical pressure on the brachial (axillary) plexus. A blindfold should be applied to protect the corneas from physical damage and minimize visual stimulus. Corneal edema, presumptively associated with prolonged exposure to ultraviolet radiation, has been reported in tapirs (Janssen 2003). Gauze or cotton should be inserted into the ears, to decrease auditory stimulus. Premature arousal can occur with excessive noise, particularly when using alpha-2 agonist and/or opioid combina-

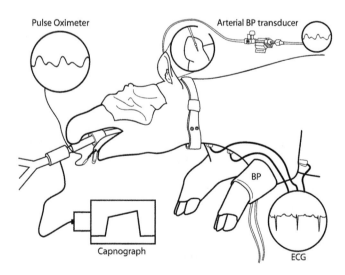

Figure 53.6. Vigilance monitoring of the tapir. Seen here: lingual transmittance pulse oximeter and associated plethesomographic waveform; side-stream (diverting) capnography and capnogram; noninvasive, oscillometric arterial blood pressure monitory (BP cuff); invasive (direct) arterial blood pressure monitoring through a blood pressure transducer with associated arterial waveform; base-apex lead electrocardiogram (illustration courtesy of MGS Studio).

tions. Minimally, heart rate, peripheral pulse strength, respiratory rate, and body temperature should be monitored as with any other large animal.

Pulse oximetry is best accomplished by applying the probe to the tongue, cheek, or ear, or by direct contact with the rectal, preputial, or vaginal mucosa. Although the oxygen–hemoglobin disassociation curve has not been determined for tapirs, the curve for horses (p50 = 25 mmHg) indicates that a 90% saturation reading on the pulse oximeter is approximately equal to an arterial partial pressure of oxygen of 60 mmHg, which is distinctly hypoxemic (Clerbaux et al. 1993). Therefore, saturation levels as measured by a pulse oximeter should be maintained well above 90% (i.e., 95–100%). The use of a capnograph is recommended, and with the advent of portable units, it is a useful monitoring device even in field situations. When intubation is impractical or not feasible, the capnograph can be attached to a tightly fitting rubber hose or endotracheal tube placed nasally to monitor respiratory trends, even if the absolute values are not reliable.

Blood gases can be monitored by sampling the facial, auricular, or medial saphenous arteries (Fig. 53.4). In one of the authors' experience, anesthesia induced with a butorphanol, and detomidine protocol in Baird's tapirs results in a time-dependent elevation in PaCO2 and decrease in PaO2, which is consistent with the effects seen during sedation with these drugs in the domestic horse (Nyman et al. 2009). Even in healthy animals, heavy sedation and general anesthesia frequently lead to a fall in the arterial partial pressure of oxygen (PaO$_2$). This is particularly true of larger animals, but only in part due to hypoventilation. Importantly, ventilation to perfusion mismatching increases dramatically in anesthetized large animals (Muir & Hubbell 1991). To compensate for hypoxemia, the use of nasal oxygen (10–15 L/min) or intubation and assisted ventilation should be considered.

As blind intubation of the tapir is accomplished with relative ease (adult tapir: 16- to 20-mm internal diameter endotracheal tube), intubation with tracheal insufflation of oxygen, or positive pressure ventilation (20–30 cm H$_2$O) are reasonable solutions. Improved oxygen saturation and ventilation may be accomplished in the field using a demand valve driven by 100% oxygen, or a manual resuscitator bag with supplemental oxygen attachment (Ambu A/S, Ballerup, Denmark, http://www.ambu.com). Only one report of the aforementioned protocols assessed the cardiopulmonary effects in detail (Foerster et al. 2000). In that report, hypoxemia was noted and supplemental oxygen was recommended.

Blood pressure can be measured indirectly, through the use of blood pressure cuffs on the limbs. Direct blood pressure measurements can be achieved most readily with the use of a 22-gauge catheter placed in the readily accessible auricular artery. A study that compared the usefulness and accuracy of indirect versus direct blood pressure monitoring methods in tapirs found that indirect blood pressure measurements using an oscillometer blood pressure monitor correlated with direct readings, indicating that this is a valid method to measure blood pressure in tapirs (Bailey et al. 2000) as measured within the limits of pressure ranges examined (field conditions).

Base-apex lead electrocardiograph application simply requires a positive lead caudal to the heart apex and a negative lead cranial to the heart base. Those unaccustomed to the base-apex lead are often perplexed by its classic description. A less confusing base-apex lead places the left leg lead caudal to the heart apex (left sternal boarder), the right arm and left arm leads cranial to the heart base on the neck in the right jugular furrow, with the ECG monitor set for lead II (often the default setting). This produces a base-apex lead electrocardiogram similar in appearance to the standard lead II. Species with a diffuse Purkinje fiber network produce a unique mean electrical axis. A simple rule of thumb states that if the animal is small or its ancestors were small, it is likely to have a type I heart with a less diffuse Purkinje network, caudally oriented mean electrical axis, and primarily positive wave form in lead II, such as seen in dogs and cats. If the animal is large or its ancestors were large, it is likely to have a type II heart with a diffuse Purkinje network, cranially oriented mean electrical axis, and primarily negative wave form in lead II, such as seen in the horse and the tapir (Fig. 53.6) (Muir & Hubbell 1991).

Temperature is typically monitored through a rectal thermometer. The depth of anesthesia can be monitored subjectively much as in a horses. Ideally, at a moderate plane of anesthesia, muscles should be relaxed even when stimulation is applied, the animal should breath in a regular manner with chest excursions that approximate a conscious animal, the position of the eye should be central, and there may be a very slight palpebral reflex. The corneal reflex should remain until very deep planes of anesthesia.

The use of atropine has been advocated by some veterinarians as an adjunct to anesthesia induced with alpha-2 agonists in tapirs to counteract bradycardia and reduce respiratory and salivary secretions. Atropine should be used judiciously at the clinician's discretion, as systemic usage in domestic equids has been associated with decreased gastrointestinal motility (Ducharme & Fubini 1983), and this effect would be difficult to document in free-ranging animals. In addition, the use of atropine could be contraindicated in hypertensive animals.

RECOVERY

To avoid rough recoveries and to minimize the cardiopulmonary effects of anesthetic agents, protocols that

allow for their antagonism are preferred. Protocols that include alpha-2 adrenergic agonists are typically antagonized well and lead to smooth, uneventful recoveries. If supplemental ketamine (or related drugs) is used, it is recommended that the reversal agent not be administered until at least 30 minutes have elapsed, to allow for redistribution of the drug. In free-ranging situations, maintaining containment of the tapir (in trap, or pit fall) can allow the animal to fully recover before release. In cases where this was not possible, authors reported following the recovered animals for a period of time to monitor signs of ataxia, depression, or renarcotization (Foerster et al. 2000). In captivity, animals should be maintained in a quiet, dark, enclosed area until fully recovered and away from water sources if the facilities allow it. Individual captive tapirs habituated to their caretakers can be enticed to remain adjacent to keepers by showing them food or other positive rewards (scratching) until fully recovered. Attempts at physical restraint by humans are not recommended once a tapir is standing, as even a partially sedated tapir can be extremely dangerous and capable of biting when cornered or aggravated. Aggressive individuals may try to fight or even chase humans during recovery.

In all cases, tapirs should be allowed to recover in the shade. The low surface area to body mass ratio of tapirs may predispose them to overheat if recovering in direct sunlight. Tapirs that are recovering from anesthesia typically begin by twitching their ears, moving the tongue in and out of the mouth, which is followed by return to sternal recumbency. From sternal recumbency, they may first sit on the hindquarters, or fully stand. Many tapirs begin walking in reverse as they gradually regain orientation to their environment. Horses recovering from inhalation anesthetics often experience dysphoria and are prone to self-inflicted trauma; therefore, additional sedatives or tranquilizers are often administered prior to recovery to buy time for inhalation anesthetic washout (Martinez et al. 2006; Muir & Hubbell 1991). Tapirs undergoing prolonged surgical procedures (beyond metabolism of injectable induction agents) may need similar treatment. If sedatives are administered, horses, as with tapirs, tend to roll to sternal recumbency and sit in a controlled pause for several minutes prior to standing directly. Ideally, the horse stands steady or walks with intent with limited ataxia. Ataxia has been reported in tapirs recovering from anesthetic protocols that included ketamine, emphasizing the need for containment and monitoring. Occasional reports of tapirs returning to a deeper plane of sedation hours after antagonism of alpha-2 agonist protocols using medetomidine or detomidine suggest that these alpha-2 agonists may be longer lived in tapirs than the agents used to antagonize them (atipamezole or yohimbine). A recent study supports the occurrence of similar effects in domestic horses following antagonism of sublingual detomidine (Knych & Stanley 2011).

REFERENCES

Andersen MS, Clark L, Dyson SJ, Newton JR. 2006. Risk factors for colic in horses after general anesthesia for MRI or nonabdominal surgery: absence of evidence of effect from perianaesthetic morphine. *Equine Veterinary Journal* 38(4):368–374.

Aubin M, Mama K. 2002. Field anesthetic techniques for use in horses. *Compendium on Continuing Education for the Practicing Veterinarian* 24(5):411–416.

AZA Tapir TAG. 2013. *Tapir (Tapiridae) Care Manual.* Silver Spring: Association of Zoos and Aquariums.

Bailey J, Foerster SH, Foerster CR. 2000. Evaluation of oscillometric blood pressure monitoring during immobilization of free-ranging Baird's tapirs (Tapirus bairdii) in Costa Rica. *Veterinary Anaesthesia and Analgesia* 28(2):97–110.

Blanco Márquez PA, Blanco Márquez VJ. 2004. Anaesthetic protocols used on *Tapirus terrestris* in Venezuela. Second International Tapir Symposium, Panama 2004: Conference Report (IUCN, IUCN/SSC-TSG, AZA, Houston Zoo, CI, eds.), Panama City.

Clerbaux T, Gustin P, Detry B, Cao ML, Frans A. 1993. Comparative study of the oxyhaemoglobin dissociation curve of four mammals: man, dog, horse and cattle. *Comparative Biochemistry and Physiology. Comparative Physiology* 106(4):687–694.

Ducharme NG, Fubini SL. 1983. Gastrointestinal complications associated with the use of atropine in horses. *Journal of the American Veterinary Medical Association* 182:229–231.

Foerster SH, Bailey JE, Aguilar R, Loria DL, Foerster CR. 2000. Butorphanol/xylazine/ketamine immobilization of free-ranging Baird's tapirs in Costa Rica. *Journal of Wildlife Diseases* 36(2):335–341.

Haddad V, Assuncao MC, de Mello RC. 2005. A fatal attack caused by a lowland tapir (*Tapirus terrestris*) in southeastern Brazil. *Wilderness and Environmental Medicine* 16(2):97–100.

Hernandez-Divers SM, Foerster CR. 2001. Capture and immobilization of free-living Baird's tapirs (*Tapirus bairdii*) for an ecological study in Corcovado National Park, Costa Rica. In: *Zoological Restraint and Anesthesia* (D Heard, ed.). Ithaca: International Veterinary Information Service. http://www.ivis.org (accessed February 8, 2014), B0184.1201.

Hernandez-Divers SM, Aguilar R, Leandro-Loria D, Foerster CR. 2005. Health evaluation of a radiocollared population of free-ranging Baird's tapirs (*Tapirus bairdii*) in Costa Rica. *Journal of Zoo and Wildlife Medicine* 36(2):176–187.

Janssen DL. 2003. Tapiridae. In: *Zoo and Wild Animal Medicine: Current Therapy 5* (ME Fowler, RE Miller, eds.), pp. 569–577. Philadelphia: W.B. Saunders.

Janssen DL, Rideout B, Edwards ME. 1996. Medical management of captive tapirs (*Tapirus spp.*). Proceedings American Association Zoo Veterinarians, Puerto Vallarta, Mexico, pp. 576–581.

Klingel H, Thenius E. 1990. Odd-toed ungulates. In: *Grzimek's Encyclopedia of Mammals*, Vol. 4 (SP Parker, ed.), pp. 547–556. New York: McGraw-Hill.

Knych HK, Stanley SD. 2011. Effects of three reversal agents on detomidine-induced changes in behavior and cardiac and selected blood parameters in the horse. Proceedings American Association Equine Practitioners, San Antonio, TX, p. 64.

Kreeger TJ. 1997. *Handbook of Wildlife Chemical Immobilization.* Laramie: International Wildlife Veterinary Services Inc.

Kusuda S, Ikoma M, Morikaku K, Koizumi J, Kawaguchi Y, Kobayashi K, Matsui K, Nakamura A, Hashikawa H, Kobayashi K, Ueda M, Kaneko M, Akikawa T, Shibagaki S, Doi O. 2007. Estrous cycle based on blood progesterone profiles and changes in vulvar appearance of Malayan tapirs (Tapirus indicus). *The Journal of Reproduction and Development* 53(6):1283–1289.

Lambeth RR, Dart AJ, Vogelnest L, Dart CM, Hodgson DR. 1998. Surgical managementmanangement of an abdominal abscess in a Malayan tapir. *Australian Veterinary Journal* 76(10):664–666.

Mama KR, Steffey EP, Pascoe PJ. 1995. Evaluation of propofol as a general anesthetic for horses. *Veterinary Surgery* 24:188–194.

Mama KR, Steffey EP, Pascoe PJ. 1996. Evaluation of propofol for general anesthesia in premedicated horses. *American Journal of Veterinary Research* 57(4):512–516.

Mangini PR, Velastin GO. 2001. Chemical restraint of two wild *Tapirus pinchaque* (mountain tapir) case report. *Archives of Veterinary Science Curitiba* 6:6.

Mangini PR, Velastin GO, Medici EP. 2001. Protocols of chemical restraint used in 16 wild *Tapirus terrestris. Archives of Veterinary Science Curitiba* 6:6–7.

Martinez EA, Wagner AE, Driessen B, Trim C. 2006. Guidelines for Anesthesia in Horses. Prepared by the American College of Veterinary Anesthesiologists Equine Standards Committee. http://www.acva.org (accessed February 8, 2014).

Matthews N, Peck K, Mealey K, Taylor T, Ray A. 1997. Pharmacokinetics and cardiopulmonary effects of guaifenesin in donkeys. *Journal of Veterinary Pharmacology and Therapeutics* 20:442–446.

Medici EP, Veloso Nunes AL, Mangini PR, Vaz Ferreira JR. 2001. Order Perissodactyla, family Tapiridae (tapirs). In: *Biology, Medicine, and Surgery of South American Wild Animals* (ME Fowler, ZS Cubas, eds.), pp. 363–375. Ames: Iowa State University Press.

Miller CL, Templeton RS, Karpinski L. 2000. Succesful treatment of oral squamous cell carcinoma with intralesional fluorouracil in a Malayan tapir (*Tapir indicus*). *Journal of Zoo and Wildlife Medicine* 31(2):262–264.

Miller-Edge M, Amsel S. 1994. Carfentanil, ketamine, xylazine combination (CKX) for immobilization of exotic ungulates: clinical experience in bongo (*Tragelaphus euryceros*) and mountain tapir (*Tapirus pinchaque*). Proceedings American Association Zoo Veterinarians, Pittsburgh, PA, pp. 192–195.

Muir WW, Hubbell JAE. 1991. *Equine Anesthesia. Monitoring and Emergency Therapy.* St. Louis: Mosby-Year Book.

Nowak RM. 1991. *Walker's Mammals of the World*, 5th ed. Baltimore: Johns Hopkins University Press.

Nyman G, Marntell S, Edner A, Funkquist P, Morgan K, Hedenstierna G. 2009. Effect of sedation with detomidine and butorphanol on pulmonary gas exchange in the horse. *Acta Veterinaria Scandinavica* 51:22.

Parás GA, Forester CR, Hernandez SM. 1996. Immobilization of free ranging Baird's tapir (*Tapirus bairdii*). Proceedings American Association Zoo Veterinarians, Puerto Vallarta, Mexico.

Peters A, Raidal SR, Blake AH, Atkinson MM, Atkinson PR, Eggins PR. 2012. Haemochromatosis in a Brazilian tapir (*Tapirus terrestris*) in an Australian zoo. *Australian Veterinary Journal* 90:29–33.

Pollock C, Ramsay E. 2003. Serial immobilization of a Brazilian tapir (*Tapirus terrestris*) with oral detomidine and oral carfentanil. *Journal of Zoo and Wildlife Medicine* 34(4):408–410.

Pukazhenthi BS, Togna GD, Padilla L, Smith D, Sanchez C, Pelican K, Sanjur OI. 2011. Ejaculate traits and sperm cryopreservation in the endangered Baird's tapir (*Tapirus bairdii*). *Journal of Andrology* 32(2):260–270.

Reid DF, Welsh E, Monteiro AM, Lerche P, Nolan A. 1997. A pharmacodynamic study of propofol or propofol and ketamine infusions in ponies undergoing surgery. *Research in Veterinary Science* 62(2):179–184.

Steffey EP, Kelly AB, Hodgson DS, Grandy JL, Woliner MJ, Willits N. 1990a. Effect of body posture on cardiopulmonary function in horses during five hours of constant-dose halothane anesthesia. *American Journal of Veterinary Research* 51:11–16.

Steffey EP, Woliner MJ, Dunlop C. 1990b. Effects of five hours of constant 1.2 MAC halothane in sternally recumbent, spontaneously breathing horses. *Equine Veterinary Journal* 22(6):433–436.

Trim CM, Lamberski N, Kissel DI, Quandt JE. 1998. Anesthesia in a Baird's tapir (*Tapirus bairdii*). *Journal of Zoo and Wildlife Medicine* 29(2):195–198.

Velastin GO, Mangini PR, Medici EP. 2004. Utilização de associação de tartarato de butorfanol e cloridrato de medetomidina na contenção de *tapirus terrestris* em vida livre: relato de dois casos. Anais XXVIII Congresso da Sociedade de Zoológicos do Brasil. 1: T063.

Witmer LM, Sampson SD, Solounias N. 1999. The proboscis of tapirs (*Tapirus terrestris*): a case study in novel narial anatomy. *Journal of Zoology* 249:249–267.

54 Rhinoceroses

Robin W. Radcliffe and Peter vdB. Morkel

THE RHINOCEROTIDAE

Introduction

Like the fabricated creature in Albretch Durer's famous lithograph, the rhinoceros has long been a source of mystery, myth, and intrigue. Part unicorn and part armored beast, the current knowledge of rhinoceros anesthesia likewise represents a melding of pure art and hard science. Today, rhinoceros anesthesia is relatively commonplace, yet no less demanding in practice.

The Rhinocerotidae are truly living fossils—a remnant and archaic mammalian family represented by only five extant species in four genera restricted to Africa and Asia. The relic survivors belie a one-time place of dominance among vertebrate organisms, with over 150 fossil rhinoceros species discovered by paleontology across four continents (Prothero 2005). Today, however, four of the five rhinoceroses are critically endangered from poaching and loss of habitat (Emslie & Brooks 1999; Foose & van Strien 1997).

Field anesthesia made possible the rhinoceros conservation success stories of the twentieth century (Harthoorn & Lock 1960; Meadows 1996; Player 1972) and remains a critical tool for proactive rhinoceros management programs incorporating translocation, ear-notching, radiotelemetry, microchip implantation, and other techniques designed to secure the conservation of both African and Asian species (Dinerstein 2003; Dinerstein et al. 1990; Kock et al. 1990, 1995). Historical and current rhinoceros anesthesia protocols are based on highly effective reversible opioid combinations, yet new anesthesia techniques continue to improve efficacy and safety for both animals and human personnel (Bush et al. 2005, 2011).

Taxonomy and Evolutionary History

The odd-toed ungulates of the order Perissodactyla include three living families: the rhinoceroses, horses, and tapirs. As the order name denotes, all Perissodactylids bear weight on one (equids) or three (rhinoceroses and tapirs) digits. Rhinoceroses and tapirs are among the most primitive of the world's large mammals and are further grouped into the suborder, Ceratomorpha, based upon a similar ancient body plan. The stout body of the rhinoceros is graviportal or designed for weight bearing with limb modifications to support large mass rather than the long angular limbs of equids in the suborder, Hippomorpha, specialized for speed.

The Perissodactyla enjoyed a period of extraordinary diversity in the Eocene epoch 34 to 55 million years ago before climate change presumably limited specie radiation, culminating in extinction of 10 of the 14 perissodactyl families by the end of the Oligocene (Radinsky 1969). Prehistoric rhinoceroses in particular, as interpreted from fossil evidence, represented a far expanded group of organisms than exist today and included both horned and hornless forms. In fact, rhinoceroses were once the most common large herbivore in North America for most of the last 50 million years (Prothero & Schoch 2002). An extinct hornless rhinoceros, named Paraceratherium (also called Indricotherium), is known to science as the largest land mammal that ever lived, measuring over 6 meters at the shoulder and weighing an estimated 20 tons (Prothero 2005; Prothero & Schoch 2002).

Biology and Morphology

The Rhinocerotidae are large terrestrial herbivores that have evolved either a browsing (black, Sumatran, and Javan) or grazing (white and greater one-horned) strategy in order to process large quantities of fibrous feeds or simple grasses, respectively. As such, they share bulky elongated skulls, dental patterns largely devoid of canines and incisors (retained to various degree in the Asian species), and prehensile or wide, flat lips in

Zoo Animal and Wildlife Immobilization and Anesthesia, Second Edition. Edited by Gary West, Darryl Heard, and Nigel Caulkett.
© 2014 John Wiley & Sons, Inc. Published 2014 by John Wiley & Sons, Inc.

the browsers and grazers, respectively. Like the equids, fermentation takes place in the cecum and colon. The rhinoceros gut is less efficient than that of ruminants since the microfloral protein formed in the hindgut is largely unavailable to the animal. As a result, rhinoceros must eat more, have a relatively fast passage of gut contents, and possess limited time to reabsorb water from the feces. Therefore, rhinoceros must drink every day or every second day, making it a water-dependent species rarely found more than 15 km from a water source.

Despite their often conspicuous absence in many fossil rhinoceros, the single horn (*Rhinoceros* sp.) or pair of horns (*Ceratotherium, Diceros*, and *Dicerorhinus* sp.) is certainly the most distinguishing feature of the living Rhinocerotidae, giving name to the group literally as the *nose-horned beasts* (Prothero & Schoch 2002). Rhinoceros horns differ from true horns of the Artiodactyla by having no central core of bone. Instead, the tubular hair-like keratin filaments are compressed in a linear fashion and set upon a bony protuberance of the skull. Underneath the horns, the skull incorporates extensive nasal bones and sinuses—structures inordinately prone to complications from trauma during capture and translocation.

Rhinoceros skin is thick (several centimeters of primarily collagenous dermis; Cave & Allbrook 1958; Shadwick et al. 1992), with the Asian species sporting subdermal plates and heavy skin folds, making skin anatomy an important consideration for remote drug delivery in the rhinoceros. The greater one-horned rhinoceros of Asia is perhaps best known for the exaggerated armor-like plates or folds first popularized in the famous Durer woodcutting of the Middle Ages. The epidermis, however, is very thin (1 mm) and heavily keratinized, incorporating extensive vasculature, which may predispose the rhinoceros to pressure necrosis, particularly in calves (Cave & Allbrook 1958; Gandolf et al. 2006). Significant body hair is an antiquated trait retained in but one living species, the Sumatran or "hairy rhinoceros," so-called for its shaggy coat of hair (Fig. 54.1). Wild *Dicerorhinus* have shorter more bristly coats than their captive relatives, a trait providing protection for the skin from the numerous biting insects that share its environment. Hair, a primordial trait of many fossil rhinoceros including the wooly rhinoceros *Coleodonta* and massive one-horned hairy *Elasmotherium*, eloquently links the Sumatran rhinoceros with its long and prosperous past.

RHINOCEROS IMMOBILIZATION AND CAPTURE

Rhinoceros Capture Beginnings

Before widespread application of chemical capture techniques, early African rhinoceros capture operations utilized ropes and a chase vehicle (made famous in the

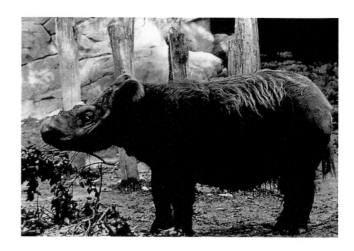

Figure 54.1. The distinctive hair coat of a Sumatran rhinoceros—a feature linking the primitive Dicerorhinus genus with its prehistoric past (image courtesy of Mohd Khan bin Momin Khan, Malaysia Department of Wildlife and National Parks).

film *Hatari* staring John Wayne and Hardy Kruger). Although dangerous to the operator and stressful to the animal, some teams in East Africa became remarkably proficient at this form of capture. Chemical capture of rhinoceros was first attempted with the dissociative anesthetic, phencyclidine, and the curariform muscle relaxant, gallamine triethiodide. In 1960, during Operation Noah, many black rhinoceros (*Diceros bicornis*) were saved from the rising waters of the newly constructed Lake Kariba, bordering Zambia and Zimbabwe, using these novel techniques (Child & Fothergill 1962; Condy 1964; Harthoorn & Lock 1960; Meadows 1996). Phencyclidine and gallamine were succeeded by the easily reversible opioids, first morphine and diethylthiambutene, followed quickly by the more potent opioids, including etorphine HCl (M99) (Keep et al. 1969; King 1969; King & Carter 1965). Over the past 50 years, etorphine has become the standard opioid for capture of the African and Asian rhinoceros, with fentanyl citrate (Sublimaze), carfentanil citrate (Wildnil) and thiafentanil oxalate (A3080) proving useful alternatives. Pioneering investigation by early practitioners, such as Toni Harthoorn, Eddie Young, Ian Hofmeyr, Ian Player, and many others, provided the foundation upon which future rhinoceros chemical capture methods including the present work are based (Harthoorn 1976; Player 1972; Young 1973).

Remote Drug Delivery: Equipment and Darting Techniques

An assortment of remote drug delivery equipment is available for rhinoceros capture, including new developments, yet some of the early systems are still in common practice today, attesting to their simple and durable design. In captive and boma situations, all darting systems can be utilized, but nylon darts (Daninject or Telinject with 60 × 2-mm smooth needles) are preferred, as they are quiet and relatively atraumatic. The authors prefer to hand-inject (using appropriate human protective safety measures) or pole-syringe captive rhinoceroses including animals held in bomas to eliminate the excitement phase associated with projectile darting.

For field capture of rhinoceros on the ground or from a helicopter a robust and reliable darting method, such as the Cap-Chur system, is preferable. Dart barrels made of aluminum or stainless steel are the most reliable for field use, especially since power settings and impact energy are high, wind or down drafts from the helicopter can be significant, and the operator is often forced to shoot through vegetation. The dart needle should be 5- to 6-cm long for adult rhinoceros. Rhinoceros skin can plug the lumen of a dart needle unless the needle has a relatively thick wall and narrow lumen (Cap-Chur NCL needles) or the tip is bent over (Fauncap dart needles) or the point is sealed and side ports are provided. The needle must have a bead, low barb, or small collar about 25 mm from the base to hold the dart in the thick skin. A novel spiral-threaded needle was developed by Deon Joubert specifically for use on thick-skinned pachyderms; the dart needle can be easily removed by screwing it out of the animal, thereby reducing skin and tissue trauma (Fig. 54.2; Joubert

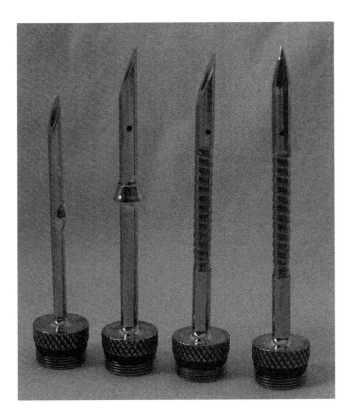

Figure 54.2. Robust dart needles for the capture of free-ranging rhinoceroses demonstrating the various design configurations of needle tip and barb. The spiral-threaded needles on the right are less traumatic and can be screwed back out of thick rhinoceros skin (photo courtesy of Joubert Capture Equipment, South Africa).

Capture Equipment, Hadison Park, Kimberley, South Africa).

Proper dart placement is essential to ensure good drug deposition. The dart should be placed perpendicular to the skin for deep intramuscular injection (the thick skin of a rhinoceros often makes an angled shot ineffective). When darting from the helicopter, the muscles of the rump or the upper part of the hind leg offer the best target. In the boma or on foot, any large muscle mass can be used for dart placement although the neck and shoulder are preferable.

Recumbency and Positioning

Recumbency and positioning are critical considerations for safe anesthesia of rhinoceros whether in a zoological setting or in the wild. Prior to induction in captivity, thick padding or heavy mats should be utilized to protect recumbent animals from the concrete floors common in these environments. Myositis and neuropathy are serious potential complications. Traditionally, rhinoceroses immobilized in the field are maintained in or moved into sternal recumbency; however, irreversible muscle damage has developed in this position (especially if the rhinoceros goes down on a slope facing upwards with the full weight on its hind legs) as a result of occlusion of the blood supply to the limbs. Although uncommon, problems even occur with careful "placement" of the legs in an apparently natural position. With the rhinoceros on its side, blood flow to the limbs is improved and circulation to the muscles allows delivery of oxygen and dissipation of carbon dioxide and heat generated while running. With the animal in lateral recumbency, the legs should be physically "pumped" up and down by hand every 20 minutes to aid circulation. The weight must be taken off the lower legs to "pump" them effectively; this is accomplished by two or more people lifting the upper legs and rolling the animal partially onto its back about 45 degrees from horizontal. We recommend that all black rhinoceros that have undergone any degree of exertion be placed in lateral recumbency for at least a few minutes.

The decision to move white rhinoceroses onto their sides should be based on several factors, including the degree of exertion, presence of muscle tremors, and duration of recumbency. White rhinoceroses often experience significant muscle rigidity, paddling, and even convulsions under opioid anesthesia; these effects are exacerbated by lateral positioning but tend to resolve with time. Therefore, white rhinoceroses should be positioned initially in sternal recumbency until complete relaxation is achieved (Kock et al. 1995).

The position in which a rhinoceros is placed during recumbency is also an important consideration for respiratory function. It has been observed that oxygen saturation of the blood is higher in sternal than lateral posture. Consistent with observations in domestic animals and humans, the black rhinoceros has greater dead space in lateral compared with sternal posture as indicated by a lower end-tidal carbon dioxide and higher dead space ratios and volumes in lateral (Morkel et al. 2010). The most appropriate posture for rhinoceroses during anesthesia must be based on the circumstances of each capture and should strike a balance between maintaining respiratory function while providing optimal circulation to the limbs.

Eyes and Ears

The eyes of the recumbent rhinoceros must be shielded with a large towel or appropriate-sized blindfold to prevent retinal damage from direct sunlight, dirt accumulation and corneal abrasion from the environment. For black rhinoceroses undergoing translocation, the use of a muslin cloth wrapped tightly around the face several times and secured to the horn with cable ties is preferred to a simple blindfold (Fig. 54.3). This technique serves to fix the eyes in a closed position and quiets the rhinoceros during crate transport. Before blindfolding, foreign material should be washed from the eyes using physiologic saline. The ear canals are plugged with cotton wool or a cloth while the rhinoceros is anesthetized, leaving tabs for quick removal. Alternatively, when a large number of rhinoceroses are to be immobilized, two cloth-covered cotton wool plugs can be joined with cord so they remain together. If the rhinoceros is being transported, its ears should remain blocked for the entire trip. Caution should be used upon removal of the earplugs as the sudden auditory stimulation can result in excitement or aggression.

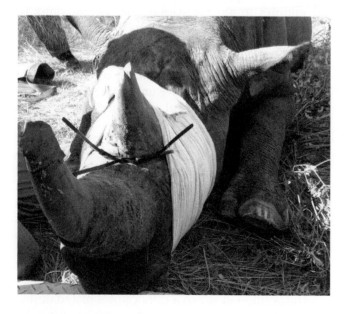

Figure 54.3.   Attachment of the "mutton cloth" blindfold to aid in crate transport of the black rhinoceros (*Diceros bicornis*). Note the use of cable ties in front of the caudal horn to secure the blindfold over both eyes.

Anesthesia Monitoring

A thorough clinical examination with monitoring of vital functions (respiration, temperature, heart rate, capillary refill time) must be conducted regularly for the duration of anesthesia. The focus should be on respiration and blood oxygenation while temperature and heart rate are usually of lesser importance. These functions are very much dependent on the degree of exertion and excitement before and during induction and must be kept in mind during your evaluation. Careful monitoring is especially important in old, debilitated, very young, and heavily pregnant animals. Any residual dart contents should be checked to see if they were injected, especially if more than one dart was used, as the success of drug delivery may dictate protocols for anesthetic monitoring and antidote administration.

Pulse oximetry (SpO_2) provides an indirect measure of oxygen saturation of hemoglobin (SaO_2) and is a valuable aid to help monitor blood oxygenation and pulse in anesthetized rhinoceros. However, it should not be a replacement for thorough patient monitoring. Without simultaneous correlation with arterial blood gases, pulse oximetry is a tool best used to monitor trends in oxygen saturation. SpO_2 values often fluctuate so the pulse oximeter should be observed for at least 1 minute; if the SpO_2 does not consistently read above 80% or is declining, an intervention is warranted. Based on lower oxygen affinity of white rhinoceros hemoglobin, it has been suggested that SaO_2 levels (ranging from lows of 40% up to 98%; Atkinson et al. 2002; Kock et al. 1995) in rhinoceros underestimate true oxygen saturation of hemoglobin when calculations are made using human formulae (Bush et al. 2004). The sensor clip is attached to the pinnae of the ear after careful scraping with a sharp blade to remove the epidermis or on mucosal folds of the penis, vulva, or rectum. A cloth is placed over the sensor as ambient light can affect the reading. In animals with excessive muscle rigidity or tremors, as is common in immobilized white rhinoceroses, the sensor may fail to obtain an accurate reading. A reflectance probe held against the nasal mucosa works well (applied beyond the pigmented area) and has also been used with varying success on the inner surface of the lips, against the gums and in the rectum or vagina.

Respiratory Gases: Oxygen and Carbon Dioxide   Respiratory depression is perhaps the most significant life-threatening complication encountered during routine anesthesia of the rhinoceros (Atkinson et al. 2002; Bush et al. 2004, 2005; Fahlman et al. 2004; Heard et al. 1992; Kock et al. 1995). Large recumbent animals experience cardiopulmonary depression and perfusion-ventilation inequalities because of large size and abdominal organs pressing upon the diaphragm. Severe respiratory compromise with hypoxemia, hypercapnia and acidosis is more common with long captive procedures or under field conditions where higher doses of opioids are used to shorten induction times (Heard et al. 1992; Kock et al. 1995). Among the African species, these physiologic changes are more prevalent in the white than black rhinoceros (Bush et al. 2004, 2005).

Respiration is the first and most critical function to be monitored in rhinoceros under anesthesia. In the field situation, it is valuable to have a reliable person who does nothing but watch the respirations, noting rate and depth. Be sure there is a free flow of air in and out of both nostrils and that the blindfold does not restrict airflow. The lower nostril, in particular, should remain clear of obstruction so passive regurgitation of stomach contents is free to drain. A cloth sack can be placed under the head to limit inhalation of dust or other debris. Respiratory rate and depth are noted by observing chest movement. When monitoring breaths on a bouncing vehicle as with immobilized rhinoceros transported on a sledge where it is difficult to watch chest movement, a finger can be hooked in the nostril or a hand held close to the nares to feel for the warm exhaled air. Breathing should be deep and regular. Respiratory rate is approximately 10–15 breaths per minute on induction, going down to 4–8 bpm about 10 minutes post induction when using potent opioids. Respiration must be monitored for at least 30–60 seconds to obtain an accurate picture of ventilatory pattern as immobilized rhinoceroses often give two or three quick breaths followed by a period of apnea. Rhinoceroses often develop apnea when moved into a different position. Animals should be rolled slowly and watched for breathing. A painful stimulus often incites the apneic rhinoceros to take a breath. Observation of venous blood color during venipuncture provides a reliable early indicator of blood oxygenation. Dark red, almost black blood indicates poor oxygenation, while a lighter red color is normal and correlates well with mucous membrane color.

If breathing is slow, the rhino develops apnea or blood oxygenation is poor (SpO_2 consistently less than 80%); partial reversal with nalorphine HBr (Nalline), nalbuphine (Nubain), or butorphanol (Torbugesic) or complete reversal with naltrexone HCl [Trexonil] or diprenorphine are indicated. Nalorphine given intravenously produces a marked and sustained improvement in the quality of respiration (Table 54.2 and Table 54.3). Its use has been associated with an approximate 20% increase in the hemoglobin saturation of oxygen (SaO_2) based on pulse oximetry (Kock et al. 1995). Although widely reported to improve oxygenation (Rogers 1993a, 1993b), recent investigation suggests nalorphine produces negligible change to oxygen partial pressures (PaO_2) in the anesthetized rhinoceros (Bush et al. 2004; Fahlman et al. 2004). Since black rhinoceros stand up readily with very small volumes of nalorphine, we recommend dosing at 5-mg nalorphine for adult black

rhinoceros and 25–30 mg for white rhinoceros under field conditions. It is very safe to use nalorphine in white rhinoceros, as this species rarely rises without stimulation and even if arousal does occur adult animals are relatively harmless in a semi-narcotized state. Intravenous doxapram HCl (Dopram; black rhinoceros 200 mg, white rhinoceros 400 mg) provides a smaller, transient improvement in respiratory rate and depth. Doxapram must be used with caution in white rhinoceroses, as it causes central nervous system excitation and exacerbates muscle tremors; effects are best noted if used in conjunction with nalorphine and supplemental oxygen.

Nasal or tracheal insufflation of oxygen (O_2; 15–30 L/ min) can produce a rapid and significant increase in blood oxygen saturation in immobilized rhinoceros. Although it did not correct systemic acidosis or hypercapnia, O_2 insufflation did substantially improve oxygenation and anesthetic safety (Bush et al. 2004; Fahlman et al. 2004). A variety of factors influence pulmonary blood gas exchange, including dose of anesthetic drug, position of the rhinoceros during immobilization, body temperature, oxygen delivery, and size of the animal. Oxygen supplementation at the flow rates commonly used for rhinoceros appears to produce a more profound improvement of patient oxygenation (PaO_2 108–194 mm Hg) in subadult African rhinoceroses compared with adults, perhaps indicating greater ventilation-perfusion mismatch with larger body size (Fahlman et al. 2004).

A control valve and flow meter are attached to the O_2 bottle, and oxygen is administered via a flexible silicon or rubber nasogastric tube (edges rounded to prevent damage to nasal mucosa), measuring 2-m long and 9- to 14-mm inside diameter (Fig. 54.4). Concurrent monitoring of the respiratory rate and depth, and

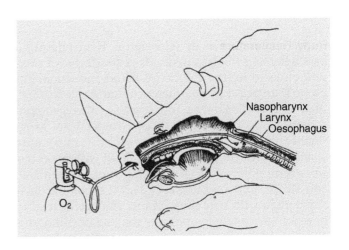

Figure 54.4. Illustration of the nasogastric tube tracheal insufflation technique for oxygen delivery in a recumbent white rhinoceros (*Ceratotherium simum*) under field conditions (adapted from Bush et al. 2004; illustration courtesy of the South African Veterinary Association).

blood oxygenation remains essential. Administration of a partial antagonist (nalorphine, nalbuphine, or butorphanol) will increase the rate and depth of respiration and improve the efficacy of oxygen delivery. Oxygen supplementation is a practical solution to enhance pulmonary gas exchange in immobilized rhinoceros and if used wisely one bottle is sufficient for many animals. Therefore, we recommend immediate intranasal or tracheal insufflation of oxygen at a high flow rate in all recumbent rhinoceroses. Within a few minutes, vital statistics will provide information about respiratory function, and in most situations, all physiologic parameters are satisfactory and the flow can be reduced or discontinued. A small percentage of animals, however, will develop a physiologic crisis where continued oxygen supplementation is critical. Aluminum oxygen bottles are now available that are small and lightweight, making them convenient for helicopter use.

Capnography offers a useful adjunct to monitoring with pulse oximetry, and many portable devices combine measurement of end-tidal carbon dioxide with oxygen saturation of hemoglobin. Capnography is common practice in human anesthesia as an aid to confirm placement of endotracheal tubes and for early warning of hypoventilation. In expired respiratory gases, capnography provides a direct measure of CO_2 eliminated from the lungs. It also gives an indirect measure of CO_2 production in the tissues and circulatory transport of CO_2 to the lungs. Capnography is a rapid noninvasive technique that offers reliable information about tissue CO_2 production, circulation, pulmonary perfusion, and alveolar ventilation and respiratory patterns. For rhinoceros capture, capnography is gaining acceptance by practitioners as a tool to help enhance anesthetic safety by offering a quick method to detect ventilatory or circulatory failure (Morkel et al. 2010).

Body Temperature Body temperature is an important parameter and the best indicator of the degree of exertion endured by the rhinoceros before induction. For every 1° increase in body temperature above normal, there is approximately a 10% increase in oxygen consumption. A rhinoceros's body temperature varies slightly during the day as the ambient temperature changes. Black rhinoceros immobilized without excessive exertion have a rectal temperature of between 36.5 and 38.5°C, and anything over 38.5°C should be liberally doused with cool water. Young rhinoceros tend to have a higher body temperature than adult rhinoceros after running a comparable distance. Although drenching with water is important, it will not have a dramatic effect in lowering the core body temperature, as there is considerable thermal inertia in such a large mammal. It helps to fan the rhinoceros with branches or a portable leaf blower after the animal has been wetted with

water. Holding leafy branches over the rhinoceros to provide shade can help lower the temperature, but it is important that people do not crowd around an immobilized rhinoceros and prevent air movement. A beach umbrella is the most efficient way to make shade—it is cheap, light, and easy to transport and can be folded to fit in the helicopter. A rhinoceros with a body temperature over 39°C must be processed quickly, while a temperature greater than 41°C mandates immediate delivery of the antidote.

The rhinoceros, like other large mammals, is prone to hyperthermia during capture and translocation. The black rhinoceros appears to suffer a greater level of hyperthermia-related morbidity and mortality in the peri-capture period than the white rhinoceros. The goal of the capture team should be to minimize exertion and speed induction. The rise in body temperature can be documented while the animal is in recumbency following excessive exertion; however, a second phase apparently unrelated to the level of exertion appears to occur upon crating. The mechanism of this hyperthermic response observed at variable periods after the rhinoceros enters the crate is not well understood, but could result from postreversal agitation and muscle activity, a physiologic stress response, inadequate airflow inside the crate, or a combination of factors or mechanisms. Simultaneous comparison of rectal and muscle temperatures in recumbent rhinoceroses demonstrates a 1°F (0.5°C) higher temperature in the muscle (Morkel et al. 2012). Since equilibration between rectal and muscle temperatures occurs slowly with time, a deep muscle thermistor can be a useful aid to measuring core body temperature. The probe is readily inserted into the dart site; however, caution must be taken to avoid exposure to dangerous immobilizing drugs.

Additional options for temperature measurement in the rhinoceros include use of a handheld infrared thermometer (Fluke Hart Scientific Inc.) in the ear canal. In a recent pilot study, deep infrared ear temperatures were comparable with deep muscle temperatures, giving a reliable and rapid assessment of core body temperature. Surprisingly, the use of cotton or wool earplugs resulted in ear canal temperature above deep muscle temperature and suggests that the inner ear in the rhinoceros may be an important site for cooling. In animals predisposed to hyperthermia (prolonged capture, high environmental temperature, etc.), rhinoceroses may benefit from removal of the earplugs and perhaps even application of some cooling mechanism to this site, such as a cold pack (Morkel et al. 2010, 2012). Another tool that has been adopted to enhance temperature monitoring in rhinoceroses is the temperature microchip (LifeChip Inc.). After reaching equilibrium when implanted under the skin or into a muscle, chip temperatures were slightly lower than rectal temperatures.

Pulse and Blood Pressure Heart rate is best obtained using a stethoscope while the pulse is readily palpable on the inside of the ear (medial auricular artery) or under the base of the tail (caudal artery). Pulse quality should be evaluated subjectively and compared with the pulse oximeter reading. It is often quite easy to visualize heart compressions by watching the chest wall or by feel with a hand placed over the cardiac window. The heart rate is usually 55–80 beats per minute, although it will be higher in rhinoceros that have undergone marked exertion, especially in young animals (up to 140 bpm). Cardiovascular function and peripheral perfusion are assessed by capillary refill time (CRT) and is measured by blanching the rhinoceros's gum for several seconds and then releasing. The observed delay or refill time should not exceed 2 seconds.

Hypertension is prevalent under etorphine anesthesia in black and white rhinoceros (Hattingh et al. 1994; Heard et al. 1992; LeBlanc et al. 1987). One report in white rhinoceros anesthetized under field conditions noted an apparent reduction in blood pressures when azaperone tartrate (Stresnil) replaced fentanyl in etorphine-based combinations, an effect observed despite the higher dose of etorphine used in the cocktails containing azaperone (Hattingh et al. 1994). These conclusions are questionable since fentanyl itself is a potent opioid with prominent hypertensive effects; possessing an activity approximately 1/15 that of etorphine, fentanyl was likely a confounding factor in the study. Although no definitive mechanism has been identified, increased sympathetic nervous system action, peripheral vasoconstriction, and hypoxemia are purported factors in etorphine-induced hypertension in both rhinoceroses and equids (Daniel & Ling 1972; Heard et al. 1992). Opioid-related hypoxemia may induce sympathetic system stimulation and hypertension. Elevated heart rate is a good indicator of hypoxia; once hypoxia resolves, the sympathetic response and associated hypertension disappear.

RHINOCEROS ANESTHESIA IN CAPTIVITY

Guidelines for Anesthesia of Captive Rhinoceroses

The large size of the rhinoceros belies an unexpected sensitivity to the opioid class of pharmacologic agents (Raath 1999). Surprisingly, the same dose of carfentanil citrate used to immobilize a 20-kg blackbuck (*Antelope cervicapra*) would also fully immobilize a 2200-kg white rhinoceros (*Ceratotherium simum*) making the rhinoceros over 100 times more opioid sensitive per unit mass than the average artiodactylid. This inordinate sensitivity of the rhinoceros family to the opioid class—while responsible for the undesirable changes observed in cardiopulmonary function—also makes it possible to adapt less potent mixed agonist-antagonist opioid agents into anesthetic protocols for both captive and wild rhinoceroses (Bush et al. 2005; Radcliffe et al. 2000a; Walzer et al. 2000).

Planning for anesthetic events should include preparation of the subject and environment where these variables can be controlled. Depending on the purpose for anesthesia, it is generally desirable to fast the animal for 12–48 hours prior to anesthesia (Radcliffe et al. 2000b). However, fasting is certainly not essential as evidenced by the many successful field operations where capture of wild rhinoceroses is conducted in the absence of preanesthetic fasting. Water access should be denied for at least 12 hours, and all water sources removed from the environment prior to drug delivery as regurgitation has been noted in white rhinoceros (Raath 1999). Both passive and active regurgitation of stomach contents are known, with the latter being very rare but quite spectacular. Passive regurgitation is common in immobilized rhinoceroses, presumably secondary to drug or hypoxemia-induced relaxation of the cardiac sphincter (Fig. 54.5). Because of the risks of regurgitation and inhalation pneumonia, great care must be taken with positioning of the head and nostrils, especially with animals in lateral recumbency.

Habitual patterns of behavior are important aspects of captive rhinoceros husbandry, facilitating close medical management. Anesthesia techniques should be adapted as part of these conditioning protocols. Regular visits by animal health staff to rhinoceros barns or bomas for acclimatization to the sights, sounds, and smells of the veterinary profession will help limit the stress of such procedures. In boma situations, it is helpful to learn the nature of each animal, including its likes and dislikes, while also listening carefully to the keeper in charge of caring for the animal.

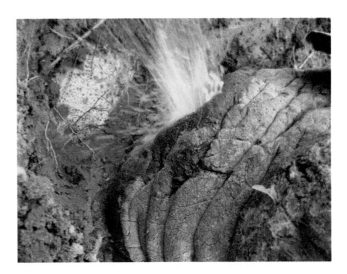

Figure 54.5. Passive regurgitation from the nares of a black rhinoceros (*Diceros bicornis*) forcefully expelled at expiration. The rhino is positioned in sternal recumbency to help the reflux drain away from the airway.

African Rhinoceros Captive Anesthetic Regimens

White Rhinoceros (*Ceratotherium simum*) The adult white rhinoceros is large and generally placid in captivity. Anesthesia with potent opioids is often associated with marked hypermetria, muscle rigidity, trembling, head shaking, and limb paddling (Fig. 54.6). These effects are undesirable and can be prevented by pre-anesthetic administration of the sedative or tranquilizer component of the cocktail. In captive animals, initial dosing with intramuscular azaperone or detomidine 20–30 minutes prior to induction with etorphine helps preclude muscle spasms and rigidity. With wild rhinoceroses, positioning in sternal recumbency until complete relaxation is achieved was deemed important in field practice (Kock et al. 1995).

Mixtures of etorphine or carfentanil combined with a sedative are standard agents for anesthesia of the captive white rhinoceros (Table 54.1). Doses ranging from 0.8 mg up to 3 mg of etorphine and 1.2 mg carfentanil are common, with supplemental opioids given IM or IV to extend anesthesia (Heard et al. 1992; Walzer et al. 2000). Following immobilizing doses of etorphine or carfentanil, other agents provide additional muscle relaxation and a deeper plane of anesthesia, including intravenous alpha-2 agents, propofol, guaifenesin, ketamine, and midazolam (Klein et al. 1997; Kock et al. 2006; Walzer et al. 2000; Zuba & Burns 1998). Muscle relaxation is critical for deep ventilation and to counteract the associated risk of oxygen depletion from muscle tremors and hyperthermia inherent with use of potent opioids. Lower opioid doses are indicated in zoo-conditioned animals, yet the potent opioids are still associated with significant cardiopulmonary changes, especially as procedure length increases (Heard et al. 1992). One captive white rhinoceros immobilized with etorphine remained hypoxemic despite maintenance of inhalation anesthesia using intermittent partial positive pressure ventilation (Cornick-Seahorn et al. 1995). Hypertension is common, while hypoventilation, pulmonary shunting, and atelectasis induce hypoxia and hypercapnia (Bush et al. 2004; Heard et al. 1992).

Butorphanol combinations are replacing use of more potent opioids for rhinoceros anesthesia in many zoological settings, as safe and reliable anesthetic planes can be achieved for most procedures including surgery (Radcliffe et al. 2000a, 2000b, 2000c). While not appropriate for all applications (i.e., fractious, nonconditioned animals or those with access to large areas), butorphanol combinations are highly effective. The author has used a mixture of butorphanol and azaperone for standing sedation and recumbent anesthesia in all four rhinoceros species maintained in captivity (white, black, greater one-horned, and Sumatran) with safe, predictable results (Radcliffe & Morkel 2007; Radcliffe et al. 2000a, 2000c). Butorphanol doses for white rhinoceros range from 50 to 120 mg for an adult and

10 to 20 mg for a calf or juvenile animal, while azaperone doses range from 100 to 160 mg for an adult with supplemental doses given up to a maximum of 300 mg (Table 54.1 and Table 54.4). Intravenous butorphanol supplementation is effective at inducing recumbency in white rhinoceroses after initial drug delivery, if needed and desirable. Intravenous dosing of azaperone without prior sedation has been associated with adverse extrapyramidal reactions in the horse and white rhinoceros and should be avoided (Radcliffe et al. 2000a).

Inhalation anesthesia is possible in captive rhinoceroses where more invasive procedures requiring surgery or longer anesthesia times are indicated. Intubation in the rhinoceros is accomplished by hand or with an endoscope to guide placement of the endotracheal tube or a guide catheter into the airway. Unlike the horse, rhinoceroses have a unique, blind diverticulum in the dorsocaudal pharynx above the glottis. The anesthetist must be careful not to pass the tube into the diverticulum during intubation (Radcliffe et al. 1998).

A white rhinoceros was safely anesthetized to treat a surgical colic by sedation with butorphanol (80 mg) and detomidine (50 mg), followed by IV glyceryl guaiacolate (50 g) and three boluses of ketamine (200 mg per bolus) for induction (Valverde et al. 2010). Anesthesia was maintained for an additional 6 hours using isoflurane in oxygen delivered at 1–2% using a circle breathing system. Positioning for surgery and recovery were challenging, but made possible through use of inflatable mats and expertise of the local fire department. Although the rhino eviscerated 3 days post surgery, the anesthesia and recovery were considered a success. Inhalation anesthesia together with a sling system facilitated laparoscopic-assisted transvaginal oocyte recovery in a black rhinoceros (Portas et al. 2006). Abdominal laparoscopy with insufflation of the abdomen is possible in rhinoceroses without general anesthesia by using a standing approach (Radcliffe et al. 2000b).

Black Rhinoceros (*Diceros bicornis*) Black rhinoceros appear predisposed to excitation during induction with etorphine, especially with remote drug delivery in zoological environments (Portas 2004). Using appropriate human safety practices, the stress of darting can be avoided by hand-injection, thereby alleviating much of the undesirable excitatory phase black rhinoceroses experience while also significantly reducing the total dose of opioid agents required (Radcliffe & Morkel 2007; Table 54.1). In bomas, to limit the "undesirable excitatory phase," great care should be taken to minimize the number of people and unusual objects close to the boma. Noise and movement should be avoided and, once recumbent, the rhinoceros's eyes should be covered and ears blocked as soon as possible. Significant induction risks include lacerations, limb and foot

Table 54.1. Suggested doses for chemical restraint of adult *captive* rhinoceroses producing anesthetic planes from sedation to recumbency

Rhino Species	Standing Sedation			Recumbency		
	Protocol	Reversal	Reference and Comments	Protocol	Reversal	Reference and Comments
White rhinoceros	50- to 70-mg butorphanol (BT) + 100-mg azaperone IM hand-injection plus constant rate infusion (CRI)	Naltrexone at 2.5 mg per mg BT IM or IV	Radcliffe et al. (2000a, 2000b); use CRI in long procedures	70- to 120-mg butorphanol + 100- to 160-mg azaperone IM hand-injection	Naltrexone at 2.5 mg per mg BT IM or IV	Radcliffe et al. (2000a); supplemental IV dosing or CRI
	120- to 150-mg butorphanol + 5- to 7-mg medetomidine (MED) IM dart (Give 1- to 2-mg nalorphine IV to keep standing)	Naltrexone at 1 mg per mg BT Atipamezole at 5 mg per mg MED	Citino (2008)	120- to 150-mg butorphanol + 5- to 7-mg medetomidine (IM dart; recumbency ~20 minutes)	Naltrexone at 1 mg per mg BT Atipamezole at 5 mg per mg MED	S. Citino, unpubl. data; improved analgesia for surgery
	0.8- to1.5-mg etorphine (M99) IM dart	Naltrexone at 40 mg per mg M99	Portas (2004)	2- to 3-mg etorphine + 20- to 40-mg azaperone IM dart	Naltrexone at 40 mg per mg M99	Portas (2004)
				1.2-mg carfentanil IM dart	Naltrexone at 100 mg per mg M99	Portas (2004)
Black rhinoceros	25- to 50-mg butorphanol IV or IM hand-injection	Naltrexone at 2.5 mg per mg BT IM or IV	Radcliffe et al. (2000c) and unpubl. data; use for subadults and crating	1- to 1.5-mg etorphine + 100-mg azaperone IM hand-injection	Naltrexone at 50 mg per mg M99 1/2IV 1/2IM	R. Radcliffe, unpubl. data; lower M99 doses with hand-injection
	1.5- to 2-mg etorphine + 2- to 3-mg medetomidine (Give 1- to 2-mg nalorphine IV to keep standing) IM dart	Naltrexone at 30 mg per mg M99 Atipamezole at 5 mg per mg MED	Citino (2008)	1.5- to 2-mg etorphine + 2- to 3-mg medetomidine (IM dart; recumbency ~15 minutes)	Naltrexone at 30 mg per mg M99 Atipamezole at 5 mg per mg MED	S. Citino, unpubl. data; enhanced analgesia for dental surgery
	2- to 2.5-mg etorphine + 10-mg detomidine (DET) + 15-mg butorphanol IM dart	Naltrexone at 40 mg per mg M99 Atipamezole at 5 mg per mg DET	Portas (2004)	2.5- to 3-mg etorphine + 60 mg azaperone IM dart	Naltrexone at 20-40 mg per mg M99	Portas (2004)

(Continued)

Table 54.1. (Continued)

Rhino Species	Standing Sedation			Recumbency		
	Protocol	Reversal	Reference and Comments	Protocol	Reversal	Reference and Comments
Greater one-horned rhinoceros	100-mg butorphanol + 100-mg azaperone IM hand injection	Naltrexone at 2.5 mg per mg BT IM or IV	R. Radcliffe and N. Lung, unpubl. data	3.5- to 3.8-mg etorphine + 14-mg detomidine + 400-mg ketamine IM pole-syringe	150- to 300-mg Naltrexone 1/2IV 1/2IM; No reversal DET	Atkinson et al. (2002)
Sumatran rhinoceros	25- to 40-mg butorphanol IM hand-injection _Note:_ Sumatran rhinoceros are easily conditioned to chute restraint and can be hand-injected. Even wild rhinos can be tamed quickly with feed and walked into a crate without use of drugs!	Naltrexone at 2.5 mg per mg BT IM or IV	Radcliffe et al. (2002); use azaperone in longer procedures	30- to 50-mg butorphanol + 50- to 60-mg azaperone IM hand-injection	Naltrexone at 2.5 mg per mg BT IM or IV	Radcliffe et al. (2004); higher doses for recumbency
				1-mg etorphine + 60-mg azaperone IM hand-injection	Naltrexone at 50 mg per mg M99 1/2IV 1/2IM	R. Radcliffe, unpubl. data; azaperone 20 minutes < M99 or suppl. midazolam
				10-mg butorphanol + 10-mg detomidine IM dart Wait 20 minutes 1.2-mg etorphine 5-mg acepromazine IM dart	150-mg naltrexone IV + 20-mg atipamezole IV	Walzer et al. (2010); 530-kg adult male; ketamine boluses (50mg each) to extend anesthesia

Sources: Citino SB. 2008. Use of medetomidine in chemical restraint protocols for captive African rhinoceroses. Proceedings of the American Association of Zoo Veterinarians and Association of Reptilian and Amphibian Veterinarians, pp. 108–109; R. Radcliffe unpubl. data; Atkinson MW, Bruce H, Gandolf AR, Blumer ES. 2002. Repeated chemical immobilization of a captive greater one-horned rhinoceros (_Rhinoceros unicornis_), using combinations of etorphine, detomidine, and ketamine. _Journal of Zoo and Wildlife Medicine_ 33(2):157–162; Portas TJ. 2004. A review of drugs and techniques used for sedation and anaesthesia in captive rhinoceros species. _Australian Veterinary Journal_ 82(9):542–549; Walzer C, Goritz F, Hermes R, Nathan S, Kretzschmar P, Hildebrandt T. 2010. Immobilization and intravenous anesthesia in a Sumatran rhinoceros (_Dicerorhinus sumatrensis_). _Journal of Zoo and Wildlife Medicine_ 41:115–120.

injuries, head trauma, damage to nasal sinuses, horn avulsion, and even death. With careful animal conditioning and procedure planning, the risks of induction excitation are easily minimized. Likewise, antagonism of narcotic anesthesia in the black rhinoceros is characterized by rapid and powerful recoveries mandating extra care; never stand in front of a narcotized rhinoceros as arousal is often sudden and unpredictable (Kock et al. 2006).

As in the other rhinoceros species, potent opioids (primarily etorphine) have historically been used for anesthesia of captive black rhinoceros with predictable results (Portas 2004). Zoo-conditioned animals require much lower doses of etorphine (1–1.5 mg) than their wild counterparts, especially when administered by hand-injection or pole-syringe (Table 54.1). Butorphanol alone or in combination with azaperone or detomidine HCl (Dormosedan) has also been used in the black rhinoceros, although its use is primarily limited to subadult animals, crating and translocation procedures, or well-conditioned animals since black rhinoceros are easily excitable and may override drug effects (Radcliffe et al. 2000c). In addition to reversing the respiratory depressant effects at the μ receptors, butorphanol also antagonizes the powerful μ sedative effects, thereby greatly lightening anesthesia. For butorphanol use in the black rhinoceros, expect light planes of anesthesia and the need for frequent redosing. A more thorough discussion of mixed agonist-antagonist opioid cocktails and newer alpha-2 agents for use in both captive and field immobilization protocols for the African rhinoceroses can be found in the New Techniques section of this chapter and Table 54.1 and Table 54.2.

Asian Rhinoceros Captive Anesthetic Regimens

Indian or Greater One-Horned Rhinoceros (Rhinoceros unicornis)
Despite the common occurrence of Indian rhinoceroses in zoological parks and a propensity for foot problems necessitating chronic care, few published accounts of anesthesia in captive greater one-horned rhinoceros exist (Atkinson et al. 2002; Portas 2004). One report combined injectable and inhalation anesthesia in a female *Rhinoceros unicornis* for ovariohisterectomy using etorphine and isoflurane in oxygen. The 7-hour long anesthesia (much of it in dorsal recumbency) was considered effective despite the animal succumbing to postsurgical complications (Klein et al. 1997). The most complete summary of captive anesthesia in this species, however, describes serial opioid-based anesthesia to facilitate long-term medical foot care in one animal. A combination of etorphine-detomidine (3–3.6 and 10–14 mg IM, respectively) was given by projectile dart or etorphine-detomidine-ketamine (3.5–3.8, 14, and 400 mg IM, respectively) administered by pole-syringe (Atkinson

et al. 2002). Use of the pole-syringe for drug delivery was preferred because darting was limited by a small target area among the peculiar anatomic neck folds and by drug selection for small dart volumes. While both drug combinations proved efficacious, subjective assessment suggested that the etorphine-detomidine-ketamine protocol produced more rapid induction, lowered the need for supplemental ketamine, and shortened reversal times (Atkinson et al. 2002).

The author has used butorphanol and azaperone (100 mg of each drug mixed in a syringe and given by hand-injection) to induce standing sedation in the Indian rhinoceros (R. Radcliffe and N. Lung, unpubl. data., 2004). A combination of butorphanol and detomidine (120 and 80 mg, respectively) produced sternal recumbency for surgical repair of a rectal prolapse (Bertelsen et al. 2004). As in the white rhinoceros, these protocols provide adequate muscle relaxation, sedation, and analgesia while being completely reversible with the pure opioid antagonists naltrexone or naloxone hyrdochloride (Narcan). Naltrexone is preferred unless short immobilization intervals are anticipated since renarcotization is common using naloxone alone; naloxone provides complete reversal for a short duration (approximately 30–60 minutes) and is only suggested if repeat procedures are planned for the same day (Bertelsen et al. 2004; Gandolf et al. 2000; Portas 2004; Radcliffe et al. 2000a).

Javan or Lesser One-Horned Rhinoceros (Rhinoceros sondaicus)
Rhinoceros sondaicus is the only rhinoceros not presently represented by captive specimens and was only extraordinarily displayed in zoological gardens during the seventeenth, eighteenth, and nineteenth centuries (Rookmaaker 1998). Although historical records indicate that at least 22 Javan rhinoceros were captured between 1647 and 1939, only four survived long enough to reach zoo exhibits in Adelaide, Calcutta, and London (Rookmaaker 1998). The entire surviving wild population of Javan rhinoceros can be found in Ujung Kulon National Park in West Java (*n* ∼ 40) and Cat Tien National Park in Vietnam (*n* ∼ 3?). No accounts of Javan rhinoceros anesthesia exist, but techniques presumably would be analogous to approaches used for the Sumatran rhinoceros (*Dicerorhinus sumatrensis*) or greater Asian one-horned rhinoceros (*Rhinoceros unicornis*) with size difference being a notable exception.

Sumatran Rhinoceros (Dicerorhinus sumatrensis)
Few reports of Sumatran rhinoceros anesthesia exist since captive specimens are rare. Etorphine (0.98–1.23 mg or 1 mg) combined with acepromazine (PromAce; 4–5 mg) or azaperone (60 mg) has been used to anesthetize captive Sumatran rhinoceroses (Portas 2004; Radcliffe & Morkel 2007). One adult male was immobilized on two occasions using a two-stage darting protocol. The

Table 54.2. Suggested doses for chemical restraint of adult *wild* rhinoceroses including supplemental agents used for respiratory support

Rhino Species	Immobilization			Respiratory Support	
	Protocol	Reversal	Reference and Comments	Protocol	Reference and Comments
White rhinoceros	2- to 3.5-mg etorphine (M99) + 40- to 90-mg butorphanol (BT) + 25- to 50-mg midazolam (MDZ) IM dart. Detomidine, medetomidine, midazolam, or azaperone can be added to this mix: (a) for better muscle relaxation and often better blood oxygenation—DMM; (b) to speed induction—DMMA.	Naltrexone at 40 mg per mg M99 IV (full reversal) OR 2- to 2.5-mg diprenorphine (M50:50) per mg M99 IV (reverses M99, but not BT)	Bush et al. (2005, 2011); reduces respiratory depression, hypoxia, tachycardia, muscle rigidity, and tremors, but with slower induction and an animal that may stay on its feet. Avoid butorphanol in combination with etorphine in rough terrain where a quick induction is safer.	• Produces immobile rhino in ~10 minutes and crating *without* partial opioid reversal • In case of inadvertent overdose or cardiopulmonary suppression, give diprenorphine to reverse the M99 while preserving the sedative effects of the BT	Bush et al. (2005, 2011) and unpubl. data; reverse part or all of opioid effects based on desired outcome
	3- to 4.5-mg etorphine + 40- to 60-mg azaperone (replace azaperone with 10- to 20-mg detomidine if no transport) IM dart Consider 5- to 20-mg midazolam slowly IV for muscle relaxation	For crate reversal: 2.4-mg M50:50 per 1-mg M99 plus 1- to 2-mg naltrexone IV if pushing. NTX will be a relatively "lively" wake up and one must be adequately prepared (i.e., animal close to crate, rope properly attached to head, and well-organized team) For field/boma reversal: naltrexone at 40 mg per mg M99 IV (full reversal)	Kock et al. (1995, 2006) Rogers (1993a); still considered standard translocation protocol P. Morkel, unpubl. data Kock et al. (1995)	All white rhino: • 20-mg butorphanol per mg M99 (20X M99 considered minimum dose for white rhinoceros, reduce to 10X or 15X if light) OR • 20- to 30-mg nalorphine IV OR • 20- to 40-mg nalbuphine IV AND/OR • 1-mg M50:50	Kock et al. (1995, 2006) M. Hofmeyr and P. Morkel, unpubl. data; Butorphanol is being used with greater frequency for its partial agonist properties in white rhinoceros across Africa

752

Species	Drug/dose	Notes	Reversal	Additional notes	Source
Black rhinoceros	4-mg etorphine + 40- to 60-mg azaperone (Replace azaperone with 100-mg xylazine or 10-mg detomidine) + 5000 IU hyaluronidase IM dart. Azaperone can be increased to 200 mg for a quicker induction if no transport. Can also combine azaperone with alpha-2 agonists. 2- to 2.5-mg thiafentanil (A3080) + 2- to 2.5-mg etorphine IM dart. Can also use thiafentanil alone at etorphine doses (i.e., up to 5 mg) but watch the respirations	Morkel (1989); higher M99 doses for *Diceros bicornis* Kock (1992); Kock et al. (2006) Hyaluronidase is always recommended to speed induction, especially as black rhino (unlike white rhino) often run themselves into trouble Rogers (1993b)	For crate reversal: 20-mg butorphanol per mg M99 OR 5- to 20-mg nalorphine per mg M99 or 1–1.8-mg M50:50 IV For field/boma reversal: naltrexone at 40 mg per mg M99 IV (full reversal) Same	• Give 5-mg butorphanol IV to increase respiration and heart rate and lighten the anesthesia. A 10-mg dose will considerably lighten anesthesia and rhino may stand. Animal less likely to stand if kept in lateral position and rhino can be easily pushed down, if necessary • *Note: Do not use the white rhino respiratory protocol in black rhino as it will cause arousal* • *Instead:* 5 mg nalorphine IV; titrate to effect • *Important* to have animal lateral and "pump" legs every 20 minutes	M. Hofmeyr, unpubl. data; P. Morkel unpubl. data; Kock et al. (2006)
Greater one-horned rhinoceros	2- to 2.5-mg etorphine + 10-mg acepromazine IM dart OR 0.7-mg carfentanil (CF)	Dinerstein et al. (1990); One sudden arousal noted; Induction times longer for breeding males	Diprenorphine at 2.5 mg per mg M99 IV Naltrexone at 100 mg per mg Carfentanil IV	• Cardiopulmonary depression not reported; 6–10 breaths per min • Surround target rhino with 10–15 trained elephants	Dinerstein et al. (1990)
Sumatran rhinoceros	2-mg etorphine + 80-mg azaperone + 5000 IU hyaluronidase IM dart OR Use M99:BT:MDZ 80-mg butorphanol + 80-mg azaperone IM dart	Author suggestion (extrapolated from captive animals)	Naltrexone at 50 mg per mg M99 IM or IV	• Treat like black rhino; muscle rigidity and tremors common • Use 5-mg midazolam to relax • Use 5-mg nalorphine for partial reversal of respiratory depression • If rhino is approachable give 25- to 40-mg butorphanol IV rather than via dart • Sumatran rhinoceros are easily tamed and can even be fed into a crate; a temporary boma can be erected to facilitate capture and crating	Radcliffe et al. (2004) and unpubl. data
		Use for compromised animal in snare	Naltrexone at 2.5 mg per mg BT IM or IV		Radcliffe et al. (2004) and unpubl. data

Sources: P. Morkel, unpubl. data; R. Radcliffe, unpubl. data; Bush M, Citino SB, Grobler D. 2005. Improving cardio-pulmonary function for a safer anesthesia of white rhinoceros (*Ceratotherium simum*): use of opioid cocktails to influence receptor effects. Proceedings of the American Association of Zoo Veterinarians, American Association of Wildlife Veterinarians and American Zoo and Aquarium Association Nutrition Advisory Group, pp. 259–260; Bush M, Citino SB, Lance WR. 2011. The use of butorphanol in anesthesia protocols for zoo and wild mammals. In: *Fowler's Zoo and Wild Animal Medicine Current Therapy 7* (RE Miller, ME Fowler, eds.), Chapter 77, pp. 596–603; Kock MD, Meltzer D, Burroughs R, eds. 2006. *Chemical and Physical Restraint of Wild Animals: A Training and Field Manual for African Species.* Zimbabwe Veterinary Association Wildlife Group and International Wildlife Veterinary Services; Rogers PS. 1993a. Chemical capture of the white rhinoceros (*Ceratotherium simum*) OR 1993b. Chemical capture of the black rhinoceros (*Diceros bicornis*). In: *The Capture and Care Manual* (AA McKenzie, ed.). Pretoria: Wildlife Decision Support Service and South African Veterinary Foundation.

first doses were considered inadequate and the authors subsequently recommended 10-mg butorphanol plus 10-mg detomidine IM followed 20 minutes later with 1.2-mg etorphine and 5-mg acepromazine IM, plus 50-mg supplemental doses of ketamine IV to extend the anesthesia period (Walzer et al. 2010). Darting of this animal likely contributed to long induction times (up to 40 minutes)—Sumatran rhinoceros are easily conditioned for hand injection in a chute. As with the African species, muscle rigidity and cardiopulmonary depression are common with use of the potent opioids, and preanesthetic administration of a tranquilizer is prudent to limit muscle tremors and improve respiratory function. Total azaperone doses should be kept to 100 mg or less as ataxia has been noted upon recovery with higher doses in this species. Butorphanol has been combined with detomidine for standing sedation while the author routinely uses a mixture of butorphanol and azaperone for standing sedation and full recumbent procedures (Table 54.1; Radcliffe et al. 2004).

As with the African species, butorphanol combinations are preferred in captive Sumatran rhinoceros to preclude the adverse cardiopulmonary changes associated with use of more potent opioids. For adult animals, butorphanol at a dose of 60–80 µg/kg with azaperone at 80–100 µg/kg and a range of 30- to 50-mg and 50- to 60-mg butorphanol and azaperone, respectively, is recommended with higher butorphanol doses being used on occasion to induce recumbency. Antagonism of the butorphanol effects is accomplished with naltrexone at a dose of 2.5 times the dose of butorphanol (Table 54.1; Radcliffe et al. 2004). Other tranquilizers may be used in place of azaperone, such as the alpha-2 agonists, but care should be exercised as hypoxemia has been reported with use of these sedatives. Local anesthetics may facilitate invasive procedures; however, use of more potent narcotics such as etorphine or other pharmacologic agents, such as ketamine and medetomidine, may be indicated to induce surgical anesthesia.

New Captive Anesthesia Techniques

Although much has been learned about rhinoceros anesthesia, limitations still hinder safe and reliable procedures for these large mammals, especially where prolonged recumbency or surgery is required (Heard et al. 1992; Klein et al. 1997). Standing restraint where possible using mixed agonist-antagonists show promise (Radcliffe et al. 2000a, 2000b). For the black rhinoceros, where potent opioids are still often preferred over mixed agonists, challenges include marked respiratory depression, inadequate muscle relaxation, need for frequent redosing, and incomplete analgesia in painful procedures. The incorporation of the potent alpha-2 agonist medetomidine with etorphine or butorphanol enhances sedation and analgesia in captive rhinoceroses (Citino 2008). Because alpha-2 agonists exacerbate respiratory depression and hypotension, contribute to dehydra-

tion, and alter thermoregulatory mechanisms they must be used with caution in rhinoceroses of unknown health status, especially old and debilitated animals. However, under captive conditions, where the health of an animal is known and a specific type of anesthesia is desirable, alpha-2 agents are effective supplements.

For the black rhinoceros, medetomidine (2–3 mg representing 2–2.9 µg/kg IM; 20 mg/mL solution) is combined with etorphine (1.5–2 mg representing 1.5–1.7 µg/kg IM; Citino 2008) and given by dart. The investigators were able to begin safe animal manipulations at approximately 9 minutes, with full recumbency achieved in 15 minutes. This combination facilitated very painful procedures, including molar extraction and foot surgery with the additional supplement of an intravenous guaifenesin-ketamine drip (1 g of ketamine in one liter 5% GGE solution) to enhance peripheral analgesia. Relaxation was excellent with easy access to the oral cavity for dental surgery. Physiologic parameters were considered normal with concomitant nasal oxygen insufflation. Recovery from anesthesia was smooth and rapid with no evidence of resedation or renarcotization using naltrexone at 30 mg per mg etorphine and atipamezole HCl (Antisedan) at 5 mg per mg medetomidine.

For white rhinoceros, where butorphanol has proven so effective in captive settings, the same investigator is using medetomidine (5–7 mg representing 2.47–2.81 µg/kg IM) and butorphanol (120–150 mg IM representing 62.5–64.9 µg/kg IM) to provide enhanced muscle relaxation and analgesia properties (Citino 2008). The animals can be manipulated within approximately 11 minutes of intramuscular drug delivery with full recumbency in 20 minutes. The addition of medetomidine into these protocols has significantly improved muscle relaxation and analgesia properties for such painful ophthalmic procedures as eye enucleation and conjunctival flap surgery. As with the black rhinoceros, a 5% guaifenesin-ketamine drip was deemed useful for long procedures and to enhance peripheral analgesia. Antagonism was complete using naltrexone at 1 mg per mg butorphanol (204–262 µg/kg naltrexone) and atipamezole at 5 mg per mg medetomidine (25.4–31.2 µg/kg atipamezole).

RHINOCEROS ANESTHESIA IN THE WILD

Guidelines for Anesthesia of Wild Rhinoceroses

Field anesthesia of Asian and African rhinoceroses is often undertaken to facilitate urgent conservation actions, such as dehorning, ear-notching, microchip application, radio-collaring, and horn transmitter implantation or translocation to safe areas (Dinerstein et al. 1990; Flamand et al. 1984). Ideally, rhinoceros capture operations should be conducted when temperatures are lower than 25°C, usually in the early morning or late afternoon. Darting free-ranging rhinoceros when ambient temperatures are high increases the risk of elevated body temperatures and associated physiological stress. If working in the late afternoon, a rhinoceros should not be darted unless there is sufficient daylight remaining (an hour is a minimum time to process the animal and deal with potential problems; Rogers 1993a, 1993b). If a rhinoceros has run hard enough for its skin to become dark with sweat, the rhinoceros's body temperature will often exceed 39°C. Such an animal should not be darted or if it has already been darted, it must be drenched with water and processed quickly. If the temperature of an immobilized rhinoceros rises above 41°C, the antidote should be administered immediately and the animal released.

With good dart placement, recumbency should follow within 3–6 minutes post drug delivery (Kock et al. 2006; Morkel 1989, 1994). Induction is usually quicker in young rhinoceroses and longer in large bulls and heavily pregnant cows. If there are no signs at about 6 minutes, the rhinoceros should be darted again. Induction times of less than 3 minutes may indicate an overdose and it is important to get to such an animal quickly so that the respiration and other vital functions can be monitored; oxygen combined with a partial antagonist should be given, if necessary. In protocols incorporating thiafentanil, rapid inductions are expected and less of a concern. Intravenous opioid use should be avoided due to risks of apnea; however, if necessary, give the opioid slowly while keeping a close eye on respiration. For the same reason, caution must be exercised when giving midazolam or alpha-2 agonists by the intravenous route.

As a rhinoceros becomes affected by etorphine, its pace shortens, the forelegs are lifted higher in a classic "Hackney gait," and the head is elevated (Fig. 54.6).

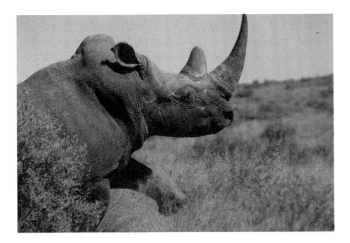

Figure 54.6. Typical induction posture in adult white rhinoceros (*Ceratotherium simum*) under the effects of etorphine, illustrating characteristic head elevation, raised hackney action of forelimbs and muscle rigidity (image courtesy of Rolfe Radcliffe, Living Fossil Productions).

The rhinoceros then starts to blunder through bushes and slows down before going into lateral or sternal recumbency. In rough terrain, rhinoceros have a tendency to run downhill once they are heavily narcotized and may easily injure themselves by running into a gully or water source. With a quick induction, rhinoceroses tend to go down in sternal recumbency. Occasionally, the forelegs collapse first and the hindquarters remain elevated. In this situation, the full weight of the abdominal organs press on the diaphragm, and respiration may be compromised, especially in heavily pregnant females, who have the weight of the fetus, adding additional pressure. Such animals must be immediately pushed onto their sides. Usually, a rhinoceros will become fully recumbent; however, if it is still on its feet, the brake rope can be placed around one of its rear legs, the blindfold over its eyes, and cotton wool in its ears.

On arrival at an immobilized rhinoceros, a quick estimate of its age and body condition should be made. Older or debilitated rhinoceros need special care. Nothing should impede respiration or push against the rhinoceros's belly, chest, or nostrils. On a slope, the rhinoceros should face uphill to alleviate pressure against the diaphragm. Field personnel must work quickly while the rhinoceros is recumbent—it helps to prepare a prioritized checklist before beginning each field capture exercise (Flamand et al. 1984; see also *Practical Strategies for Rhinoceros Field Anesthesia*).

African Rhinoceros Wild Anesthetic Regimens
White Rhinoceros (*Ceratotherium simum*) With the high doses of opioids used to speed induction under field conditions, the safe anesthesia of wild white rhinoceroses represents one of the most challenging branches of rhinoceros anesthesia (Table 54.2). Hypoxia, hypercapnia, hypertension, tachycardia, and acidosis are common physiologic abnormalities reported in anesthetized white rhinoceros (Bush et al. 2004; Heard et al. 1992). A variety of techniques have been adopted to help alleviate the significant opioid-induced cardiopulmonary depression in African rhinoceroses. These include use of partial agonist-antagonist agents to reverse the μ-regulated opioid respiratory depression, respiratory stimulants, such as doxapram, nasal or tracheal insufflation of oxygen, and incorporation of mixed agonist-antagonist agents into more potent opioid-based protocols to influence receptor effects (Bush et al. 2004, 2005; Fahlman et al. 2004; Kock et al. 1995; Radcliffe et al. 2000a).

Opioid doses for field anesthesia of adult white rhinoceroses range from 3 to 4.5 mg of etorphine plus 40- to 60-mg azaperone or 10- to 20-mg detomidine (Table 54.2; Bush et al. 2004; Kock et al. 1995; Rogers 1993a). Hyaluronidase (Hylase; 5000 IU) is often incorporated into darting protocols for rhinoceros to shorten induction times (Morkel 1989). White rhinoceroses stopped moving 2–3 minutes sooner with hyaluronidase, but often remained standing (Kock et al. 1995). Fentanyl was once incorporated into drug cocktails for white rhinoceros but is rarely used today (1 mg of etorphine being equipotent to 15 mg of fentanyl; Rogers 1993a). The parasympatholytic agent, hyoscine, was historically combined with opioids for its sedative and amnesic properties, as well as to induce "temporary blindness" by pupillary dilation (Player 1972; Rogers 1993a). However, its use is no longer widely accepted because of undesirable side effects and is now considered obsolete (Kock et al. 1995; Raath 1999).

An extensive study of white rhinoceros anesthesia incorporating several drug protocols and 141 immobilizations over a 2-year period was conducted in Zimbabwe to enable dehorning operations (Kock et al. 1995). Initial immobilization mortality was quite high at 7% and was primarily attributed to hypoxemia and cardiovascular collapse. Subsequent captures utilized lower opioid immobilizing doses and simultaneously incorporated routine use of nalorphine (10–20 mg) or nalbuphine HCl (20–40 mg) to help improve respiration—especially in longer procedures, where mortality was most prevalent. Of the various drug combinations tested (etorphine alone and in combination with fentanyl, xylazine, or detomidine), the etorphine-detomidine combination was considered superior because it was empirically judged as smoother and more rapid (no statistical significance). Pulse rates and creatinine phosphokinase (CPK) levels were significantly lower with the etorphine-detomidine combination, suggesting improved cardiac function and less muscle damage, respectively (Kock et al. 1995). Good muscle relaxation was observed without the rigidity and paddling common with use of potent opioids in the white rhinoceros. The ratio of etorphine to tranquilizer was critical and dose dependent, likely reflecting differences in drug pharmacology and onset of action.

An effective alternative for mitigating muscle rigidity in wild white rhinoceroses is the use of midazolam (Radcliffe & Morkel 2007; Table 54.2). Since immobilized white rhinoceros are often first encountered in a standing position with a rigid body posture, intravenous midazolam at 5–20 mg is effective in inducing good muscle relaxation and recumbency. The Zimbabwe workers noted that even small incremental increases in etorphine in the initial immobilizing dose or redosing with etorphine resulted in poorer muscle relaxation and increased head shaking, jerking, and limb paddling (Kock et al. 1995). Midazolam has excellent muscle relaxation properties and is a useful adjunct in these situations.

Black Rhinoceros (Diceros bicornis) Capture-related stress is a significant factor in field immobilization of the black rhinoceros, resulting in morbidity and mor-

tality in the postcapture period (Keep 1973; McCulloch & Achard 1969). Rapid immobilization using high opioid doses in combination with hyaluronidase is the single most critical factor in reducing stress during black rhinoceros capture operations (Kock 1992; Morkel 1989, 1994). Furthermore, higher etorphine doses and use of hyaluronidase were associated with significantly shorter induction times, lower body temperatures, shorter distances moved, and reduced muscle damage, as evidenced by lower CPK and lactate dehydrogenase levels (Kock 1992). Although two accounts list 3-mg etorphine as a standard opioid immobilizing dose for wild black rhinoceros (Kock et al. 1990; Rogers 1993b), subsequent study suggests that 3 mg of etorphine is inadequate due to prolonged induction periods and associated capture stress (Kock 1992). Based on review of published material and considerable author experience, 4 mg of etorphine is recommended as a good standard dose for an adult black rhinoceros bull or cow in good body condition (Table 54.2; Morkel 1989, 1994).

A scaled-down opioid dose should be utilized in young animals or those in poor body condition; however, in all other circumstances, a low dose of etorphine is contraindicated for free-range capture of the black rhinoceros (Kock et al. 2006). Azaperone is incorporated into etorphine-based African rhinoceros immobilization protocols at 40–60 mg total dose (Table 54.2). Concentrated (100 mg/mL) azaperone solutions should be carefully examined before use as they often crystallize under field conditions. Xylazine or Detomidine (100 or 10 mg per adult, respectively) can be substituted for azaperone based on individual preference.

A disparity is evident in the opioid dose required for immobilization of the various subspecies of black rhinoceros. The desert subspecies (Diceros bicornis bicornis) needs a slightly higher dose than the other subspecies. While 5 or even 6 mg etorphine may be necessary for an adult D. b. bicornis in good condition, 4 mg is usually more than adequate for a comparable response in animals of the Diceros bicornis minor or Diceros bicornis michaeli subspecies. Not only is there variation between subspecies, but there also appears to be some difference among individuals. The capture veterinarian must therefore be aware of these vagaries in dose response and be prepared to respond if an animal reacts unfavorably.

Asian Rhinoceros Wild Anesthetic Regimens
Indian or Greater One-Horned Rhinoceros (Rhinoceros unicornis) Techniques for field anesthesia of the greater one-horned rhinoceros were developed to meet research needs, including the elucidation of basic ecology, genetics, social organization, and dispersal biology (Dinerstein 2003; Dinerstein et al. 1990). Furthermore, translocation programs are proving essential for reaching long-term population management goals

for *R. unicornis* in India and Nepal. Capture of wild greater one-horned rhinoceros is usually conducted from atop trained elephants to facilitate finding and darting of rhinoceroses among the dense tall-grass habitats in the floodplain grasslands and riverine forests, where these rhinoceroses flourish. In addition to providing an elevated platform, elephants (10–15 animals) are used to surround the target rhinoceros before and after darting to facilitate observation of the animal during induction and to prevent escape into open water (Dinerstein et al. 1990).

Adult greater one-horned rhinoceros weigh an estimated 2000 kg, with males slightly larger than females. Dinerstein and colleagues immobilized 39 animals (representing 51 events) using a combination of etorphine and acepromazine (2–2.5 and 10 mg, respectively) delivered via remote intramuscular injection either in the shoulder or rump using Cap-Chur darts with 5-cm needles (Table 54.2; Dinerstein et al. 1990). One adult female was immobilized with carfentanil (0.7 mg), and all animals were successfully reversed in the field using diprenorphine HCl (M50:50). Induction times were found to be significantly longer in breeding versus nonbreeding males, with the former group rarely moving far from the site of darting. A large disparity in induction times was noted across all age and sex groups, presumably related to variable drug delivery from dart placement among the thick skin folds characteristic of the species (Dinerstein et al. 1990).

Javan or Lesser One-Horned Rhinoceros (*Rhinoceros sondaicus*) There have been no published reports describing field capture or anesthesia of the Javan rhinoceros. As with the Sumatran rhinoceros, pitfall trap methodologies rather than stockade style traps are recommended for capture of lesser one-horned rhinoceroses in the rainforest environment, provided the risks of flooding can be controlled (Nardelli 1987b; Sadmoko 1990). Field anesthesia is also possible—especially where animals are pushed out of the forest by human activities—and should be based on extrapolation of the best available information from the other Asian species.

Sumatran Rhinoceros (*Dicerorhinus sumatrensis*) Several intensive operations have been conducted to capture wild Sumatran rhinoceroses using corral or stockade traps with little or no success (Abdullah 1987; Sadmoko 1990). In one instance, an adult female Sumatran rhinoceros suffered severe head injuries and acute death following capture in a stockade trap from apparent panic-related self-trauma (Nardelli 1987a). Planned capture of wild Sumatran rhinoceros in the forests of Southeast Asia has been most effective by use of the pitfall trap. Pitfall traps measured 10′ × 4′ × 8′ (length × width × depth) and incorporated strong plywood walls to preclude landslides and a breakaway

false ceiling that drops the animal into the excavated pit beneath (Fig. 54.7). Site selection favoring heavily used rhinoceros trails was considered the single most important criteria for success or failure of the pitfall trap (Abdullah 1987). Nevertheless, pitfalls suffer from significant problems. In many Sumatran rhinoceros areas, poor drainage results in flooding of the pit despite careful preventive measures. Interference from nontarget species is also a common hazard; tapir, elephants, cattle, and even human beings have fallen into pitfall traps despite sign boards erected for the benefit of man (Abdullah 1987)!

Due to the dense nature of the rainforest environment and rare sighting of individual rhinoceroses therein, routine chemical capture techniques developed for Asian and African rhinoceros are too dangerous, as an animal may be lost in the darting process. Increasingly, however, animals are being pushed from the jungle by human encroachment, and once beyond the protective boundary of the forest, are immediately threatened. In these circumstances, pitfall capture methods are not feasible and chemical capture techniques are indicated. Therefore, the capture process for an "at-risk" Sumatran rhinoceros found wandering within a Southeast Asian village or otherwise outside a protected area should be approached with careful planning of some urgency. Once the appropriate National Park, Rhinoceros Protection Unit (RPU) and Sanctuary staff have been contacted, the following stepwise approach to capture and translocation is suggested (Radcliffe et al. 2004).

Guidelines for Capture of Displaced Sumatran Rhinoceroses

Secure Immediate Area In the event a wild Sumatran rhinoceros is found wandering outside a protected area, the first priority should be to secure the area from villagers and would-be poachers to prevent the animal from being shot or otherwise harmed before capture or relocation of the rhinoceros is possible.

Determine Relocation Strategy If possible, a small core-group of decision makers should be formed to make immediate assessment of the risks and benefits of rhinoceros relocation. If the rhinoceros were unharmed and close to a protected area (<10 km), then it may be desirable to move the rhinoceros without capture by pushing it back toward the forest. If the animal was injured or otherwise in need of medical attention or far (>10 km) from the forest, a decision should be made to capture the animal.

Make a Plan for Rhinoceros Capture Considering the high risks associated with capture by the "chase to exhaustion" method (i.e., rhinoceros is captured following an extensive stressful chase without the use of routine chemical capture methods), this approach

Rhinoceros Pitfall Trap

Skala 1 : 100

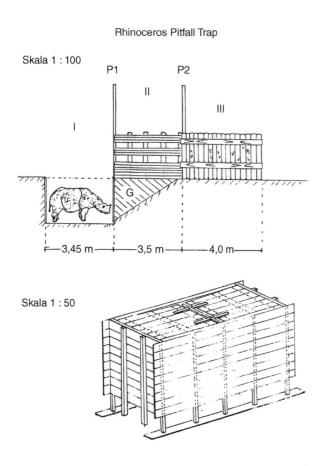

Skala 1 : 50

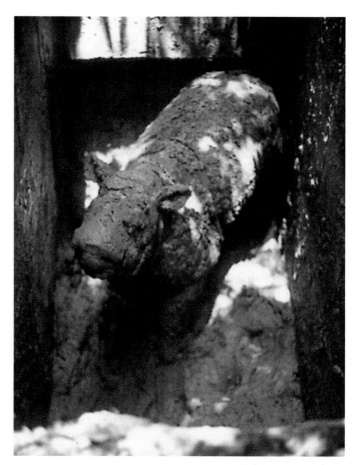

Figure 54.7. Diagrammatic sketch of pitfall capture method used in Indonesia's Riau Province for capture of wild Sumatran rhinoceros (*Dicerorhinus sumatrensis*) (sketches adapted from Sadmoko 1990; image courtesy of Mohd Khan bin Momin Khan, Malaysia Department of Wildlife and National Parks).

should only be attempted as a last resort (Fig. 54.8). The following are suggested guidelines and methodology for capture of at-risk Sumatran rhinoceroses outside a protected area.

Capture Method 1: Field Capture Using Chemical Restraint If a trained capture team is available (i.e., within 5 hours' travel time), then it may be wise to have the RPU ranger staff carefully monitor and secure the rhinoceros and surrounding area from a distance without pushing the animal to run as the rangers await the capture team. A rapid induction and recumbency will be essential for safe capture of a tropical ungulate species, such as the Sumatran rhinoceros, that may risk drowning or suffer from capture myopathy.

For field anesthesia of the Sumatran rhinoceros, a combination of equal parts butorphanol and azaperone (80 mg each) is recommended for simplicity, and its inherent safety for both rhinoceros and people alike (Table 54.2; Radcliffe et al. 2004). However, if a well-trained veterinary capture team is available then use of more potent opioids, such as etorphine combined with azaperone and hyaluronidase (2 mg, 80 mg, and

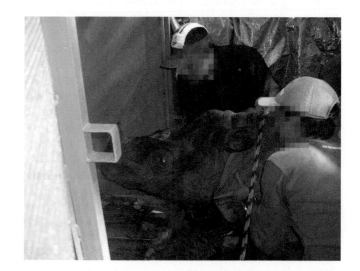

Figure 54.8. Like the other rhinoceros species, the Sumatran rhinoceros (*Dicerorhinus sumatrensis*) is prone to capture myopathy. Here, a wild "hairy" rhinoceros is restrained with a girth rope in hopes of moving the animal into a temporary boma. Hyperthermia is best avoided by limiting chase periods and liberal application of water (image courtesy of Sugiyo, Wildlife Conservation Society, Indonesia Program).

5000 IU, respectively) or the newer etorphine-butorphanol-midazolam protocols, may be considered depending on the situation (Bush et al. 2011). If the rhinoceros is already compromised from a chase or is restrained by a snare, the use of the safer butorphanol protocol is preferable to the potent opioids (Table 54.2). The butorphanol-azaperone combination may require confinement within a temporary boma or some additional restraint via a body or head rope to facilitate crating in healthy animals.

Capture Method 2: Field Capture by Erecting Temporary Boma The Sumatran rhinoceros is perhaps the only species of rhinoceros that can be captured by human physical restraint alone, albeit after much chasing and associated capture stress. Therefore, if a trained capture team is not available and the rhinoceros is in immediate peril, physical capture can be a feasible option. To begin, the animal can be followed from a safe distance and without excessive chasing until the rhinoceros is located within an area where it is resting and approachable (i.e., in water or other suitable location; Fig. 54.9). Large rolls of shade cloth or tarpaulin are then carefully erected without disturbance to form a temporary boma surrounding the rhinoceros that will facilitate sedation, crating, and transport. Once the animal is restricted

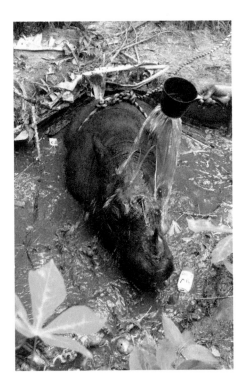

Figure 54.9. A wild Sumatran rhinoceros (*Dicerorhinus sumatrensis*) undergoing "hand translocation" without use of chemical restraint after displacement from a protected forest reserve in Indonesia. Although this animal survived significant capture-related morbidity, chemical capture techniques are preferred if trained staff are readily available (image courtesy of Chandra Putra, Way Kambas National Park, Sumatra).

within the confines of the "artificial boma," hand-injection or pole-syringe delivery of the butorphanol-azaperone combination will facilitate safe crating and transfer. The boma method is not likely to eliminate the long chase periods and accompanying stress, but it was effective in the recent capture and relocation of a young adult Sumatran rhinoceros in Indonesia (Fig. 54.7).

RHINOCEROS CRATING AND TRANSPORT

The moving or translocation of rhinoceroses is a specialized branch of rhinoceros anesthesia that has been practiced since the first African rhinoceroses were saved from the rising waters of Lake Kariba. The crating and relocation of rhinoceroses is now standard practice as urgent conservation measures, including enhanced animal monitoring and protected area management, have become effective tools in the fight against poaching (Flamand et al. 1984; Henwood 1989; Hitchens et al. 1972).

Walking a Rhinoceros

If a crate cannot be placed directly in front of the anesthetized animal, the rhinoceros can be "walked" a distance and guided into the crate (Fig. 54.10 and Table 54.3). When the rhinoceros becomes recumbent, the blindfold, cotton wool, head rope, and brake rope are applied. Four to six people are stationed on each rope, two people on each shoulder, one person to the side leading the team and two people walking in front of the rhinoceros, clearing obstacles in its path. The rhinoceros is given small incremental doses of intravenous nalorphine or diprenorphine depending on species; doses vary, but as little as 20- to 25-mg nalorphine may be needed in total (Table 54.3; Kock et al. 2006). Alternatively, butorphanol can be given IV at 10 times the etorphine dose to walk a white rhinoceros into a crate. Regardless of antidote used, a prodder is

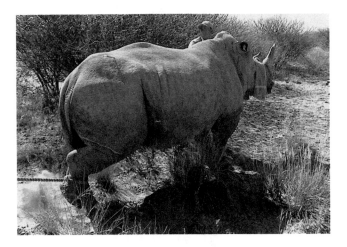

Figure 54.10. "Walking" an etorphine-immobilized white rhinoceros (*Ceratotherium simum*) using ropes and trained personnel to guide and stabilize the narcotized animal.

Table 54.3. Suggested opioid reversal protocols for walking, crate loading and transport of adult African rhinoceroses

Opioid Use for Crating and Translocation of African Rhinoceros

Method	Use	Reversal Drug or Opioid	Technique for Crating or Translocation
Butorphanol or nalorphine walking and crating method	For opiate (M99) immobilized rhinoceros	*White rhino* *Walking:* 10- to 20-mg BT per mg M99 Add 1- to 2-mg M50:50 for adult bulls for walking or crating (Hofmeyr) OR 1-mg M50:50 plus 20-mg nalorphine. Give further incremental 10–20mg Nalorphine IV up to 75mg (Kock et al. 2006) *Crating:* 10- to 20-mg BT per mg M99 OR Diprenorphine (M50:50) at 2.4× etorphine dose IV. Add 1- to 2-mg naltrexone to prevent pushing in crate. Can combine the naltrexone with diprenorphine—expect a relatively lively wake up so be properly prepared with head rope, position of crate, and so on! *Black rhino* *Walking:* Start with 5-mg nalorphine IV. Give incremental 5-mg doses every 5–10 minutes up to 20- to 40-mg (Kock et al. 2006) *Crating:* 15-mg butorphanol IV per mg M99 with rhino's head in crate door (Hofmeyr) Add 1- to 2-mg M50:50 to preclude pushing OR 10- to 20-mg nalorphine per mg etorphine. 1- to 2-mg M50:50 IV may be necessary to prevent pushing (Morkel) OR Blindfold with tight muslin cloth and wake up with 1- to 2-mg IV M50:50 *Avoid* myopathy in crating process by ensuring rhino does not squat in crate; use prodder plus repeat 1- to 2-mg M50:50 or 5-mg butorphanol doses	• Blindfold rhino; after cleaning eyes of mud or other debris, wrap a 4-m piece of muslin (mutton) cloth to cover eyes completely; attach three zip ties to secure muslin cloth forward of posterior horn. (*Note:* The blind fold option is really for black rhino and although it can be used on white rhino as well there is much less need for it.) • Position rhino's head close to or inside crate door: black rhino very important to have head in door—white rhino not critical; keep ears plugged until crated or leave in for transport • Place *head rope*; use 20-m soft nylon behind posterior horn with knot on side of head passing rope end through hole in crate • Place *break rope* on rear leg just below hock; use 8 meter nylon rope • Position 8 people on head rope and 4 people on break rope. Can use a 4 × 4 pick-up truck for back-up on rope if not enough people for head rope • *Reverse; wait 90–120 seconds.* Use electric prodder or water in ear to stimulate rhino to stand if it does not do so by itself • *Walk* rhino into crate by pulling on head rope, slow rhino with break rope, or go slowly with head rope; guide rhino by ground personnel; slide and secure pipes in crate (most crates have horizontal pipes, some only have the doors) • If black rhino pushes in crate, give 1-mg naloxone or 0.6- to 1.2-mg diprenorphine iv; if white rhino pushes, give 1- to 2-mg naltrexone iv; use prodder on head or shoulders and not on hindquarters since rhino will tend to push/squat more with stimulation of hindquarters.

Method	Use	Dosages	Comments
Butorphanol alone Crating method	For awake rhinoceros in zoo or boma environment	*White rhino:* 50-mg butorphanol IV (Radcliffe) *Black rhino:* 25- to 500-mg butorphanol IV at time of crating for conditioned animals (Radcliffe) Boma black rhinos: Start with 10-mg Butorphanol IV and increase in 5 mg increments (Hofmeyr)	• Butorphanol is a useful agent for crating and transport of crate-conditioned rhinos in zoological settings—combine with azaperone as needed • Butorphanol provides excellent sedation without concerns of excessive head pressing in crate and occlusion of nostrils in corner • No reversal required for butorphanol once rhino is in crate
Diazepam:nalorphine Crating method	For field immobilized rhinoceros	*White and black rhino* 10- to 15-mg Diazepam IV 10 minutes before "waking" rhino with reversal protocol (Morkel) Use standard crating methodologies earlier for white and black rhinos after giving diazepam	• Give diazepam to recumbent rhino and wait 10 minutes • Use same crating procedure as earlier using diprenorphine alone (white rhino) or nalorphine combined with diprenorphine (black rhino) • This protocol eliminates much of the pushing often observed in the crate following diprenorphine or nalorphine reversal procedures • Diazepam provides good sedation for ~8 hours especially in white rhino
Etorphine:azaperone Boma crating	For loading and transport of boma rhinos	*White rhino* *Boma crating:* 1- to 2.5-mg etorphine IM (higher dose for adult bull) plus butorphanol at 10X M99 dose plus 20-mg (subadult) or 40-mg (adult) azaperone *Note:* Butorphanol can also be given at time of recumbency rather than in the original dart, particularly if rhino requires medical care or other procedures under recumbency (Buss) *White or black rhino* 0.7- to 1.2-mg etorphine IM (Kock et al. 2006) OR 0.3- and 0.5-mg M99 for black and white rhino, respectively, without need to reverse *Crate sedation:* 0.05- to 0.15-mg etorphine IM plus 100- to 200-mg azaperone (can put in same syringe) IM or 10 to 30mg diazepam IM (not in same syringe) *Transport:* 50- to 150-mg zuclopenthixol acetate IM	• Use low doses etorphine to crate rhinos from boma; combine with Azaperone in black rhino; wave white flag on pole to lure rhino into crate • Etorphine is the *only agent* to calm an excitable rhino inside a crate • Butorphanol is replacing nalorphine and diprenorphine for both respiratory support and arousal for crate loading in both white and black rhinoceros—use small incremental doses (5mg or less) in black rhinos as reversal is more dramatic and produces a lively rhino • For crate sedation: Nalorphine sedation wears off ~5 hours post crating; thereafter give etorphine every 2 hours for duration of trip • If rhino is not excitable, give azaperone up to 200mg per 6 hours • *Note:* More etorphine is not effective within 3–4 hours of diprenorphine use and 8–24 hours following reversal with naltrexone • Avoid perphenazine in white rhino (if going to boma) as it causes anorexia; low dose OK if going straight to field

Sources: P. Buss, unpubl. data; M. Hofmeyr, unpubl. data; P. Morkel, unpubl. data; R. Radcliffe, unpubl. data; Kock MD, Meltzer D, Burroughs R, eds. 2006. *Chemical and Physical Restraint of Wild Animals: A Training and Field Manual for African Species.* Zimbabwe Veterinary Association Wildlife Group and International Wildlife Veterinary Services; Rogers PS. 1993a. Chemical capture of the white rhinoceros (*Ceratotherium simum*) or Rogers PS. 1993b. Chemical capture of the black rhinoceros (*Diceros bicornis*). In: *The Capture and Care Manual* (AA McKenzie, ed.). Pretoria: Wildlife Decision Support Service and South African Veterinary Foundation.

judiciously applied to the feet just above the nail, or to the muzzle or perineal area to get the rhinoceros to stand and keep it moving. After each dose, wait a few minutes (up to 10 minutes) and check the rhinoceros's response to the prodder or by squirting water in the ear. If there is no response, give another dose of antagonist. Once the rhinoceros stands, it should begin to stagger forward and can then be readily guided with the head rope and by the people on the sides. If the rhinoceros moves too fast, go slowly with the head rope and pull the brake rope to slow the moving rhinoceros. Particularly with young and fractious individuals, it is important to slow the rhinoceros as it approaches the crate so it does not traumatize itself upon entrance. A rhinoceros that charges too quickly into the crate can strike the far wall with such force to avulse the horn or crush the nasal bones. To preclude problems with loading, 10- to 15-mg intravenous diazepam 10 minutes before waking the rhinoceros helps to keep animals calm when aroused in the crate.

Black Rhinoceros Crating

The recent decline in availability and manufacture of the partial agonist-antagonist nalorphine in southern Africa has necessitated use of alternative techniques for partial reversal and crating of black rhinoceros in the field. Initial trials using similar agents, such as nalbuphine and butorphanol, have worked (sometimes quite well), although they have also been associated with irregular outcomes and responses in the black rhinoceros. Nalbuphine provides a satisfactory partial reversal that facilitates crating of black rhinoceros, but appears to predispose crated animals to dog-sitting and squatting that can lead to serious myopathy and inability to stand (Fig. 54.11). Butorphanol given in higher doses

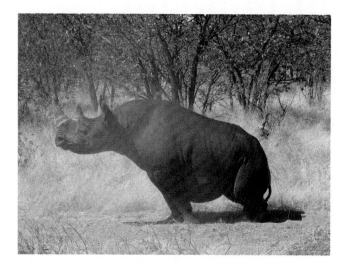

Figure 54.11. Posttranslocation myopathy in a black rhinoceros; capture complications are more prevalent in animals that experience excessive chase periods, hyperthermia, or struggle to stand upon crating (image courtesy of Birgit Kötting, Etosha Ecological Institute, Namibia).

(25–30 mg for an adult animal) also provides a reliable partial reversal for crating of black rhinoceros. However, such animals seem prone to head pressing in the crate and require constant supervision.

A novel approach to crating the black rhinoceros currently practiced in Namibia combines diprenorphine together with methods to limit noise and visual stimulus during transport. A muslin (mutton) cloth works well for both white and black rhinoceros (Fig. 54.3). Animals remain remarkably tranquil, although some degree of chemical tranquilization is still necessary. The beauty of blindfolding is that a physical rather than a chemical means is used to calm the animal. The cloth must be placed with great care to avoid damage to the eyes or loss of the blindfold during crate transport. One must brush or blow any dirt from around the eyes and flush the eyes with saline, if necessary. Tying the blindfold properly takes two people—the secret is to start with a 4-m length of muslin cloth and place the middle point on the forehead directly behind the back horn. Both ends of the cloth are pulled tightly on either side of the head, making sure both eyes are closed in a normal manner. The cloth is wrapped under the jaw around the opposite side behind the back horn where it is tied securely. While wrapping, the cloth should be "spread" to cover the eye properly and hooked behind the jaw. Three heavy-duty cable ties 40 cm in length are used to secure the blindfold to the rhinoceros. Two ties are threaded through holes in the cloth fashioned above and forward of the eye and closed to form a loop. A third cable tie is threaded through the two loops in front of the back horn and pulled tight. The cable ties serve to pull the cloth forward securely over the eyes. If the cloth becomes loose during the journey, simply pull on a cable tie to tighten the blindfold.

Reversal and crating is then routine: a heavy hemp rope is secured around the head with blindfold and threaded through the front of the crate. This rope will provide the forward pull upon standing and will direct the rhinoceros into the forward part of the crate. A second rope is secured to one rear leg and is used as a "break rope" to simultaneously slow the momentum of the rhinoceros so it does not collide with the front of the crate, where horn or nasal trauma may result. A relatively high dose of diprenorphine (black rhinoceros adult, 1.5–2 mg; subadult, 1 mg) is given intravenously after positioning immediately in front of the crate door. Two minutes are allowed to pass while all staff is quiet and the animal undisturbed. Upon standing, the rhinoceros is pulled forward into the crate while the break rope on the back leg slows the rhinoceros. Once inside the crate, the rhinoceros is secured by sliding three pipes into place at the rear of the crate and the rear doors closed. This protocol consistently produces a lively and relatively awake rhinoceros inside the crate that remains calm because of the combined use of a secure blindfold and earplugs.

Rhinoceroses blindfolded with muslin cloth travel well and can be given other sedatives, including azaperone (60–100 mg) or additional opioids (etorphine or butorphanol) during transport as needed. From about 4 hours onward, an additional 0.05- to 0.1-mg etorphine (usually with about 60 mg azaperone) is administered, and is usually repeated every 2 hours. The veterinarian (or someone with a high level of experience with opiates) must remain with the animal for the entire trip to evaluate and top-up as needed. "Straightening" with a prodder applied lightly to the forehead, neck, or shoulder is often necessary in the first few hours. The mutton-cloth can be kept on for as much as 36 hours. It is essential to put the cloth on tightly and to make sure it is 100% clean and that no sand or dirt gets into the rhinoceros's eyes.

The beauty of the tight blindfold and blocked ears is that you can wake up the rhinoceros to a large degree (and therefore prevent pushing), but because the animal can't see or hear, it is very unresponsive and rarely gets excited—the effect is quite remarkable. However, the muslin cloth blindfold is inadequate by itself for crate transport, and additional tranquilization using repeated ultra low doses of etorphine and azaperone is essential along the road.

Tranquilization during Transport

All black rhinoceros require tranquilization during transport (even most crate-conditioned animals) to preclude excessive struggle and associated trauma (Table 54.3). Other rhinoceros species tolerate transport better than black rhinoceroses, but still often benefit from some sedation. The veterinarian must always travel with the rhinoceros and be prepared to give additional sedatives or even narcotics if needed. It is imperative that the veterinarian anticipates the animal's tranquilization needs as waiting until the rhinoceros is alert and bouncing around, will risk unnecessary trauma to both animal and attendant. Additionally, a cool animal is generally more relaxed than an overheated one.

Rhinoceroses settle into the rhythm of transport quite well after just a few hours. However, as the short-acting tranquilizers begin to wear off, the animal may become excited if suddenly startled (i.e., from stopping, off-loading, etc.). The rhinoceros can be redosed with tranquilizers while the vehicle is in motion or alternatively, stop, inject, and start moving again immediately. In most instances, hand-injection is the best method to deliver additional tranquilizer. A 20-gauge, 1.5-in needle is inserted into the lateral muscles of the neck while avoiding the nuchal region. Beware of the head and horn during neck injections. For restless individuals, the gluteal region also works well. Once the rhinoceros has settled, attach the syringe and inject the drug. A pole-syringe can also be used, but hand injection is preferred because it precludes the startled response resulting from the jab of the pole. Beware of

coring where the rhinoceros's skin may block the needle lumen. An intramuscular injection takes 5–10 minutes for first effect; for a faster response, an intravenous injection into the ear vein is sometimes possible, although care must be taken to avoid the dangerous area around the animal's head and horn.

Resting by the rhinoceros during transport can be beneficial or a potential problem, depending on the rhinoceros's position and duration of recumbency. If the rhinoceros lies down while the vehicle is moving, the rocking and bouncing action of the truck helps to facilitate limb circulation. Beware, however, if the rhinoceros lies down for a long period (>60 minutes) in a stationary vehicle, unless you are very comfortable with its position. Rhinoceroses heavily sedated with opioids often struggle to work out a way to lie down; however, if they manage to do it once, they will lie down more easily thereafter.

Short-acting tranquilizers, such as azaperone, xylazine or detomidine, and diazepam or midazolam, are useful agents to produce a calming effect in rhinoceroses during transport. Azaperone is the tranquilizing agent of choice at 100–250 mg per adult and can be repeated every six hours as needed (Kock et al. 2006; Rogers 1993a, 1993b). A forty mg per mL azaperone solution is a convenient preparation and mixes well with etorphine for intramuscular administration to a fractious, crated rhinoceros. The administration of opioids, either alone or in combination with intramuscular azaperone or diazepam, is the only effective way to preclude an excited black rhinoceros from traumatizing itself inside a crate (Table 54.3). Etorphine and azaperone (0.05–0.15 mg and 100–200 mg, respectively) are delivered by hand injection or pole-syringe with sedation achieved in 5–10 minutes for durations of 2 hours or more.

Long-acting tranquilizers can help to calm an animal, however, are inadequate by themselves to sedate an excited animal during transport. Zuclopenthixol acetate (Clopixol Acuphase; 25–150 mg per adult rhinoceros up to 400 mg) takes about an hour to provide sedative effects after administration, while perphenazine enanthate (Trilafon; 200–400 mg per adult) takes about 12 hours for first noticeable effects (Kock et al. 2006; Swan 1993; Table 54.3). Perphenazine works well for the translocation of black rhinoceros while caution should be exercised in white rhinoceros as its use has been implicated in anorexia (Kock et al. 2006; Portas 2004).

Black Rhinoceros Off-Loading from Crate

Black rhinoceros, and especially juveniles and sub-adults, are notorious for being aggressive and sometimes even self-destructive to themselves and the crating equipment (trucks, crates, etc.) at offloading sites. In Namibia, where rhinoceros are often moved from veldt to veldt without the use of bomas and adaptation periods, the capture team uses a technique for off-loading that is effective and largely eliminates the aggressive phase. At the off-loading site, the rhinoceros is resedated inside the crate using a low dose of etorphine (adult, 0.1–0.2 mg) combined with azaperone (adult, 80–120 mg) and allowed to narcotize over a several minute period. Once the rhinoceros is head pressing or otherwise sedated, the muslin blindfold and earplugs are removed and the etorphine antagonist administered. A standard dose of 12–18 mg of diprenorphine for an adult animal is administered by intramuscular (not IV) injection and the crate doors are opened. As the rhinoceros regains first levels of awareness, it walks slowly from the crate even while still sedated and partially narcotized. These black rhinoceroses tend to walk directly away from the crate and into the veldt without the characteristic aggression and attack of the crate or related equipment. As the animal continues to walk away from the off-loading site, it becomes more fully aware of its surroundings and ambulates from the site in a normal fashion. This protocol has largely eliminated the aggression and self-trauma that is often characteristic of black rhinoceros at off-loading.

ALTERNATIVE RHINOCEROS ANESTHESIA TECHNIQUES

Antidote Choice

Following intravenous antidote administration, a rhinoceros will stand within 60–80 seconds. Response to the antidote is first noted as an increase in the depth and rate of respiration and movement of the ears and eyes. Rhinoceroses get to their feet quickly and are immediately strong and aggressive. A rhinoceros should always be moved into sternal recumbency before giving the antidote or it may *bash* its head on the ground as it attempts to rise from the lateral position. Intramuscular dosing of the antidote is often preferred for arousal of rhinoceros cow–calf combinations so that the pair awake slowly and have time to join together without dashing off in opposite directions. If intravenous dosing is desired with recovery of cow–calf pairs, the cow is injected first, thirty seconds before the calf.

Out of tradition, opioid antagonists are dosed using empirically derived ratios rather than on a mg per kg basis; for the pure opioid antagonist, naltrexone, dosage ratios of 20–50 times the etorphine mg dose and 90–100 times the carfentanil mg dose are considered standard for captive rhinoceros (Allen 1996; Kock et al. 2006; Swan 1993). Renarcotization has been reported in the white rhinoceros, but it is a rare occurrence in the black rhinoceros (Kock et al. 1990; Portas 2004). Field workers frequently use lower naltrexone doses (12.5 : 1 naltrexone to etorphine ratio) without a problem (Kock et al. 1995); however, sedative signs at these doses have been reported in white rhinoceroses and a minimum of 40 : 1 is therefore recommended to preclude renarcotization

(Kock et al. 1995; Portas 2004; Rogers 1993a). While naltrexone is considered the agent of choice for complete reversal of narcotic anesthesia, a number of scenarios arise under both captive and field conditions where a full reversal of an opioid-based procedure is undesirable.

The choice of antagonist and its desired action is dependent on two factors: species and location. Black rhinoceros are reversed into a crate with nalorphine, nalbuphine, or butorphanol, alone or in combination (Kock et al. 2006; Radcliffe & Morkel 2007: Table 54.2 and Table 54.3). In the boma, *Diceros bicornis* are reversed with naltrexone, although very nervous or aggressive individuals may benefit from reversal with diprenorphine for its sedative properties. *Diceros bicornis* are completely reversed in the field using naltrexone; however, because it is expensive, a combination of naltrexone and diprenorphine is often used for field reversal. In this case, the standard diprenorphine dose (2–2.5 times the etorphine dose; Swan 1993) is administered by intramuscular injection together with 50–100 mg of naltrexone.

In marked contrast to black rhinoceroses, white rhinoceroses are reversed into a crate using diprenorphine, with perhaps 1–2 mg of naltrexone. In the boma and in the field, *Ceratotherium simum* are similarly reversed with naltrexone. Diprenorphine is often used for translocation of *Ceratotherium simum*, since its partial agonist-antagonist actions provide significant narcosis during travel. However, diprenorphine has minimal agonist effects in *Diceros bicornis* and therefore should be used judiciously for transport in this species. For any partial antagonism in a crate situation, it is critical that the rhinoceros be monitored very carefully to prevent excessive head pressing and occlusion of the airway or damage to the neck and limbs. A cattle prodder is a vital piece of equipment in managing sedated rhinoceroses during travel.

Other Drugs and Immobilization Doses

Rhinoceros can also be immobilized with the other potent opioids carfentanil, fentanyl and thiafentanil. The following drug dosages are indicated for adult free-ranging rhinoceroses in good condition:

- Carfentanil at 1–1.2 and 0.9 mg (captive adult white and black rhinoceros, respectively; Portas 2004; Rogers 1993a) and 3 mg for wild adult rhinoceros (De Vos 1978; Hofmeyr et al. 1975). Carfentanil produces a quick induction and it is not necessary to combine with azaperone or xylazine.
- Etorphine at 1.8-mg plus 30-mg fentanyl (black rhinoceros; Kock et al. 2006; Rogers 1993b).
- Fentanyl alone at 60 mg (black rhinoceros; Rogers 1993b).
- Thiafentanil can be mixed equally with etorphine. The adult rhinoceros dose is 2- to 2.5-mg thiafentanil

plus 2- to 2.5-mg etorphine. This mixture gives a faster induction time than etorphine alone. The usual antidotes for etorphine work well.

Rhinoceros Anesthesia Complications

With opioid-induced cardiopulmonary depression common in anesthetized rhinoceros, the need may arise to deliver artificial ventilation. For emergency respiratory support in a rhinoceros, the animal is first pushed onto its side. A large person forces the knee and lower leg (with foot placed firmly on the ground) into the abdomen to vigorously force the abdomen diagonally upward and forward against the diaphragm. This moves the diaphragm, forcing air into and out of the lungs and keeps the animal alive while the intravenous opioid antagonist takes effect. When one leg is tired, use the other leg and recruit additional people to assist. Jumping on the ribs or back of the rhinoceros is ineffective and does nothing but fracture ribs and inflict unnecessary trauma.

Myopathies are common in rhinoceros that experience excessive chase periods or hyperthermia during capture. An especially critical period occurs at the time of crate loading and initial transport during field translocation of rhinoceroses. If stimulated to rise too early after partial reversal, animals may enter the crate and assume a rigid, semi-squatting position with their hind legs. This is undesirable and must be resolved quickly before the muscles are irreversibly damaged (Fig. 54.11). Use of the electric prodder on the head can often stimulate the animal to rise and stand, but avoid prodding the hindquarters as this can exacerbate the problem. If this does not work, consider prompt intravenous administration of diprenorphine or nalorphine. A sling can also be placed under the belly of the animal, just in front of the rear legs to lift the hindquarters (using the crane on the recovery truck) until the strength has returned to the hind limbs.

A very small percentage of black rhinoceros develop an adverse reaction that the author refers to as the "fat nose syndrome" (Radcliffe & Morkel 2007). Essentially, the nostrils close up and appear edematous with a much-reduced opening to the nares. The anesthetist is often forced to hold open or pull the nostrils apart. This unusual response may indicate a hypersensitivity reaction; morphine is known to cause histamine release in humans and, perhaps etorphine—derived from the same group of opium alkaloids—can produce the same uncommon effect in susceptible rhinoceroses.

New Field Anesthesia Techniques

Today's understanding of Rhinocerotidae anesthesia is truly the embodiment of many courageous pioneers who have led by exciting experimentation and hard-won experience (Harthoorn & Lock 1960; Kock et al. 2006; Player 1972; Young 1973). Yet with the immense challenges inherent in practical anesthesia of these complex mammals, innovative procedures are welcome. The newest ideas for rhinoceros anesthesia are arising from a combination of practical experience and a desire to explore the depths of pharmacology. Nowhere are such explorations more exciting than the emerging science of mixed opioid receptor action on central nervous system activity (Chindalore et al. 2005). Various opioid receptor affinities and their pharmacologic action are well described in humans but remain little understood in animals—including the rhinoceros—which is certain to be unique in many respects. Indeed, the most exciting of these novel investigations is, at least for rhinoceros capture specialists, the incorporation of mixed agonist-antagonist opioid cocktails as part of routine field capture methodologies for the African rhinoceros (Bush et al. 2005).

Recent work by Bush and colleagues in white rhinoceroses combines a mixture of concentrated butorphanol (40–90 mg; 30-mg/mL solution) with etorphine and midazolam (2–3.5 mg and 25–50 mg, respectively; Table 54.2; Bush et al. 2005, 2011). The addition of butorphanol to the anesthetic combination of etorphine and midazolam produces enhanced muscle relaxation and oxygenation with improved physiological parameters compared with the standard protocol of etorphine and azaperone in the white rhinoceros. Butorphanol is a mixed opioid agonist-antagonist; its agonist κ receptor produces analgesia and marked sedation, while the weak μ receptor antagonism reduces respiratory depression and rigidity. The weak σ (non-opioid) receptor agonist stimulates respiratory drive. Etorphine is a μ agonist causing respiratory depression and muscle rigidity—these adverse μ agonist actions are reversed by butorphanol and significantly reduce the cardiopulmonary depression typical of the pure opioids alone. In black rhinoceroses, the butorphanol antagonism of μ-opiate actions will result in a lively rhinoceros not suitable for handling without additional sedation.

Besides the marked improvement in oxygen saturation, there is a decrease in heart rate closer to normal, making the heart a more effective pump. Blood gas values reveal a more normal pH and PCO_2, while blood pressures remain lower than with the standard pure opioid agonist protocols. Administering diprenorphine, a μ antagonist, intravenously 12 minutes into the anesthetic episode reverses etorphine, but not butorphanol, further counteracting adverse μ effects of etorphine while preserving butorphanol sedation effects. Therefore, if inadvertent opioid overdosage should occur, compromised physiological parameters can be rapidly corrected without losing control of the animal. These discoveries may help to bring field rhinoceros capture into the realm of safety realized with captive animals where butorphanol-based protocols are now standard replacements for more potent opioids (Portas 2004; Radcliffe et al. 2000a).

RHINOCEROS CALF ANESTHESIA

Captive Calf Protocols

Anesthesia of captive white and black rhinoceros calves is safely accomplished with butorphanol alone or in combination with detomidine (Gandolf et al. 2006; Langan et al. 2001; Radcliffe et al. 2000c). Due to high sensitivity to opioid agents, rhinoceros calves respond very well to sedation and anesthesia with mixed agonist-antagonists, precluding many of the adverse cardiopulmonary depressant effects observed with more potent pure agonists of this class. Furthermore, a rapid onset of action is attained by intravenous delivery or a slower induction by intramuscular administration, with both methods proving safe and effective for serial anesthesia (Gandolf et al. 2006; Table 54.4). The combination of the alpha-2 agonist, detomidine, along with the butorphanol was thought to enhance muscle relaxation and depth of anesthesia with intramuscular use in white rhinoceros calves. Complete reversal is achieved using naltrexone at four to five times the butorphanol mg dose and yohimbine HCl (Yobine) or atipamezole at 0.125 mg/kg for antagonism of the alpha-2 agent.

Cow and Calf Field Capture

Field immobilization of juvenile rhinoceros is not without inherent risk as calves may separate from their dams after darting or become recumbent at different times despite concurrent drug delivery (Fig. 54.12). Additionally, calves are more susceptible to capture stress, hyperthermia, and postcapture morbidity and mortality in boma situations (Kock et al. 1995). Translocation of cows with calves less than 18 months of age can be traumatic and is best avoided, while movement of very young calves 2–3 months old is particularly high risk. Even with successful translocation, it can be difficult to reunite the cow and calf as the stress of capture and confinement often results in adult aggression directed toward the calf or the cow drying up. Methods for opioid sedation (0.2- and 0.05-mg etorphine for a cow and calf, respectively) have been used to facilitate boma reintroduction of cow-calf combinations (Kock et al. 2006). The wild black rhinoceros cow is solitary by nature and usually retreats to a quiet spot to calve and will stay there for the first month afterwards. Therefore, if a black rhinoceros gives birth in a boma, she rarely manages to raise the calf.

Opioid doses lower than those reported for adult animals are utilized for juvenile rhinoceros, with subadults receiving approximately one-half the adult dose. For example, when combined with a tranquilizer subadult African rhinoceros (age ~2.5 years) should receive 1.75- to 2-mg etorphine while very young calves (age 2–3 months) can be immobilized with as little as 0.5–1 mg etorphine (Rogers 1993a, 1993b; Table 54.4). A marked difference is observed in the escape behavior of African rhinoceros cow-calf pairs and should be anticipated during the chase and capture. White rhinoceros calves run ahead of their mothers while black rhinoceros calves run close at their mothers' heels (Kock et al. 2006).

When darting a cow with a calf from a helicopter, a fixed-wing aircraft is desirable to circle the capture site to assist with spotting. As a general rule, the cow is darted first, and about a minute, later the calf is darted (Kock et al. 2006). If the timing and darting are good, the pair will often go down together. Should the pair split up, the fixed-wing aircraft can stay with one animal. In open country where visibility is good, the calf can be darted once the cow shows early signs of narcosis. In more thickly vegetated country, where it is difficult to observe two separated animals, it is better to wait until the cow shows marked effects or is even recumbent before darting the calf. If the calf splits from its mother, the position of the immobilized mother can be taken by GPS or marked with a smoke grenade or toilet paper and the calf followed. Losing sight of a darted rhinoceros must be avoided, and it is therefore mandatory to have experienced trackers as part of the ground team. When darting a cow-calf pair on foot, the calf will usually stay close to its immobilized mother. If approached carefully, the calf can be darted and will generally become recumbent close to its mother; note that black rhinoceros calves are skittish and run off more easily than white rhinoceros calves.

Wild subadult greater one-horned rhinoceroses have been immobilized using the same dosage as adult animals (2- to 2.5-mg etorphine plus 10-mg acepromazine; Dinerstein et al. 1990). However, subadult animals proved more difficult to capture and often evaded darting attempts by outrunning the trained elephants that are commonly utilized for field immobilization of greater one-horned rhinoceroses in the tall grassland habitats of India and Nepal. Indian rhinoceros calves were immobilized with 0.5- to 1-mg etorphine and 5-mg acepromazine using shorter 2.5-cm Cap-Chur needles. As with capture of African rhinoceros cow-calf pairs, it is recommended that greater one-horned cows be immobilized before their calves. Calves did not run away and were easier to capture if the mother was immobilized first to avoid trampling risk to calves or aggression toward the ground crew (Dinerstein et al. 1990).

Conclusion

During the Indian Mutiny, a British soldier fired a bullet into the regiment's cherished mascot, a rhinoceros. In a spirit of scientific inquiry, the soldier tested the long-held belief—a conviction still strongly held by many since Durer's famous rhinoceros—that its skin was held together with rivets like a knights armor and impenetrable to any volley man could throw its way.

Table 54.4. Suggested doses for immobilization and anesthesia of rhinoceros calves in both *captive* and *wild* environments.

Rhino Species	Captive Calves			Wild Calves		
	Protocol	Reversal	Reference and Comments	Protocol	Reversal	Reference and Comments
White rhinoceros	10- to 20-mg butorphanol (BT) IV for 66- to 159-kg calf (Dose 0.13–0.15 mg/kg IV)	Naltrexone at 5 mg per mg BT	Gandolf et al. (2006) Heavy sedation Light anesthesia Mild resedation noted 8 hours post-reversal in one calf	*Calf:* 0.1- to 1-mg etorphine (M99) *Juvenile:* 1- to 2.5-mg etorphine *Subadult:* 2.5- to 3.5-mg etorphine (*Note:* Above ranges represent calves of all sizes.) *Note:* All white rhinos, including calves, get IV butorphanol at 10–20× the mg M99 dose ASAP upon recumbency to provide respiratory support OR 1-mg M50:50 plus 10-mg Nalorphine IV	Diprenorphine at 2.5 mg IV per mg M99 for transport Naltrexone at 40 mg per mg M99	Kock et al. (2006) from SANP *Note:* Always dart mother rhino 30–60 seconds *before* calf (Primarily for black rhino who easily split. In the case of white rhino, the calf rarely leaves the mother's side so one can wait longer or until mother goes down before darting the calf)
	2.5- to 5-mg butorphanol + 1.5- to 1.8-mg detomidine (DET) IM for 69–122 kg calf (Dose 0.03 mg/kg BT plus 0.07 mg/kg DET)	Naltrexone at 4 mg per mg BT Yohimbine at 0.125 mg/kg	Gandolf et al. (2006) Surgical anesthesia	*Calf:* 0.1- to 1-mg etorphine + 5- to 20-mg azaperone *Subadult:* 2.5- to 3.5-mg etorphine + 30- to 60-mg azaperone	Diprenorphine at 3 mg IV per mg M99	Rogers (1993a)
Black rhinoceros	25-mg butorphanol IV for ~500 kg subadult calf	Naltrexone at 5 mg per mg BT	Radcliffe et al. (2000c) Heavy standing sedation	*Calf:* 0.1- to 1-mg etorphine *Subadult:* 2.5- to 3.5-mg etorphine *Calf:* 0.1- to 1-mg etorphine + 10- to 50-mg azaperone *Subadult:* 1.75- to 3.5-mg etorphine + 100-mg azaperone *Note:* Do not use the M50:50 plus nalorphine protocol in black rhinos as it will cause arousal *Instead:* 5-mg butorpahnol or nalorphine IV; titrate to effect	Naltrexone at 40 mg IV per mg M99 Diprenorphine at 3 mg IV per mg M99	Kock et al. (2006) from SANP Rogers (1993b) Kock et al. (2006) *Note:* Always dart mother rhino 30–60 seconds *before* calf
Greater one-horned rhinoceros	Butorphanol IV or IM Use white rhino as model	Naltrexone at 5 mg per mg BT	Author suggestion based on use in African rhino calves	*Calf:* 0.5- to 1-mg etorphine + 5-mg acepromazine *Subadult:* 2- to 2.5-mg etorphine + 10-mg acepromazine	Diprenorphine at 2.5 mg IV per mg M99	Dinerstein et al. (1990) Same dose used for adult/subadult

Sources: Dinerstein E, Shrestha S, Mishra H. 1990. Capture, chemical immobilization, and radio-collar life for greater one-horned rhinoceros. *Wildlife Society Bulletin* 18(1):36–41; Atkinson MW, Bruce H, Gandolf AR, Blumer ES. 2002. Repeated chemical immobilization of a captive greater one-horned rhinoceros (*Rhinoceros unicornis*), using combinations of etorphine, detomidine, and ketamine. *Journal of Zoo and Wildlife Medicine* 33(2):157–162; Gandolf AR, Wolf TM, Radcliffe RW. 2006. Serial chemical restraint for treatment of decubitus ulcers in two neonatal white rhinoceroses (*Ceratotherium simum*). *Journal of Zoo and Wildlife Medicine* 37(3):387–392; Kock MD, Meltzer D, Burroughs R, eds. 2006. *Chemical and Physical Restraint of Wild Animals: A Training and Field Manual for African Species.* Zimbabwe Veterinary Association Wildlife Group and International Wildlife Veterinary Services.

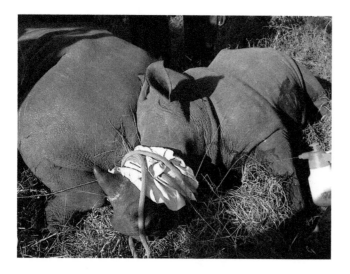

Figure 54.12. Anesthesia of rhinoceros calves is challenging, particularly under field conditions where darting of the cow–calf pair must be well coordinated in order to limit stress on both parent and offspring.

To the surprise of royalty and commoners alike, the rhinoceros quickly expired.

The future of the world's rhinoceroses will remain tenuous as human conflicts over shared resources escalate and rhinoceros horn continues to be cherished by traditional Asian societies for supposed unicorn-like mythical properties. Nevertheless, it is comforting to know that man—while solely responsible for the current crisis—is also simultaneously making strides to save the relic rhinocerotoids from their greatest enemy, ourselves. Safe anesthesia of wild and captive rhinoceroses alike will help scientists realize these conservation goals. Let us not make the same mistake as the British soldier and believe, naïvely, that the *armored* rhinoceros is invincible to the actions of our kind.

Practical Strategies for Rhinoceros Field Anesthesia

- Darts should be tested and prepared ahead of time leaving only the drug loading process to complete immediately prior to capture. Load the dart once you have visualized the rhinoceros—tailoring the dose for size, age, and condition of the animal. The rhinoceros should not be chased while the dart is being loaded. When darting from a helicopter, get the dart in quickly and back off until drugs considerably affect the rhinoceros.
- Dart sites must be given special care in rhinoceroses because of the propensity for abscess formation. Rhinoceros skin is thick and tough, making drainage of subcutaneous infections unlikely without appropriate wound care. Intramammary antibiotic preparations are common; however, the authors prefer infusion of 500-mg oxytetracycline directly into the dart wound. Oxytetracycline is a broad-spectrum antibiotic in high concentration, stable at room temperatures, viscous (does not easily run back out of wound) and readily available.
- Tranquilizers are often combined with potent opioids to improve muscle relaxation in recumbent animals and to help sedate and calm the rhinoceros during transport.
- The addition of hyaluronidase, a hydrolytic enzyme that increases tissue permeability, greatly improves drug absorption and can markedly shorten the induction time.
- A lower opioid dose must be used for rhinoceroses that are in bomas, debilitated, old, or where you

cannot get to the immobilized animal quickly (e.g., when darting on foot). *Be very careful with animals in poor body condition.* In most other situations, underdosing of opioids is contraindicated for free-range capture of rhinoceroses.
- In general, any need for repeat darting of animals following partial or incomplete injection of immobilizing agents should redeliver the original full immobilizing dose. This is a useful rule for captive animals as well since repeat darting is often associated with excitation and prolonged drug effects if titration is attempted.
- A rapid induction shortens the period the rhinoceros is moving in a semi-narcotized state and thereby lessens the chance that the rhinoceros will injure itself by encountering a hazard. This is especially true when immobilizing rhinoceroses in rough terrain. A quick induction also limits the exertion and the physiological stress associated with increased body temperature, heart rate, oxygen consumption, and related physiologic changes. Caution must be used, however, as very rapid induction times are often associated with marked respiratory depression, especially in the more susceptible white rhinoceros.
- *Nalorphine (Nr), nalbuphine (Nb),* and *butorphanol (B)* are useful in African rhinoceros (Table 54.2 and Table 54.3):
  - To *improve respiration,* give 5-mg *Nr* IV for black rhinoceros and 20- to 30-mg *Nr* for white rhinoc-

eros. Black rhinoceroses are very sensitive to *Nr* and *B*, so administer small incremental 5 mg doses given intravenously to effect. *Nb* and *B* may be used at approximately twice the *Nr* dose (20–40 mg) in a similar fashion for improving respiration in the white rhinoceros.

- To *walk a rhinoceros*, start with 10-mg *Nr* IV in black rhinoceros up to a total dosage of 20- to 40-mg *Nr* in 5 mg increments. For white rhinoceros standard practice is now to give *B* at 10× (up to 20×) the etorphine (M99) dose (10- to 20-mg *B* per mg M99). *B* can be incorporated into the initial dart or given at the time of loading. Others

give 1-mg diprenorphine plus 20-mg *Nr* IV followed by small incremental doses of 10- to 20-mg *Nr* up to 75 mg.

- For *transport*, wake the black rhinoceros up into the crate with 10–20 mg of *Nr* IV per 1 mg of M99. May also need to give 1- to 2-mg diprenorphine IV if animal is pushing or collapsing in crate. Wake white rhinoceros with 10 to 20 mg of *B* per mg M99 or give diprenorphine at 2.4 times M99 dose (generally a "lively" wake up). Can also give 1–2 mg of naltrexone with diprenorphine or later in transport to prevent pushing in crate.

REFERENCES

Abdullah MT. 1987. Rhino trapping in Malaysia. Proceedings of the 4th International Union for Conservation of Nature/Species Survival Commission's Asian Rhino Specialist Group. Jakarta, Indonesia. Rimba Indonesia. Vol. XXI No. 1: 27–30.

Allen JL. 1996. A comparison of nalmefene and naltrexone for the prevention of renarcotization following carfentanil immobilization of nondomestic ungulates. *Journal of Zoo and Wildlife Medicine* 27(4):496–500.

Atkinson MW, Bruce H, Gandolf AR, Blumer ES. 2002. Repeated chemical immobilization of a captive greater one-horned rhinoceros (*Rhinoceros unicornis*), using combinations of etorphine, detomidine, and ketamine. *Journal of Zoo and Wildlife Medicine* 33(2):157–162.

Bertelsen MF, Olberg R, Mehren KG, Smith DA, Crawshaw GJ. 2004. Surgical management of rectal prolapse in an Indian rhinoceros (*Rhinoceros unicornis*). *Journal of Zoo and Wildlife Medicine* 35(2):245–247.

Bush M, Citino SB, Grobler D. 2005. Improving cardio-pulmonary function for a safer anesthesia of white rhinoceros (*Ceratotherium simum*): use of opioid cocktails to influence receptor effects. Joint Proceedings of the American Association of Zoo Veterinarians, American Association of Wildlife Veterinarians and Association of Zoos and Aquarium's Nutrition Advisory Group, pp. 259–260. Omaha, NE.

Bush M, Citino SB, Lance WR. 2011. The use of butorphanol in anesthesia protocols for zoo and wild mammals. In: *Fowler's Zoo and Wild Animal Medicine Current Therapy 7* (RE Miller, ME Fowler, eds.), Chapter 77, pp. 596–603. New York: Elsevier.

Bush MR, Raath JP, Grobler D, Klein L. 2004. Severe hypoxaemia in field-anaesthetised white rhinoceros (*Ceratotherium simum*) and effects of using tracheal insufflation of oxygen. *Journal of the South African Veterinary Association* 75(2):79–84.

Cave AJ, Allbrook DB. 1958. Epidermal structures in a rhinoceros (*Ceratotherium simum*). *Nature* 182(4629):196–197.

Child G, Fothergill R. 1962. Techniques used to rescue black rhinoceros (Diceros bicornis) on Lake Kariba, Southern Rhodesia. *Kariba Studies* 2:37–41.

Chindalore VL, Craven RA, Peony Yu K, Butera PG, Burns LH, Friedmann N. 2005. Adding ultralow-dose naltrexone to oxycodone enhances and prolongs analgesia: a randomized, controlled trial of oxytrex. *The Journal of Pain* 6(6):392–399.

Citino SB. 2008. Use of medetomidine in chemical restraint protocols for captive African rhinoceroses. Joint Proceedings of the American Association of Zoo Veterinarians and Association of Reptilian and Amphibian Veterinarians, pp. 108–109. Los Angeles, CA.

Condy JB. 1964. The capture of black rhinoceros (*Diceros bicornis*) and buffalo (*Syncerus caffer*) on Lake Kariba. *Rhodesian Journal of Agricultural Research* 2:31–34.

Cornick-Seahorn JL, Mikota SK, Schaeffer DO, Ranglack GS, Boatright SB. 1995. Isoflurane anesthesia in a rhinoceros. *Journal of the American Veterinary Medical Association* 206(4): 508–511.

Daniel M, Ling CM. 1972. The effect of an etorphine-acepromazine mixture on the heart rate and blood pressure of the horse. *The Veterinary Record* 90:336–339.

De Vos V. 1978. Immobilization of free-ranging wild animals using a new drug. *The Veterinary Record* 103:64–68.

Dinerstein E. 2003. *The Return of the Unicorns: The Natural History and Conservation of the Greater One-Horned Rhinoceros*. New York: Columbia University Press.

Dinerstein E, Shrestha S, Mishra H. 1990. Capture, chemical immobilization, and radio-collar life for greater one-horned rhinoceros. *Wildlife Society Bulletin* 18(1):36–41.

Emslie R, Brooks M. 1999. *African Rhino: Status Survey and Action Plan*. Cambridge: IUCN Publications.

Fahlman A, Foggin C, Nyman G. 2004. Pulmonary gas exchange and acid-base status in immobilized black rhinoceros (*Diceros bicornis*) and white rhinoceros (*Ceratotherium simum*) in Zimbabwe. Joint Proceedings of the American Association of Zoo Veterinarians, American Association of Wildlife Veterinarians and Wildlife Disease Association, pp. 523–525. San Diego, CA.

Flamand JRB, Rochat K, Keep ME. 1984. An instruction guide to the most commonly and most successfully used methods in rhino capture, handling, transport, and release. In: *The Wilderness Guardian* (T Cornfield, ed.), pp. 585–596. Nairobi: Nairobi Space Publications.

Foose TJ, van Strien N. 1997. *Asian Rhinos: Status Survey and Conservation Action Plan*. Cambridge: IUCN Publications.

Gandolf AR, Willis MA, Blumer ES, Atkinson MW. 2000. Melting corneal ulcer management in a greater one-horned rhinoceros (*Rhinoceros unicornis*). *Journal of Zoo and Wildlife Medicine* 31(1): 112–117.

Gandolf AR, Wolf TM, Radcliffe RW. 2006. Serial chemical restraint for treatment of decubitus ulcers in two neonatal white rhinoceroses (*Ceratotherium simum*). *Journal of Zoo and Wildlife Medicine* 37(3):387–392.

Harthoorn AM. 1976. The chemical restraint of the principal groups of wild animals; family Rhinocerotidae. In: *The Chemical Capture of Animals: A Guide to the Chemical Restraint of Wild and Captive Animals*, pp. 195–202. London: Baillière Tindall.

Harthoorn AM, Lock JA. 1960. The rescue of the rhinoceroses at Kariba Dam. *Oryx* 5(6):351–355.

Hattingh J, Knox CM, Raath JP. 1994. Arterial blood pressure and blood gas composition of white rhinoceroses under etorphine anesthesia. *South African Journal of Wildlife Research* 24:12–14.

Heard DJ, Olsen JH, Stover J. 1992. Cardiopulmonary changes associated with chemical immobilization and recumbency in a white rhinoceros *(Ceratotherium simum)*. *Journal of Zoo and Wildlife Medicine* 23:197–200.

Henwood RR. 1989. Black rhino *Diceros bicornis* capture, transportation and boma management by the Natal Parks Board. *Koedoe* 32(2):43–47.

Hitchens PM, Keep ME, Rochat K. 1972. The capture of the black rhinoceros in Hluhluwe Game Reserve and their translocation to the Kruger National Park. *Lammergeyer* 17:18–30.

Hofmeyr JM, Ebedes H, Freyer REM, de Bruine JR. 1975. The capture and translocation of the black rhinoceros *Diceros bicornis* Linn. in South West Africa. *Madoqua* 9(2):35–44.

Keep ME. 1973. The problems associated with the capture and translocation of black rhinoceros in Zululand, Republic of South Africa. *Lammergeyer* 18:15–20.

Keep ME, Tinley JL, Rochat K, Clark JV. 1969. The immobilization and translocation of black rhinoceros *Diceros bicornis* using etorphine hydrochloride (M99). *Lammergeyer* 10:4–11.

King JM. 1969. The capture and translocation of the black rhinoceros. *East African Wildlife Journal* 7:115–130.

King JM, Carter BH. 1965. The use of the oripavine derivative M99 for the immobilization of the black rhinoceros *(Diceros bicornis)* and its antagonism with the related compound M285 or nalorphine. *East African Wildlife Journal* 3:19–26.

Klein LV, Cook RA, Calle PP, Raphael BL, Thomas P, Stetter MD, Donawick WJ, Foerner JJ. 1997. Etorphine-isoflurane-O₂ anesthesia for ovariohisterectomy in an Indian rhinoceros *(Rhinoceros unicornis)*. Proceedings of the American Association of Zoo Veterinarians, pp. 127–130. Houston, TX.

Kock MD. 1992. Use of hyaluronidase and increased etorphine (M99) doses to improve induction times and reduce capture-related stress in the chemical immobilization of the free-ranging black rhinoceros *(Diceros bicornis)* in Zimbabwe. *Journal of Zoo and Wildlife Medicine* 23(2):181–188.

Kock MD, La Grange M, du Toit R. 1990. Chemical immobilization of free-ranging black rhinoceros *(Diceros bicornis)* using combinations of etorphine (M99), fentanyl, and xylazine. *Journal of Zoo and Wildlife Medicine* 21(2):155–165.

Kock MD, Morkel P, Atkinson M, Foggin C. 1995. Chemical immobilization of free-ranging white rhinoceros *(Ceratotherium simum simum)* in Hwange and Matobo National Parks, Zimbabwe, using combinations of etorphine (M99), fentanyl, xylazine and detomidine. *Journal of Zoo and Wildlife Medicine* 26(2):207–219.

Kock MD, Meltzer D, Burroughs R, eds. 2006. *Chemical and Physical Restraint of Wild Animals: A Training and Field Manual for African Species*. Greyton: Zimbabwe Veterinary Association Wildlife Group and International Wildlife Veterinary Services.

Langan J, Ramsay E, Schumacher J, Chism T, Adair S. 2001. Diagnosis and management of a patent urachus in a white rhinoceros calf *(Ceratotherium simum)*. *Journal of Zoo and Wildlife Medicine* 32:118–122.

LeBlanc PH, Eicker SW, Curtis M, Beehler B. 1987. Hypertension following etorphine anesthesia in a rhinoceros *(Diceros simus)*. *Journal of Zoo and Wildlife Medicine* 18:141–143.

McCulloch B, Achard PL. 1969. Mortalities associated with the capture, translocation, trade, and exhibition of black rhinoceros. *International Zoo Yearbook* 9:184–191.

Meadows K. 1996. *Rupert Fothergill: Bridging a Conservation Era*. Bulawayo: Thorntree Press (Pvt) Ltd.

Morkel P. 1989. Drugs and dosages for capture and treatment of black rhinoceros *(Diceros bicornis)* in Namibia. *Koedoe* 32(2):65–68.

Morkel P. 1994. Chemical immobilization of the black rhino *(Diceros bicornis)*. Proceedings of a Symposium on "Rhinos as Game Ranch Animals". South African Veterinary Association. Onderstepoort, Republic of South Africa. pp. 128–135.

Morkel P, Radcliffe RW, Jago M, du Preez P, Felippe MJB, Nydam DV, Taft A, Lain D, Miller MM, Gleed RD. 2010. Acid-base balance and ventilation during sternal and lateral recumbency in field immobilized black rhinoceros *(Diceros bicornis)* receiving oxygen insufflation: a preliminary report. *Journal of Wildlife Diseases* 46(1):236–245.

Morkel P, Miller MM, Jago M, Radcliffe RW, du Preez P, Olea-Popelka F, Sefton J, Taft A, Nydam DV, Gleed RD. 2012. Serial temperature monitoring and comparison of rectal and muscle temperatures in immobilized free-ranging black rhinoceros *(Diceros bicornis)*. *Journal of Zoo and Wildlife Medicine* 43(1):120–124.

Nardelli F. 1987a. The conservation of the Sumatran rhinoceros *(Dicerorhinus sumatrensis)*: a situation report and proposal for future directions. Proceedings of the 4th International Union for Conservation of Nature/Species Survival Commission's Asian Rhino Specialist Group, XXI(1):31–38. Jakarta, Indonesia; Rimba Indonesia.

Nardelli F. 1987b. The conservation of the Javan rhinoceros *(Rhinoceros sondaicus* Desm.): a proposal and plan for capture operations. Proceedings of the 4th International Union for Conservation of Nature/Species Survival Commission's Asian Rhino Specialist Group XXI(1):64–69. Jakarta, Indonesia; Rimba Indonesia.

Player I. 1972. *The White Rhino Saga*. New York: Stein and Day.

Portas TJ. 2004. A review of drugs and techniques used for sedation and anaesthesia in captive rhinoceros species. *Australian Veterinary Journal* 82(9):542–549.

Portas TJ, Hermes R, Bryant BR, Goritz F, Thorne AR, Hildebrandt TB. 2006. Anesthesia and use of a sling system to facilitate transvaginal laparoscopy in a black rhinoceros *(Diceros bicornis minor)*. *Journal of Zoo and Wildlife Medicine* 37:202–205.

Prothero DR. 2005. *The Evolution of North American Rhinoceroses*. New York: Cambridge University Press.

Prothero DR, Schoch RM. 2002. *Horns, Tusks and Flippers: The Evolution of Hoofed Mammals*. Baltimore: The Johns Hopkins University Press.

Raath JP. 1999. Anesthesia of white rhinoceroses. In: *Zoo and Wild Animal Medicine: Current Therapy 4* (ME Fowler, RE Miller, eds.), Philadelphia: W.B. Saunders.

Radcliffe RM, Hendrickson DA, Richardson GL, Zuba JL, Radcliffe RW. 2000b. Standing laparoscopic-guided uterine biopsy in a southern white rhinoceros *(Ceratotherium simum simum)*. *Journal of Zoo and Wildlife Medicine* 31(2):201–207.

Radcliffe RW, Morkel P. 2007. Chapter 48: Rhinoceros anesthesia. In: *Zoo Animal and Wildlife Anesthesia and Immobilization*, 1st ed. G West, N Caulkett, D Heard, eds.), pp. 543–566. Ames: Blackwell Publishing.

Radcliffe RW, Schumacher J, Hartsfield SM, Merritt AM, Murray MJ. 1998. Idiopathic distal esophageal dilation in a southern black rhinoceros *(Diceros bicornis minor)*. *Journal of Zoo and Wildlife Medicine* 29:465–469.

Radcliffe RW, Ferrell ST, Childs SE. 2000a. Butorphanol and azaperone as a safe alternative for repeated chemical restraint in captive white rhinoceros *(Ceratotherium simum)*. *Journal of Zoo and Wildlife Medicine* 31(2):196–200.

Radcliffe RW, Paglia DE, Couto CG. 2000c. Acute lymphoblastic leukemia in a juvenile southern black rhinoceros *(Diceros bicornis minor)*. *Journal of Zoo and Wildlife Medicine* 31(1):71–76.

Radcliffe RW, Citino SB, Dierenfeld ES, Foose TJ, Paglia DE, Romo JS. 2004. Intensive management and preventative medicine protocol for the Sumatran rhinoceros *(Dicerorhinus sumatrensis)*. Unpublished report prepared for the International Rhino Foundation, Yulee, FL.

Radinsky LM. 1969. The early evolution of the Perissodactyla. *Evolution* 23(2):308–328.

Rogers PS. 1993a. Chemical capture of the white rhinoceros (*Ceratotherium simum*). In: *The Capture and Care Manual* (AA McKenzie, ed.), pp. 512–529. Pretoria: Wildlife Decision Support Service and South African Veterinary Foundation.

Rogers PS. 1993b. Chemical capture of the black rhinoceros (*Diceros bicornis*). In: *The Capture and Care Manual* (AA McKenzie, ed.), pp. 553–556. Pretoria: Wildlife Decision Support Service and South African Veterinary Foundation.

Rookmaaker LC. 1998. *The Rhinoceros in Captivity*. Den Haag: SPB Academic Publishing.

Sadmoko AS. 1990. Study on capture techniques of Sumatran rhinoceros (*Dicerorhinus sumatrensis*, Fischer, 1814) in Riau Province. Department of Forest Resource Conservation, Faculty of Forestry; Bogor Agricultural University (IPB). Bogor, Indonesia (text in Bahasa Indonesian).

Shadwick RE, Russell AP, Lauff RF. 1992. The structure and mechanical design of rhinoceros dermal armour. *Philosophical Transactions of the Royal Society of London. Series B, Biological Sciences* 337(1282):419–428.

Swan GE. 1993. Drug antagonists. In: *The Capture and Care Manual* (AA McKenzie, ed.), pp. 47–56. Pretoria: Wildlife Decision Support Service and South African Veterinary Foundation.

Valverde A, Crawshaw GJ, Cribb N, Bellei M, Gianotti G, Arroyo L, Koenig J, Kummrow M, Costa MC. 2010. Anesthetic management of a white rhinoceros (*Ceratotherium simum*) undergoing an emergency exploratory celiotomy for colic. *Veterinary Anaesthesia and Analgesia* 37:280–285.

Walzer C, Goritz F, Pucher H, Hermes R, Hildebrandt T, Schwarzenberger F. 2000. Chemical restraint and anesthesia in white rhinoceros (*Ceratotherium simum*) for reproductive evaluation, semen collection and artificial insemination. Joint Proceedings of the American Association of Zoo Veterinarians and International Association for Aquatic Animal Medicine, pp. 98–101. New Orleans, LA.

Walzer C, Goritz F, Hermes R, Nathan S, Kretzschmar P, Hildebrandt T. 2010. Immobilization and intravenous anesthesia in a Sumatran rhinoceros (*Dicerorhinus sumatrensis*). *Journal of Zoo and Wildlife Medicine* 41:115–120.

Young E. 1973. *The Capture and Care of Wild Animals*. Cape Town: Human and Rousseau Publishers (Pty) Ltd.

Zuba JR, Burns RP. 1998. The use of supplemental propofol in narcotic anesthetized non-domestic equids. Joint Proceedings of the American Association of Zoo Veterinarians and American Association of Wildlife Veterinarians, pp. 11–18. Omaha, NE.

55 Nondomestic Suids

Luis R. Padilla and Jeff C. Ko

INTRODUCTION

A large amount of information has been published on anesthesia and immobilization techniques of domestic swine. In contrast, studies pertaining to anesthesia of free-ranging or nondomestic suid species are limited in the documentation of physiological responses to anesthetic drugs, focusing instead on efficacy, induction and recovery times, and subjective descriptions of anesthetic quality. The domestic pig is still the most appropriate physiological model for anesthesia of other species, but readers seeking protocols for anesthesia of captive domestic pigs are referred to specific literature reviews on the subject (Swindle 1998; Thurmon & Smith 2007). We have included specific comments on Vietnamese potbellied pigs, since these are common exhibit animals in zoological institutions.

TAXONOMY

The suborder Suiformes includes the families Suidae and Tayassuidae, which encompass all pigs, hogs, babirussa, and peccaries. The generic term "suid" is commonly used to refer to members of both families. Table 55.1 is a list of known suid species, and adult weight ranges have been listed where available. The family Suidae includes pigs, hogs, and babirussa, and total 14 species in 5 genera. The Eurasian wild boar (*Sus scrofa*) is the wild ancestor of the domestic pig. Numerous breeds of the domestic pig (*Sus scrofa*) exist, and in many places, feral populations have been established in a free-ranging state, blurring the distinction between wild boar and domestic pig. The family Tayassuidae includes the peccaries or javelinas, currently found in three genera with one species each. A third family in the suborder Suiformes, Hippopotamidae, is the subject of a separate chapter in this book.

The main anatomical differences between the Tayassuidae and Suidae families are in dentition, tail length, hind limb anatomy, and the presence of a scent gland dorsally in the lumbosacral region in peccaries. Sexual size dimorphism is more prominent in the Suidae than the Tayassuidae. The babirussa (*Babyrousa babyrussa*) has distinct features from the other members of the Suidae family, including a complex, sacculated stomach suggestive of foregut fermentation (Leus et al. 1999), and remarkable canines in the males.

GENERAL CONSIDERATIONS OF SUID BIOLOGY AND PHYSIOLOGY

All suids can be dangerous animals when approached. Most species have powerful jaws with sharp dentition, and individuals can be extremely fast and capable of inflicting severe wounds on humans. Canines grow as sharp tusks in many species, which is accentuated in males of the Suidae family. In addition, the short, strong limbs and a muscular neck, limit the possibility of physical restraint to juveniles or very small individuals. Many individuals will fight aggressively when cornered or restrained, and sows can be very protective of their offspring. Suids can be capable climbers and agile jumpers that can escape from many situations or evade restraint.

Physiological or social stress should be minimized prior to anesthetic induction in order to achieve the desired results. Gregarious, social individuals are likely to be highly stressed if isolated prior to anesthesia. If prolonged isolation is necessary, stress can be decreased by allowing visual contact between group mates. During anesthetic induction, it is preferable to isolate the target animal from the rest of a group to minimize the risk of inadvertent trauma or misdirected aggression from companions.

Zoo Animal and Wildlife Immobilization and Anesthesia, Second Edition. Edited by Gary West, Darryl Heard, and Nigel Caulkett.
© 2014 John Wiley & Sons, Inc. Published 2014 by John Wiley & Sons, Inc.

Table 55.1.   Species of suids by family and weight ranges

Species	Adult Weight	Common Name	Comments
Family Suidae			"True" pigs
Sus scrofa	40–300 kg	Eurasian wild boar	Domesticated into farmed pigs, many wild "races" exist
	32–100 kg	Vietnamese potbellied pig	Breed of domestic pig, commonly seen in zoos
Sus salvanius	6–10 kg	Pygmy hog	
Sus bucculentus		Vietnamese warty pig	
Sus verrucosus	35–185 kg	Javan warty pig	
Sus barbatus	100–200 kg	Bearded pig	
Sus philippensis		Philippine warty pig	Three subspecies are recognized, although at least one may be a full species.
Sus cebifrons	20 – 80 kg	Visayan warty pig	
Sus celebensis	40–70 kg	Sulawesi warty pig	
Potamochoerus porcus	45–120 kg	Red river hog	
Potamochoerus larvatus	50–115 kg	African bush pig	
Hylochoerus meinertzhageni	100–275 kg	Giant forest hog	
Phacochoerus africanus	50–150 kg	Common warthog	
Phacochoerus aethiopicus	45–140 kg	Desert warthog	
Babyrousa babyrussa	40–100 kg	Babirusa	
Family Tayassuidae			Peccaries or Javelinas
Catagonus wagneri	30–45 kg	Chacoan peccary	
Tayassu (Pecari) tajacu	15–35 kg	Collared peccary	
Tayassu pecari	25–40 kg	White-lipped peccary	

Domestic pigs should be fasted for 24 hours (Moon & Smith 1996), and nondomestic suids should be fasted for 12–18 hours (Calle & Morris 1999) or longer. In addition to being at risk for vomiting and aspiration, inadequately fasted pigs are prone to gastric distension, which may physically compromise ventilation by altering pleural pressure and chest wall mechanics (Mutoh et al. 1991). When food is withheld, suids may consume other things accessible to them, including shavings, bedding material, orground and wall substrates.

Suid skin is tough, tight, and not very pliable, and contains a significant subcutaneous adipose tissue layer. Areas with thick fat deposits are less desirable for reliable injections, as administration into the adipose tissue layers will result in variable or altered responses when compared to true intramuscular injections, which should not be mistaken for decreased drug efficacy or variable species susceptibility. The amount and distribution of fat varies with age, between species, subspecies, and breeds. Injection into leaner muscle masses, such as the semimembranosus, semitendinosus, or the dorsal prescapular muscle mass (Calle & Morris 1999), will result in more predictable effects. The choice of needle length is crucial to obtaining deep muscle injections, and a minimum length of 1.5 in (3.8 cm) is suggested to assure intramuscular placement in adult animals.

Suids are prone to hyperthermia. All species have a relatively low surface area in a proportionately large-volume body with a significant layer of subcutaneous body fat, and limited sweating capabilities for heat dissipation. Physical excitement or increased exertional activity prior to successful immobilization may result in muscular heat generation and elevations in core body temperature. Severe elevations in body temperature can be treated by cooling the skin surface with alcohol baths or placing ice packs around large vessels (Moon & Smith 1996), using cool intravenous fluids, or, in extreme cases, using cold water enemas. Close temperature monitoring and good clinical judgment must be used to prevent overtly aggressive rapid cooling and hypothermia.

Although hyperthermia can occur in any suid species, the syndrome known as malignant hyperthermia only occurs in domestic swine. The malignant hyperthermia syndrome of swine is a well-documented, autosomal recessive condition of domestic pigs resulting in abnormal skeletal muscle function due to defective calcium handling (Moon & Smith 1996). Large white breeds of domestic swine are considered most susceptible, but it can occur in any breed or mixed-breed individual, including miniature pot-bellied pigs (Claxton-Gill et al. 1993). Manifestations of hyperthermia and muscle rigidity can be induced by stress, elevated ambient temperatures, inhalant and injectable anesthetics, paralytic agents, and other drugs. The body temperature of affected pigs can increase as high as 110°F (43.3°C) (Moon & Smith 1996), and muscle rigidity, tachycardia, tachypnea, hypoxemia, and cardiac arrhythmias can develop. Serum chemistries may show elevations in potassium, ionized calcium, myoglobin, and creatine kinase. Clinicians suspecting this condition should immediately institute supportive symptomatic therapy and discontinue inhalant anesthetics. Dantrolene is an effective treatment for this condition (Gronert 1980), and can be used prophylactically in pigs considered at risk. Azumolene, a dantrolene analog, has greater water solubility, and may be a more practical treatment option (Dershwitz & Sréter 1990). Other drugs that cause muscle relaxation might be used in managing hyperthermia by reducing continued muscle activity.

Neonatal suids are prone to hypothermia during the first few days after birth. Managers should provide supplemental heat sources and protection from environmental temperature fluctuations. Sows, in particular inexperienced ones, should be monitored to ensure adequate maternal care is provided, and that denning sites are safe for the piglets.

TRAPPING AND PHYSICAL RESTRAINT

Manual restraint of nondomestic suids should be reserved for juveniles or small domesticated individuals. Juvenile suids and small pigs can be restrained with one hand under the sternum and one hand over the back. The handler should anticipate that loud vocalizations may occur in response to physical restraint and manipulations. Prolonged or rough handling should be avoided, especially during hot weather, as it can result in hyperthermia. Juvenile and neonates may vocalize and struggle to the point of exhaustion and collapse during prolonged or strenuous restraint.

The use of snares, ropes, and similar physical restraint devices used in domestic swine production is not generally recommended in nondomestic suid species due to the high probability of injury to restrainer or animal, but can be done by experienced personnel. A description of translocations of collared peccaries detailed the use of a pole snare loop placed behind the upper canines and drawn tight while a second person physically restrained the hind legs (Porter 2006). This restraint was sufficient for placing ear tags and loading onto a trailer for relocation.

A variety of net restraint devices have been designed for domestic swine restraint, and have been modified for the capture of free-ranging suids. Warthogs have been captured using a funnel-shaped net set at the entrance of their sleeping burrows, occasionally resulting in the capture of multiple individuals as they emerge (Cumming 1975). Modified deer traps, "box traps," and corral traps have been used for capturing free-ranging suids with variable rates of success.

VASCULAR ACCESS

The subcutaneous adipose tissue layer and the tight skin of most suids can make vascular access a challenging task. Sedation or anesthesia should be used to facilitate blood collection in nondomestic species, except in very small individuals. Blood can be collected from the jugular, femoral, cephalic, saphenous, tail (coccygeal), and auricular veins. Catheter placement is possible in the cephalic, saphenous, and auricular veins. Although other sites are described in this section, they are not

recommended in most situations due to inherent technique risks.

Blood collection from the femoral vein can be done in most species, although the amount of adipose tissue and thick muscle mass can make it difficult in certain individuals. Caution must be taken to avoid lacerating the femoral artery. The femoral vein can be accessed with the animal on dorsal recumbency and slightly extending the hind leg caudally. The clinician palpates between the muscle bellies to find the femoral groove and a long needle (1 in or longer, depending on the size and body condition of the animal) is advanced with slight negative pressure. After successful collection, pressure should be applied to minimize hematoma formation. Venipuncture on this site can be painful, and some individuals may show some lameness after recovery, associated with deep hematoma formation or soft tissue trauma. With aggressive repositioning of the needle, there is also a risk of creating an iatrogenic arteriovenous fistulation.

The cephalic and lateral saphenous veins can sometimes be palpated under the skin. In individuals of some species, such as warthogs and red-river hogs, these veins are easily palpated and accessible, but in others, the veins can roll under the skin. A clinician familiar with the orientation of these veins might be able to blindly advance a small needle and obtain a blood sample. Blind catheterization of these veins is possible, although it is recommended that a scalpel blade be used to puncture the thick skin and avoid damaging the catheter stylette, or that a true "cut down" procedure be used for optimum visualization and securing an intravenous catheter in place.

The coccygeal or tail vein is a marginally adequate venipuncture site for collecting small volumes of blood in most species. In peccaries, the tail is relatively shorter, and venipuncture is more challenging, but small volume samples (at 1–3 mL) can still be collected if the needle is heparinized. The vein is located on the ventral mid-point of the tail. An individual can be placed on lateral recumbency and the vein is approached ventrally at the base of the tail, using a 21- to 23-gauge needle. If too much negative pressure is used, the vein can be easily collapsed.

Suids have thick, muscular necks, and the jugular vein is not palpable or externally visible. Redundant folds of skin around the neck, or extensive adipose tissue stores, may limit access to the jugular vein. However, if accessed, the jugular vein is large in all species. A long needle advanced cranially in the direction of the jugular furrow, with a slightly medial orientation while applying negative pressure, can be successful at venipuncture.

Anterior vena cava puncture is widely used for blood collection in domestic pig production, but is not without potentially detrimental effects, and its application should be judiciously employed by clinicians on a case-by-case basis. Risks of improper anterior vena cava puncture include blood vessel laceration and cardiac tamponade (Moon & Smith 1996). In small pigs, or with improper restraint, an overtly aggressive clinician may accidentally induce a pneumothorax, hemothorax, or other intrathoracic lacerations if using an improper length needle. A technique has been described for chemically restrained collared peccaries, and has been used in large numbers of anesthetized collared peccaries (*T. tajacu*) to obtain large (>20 mL) volumes of blood, with no fatalities (Lochmiller et al. 1984). After placing a peccary in dorsal recumbency in a "V-shaped" trough, the head is extended slightly to stretch the sternocephalicus musculature. The site of needle entry is found by placing a thumb against the anterior portion of the manubrium of the sternum. The needle is inserted at a point equal to the width of the thumb anterior and lateral to the edge of the sternocephalicus muscle. The needle is directed caudally and angled dorsomedially at a 30–40° angle formed by the point of the sternum. In an adult peccary, the authors preferred a 21-gauge, 1.5-in long needle.

The auricular veins on the ears of domestic pigs are a common site for intravenous access, catheter placement, and blood collection. The veins are present on the dorsolateral aspect of the ear. Their usefulness in exotic suid species varies, but should be considered for quick vascular access or when injecting small volumes. Large-eared species, such as red river hogs and warthogs, may have prominent veins, but they are of negligible size in other species (babirussa, warty pigs and peccaries). Using a warm compress or topical alcohol may induce superficial vasodilation, and applying pressure at the base of the ear may help identify the veins. A butterfly catheter can be secured around the flat (posterior) part of the ear, or a short catheter can be glued in place with the inside of the ear rolled around gauze to provide rigidity and support in securing the catheter. A clinician should keep in mind that most suid species have very sensitive ears, and even seemingly minor manipulations have resulted in auricular discomfort (abnormal ear posture and rubbing ear on surfaces) for days after a procedure.

Orbital sinus puncture is used in some research laboratories for blood collection in domestic pigs, and a variation has been used and described for anesthetized collared peccaries (Lochmiller et al. 1984). A peccary is placed in dorsal recumbency, with the head extended and stabilized by holding the snout. A 16-gauge, 1-in long needle without a syringe is placed at the medial canthus of the eye, medial to the nictitating membrane. The needle is advanced approximately 2 cm at a slightly ventral, posterior angle through the conjunctiva, until the orbital sinus is reached. Blood will flow through the needle and can be freely collected in a tube placed under the hub. When collection is completed, the needle is removed and pressure is applied to the closed eyelid to stop blood flow. As described, this technique may have value in research settings, but is not likely to be popular with zoo staff or pet owners, and potential complications exist. Orbital sinus puncture is not recommended for venipuncture in most situations, since more readily accessible sites exist.

ENDOTRACHEAL INTUBATION AND ANESTHETIC MONITORING AND SUPPORT

Sternal recumbency is recommended for ease of endotracheal intubation, but lateral recumbency is more practical for very large individuals, animals with large tusks, obese and brachycephalic animals. Some clinicians may prefer positioning individuals withlarge abdominal girth in lateral or dorsal recumbency. In these cases, suspending the head slightly at the end of an elevated table or platform may facilitate positional manipulation. A common hurdle to successful endotracheal intubation is the difficulty in opening the mouth sufficiently to visualize and advance an endotracheal tube. This might be facilitated with a deeper plane of anesthesia or different drug combinations, but one must consider that the mouth does not open widely in some species, even in extremely relaxed individuals. In addition, the larynx of most suids is difficult to reach due to the elongated shape of the head and distal location in most species.

Using soft gauze strips behind the upper and lower canines, an assistant can open the mouth and simultaneously position and extend the head slightly. Anatomical idiosyncrasies in suids make endotracheal intubation challenging, but familiarization with the anatomy and visualization of the tortuous route to the airway will facilitate success. A long laryngoscope blade can be used to push the epiglottis and expose the larynx. A long stylette can be passed into the larynx and the endotracheal tube can be threaded over the stylette or guided through the eye of Murphy while rotating at the point of contact with the larynx. If advanced too aggressively, a stylette can damage the laryngeal mucosa, resulting in edema and subsequent airway obstruction. A stylette that is advanced too far into the trachea may damage the peribronchial tissues, causing a pneumothorax (Thurmon et al. 1996). If the larynx is physically stimulated, laryngospasms, apnea and subsequent cardiovascular collapse may occur as part of the laryngochemical reflex (Ko et al. 1993a). The reflex occurs commonly in domestic pigs, but the response can be ameliorated with a topical anesthetic, such as lidocaine or cetacaine, applied on the larynx prior to attempts at intubation.

The endotracheal tube can be advanced into the larynx with the normal curvature of the tip pointing ventrally. The tube will encounter resistance as it reaches the posterior floor of the larynx, and rotating the tube slightly at this point facilitates advancement.

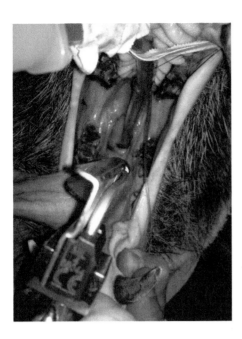

Figure 55.1. Intubation of a Chacoan peccary (*Catagonus wagneri*) utilizing a Miller laryngoscope blade (photo by Gary West).

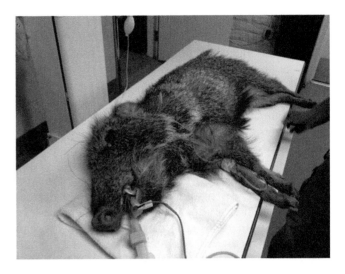

Figure 55.2. An anesthetized Chacoan peccary (*Catagonus wagneri*) being monitored with mainstream capnography and pulse oximetry. An intravenous catheter had been placed in a cephalic vein (photo by Gary West).

Suids are obligate nasal breathers, and caution should be used when securing the endotracheal tube. Tying a tube too tightly around the nose or muzzle may cause significant congestion of upper respiratory passages, leading to difficulty breathing during and after recovery. This consideration should be emphasized in brachycephalic individuals, such as potbellied pigs (Fig. 55.1).

When endotracheal intubation is not feasible, the intranasal route is an easy and practical way to administer supplemental oxygen or anesthetic gas to suids, but should not be used for positive ventilation. Attempts at ventilating domestic pigs through nasal intubation have resulted in significant gastric distension, anterior displacement of the diaphragm, and decreased functional lung capacity (Thurmon et al. 1996). Improper intubation (i.e., esophageal instead of endotracheal) may result in similar complications.

The same monitoring equipment used in other mammalian species can be used in anesthetized suids (Fig. 55.2). However, the clinician should not rely on monitoring equipment alone, and visual or palpable assessment of respirations, pulse or heart rate, and mucous membrane coloration and capillary reflex times should not be ignored. Ocular positioning is not an adequate indicator of anesthetic depth in suids due to the shallowness of the orbital socket.

A pulse oximetry probe can be placed on the tongue, ear, or vulvar or preputial folds. A rectal probe can be used, but mucosal contact must be confirmed by removal of feces. Interpretation of pulse oximetry values is more accurately done if respiration and

ventilations are concurrently monitored. Capnography is a useful indicator of physiologic state of anesthetized suids. In domestic pigs, elevations in end-tidal CO_2 are seen early in the onset of malignant hyperthermia before other signs appear (Moon & Smith 1996), and early recognition of elevations in end-tidal CO_2 may help identify other physiological derangements that are significant to anesthetic management. Capnography trends can be monitored nasally in nonintubated animals by tightly fitting a tube inside the nostril and attaching the reading device to the end. Most suids tend to hypoventilate under anesthesia, which may be a reflection of the most popular anesthetic protocols used, a large (possibly full) stomach, obesity in most captive animals, or a combination of these. End-tidal CO_2 readings higher than 45 mmHg warrant ventilatory support, and possibly oxygen supplementation. Positive pressure mechanical ventilation should not exceed what is necessary for minimal visible chest expansion, and caution should be used to avoid exceeding 20 cm H_2O, which has been seen to cause spontaneous pneumothorax in healthy pot-bellied pigs (Lukasik & Moon 1996).

Indirect blood pressure monitoring is recommended. Placing direct, invasive blood pressure monitors in anesthetized suids is impractical and time consuming for most nondomestic species, mostly due to difficulties in arterial catheterization. Although no specific studies have been done in any exotic suid species, a close correlation between oscillometric methods of blood pressure monitoring and direct arterial blood pressure methods have been shown in domestic pigs, and trends seen in indirect blood pressure readings are more useful than absolute numbers recorded (Moon & Smith 1996). If a commercially available indirect blood pressure monitor is not available, a simple method is to use a Doppler flow probe on the second digit to locate a pulse and place a cuff with a sphyngomanometer proximally over the metatarsus. A study done on domestic sows showed that similar cuff placement with a pulse oximetry probe positioned distally on the second digit (instead of a Doppler flow probe), correlated closely with direct arterial blood pressure (Caulkett et al. 1994). Cuffs placed on the legs should be of a width between 40% and 60% of the limb circumference (Moon & Smith 1996). Cuff placement on the legs can be above or below the carpus or tarsus, but the cuff bladder should be over the medial aspect of the leg. If the cuff is placed on the tail, the bladder should face ventrally (Moon & Smith 1996).

Traditional electrocardiography "alligator" clips may be difficult to attach to the tight suid skin. Instead, 25-gauge needle electrodes can be inserted subcutaneously, or patch electrodes can be adhered to the skin after degreasing with acetone, as has been described for domestic swine (Moon & Smith 1996). Temperature can be measured easily rectally, or with an esophageal probe.

ANESTHETIC COMBINATIONS

General Principles

The majority of immobilization scenarios for nondomestic suids will be to facilitate routine, minimally invasive procedures (such as relocation, physical exam, hoof trimming, blood collection, and placement of radio collars), where a light plane of anesthesia or deep sedation will suffice. After induction, deeper planes of anesthesia can be achieved with inhalant anesthetics or supplemental doses of injectable anesthetics.

Many injectable anesthetic protocols have been reported and are summarized in Table 55.2. Most balanced combination protocols have fewer side effects than any single-drug protocol, since the different drugs may potentiate anesthetic effects and decrease the effective necessary dose of any single drug. In choosing a balanced anesthetic combination, it has been suggested that suids may be relatively more resistant to opioids and alpha-2-adrenergic agonists than other species, but relatively more sensitive to the effects of benzodiazepines (Moon & Smith 1996). However, this assumption should be taken with caution when extrapolating to different suid species, as significant species and individual variation exists, and there have been reports of individuals with profound sensitivity to opioids.

Sedatives and Preanesthetic Medications

Preanesthetic sedatives can be used to decrease anesthetic drug doses, facilitate administration of the induction agent, or ease preanesthetic anxiety. Oral diazepam or midazolam has been given to suids prior to anesthetic induction, resulting in calmer individuals prior to immobilization, facilitating darting, and minimizing complications (such as hyperthermia) associated with preanesthetic excitement.

Oral alpha-chloralose was historically used to capture feral pigs in the United States. The sites would be prebaited with food for several days to attract pigs to the area, before adding drug-laced bait for the capture. Different mixtures are used to enhance the adherence of alpha-chloralose to bait, such as corn. The minimum effective dosage for hog capture has been reported as 2.2 g/40 kg of body weight. and the maximum safe dosage for feral hog capture has been reported as 2.2 g/10 kg of body weight (Carpenter & Brunson 2007).

The use of xylazine (1.1–2.1 mg/kg IM) prior to anesthetic induction with tiletamine-zolazepam has been reported in babirussa (James et al. 1999), and midazolam (0.15 mg/kg IM) and medetomidine (0.02–0.07 mg/kg IM) have been similarly used prior to induction of anesthesia with other agents. However, the use of preanesthetic drugs is impractical in animals that cannot be confined or where the anxiety of multiple injections clearly outweighs the practicality of a single darting event.

The use of anticholinergics as adjunct premedications with a sedative before anesthesia has been advocated in domestic pigs (Moon & Smith 1996), and should be considered in Vietnamese potbellied pigs. Anticholinergics decrease the likelihood of bradycardia, avoid bronchoconstriction, minimize airway secretions, and decrease salivation. Atropine (0.04 mg/kg) or glycopyrrolate (0.005–0.02 mg/kg) can be administered intramuscularly as part of premedicants. Glycopyrrolate is a more potent antisialogogue than atropine, but is also longer acting. Caution should be used when administering anticholinergics in conjunction with drugs that can cause peripheral hypertension, such as alpha-2 adrenergic agonists.

Anesthetic and Sedation Protocols

Butyrophenones and Phenothiazines Azaperone is a short-acting butyrophenone neuroleptic designed for intramuscular injection with a wide safety margin in domestic swine. Although its main use has been to decrease aggression in domestic swine, azaperone can be used alone as a reliable sedative, or as an anesthetic adjunct with dose-dependent effects. Doses of 0.25–0.5 mg/kg produce mild sedation without ataxia in domestic pigs (Braun 1993). Doses of 0.5–2.0 mg/kg reduce intraspecies aggression and cause mild ataxia, while doses of 2–4 mg/kg result in significant sedation and possible recumbency in adult pigs (Braun 1993). However, doses exceeding 2 mg/kg are also more likely to cause negative drug effects, which are similar to those caused by phenothiazines, including hypotension,

Table 55.2. Common immobilization protocols used in nondomestic suids

Drug Combination	Dose (mg/kg)	Species Documented	Comments	References
Ketamine (K)	20 (K)	Collared peccaries	Not recommended. Induction and recoveries are prolonged and violent, and high mortality possible	Gallagher et al. (1985); Hellgren et al. (1985)
Ketamine (K)/xylazine (X)	7.7 (K)/4.3 (X)	White-lipped peccaries	Field use for radio-collaring 17 free-ranging animals, but no physiologic parameters reported. Recoveries were prolonged (1–3 hours) with no mention of antagonism	Reyna-Hurtado et al. (2009)
Ketamine (K)/Tiletamine-zolazepam (TZ)/Medetomidine (M)	3.9 (K)/0.63 (TZ)/0.03 (M)	Chacoan peccaries	Prolonged recoveries despite atipamezole antagonism, residual ataxia	Sutherland-Smith et al. (2004)
Tiletamine-zolazepam (TZ)	2–5 (TZ)	Multiple species	Smooth induction, poor muscle relaxation, prolonged recoveries might be rough. Duration of recovery is dose dependent, not induction	Allen (1992); Calle and Morris (1999)
	2.18 (TZ)	Chacoan peccaries	Prolonged recoveries, poor relaxation	
Tiletamine-zolazepam (TZ)/Xylazine (X)	2.35 (TZ)/2.35 (X)	Collared peccaries	Prolonged recoveries, but study did not antagonize xylazine; fatality associated with a double dose	Gabor et al. (1997)
	1.23(TZ)/1.23 (X)	White-lipped peccaries	Dose of 1.51 TZ and 1.51 X not successful in Collared peccaries	Selmi et al. (2003)
	1.2–2.1 (X)/1.8–3.3 (TZ)	Babirussa	(X) administered as a premedicant, followed by TZ 20 minutes later. Antagonism with 0.14-mg/kg yohimbine and 1-mg flumazenil for every 20-mg zolazepam. Bradycardia seen in some cases. Concurrent administration of TZ and X can be used at similar doses with same effects	James et al. (1999)
Tiletamine-zolazepam (TZ)/romifidine (R)	3 (TZ)/0.5 (X); 3.3 (TZ)/1.6 (X); 3–6 (TZ)/0.1 (R)	Warthogs; Feral pigs; Wild pigs	Recoveries >90 minutes	Sonntag et al. (2004); Sweitzer et al. (1997); Siemon et al. (1992)
Tiletamine-zolazepam (TZ)/butorphanol (B)	1.46 (TZ)/0.14 (B)	White-lipped peccaries	Similar doses ineffective for collared peccaries	Selmi et al. (2003)
	1.26 (TZ)/0.36 (B)	Babirussa; Bearded pigs	Reverse with naltrexone, poor overall relaxation	Padilla (2004)
Medetomidine (M)/butorphanol (B)/ketamine (K)	0.06–0.1 (M)/0.3–0.4 (B)/0.6–1.1 (K)	Multiple species	*Preferred combination can be used in all suid species.* Antagonize medetomidine with atipamezole, butorphanol with naltrexone. Lower dose range used in calm, captive individuals.	Morris and Shima (2003) (upper range of doses)
Medetomidine (M)/butorphanol (B)/midazolam (Mz)	0.04–0.07 (M)/0.15–0.3 (B)/0.08–0.3 (Mz)		Midazolam or medetomidine can be administered as a premedicant 10–15 minutes prior to rest of anesthetic cocktail, or all can be administered concurrently	
Detomidine (D)/butorphanol (B)/midazolam (Mz)	0.06–0.125 (D)/0.3–0.4 (B)/0.2–0.4 (Mz)	Multiple species	Dexmedetomidine can be used as a substitute for medetomidine. See text. Antagonize detomidine with atipamezole or yohimbine, and naltrexone.	Morris et al. (1999)
Xylazine (X)/butorphanol (B)/midazolam (Mz)	2–3 (X)/0.3–0.4 (B)/0.3–0.4 (Mz)	Multiple species	Detomidine or midazolam can be administered as a premedicant or concurrently. Animals may resedate within hours after antagonism.	Morris et al. (1999)
Detomidine (D)/butorphanol (B)/tiletamine-zolazepam (TZ)	0.06–0.125 (D)/0.3–0.4 (B)/0.6 (TZ)	Multiple species	Antagonize with atipamezole or yohimbine, and naltrexone.	Morris et al. (1999)
Xylazine (X)/butorphanol (B)/tiletamine-zolazepam (TZ)	2–3 (X)/0.3–0.4 (B)/0.6 (TZ)	Multiple species	Xylazine or midazolam can be administered as a premedicant or concurrently	Morris et al. (1999)

779

bradycardia, and decreased cardiac output and contractility. Priaprism has been reported in adult boars (Moon & Smith 1996).

Although the use of azaperone in exotic suid immobilization protocols has not extensively documented, it has a lot of potential as an anesthetic adjunct in nondomestic species, and has been used reliably in Vietnamese potbellied pigs. The recommended dose for potbellied pig sedation is 0.25 to 2.0 mg/kg IM, and doses of 2.0–8.0 mg/kg are suggested for anesthesia (Calle & Morris 1999). Caution should be used at the higher range of the suggested dose, as prolonged recoveries may be seen.

Acepromazine is a phenothiazine compound used as a sedative adjunct in domestic pigs, but considered an inadequate sedative when used by itself (Moon & Smith 1996). Its negative side effects are dose dependent and can be severe, including hypotension, decreased heart rate, hypothermia, and decreased respiratory rate. However, acepromazine can be used to manage hyperthermia (Moon & Smith 1996) and hypertension, or as a mild sedative adjunct.

Ketamine Combinations Ketamine has been used extensively in suid immobilizations. Ketamine should not be used as a sole anesthetic agent due to the poor quality of anesthesia, extreme muscle rigidity, and rough recoveries, but is the base for balanced anesthetic protocols, and understanding its effects is important for the formulation of these combinations. To produce immobilization, ketamine alone requires relatively high doses (15–25 mg/kg), and the muscle rigidity precludes endotracheal intubation. Despite a relatively minor cardiorespiratory depressant effects (Tranquilli et al. 1983), ketamine can increase systemic and pulmonary arterial blood pressure, cause tachycardia, and increase in cardiac output and myocardial oxygen consumption. Recoveries are rough, including hypersensitivity to stimulus and increased activity of the limbs (paddling), which may lead to hyperthermia, predisposing suids to self-trauma, pulmonary edema, and even death.

Domestic pigs absorb ketamine rapidly, and almost completely, after intramuscular injection (Loscher et al. 1990). Anesthetic recovery in pigs occurs as ketamine is redistributed from the brain to other tissues, with drug excretion and metabolism being less critical for anesthetic duration. This is a significant consideration when choosing drugs for individuals with compromised organ function, since prolonged excretion is unlikely to affect duration of anesthesia. The elimination half-life of ketamine in healthy pigs is approximately 2 hours after intramuscular or intravascular administration.

Ketamine has been used safely as a sole anesthetic agent in numerous peccary immobilizations (Hellgren et al. 1985). In collared peccaries (*Tayassu tajacu*),

ketamine was used without detrimental, permanent effects at 20 mg/kg (Hellgren et al. 1985) administered intramuscularly. Prolonged recoveries (>120 minutes) should be expected when peccaries are immobilized with 15–25 mg/kg ketamine administered intramuscularly, and heat stress may be seen in relation to ambient weather (Gallagher et al. 1985).

Some of the negative effects of ketamine anesthesia can be ameliorated with anesthetic adjuncts, which also decrease the ketamine dose required to achieve effective immobilization. Alpha-2-adrenergic agonists, such as xylazine, detomidine, medetomidine, or dexmedetomidine, are popular adjuncts to ketamine as a suid anesthetic. These combinations offer the advantage of being reversible to result in faster recoveries, but the reversal of the alpha-2-adrenergic agonists is independent of the patient's ability to metabolize and clear ketamine. If the alpha-2 adrenergic agonist is reversed before ketamine is fully metabolized, recoveries can be undesirable, characterized by hyperkinesia of all limbs while recumbent, severe and prolonged ataxia, and distress vocalizations. It has been shown cardiac output decreased significantly for 30 minutes after administration of a ketamine (10 mg/kg) and xylazine (1 mg/kg) combination in domestic pigs, and arterial PO_2 decreased for 10 minutes while total vascular resistance was significantly increased (Trim & Gilroy 1985). It is likely that other alpha-2-adrenergic agonists in combination with ketamine have similar effects in exotic suids, and should be used with caution, but the more specific receptor affinity of the newer generation drugs is likely to result in less undesirable effects.

The wide availability of ketamine and xylazine has made this combination a popular choice used by field biologists studying wild or feral suids. Xylazine decreases the induction dose of ketamine, and can be antagonized with atipamezole or yohimbine. Although the effects of anesthetic monitoring were not reported, Reyna-Hurtado et al. (2009) reported safely immobilizing 17 white-lipped peccaries (*Tayassu pecari*) using a combination of ketamine (7.7 mg/kg) and xylazine (4.3 mg/kg) delivered by dart rifle. The animals recovered in 1–3 hours, and the authors did not report administering any antagonists.

Ketamine, used in conjunction with benzodiazepines (diazepam, climazolam, or midazolam) offers better relaxation and smoother recoveries that ketamine alone. Midazolam is a more reliable intramuscular sedative than diazepam because it is water soluble. Recoveries after ketamine-benzodiazepine combinations can be prolonged, usually taking several hours. Recovery times can be shortened by the administration of flumazenil.

Tiletamine-Zolazepam Combination A commercially available 1:1 formulated ratio of tiletamine-zolazepam combination has been used extensively in exotic suids (Calle & Morris 1999), and can be used safely in any species if the recovery effects are anticipated and properly managed. Kumar et al. (2006) reported the half-lives for tiletamine and zolazepam in the terminal elimination phase in domestic pigs anesthetized with a 10 mg/kg combined dose as 3.7 and 8.4 hours, respectively. These prolonged half-lives are significantly prolonged when compared with other domestic species (Lin et al. 1993). The authors also commented on the observation of a secondary peak in a concentration-time profile of zolazepam, which could be attributed to enterohepatic recycling or differential absorption rates from the injection site.

Despite the prolonged recovery times and possible undesirable effects, the combination of tiletamine-zolazepam offers the advantages of relatively low cost, wide availability, and a relatively wide margin of safety. Commercially available formulations can be reconstituted to different concentrations, allowing for smaller volumes of induction. Induction times are rarely affected by increasing dose, but recovery times can be prolonged at higher doses. The dissociative anesthetic portion of this combination, tiletamine, is considered more potent than ketamine. Zolazepam, the benzodiazepine part of the combination, is likely responsible for prolonged recoveries. The use of flumazenil (1-mg flumazenil for 20-mg zolazepam IV or IM; Calle & Morris 1999) as a benzodiazepine antagonist may shorten recovery times, but the effects may be of short duration and animals may relapse into a more sedate state as the flumazenil is metabolized.

Tiletamine-zolazepam anesthesia is characterized by relatively fast inductions, moderate muscle relaxation that is inadequate for endotracheal intubation, and prolonged, sometimes violent, recoveries. Most suids retain some degree of hyperresponsive reflexes, such as exaggerated limb withdrawal when stimulated. Heart rate and arterial blood pressure may increase. Respiration rate may decrease initially, but minute ventilation is well maintained. Recoveries may show repetitive motion of the legs (paddling) prior to standing, excessive salivation, altered thermoregulation, increased vocalizations, and prolonged ataxia (Moon & Smith 1996). Deaths have been occasionally reported after using tiletamine-zolazepam, due to complications of rough recoveries (Morris & Shima 2003).

Chacoan peccaries (Catagonus wagneri) were immobilized reliably and safely with tiletamine-zolazepam at a mean dose of 2.18 mg/kg intramuscularly (Allen 1992). Anesthesia was induced in 7.6 minutes, but recoveries were prolonged (90–240 minutes), and some animals retained a dull mentation for up to 8 hours after immobilization. A more recent study (Sutherland-Smith et al. 2004) mentions that Chacoan peccaries anesthetized with 3.2 mg/kg tiletamine-zolazepam took longer than 8 hours to recover, which may be a function of higher doses resulting in prolonged recoveries, as had been previously suggested (Allen 1992).

Tiletamine-Zolazepam/Alpha-2 Adrenergic Agonist Combinations The addition of alpha-2 adrenergic agonists adjuncts to tiletamine-zolazepam anesthetic protocols allows the usage of lower doses of tiletamine-zolazepam to achieve desired effects while improving overall muscular relaxation. The negative cardiovascular side effects involved with this addition are offset by the benefits of faster, smooth recoveries and better relaxation, often allowing for endotracheal intubation.

Xylazine has been a popular, inexpensive, and widely used adjunct to tiletamine-zolazepam immobilization protocols in nondomestic suid immobilizations. Commercially available formulations of tiletamine-zolazepam can be reconstituted with xylazine (Gabor et al. 1997), and immobilization protocols can be predetermined by volume per weight to simplify dose calculations in the field. In domestic pigs, it has been shown that the addition of xylazine to tiletamine-zolazepam-based immobilization protocols increases relaxation to facilitate intubation (Ko et al. 1993b). Increasing the xylazine dose in xylazine-tiletamine-zolazepam anesthesia of domestic pigs enhances the quality of anesthesia, sedation, and muscle relaxation without prolonging recovery times (Ko et al. 1995).

Wild feral pigs (Sus scrofa) in North America have been reliably immobilized with a xylazine (1.6 mg/kg) and tiletamine-zolazepam (3.3 mg/kg) intramuscular combination delivered to trapped pigs by blowdart (Sweitzer et al. 1997). Animals recovered and were released within 120 minutes of initial injection. Authors reported slight decreases in heart rates and body temperatures, but adequate respiration rates and blood oxygen saturation levels. Immobilization of a large number (n = 107) of collared peccaries (Tayassu tajacu) has been described using a tiletamine/zolazepam (2.35 mg/kg) and xylazine (2.35 mg/kg) combination, although the authors reported it as a combined average dose of 4.7 ± 0.9 mg/kg (Gabor et al. 1997). One fatality was reported in a peccary receiving an overdose (9.78 mg/kg combined dose). Recovery times in peccaries were prolonged, being described as conscious at 64 ± 29 minutes and first standing at 92 ± 33 minutes from injection, but xylazine was not antagonized in the study. Selmi et al. (2003) used intramuscular tiletamine-zolazepam (1.23 ± 0.26 mg/kg) in combination with xylazine (1.23 ± 0.26 mg/kg) successfully in white-lipped peccaries, but similar doses (1.51 ± 0.29 mg/kg tiletamine-zolazepam and 1.51 ± 0.29 mg/kg of xylazine) were unsuccessful at providing immobilization in collared peccaries, undermining that species-specific differences must be taken into account.

A combination of 3.9 mg/kg ketamine, 0.63 mg/kg tiletamine-zolazepam, and 0.03 mg/kg medetomidine was used to immobilize captive Chacoan peccaries (*Catagonus wagneri*) (Sutherland-Smith et al. 2004). Sufficient immobilization for handling was achieved at 12.6 ± 3.7 minutes, and good muscle relaxation was produced, although animals that were approached too soon after recumbency would be aroused and stumble away. Heart and respiratory rates declined, but oxygen saturation increased during anesthesia. Atipamezole was used to antagonize the medetomidine, but recoveries were still very prolonged (55–455 minutes) and showed residual ataxia.

In babirussa, xylazine (1.2–2.1 mg/kg IM) premedication followed by tiletamine and zolazepam (1.8–3.3 mg/kg) produced good relaxation, smooth inductions, and sufficient immobilization for minimally invasive procedures, although additional drugs were necessary to deepen or prolong anesthesia (James et al. 1999). The authors report bradycardia in some animals (range of 35–111 beats per minute) while maintaining good oxygen saturation and stable respiratory rates (James et al. 1999). Female babirussa required slightly higher induction doses to reach similar effects. A small study (Sonntag et al. 2004) showed that warthogs can be immobilized safely with tiletamine-zolazepam (3.0 mg/kg) and xylazine (0.5 mg/kg), although recoveries were prolonged (>90 minutes).

Romifidine has not been used extensively in suids, but one report describes its use (0.1 mg/kg) as an anesthetic adjunct to tiletamine-zolazepam (3–6 mg/kg) in wild boars (Siemon et al. 1992). Since these doses of tiletamine-zolazepam alone may be sufficient to sedate swine, the benefits of romifidine are likely to be supplemental and improve overall relaxation.

Tiletamine–Zolazepam/Butorphanol Tiletamine-zolazepam (1.46 mg/kg) has been used successfully in conjunction with butorphanol (0.14 mg/kg) to immobilize white-lipped peccaries (*Tayassu pecari*), but similar doses are ineffective to immobilize collared peccaries (Selmi et al. 2003). However, similar doses of tiletamine-zolazepam (1.26 mg/kg IM) combined with higher doses of butorphanol (0.36 mg/kg) resulted in adequate immobilization of babirussa for elective procedures (Padilla 2004), and similar doses can be used in peccaries and warthogs, although relaxation is inadequate for intubation. Caution is prudent when using higher doses of butorphanol, as some practitioners have reported profound sensitivity and characteristic opioid effects (respiratory depression and muscle tremors) in certain individuals, notably babirussa. Antagonism of opioid effects with naltrexone or naloxone may shorten recoveries.

Medetomidine- and Dexmedetomidine-Based Anesthesia Medetomidine has been shown to induce deeper planes of sedation than xylazine in domestic pigs (Sakaguchi et al. 1992a), making it a useful and more complete anesthetic agent for suid immobilization. At higher doses of medetomidine (>0.08 mg/kg), depth of sedation does not seem to increase significantly in domestic pigs, but the duration of sedation does. The study also showed better analgesia with medetomidine when compared with xylazine. The anesthetic properties of medetomidine can be potentiated in domestic pigs by administering butorphanol concurrently at 0.2 mg/kg (Sakaguchi et al. 1992b), and the combination is safe when administered to atropinized pigs (Sakaguchi et al. 1993). Medetomidine effects in domestic pigs can be antagonized with atipamezole at two to four times the medetomidine dose (Nishimura et al. 1992), although most clinicians prefer to use a 5:1 atipamezole:medetomidine ratio for antagonism (Morris & Shima 2003).

Medetomidine effects can also be potentiated when used in combination with midazolam (Nishimura et al. 1993). The cardiopulmonary effects of a medetomidine (0.04 mg/kg) and midazolam (0.2 mg/kg) combination in swine include a rapid increase in arterial and pulmonary arterial pressure due to peripheral vasoconstriction (Nishimura et al. 1994). The antagonism of medetomidine with atipamezole resulted in a decrease in peripheral vascular resistance, decrease in blood pressure and increased cardiac output and heart rate (Nishimura et al. 1994).

The ability to potentiate medetomidine with both butorphanol and midazolam has made the combination of the three a very popular anesthetic choice in nondomestic suids. A 0.07 mg/kg medetomidine, 0.3 mg/kg butorphanol, and 0.3 mg/kg midazolam protocol has been extensively used in captive suids of multiple species (Morris & Shima 2003) and is the preferred protocol across suid species at most captive zoological institutions (Morris et al. 1999). Medetomidine can be administered 5–15 minutes prior to the rest of the drugs, having a premedicant effect. This protocol offers the advantages of being almost entirely reversible and producing consistently good results across species (Morris & Shima 2003). However, at the doses published, significant bradycardia and hypoxemia are common side effects, and unexplained severe hypoglycemia has been seen in fasted and unfasted suids at one institution (Morris & Shima 2003). Lingering sedation from which suids can be aroused is often seen at high doses using this drug combination for immobilization. Lower doses, as low as 0.04 mg/kg medetomidine, 0.08 mg/kg midazolam, and 0.15 mg/kg butorphanol, have been used successfully in babirussa, red river hogs, and warthogs, and might be used in other species. These lower ranges were derived from the domestic swine literature (Nishimura et al. 1994; Sakaguchi et al. 1992b), and may reflect variations in individual temperament and species susceptibility. For most animals, a large volume of induction drugs is needed, although the recent availability of highly concentrated or compounded formulations of medetomidine, midazolam, and butorphanol allows smaller volumes of induction. Clinicians have also reported sudden arousals when suids are approached too soon after recumbency or when stimulated, and recently, there have been anecdotal reports of profound sedation within hours after initial antagonism. These anecdotal reports may be due to a recycling of the medetomidine when used at higher doses.

Dexmedetomidine is a dextroisomer of medetomidine, and responsible for the anesthetic effects seen with medetomidine. When compared to medetomidine, dexmedetomidine has not been available as long for veterinary usage. In addition, because it is only commercially available as a 0.5 mg/mL formulation in the United States, its application to nondomestic suid anesthesia has been limited by volume. Medetomidine (which is available in more concentrated, often compounded, formulations) is still more widely used and practical in the anesthesia of non-domestic suid species. Dexmedetomidine can replace medetomidine in balanced anesthetic combinations at a dose range of 0.02–0.04 mg/kg (which is roughly 50% of the mg/kg dosage used for medetomidine) in most species. The manufacturer of 0.5 mg/mL dexmedetomidine recommends antagonism with 5 mg/mL atipamezole at a 1 : 1 volume (or 10 : 1 atipamezole to dexmedetomidine in a mg : mg basis). When compared with medetomidine, dexmedetomidine produces similar anesthetic effects, although controlled comparisons are limited and primarily anecdotal in non-domestic suid species. In a recent study done in propofol-sedated domestic swine, dexmedetomidine administered intravenously at rates of 0.2, 0.4, and 0.7 μg/kg/h resulted in decreased bispectral index, mean arterial pressure, heart rate cardiac output, and mixed venous oxygen saturation, although the effects were dose dependent (Sano et al. 2010). This study suggests that relatively low doses of dexmedetomidine may be adequate as an adjunct in balanced anesthetic protocols. Due to limited reports of its use in nondomestic suid species, dexmedetomidine-based protocols are not included in Table 55.2.

Variations of the medetomidine-based protocols have been described. A combination of butorphanol (0.3–0.4 mg/kg), detomidine (0.06–0.125 mg/kg), or xylazine (2–3 mg/kg) and midazolam (0.3–0.4 mg/kg) has been used in Vietnamese potbellied pigs, Eurasian wild boars, red river hogs, warthogs, bearded pigs, and babirussa (Calle & Morris 1999). This protocol is characterized by rapid, smooth induction with excellent relaxation. In these combinations, medetomidine has been replaced by xylazine or detomidine, and it is likely that the other two drugs (midazolam and butorphanol) result in similar potentiation of the alpha-2 agonist effects. Another variation has been the substitution of tiletamine-zolazepam (0.6 mg/kg) for midazolam, used in some species with similar results (Calle & Morris

1999) and having the distinct advantage of smaller induction volumes. The authors suggest that some species are more sensitive to this drug combination based on temperament (red river hogs, babirussa, and potbellied pigs), and lower dosages of butorphanol can be used. Bearded pigs, warthogs, and Eurasian boars may require the higher end of the suggested dosage range.

Propofol Because propofol must be administered intravenously, it is an impractical choice for induction of anesthesia in exotic suids, but some individuals could be potentially conditioned to tolerate intravenous injections and anesthetic induction with propofol. More commonly, propofol has been used as an anesthetic supplement to reach a deeper plane of anesthesia after induction with different agents, or used for maintenance of anesthesia as a continuous intravenous infusion. At higher infusion rates, heart rate and cardiac index decrease in domestic pigs (Moon & Smith 1996). Propofol can be a significant respiratory depressant if administered rapidly, or if high doses are used.

Inhalant Anesthetics The use of inhalant anesthetic gases as induction agents is impractical in most exotic suid species. However, inhalant anesthetics can be used in small or severely debilitated animals, for supplementation or maintenance of anesthesia after induction with an injectable agent. Sevoflurane is the safest inhalant anesthetic agent currently available. Minimum alveolar concentrations (MAC) for domestic pigs are estimated at 0.9–1.25 for halothane, 1.5–2.0 for isoflurane and 2.0–2.7 for sevoflurane (Thurmon et al. 1996). A study done on newborn swine comparing halothane, isoflurane, and sevoflurane showed that mean systemic arterial pressure and heart rate decreased the least with sevoflurane when compared with awake piglets, but heart rate decreased the least with isoflurane (Lerman et al. 1990). Mean measurements of systemic arterial pressure were also lower in isoflurane- and halothane-anesthetized piglets than when sevoflurane was used. Sevoflurane is associated with faster recoveries than other inhalants. Caution should be used with domestic pigs known to be susceptible to malignant hyperthermia, as this condition can be triggered by inhalants, and traditionally associated with halothane usage.

Long-Acting Tranquilizers Limited objective information is available on the use of long-acting tranquilizers in suids. Perphenazine, a long-acting phenothiazine, has been used at 30–50 mg per warthog prior to translocations (Ebedes 1993). Two young warthogs overdosed with perphenazine at 5 mg/kg died 3 days later. Although it is unclear if the animals died directly from the overdose, the warthogs were anorexic after drug administration (Ebedes 1993).

CONCLUSIONS

Balanced anesthetic protocols using multiple drug combinations allow for less detrimental side effects with better anesthetic qualities. Although the combination of butorphanol-medetomidine and midazolam is a reliable and safe combination for inducing anesthesia in most captive nondomestic suids, it is not applicable or practical in all situations. Clinicians should choose an anesthetic protocol that is likely to achieve the desired level of anesthesia while balancing against the detrimental effects most likely to be significant for an individual patient.

As newer monitoring equipment becomes available and is applied to document the physiological effects in nondomestic suid anesthetic episodes, the literature should evolve into more scientific and objective descriptions of different anesthetic protocols. Ultimately, this will help in refining techniques applicable to the captive and free-ranging management of these species.

REFERENCES

Allen JL. 1992. Immobilization of giant Chacoan peccaries (*Catagonus wagneri*) with a tiletamine hydrochloride/zolazepam hydrochloride combination. *Journal of Wildlife Diseases* 28(3):499–501.

Braun W. 1993. Anesthetics and surgical techniques useful in the potbellied pig. *Veterinary Medicine* 88:441–447.

Calle PP, Morris PJ. 1999. Anesthesia of non-domestic suids. In: *Zoo and Widlife Medicine: Current Therapy*, 4th ed. (ME Fowler, RE Miller, eds.), pp. 639–646. Philadelphia: W.B. Saunders.

Carpenter RE, Brunson DB. 2007. Exotic and zoo animal anesthesia. In: *Lumb and Jones Veterinary Anesthesia and Analgesia*, 4th ed. (WJ Tranquilli, JC Thurmon, KA Grimm, eds.), pp. 785–805. Ames: Blackwell Publishing.

Caulkett NA, Duke T, Bailey JV. 1994. A comparison of systolic blood pressure measurement obtained using a pulse oximeter, and direct systolic pressure measurement in anesthetized sows. *Canadian Journal of Veterinary Research* 58(2):144–147.

Claxton-Gill MS, Cornick-Seahorn JL, Gamboa JC. 1993. Suspected malignant hyperthermia syndrome in a miniature potbellied pig anesthetized with isoflurane. *Journal of the American Veterinary Medical Association* 203(10):1434–1436.

Cumming DHM. 1975. A technique for the capture of the warthog, *Phacochoerus aethiopicus* Pallas. *African Journal of Ecology* 13(2):113–120.

Dershwitz M, Sréter FA. 1990. Azumolene reverses epidosed of malignant hyperthermia in susceptible swine. *Anesthesia and Analgesia* 70(3):253–255.

Ebedes H. 1993. The use of long-acting tranquillizers in captive wild animals. In: *The Capture and Care Manual: Capture, Care, Accommodation, and Transportation of Wild African Animals* (AA McKenzie, ed.), pp. 71–99. Pretoria: South African Veterinary Foundation.

Gabor TM, Hellgren EC, Silvy NJ. 1997. Immobilization of collared peccaries (*Tayassu tajacu*) and feral hogs (*Sus scrofa*) with Telazol® and xylazine. *Journal of Wildlife Diseases* 33(1):161–164.

Gallagher JF, Lochmiller RL, Grant WE. 1985. Immobilization of peccaries with ketamine hydrochloride. *Journal of Wildlife Management* 49(2):356–357.

Gronert GA. 1980. Malignant hyperthermia. *Anesthesiology* 53(5):395–423.

Hellgren EC, Lochmiller RL, Amoss MS, Grant WE. 1985. Endocrine and metabolic responses of the collared peccary (*Tayassu tajacu*) to immobilization with ketamine hydrochloride. *Journal of Wildlife Diseases* 21(4):417–425.

James SB, Cook RA, Raphael BL, Stetter MD, Kalk P, MacLaughlin K, Calle PP. 1999. Immobilization of babirusa (*Babyrousa babyrussa*) with xylazine and tiletamine/zolazepam and reversal with yohimbine and flumazenil. *Journal of Zoo and Wildlife Medicine* 30(4):521–525.

Ko JCH, Thurmon J, Tranquilli W, Benson GJ, Olson W. 1993a. Problems encountered when anesthetizing potbellied pigs. *Veterinary Medicine* 88:435–441.

Ko JCH, Williams BL, Smith VL, McGrath CJ, Jacobson JD. 1993b. Comparison of telazol, telazol-ketamine, telazol-xylazine and telazol-xylazine-ketamine as chemical restraint and anesthetic induction combination in swine. *Laboratory Animal Science* 43(5):476–480.

Ko JCH, Williams BL, Rogers ER, Pablo LS, McCaine WC, McGrath CJ. 1995. Increasing xylazine dose-enhanced anesthetic properties of Telazol-xylazine combination in swine. *Laboratory Animal Science* 45(3):290–294.

Kumar A, Mann HJ, Remmel RP. 2006. Pharmacokinetics of tiletamine and zolazepam (Telazol®) in anesthetized pigs. *Journal of Veterinary Pharmacology and Therapeutics* 29(6):587–589.

Lerman J, Oyston JP, Gallagher TM, Miyasaka K, Volgyesi GA, Burrows FA. 1990. The minimum alveolar concentration (MAC) and hemodynamic effects of halothane, isoflurane, and sevoflurane in newborn swine. *Anesthesiology* 73(4):717–721.

Leus K, Goodall GP, Macdonald AA. 1999. Anatomy and histology of the babirusa (*Babyrousa babyrussa*) stomach. *Comptes Rendus de l'Academie des Sciences. Serie III, Sciences de la Vie* 322(12):1081–1092.

Lin HC, Thurmon JC, Benson GJ, Tranquilli WJ. 1993. Telazol – a review of its pharmacology and use in veterinary medicine. *Journal of Veterinary Pharmacology and Therapeutics* 16(4):383–418.

Lochmiller RL, Hellgren EC, Robinson RM, Grant WE. 1984. Techniques for collecting blood from collared peccaries, *Dicotyles tajacu* (L.). *Journal of Wildlife Diseases* 20(1):47–50.

Loscher W, Ganter M, Fassbender CP. 1990. Correlation between drug and metabolite concentrations in plasma and anesthetic action of ketamine in swine. *American Journal of Veterinary Research* 51(3):391–398.

Lukasik VM, Moon PF. 1996. Two cases of pneumothorax during mechanical ventilation in Vietnamese potbellied pigs. *Veterinary Surgery* 25(4):356–360.

Moon PF, Smith LJ. 1996. General anesthetic techniques in swine. *The Veterinary Clinics of North America. Food Animal Practice* 12(3):663–691.

Morris PJ, Shima AL. 2003. Suidae and Tayassuidae (wild pigs, peccaries). In: *Zoo and Wild Animal Medicine*, 5th ed. (ME Fowler, RE Miller, eds.), pp. 586–602. St. Louis: Saunders.

Morris PJ, Bicknese B, Janssen DL, Sutherland-Smith M, Young L. 1999. Chemical immobilization of exotic swine at the San Diego Zoo. Proceedings of the American Association of Zoo Veterinarians, pp. 150–153.

Mutoh T, Lamm WJ, Embree LJ, Hildebrandt J, Albert RK. 1991. Abdominal distension alters regional pleural pressures and chest wall mechanics in pigs *in vivo*. *Journal of Applied Physiology* 70(6):2611–2618.

Nishimura R, Kim H, Matsunaga S, Sakaguchi M, Sasaki N, Tamura H, Takeuchi A. 1992. Antagonism of medetomidine sedation by atipamezole in pigs. *Journal of Veterinary Medical Science* 54(6):1237–1240.

Nishimura R, Kim H, Matsunaga S, Hayashi K, Tamura H, Sasaki N, Takeuchi A. 1993. Sedative effect induced by a combination of medetomidine and midazolam in pigs. *Journal of Veterinary Medical Science* 55(5):717–722.

Nishimura R, Kim HY, Matsunaga S, Hayashi K, Tamura H, Sasaki N, Takeuchi A. 1994. Cardiopulmonary effects of medetomidine-midazolam and medetomidine-midazolam-atipamezole in laboratory pigs. *Journal of Veterinary Medical Science* 56(2): 359–363.

Padilla LR. 2004. Immobilization of babirussa (*Babyroussa babyroussa*) using a butorphanol-tiletamine-zolazepam combination. Proceedings of the American Association of Zoo Veterinarians, pp. 610–611.

Porter BA. 2006. Evaluation of collared peccary translocations in the Texas Hill Country. Master's Thesis, Texas A&M University.

Reyna-Hurtado R, Rojas-Flores E, Tanner GW. 2009. Home range and habitat preferences of white-lipped peccaries (*Tayassu pecari*) in Calakmul, Campeche, Mexico. *Journal of Mammalogy* 90(5):1199–1209.

Sakaguchi M, Nishimura R, Sasaki N, Ishiguro T, Tamura H, Takeuchi A. 1992a. Sedative effects of medetomidine in pigs. *Journal of Veterinary Medical Science* 54(4):643–647.

Sakaguchi M, Nishimura R, Sasaki N, Ishiguro T, Tamura H, Takeuchi A. 1992b. Enhancing effect of butorphanol on medetomidine-induced sedation in pigs. *Journal of Veterinary Medical Science* 54(6):1883–1185.

Sakaguchi M, Nishimura R, Sasaki N, Ishiguro T, Tamura H, Takeuchi A. 1993. Cardiopulmonary effects of a combination of medetomidine and butorphanol in atropinized pigs. *Journal of Veterinary Medical Science* 55(3):497–499.

Sano H, Doi M, Yu S, Kurita T, Sato S. 2010. Evaluation of the hypnotic and hemodynamic effects of dexmedetomidine on propofol-sedated swine. *Experimental Animals* 59(2): 199–205.

Selmi AL, Mendes GM, Figueiredo JP, Guimarães FB, Selmi GRB, Bernal FEM, McMannus C, Paludo GR. 2003. Chemical restraint of peccaries with tiletamine/zolazepam and xylazine or tiletamine/zolazepam and butorphanol. *Veterinary Anaesthesia and Analgesia* 30(1):24–29.

Siemon A, Wiesner H, vin Hegel G. 1992. Die Verwendung von Tiletamin/Zolazepam/Romifidine zur Distansimmobilisation von Wildschweinen. *Tierarztliche Praxis* 20(1):55–58.

Sonntag S, Hackenbroich C, Böer M, Bonath KH. 2004. Tiletamine-zolazepam-xylazine immobilization in warthogs (*Phacochoerus aethiopicus*). Proceedings European Association of Zoo and Wildlife Veterinarians, pp. 105–106. Ebeltoft, Denmark.

Sutherland-Smith M, Campos JM, Cramer C, Thirstadt C, Toone W, Morris PJ. 2004. Immobilization of Chacoan peccaries (*Catagonus wagneri*) using medetomidine, Telazol®, and ketamine. *Journal of Wildlife Diseases* 40(4):731–736.

Sweitzer RA, Ghneim GS, Gardner IA, Van Vuren D, Gonzales BJ, Boyce WM. 1997. Immobilization and physiological parameters associated with chemical restraint of wild pigs with Telazol® and xylazine hydrochloride. *Journal of Wildlife Diseases* 33(2): 198–205.

Swindle MM. 1998. *Surgery, Anesthesia and Experimental Techniques in Swine*. Ames: Iowa State University Press.

Thurmon JC, Smith GW. 2007. Swine. In: *Lumb and Jones Veterinary Anesthesia and Analgesia*, 4th ed. (WJ Tranquilli, JC Thurmon, KA Grimm, eds.), pp. 747–763. Ames: Blackwell Publishing.

Thurmon JC, Tranquilli WJ, Benson GJ. 1996. *Lumb and Jones Veterinary Anesthesia*, 3rd ed. Baltimore: Williams and Wilkins.

Tranquilli WJ, Thurmon JC, Benson GJ. 1983. Organ blood flow and distribution of cardiac output in hypocapneic ketamine-anesthetized swine. *American Journal of Veterinary Research* 44 (8):1578–1582.

Trim CM, Gilroy BA. 1985. Cardiopulmonary effects of a xylazine and ketamine combination in pigs. *Research in Veterinary Science* 38(1):30–34.

56 Hippopotamidae

Michele Miller, Gregory J. Fleming, Scott B. Citino, and Markus Hofmeyr

INTRODUCTION

With the use of newer and different drug combinations, higher concentrations of injectable agents, and improved techniques, safer and more effective sedation and general anesthesia can be successfully achieved in both species of hippopotami. However, they continue to present unique challenges due to their physical size, physiology, aquatic nature, and potential danger to staff. This chapter will describe both historical as well as newly developed techniques for captive and free-ranging common and pygmy hippo anesthesia.

TAXONOMY AND ANATOMY RELATED TO IMMOBILIZATION

The two extant species of hippopotamus, Nile hippo (*Hippopotamus amphibious*) and pygmy hippo (*Choeropsis liberiensis*), belong to different genera and both are indigenous to Africa. *Hippopotamus amphibious* has a weight range of 1179–2500 kg, with adult males typically larger than females (Miller 2003). Length along the back ranges 119–302 cm, with an average of 270 cm. Captive hippos tend toward obesity, which may complicate anesthesia due to pressure on the diaphragm during recumbency. If a scale is not available, weight estimates should be carefully considered since this may have significant impacts on anesthetic effects.

Nile hippos have an hourglass-shaped skull with nostrils and eyes set on the top of the head to allow access above water without lifting their entire head. Nostrils have a valve-like closure that activates when submerged and opens upon surfacing, even when sleeping.

The pygmy hippo, *Choeropsis liberiensis*, ranges in weight from 160 to 350 kg. They are approximately 70–80 cm high at the shoulder and 140–160 cm in length (Eltringham 1999). Males are usually only slightly larger than females. Their skull is more of a pear shape, with eyes set on the sides rather than top of the head. Both hippo species have opening jaw angles of greater than 90°, facilitating oral exams and intubation, although the heavy masseter muscles and weight of the skull may make opening the mouth of an anesthetized hippo difficult without accessory items or repositioning.

Hippos have a four-compartment stomach and are considered "pseudoruminants." The slow gastrointestinal transit time may lead to increased pressure on the diaphragm due to gastrointestinal contents during recumbency. Some studies suggest that the stomach content represents two nights' feeding (Eltringham 1999). Therefore, a minimum of 12–24 hours fasting is recommended for captive hippos, with overnight water restriction, to minimize abdominal content fill (Loomis & Ramsay 1999; Ramsay et al. 1998).

Both species of hippopotamus are semi-aquatic mammals, spending their days in or near water, coming out to feed primarily between dusk and dawn. The common hippo, widely distributed in sub-Saharan Africa, is a social animal, lives in pods ranging in size from a few to over 100 animals led by a dominant bull with a harem of cows and their offspring.

Pygmy hippos are found only in West Africa and are solitary by nature. They can be aggressive toward conspecifics, especially when housed together in captive situations. Similar to the Nile hippo, they thermoregulate by spending time in water during the day.

ANATOMY AND PHYSIOLOGY RELATED TO CAPTURE AND IMMOBILIZATION

Skin and Thermoregulation

Due to their large volume to surface area ratio, thermoregulation is a critical function for hippos and should

Zoo Animal and Wildlife Immobilization and Anesthesia, Second Edition. Edited by Gary West, Darryl Heard, and Nigel Caulkett.
© 2014 John Wiley & Sons, Inc. Published 2014 by John Wiley & Sons, Inc.

be carefully monitored during an immobilization. Hippo skin is uniquely designed to assist in control of temperature and water loss. Although it appears thick, the epidermal layer is thin, with a thick dermis containing blood vessels and subdermal glands, which secrete froathy white or reddish viscous material (Eltringham 1999). The role of the secretions is incompletely understood but is speculated to assist in evaporative cooling and wound healing. Increased secretions are often observed during times of excitement. These secretions increase the difficulty of handling a recumbent hippo.

CARDIOVASCULAR SYSTEM

Vascular Access Sites for Blood Collection
The pigmented epidermis and thick dermal connective tissue surrounding peripheral blood vessels make visualization difficult. In young or some free-ranging animals, veins may be visible due to increased blood pressure after exertion or lean body condition. Other methods for locating blood vessels include Doppler and ultrasound probes, or blind approximation. Most peripheral veins on hippos are relatively thin-walled and may easily collapse with negative pressure from a syringe (Fig. 56.1).

One technique is to collect blood by allowing it to drip from the hub of a needle into an open tube containing the appropriate anticoagulant. In some cases, if a good blood flow is obtained, the use of an extension set may assist with the long blood draw times. Clotting is a potential problem, and pretreatment of tubing or syringes with anticoagulant is recommended.

Peripheral veins that can be accessed include cephalic, median (located on the medial aspect of the antebrachium), palmar and plantar digital (located on the caudal aspect of the distal limb), medial saphenous, ventral abdominal, interdigital (located midway

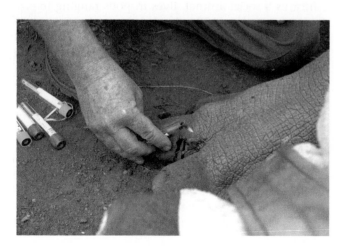

Figure 56.1. Blood collection from hub of needle using a digital vein on the forelimb of a Nile hippopotamus.

between the toes just proximal to the webbing), and sublingual veins (Miller 2007; Stalder et al. 2012). In young or small individuals, blood can be collected from the vena cava using a technique similar to a domestic pig. Auricular veins tend to collapse, yield minimal blood volume, and are very sensitive, even under anesthesia. The ventral tail artery, on the midline at the base of the tail, lies very close to the ventral tail vein. Both the artery and vein are sensitive to movement of the needle and can constrict, preventing any further blood collection.

Samples should be prioritized due to potentially limited volume due to collection difficulties. Ideally, dedicated personnel should be assigned to acquire the most essential samples to minimize time required during the immobilization.

Vascular Access for Fluid and Drug Administration
Intravenous catheterization is typically reserved for critically ill or young animals, since it requires a surgical cut-down for placement. Fluid replacement therapy alternatives include nasogastric tube, enema, or intraperitoneal fluids. Intravenous medications may be diluted in isotonic fluids and administered intraperitoneally with caution.

Intraosseous catheters can be used in juvenile or small hippos as an alternative to intravenous fluid or drug administration. Spinal needles or intraosseous biopsy needles placed in the greater trochanter of the femur have been used successfully in one case of a juvenile Nile hippo.

In anesthetized Nile hippos, the paired sublingual veins can be palpated and catheterized. The vein on the ventral aspect of the tongue can be accessed with a 20-gauge butterfly catheter or a conventional intravenous catheter. This vessel can be used for injection of intravenous fluids, anesthetic drugs, or collection of venous blood samples (Stalder et al. 2012).

Cardiovascular System Monitoring
Auscultation and palpation of pulses are difficult due to size in most adult hippos. However, positioning may facilitate success and periodic attempts should be made. Using one of the new electronic stethoscopes can enhance audible detection of heart sounds. Positioning the animal leaning slightly left will also place the heart closer to the thoracic wall. The stethoscope should be placed near the left elbow in the axilla when the animal is in sternal recumbency. Pulses can sometimes be palpated interdigitally or occasionally near the cephalic, medial saphenous, and sublingual vessels. Doppler probes placed directly on the cornea using copious amounts of gel have also been used to monitor heart rates in immobilized hippos. Heart rates vary significantly depending on the level of exertion and excitement prior to anesthesia, drugs, and dosages

administered. Typical heart rates in immobilized animals are 20–60 beats per minute, but trends are more critical than actual numbers.

RESPIRATORY SYSTEM

With some drug combinations (nonpotent narcotic combinations), anesthetized hippos appear to exhibit a respiratory pattern similar to a "dive reflex" in which they may take several breaths in short succession then breath hold (Stalder et al. 2012). This may result in erratic minute respiratory rates, oxygen saturation, and end-tidal CO_2 values (Fleming et al. 2010). Hippos anesthetized with potent opioids are often apneic and tend not to show this dive response. Therefore, it is critical to visually monitor respiratory cycles over several minutes and assess trends since apnea, hypoxemia, and hypercapnia are common complications.

Nasal Insufflation

When feasible, nasal insufflation with oxygen using a 12-mm endotracheal tube for a common hippo (and smaller for pygmy hippo) can increase both dead space and alveolar oxygen partial pressures, resulting in increased arterial oxygen (Ramsay et al. 1998). Supplemental inhalant anesthetics can also be administered by nasal insufflation. This may reduce the need for additional injectable anesthetic drugs during prolonged procedures. Typically, 0.5–2.5% isoflurane administered through a nasal tube can provide sufficient analgesia and restraint.

Intubation

For extended procedures or when using inhalant agents for supplemental or maintenance anesthesia, intubation is recommended. Necessary equipment and personnel should be available to assist in repositioning the animal to open the jaws, although some drugs combinations provide adequate muscle relaxation for manual opening. This is usually easier in lateral recumbency. An inflated tire inner tube from a small vehicle may be used under the head to keep the head in line with the body and keep the airway straight. Ropes or straps placed behind the canines can be used to open the mouth and place different-size wooden wedges, with rope pull strings between the upper and lower molar arcades to keep the mouth open. This technique allows for easier access to the oral cavity. Rope handles, or pulls, should be attached to each rope block for ease of removal. Other equipment may be needed, including poles with nooses ("rabies poles"), ropes, duct tape, ratchet straps, and headlamps or flashlights for visualizing tube placement. Due to the redundant folds of buccal and oropharyngeal tissue, fleshy tongue, and long soft palate, it is easier to place an endotracheal tube in an adult hippo by blind manual insertion than using a laryngoscope, which are typically too short.

Adult common hippos usually require 24- to 30-mm endotracheal tubes (ETT) and 14-mm ETT for pygmy hippos. The smaller narrow oral cavity of the pygmy hippo makes intubation slightly more difficult but can be accomplished by manual palpation of the glottis and insertion of the tube in a similar manner. A large-animal anesthesia machine should be used with the flow rate set at approximately 5–10 mL/kg/min. For nonemergency procedures, ensure that there are adequate supplies of oxygen cylinders and inhalant anesthetics during the planning phase. If a large animal anesthetic machine is not available, a high pressure demand valve may be used to insufflate the lungs. A double-demand valve system developed for elephant anesthesia could also be used for hippo anesthesia (Horne et al. 2001).

Respiratory System Monitoring

Respiratory monitoring is one of the most important components of hippo anesthesia since it is the area where complications most commonly occur (Miller 2007; Ramsay et al. 1998). The most common method of monitoring is visualization of thoracic excursions or anesthetic bag movements, although nostril air flow can also provide information on depth as well as rate of breaths. Respiratory rates are influenced by drug combinations, but ideal ranges are 4–20 breaths/min.

Respiratory complications include apnea, hypoventilation, hypoxemia, hypercapnia, and respiratory acidosis (Flach et al. 1998; Fleming et al. 2010; Loomis & Ramsay 1999; Miller 2003). Administration of doxapram, supplemental oxygen, partial or complete reversal should be considered to address respiratory issues, depending on the degree of other physiological impairments (Dumonceaux et al. 2000; Ramsay et al. 1998).

THERMOREGULATION AND BODY TEMPERATURE

Since thermoregulation is critical when taking a hippo out of water for a period of time, temperature monitoring should ideally be performed throughout the procedure. Water, ice, a hose for enema, methods to provide evaporative cooling (e.g., fans), and shade should be available to control temperature and cool the animal if necessary. Expected body temperatures of anesthetized hippo are 35–38°C (using a thermometer inserted 6 in into the rectum). However, due to the large mass of the hippo, this may not reflect core temperature. Readings over 39°C should be considered hyperthermic and cause for concern (Stalder et al. 2012).

SPECIFIC USE OF ANESTHETIC MONITORING EQUIPMENT ON HIPPOS

As mentioned earlier, commonly used anesthetic monitoring equipment can be used on immobilized hippos but may be limited to certain locations or placement due to anatomy. This section describes techniques to improve accuracy and success.

Pulse Oximetry

Pulse oximetry can be used to measure heart rates but should not be the sole method due to unreliability associated with probe placement (difficult to keep in place), possible vasoconstriction due to drugs, poor reflectance through the dense dermal connective tissue, and interference by skin secretions. However, oxygen saturation readings above 90% can be achieved in anesthetized hippopotamus (Dumonceaux et al. 2000). Auricular pulse oximetry may be attempted by using a dull knife blade (common butter knife) to scrape off the auricular dermal pigmentation and then apply the pulse oximeter probe. Cooler environmental temperatures may also cause auricular vasoconstriction, resulting in decreased sensitivity of pulse oximetry readings.

Other sites that have been used to obtain pulse oximeter readings in hippos include conjunctiva/ nictitating membrane, oral mucous membrane, vulva, prepuce, and rectal mucosa (Miller 2007; Morris et al. 2001). One technique is to remove the sensors from the "C" or "V" clamp and tape or hold them side-by-side in close proximity to function as reflectance probes when using them at some of these sites (e.g., conjunctival membrane) and shield them from light. Depending on the site, readings may range from 70% to 90%, but trends should be monitored and interpreted in conjunction with other observations, such as color of mucous membranes and capillary refill time.

Capnography

Capnography can be useful for measuring both respiratory rate and end tidal CO_2. The capnograph can be attached to a small (9–12 mm) endotracheal tube that is placed into one of the nostrils. This will provide adequate flow rate for the capnograph to work. $ETCO_2$ during the first breath after breath holding may be 70–80 mmHg, which usually decreases to levels around 40–50 mmHg after a few breaths. Animals that have a regular respiratory pattern should have values ranging 35–55 mmHg when breathing air.

Temperature Monitoring Devices

A constant-reading digital thermometer with a long flexible probe placed rectally may provide the most accurate readings. Another method for assessing temperature is to use a thermometer placed in the muscle at the dart site. Small digital thermometers, if used, should be placed in direct contact with the rectal mucosa to improve accuracy.

Blood Gas Analysis

Blood gas measurements provide a more complete analysis of cardiorespiratory function, when available.

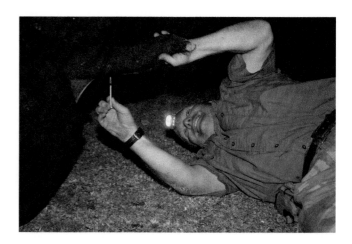

Figure 56.2. Sample collection for arterial blood gas analysis using ventral tail artery from a Nile hippopotamus.

The ventral tail artery is the ideal site for obtaining arterial blood gas samples. When performing arterial sampling, it is best to utilize a 1-cc syringe. When the artery is penetrated, the syringe will fill by arterial pressure alone, ensuring proper placement and not a venous sample. Repeated samples from the ventral tail artery are possible. Ventral tail blood samples may be more difficult to obtain in obese captive animals as their tails become enlarged with adipose stores, making vessel location difficult (Fig. 56.2).

Portable veterinary blood gas analyzers have been used with hippos. Although normal values have not been established, reference ranges for other large ungulates can be extrapolated to these species. Morris et al. (2001) reported average venous blood values from an immobilized juvenile common hippo as follows: pH = 7.4 ± 0.1, PCO_2 = 61.5 ± 8.1 mmHg, PO_2 = 71 ± 30 mmHg.

PLANNING FOR A HIPPO IMMOBILIZATION PROCEDURE

Any procedure requiring extensive equipment, supplies, and personnel should be planned well in advance to increase a successful outcome. It is important that all involved staff have clearly defined roles and responsibilities. Regular communication and checklists can be helpful to determine progress. Defined priorities and contingency plans should be discussed prior to the procedure. Safety for animal and personnel must be included in the planning.

Induction

Most hippos are darted with immobilization drugs. Less commonly used options are pole syringe, hand injection, or oral administration (Clyde et al. 1998; Dumonceaux et al. 2000; Weston et al. 1996; Zoli

Gymesi, pers. comm.). Preferred dart sites due to thinner skin thickness are just behind the ear, caudal thigh, and biceps area. In common hippos, a 60- to 64-mm needle is used and must be at right angles to the skin to ensure an intramuscular injection. A 38- to 40-mm needle should be adequate for adult pygmy hippos. Longer 75-mm needles are available and may provide some extra penetration if the dart is not at right angles to the skin for use in the common hippo. Administration in crates, some chutes, or from remote sites may limit choice of injection sites. Intradermal injection of drugs will result in a slower or incomplete induction, which can result in sudden arousal with stimulation. Signs of induction usually include head lowering, sweating, salivation, ataxia, "dog-sitting," and recumbency. Tail tone in anesthetized hippos may be one measure of anesthetic depth. When reaching a safe anesthetic plane for handling, the tail will be limp and easily manipulated with nonpotent narcotic combinations. However, with potent opioids, tail movement may be maintained despite being at an adequate anesthetic plane. Adequate time after recumbency should be allowed before approaching since stimulation and arousal is possible especially with the nonpotent opioid combinations (Clyde et al. 1998; Morris et al. 2001).

During induction, a hippo may raise its head to take a breath as if in water. This behavior occurs at the start of the anesthesia. Once the animal reaches a deeper plane, this behavior ceases in most individuals.

Placing a blindfold and ear plugs minimizes external stimuli. For added safety, a "muzzle" or ratchet strap can be placed around the jaw just caudal to the canines to prevent accidental opening of the mouth when working around the head.

Positioning

Hippos should be left in their initial position until they reach an adequate plane of anesthesia since movement can also stimulate arousal. The short limbs and barrel-shaped body of a hippo make positioning and transport difficult during anesthesia. Weight on limbs is a concern during extended procedures due to the potential for neuropathy, compromised tissue perfusion, and myopathy. Ideally, limbs should be positioned to optimize circulation and minimize weight on pressure points, such as elbows and hocks, by placing the animal on a soft or padded surface. If the procedure requires an extended period of recumbency, "pumping" or massaging the limbs periodically can aid perfusion, if positioning permits.

Positioning to optimize cardiorespiratory function especially during prolonged procedures is critical. Abdominal contents create pressure on the diaphragm and compromise respirations if left in sternal for longer procedures unless ventilation is assisted (Morris et al. 2001; Ramsay et al. 1998). Therefore, attempts to roll the hippo laterally should be made if respiratory compromise is suspected. This may also assist with increasing perfusion to extremities. Rolling hippos back up into a sternal position is difficult due to their body shape and size.

Recovery

Once the anesthetic procedure is completed, all personnel and equipment should be removed to a safe distance. The hippo should be left in a sternal or semi-sternal position for recovery, although if this is not possible, recovery from lateral position has been performed (Miller 2007; Morris et al. 2001).

Reversal drugs should be administered intramuscularly for ease and to minimize time. Intramuscular reversal can be achieved by inserting a 3-in spinal needle then into the neck fold or the triceps muscle. This deep insertion should increase the likelihood of intramuscular versus intradermal administration. The tongue muscle may be used for intramuscular injection of reversal drugs (Fleming et al. 2010). However, care must be taken if large drug volumes are injected (e.g., atipamezole) due to swelling and trauma.

Recovery times depend on the drugs used and a successful deep intramuscular injection. Immediate short-term ataxia is often observed. In captive hippos immobilized with butorphanol-detomidine, access to water was allowed as soon as 2 hours post anesthesia (Morris et al. 2001).

Anesthetic Records

Detailed records are critical to advancing knowledge of safe and effective immobilization techniques for hippopotamus. Reviews of records reveal trends and additional areas for investigation as well as potential answers when complications occur. Minimum data should include animal information, date, weight (or estimate), drugs administered (dose, route, and time), time to initial effect, time to recumbency, heart rates, respiratory rates, temperatures, other monitoring parameters, any complications, antagonists administered (dose, route, time), and recovery time and effect. Standardized forms are available through many computerized medical records programs. Final reports should become part of the individual animal's medical record.

Safety

Both hippo species are extremely dangerous and can inflict mortal wounds to humans if charged or trapped in a pen. If the hippo is to be moved or handled without anesthesia, then this must occur from a protected position. Push boards can be used in habituated pygmy or young Nile hippo, but care needs to be taken that adequate escape routes exist if the animal cannot be managed with the board.

Under field conditions, a heavy-caliber rifle (0.375 or bigger) must be on hand to deal with emergency dangerous situations. If there is any concern regarding immobilization, administering supplemental drugs before handling the animal reduces the risk of spontaneous arousal and can help facilitate body repositioning. Other safety measures, such as placing a jaw strap, using a blindfold and earplugs, reducing noise levels, and minimizing stimulation have been covered but are crucial for personnel safety. Continuous monitoring of anesthetic depth should also be considered part of the safety procedures and staff made aware of any changes.

HISTORICAL REVIEW OF HIPPO IMMOBILIZATION

Common Hippo

Due to the historically high mortality rate associated with hippo anesthesia, there have been few published reports prior to the 1970s. As with other large ungulates, potent narcotics were initially used alone or with xylazine or acepromazine. Frequent complications included apnea, cyanosis, bradycardia, and death. In one review of Nile hippo immobilizations, 6/16 (37.5%) resulted in complications (Ramsay et al. 1998). However potent opioids have been used successfully. Etorphine at 0.001–0.005 mg/kg (total dose 2–6 mg) with or without xylazine (0.061–0.083 mg/kg; total dose 100–150 mg) intramuscularly will induce general anesthesia (Ramsay et al. 1998). This combination can be reversed with 100-mg naltrexone to 1-mg etrophine IM and yohimbine 0.1–0.3 mg/kg IM. Close monitoring for adverse signs is essential when using narcotics in hippos and preparation for complete reversal considered if signs worsen.

Administration of nasal oxygen or intubation with intermittent positive pressure ventilation appears to improve oxygen saturation, especially with the narcotic combinations (Dumonceaux et al. 2000; Loomis & Ramsay 1999; Ramsay et al. 1998). Doxapram administration intramuscularly also has been used to mitigate respiratory depression.

In more recent years, the use of restraint devices and husbandry training has facilitated medical procedures with captive hippos so that only restraint or minor sedation can be used (Krueger et al. 1996). Azaperone and acepromazine provide mild sedation but no analgesia (Burroughs et al. 2006; Loomis & Ramsay 1999).

Detomidine and butorphanol combinations can be administered for minor procedures requiring analgesia and sedation, or as induction agents for immobilization based on dosage. Other drugs can also be added to change or extend the level of anesthesia. Typical dosages are 0.02- to 0.06-mg/kg detomidine with 0.06- to 0.20-mg/kg butorphanol IM. Supplemental doses can be administered at a ratio of 1:3 detomidine:butorphanol based on effect (Morris et al. 2001). Initial effects may be observed as early as 10–20 minutes depending on injection placement with recumbency at 20–30 minutes. However, full effect may take longer and stimulation may cause arousal. Therefore, invasive, painful, or prolonged procedures should be supplemented with isoflurane, ketamine (0.1–1 mg/kg IM), propofol, low dose etorphine, or supplemental detomidine (or medetomidine) and butorphanol (Miller 2007; Morris et al. 2001). Propofol can be administered as a bolus at 0.5 mg/kg or 50–100 µg/kg/min as an infusion IV.

Inhalant anesthetics are useful alternatives to injectable drugs for extending general anesthesia. Ideally, this should be provided through intubation, although it can be effective by nasal insufflations (Dumonceaux et al. 2000). Staff and environmental safety should be considered when using this later method.

Reversal of the detomidine-butorphanol combination is accomplished with naltrexone at a 20:1 ratio of butorphanol (in milligrams) or 0.4–0.6 mg/kg IM (Morris et al. 2001). Atipamezole at five times the milligram dose of medetomidine or detomidine IM, or yohimbine 0.1–0.3 mg/kg IM or IV, antagonizes the effects of the alpha-2 agonists (Clyde et al. 1998). Arousal is relatively rapid, usually within 5–20 minutes, unless the hippo has received supplemental drugs.

Pygmy Hippo

There are fewer historical anesthetic reports in pygmy hippos. Nonetheless, they present the same types of challenges as their larger counterparts. In order to minimize the need for immobilization, many facilities have instituted training programs and modified structures to permit minor medical procedures, such as wound treatment, to be performed.

There have been a few anesthetic events using narcotics in pygmy hippos combining etorphine or carfentanil with xylazine (Miller 2003). The commercial combination of etorphine and acepromazine has also been used. However, similar complications were observed in pygmy hippos, and use of potent opioids has fallen out of favor.

For minor sedation or as an adjunct for initial induction, oral detomidine or diazepam, and injectable midazolam (0.1 mg/kg IM) have shown promising results (Weston et al. 1996; K. Mehren, pers. comm.).

Although there are fewer reports, the experience with butorphanol-detomidine in pygmy hippos has been generally good. Since the introduction of concentrated medetomidine, the combination of medetomidine-butorphanol has been more commonly used. The ratio of alpha-2 agonist to butorphanol is approximately 1:5, which is different than that used in the Nile hippo (Miller 2007). This resulted in dosages of 0.04–0.06 mg/kg of medetomidine or detomidine and 0.1–0.2 mg/kg of butorphanol IM (P. Morris, pers. comm.). Anesthesia can be extended with supplemental doses of ketamine or gas anesthesia. Reversal agents are similar to those used in the common hippo.

For prolonged, painful or invasive procedures, intubation and maintenance on isoflurane is recommended.

If this is not feasible, other alternatives include using local blocks combined with supplemental ketamine or additional medetomidine-butorphanol as needed. However, this requires continuous monitoring and recalculation of reversal agents.

NEW ADVANCES IN HIPPO RESTRAINT AND IMMOBILIZATION

General Anesthesia of Captive Common Hippos

The recent development of a reversible combination of medetomidine (0.04–0.05 mg/kg), butorphanol (0.05–0.10 mg/kg) and azaperone (0.05 mg/kg, to a max of 125 mg total) has been used successfully in both wild ($n = 20$) and captive common hippos ($n = 5$) (Fleming et al. 2010). This combination was derived from standing sedation dose for captive elephants (Neiffer et al. 2005) (Table 56.1).

Procedures on captive hippos were possible to perform that lasted as long as 3 hours using butorphanol-alpha-2 agonist induction with isoflurane supplementation. An additional dose of 1–2 mg/kg of ketamine in a second dart may provide some additional anesthesia and provide a higher level of safety. Reversal drugs were naltrexone at 0.12 mg/kg IM (3× butorphanol dosage) and atipamazole at 0.36 mg/kg IM (3× medetomidine dosage). In captive hippo, if the animal is not standing by 45–60 minutes, it is advisable to give an additional dose of naltrexone and atipamezole by dart. Yohimbine (0.1 mg/kg) can also be used but does not appear to be as effective as atipamezole in reversing medetomidine.

Table 56.1. New anesthetic combination dosages for captive hippos[a]

Immobilizing Drugs		Reversals
Nile hippos		
Butorphanol	0.04 mg/kg	Naltrexone (3–5× butor dosage)
Azaperone	0.05–0.1 mg/kg	
Medetomidine	0.06–0.08 mg/kg	Atipamezole (3–5× medet dosage)
Ketamine	1 mg/kg	
Pygmy hippos		
Medetomidine	0.035 mg/kg	Atipamezole (3–5× medet dosage)
Butorphanol	0.20 mg/kg	Naltrexone (3–5× butor dosage)
Detomidine	0.07 mg/kg	Atipamezole (3–5× detom dosage)
Butorphanol	0.15 mg/kg	Naltrexone (3–5× butor dosage)
Ketamine	0.88 mg/kg	

[a]Dosages may require supplemental drugs depending on individual circumstances.

In a recent study, 10 captive hippopotamus were kept anesthetized for castration using a combination of medetomidine (60–80 μg/kg) and ketamine (1 mg/kg) administered IM, with supplemental ketamine (0.1–0.4 mg/kg IV) three to five times in the sublingual vein (Stalder et al. 2012). Transient periods of apnea were noted in 6 of 10 animals. This protocol provided approximately 97 minutes ± 35 minutes of anesthetic time. Reversal with atipamezole 0.3 mg/kg (50% IV, 50% IM) resulted in standing animals in 5–7 minutes.

Capture and Immobilization of Free-Ranging Common Hippos

Wild hippos frequently use trails from the water to feeding sites that can be used for camera trapping and capture (D. Cooper, pers. comm.). Knowledge of these locations provides potential capture sites. Generally, trap capture of Nile hippo is done at the edge of the pool or dam that they live in, and alfalfa hay is used as the bait into the capture corral, which can be closed remotely trapping the hippo inside. This method is time-consuming, but usually the only way in which large numbers of common hippo are captured safely and cost-effectively in Africa.

Free-ranging hippos create another level of complexity due to their tendency to be in or near water and other hippos during daytime hours when capture usually is planned. Immobilization of free-ranging Nile hippos can be accomplished by darting at night when the animal is at least 1 km from the water. A combination of medetomidine (0.04–05 mg/kg), butorphanol (0.05–0.10 mg/kg), and azaperone (0.05 mg/kg to a max of 125 mg) was utilized. If darted, and left alone, undisturbed hippos usually will only run 10–30 m and then resume grazing. Free-ranging hippo should only be darted in or close to water, if they are on their own, or can be separated from the pod. Once in the pod, the animal can become lost or pushed under water when anesthetized. Helicopter darting is an effective way to dart single or individuals that have broken away from the pod. From a helicopter, the gluteus muscles or the muscles along the spine are ideal targets for perpendicular darts. Longer needles are required due to the thicker skin over the dorsum; recommended lengths are 75–80 mm.

Preliminary studies done on captured hippos showed they would stop running or walking at 5 minutes, rest their head, dog sit, and then become recumbent within 10 minutes if the dart went deeply intramuscular. If the drug went subcutaneous, induction could take as long as 45 minutes and require supplemental doses for safe handling.

Several hippos immobilized with both the medetomidine, butorphanol, and azaperone combination (Fleming et al. 2010), and medetomidine and ketamine combination (Stalder et al. 2012) had transient apnea and exhibited the breath-holding behavior for approximately 20–30 minutes post darting. With regular respirations, SPO₂ values were in the high 90s and ETCO₂ were between 30 and 50 mmHg. Higher ETCO₂ and lower SPO₂ values were initially recorded during the initial breath-holding phase. Other physiologic values followed a similar trend suggestive of acidosis (PCO₂ 35–70 mmHg, PO₂ 35–75 mmHg, SO₂ 82–95%, pH 7.15–7.35, and rectal temperature 35–38°C). Procedure length was variable but averaged about 80 minutes in the field without any anesthetic supplementation.

Recovering hippos in field conditions may have additional challenges such as water or other topographical challenges that should be considered. A large rubber mat can be slid under the hippo and used to move the animal prior to reversal.

New Advances in Captive Pygmy Hippo Immobilization

The frequency of immobilization of captive pygmy hippos has increased since development of the newer anesthetic combinations. Drugs can be administered by either pole syringe, hand syringe, orally, or dart. Successful dental and other procedures can be accomplished under general anesthesia using the following dosages. Oral premedication with midazolam (0.1 mg/ kg), diazepam (0.5 mg/kg), and detomidine (0.045 mg/ kg) have been used prior to immobilization with alpha-2-agonist-butorphanol combinations (with or without ketamine) (J. Napier, Z. Gyimesi, and E. Baitman, pers. comm.). In general, no obvious drug effect was reported, although some synergistic effects may have occurred since overall ratings for the procedures were good to excellent. Ranges for intramuscular detomidine-butorphanol-ketamine combinations were as follows: detomidine (0.07–0.08 mg/kg); butorphanol (0.15–0.20 mg/kg); ketamine (0.8–2.0 mg/kg). Other successfully used drugs were medetomidine (0.035 mg/kg) and butorphanol (0.2 mg/kg) given IM (Z. Gyimesi, pers. comm.). Nasal insufflation and intubation with administration of isoflurane have also been used to supplement oxygen and anesthesia in pygmy hippos.

The alpha-2 agonists were reversed with atipamezole at five times the dosage of medetomidine or detomidine administered IM. Naltrexone was typically used to butorphanol at a ratio of 5–16 times the dosage of the opioid. Recovery times were reported as mild sedation at 2–17 minutes after administration of the reversal agents.

Capture of Free-Ranging Pygmy Hippos

Pygmy hippos browse on a variety of natural leaves, as well as crop leaves, such as sweet potato and okra. Similar to their larger counterparts, they use trails to travel to and from the water and these provide opportunities for camera and pit traps (A. Conway, pers. comm.). Few attempts have been made to capture free-ranging pygmy hippos in recent years. Since free-ranging pygmy hippos live in dense vegetation along rivers, darting is not a feasible option. Successful capture of a pygmy hippo in Sierra Leone has been accomplished using a pit trap system (A. Conway, pers. comm.). Pit traps are dug along trails with dimensions of 2 m deep, 2 m long, and 1 m wide. Rice bags containing dirt are placed at the bottom to prevent injury, and a series of small branches are used to support a reed mat to cover the entrance of the pit, which is covered by leaves. The hippo stepping on the mat results in the animal falling into the trap. Immobilization after restraint is feasible. Although not field-tested, a recommended protocol for this procedure would be 0.375-mg/kg medetomidine, 0.9-mg/kg butorphanol, 0.5-mg/ kg ketamine, and ±0.4-mg/kg azaperone IM. The total volume for an adult pygmy hippo would fit in a 3-mL dart. Reversal agents should be naltrexone at three to five times the butorphanol dosage and atipamezole at five times the medetomidine dosage IM.

REFERENCES

Burroughs R, Morkel P, Kock MD, et al. 2006. Chemical immobilization-individual special requirements, hippopotamus. In: *Chemical and Physical Restraint of Wild Animals* (MD Kock, D Meltzer, R Burroughs, eds.), pp. 177–179. Greyton: IWVS (Africa).

Clyde VL, Wallace RS, Pocknell AM. 1998. Dermatitis caused by group G beta-hemolytic *Streptococcus* in Nile hippos (*Hippopotamus amphibious*). Proceedings of the American Association of Zoo Veterinarians, pp. 221–225.

Dumonceaux G, Citino SB, Burton M, et al. 2000. Chemical restraint and surgical removal of a perineal mass from a Nile hippopotamus (*Hippopotamus amphibious*). Proceedings of the American Association of Zoo Veterinarians, pp. 288–290.

Eltringham SK. 1999. *The Hippos*. San Diego: Academic Press.

Flach E, Furrokh IK, Thorton SM, et al. 1998. Caesarean section in a pygmy hippopotamus (*Choeropsis liberiensis*) and the management of the wound. *The Veterinary Record* 143:611–613.

Fleming GJ, Hofmeyr M, Citino SB, et al. 2010. Reversible chemical restraint of the Nile Hippo. Proceedings of the American Association of Zoo Veterinarians and American Association of Wildlife Veterinarians.

Horne WA, Tchamba MA, Loomis MR. 2001. A simple method of providing intermittent positive-pressure ventilation to etorphine-immobilized elephants (*Loxodonta africana*) in the field. *Journal of Zoo and Wildlife Medicine* 32:519–522.

Krueger S, Shellabarger W, Reichard T. 1996. Hippopotamus training: implications for veterinary care. Proceedings of the American Association of Zoo Veterinarians, pp. 54–58.

Loomis MR, Ramsay EC. 1999. Anesthesia for captive nile hippopotamus. In: *Zoo and Wild Animal Medicine: Current Therapy*, 4th ed. (ME Fowler, RE Miller, eds.), pp. 638–639. Philadelphia: W.B. Saunders.

Miller M. 2003. Hippopotamidae (Hippopotamus). In: *Zoo and Wild Animal Medicine—Current Therapy*, 5th ed. (ME Fowler, RE Miller, eds.), pp. 602–612. St Louis: W.B. Saunders.

Miller M. 2007. Hippopotami. In: *Zoo Animal and Wildlife Immobilization and Anesthesia* (G West, D Heard, N Caulkett, eds.), pp. 579–584. Ames: Blackwell.

Morris PJ, Bicknese B, Janssen D, et al. 2001. Chemical restraint of juvenile east African river hippopotamus (*Hippopotamus amphibious kiboko*) at the San Diego Zoo. In: *Zoological Restraint and Anesthesia* (D Heard, ed.). Ithaca: International Veterinary Information Service. http://www.ivis.org (accessed February 8, 2014).

Neiffer DL, Miller MA, Weber M, et al. 2005. Standing sedation in African elephants (*Loxodonta africana*) using detomidine and butorphanol combinations. *Journal of Zoo and Wildlife Medicine* 36:250–256.

Ramsay EC, Loomis MR, Mehren GK, et al. 1998. Chemical restraint of the nile hippopotamus (*Hippopotamus amphibius*) in captivity. *Journal of Zoo and Wildlife Medicine* 29:45–49.

Stalder GL, Petit T, Horowitz I, et al. 2012. Anesthesia in ten captive common hippopotami(*Hippopotamus amphibius*) by medetomidine/ketamine combination. *Journal of the American Veterinary Medical Association* 241:110–116.

Weston HS, Gafella AM, Burt L, et al. 1996. Immobilization of a pygmy hippopotamus (*Choeropsis liberiensis*) for the removal of an oral mass. *Proceedings of the American Association of Zoo Veterinarians* 1996, pp. 576–581.

57 Camelids

Khursheed R. Mama and Chris Walzer

INTRODUCTION

Anesthesia may be required for diagnostic and corrective procedures in veterinary hospitals, in zoological parks, in the field, or in the animal's natural habitat. This chapter will attempt to provide information relevant to anesthetic management of camelids so as to maximize chances of a favorable outcome.

It is important to recognize that camelids are native to very different geographical areas, ranging from the high altitude of the Andes to the deserts of India, Africa, and the Middle East. As such, even though they are all camelids, their physiological adaptations differ. For example, camels are well adapted to drought conditions and may store and draw on water reserves. Llamas and alpacas have a left-shifted oxygen hemoglobin dissociation curve (Chiodi 1970), and their red blood cell configuration and hemoglobin content differs from many other mammalian species (Fowler & Zinkl 1989; Van Houten et al. 1992). These are likely adaptations for survival at high altitudes, where the oxygen tension is low.

PATIENT RESTRAINT AND HANDLING

Fasting prior to general anesthesia is recommended to minimize regurgitation, aspiration, and bloating. Depending on the nature of the procedure and anticipated duration of recumbency, a 12- to 18-hour fasting period is recommended in adult llamas and alpacas; a 24- to 36-hour fast has been recommended for camels. Many recommend withholding water in addition to feed for at least a portion of that time. Fasting of nursing juveniles is not necessary and may increase their stress and likelihood of metabolic derangement.

Camelids may be trained to a halter and led using this. A towel may be hung loosely over the nostrils and mouth in the event that an animal attempts to spit at the handler. A small corral may be used to facilitate catching an individual animal from a herd. An arm placed around the neck of llamas and alpacas will help restrain the patient until a halter can be placed. Chutes designed especially for llamas and alpacas greatly facilitate restraint for procedures, such as catheter placement. Domesticated camels may be restrained in stocks designed for horses or eased to sternal recumbency using a rope placed around the forelimb. They may also be trained to a seated ("cushed") position by their handler.

INSTRUMENTATION

Intravenous catheterization and endotracheal intubation have historically been considered challenging in camelids. Success can be maximized with proper knowledge of the anatomy and availability of appropriate equipment.

The most common site for venous access in camelids is the jugular vein. The greatest challenge in placing a jugular catheter in adult camelids is lack of animal compliance. Many patients will "cush" and rise during the procedure, making for a moving target. Restraint in an appropriate chute or stanchion can help significantly. The other difficulty faced when placing a jugular catheter is locating the vein. Many camelids, especially males, have thick (up to 1 in) skin in the proximal portion of their neck and balloting the vein can prove challenging especially as the vein is fairly deeply located. Knowledge of the anatomical landmarks is

Zoo Animal and Wildlife Immobilization and Anesthesia, Second Edition. Edited by Gary West, Darryl Heard, and Nigel Caulkett.
© 2014 John Wiley & Sons, Inc. Published 2014 by John Wiley & Sons, Inc.

therefore important. In the proximal neck, the jugular vein is located at the bisection of a line drawn caudally from the lower jaw with a line drawn ventrally from the base of the ear (Davis et al. 1996). Despite difficulty palpating the vessel in the proximal portion of the neck, many prefer this site for catheter placement due to better separation between the jugular vein and carotid artery (Davis et al. 1996; Riebold et al. 1989). This approach should also be considered when performing venipuncture for administration of drugs as cerebral injury has been reported following inadvertent intracarotid injection of anesthetic drugs (Valentine et al. 2009), and it can be difficult to differentiate arterial from venous blood in South American camelids due to the brightness of venous blood (Grint & Dugdale 2009). Distention of the vein is best accomplished by holding off behind the palpable ventral projection of the C6 vertebra. If one is still unable to palpate the vein, a narrow gauge (25 or 23) inch to inch and a half needle may be used to locate the same prior to catheter placement.

Once the vein is located and the site appropriately prepared, an incision through all the layers of the skin is recommended in the adult camelid. This incision is best made with a scalpel blade after subcutaneous local anesthetic (1–2 mL of 2% lidocaine) is infiltrated at the site (Heath 1989). In order not to accidentally lacerate the vessel, do not distend the vein while making this incision through which the catheter may then be placed. Continue to distend the vein while the catheter is advanced to minimize the chances of it getting caught on valves within the same. Valves have been anecdotally reported to impede threading the jugular catheter. Secure the catheter so that it does not "kink" at the point of entry through the skin.

Alternate sites for catheter placement include the lateral thoracic vein in adult camels and the cephalic or saphenous vein in juvenile patients. Auricular vessels may be used in anesthetized patients. The size of the catheter used should be appropriate for the size of animal with consideration given to the reason for its placement. For example, a large-gauge catheter similar to that placed in adult patients is generally unnecessary in a 10-kg cria. Alternatively, if significant hypotension is expected in an adult patient due to the disease process or because of anticipated hemorrhage, at least one large-gauge catheter is recommended.

The technique for endotracheal intubation varies with the camelid species in question. For llamas and alpacas, visual orotracheal intubation is facilitated by appropriate equipment and positioning. Ideally, the animal should be placed in sternal recumbency with the head extended. A ruminant mouth gag or strips of tape/gauze may be used to spread the jaws and facilitate visualization using a long, but narrow laryngoscope blade. Intubation may be performed directly using an endotracheal tube or either directly or retrograde by first placing a flexible guide to help direct the endotracheal tube into the trachea (Sanchez et al. 1993). Topical local anesthetic (lidocaine) is used to facilitate intubation in the lightly anesthetized patient. The tube is generally secured behind the ears after the cuff is inflated. Passage of the tube via the nasal passage (nasotracheal intubation) may also be performed in llamas and alpacas. (Riebold et al. 1994) The tube is passed into the trachea via the ventral medial nasal meatus after proper lubrication. While this usually necessitates a smaller tube (e.g., 8- or 9-mm internal diameter vs. 12- or 14-mm internal diameter in an adult llama) than via the oral route and there is a potential for hemorrhage during placement, the tube may be left in place until the animal is fully recovered without fear of the patient chewing it. Vasoconstrictors, such as phenylephrine, may be administered topically to minimize hemorrhage during nasotracheal tube placement. Since camelids are nasal breathers, this method helps minimize the risk of upper airway obstruction in the recovery period. This technique may also be utilized to minimize the need to work around the endotracheal tube during procedures involving the oral cavity.

In adult camels, intubation is usually performed blindly or by manual palpation of the arytenoid cartilages. After the patient is adequately anesthetized, a large animal mouth gag may be used to facilitate introduction of the arm into the oral cavity. If the oral cavity is too narrow, a guide tube may first be inserted into the trachea. Caution must be exercised to prevent laceration of the endotracheal tube on the rear teeth. Depending on the size of the patient, a range of tubes from 16- to 26-mm internal diameter may be necessary (Alsobayil & Mama 1999) (Fig. 57.1).

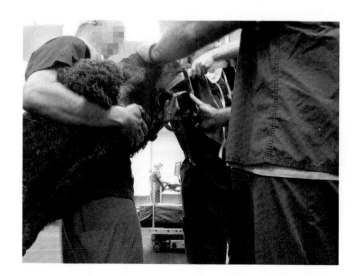

Figure 57.1.   Direct manual intubation of a dromedary camel (photo courtesy of Gary West).

ANESTHETIC TECHNIQUES

Regional and general anesthetic techniques may be used in camelids. General anesthesia may be achieved with injectable agents, inhaled agents, or a combination of these. For the reader who wishes to pursue this further, detailed reviews of anesthetic drugs and techniques for camelids are available (Ali 1988; Alsobayil & Mama 1999; Fowler 1989; Mama 2000). Regardless of the drugs selected, keep in mind that the range of body weights is very broad among camelids, ranging from an 8- to 10-kg newborn cria to a 500-kg camel. Hence, it is important to try to get an accurate weight and calculate dosage based on this. Fiber in adult llamas and alpacas can be very misleading, and when a scale is not available, palpation of the patient may assist in determining weight. Typically, adult alpacas weigh 40–60 kg, and whereas body weight in adult llamas may range from 120 to 300 kg. Body weight also influences equipment requirements, ranging from endotracheal tubes and the anesthetic machine to the type of padding used.

Regional Anesthesia

Regional administration of local anesthetics can facilitate surgical intervention and minimize the need for administration of drugs with systemic effects. Local anesthetics may be used to facilitate a host of procedures. Blocking individual nerves, for example, the mandibular nerve, for dental procedures involving the lower jaw are commonly utilized in awake or sedated patients and as an adjunct to general anesthesia. The anatomy and location of the mandibular and mental foramina to facilitate regional anesthesia at these nerves has been well described (Zhu et al. 2009). Paravertebral blocks similar to those described in both horses and cattle have been used in camelids. (Fowler 1989; Said 1964) as have epidural techniques.

Caudal epidural administration of 12–15 mL of 2% lidocaine in a sternally recumbent adult camel provides anesthesia of the perineum and udder or scrotum for 1–2 hours without influencing motor control (White 1986). Lidocaine (0.22 mg/kg) and xylazine (0.17 mg/kg) have been used to facilitate diagnostic and surgical procedures involving the rectum, vagina and perineum in llamas (Grubb et al. 1993). The onset of anesthesia was 3–4 minutes following either lidocaine or xylazine and lidocaine, but the duration varied significantly lasting about 1 hour in the lidocaine group and 6 hours in the group receiving both drugs. Analgesia following xylazine alone was evident after about 20 minutes and lasted 3 hours. Mild sedation is reported in animals receiving xylazine. Clinical evaluation of efficacy of caudal epidural analgesia with lidocaine, or a combination of lidocaine and xylazine in alpacas undergoing castration, revealed that while a combination or epidural xylazine and lidocaine had the best efficacy, incomplete blockade of the spermatic cord was observed in many animals (Padula 2005). Epidural morphine at doses similar to those used in other species may provide longer-term analgesia and may have value for postoperative analgesia for procedures involving the hind limbs or caudal abdomen and perineum.

Drugs for Sedation and Field Anesthesia in Domesticated Camelids

Many techniques and drugs for sedation and anesthesia have been used in camelids and for detailed information on the same and individual drug effects, the reader is referred to more comprehensive reviews and references therein. (Ali 1988; Alsobayil & Mama 1999; Fowler 1989; Mama 2000). This section of the manuscript will highlight commonly used techniques for domesticated animals.

Intramuscular (IM) and intravenous (IV) administration of xylazine or xylazine and ketamine has been extensively described for use in llamas, alpacas and camels (Bolbol 1991; DuBois et al. 2004; Fowler 1989; Gavier et al. 1988; Prado et al. 2008a; White et al. 1987). While these drugs alone and in combination do provide effects ranging from sedation to short-term anesthesia, the degree (level of sedation or anesthesia) and duration (may range from 10 to 60 minutes) of response in individual animals is variable. The addition of butorphanol to an IM combination of xylazine and ketamine has also been evaluated in llamas and alpacas. Xylazine (0.03 or 0.04 mg/kg, IM), butorphanol (0.3 and 0.4 mg/kg, IM), and ketamine (3 or 4 mg/kg, IM) was administered to seven male llamas and seven male alpacas based on dose recommendations from Dr. LaRue Johnson (Mama et al. 2000). Most animals became recumbent in an average of 4.3 (llamas) and 6.7 (alpacas) minutes. Induction quality was good, with animals generally showing some degree of ataxia before assuming a sternal or lateral position. Despite receiving lower drug doses, llamas appeared more deeply anesthetized and remained recumbent for a longer duration (mean time to standing 63 minutes) than did alpacas (mean time to standing 22 minutes). All animals recovered without apparent complications, but hypoxemia (average PaO_2 of 45–55 mm Hg, barometric pressure 640 mm Hg), and mild hypoventilation (average $PaCO_2$ was 46–49 mm Hg), associated with recumbency, was commonly seen in this study. Direct mean auricular arterial blood pressure was well maintained, averaging 131 mm Hg in llamas and 144 mm Hg in alpacas; heart rate ranged from 29 to 37 beats/min in llamas and 37 to 49 beats/min in alpacas.

Other alpha-2/dissociative and/or benzodiazepine combinations include xylazine and tiletamine/zolazepam or medetomidine and ketamine (DuBois et al. 2004; Hammer et al. 1999; Waldridge et al. 1997) and medetomidine, butorphanol and ketamine (Georoff et al. 2010). Selection of a specific alpha-2 or dissociative agent is in large part based on drug availability, circumstance, and familiarity on the part of the veterinarian. Effects may vary in duration and magnitude but tend to be qualitatively similar between the different agents.

Butorphanol (0.1 mg/kg, IM) has also been used in combination with intratesticular lidocaine (2%, 2–5 mL/testicle) for chemical restraint to facilitate standing castration in over 100 llamas (Barrington et al. 1993). The authors' impression was that the animals receiving butorphanol appeared less stressed than those receiving only intratesticular lidocaine.

Similar drug combinations are utilized for anesthesia in field conditions for camels. White et al. (1987) describe the use of intramuscular xylazine and ketamine individually and in combination. Behavioral responses and measured cardiovascular parameters of the combination were thought to be improved over individually administered drug. Detomidine and medetomidine have also been used alone to provide sedation or in combination with ketamine for anesthesia. In studies evaluating the effect of these drugs on platelet function and coagulation, xylazine, but not detomidine or ketamine, was shown to decrease platelet numbers which might be of relevance for procedures in which bleeding is anticipated (Almubarak 2007). The effects of the alpha-2 drugs may be reversed with yohimbine or atipamezole at the conclusion of the procedure to facilitate a more rapid recovery (Riebold et al. 1986; Waldridge et al. 1997). While tolazoline has also been used successfully in the research environment for reversal of alpha-2 effects (DuBois et al. 2004; Prado et al. 2008a), there have been anecdotal reports suggesting complications following its administration is possible in camelids.

The phenothiazine tranquilizers are a class of drug that seem to be more widely used in camels than in llamas and alpacas. While acepromazine is the tranquilizer most veterinarians are familiar with, other drugs in this class include proprionyl promazine, chlorpromazine and triflupromazine. These drugs tend to have prolonged effects and are not reversible, but in many circumstances, camels are quieted and seem generally less responsive to their surroundings (Alsobayil & Mama 1999). Prado et al. (2008b) report no sedation with acepromazine or acepromazine and butorphanol in young llamas. However, they did demonstrate a longer period of antinociception during anesthesia maintained with Telazol following these treatments.

Drugs for Sedation and Field Anesthesia in Nondomesticated Camelids

Conservation efforts often require capture and handling of animals. Wildlife capture and anesthesia is a complex operation that can cause significant injury or death. Although skill, experience, and appropriate veterinary training can minimize the risk, it is necessary to evaluate whether the procedure is necessary and whether the potential gains in knowledge for conservation of the species outweigh the risks (Osofsky & Hirsch 2000). Many of the aforementioned techniques may be used at modified dosages to provide chemical restraint for nondomesticated camelids. Additional suggestions are provided in the subsequent text.

Wild South American Camelids (SAC) Traditionally, SAC are physically restrained for fiber (wool) harvest using various herding techniques (Bonacic et al. 2006). There are very few reports in the literature detailing the capture and field anesthesia of wild SAC for conservation purposes. One describes the use of tiletamine and zolazepam for immobilization of guanacos in a Chilean national park, but results of this combination were thought to be largely unsatisfactory (Karesh et al. 1998; Sarno et al. 1996). Recently, Georoff et al. (2010) describe use of a combination of IM medetomidine, butorphanol, and ketamine followed by reversal with atipamezole and naltrexone in captive (zoological park) guanacos. They report a reliable onset of anesthesia and effective reversal with no noted behavioral side effects. Due to these favorable qualitative aspects, further evaluation in the field situation is warranted. However, bradycardia, hypertension, and hypoxemia as reported by authors will need to be managed during drug-induced recumbency.

As with guanacos, descriptions of field anesthesia for the smallest SAC, the vicuna (*Vicugna vicugna*) are extremely limited. Ketamine (7.8 mg/kg) and xylazine (1.2 mg/kg) sometimes in combination with midazolam (0.35 mg/kg) and atropine (0.07 mg/kg) has been used successfully in the field setting to collect semen via electroejaculation (Hoyos 2009; Urquieta et al. 1992).

Wild Bactrian camel (*Camelus ferus*) The range of the wild Bactrian camel has been reduced to only three locations worldwide: two in China (Lop Nuur and Taklamakan Desert) and one in Mongolia (Great Gobi A SPA). The population is listed by IUCN as critically endangered and there remain an estimated ~600 animals in China and between 350 and 1950 in the Great Gobi A SPA (Walzer et al. 2008).

Potent opioids, such as etorphine, have been used in camels either alone or in combination with acepromazine, ketamine, xylazine, detomidine, butorphanol and tiletamine, and zolazepam (Blumer et al. 1999; deMaar et al. 1998; Walzer et al. 2005). Pacing is commonly described prior to recumbency when potent opioids are used without a tranquilizer. Significant respiratory depression is a potential complication. Availability of a mechanical breathing device and oxygen supplementation are therefore highly recommended when potent opioids are utilized. Alpha-2 agents, when used, and potent opioids may be reversed at the conclusion of the procedure.

As has been described for other species such as the Asiatic wild ass (*Equus hemionus*) and Przewalski's horse (*Equus ferus prezwalskii*) a chase method (in this instance the animal was darted from a moving jeep) was used to capture a single wild Bactrian camel for radio collaring. This method is similar to that traditionally employed by poachers (Blumer et al. 1999; Walzer 2003). However, whereas poachers use a shot gun, veterinary and conservation personnel typically use a CO_2-powered dart gun (Daninject JM,TM Dan-Inject ApS, Børkop, Denmark) often with a short (4-cm) barrel to facilitate mobility in the confines of the chase vehicle (jeep). When using the chase technique personnel must be sensitive to ambient conditions and to limiting chase time to 15 minutes (or less) to prevent hyperthermia. Additionally, when tracking the animal post injection in the rump, caution must be exercised so it is not disturbed until fully immobilized. Animals are then typically approached from the rear.

Walzer and Kaczensky (2005) describe using the chase technique to induce anesthesia in one male and two female camels with etorphine (4.4 mg), butorphanol (10 mg), detomidine (13 mg), and tiletamine-zolazepam (160 mg). Because ambient temperature varied between −15 and −30°C during the day, all drug combinations were supplemented with propylene glycol to prevent freezing. Anesthesia was reversed with naltrexone (200 mg IV), a long acting opioid antagonist and atipamezole (25 mg IV).

During subsequent expeditions, 10 additional camels were immobilized using the method described above. In 9 of 10 camels, anesthesia and subsequent recovery was uneventful, but one animal, an old bull (>15 years), died during capture. While the cause is unknown, the animal was extremely bloated and appeared to have regurgitated when located approximately 40 minutes post injection (Walzer et al. 2008).

Based on these experiences, the author (Walzer) currently recommends a combination of etorphine (4.4 mg IM), butorphanol (10 mg IM), and detomidine (15 mg IM) for the immobilization of wild adult camels. Butorphanol is used in this combination to a potentially alleviate the marked respiratory depression induced by the etorphine at the μ receptor while potentiating sedation at the κ and σ opioid receptors. This combination can be varied as necessary for the circumstance. For example, the addition of tiletamine-zolazepam provides a more rapid transition to sternal recumbency. Alternatively, by decreasing the etorphine dose by 1 mg and omitting tiletamine and zolazepam, the animal appears sedated but often remains standing or in sternal recumbency. This can be helpful when locating the animal in the steppe landscape, but can also lead to prolonged pacing phase in which the animal can cover a greater distance and potentially injure itself.

While not specific to anesthesia management, a unique drug that has received some consideration for

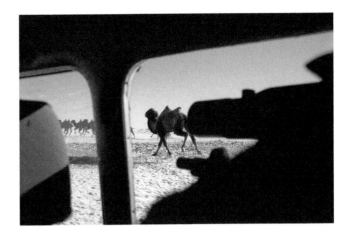

Figure 57.2. Pursuing a herd of wild Bactrian camels in the Great Gobi "A" Strictly Protected Area in Mongolia in order to place a dart (photo courtesy of Petra Kaczensky).

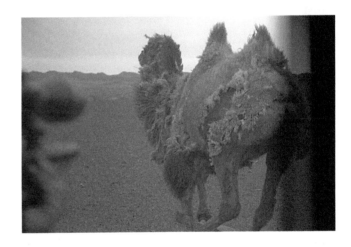

Figure 57.3. Applying a dart to the hindquarters of a wild Bactrian camel from a jeep in the Great Gobi "A" Strictly Protected Area (photo courtesy of Petra Kaczensky).

handling and transportation of camels is reserpine, an indole alkaloid that *irreversibly* blocks uptake of norepinephrine and dopamine (Al-Ani 2004). Its availability in many developed nations, however, is limited, due to significant side effects (Fig. 57.2, Fig. 57.3, Fig. 57.4, Fig. 57.5, and Fig. 57.6).

Anesthetic Techniques for a Hospital Environment

Anesthetic Induction and Short-Term Maintenance The hospital setting provides a more controlled environment and allows one to better titrate drugs to achieve sedation, short-term anesthesia or to transition a patient to inhalation anesthesia. The placement of an intravenous catheter facilitates this titration of the drugs to a given end-point for an individual patient.

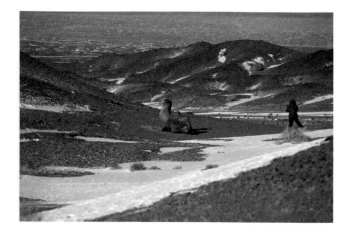

Figure 57.4. Applying a supplemental anesthetic dose to an immobile but not approachable wild Bactrian camel in the Great Gobi "A" Strictly Protected Area in Mongolia (photo courtesy of Petra Kaczensky).

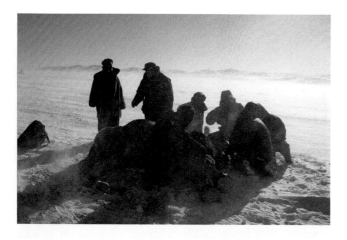

Figure 57.5. Team working in subzero conditions collecting biological samples and placing a satellite radio collar on a wild Bactrian camel (photo courtesy of Petra Kaczensky).

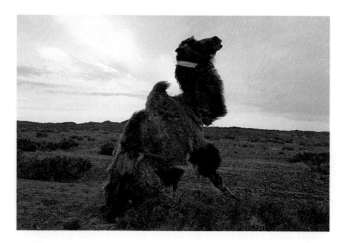

Figure 57.6. A satellite radio-collared, wild Bactrian camel, shakily rising to its feet some 30 seconds after anesthesia reversal with intravenous naltrexone and atipamezole (photo courtesy of Chris Walzer).

Most induction combinations include either ketamine (2–5 mg/kg titrated to effect) or propofol (2 mg/kg titrated to effect) in conjunction with a centrally acting muscle relaxant, such as guaifenesin (25–75 mg/kg), diazepam, or midazolam (0.02–0.1 mg/kg). Use of chloral hydrate alone or with magnesium sulfate has also been described for induction and short term anesthesia maintenance in camels (Ali 1988). Alpha-2 agonists, such as xylazine and medetomidine, may also be used, especially in larger and more unruly animals. These may be administered IM to facilitate catheterization or IV prior to ketamine or propofol. Keep in mind that the dose for xylazine in camelids is in between that reported for cattle (0.03–0.1 mg/kg) and horses (0.3–1.0 mg/kg).

Ketamine combinations have been routinely used for anesthetic induction in camelids. Typically, animals become recumbent about 45 seconds following IV administration, and intubation conditions are good in most circumstances if one is fairly efficient. Additional drugs may be safely administered if the patient maintains pharyngeal tone or is swallowing. A retrospective study describes successful anesthesia maintenance in dromedary camels for a variety of surgical procedures with repeated doses of xylazine and ketamine (Al-Mubarak et al. 2008).

While propofol combinations are not used as frequently, studies do report its safety and efficacy in camelids. For example, propofol was used in camels premedicated with xylazine and diazepam to induce and maintain short-term anesthesia (Fahmy et al. 1995). The same dose has also been used for induction in llamas (Duke et al. 1997).

Inhalation anesthetic induction has been successfully used in llamas and alpacas on occasions where intravenous catheterization prior to anesthetic induction has proved challenging. While regurgitation and aspiration concerns are valid, fasted animals are less likely to manifest these complications. However, this process can be quite time consuming; anesthetic induction was reported to take an average of 17–19 minutes from time of first isoflurane breath to orotracheal intubation in unpremedicated healthy adult llamas (Mama et al. 1999, 2001). This time may be significantly reduced in debilitated patients, and in those receiving premedication.

Anesthetic Maintenance When available, inhalation anesthetic techniques are used to maintain anesthesia in patients undergoing highly invasive surgical procedures (e.g., celiotomy and fracture repair). Halothane, isoflurane, and sevoflurane have all been used been used to maintain anesthesia in camelids, but studies are limited. One report provides the minimum alveolar concentration (MAC) of isoflurane in llamas 1.05 ± 0.17% (Mama et al. 1999), whereas another provides the same information for sevoflurane in both llamas

(2.29 ± 0.14%) and alpacas (2.33 ± 0.09%) (Grubb et al. 2003). These values are similar to those reported in other species and one presumes that adult camels would be similar. A small animal anesthetic machine and breathing circuit are appropriate for llamas and alpacas, whereas a large animal breathing circuit is necessary for adult camels.

Cardiopulmonary and behavioral responses are described with inhalation agents in anesthetized camelids. In adult llamas, a decrease in mean arterial blood pressure and an increase in heart rate were observed with increasing isoflurane dose during both spontaneous and controlled ventilation. Cardiac output and $PaCO_2$ were higher during spontaneous ventilation than during controlled ventilation (Mama et al. 2001). The broadest base of experience in camels is with halothane. Following anesthetic induction with injectable agents, anesthesia has been successfully maintained with halothane vaporizer settings between 1% and 3% (Singh et al. 1994; White et al. 1986). Blood pressure is reported to be in the same range as for other domestic species, but with a tendency toward higher values much like those observed in cattle. Rapid shallow breaths and rising $PaCO_2$ values are also described. During inhalation-induced recumbency, spontaneous behaviors (e.g., swallowing and limb movement) decreased with increasing anesthetic depth. Jaw tone and palpebral reflex activity also decreased as isoflurane dose increased. Recovery from anesthesia was also reported to be uneventful (Mama et al. 1999, 2001; Singh et al. 1994; White et al. 1986).

Inhalation anesthetics are the mainstay for anesthetic maintenance, but the need for specialized delivery equipment generally limits the use of this technique to the hospital environment. While expensive, the advent of short-acting, rapidly cleared IV drugs, such as propofol, provides veterinarians with the option of maintaining general anesthesia using continuous infusions. Two intravenous infusion doses of propofol (0.2 mg/kg/min and 0.4 mg/kg/min) used for anesthetic maintenance in llamas have been assessed after a 2 mg/kg induction dose (Duke et al. 1997). The infusions were maintained for 60 minutes during which time llamas receiving the higher dose appeared adequately anesthetized and generally unresponsive to external stimuli, whereas llamas receiving the lower dose were noise sensitive and made some weak attempts to raise their head. Animals stood an average of 13–22 minutes following termination of the low and high dose infusion, respectively, and showed little to no ataxia.

During anesthetic maintenance with both infusions of propofol the heart rate was increased (to approximately 90 beats/min) over predrug values (of approximately 55 beats/min). Mean carotid arterial pressure was similar to predrug values and ranged from an average of 103 to 147 mmHg during drug-induced recumbency. The $PaCO_2$ increased and PaO_2 decreased

in recumbent animals but were felt to be within a clinically acceptable range. Three llamas did, however, become dyspneic and required placement of a nasopharyngeal tube to ensure a patent airway.

Combinations of inhalation agents and injectable drugs may also be of benefit in managing general anesthesia. In one study, authors describe a mean reduction in isoflurane dose requirement of 37% when receiving 40 μg/kg/min of ketamine by IV infusion (Schlipf et al. 2005). Another report describes a small but not statistically significant decrease in bispectral index values following 0.1 mg/kg IV of butorphanol in isoflurane-anesthetized alpacas, indicating a potential benefit (Garcia-Pereira et al. 2007). Except for a decrease in systemic vascular resistance, cardiovascular parameters were largely unchanged after butorphanol; as animals were ventilated, effects on respiration could not be assessed. Larenza et al. 2008 describe the successful use of a more complex protocol using fentanyl s-ketamine, midazolam, and isoflurane in an alpaca with increased anesthetic risk. Respiratory function was, however, negatively affected.

Muscle Relaxation during General Anesthesia When muscle relaxation provided by the anesthetic agents alone is not adequate (e.g., intraocular surgery and reduction/repair of a displaced long bone fracture), drugs that block the neuromuscular junction (peripherally acting muscle relaxants) are used as adjuncts during general anesthesia. The efficacy of atracurium, administered via intermittent IV bolus (0.15 mg/kg initial dose, followed by 0.08 mg/kg) or IV infusion (0.15 mg/kg initial dose, followed by 0.4 mg/kg/h), has been evaluated in halothane anesthetized, mechanically ventilated llamas (Hildebrand & Hill 1993). Another report suggests that both succinylcholine and gallamine may be used successfully to supplement relaxation during general anesthesia in camels (Held & Paddleford 1982). When using these agents, it is essential to be aware that they provide no analgesic or sedative properties and that ventilation will be significantly depressed.

ANESTHETIC RECOVERY

Although the occasional patient may have a violent recovery, in general, camelids recover well from anesthesia. When possible, it is ideal to place the camelid in a sternal posture with the head elevated. This allows both for eructation and helps minimize any nasal edema. Oxygen insufflation during this period is also beneficial. If the patient is orotracheally intubated, the endotracheal tube should be protected so it does not get lacerated by the molars. In the alpaca and llama this is relatively easy to do with a partially used 2-in roll of tape which can be placed over the tube in the mouth with a tab hanging out. It is important not to remove the endotracheal tube until one is sure that the patient can control their airway. Camelids frequently show early arousal and chew their tube and raise their head briefly and then seemingly "fall asleep" again. Removal of the tube in this early period therefore can result in airway obstruction. Often, this is silent and only evident when observing the chest move inward (as opposed to outward) during inspiration. Intervention is critical and may be as simple as extending the head and trying to get the patient to swallow and providing oxygen; in extreme cases, reintubation is necessary.

ANALGESIC TECHNIQUES

While efficacy of local and regional anesthetic techniques is reported in camelids (Barrington et al. 1993; Grubb et al. 1993), there is very little published regarding benefits or side effects of systemically administered analgesics in these animals. Hence, much of the use is based on personal preference and extrapolation from other species. Evaluation is further confounded by difficulty in assessing clinical signs of and hence resolution of pain. While no animal should suffer because of pain, one should continue to obtain evidence for efficacy of analgesic drugs to ensure appropriate therapy for the patient.

Nonsteroidal anti-inflammatory drugs and opioids have been used and studied to a limited extent in South American Camelids (llamas). The pharmacokinetics of ketoprofen, phenylbutazone, and flunixin meglumine are described in llamas (Navarre et al. 2001a, 2001b, 2001c). However as authors state, the determination of serum or plasma concentrations associated with analgesia are only extrapolated from other species; serum concentrations between 0.4 and 0.6 μg/mL of ketoprofen are considered effective in humans, and a target of 5–15 μg/mL is suggested for phenylbutazone in horses. As plasma or serum concentrations may not truly represent therapeutic effects at the site of the lesion within the tissue, relating kinetic data to clinical efficacy is further confounded. However, these drugs continue to be used in camelids with apparent clinical success.

Use of the opioids in the clinical environment is perhaps more controversial. While potent opioids have been used to provide immobilization, information on the use of these drugs as analgesics is limited. There is one report suggesting use of intramuscular butorphanol (0.1 mg/kg) is of some benefit in animals experiencing somatic pain; the short half-life following intravenous butorphanol was thought to limit its clinical usefulness (Carroll et al. 2001). Mixed results were described by authors assessing analgesia produced by morphine in healthy llamas. A dose of 0.25 mg/kg IV produced the most consistent increase in tolerance to a cutaneous electrical stimulus in this report (Uhrig et al. 2007). While studies such as these may not represent the true clinical condition, the variability in response when compared with the effects of these drugs in

studies conducted in other species (e.g., dog) suggest the need for further evaluation.

MONITORING DURING ANESTHETIC-INDUCED RECUMBENCY

Monitoring anesthetic depth in camelids can be challenging as they maintain ocular reflexes at seemingly all planes of anesthesia. In addition to a brisk palpebral, the globe also tends to rotate periodically during anesthesia and to the inexperienced individual, this is quite disconcerting, but seems to bear little correlation with movement in response to a noxious stimulus. Eyelid aperture (or the distance between eyelids) has been correlated and widens with increasing inhalant anesthetic depth in llamas (Mama et al. 2001). Jaw tone is another useful method for monitoring anesthetic depth in the smaller camelids. Assessment of prepucial and rectal tone, drooping of the lower lip, relaxation of neck, and abdominal and tail musculature have been advocated by some as another means to assess depth of anesthesia and muscle relaxation (Alsobayil & Mama 1999).

Guidelines for monitoring physiologic responses during drug-induced recumbency are much the same as for any other species. The degree of monitoring should be appropriate for the patient's health status and with regard to the procedure; monitoring a young animal undergoing a castration will differ significantly from a patient needing abdominal exploratory surgery.

Monitoring for short-term chemical restraint in a field situation may include auscultation of the heart and lungs, palpation of the pulse, and evaluation of mucous membrane color and refill time. Changes in muscle tone or gross movement are commonly used to assess anesthetic depth. For longer procedures or those in which the animal may be at more risk, noninvasive battery-powered monitors, such as a pulse oximeter and Doppler or oscillometric blood pressure monitor, may easily be placed. A rectal thermometer is used to monitor body temperature if deemed necessary. While it is recommended that record notations be made at 5-minute intervals, it is ideal to observe the patient continuously.

In a referral hospital setting, monitoring is generally more extensive as patients are often significantly compromised. Typically, in addition to pulse palpation and observation of mucous membranes, the cardiovascular system is evaluated using an electrocardiogram (ECG) to assess heart rate and rhythm, and an arterial catheter is placed for direct (invasive) blood pressure monitoring. ECG leads function best when clips are placed in areas with less fiber (axilla and flank or upper lip/base of the ear). Depending on the procedure, leads should be placed on either side of the heart or cranial and caudal to the heart. Arterial catheters (20- or 22-gauge 3–5 cm) are commonly placed in the auricular or medial saphenous artery, but the carpal, cranial tibial, or middle coccygeal artery may also be used in camels. Heart rate ranges from 60 to 120 beats per minute in llamas and alpacas during inhalation anesthesia, but may be significantly lower if alpha-2 agonists are used. In camels, heart rate is more typically 40–50 beats per minute, but bradycardia and second-degree AV block may be observed with use of alpha-2 agonists (White et al. 1987). Blood pressure in llamas and alpacas seems to be quite labile and may vary from a mean pressure of 50–60 mmHg to 100 mmHg for seemingly no apparent reason. Despite this, studies have shown that there is a trend and blood pressure decreases with increasing inhalation anesthetic depth, as has been shown for other species (Mama et al. 2001).

A thermistor probe is placed nasally or rectally for evaluation of body temperature and either a pulse oximeter (SpO_2) and capnograph or arterial blood gases ($PaCO_2$, PaO_2) are used to evaluate pulmonary function. Values are similar to those observed in other domestic species or in the range of 95–100% for SpO_2 and 40–50 mmHg for end tidal and $PaCO_2$. PaO_2 values are influenced by the inspired oxygen and may range from 80 to 100 mmHg at sea level for a patient breathing room air to 500 mmHg for a patient breathing 100% oxygen. Keep in mind that altitude will significantly decrease these values.

For critically ill patients, glucose, electrolyte, and acid–base monitoring, and measurement of PCV and TP can add useful information. Note that unlike most other species, apparently healthy llamas and alpacas frequently have a packed cell volume (PCV) ranging upwards from the mid-20s.

Monitoring abdominal distention and for the presence (and volume) or absence of regurgitation, and for degree of nasal edema during drug-induced recumbency are also important as they may indicate the need for intervention to ensure a favorable outcome (Fig. 57.7 and Fig. 57.8).

SUPPORT DURING ANESTHETIC-INDUCED RECUMBENCY

As with monitoring, supportive care should also be related to patient's needs with some exceptions. For example, the eye should always be protected and lubricated in camelids as they tend to protrude from the head and are easily traumatized. Attention should always be given to patient positioning so as not to cause neural or muscle damage; lower forelimb pulled forward in lateral recumbency and upper limbs supported in a natural position (not hanging). In dorsal recumbency, the limbs should be flexed. For longer procedures or larger patients, padding becomes increasingly important. Air or foam mattresses and water beds have all been utilized successfully.

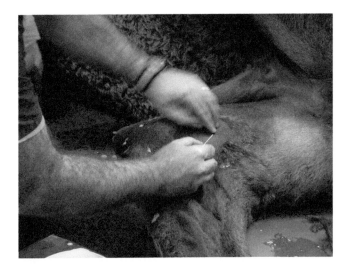

Figure 57.7. Placement of an arterial catheter in the medial saphenous artery (photo courtesy of Gary West).

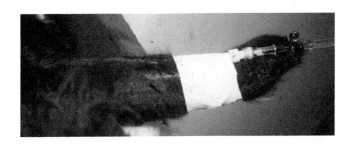

Figure 57.8. Placement of an arterial catheter in the auricular artery of a llama.

In cool environments or in young and small patients, external heat should be provided, whereas active cooling may be necessary in warm environments. Circulating air or water blankets or radiant heat lamps may be used for warmth, whereas providing shade or using a fan or simply hosing the patient with water will help keep the patient cool.

A balanced electrolyte solution should be administered intravenously to patients undergoing inhalation anesthesia or those in whom recumbency is expected to last greater than 1 hour. An administration rate of 5 mL/kg/h is suggested for most patients. Dehydrated patients should receive a fluid volume appropriate for the perceived level (e.g., 5% of a 100-kg animal is equivalent to 5 L). If heart rate or blood pressure values fall out of the normal range, additional intervention may be necessary. This may include anticholinergics, such as atropine, and inotropes/vasopressors, such as ephedrine, dobutamine, or phenylephrine. A recent study describes the use of both dobutamine (4 and 8 µg/kg/min) and norepinephrine (0.3 and 1 µg/kg/min) in isoflurane-anesthetized alpacas. Both drugs increased cardiac output and appeared safe and effective at the lower dose studied for each drug. At higher doses, increased arrhythmogenicity was observed for dobutamine, and excessive vasoconstriction was a noted side effect for norepinephrine (Vincent et al. 2009).

In critically ill patients, electrolytes may need to be adjusted and acid–base balance corrected. In very young patients, glucose supplementation may be necessary. Methods for calculating and adjusting these values are available.

While oxygen is routinely used in patients during inhalation anesthesia, this is less common when using injectable techniques. Since llamas and alpacas have been shown to become hypoxic during injectable anesthetics, oxygen supplementation is highly recommended especially for patients at altitude. Camels are also prone to hypoxemia due to their body mass, and oxygen supplementation should always be considered during recumbency. Availability of lightweight aluminum tanks and flow meters has made this easier to achieve in field conditions. The flow meter is connected to a small flexible hose placed in the ventromedial nasal meatus up to the medial canthus of the eye. An ambu bag should be available in case of a need to ventilate a patient in the field. For a patient connected to a breathing circuit, manual or mechanical ventilation is easily accomplished.

While uncommon in llamas and alpacas, recumbent camels may bloat, and placement of a "bloat" tube may be necessary to help relieve this and minimize the influence on venous return and pulmonary function. Because these animals are obligate nasal breathers, nasal edema can be problematic following extubation. When possible, the head should be positioned to allow drainage of regurgitant fluid while still minimizing edema. Alternatively, vasoconstrictors, such as phenylephrine, may be diluted and gently placed in the nasal passages prior to extubation. If food material is observed from the nose, gentle lavage (after ensuring the endotracheal tube cuff is sealed) is recommended.

SUMMARY

Chances of a favorable outcome are increased with an understanding of basic physiological differences between camelids and other species, and selection of appropriate drug, monitoring, and supportive techniques (Table 57.1 and Table 57.2).

Table 57.1. Drug protocols for sedation and anesthesia in domesticated healthy adult camelids[a]

Drug or Drug Combination	Dose (mg/kg) and Route of Administration	Approximate Onset (Minute) of Action and Anticipated End Point	Approximate Duration of Anesthetic Action	Anticipated Recovery for Drugs Resulting in General Anesthesia
Sedation				
Acepromazine	0.05–0.1, IM	5–15, tranquilization	1–4 hours	N/A
Xylazine	0.25, IM	15, sedation	1–4 hours	N/A
	0.1–0.2, IV	5, sedation	1–4 hours	N/A
Anesthesia				
Xylazine	0.1–0.2, IM	5–10, recumbency	10–20 minutes	45 minutes to 2 hours
Ketamine	2–3, IM			
Xylazine	0.03–0.05, IM	5–10, recumbency	10–20 minutes	20 minutes to 1 hour
Butorphanol	0.3–0.5, IM			
Ketamine	2–4, IM			
Xylazine	0.1–0.2, IM	45 seconds after guaifenesin and ketamine, recumbency	10–20 minutes	45 minutes to 2 hours
Guaifenesin	50–100, IV			
Ketamine	1–2, IV			
Xylazine	0.1–0.2, IM	45 seconds after diazepam and ketamine, recumbency	10–20 minutes	45 minutes to 2 hours
Diazepam	0.1–0.25, IV			
Ketamine	1–2, IV			
Xylazine	0.1–0.25, IV	1 minute after propofol, recumbency	10–20 minutes	45 minutes to 2 hours
Diazepam	0.25, IV			
Propofol	2, IV			
Maintenance				
Halothane	Vaporizer set between 0.8% and 1.5%	Administered to effect	Administered to effect	30–90 minutes following discontinuation
Isoflurane	Vaporizer set between 1% and 2%	Administered to effect	Administered to effect	20–60 minutes following discontinuation
Sevoflurane	Vaporizer set between 2% and 3%	Administered to effect	Administered to effect	20–60 minutes following discontinuation

[a]Dosages are approximate and may need adjustment for the individual patient and scenario.

Table 57.2. Drug protocols for sedation and anesthesia in domesticated neonatal camelids[a]

Drug or Drug Combination	Dose (mg/kg) and Route of Administration	Approximate Onset of Action and Anticipated End Point	Approximate Duration of Anesthetic Action	Anticipated Recovery for Drugs Resulting In General Anesthesia
Sedation				
Butorphanol	0.05–0.1, IV	30 seconds–1 minute	10–20 minutes	N/A
Diazepam	0.05–0.2, IV	30 seconds–1 minute	10–20 minutes	N/A
Anesthesia				
Isoflurane	1–3% by mask, to recumbency	Variable but within 5 minutes	While being administered	15–30 minutes after discontinuation
Sevoflurane	2–4% by mask, to recumbency	Variable but within 5 minutes	While being administered	15–30 minutes after discontinuation
Diazepam Ketamine	0.05–0.1, IV 1–2, IV	30–45 seconds after administration	10–20 minutes	30 minutes
Diazepam Propofol	0.05–0.1, IV 1–2, IV	30–45 seconds after administration	5–15 minutes	20–30 minutes

[a]Dosages are approximate and may need adjustment for the individual patient and scenario.

REFERENCES

Al-Ani FK. 2004. Anesthesia and surgery. In: *Camel: Management and Diseases*, p. 342. Amman: Al-Shraq Printing Press.

Ali BH. 1988. A survey of some drugs commonly used in the camel. *Veterinary Research Communications* 12:67–75.

Almubarak AI. 2007. Effects of some anaesthetics and chemical restraints on blood clotting in camels. *Journal of Animal and Veterinary Advances* 6(1):33–35.

Al-Mubarak AI, Abdin-Bey MR, Ramadan RO. 2008. A retrospective clinical evaluation of xylazine-ketamine total intravenous anaesthesia (TIVA) in dromedary camels. *Journal of Camel Practice and Research* 15(2):201–203.

Alsobayil FA, Mama KR. 1999. Anesthetic management of dromedary camels. *Compendium of Continuing Education Food Animal Supplement* 21(3):102–111.

Barrington GM, Meyer TF, Parish SM. 1993. Standing castration of the llama using butorphanol tartrate and local anesthesia. *Equine Practice* 15:35–39.

Blumer ES, Namshir Z, Tuya T, et al. 1999. Field studies of wild Bactrian camels (*Camelus bactrianus ferus*) in Mongolia. Proceedings of the American Association of Zoo Veterinarians, pp. 187–190.

Bolbol AE. 1991. Clinical use of combined xylazine and ketamine anaesthesia in the dromedary. *Assuit Veterinary Medical Journal* 25:186–192.

Bonacic C, Feber RE, Macdonald DW. 2006. Capture of vicuna (*Vicugna vicugna*) for sustainable use: animal welfare implications. *Biological Conservation* 129:543–550.

Carroll GL, Boothe DM, Hartsfield SM, et al. 2001. Pharmacokinetics and pharmacodynamics of butorphanol in llamas after intravenous and intramuscular administration. *Journal of the American Veterinary Medical Association* 219(9):1263–1268.

Chiodi H. 1970. Comparative study of blood gas transport in high altitude and sea level camilidae and goats. *Respiration Physiology* 11:84–93.

Davis IA, McGaffin JR, Kuchinka GD. 1996. Intravenous catheterization of the external jugular vein in llamas. *Compendium of Continuing Education Food Animal Supplement* 18(3):330–335.

deMaar TWJ, Bohuis H, Mugo MJ. 1998. Field anesthesia of camels (*Camelus dromedarius*) and the use of medetomidine/ketamine with atipamezole reversal. Proceedings AAZV and AAWV Joint Conference, pp. 54–57.

DuBois WR, Prado TM, Ko JH, et al. 2004. A comparison of two intramuscular doses of xylazine-ketamine combination and tolazoline reversal in llamas. *Veterinary Anaesthesia and Analgesia* 31:90–96.

Duke T, Egger CM, Ferguson JG, et al. 1997. Cardiopulmonary effects of propofol infusion in llamas. *American Journal of Veterinary Research* 58(2):153–156.

Fahmy LS, Farag KA, Mostafa MB, et al. 1995. Propofol anaesthesia with xylazine and diazepam premedication in camels. *Journal of Camel Practice and Research* 2(2):111–114.

Fowler ME. 1989. Anesthesia. In: *Medicine and Surgery of South American Camelids* (ME Fowler, ed.), pp. 51–63. Ames: Iowa State University Press.

Fowler ME, Zinkl JG. 1989. Reference ranges for hematologic and serum biochemical values in llamas (*Lama glama*). *American Journal of Veterinary Research* 50(12):2049–2053.

Garcia-Pereira FL, Greene SA, Keegan RD, et al. 2007. Effects of intravenous butorphanol on cardiopulmonary function in isoflurane-anesthetized alpacas. *Veterinary Anaesthesia and Analgesia* 34:269–274.

Gavier D, Kittleson MD, Fowler ME, et al. 1988. Evaluation of a combination of xylazine, ketamine and halothane for anesthesia in llamas. *American Journal of Veterinary Research* 49:2047–2055.

Georoff TA, James SB, Kalk P, et al. 2010. Evaluation of medetomidine-ketamine-butorphanol anesthesia with atipamezole-naltrexone antagonism in captive male guanacos (*Lama guanicoe*). *Journal of Zoo and Wildlife Medicine* 41(2):255–262.

Grint N, Dugdale A. 2009. Brightness of venous blood in South American Camelids: implications for jugular catheterization. *Veterinary Anaesthesia and Analgesia* 36:63–66.

Grubb TL, Riebold TW, Huber MJ. 1993. Evaluation of lidocaine, xylazine and a combination of lidocaine and xylazine for epidural analgesia in llamas. *Journal of the American Veterinary Medical Association* 203:1441–1444.

Grubb TL, Schlipf JW, Riebold TW, et al. 2003. Minimum alveolar concentration of sevoflurane in spontaneously breathing llamas and alpacas. *Journal of the American Veterinary Medical Association* 223(8):1167–1169.

Hammer S, Gualy M, Bonath KH. 1999. Medetomidine/ketamine-anesthesia of llama (*Lama glama*) under field conditions and its influence on haemodynamics, respiration and metabolism. Proceedings of the 3rd European Symposium and Supreme European Seminar, pp. 267–268.

Heath RB. 1989. Llama anesthetic programs. *The Veterinary Clinics of North America. Food Animal Practice* 5:71–80.

Held JP, Paddleford RR. 1982. Clinical use of succinylcholine and gallamine in the camel (*Camelus bactrianus*) during general anesthesia. *Journal of Zoo Animal Medicine* 13:84–87.

Hildebrand SV, Hill T. 1993. Neuromuscular blockade by use of atracurium in anesthetized llamas. *American Journal of Veterinary Research* 54:429–433.

Hoyos MAE. 2009. Reproducción en la vicuna macho (Vicugna vicugna): evaluacion del método de contención química, colección de semen, análisis del eyaculado y biometría testicular. Master's Thesis, Universidad Nacional Mayor de San Marcos.

Karesh W, Uhart M, Dierenfeld E et al. 1998. Health evaluation of free-ranging guanaco (*Lama guanicoe*). *Journal of Zoo and Wildlife Medicine* 29:134–141.

Larenza MP, Zanolari P, Jaggin Shmucker N. 2008. Balanced anesthesia and ventilation strategies for an alpaca (*Lama pacos*) with an increased anesthetic risk. *Schweizer Archiv fur Tierheilkunde* 150(2):77–81.

Mama KR. 2000. Anesthetic management of camelids. In: *Recent Advances in Anesthetic Management of Large Domestic Animals* (EP Steffey, ed.). Ithaca: International Veterinary Information Service. http://www.ivis.org/advances/steffey_anesthesia/mama_camelids/ivis.pdf (accessed on March 12, 2014).

Mama KR, Wagner AE, Parker DA, et al. 1999. Determination of minimum alveolar concentration of isoflurane in llamas. *Veterinary Surgery* 28:121–125.

Mama KR, Aubin ML, Johnson LW. 2000. Experiences with xylazine butorphanol and ketamine for short term anesthesia in llamas and alpacas. Proceedings of the World Congress of Veterinary Anaesthesia, 104.

Mama KR, Wagner AE, Steffey EP. 2001. Circulatory, respiratory and behavioral responses in isoflurane anesthetized llamas. *Veterinary Anaesthesia and Analgesia* 28(1):12–17.

Navarre CB, Ravis WR, Campbell J, et al. 2001a. Stereoselective pharmacokinetics of ketoprofen in llamas following intravenous administration. *Journal of Veterinary Pharmacology and Therapeutics* 24:223–226.

Navarre CB, Ravis WR, Nagilla R, et al. 2001b. Pharmacokinetics of phenylbutazone in llamas following single intravenous and oral doses. *Journal of Veterinary Pharmacology and Therapeutics* 24:227–231.

Navarre CB, Ravis WR, Nagilla R, et al. 2001c. Pharmacokinetics of flunixin meglumine in llamas following a single intravenous dose. *Journal of Veterinary Pharmacology and Therapeutics* 24: 361–364.

Osofsky SA, Hirsch KJ. 2000. Chemical restraint of endangered mammals for conservation purposes: a practical primer. *Oryx* 34:27–33.

Padula AM. 2005. Clinical evaluation of caudal epidural anaesthesia for the neutering of alpacas. *The Veterinary Record* 156: 616–617.

Prado TM, DuBois WR, Ko JCH, et al. 2008a. A comparison of two combinations of xylazine-ketamine administered intramuscularly to alpacas and of reversal with tolazoline. *Veterinary Anaesthesia and Analgesia* 35:201–207.

Prado TM, Doherty TJ, Boggan EB, et al. 2008b. Effects of acepromazine and butorphanol on tiletamine-zolazepam anesthesia in llamas. *American Journal of Veterinary Research* 69(2): 182–188.

Riebold TW, Kaneps AJ, Schmotzer WB. 1986. Reversal of xylazine-induced sedation in llamas, using doxapram or 4-aminopyridine or yohimbine. *Journal of the American Veterinary Medical Association* 189(9):1051–1061.

Riebold TW, Kaneps AJ, Schmotzer WB. 1989. Anesthesia in the llama. *Veterinary Surgery* 18:400–404.

Riebold TW, Engel HN, Grubb TL, et al. 1994. Orotracheal and nasotracheal intubation in llamas. *Journal of the American Veterinary Medical Association* 204(5):779–783.

Said AH. 1964. Some aspects of anaesthesia in the camel. *The Veterinary Record* 76:550–554.

Sanchez TF, Janssen DD, Morris PJ, et al. 1993. Assisted intubation techniques in llama (*Lama glama*): retrograde intubation. Proceedings Am Assoc of Zoo Vets, pp. 161–167.

Sarno RJ, Hunter RL, Franklin WL. 1996. Immobilization of guanacos by use of tiletamine/zolazepam. *Journal of the American Veterinary Medical Association* 208(3):408–409.

Schlipf JW, Eaton K, Fulkerson P, et al. 2005. Constant rate infusion of ketamine reduces minimal alveolar concentration of isoflurane in alpacas. *Veterinary Anaesthesia and Analgesia* 32:7.

Singh R, Peshin PK, Patil B, et al. 1994. Evaluation of halothane as an anesthetic in camels (*Camelus dromedaries*). *Zentralbl Veterinarmed A* 41:359–368.

Uhrig SR, Papich MG, KuKanich B, et al. 2007. Pharmacokinetics and pharmacodynamics of morphine in llamas. *American Journal of Veterinary Research* 68(1):25–34.

Urquieta B, Schiappacasse FM, Raggi SL, et al. 1992. Sedation, immobilization and anesthesia with xylazine-ketamine in vicuna (*Vicugna vicugna*). *Avances en Ciencias veterinarias* 7: 177–184.

Valentine BA, Riebold TW, Wolff PL, et al. 2009. Cerebral injury from intracarotid injection in an alpaca (*Vicugna pacos*). *Journal of Veterinary Diagnostic Investigation* 21:149–152.

Van Houten D, Weiser MG, Johnson L, et al. 1992. Reference hematologic values and morphologic features of blood cells in healthy adult llamas. *American Journal of Veterinary Research* 53(10):1773–1775.

Vincent CJ, Hawley AT, Rozanski EA, et al. 2009. Cardiopulmonary effects of dobutamine and norepinephrine infusion in healthy anesthetized alpacas. *American Journal of Veterinary Research* 70(10):1236–1242.

Waldridge BM, Lin HC, De Graves FJ, et al. 1997. Sedative effects of medetomidine and its reversal by atipamezole in llamas. *Journal of the American Veterinary Medical Association* 211(12): 1562–1565.

Walzer C. 2003. Equidae. In: *Zoo and Wild Animal Medicine, Current Therapy* (ME Fowler, RE Miller, eds.), pp. 578–586. Philadelphia: W.B. Saunders.

Walzer C, Kaczensky P. 2005. Wild camel training and collaring mission for the Great Gobi a strictly protected area in Mongolia. Final report for UNDP for the short-term international expert contracts. http://www.savethewildhorse.org/files/Downloads/PDF/Studies/2005_12_22_report_camel_collaring%5B1%5D.pdf (accessed November 13, 2011).

Walzer C, Kaczensky P, Enkhbileg D, et al. 2008. Through the eye of the deaert to capture and collar wild Bactrian camels (*Camelus ferus*). Proceedings AAZV-AARV Joint Conference, pp. 90–94.

White RJ. 1986. Anaesthetic management of the camel. In: *The Camel in Health and Disease* (A Higgens, ed.), pp. 136–148. Philadelphia: Balliere Tindall.

White RJ, Bark H, Balis S. 1986. Halothane anaesthesia in the dromedary camel. *The Veterinary Record* 119:615–617.

White RJ, Bali S, Bark H. 1987. Xylazine and ketamine anesthesia in the dromedary camel under field conditions. *The Veterinary Record* 120:110–113.

Zhu L, Want JL, Zhang H. 2009. A survey on the mandible of Bactrian camel (*Camelus bactrianus*) and Yak (*Bos grunniens*); implications for regional anaesthesia of the mandible. *Journal of Camel Practice and Research* 16(2):237–239.

58 Giraffidae

Scott B. Citino and Mitchell Bush

TAXONOMY AND BIOLOGY

Giraffids were once very diverse and widespread throughout Africa, Asia, and Europe. Presently, only two genera with one species per genera are extant within the family *Giraffidae*: the giraffe, *Giraffa camelopardalis*, and the okapi, *Okapia johnstoni*. Historically, nine subspecies of giraffe have been described based on body size, color, coat pattern, and geographic distribution (Dagg & Foster 1976; Nowak & Paradiso 1983). Recent mitochondrial DNA and nuclear microsatellite analysis show that there are at least six genealogically distinct lineages of giraffe with little evidence of interbreeding between them, and five of the six lineages also contain genetically discrete populations, yielding at least 11 genetically distinct populations (Brown et al. 2007). Shared characteristics of giraffids include long legs with forelegs longer than rear legs, elongated necks, large eyes and ears, long, dark, prehensile tongues, lack of a gallbladder in most animals, thick skin with coat patterns that provide camouflage, and the presence of skin-covered ossicones that arise over the parietal bones in giraffe and the frontal bones in okapi (Bush 2003; Dagg & Foster 1976; Nowak & Paradiso 1983). Giraffids are browsing ruminants that are highly selective feeders. Their stature allows them to exploit feeding niches unavailable to other terrestrial herbivores. Giraffe dwell primarily in *Acacia*-, *Commiphora*-, and *Terminalia*- dominated savannahs and semi-arid, open woodlands, while the okapi lives in the mid-elevation, equatorial hardwood forests of northeast Democratic Republic of the Congo (Dagg & Foster 1976; Nowak & Paradiso 1983). Okapi live relatively secretive, solitary lives, while giraffe are more social, living in loosely organized female herds and subadult male bachelor groupings with solitary adult males.

ANATOMY AND PHYSIOLOGY RELATED TO ANESTHESIA

The art and science of giraffe anesthesia remains a challenge due to their unique anatomy and physiology, which presents inherent risks during chemical restraint and, consequently, can result in unacceptable morbidity or mortality. Their large size and cumbersome shape limits physical control during critical times of induction and recovery, and limits manipulation once the giraffe is down. Adult giraffes range from 4.5- to 5.5-m tall and can weigh from 500 to 1950 kg, with males being larger (Bush 2003; Dagg & Foster 1976; Nowak & Paradiso 1983). Even weighing giraffe during anesthetic procedures can be difficult due to their size and shape. Formulas have been published to estimate weight from body measurements (Hall-Martin 1977). Adult okapi range in weight from 240 to 350 kg and have shoulder heights of 1.5–1.8 m, with females being larger (Nowak & Paradiso 1983; S. Citino, pers. obs. and unpubl. data, 2011). Giraffes have a characteristic long neck, which if not controlled, acts as a lever arm during inductions and recoveries, creating a danger to the giraffe and/or the support staff. Malpositioning of the neck can lead to airway obstruction and/or cramping or focal myopathies of neck muscles, which can produce fatalities (Bush et al. 2002; S. Citino, pers. obs. and unpubl. data, 2011). The giraffe's long neck also presents unique problems in regards to regulation of systemic arterial blood pressure, maintenance of cerebral circulation, and generation of respiratory dead space (Bush 1993, 2003; Bush et al. 2002; Hargens 1988; Hargens et al. 1987; Hugh-Jones et al. 1978; Langman 1973; Mitchell & Skinner 1993; Pedley et al. 1996; Warren 1974). To maintain cerebral circulation, giraffe maintain the highest mean arterial pressure at the level of the heart

Zoo Animal and Wildlife Immobilization and Anesthesia, Second Edition. Edited by Gary West, Darryl Heard, and Nigel Caulkett.
© 2014 John Wiley & Sons, Inc. Published 2014 by John Wiley & Sons, Inc.

of any animal thus far studied (approximately 200 mmHg) (Hargens 1988; Hargens et al. 1987). In dependent areas, such as the legs and feet, the mean arterial pressure may exceed 400 mmHg (Hargens 1988; Hargens et al. 1987). To prevent edema and pooling of fluids in dependent areas, giraffe have capillaries highly impermeable to plasma proteins, precapillary sphincters and pronounced arterial and arteriolar wall hypertrophy, a prominent lymphatic system, one-way valves in lymphatics and veins, and tight skin and fascial layers that provide a functional "antigravity suit," and pumping mechanism during movement (Hargens 1988; Hargens et al. 1987). Because of the giraffe's unique cardiovascular physiology, the giraffe heart may be more prone to injury from oxygen debt during periods of hypoxemia (Linton et al. 1999). Giraffe are speculated to have a large respiratory dead space generated by their long trachea, which appears to be compensated for by a smaller than expected tracheal diameter, slow deep respirations, and a large tidal volume (Bush 2003; Hugh-Jones et al. 1978; Langman et al. 1982). The long legs of giraffe make them prone to stumbling and splaying during induction and recovery, which can lead to fractures, luxations, muscle and ligament tears, and/or nerve damage. Recumbent giraffe require good footing and sufficient room to be able to rock forward with their long neck to get their long legs underneath them to stand. Giraffe and okapi have elongated skulls (elongated diastema) with narrow interdental spaces, which can make endotracheal intubation challenging, and the posterior position of the larynx impedes drainage of pharyngeal fluids and enhances the potential for aspiration (Bush et al. 2002; Dagg & Foster 1976; Nowak & Paradiso 1983). Giraffe and okapi have a tendency to regurgitate while under the influence of certain chemical restraint agents, which can lead to morbidity and mortality from aspiration pneumonia (Bush 1993, 2003; Bush et al. 2002). The thick skin of giraffids requires the use of long, robust needles to assure good intramuscular injections. Giraffe can alter their body temperature to minimize water loss and help with heat regulation (Bush 2003; Langman et al. 1982). Besides having a tendency toward hyperthermia from overexertion during field captures, giraffe are reported to sometime suffer from a malignant hyperthermia-like syndrome during anesthesia (Citino et al. 1984). Conversely, if ambient temperatures are low, giraffe and okapi tend to loose body temperature rapidly during anesthesia and can become hypothermic (S. Citino, pers. obs. and unpubl. data, 2011).

The most commonly used vascular access site in giraffids is the jugular vein. Due to thick cervical skin, the jugular vein may not always be visible but can usually be palpated and is generally more accessible closer to the head. Auricular and facial veins are also very accessible during anesthetic procedures (see Fig.

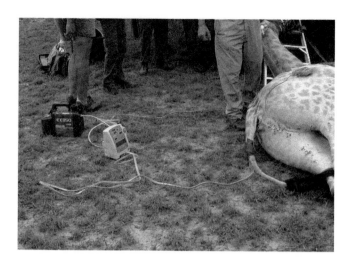

Figure 58.1. Indirect blood pressure monitoring utilizing an oscillometric blood pressure monitor and cuff on the tail of an immobilized giraffe.

58.1). Through-the-needle catheters are more effective for jugular catheterization in these species. If over-the-needle catheters are used for jugular catheterization, a stab incision or partial cut-down is generally required. The auricular artery on the dorsal ridge of the ear is most often used for arterial blood collection and for arterial catheterization for invasive blood pressure measurements. Pulse oximetry transmission sensor placement is generally most effective across a scraped ear or across vulvar, mammary, prepucial, or scrotal skin. End-tidal CO_2 adapters can be attached to an endotracheal tube or to a small tube placed in a nostril. Tail cuffs appear to work best for noninvasive blood pressure measurements. Lead placement for electrocardiography is best accomplished with needles placed through the thick skin of giraffids.

ANALGESIA

The most commonly used drugs for analgesia in giraffids are nonsteroidal anti-inflammatory drugs (NSAIDs) (Teare 2000). Flunixin meglumine (IV, IM, or PO, 1.0–2.0 mg/kg SID), phenylbutazone (PO, 1.0–3.0 mg/kg SID to BID), and ketoprofen (IV or IM, 0.5 to 2.0 mg/kg SID) have been used most often (S. Citino, pers. obs. and unpubl. data, 2011; Teare 2000). Other NSAIDS used in giraffids include etodolac (PO, 2.5–5.0 mg/kg, SID to BID), carprofen (PO, 2.0 mg/kg, SID to BID), and meloxicam (PO, 0.10 mg/kg, SID) (S. Citino, pers. obs. and unpubl. data, 2011). Gabapentin (PO, 2.0–5.0 mg/kg SID), a GABA analog, has shown promise as an analgesic for neuropathic and orthopedic pain in giraffids (S. Citino, pers. obs. and unpubl. data, 2011). Low doses of butorphanol may also be effective for some types of pain.

PHYSICAL AND MECHANICAL RESTRAINT

Only very young giraffe and okapi calves can be safely restrained manually. Mattresses or flexible padding can be wrapped around older calves, or they can be pushed into a padded corner with push boards to safely restrain them for minor procedures.

Mechanical restraint of giraffes is appropriate for minimally invasive procedures, such as blood sampling, tuberculin testing, rectal examinations, and minor hoof trimming, but giraffes can present dangers to handlers and themselves during such procedures. Giraffes have powerful kicks; can strike outward with their forelegs; and can swing and bash with their neck and head. If the footing is slippery, they can fall and injure themselves or ground support staff. Giraffe restraint devices vary from crates and walk-through chutes to small stalls or hallways with moveable walls to innovative mechanical or hydraulic squeeze chutes (Calle & Bormann 1988). All restraint devices should be designed to prevent entrapment of the neck or legs and to allow easy removal of a giraffe that goes down in the device. Successful mechanical restraint of giraffe is dependent on facility design, training, and conditioning of the giraffe, plus a well-trained staff. A well-designed chute, with a side that opens, can also be a valuable giraffe anesthesia induction device that allows close confinement, head control, and controlled progression to sternal recumbency. Mechanical restraint has been infrequently used on okapi; however, okapi have been conditioned to a special crate for venipuncture and other minor procedures (Mehrdadfar et al. 2003). Okapi are excellent kickers and the head and ossicones of males are formidable weapons.

For more extensive or invasive procedures on standing giraffe such as hoof trims, obstetrics, minor surgeries, percutaneous biopsies, and so on, chemically assisted mechanical restraint can sometimes be used. This generally involves the use of an α-2-adrenergic agonist alone or α-2-adrenergic agonist-azaperone combination given just prior to placing a giraffe into a mechanical restraint device. Xylazine (0.10–0.2 mg/kg IM), detomidine (15–40 μg/kg IM), xylazine-azaperone (0.10 to 0.12 mg/kg IM–0.20 to 0.50 mg/kg IM), and detomidine-azaperone (15 to 30 μg/kg IM–0.25 to 0.35 mg/kg IM) have been most commonly used for this purpose (Bush 2003; Bush et al. 2002; S. Citino, pers. obs. and unpubl. data, 2011). To increase sedation and analgesia, low doses of butorphanol (10–20 mg IV total) can be given to adult giraffe (S. Citino, pers. obs. and unpubl. data, 2011). Giraffe given these drugs in a restraint device can potentially become ataxic and go down, so handlers should always be prepared for this. Xylazine and detomidine can be partially reversed with yohimbine (0.10–0.20 mg/kg IV or IM) or atipamezole (0.10–0.20 mg/kg IV or IM), and butorphanol can be reversed with naltrexone (2.0 mg naltrexone/mg of butorphanol IV or IM) (Bush 2003; Bush et al. 2002; S. Citino, pers. obs. and unpubl. data, 2011). A few sudden deaths have occurred after IV administration of α-2-adrenergic and opioid antagonists in giraffes, so these drugs are preferentially given IM (S. Citino, pers. obs. and unpubl. data, 2011).

SEDATION AND TRANQUILIZATION

Standing sedation for hands-on procedures is rarely attempted in older giraffe outside of a restraint device due to the potential danger these animals pose to handlers (Table 58.1 and Table 58.2). α-2-adrenergic agonists at the suggested doses earlier can be used for safer manipulations in enclosures and chutes, for getting reluctant dam's to allow calves to nurse, and to calm animals in stressful or dangerous situations (Bush 2003; Bush et al. 2002; S. Citino, pers. obs. and unpubl. data, 2011; Fischer et al. 1997). It should always be remembered that giraffe under α-2-adrenergic agonist sedation can still kick, strike, and rapidly arouse from sedation and become very dangerous. Azaperone has also been used at 0.20–0.50 mg/kg IM as a short-acting, calming, and stress-reducing agent in giraffe (S. Citino, pers. obs. and unpubl. data, 2011). Intermediate and long-acting neuroleptics that have been used in adult giraffe include haloperidol (male, 20–30 mg IM; female, 15–20 mg IM), zuclopenthixol acetate (100–300 mg IM), and perphenazine enanthate (100–250 mg IM) (S. Citino, pers. obs. and unpubl. data, 2011; Ebedes & Raath 1995). Haloperidol has its onset in about 15 minutes and its effects last for 15–24 hours; zuclopenthixol acetate has its onset in 1–6 hours and its effects last about 3 days; and perphenazine enanthate has its onset in about 2–3 days and its effects last for 7–10 days (Ebedes & Raath 1995). Giraffe appear sensitive to these neuroleptic agents, with untoward effects, such as anorexia and extrapyramidal effects, common (S. Citino, pers. obs. and unpubl. data, 2011). Due to a significant potential for disorientation, unsteadiness on their feet, and collapse in their transport container, the use of sedatives and/or neuroleptic agents in giraffe during transport is considered risky and should only be done with great care.

Standing restraint in adult okapi for minor procedures, such as venipuncture, physical exam, obstetrics, radiography, ultrasound, and catheter placement, has been accomplished with xylazine given at 125–300 mg IM (0.50–1.20 mg/kg IM) (Citino 1996; Citino et al. 2006; Raphael 1999; Teare 2000). Xylazine can be partially reversed with yohimbine (0.10 to 0.20 mg/kg IV or IM) or tolazoline (0.50 mg/kg IV or IM) (Citino 1996, pers. obs. and unpubl. data, 2011; Raphael 1999). More complete reversal of xylazine has been achieved with the experimental α-2-adrenergic antagonist RX821002 (5.0 mg total dose IV) or combinations of yohimbine or tolazoline and atipamizole (30–100 μg/kg IV or IM)

Table 58.1. Drugs used for chemical restraint in giraffe

Drug	Dosage	Reversal Agent/Dose	Purpose
Xylazine	0.10–0.20 mg/kg IM	Yohimbine (0.10–0.20 mg/kg IV or IM) Atipamezole (0.10–0.20 mg/kg IV or IM)	Sedation or chemically assisted mechanical restraint
Detomidine	15–40 µg/kg IM	Yohimbine (0.10–0.20 mg/kg IV or IM) Atipamezole (0.10–0.20 mg/kg IV or IM)	Sedation or chemically assisted mechanical restraint
Azaperone	0.20–0.50 mg/kg IM	None	Tranquilization, calming, or stress reduction
Haloperidol	Adult male: 20–30 mg IM Adult female: 15–20 mg IM	None	Neuroleptic, untoward effects possible
Zuclopenthixol acetate	Adult: 100–300 mg IM	None	Intermediate-acting neuroleptic, untoward effects possible
Perphenazine enanthate	Adult: 100–250 mg IM	None	Long-acting neuroleptic, untoward effects possible
Xylazine (X) + azaperone (A) Butorphanol (B) if needed	X: 0.10–0.12 mg/kg IM A: 0.20–0.50 mg/kg IM B: 10–20 mg total IV	Same as above for xylazine B: Naltrexone 2.0-mg/mg butorphanol IV	Chemically assisted mechanical restraint
Detomidine (D) + azaperone (A) Butorphanol (B) if needed	D: 15–30 µg/kg IM A: 0.25–0.35 mg/kg IM B: 10–20 mg total IV	Same as above for detomidine B: Naltrexone 2.0-mg/mg butorphanol IV	Chemically assisted mechanical restraint
Etorphine (E) + xylazine (X)	X: Adult: 70–100 mg IM X: Yearling: 30–40 mg IM After sedation followed by: E: Adult: 1.5–2.5 mg IM E: Yearling: 0.5–1.25 mg IM	Same as above for xylazine E: Naltrexone 50- to 100-mg/mg etorphine IV or IM	Staged protocol for anesthesia of captive giraffe
Carfentanil (C) + xylazine (X)	X: Same as for etorphine + xylazine After sedation followed by: C: Adult: 1.2–2.1 mg IM C: Yearling: 0.20–0.90 mg IM	Same as above for xylazine C: Naltrexone 100-mg/mg carfentanil IV or IM	Staged protocol for anesthesia of captive giraffe
Thiafentanil (T) + medetomidine (M) + ketamine (K)	T: 5.8 ± 1.5 µg/kg IM M: 12.9 ± 5.1 µg/kg IM K: 0.65 ± 0.18 mg/kg IM	T: Naltrexone 30-mg/mg thiafentanil IV or IM M: Atipamezole 3–5 times the medetomidine dose IV or IM	Protocol for captive giraffe, medetomidine resedation can occur, good analgesia for surgery
Medetomidine (M) + ketamine (K)	M: 150 µg/cm Shd Hgt K: 3.0 mg/cm Shd Hgt or M: Male: 50–70 mg IM M: Female: 40–50 mg IM M: Subadult: 18–20 mg IM K: Male: 1000–1200 mg IM K: Female: 800–900 mg IM K: Subadult: 300–500 mg IM	Atipamezole (350 µg/cm) Shd Hgt or 3–5 times the medetomidine dose IM	Protocol for captive giraffe, medetomidine resedation can occur, inadequate analgesia for surgery
Etorphine	Adult: 8–15 mg IM	Naltrexone 30- to 100-mg/mg etorphine IV or diprenorphine 2.0-mg/mg etorphine IV	Protocol for free-ranging giraffe
Etorphine (E) + thiafentanil (T)	E: Adult: 4.0 mg IM T: Adult: 8–16 mg IM	Naltrexone 30–100 mg/mg opioid IV or diprenorphine 2.0 mg/mg opioid IV	Protocol for free-ranging giraffe
Thiafentanil	Adult: 8–16 mg IM	Naltrexone 30-mg/mg thiafentanil IV or diprenorphine 2.0-mg/mg thiafentanil IV	Protocol for free-ranging giraffe

(Citino 1996, pers. obs. and unpubl. data, 2011; Raphael 1999; Teare 2000). For okapi that appear resistant to xylazine alone, the addition of azaperone (0.20–0.40 mg/kg IM) may improve the standing restraint (S. Citino, pers. obs. and unpubl. data, 2011). Good standing restraint for venipuncture, catheter placement, vaginal insemination, and so on has also been achieved with xylazine (0.40–0.80 mg/kg IM) or detomidine (40–100 µg/kg IM) with butorphanol (80–200 µg/kg IM) (S. Citino, pers. obs. and unpubl. data, 2011; Teare 2000). Recently, medetomidine (60–90 µg/kg IM) with butorphanol (45–55 µg/kg IM) has successfully been used for standing restraint of okapi at one institution (J. Raines, pers. comm., 2011). Butorphanol has been reversed with naltrexone (1.0 mg/mg butorphanol IV or IM) (S. Citino, pers. obs. and unpubl. data, 2011),

Table 58.2. Drugs used for chemical restraint in okapi

Xylazine (X) And can add if needed: Azaperone (A)	X: 0.50–1.20 mg/kg IM X: Adult:125–300 mg IM A: 0.20–0.40 mg/kg IM	Partial reversal: yohimbine 0.10–0.20 mg/kg IV or IM or tolazoline 0.50 mg/kg IV or IM Better reversal: RX821002 5.0 mg IV or yohimbine or tolazoline + atimpamezole 30–100 μg/kg IV or IM	Standing restraint for minor procedures
Azaperone	0.20–0.50 mg/kg IM	None	Tranquilization, calming, or stress reduction
Haloperidol	80–100 μg/kg IM 0.90–1.5 mg/kg PO	None	Neuroleptic
Zuclopenthixol acetate	0.40–1.0 mg/kg IM	None	Intermediate-acting neuroleptic
Xylazine (X) + butorphanol (B)	X: 0.40–0.80 mg/kg IM B: 80–200 μg/kg IM	Same as above for xylazine B: Naltrexone 1.0-mg/mg butorphanol IV or IM	Standing restraint for minor procedures
Detomidine (D) + butorphanol (B)	D: 40–100 μg/kg IM B: 80–200 μg/kg IM	D: Same as for xylazine above B: Same as above for butorphanol	Standing restraint for minor procedures
Medetomidine (M) + butorphanol (B)	M: 60–90 μg/kg IM B: 45–55 μg/kg IM	M: Atipamezole 5.0-mg/mg medetomidine IV or IM B: Same as above for butorphanol	Standing restraint for minor procedures
Carfentanil (C) + xylazine (X)	X: 0.12 ± 0.02 mg/kg IM X: Adult:30–45 mg IM After sedation followed by: C: 4.7 ± 0.8 μg/kg IM C: Adult:0.9–1.5 mg IM	X: Same as for xylazine above C: Naltrexone 100-mg/mg carfentanil 1/2 IV 1/2 SQ	Staged protocol for anesthesia of captive okapi
Thiafentanil (T) + xylazine (K) or detomidine (D) + ketamine (K)	X: 0.12 ± 0.03 mg/kg IM X: Adult:30–45 mg IM Or: D:0.05± 0.01 mg/kg IM D: Adult:12–20 mg IM After sedation followed by: T: 5.3 ± 0.3 μg/kg IM T: Adult:1.4–2.0 mg IM K: 0.6 ± 0.1 mg/kg IM K: Adult:120–220 mg IM	X: Same as for xylazine above D: Same as for xylaxine above T: Naltrexone 30-mg/mg thiafentanil IM	Staged protocol for anesthesia of captive okapi. Rapid inductions with shorter working times. Characteristics of anesthesia very similar to carfentanil combinations.
Etorphine (E) + xylazine (X)	X: Adult:40–50 mg IM After sedation followed by: E: Adult:4.0–5.0 mg IM	X: Same as for xylazine above E: Naltrexone 30–50 mg/mg etorphine IV or diprenorphine 2.0-mg/mg etorphine IV	Staged protocol for anesthesia of captive okapi, greater risk of regurgitation with etorphine
Medetomidine (M) + ketamine (M) +/- Midazolam (Mi)	M: 60–155 μg/kg IM K: 1.0–3.9 mg/kg IM Mi: 0.1 mg/kg IM	Atipamezole 5 times the medetomidine dose IV or IM	Protocol for captive okapi, better restraint at the higher end of dose range
Medetomidine (M) + butorphanol (B) + ketamine (K)	M: 60–70 μg/kg IM B: 50–100 μg/kg IM K: 2.0–3.0 mg/kg IM	M: Same as above for medetomidine B: Same as above for butorphanol	Protocol for captive okapi

and medetomidine has been reversed with atipamezole at five times the medetomidine dose (J. Raines, pers. comm., 2011). Azaperone (0.20–0.50 mg/kg IM) and haloperidol (80–100 μg/kg IM) have been used to tranquilize flighty animals when moved or manipulated in enclosures (Citino 1996, pers. obs. and unpubl. data, 2011; Raphael 1999). Haloperidol (0.90–1.50 mg/kg) has also produced mild calming effects when given orally to okapi (S. Citino, pers. obs. and unpubl. data, 2011). The intermediate-acting neuroleptic zuclopenthixol acetate (0.40–1.0 mg/kg IM) has been used to reduce stress and calm animals during transport (S. Citino, pers. obs. and unpubl. data, 2011; Raphael 1999). A combination of zuclopenthixol acetate (100 mg IM 15 hours before move) and haloperidol (10–20 mg

IM to facilitate crating) was used to load and transport two okapi that were not crate trained (Redrobe 2003).

ENDOTRACHEAL INTUBATION

A 40- to 60-cm laryngoscope blade is required to visualize the glottis in adult giraffe, while a 30- to 40-cm laryngoscope blade will suffice in okapi (S. Citino, pers. obs. and unpubl. data, 2011). Adult giraffe will generally take endotracheal tubes with internal diameters of 24–30 mm, while adult okapi generally take tubes of 20 to 26 mm (S. Citino, pers. obs. and unpubl. data, 2011). Giraffids are best intubated using the "Bush technique"—visualizing the glottis with a laryngoscope, passing a tracheal exchange catheter through the glottis, threading the exchange catheter through the Murphy's eye of the endotracheal tube, and passing the tube through the glottis using the exchange catheter as a guide (Bush 1996). In large giraffe, the glottis can be digitally palpated and an endotracheal tube manually placed. Giraffids can also be intubated by passing a fiberoptic endoscope through the endotracheal tube, visually passing the endoscope into the trachea, and then using the endoscope as a stylet to place the tube. The authors recommend using a cuffed endotracheal tube to intubate giraffe that will be anesthetized for longer than 15 minutes. Oxygen can then be supplied by insufflation or jet ventilation, and respiratory support can be given with a one or two demand valve system or field ventilator (Citino et al. 2007). If giraffids are inadequately anesthetized (tongue movement and swallow reflex present), stimulation of the pharynx during endotracheal intubation can initiate active regurgitation.

ANESTHESIA OF GIRAFFE

Even with the development of newer and safer drugs and improved physiological monitoring equipment, giraffe anesthesia remains a major challenge due to their unique anatomy and physiology (Table 58.1). Despite the frequent need to capture and relocate this species *in situ*, giraffe are still considered a high risk species to chemical capture due to their large size and unique physiology and handling problems. Due to their awkward shape, weight estimation and dosage calculation is difficult, especially in the field. All of these special characteristics predispose them to life-threatening, anesthesia-related complications, including (1) vomiting/passive regurgitation leading to fatal inhalation pneumonia; (2) respiratory depression and hypoventilation with resulting hypoxemia and hypercarbia; (3) tachycardia, hypertension, bradycardia, hypotension, or other significant cardiac emergencies; (4) self-induced trauma during induction and/or following reversal; and (5) hyperthermia and/or capture myopathy secondary to prolonged and stormy induction and incomplete anesthesia reversal (Bush 1993, 2003; Bush et al. 2002; Citino et al. 1984). The historical high morbidity and mortality encountered during giraffe anesthesia, in both captive and free-ranging settings, leads to a hesitancy to anesthetize them.

Historical verbal and published reports describe the use of several drugs and drug combinations for giraffe anesthesia. Drugs used alone or in combination have included succinylcholine, gallamine, hyoscine, atropine, hyaluronidase, glycerol guaiacolate, acepromazine, azaperone, xylazine, detomidine, medetomidine, ketamine, telazol, barbiturates, butorphanol, fentanyl, etorphine, carfentanil, and thiafentanil (A3080) (Bush 1976, 1993, 2003; Bush & de Vos 1987; Bush et al. 1976, 1997, 2001, 2002; S. Citino, pers. obs. and unpubl. data, 2011; Fischer et al. 1997; Gardner et al. 1986; Geiser et al. 1992; Hirst 1966; Lamberski et al. 2004; Langman 1973; Morkel 1992, 1993; Rapley et al. 1975; Vahala 1990; Vogelnest & Ralph 1997; Wiesner & von Hegel 1989; Williamson & Wallach 1968; York 1975; York et al. 1973; J. Raath, pers. comm., 2006).

Many of the problems associated with anesthesia can be minimized in captive giraffe with careful pre-planning and forethought. An experienced staff to assist with the critical induction and recovery phases of anesthesia and for monitoring the patient is essential. Fasting of giraffids is probably overemphasized and detrimental and should occur for no longer than 12 hours, with concentrate being the primary foodstuff to withhold. Animals should be prevented from drinking large quantities of water just prior to anesthesia by withholding water for 2–6 hours depending on climatic conditions. The site and method of induction are also critical for success. The use of a well-designed chute for giraffe induction can greatly reduce risk and allow a staged and controlled induction to occur (Bush 2003; Calle & Bormann 1988; S. Citino, pers. obs. and unpubl. data, 2011). The chute must be designed so forward pressing or falling will not compromise respiration, with no potential foot, leg, or neck traps, and with a complete side that swings open to allow easy removal and positioning of the giraffe. If a suitable chute is not available a confined space with smooth, solid walls, lack of trip and fall hazards, and a catwalk for access to the animal's head during the procedure can be used. If a catwalk is absent around the induction area and a halter can be placed before or during induction, a ceiling pulley and rope apparatus can be used to suspend the giraffe's head and neck during induction to reduce falling injuries and prevent head slamming. If the giraffe must be induced in a larger area without head control, all tripping and falling hazards should be removed or minimized and methods for keeping the giraffe away from dangerous pressing points and head and neck traps should be determined. No matter where giraffe anesthesia is accomplished, good footing is mandatory to prevent slipping and splaying. Also, adequate staff and/or equipment should be present to move an animal quickly, if necessary. Since complications can occur rapidly in anesthetized giraffe, close physiologic monitoring is essential for patient safety and should include both the usual visual and tactile monitoring, as well as electronic monitoring (i.e., temperature, pulse oximetry, capnography, invasive and noninvasive blood pressure, electrocardiography, and arterial blood gas and pH measurements). Perhaps the hardest thing to do is back off from a procedure. Many procedures involving giraffe require extensive coordination to make sure that people, facilities, and equipment are ready. Unless conducting an emergency procedure, if something is not going right or if there is a factor that can be changed to enhance the success of the procedure, it should be stopped and rescheduled. Even with the most careful planning and preparation, procedural complications can still occur in captive situations but are amplified in free-ranging giraffes since there is minimal control of the situation.

There are standardized procedures for handling an anesthetized giraffe in lateral recumbency, which include supporting the neck with a board or ladder so the head is maintained above the rumen with the nose pointed down to facilitate drainage of fluids. The neck should be kept straight without kinks or angulations. The angle of the neck is altered every 10–15 minutes and the neck can be massaged to minimize muscle spasms that in the postrecovery period can be life-threatening. Padding should be placed under the giraffe, particularly under the shoulder and radius to prevent pressure trauma to the radial nerve. Oxygen should be supplied by either nasal insufflation or endotracheal tube (see Fig. 58.2, Fig. 58.3, and Fig. 58.4).

Recovery is a very critical time in a giraffe anesthetic procedure. Good footing is essential during recovery,

as is adequate space for the giraffe to rock forward and get momentum to stand. If the giraffe does not regain its feet within 45 minutes of administration of the antagonist, the prognosis is poor for the animal's recovery. The route of administration of the antagonist can greatly influence recovery. Intramuscular administration of the antagonists will generally provide a slow, controlled recovery, which is generally preferred (Bush 2003; Bush et al. 2002; S. Citino, pers. obs. and unpubl. data, 2011; Lamberski et al. 2004). Many times with IV

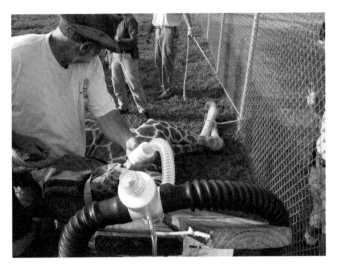

Figure 58.3. An intubated giraffe receiving supplemental oxygen and ventilatory support.

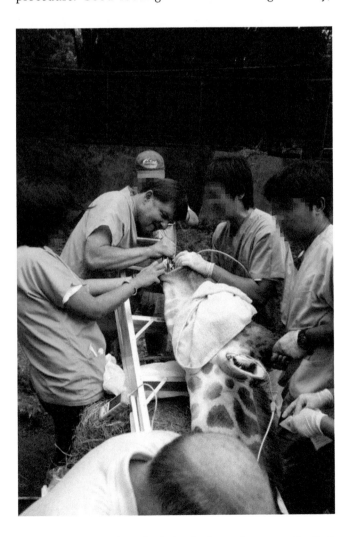

Figure 58.2. Endotracheal intubation of an anesthetized giraffe, note that the head and neck are held in a straight position.

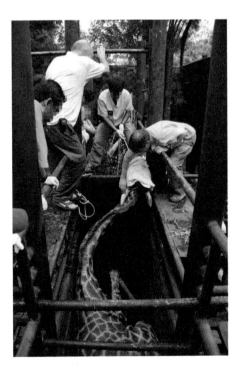

Figure 58.4. Staged induction of a captive giraffe in a chute system.

administration of antagonists, giraffe will become excited, head slam and try to stand before ready, and will fall, potentially injuring themselves.

The most widely used anesthetic regimens for giraffe have involved use of opioids alone or in combination with sedatives (e.g., xylazine), tranquilizers (e.g., azaparone), and/or absorption accelerants (e.g., hyaluronidase) and, most recently, the potent specific α-2-adrenergic agonist medetomidine with ketamine (Bush 1976, 1993, 2003; Bush & de Vos 1987; Bush et al. 1976, 1997, 2001, 2002; Geiser et al. 1992; Hirst 1966; Lamberski et al. 2004; Langman 1973; Morkel 1992, 1993; Rapley et al. 1975; Vahala 1990; Vogelnest & Ralph 1997; Wiesner & von Hegel 1989; Williamson & Wallach 1968; York 1975; York et al. 1973).

A staged protocol using etorphine and xylazine has been used commonly in the past for anesthesia of captive giraffe (Bush 1976, 1993, 2003; Bush et al. 1976, 2002). This approach tends to cause less respiratory depression since etorphine doses can be titrated to the needs of the individual animal and situation. This protocol is ideally carried out in a chute or confined area where head control can be maintained. Initially, giraffe are given xylazine (70–100 mg/adult or 30–40 mg/yearling IM). Atropine (7.0–8.0 mg/adult or 2.0–3.0 mg/yearling IM) can be given simultaneously to prevent xylazine-induced bradycardia. Five to 10 minutes after xylazine administration, signs of sedation occur (i.e., stargazing, ataxia, and tongue protrusion with slight salivation). About 15–20 minutes after the xylazine, a narcotizing dose of etorphine (1.5–2.5 mg/adult or 0.5–1.25/yearling IM) is administered. This dose may induce recumbency within 15–20 minutes. Ideally, a head halter, placed when the animal is narcotized, is used to help control the head and assist the animal to the ground, without tumbling over backwards. If the giraffe does not become recumbent after etorphine administration, it can be supplemented with etorphine (0.5–1.0 mg IM or IV), 5% guaifenesin solution IV to effect, or ketamine (100–400 mg IV), or can be physically cast. For reversal of etorphine, naltrexone (50–100 mg/mg etorphine, 1/2 IV, 1/2IM or all IM) is given and for xylazine, yohimbine (0.10–0.20 mg/kg IV or IM) or atipamezole (50–100 mg total 1/4 IV 3/4 IM or all IM) is given. It is possible to substitute carfentanil (1.2–2.1 mg/adult or 0.30–0.90/yearling IM) for etorphine in this protocol (S. Citino, pers. obs. and unpubl. data, 2011). See Fig. 58.5, Fig. 58.6, and Fig. 58.7.

Current methods for capture of free-ranging giraffe utilize high doses of opioids alone for rapid induction and no lingering drug effects during transport. Etorphine (8.0–15.0 mg/adult), thiafentanil (8.0–16.0 mg/adult), or a combination of etorphine (4.0 mg/adult) and thiafentanil (8.0–16.0 mg/adult) with or without hyaluronidase are most commonly used (S. Citino, pers. obs. and unpubl. data, 2011; Morkel 1992, 1993). Giraffe become narcotized rapidly, but many must be

cast with ropes. Once down, muscle relaxation is poor, animals require significant restraint, and most must be fully or partially reversed with diprenorphine or naltrexone to prevent severe hypoxemia while hoods, ear plugs, and ropes are applied. This anesthetic technique greatly limits what can safely be done to a giraffe while it is recumbent. Once reversed, giraffe are very active and can be a danger to themselves and the ground crew during loading for transport. This method is for capture only and requires a well-trained and experienced capture team to safely cast, restrain, and load giraffe for transport (see Fig. 58.8 and Fig. 58.9). Most recently, a combination of thiafentanil and butorphanol has been

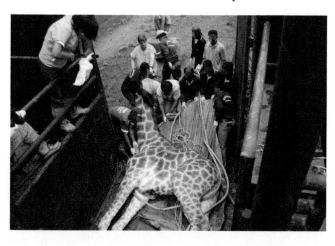

Figure 58.5. Staged induction of a captive giraffe; note that the whole side of the chute opens, allowing the giraffe to be positioned in lateral recumbency.

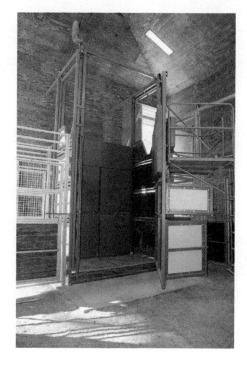

Figure 58.6. Chute system for captive giraffe. Note padding, attached deck for handlers to access the head, and one side swings open for access to the animal during induction.

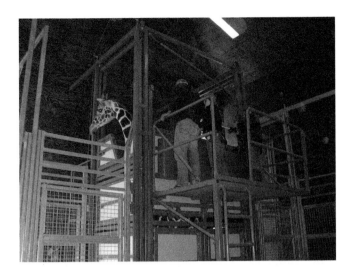

Figure 58.7. Chute system for handling captive giraffe. Note that the animals walk through the chute daily to access the outside yard.

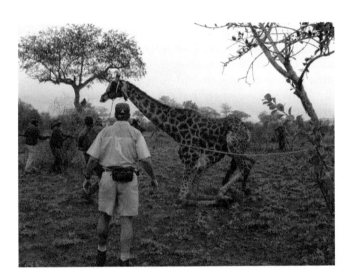

Figure 58.8. Free-ranging giraffe in Kruger National Park, South Africa shortly after reversal of thiafentanil anesthesia. Notice blindfold, halter, lead rope, body ropes, and capture crew in place for loading giraffe into field chariot for transport out of veldt. Notice potential for hind limb splaying despite good footing in the field and the requirement for the giraffe to rock forward to stand.

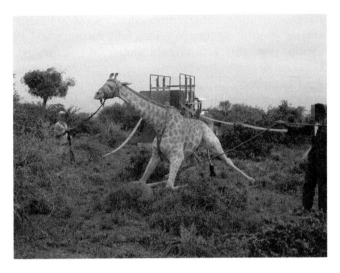

Figure 58.9. Free-ranging giraffe starting to stand after reversal of thiafentanil-medetomidine-ketamine anesthesia. Notice blindfold, earplugs, halter, and ropes in place for loading giraffe into the chariot in the background. Notice potential for rear limb splaying despite good footing in the field.

used for capture of free-ranging giraffe, with less respiratory depression, probably due to the partial mu opioid receptor antagonist effect of butorphanol (J.P. Raath and L. Venter, pers. comm., 2006.).

A nonnarcotic alternative for giraffe chemical restraint is the combination of medetomidine and ketamine. This combination has been used successfully in captive and free-living giraffes with dosages correlated to the giraffe's shoulder height. In "calm" animals, 150 μg medetomidine + 3.0 mg ketamine/cm of shoulder height provided a rapid and relatively uneventful induction (Bush 2003; Bush et al. 1997, 2001). Larger giraffes experienced a less desirable immobilization,

which may indicate the dosage correlation to shoulder height may not be appropriate in larger animals. Another retrospective study in 30 captive giraffe recommends doses of medetomidine (subadult, 18–20 mg; adult female, 40–50 mg; adult male, 50–70 mg) and ketamine (subadult, 300–500 mg; adult female, 800–900 mg; adult male, 1000–1200 mg) (Lamberski et al. 2004). A nice characteristic of this combination is smooth inductions with animals usually sitting down in sternal recumbency before rolling over laterally. With medetomidine-ketamine, an inverse relationship is observed between the level of excitement and the quality of the immobilization—the more excited the giraffe prior to and after darting, the more physical restraint is required to bring the animal to a sternal position. This combination also produces a characteristic tachypnea (50–60 breath/min) and inadequate analgesia for painful procedures. Administration of atipamezole (350 μg/cm of shoulder height or five times the medetomidine dose IM) results in a rapid and usually complete reversal. Resedation has been seen in some giraffe given medetomidine 3–28 hours after reversal, therefore giraffes should be monitored closely during this time, and additional atipamezole should be administered if signs of resedation occur (S. Citino, pers. obs. and unpubl. data, 2011; Lamberski et al. 2004). Resedation appears to occur most commonly in the Rothschild's (*Giraffa camelopardalis rothschildi*) and Southern giraffe (*Giraffa camelopardalis giraffa*) subspecies and less commonly in the reticulated (*Giraffa camelopardalis reticulata*) subspecies (S. Citino, pers. obs. and unpubl. data, 2011). Signs of medetomidine resedation include decreased awareness to surroundings, dull eyes, inappetance, lowered neck, widened stance, salivation, tongue protrusion, excessive licking, ataxia, leaning against objects, and recumbency (S. Citino, pers. obs. and unpubl. data, 2011; Lamberski et al. 2004).

A newer drug combination, thiafentanil-medetomidine-ketamine, has safely and successfully been used for chemical restraint of captive and free-ranging giraffe (Citino et al. 2006). Dosing requirements are markedly different between captive (thiafentanil 5.8 ± 1.5 µg/kg + medetomidine 12.9 ± 5.1 µg/kg + ketamine 0.65 ± 0.18 mg/kg IM), free-ranging, ground-darted (thiafentanil 6.6 ± 1.5 µg/kg + medetomidine 15.9 ± 3.7 µg/kg + ketamine 0.50 ± 0.19 mg/kg IM), and free-ranging, helicopter-darted (thiafentanil 10.0 ± 4.0 µg/kg + medetomidine 14.0 ± 9.4 µg/kg + ketamine 0.39 ± 0.20 mg/kg IM) giraffe. The degree of excitement associated with helicopter darting appears to negate the effects of medetomidine and makes this combination less suitable for helicopter darting. In calm animals, onset of action is ultra-rapid, with most animals down in 2–5 minutes. Giraffe exhibit excellent muscle relaxation and are very safe to work around with this combination. Analgesia appears very good, and there is a long duration of action, so it appears useful for surgical and prolonged major procedures (Borkowski et al. 2009; Quesada et al. 2011). A marked apneustic breathing pattern is often seen and moderate to severe hypoxemia can occur, so oxygen supplementation and/or respiratory support are recommended. Anesthesia is reversed with naltrexone (30 mg/mg thiafentanil IV or IM) and atipamezole (three to five times the medetomidine dose IV or IM). Recoveries are best when antagonists are administered IM. As with medetomidine-ketamine, evidence of medetomidine-associated resedation is seen in some giraffe postreversal requiring additional supplements of atipamezole (S. Citino, pers. obs. and unpubl. data, 2011). Resedation can be a potentially life threatening problem in giraffe, especially during transport and when giraffe are not observed closely for signs of resedation post recovery.

The reader is referred to this chapter's references for published methods of giraffe anesthesia and for more detailed descriptions of these procedures.

OKAPI ANESTHESIA

In comparison with giraffe, there are far fewer inherent problems that can occur during okapi anesthesia due to their more conventional size and shape (Table 58.2). However, complications associated with anesthesia are still one of the most significant causes of adult morbidity and mortality in the international captive population (S. Citino, pers. obs. and unpubl. data, 2011; Raphael 1999). The most common anesthesia-associated problems reported in okapi are regurgitation and aspiration of rumen contents and postanesthesia gastroin-

testinal stasis or ileus (S. Citino, pers. obs. and unpubl. data, 2011).

Chemical immobilization of okapi is most commonly accomplished with an opioid (carfentanil, etorphine, or thiafentanil) in combination with an α-2-adrenergic agonist (xylazine) or tranquilizer (acetylpromazine) (Citino 1996, pers. obs. and unpubl. data, 2011; Mortelmans 1978; Raphael 1999; Teare 2000). Okapi should not be fasted for longer than 12 hours prior to anesthesia as hypoglycemia and electrolyte imbalances can be induced (S. Citino, pers. obs. and unpubl. data, 2011). Water can be withheld for 2–6 hours, depending on climatic conditions. Inductions with opioid combinations can sometimes be stormy, with okapi stumbling, crashing, exhibiting opisthotonus, falling backwards, and flailing and head-slamming once down. It is important to induce okapi in relatively small enclosures with good footing, smooth walls, and lack of trip and fall hazards. Once an okapi is well narcotized, two to three well-trained handlers should use controlled restraint to smooth the induction and prevent injury. A padded stall with a hinged crush wall also works nicely for preventing injuries during induction. Once down, the animal is placed sternal with its head above its rumen and nose down, is blindfolded, and given oxygen by nasal insufflation. If the okapi must be placed in lateral recumbency, adequate padding should be placed under pressure points. As with most ruminants, okapi should not be rolled onto their back unless intubated, as this can stimulate regurgitation of rumen contents. Okapi should be kept warm during anesthesia as they have a tendency to become hypothermic (S. Citino, pers. obs. and unpubl. data, 2011) (Fig. 58.10, Fig. 58.11, and Fig. 58.12).

Figure 58.10. Standing sedation in a captive okapi with xylazine and butorphanol for an echocardiography examination.

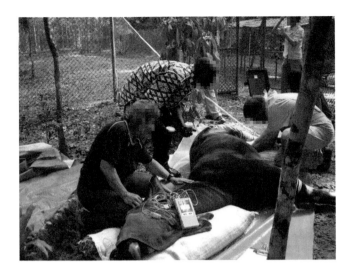

Figure 58.11. Anesthesia of an okapi in a field situation. Note that there is adequate padding of the okapi in lateral recumbency. Side-stream capnography is being used by placing a sampling adapter in the nostril, to estimate end-tidal carbon dioxide readings on exhalation.

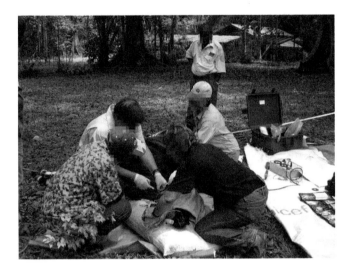

Figure 58.12. Anesthesia of an okapi in a field situation. Note that the pulse oximeter is placed on the tongue and a side-stream capnograph sampling adapter is placed in the nostril.

Over 170 successful okapi procedures without mortality have been completed using carfentanil and xylazine in a staged technique (Citino 1996, pers. obs. and unpubl. data, 2011). Xylazine (0.12 ± 0.02 mg/kg IM, adult total dose = 30–45 mg IM) is given first and is followed in 15–20 minutes with carfentanil (4.7 ± 0.8 μg/kg IM, adult total dose = 0.9–1.5 mg IM). This staged technique requires less opioid and produces a much smoother induction, with better muscle relaxation, than combining the opioid and xylazine together. The better the initial sedation from xylazine, the smoother the induction will generally be. Azaperone (50.0 mg average total adult dose) can be added to the xylazine

to increase sedation and improve inductions in problem animals. For okapi receiving significant stimuli during anesthesia (e.g., electroejaculation), ketamine (1.0–1.5 mg/kg) can be added to the carfentanil dart to potentiate the xylazine and carfentanil. If supplements are needed to prevent struggling, improve muscle relaxation, or deepen anesthesia, xylazine (2.0–5.0 mg boluses IV), ketamine (50–200 mg boluses IV), and 5% guaifenesin solution IV drips have been used. Naltrexone (100 mg/mg carfentanil 1/2 IV 1/2 SQ or IM) is used to reverse the carfentanil, and yohimbine (0.10–0.20 mg/kg IV or IM), tolazoline (100 mg IV or IM total adult dose), RX821002 (5.0 mg IV total adult dose), or atipamezole (0.125 mg/kg IV or IM) is used to reverse the xylazine. Reversals tend to be smoother when all antagonists are given IM (S. Citino, pers. obs. and unpubl. data, 2011). After reversal, two experienced handlers should stay with the okapi to prevent injury until it is standing. Renarcotization is occasionally seen in okapi anesthetized with carfentanil, so animals should be observed closely for 24 hours and supplemented with naltrexone if necessary (S. Citino, pers. obs. and unpubl. data, 2011).

Etorphine can also be used in a staged anesthetic technique with xylazine (Citino 1996; Raphael 1999; Teare 2000). As discussed earlier, xylazine (40–50 mg IM total adult dose) is first given, followed in 15 to 30 minutes by etorphine (4.0–5.0 mg IM total adult dose). There appears to be a greater risk of regurgitation with etorphine versus carfentanil in okapi (Citino 1996; Raphael 1999; Teare 2000). Etorphine is reversed with naltrexone (30–50 mg/mg of etorphine IV) or diprenorphine (2.0 mg/mg of etorphine IV).

The newest potent opioid, thiafentanil (A3080), has recently been used in staged techniques with either xylazine or detomidine for short anesthetic procedures in okapi (S. Citino, pers. obs. and unpubl. data, 2011). Xylazine (0.12 ± 0.03 mg/kg IM, adult total dose = 30–45 mg IM) or detomidine (0.05 ± 0.01 mg/kg IM, adult total dose = 12–20 mg IM) is given first and is followed in 15–20 minutes with thiafentanil (5.3 ± 0.3 μg/kg IM, adult total dose = 1.4–2.0 mg IM) and ketamine (0.6 ± 0.1 mg/kg IM, adult total dose = 120–220 mg IM). Inductions are rapid after thiafentanil-ketamine administration (2–6 minutes), and the characteristics of the anesthesia are very similar to the carfentanil-xylazine combination described earlier; however, working time with this combination is much shorter (25–40 minutes). If longer working times are required, supplemental drugs will be needed. Naltrexone (30 mg/mg of thiafentanil IM) is used to reverse the thiafentanil, and yohimbine (0.10–0.20 mg/kg IM), tolazoline (100 mg IM total adult dose), RX821002 (5.0 mg IV total adult dose), or atipamezole (0.125 mg/kg IM) is used to reverse the xylazine or detomidine. Renarcotization has not been seen in okapi anesthetized with thiafentanil.

The nonnarcotic combination of medetomidine (60–155 µg/kg IM) and ketamine (1.0–3.9 mg/kg IM) can be used to induce a deep sedation in okapi adequate for most minor procedures (Citino 1996; Raphael 1999; Teare 2000; L. Klein, pers. comm., 2011). Deep IM injection (50–60 mm needles) is required with this drug combination and the higher end of the dosage range for medetomidine (100–155 µg/kg) generally produces a better anesthesia without the need for supplementation (L. Klein, pers. comm., 2011). First signs generally occur in 1–7 minutes, and animals are recumbent in 3–34 minutes, with an average of 15–20 minutes. Induction is generally much smoother than with opioid combinations. Adding midazolam (0.1 mg/kg) to this combination seems to speed induction and makes it smoother (L. Klein, pers. comm., 2011). In contrast to opioid combinations, okapi are aware and will still kick or flee during induction with this drug combination, so should not be approached until down and relaxed. Okapi should not be reversed for 15–20 minutes post induction to reduce unsteadiness from residual ketamine. Some regurgitation can occur if animals are in lateral recumbency with their head and neck flat out, so the head should be kept elevated with nose point down. Medetomidine is reversed by atipamezole (5.0 mg/mg medetomidine IV or IM). There have been reports of postanesthesia ileus, with some fatalities, in okapi receiving medetomidine and ketamine (S. Citino, pers. obs. and unpubl. data, 2011).

Recently, a combination of medetomidine (60 to 70 µg/kg IM), butorphanol (50 to 100 µg/kg IM), and ketamine (2 to 3 mg/kg IM) has been used for anesthesia of okapi at one institution for minor surgical procedures and hoof trimming (J. Raines, pers. comm., 2011). For longer or more invasive procedures, okapi were intubated and placed on isoflurane inhalation anesthesia.

REFERENCES

Borkowski R, Citino S, Bush M, et al. 2009. Surgical castration of subadult giraffe (Giraffa camelopardalis). Journal of Zoo and Wildlife Medicine 40(4):786–790.

Brown DM, Brenneman RA, Koepfli K, et al. 2007. Extensive population genetic structure in the giraffe. BMC Biology 5:57. http://www.biomedcentral.com/1741-7007/5/57 (accessed February 12, 2014).

Bush M. 1976. Giraffe restraint and immobilization. Annual Proceedings of the American Association of Zoo Veterinarians, pp. 151–154.

Bush M. 1993. Anesthesia of high risk animals: giraffe. In: Zoo and Wild Animal Medicine-Current Therapy 3 (ME Fowler, ed.), pp. 545–547. Philadelphia: WB Saunders.

Bush M. 1996. A technique for endotracheal intubation of nondomestic bovids and cervids. Journal of Zoo and Wildlife Medicine 27(3):378–381.

Bush M. 2003. Giraffidae. In: Zoo and Wild Animal Medicine, 5th ed. (ME Fowler, RE Miller, eds.), pp. 625–633. St. Louis: Saunders.

Bush M, de Vos V. 1987. Observations on field immobilization of free-ranging giraffe (Giraffa camelopardalis) using carfentanil and xylazine. Journal of Zoo and Wildlife Medicine 18:135–140.

Bush M, Ensley PK, Mehren K, et al. 1976. Immobilization of giraffes with xylazine and etorphine hydrochloride. Journal of the American Veterinary Medical Association 169:884–885.

Bush M, Raath JP, Phillips LG, et al. 1997. Immobilization of free-ranging giraffe (Giraffa camelopardalis) using medetomidine and ketamine. Annual Proceedings of the American Association of Zoo Veterinarians, pp. 276–277.

Bush M, Grobler DG, Raath JP, et al. 2001. Use of medetomidine and ketamine for immobilization of free-ranging giraffes. Journal of the American Veterinary Medical Association 218: 245–249.

Bush M, Grobler DG, Raath JP. 2002. The art and science of Giraffe (Giraffa camelopardalis) immobilization/anesthesia. In: Zoological Restraint and Anesthesia (D Heard, ed.), pp. 1–6. Ithaca: International Veterinary Information Service. http://www.ivis.org (accessed February 12, 2014).

Calle PP, Bormann JC. 1988. Giraffe restraint, habituation, and desensitization at the Cheyenne Mountain Zoo. Zoo Biology 7:243–252.

Citino SB. 1996. Anesthesia of okapi (Okapia johnstoni). In: Okapi Metapopulation Workshop (J Lukas, ed.). Yulee: White Oak Conservation Center.

Citino SB, Bush M, Phillips LG. 1984. Dystocia and fatal hyperthermic episode in a giraffe. Journal of the American Veterinary Medical Association 185:1440–1442.

Citino SB, Bush M, Lance W, et al. 2006. Use of thiafentanil (A3080), medetomidine, and ketamine for anesthesia of captive and free-ranging giraffe (Giraffa camelopardalis). Proceedings of the American Association of Zoo Veterinarians, pp. 211–213.

Citino SB, Bush M, Rivera O. 2007. A simple, unique field ventilator for large ungulates: another use for your leaf blower. Proceedings of the American Association of Zoo Veterinarians, pp. 51–52.

Dagg AI, Foster JB. 1976. The Giraffe: Its Biology, Behavior and Ecology. New York: Van Nostrand Reinhold.

Ebedes H, Raath JP. 1995. The use of long term neuroleptics in the confinement and transport of wild animals. Proceedings of the Joint Conference of the Proceedings of the American Association of Zoo Veterinarians, Wildlife Disease Association, and American Association of Wildlife Veterinarians, pp. 173–176.

Fischer MT, Miller RE, Houston EW. 1997. Serial tranquilization of a reticulated giraffe (Giraffa camelopardalis reticulata) using xylazine. Journal of Zoo and Wildlife Medicine 28(2):182–184.

Gardner HM, Hull BL, Hubbell JAE, et al. 1986. Volvulus of the ileum in a reticulated giraffe. Journal of the American Veterinary Medical Association 189(9):1180–1181.

Geiser DR, Morris PJ, Adair HS. 1992. Multiple anesthetic events in a reticulated giraffe (Giraffa camelopardalis). Journal of Zoo and Wildlife Medicine 23(2):189–196.

Hall-Martin AJ. 1977. Giraffe weight estimation using dissected leg weight and body measurements. The Journal of Wildlife Management 41(4):740–745.

Hargens AR. 1988. Gravitational cardiovascular adaptation in the giraffe. The Physiologist 30(1 Suppl.):S15–S18.

Hargens AR, Millard RW, Pettersson K, et al. 1987. Gravitational haemodynamics and oedema prevention in the giraffe. Nature 329:59–60.

Hirst SM. 1966. Immobilization of the Transvaal giraffe Giraffa camelopardalis giraffa using an oripavin derivative. Journal of the South African Veterinary Medical Association 37:85–89.

Hugh-Jones P, Barter CE, Hime JM, et al. 1978. Dead space and tidal volume of the giraffe compared with some other mammals. Respiration Physiology 35:53–58.

Lamberski N, Newell A, Radcliffe R. 2004. Thirty immobilizations of captive giraffe (Giraffa camelopardalis) using a combination of medetomidine and ketamine. Proceedings of the Joint Conference of the Proceedings of the American Association of Zoo Veterinarians, Wildlife Disease Association, and American Association of Wildlife Veterinarians, pp. 121–123.

Langman VA. 1973. The immobilization and capture of giraffe. *South African Journal of Science* 69:200.

Langman VA, Bamford OS, Maloiy GMO. 1982. Respiration and metabolism in the giraffe. *Respiration Physiology* 50:141–152.

Linton RAF, Taylor PM, Linton NWF, et al. 1999. Cardiac output measurement in an anesthetized giraffe. *The Veterinary Record* 145:498–499.

Mehrdadfar F, Shuler J, McCaffree K. 2003. Some notes on restraint box design for okapi. *International Zoo News* 325:216–221.

Mitchell G, Skinner JD. 1993. How giraffes adapt to their extraordinary shape. *Transactions of the Royal Society of South Africa* 48(2):207–218.

Morkel P. 1992. Giraffe capture with etorphine HCl (M-99) and hyalase: a new approach. In: *The Use of Tranquilizers in Wildlife* (H Ebedes, ed.), pp. 58–59. Pretoria: Department of Agricultural Development, Sinoville Printers.

Morkel P. 1993. Chemical capture of the giraffe (*Giraffa camelopardalis*). In: *The Capture and Care Manual: Capture, Care, Accommodation and Transportation of Wild African Animals* (AA McKenzie, ed.), pp. 601–607. Pretoria: Wildlife Decision Support Services CC.

Mortelmans J. 1978. Anaesthesia in okapis. *Acta zoologica et pathologica Antverpiensia* 71:41–44.

Nowak RM, Paradiso JL. 1983. *Walker's Mammals of the World*, 4th ed., pp. 1226–1230. Baltimore: The Johns Hopkins University Press.

Pedley TJ, Brook BS, Seymour RS. 1996. Blood pressure and flow rate in the giraffe jugular vein. *Philosophical Transactions of the Royal Society of London. Series B, Biological Sciences* 351:855–866.

Quesada R, Citino SB, Easley JT, et al. 2011. Surgical resolution of an avulsion fracture of the peroneus tertius origin in a giraffe (*Giraffa camelopardalis reticulate*). *Journal of Zoo and Wildlife Medicine* 42(2):348–350.

Raphael BL. 1999. Okapi medicine and surgery. In: *Zoo and Wild Animal Medicine, Current Therapy 4* (ME Fowler, RE Miller, eds.), p. 649. Philadelphia: W.B. Saunders.

Rapley WA, Mehren KG, Bonar CJ, et al. 1975. Repair of a fractured mandible in a giraffe using rompun and M-99 immobilization. Proceedings of the American Association of Zoo Veterinarians, pp. 12–15.

Redrobe S. 2003. Novel use of two tranquilizers, zuclopethixol and haloperidol, to facilitate the transportation of two okapi (*Okapia johnstoni*). Proceedings of the American Association of Zoo Veterinarians, p. 252.

Teare A. 2000. Okapi ISIS MedARKS library disk.

Vahala J. 1990. Experiences with immobilization of giraffes (*Giraffa camelopardalis*) in captivity. *Veterinarstvi* 40(7):321–323.

Vogelnest L, Ralph HK. 1997. Chemical immobilisation of giraffe to facilitate short procedures. *Australian Veterinary Journal* 75(3):180–182.

Warren JV. 1974. The physiology of the giraffe. *Scientific American* 213:96–105.

Wiesner H, von Hegel G. 1989. The immobilization of giraffes. *Tierarztliche Praxis* 17(1):97–100.

Williamson WM, Wallach JD. 1968. M.99-induced recumbency and analgesia in a giraffe. *Journal of the American Veterinary Medical Association* 153(7):816–817.

York W. 1975. Fentanyl citrate for wild animal capture. *Journal of Zoo Animal Medicine* 6(1):14–15.

York W, Kidder C, Durr C. 1973. Chemical restraint and castration of an adult giraffe. *Journal of Zoo Animal Medicine* 4(2):17–21.

59 Cervids (Deer)

Nigel Caulkett and Jon M. Arnemo

INTRODUCTION

A variety of deer species are distributed worldwide. It is beyond the scope of this chapter to discuss each species; therefore, the emphasis will be placed on general principles, with a brief discussion of current techniques in selected species. A complete description of dose requirements for individual species can be found in Kreeger and Arnemo (2012).

SPECIES-SPECIFIC PHYSIOLOGY

Deer are prone to rumenal tympany, regurgitation, hypoxemia, hyperthermia, and capture myopathy. Maintenance in sternal recumbency will help prevent the development of rumenal tympany. If rumenal tympany is a problem, the animal may be rocked gently to stimulate eructation. A rumen tube can be used, but may predispose to regurgitation and aspiration. Generally, if rumenal tympany is severe, it is advisable to finish the procedure quickly and antagonize the anesthetic agents. If alpha-2 agonists have been used, the administration of tolazoline, yohimbine, or atipamezole will stimulate rumenal activity and relieve rumenal tympany.

Capture myopathy is a potentially serious complication that can be very difficult to treat (Spraker 1993). Capture myopathy can be acute. In the acute form of capture myopathy, the animals' oxygen demand is far in excess of oxygen supply. Animals often present with hyperthermia, cyanosis, acidosis, tachycardia, and hypotension. The animal may die during the anesthesia or soon after. If the animal survives the acute stage, it may develop subacute or chronic capture myopathy. This can have a variety of manifestations, including paraplegia, ruptured muscles, myoglobinuria, or oliguria (Spraker 1993). The treatment of acute capture myopathy is directed at symptomatic treatment for shock, correcting acid–base disturbances, maintaining normothermia, and oxygenation. Treatment is extremely difficult in a field situation and often unsuccessful. Animals with chronic capture myopathy generally need to be euthanized. It is best to prevent capture myopathy by keeping chase times to a minimum and avoiding prolonged physical restraint. A complete review of capture myopathy can be found in Chapter 15.

Trauma is not uncommon during capture. White-tailed deer can be very flighty and, as such, they are prone to self-trauma.

PHYSICAL CAPTURE AND RESTRAINT

In zoo and game-farmed situations, deer may be effectively handled in drop-floor or hydraulic squeeze chutes (Fig. 59.1).

It is always best to minimize physical restraint times to decrease the risk of trauma or stress-related complications. Long-acting neuroleptic drugs can be used to decrease the stress of repeat handling (Read et al. 2000). Free-ranging deer may be captured with the use of net guns, drive nets, or clover traps. As mentioned earlier, restraint times should be minimized, and supplemental sedation should be considered during handling (Cattet et al. 2004).

CHEMICAL RESTRAINT AND ANESTHESIA

Vascular Access

Venous access is not difficult in deer. The cephalic vein, lateral saphenous vein, and jugular vein can all be easily accessed (Fig. 59.2). The auricular artery can be easily cannulated in most species for direct blood pressure monitoring or to facilitate sampling for arterial blood gas analysis. Arterial blood samples may also be

Zoo Animal and Wildlife Immobilization and Anesthesia, Second Edition. Edited by Gary West, Darryl Heard, and Nigel Caulkett.
© 2014 John Wiley & Sons, Inc. Published 2014 by John Wiley & Sons, Inc.

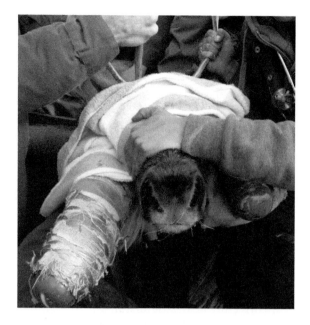

Figure 59.1. Reindeer restrained in a drop floor chute.

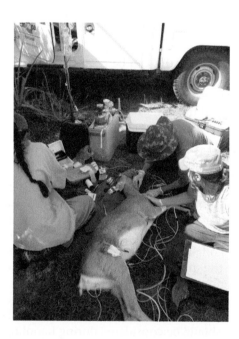

Figure 59.2. Jugular blood sampling from a pampas deer.

obtained from the femoral artery when auricular arterial catheterization proves to be difficult.

Intubation

Intubation can be difficult in cervids. The best technique is to maintain the animal in sternal recumbency with the head and neck extended upwards. Use a laryngoscope with a long flat blade and stiffen the endotracheal tube with a stylet. The epiglottis is long and mobile in cervids. The flat blade of the laryngoscope should be carefully placed on the dorsum of the

epiglottis, depressing it ventrally. The opening to the glottis can then be visualized and intubation can proceed. Animals induced with xylazine and ketamine may swallow, or close the glottic opening during intubation. The depth of anesthesia may be increased, to facilitate intubation, with an additional dose of ketamine (1–2 mg/kg) or propofol (2–4 mg/kg) (Woodbury et al. 2005).

Preanesthetic Concerns

Several factors can influence the method of anesthesia, and the means of drug administration. It is important to plan the capture carefully, as prolonged chase times can result in capture myopathy, trauma, or hyperthermia.

Elective procedures, in captive animals, should be planned for the cool hours of the day. Rumenal tympany can be a complication during anesthesia. If the procedure is elective, captive deer should be fasted for 24 hours. Deer are prone to hypoxemia during anesthesia (Moresco et al. 2001; Murray et al. 2000; Paterson et al. 2009; Read et al. 2001). Hypoxemia is exacerbated by positioning in dorsal or lateral recumbency. Alpha-2 agonist drugs, such as xylazine or medetomidine, will also exacerbate hypoxemia (Read et al. 2001). Chronically debilitated animals and animals with severe fluid deficits or blood loss are generally not good candidates for anesthesia, and will be at increased risk for complications.

MONITORING AND SUPPORTIVE CARE

Pulmonary Function

Whenever possible, deer should be positioned in sternal recumbency. The head and neck should be extended to maintain a patent airway. The animal should be monitored for hypoxemia, ideally with a pulse oximeter. A multi-site sensor applied to the tongue generally provides a good signal. Normal hemoglobin saturation should be 95–98%, below 85% is considered hypoxemic. Severely hypoxemic animals are often tachycardic. Heart rates above 150 in mature deer may result from a stress response due to hypoxemia, hypercarbia, pain, or hypotension. Supplemental inspired oxygen should be considered in hypoxemic animals. Oxygen can be easily delivered via nasal insufflation (Read et al. 2001).A nasal catheter should be placed and threaded as far as the medial canthus of the eye. A flow rate of 1–2 L/min is generally sufficient for smaller species, such as white-tailed deer (Fahlman et al. 2011). Higher flow rates may be required in larger deer species, such as red deer and moose (Paterson et al. 2009).

In order to conserve oxygen and prolong tank life, the flow should be adjusted downwards to find the minimum flow that will allow maintenance of $SpO_2 \geq 95\%$. An alternative strategy is to use a portable oxygen concentrator; these devices have proven effective in treating hypoxemia during anesthesia of reindeer (Fahlman et al. 2012).

Monitoring the Cardiovascular System

Heart rate should be monitored, at minimum, every 5 minutes. The auricular artery is easily palpated in deer. If the auricular artery cannot be palpated, a femoral pulse can be used. Blood pressure can be easily measured with an oscillometric cuff placed proximal to the carpus.

Thermoregulation

Rectal temperature should be monitored every 5–10 minutes. Deer are prone to hyperthermia (Moresco et al. 2001; Read et al. 2001). Rectal temperatures greater than 40°C are cause for concern, and attempts should be made to cool the animal. Rectal temperature in excess of 41°C is an emergency and should be treated aggressively. It is difficult to actively cool large animals and often the best option is to antagonize the immobilizing agents and allow the animal to recover. Hyperthermia, in the face of hypoxemia, is a particularly serious complication, as hyperthermia increases metabolic oxygen demand. Hyperthermic animals should receive supplemental inspired oxygen to offset hypoxemia.

PHARMACOLOGICAL CONSIDERATIONS FOR ANESTHESIA OF DEER

This section is an overview of pharmacological agents that can be used for anesthesia of deer. Attention must be paid to hunting seasons and appropriate marking of wild captured animals, to avoid consumption of drug residues in meat.

Anesthesia of Captive or Game-Farmed Deer

Game-farmed and other captive deer often have very different drug requirements compared with free-ranging animals. The following sections deal with anesthetic management of captive deer.

Sedation of Captive Deer White-tailed deer and mule deer usually require 2–3 mg/kg body weight (BW) of xylazine, IM, to produce recumbent sedation. American elk require approximately 1 mg/kg, IM, to produce recumbent sedation (Caulkett 1997). Once the xylazine has been administered, the animal should be left alone until it assumes a position of lateral recumbency or sternal recumbency with its head down. The deer can be cautiously approached and a towel should be placed over its eyes to decrease stimulation; noise should be kept to a minimum. Animals may appear to be very sedate under xylazine sedation, but they can rouse suddenly. To decrease the chance of sudden arousal, administer 1 mg/kg of ketamine into the jugular vein. Anesthesia can be maintained with 1–2 mg/kg of

ketamine IV, as required (generally at 10–15 minute intervals).

Yohimbine is effective in most cervids at a dose of 0.1–0.2 mg/kg BW. Administer 0.1 mg/kg IV and 0.1 mg/kg IM. Tolazoline is also effective, and can be used at a dose of 2–4 mg/kg. Atipamezole can be used at 1 mg IM per 10 mg of xylazine.

Local Analgesia for Velvet Antler Removal The simplest way to block velvet antler is to perform a ring block at the base of the antler pedicle. Lidocaine HCl (without epinephrine) is administered at a dose rate of 1 mL/cm of pedicle circumference (Wilson et al. 2000). The block will produce surgical analgesia in 1–2 minutes and will last approximately 90 minutes.

Inhalational Anesthesia

Inhalational anesthesia is recommended for prolonged, or very invasive procedures. Either halothane or isoflurane can be used. A small animal circle system can be used on animals weighing up to 150 kg (Fig. 59.3). Use a 3- to 6-L rebreathing bag and fresh gas flows of 10–20 mL/kg BW/min. Cervids premedicated with xylazine can usually be maintained on approximately 1% halothane or 1.3% isoflurane. Induction of captive adult cervids can often be achieved with xylazine sedation followed by IV ketamine at a dose of 2–3 mg/kg BW, using the techniques described earlier. Xylazine-tiletamine-zolazepam can also be used for induction, at the dosage quoted later. Fawns are usually easy to handle. Fawns can be induced with IV diazepam, 0.2 mg/kg, followed by 0.05 mg/kg of butorphanol IV, followed by 2–3 mg/kg of ketamine.

Airway protective reflexes are absent under inhalational anesthesia, and regurgitation and aspiration can occur; therefore, intubation is recommended. Hypoventilation may be encountered, necessitating

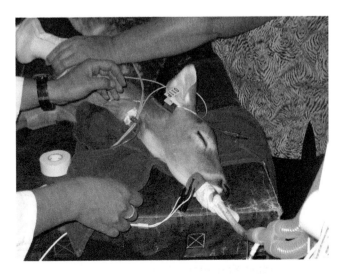

Figure 59.3. Maintenance volatile anesthesia of fawns can easily be achieved with a small animal anesthetic machine.

intermittent positive pressure ventilation. Usually, cervids maintain a relatively high blood pressure; hypotension may be encountered if rumenal tympany is present. The respiratory and hemodynamic compromise produced by rumenal tympany can be severe. The incidence of rumenal tympany can be decreased if food is withheld for 24–36 hours prior to anesthesia. Water should be withheld for 12 hours prior to anesthesia. Rumenal tympany may be resolved by passage of a stomach tube. If not, the anesthesia may be terminated, or emergency rumenal trocharization performed. Passive regurgitation can occur. Inflate the cuff on the endotracheal tube to ensure an adequate seal of the airway. The animal should be extubated when the swallowing reflex occurs, and the ETT should be removed with the cuff partially inflated. Animals that have had xylazine premedication should receive yohimbine, to reverse the effects of the xylazine, at a dose of 0.1–0.2 mg/kg BW. Divide the dose, give half IM and half IV. Postoperative analgesia can be achieved with 0.025–0.05 mg/kg BW of butorphanol.

Capture of Free-Ranging Deer

Wild deer will generally be at a greater risk for complications than captive deer. Drug requirements are higher and the risk of capture myopathy, hyperthermia, or trauma is potentially higher. There are a variety of protocols for capture of deer. This section describes some of these protocols.

Xylazine-Tiletamine-Zolazepam Xylazine-tiletamine-zolazepam is a useful mixture for capture of wild deer (Millspaugh et al. 1995; Murray et al. 2000) and for chemical immobilization and light anesthesia in game-farmed or zoo animals. The effective dose for American elk is 1 mg/kg of xylazine + 2 mg/kg of tiletamine-zolazepam. White-tailed deer and mule deer require 1.5 mg/kg of xylazine + 3 mg/kg of telazol. Excited animals often require a higher dose. This combination will provide approximately 45 minutes–1 hour of anesthesia. Anesthesia may be prolonged with IV ketamine at a dose of 1–2 mg/kg, Q 15 minutes. Once the procedure has been completed antagonism of xylazine is recommended with tolazoline or yohimbine at the earlier dosage. The major complication associated with this technique is hypoxemia. Read et al. (2000) conducted a trial to measure the respiratory effects of a xylazine-tiletamine-zolazepam mixture. All elk exhibited mild to marked hypoxemia (PaO_2 = 43 ± 11.8 mmHg) and showed marked improvement after 5 minutes of nasal insufflation of oxygen at 10L/min (PaO_2 = 207 ± 60 mmHg).

Medetomidine-Ketamine Medetomidine is a very useful alpha-2 agonist drug for wildlife anesthesia when it is formulated at a concentration of 10–30 mg/mL.

Medetomidine is 20–40 times more potent than xylazine. However, its use alone is not generally recommended as inducuction times are unacceptably long. Medetomidine is generally used in combination with ketamine. The major advantage of medetomidine-ketamine is that ketamine requirements are much lower than with xylazine. This factor allows for an earlier antagonism of the combination that is, the alpha-2 agonist can be antagonized with less risk of unmasking convulsive activity or rigidity from residual ketamine. Hypoxemia and hypertension are the major complications that may be encountered with medetomidine-ketamine (Caulkett et al. 2000). Medetomidine should always be antagonized with atipamezole at a 3–5:1 ratio. Less specific alpha-2 agonist drugs (yohimbine and tolazoline) are usually not effective.

Potent Opioids Potent opioids, such as, etorphine, carfentanil, and fentanyl, have been widely used for immobilization of several different deer species (Caulkett et al. 2000; Haigh 1990, 1991; Moresco et al. 2001). In most cases, they have been combined with xylazine, acepromazine, or other sedatives in order to achieve optimum immobilization. The choice of opioid for use in deer may be governed as much by availability as by any other factor.

Thiafentanil is another potent opioid anesthetic that has proven to be extremely useful for capture of deer. Doses in North American elk as high as 100 μg/kg provided very rapid immobilization (<1 minute in some cases), and numerous elk have been immobilized at doses near 50 μg/kg (Smith et al. 1993). A very complete overview of thiafentanil can be found in (Lance & Kenny 2011).

A variety of opioid antagonists have been used in deer. They include nalorphine, diprenorphine, naloxone, nalmefene, and naltrexone; of these products, naloxone has the shortest half-life. Narcotic recycling, or resedation, especially of animals immobilized with carfentanil or etorphine, has been reported when naloxone is used (Haigh 1991). Naltrexone has a much longer duration of action than any of the other antagonists listed (Kreeger & Arnemo 2012), and when adequate doses of naltrexone are used, recycling is generally not a problem (Haigh 1990).

Sedation of Free-Ranging Deer

Intranasal Alpha-2 Agonist Administration Intranasal drug administration has the advantage of a rapid onset time, reliability, and ease of administration. It is a useful technique to produce sedation in deer that are captured by physical means (Fig. 59.4). Xylazine administered intranasally at a dose of 1.5–2 mg/kg will produce reliable sedation, and stress reduction in American elk (Cattet et al. 2004). Onset is rapid (often less than 1 minute), and the effects can be antagonized with yohimbine.

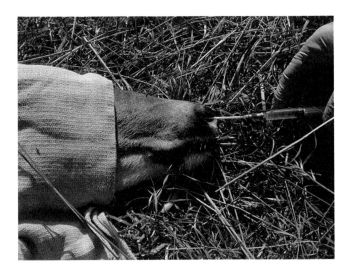

Figure 59.4. Intranasal drug administration to a white-tailed deer.

Neuroleptic Agents

Neuroleptics can be extremely useful in the management of wild and semi-domesticated deer. These drugs will facilitate transport of deer and will decrease stress in acutely captured deer. They have the potential to decrease the risk of trauma, and capture myopathy. Azaperone (0.2 mg/kg) can be used immediately post reversal to facilitate short translocations (6 hours or less). Zuclopenthixol acetate (1 mg/kg) will provide up to 4 days of tranquilization (Read et al. 2000). Animals treated with this drug demonstrate decreased flight distance, decreased indices of stress, and improved water and food consumption compared to untreated animals (Read et al. 2000).

Anesthetic Protocols for Various Deer Species

White-Tailed Deer (*Odocoileus virginianus*)& Mule Deer (*Odocoileus hemonius*) Mature white-tailed deer weigh 60–150 kg (Kreeger & Arnemo 2012). Mature mule deer weigh 75–135 kg. They are not difficult to anesthetize as long as they are kept calm during immobilization. Excited deer tend to override the sedative effects of alpha-2 agonists and often require higher doses for induction. Common complications include the following: trauma, hyperthermia, and potentially capture myopathy. Rumenal tympany is not commonly encountered during anesthesia of these species. A variety of techniques have been used to induce immobilization. Hypoxemia is not uncommon, and supplemental inspired oxygen should be considered.

White-tailed deer can be effectively anesthetized with 2.2 mg/kg of xylazine, combined with 4.4 mg/kg of tiletamine-zolazepam (Murray et al. 2000). This combination is equally effective on mule deer, and immobilization can be partially antagonized with 0.1–0.2 mg/

kg of yohimbine. Medetomidine at a dosage of 0.1 mg/ kg, combined with 2.5 mg/kg of ketamine, will produce a good quality of immobilization in mule deer and white-tailed deer (Caulkett et al. 2000). Atipamezole administered at three to five times the medetomidine dose will effectively antagonize immobilization. Thiafentanil can be used in white-tailed deer at a dosage of 0.1 mg/kg, combined with 1 mg/kg of xylazine, reversal can be achieved with 2 mg/kg of naltrexone, combined with 2 mg/kg tolazoline. In mule deer, a thiafentanil dose of 0.15 mg/kg, combined with 1 mg/kg of xylazine, is recommended (Kreeger & Arnemo 2012).

North American Elk (*Cervus canadensis*) and Red Deer (*Cervus elaphus*) Elk or red deer may be captured via physical or chemical means. If physical capture (net gunning) is used, sedation can be quickly induced with intranasal xylazine (Cattet et al. 2004). Mature elk weigh 230- to 318-kg, red deer weigh 60–180 kg (Kreeger & Arnemo 2012). Chemical immobilization can be induced with opioids or alpha-2 agonists combined with dissociatives. Hypoxemia is common in anesthetized elk; it has been described during anesthesia with carfentanil-xylazine (Moresco et al. 2001). In this study, hypoxemia was effectively treated by partial antagonism of carfentanil with a low dose of naloxone. Hypoxemia has also been characterized during immobilization with xylazine-tiletamine-zolazepam (Read et al. 2001). Elk can be immobilized with 10 μg/kg of carfentanil combined with 0.1 mg/kg of xylazine (Moresco et al. 2001). Immobilization should be antagonized with naltrexone. A mixture of 0.4 mg/kg of xylazine, combined with 3 mg/kg of tiletamine-zolazepam, is also effective (Millspaugh et al. 1995). Immobilization, with this combination, can be partially antagonized with 0.125 mg/kg of yohimbine.

Red deer are distributed throughout Europe; they are smaller than elk but considerations are similar. The drug of choice for red deer capture is 0.11 mg/kg of medetomidine, combined with 2.2 mg/kg of ketamine (Arnemo et al. 1994a). Medetomidine should be antagonized with 0.5 mg/kg of atipamezole. A good alternative is 2.5–3.0 mg/kg of xylazine, combined with 2.5–3.0 mg/kg of tiletamine-zolazepam (Janovsky et al. 2000). Atipamezole should be used to antagonize xylazine at a dose ratio of 1:8 (mg:mg). However, due to the long elimination time of tiletamine-zolazepam, recoveries are often prolonged.

American Moose and European Moose (*Alces americanus* and *Alces alces*) Anesthesia of moose is very similar to anesthesia of other deer. One of the major complicating factors with moose is their large size. Mature moose can weigh 400–800 kg (Kreeger & Arnemo 2012). All of the same precautions apply, and particular attention must be paid to the prevention of capture myopathy and hyperthermia. There are several drug choices for anesthesia of moose. Carfentanil-xylazine has been advocated, as in other deer (Seal et al. 1985). The addition of xylazine to carfentanil will decrease the incidence of muscle rigidity; unfortunately, the addition of xylazine will also increase the risk of regurgitation and aspiration pneumonia (Kreeger 2000). For this reason, if carfentanil is used in moose, it should be administered as the sole agent at a dose of 10 µg/kg. In addition to the risk of regurgitation, they are at risk for hyperthermia and capture myopathy. Thiafentanil at a dose of 0.03 mg/kg is good alternative (Kreeger et al. 2005). Reversal of immobilization can be achieved with 0.6 mg/kg of naltrexone.

European moose have been effectively immobilized with 60 µg/kg of medetomidine, combined with 1.5 mg/kg of ketamine. (Arnemo et al. 1994b). Immobilization can be antagonized with 0.3 mg/kg of atipamezole. Currently, the drug of choice for free-ranging moose is etorphine, alone, at a dose of 7.5 mg of etorphine per adult, and half this dose in calves (Arnemo et al. 2004). We have also seen good results with xylazine-tiletamine-zolazepam in moose captured for translocation from urban areas. A dose of 1.5 mg/kg of xylazine combined with 3 mg/kg of tiletamine-zolazepam has proven effective (N. Caulkett unpubl. data, 2005), but recoveries may be prolonged following xylazine reversal. Immobilization can be partially antagonized with yohimbine or tolazoline.

Caribou and Reindeer (*Rangifer tarandus*) Caribou often have high drug requirements, when compared with other deer species. Their speed and agility can make them a difficult target for remote delivery. *Rangifer* sp. range in size from 80 to 300 kg (Kreeger & Arnemo 2012), with woodland caribou being the largest subspecies. The drug combination of choice for reindeer is 0.1–0.2 mg/kg of medetomidine plus 1–2.5 mg/kg of ketamine (Arnemo et al. 2000, 2011; Kreeger & Arnemo 2012), Dose rates in *Rangifer* are very variable depending on the capture technique, the degree of human conditioning (domestic vs. wild), and the subspecies being captured.

Fallow Deer (*Dama dama*) Adult fallow weigh 40–100 kg (Kreeger & Arnemo 2012). A variety of techniques have been used to anesthetize fallow deer, often with unreliable effects. One potentially reliable drug combination for fallow deer is 0.1 mg/kg of medetomidine + 1 mg/kg of tiletamine-zolazepam (Fernandez-Moran et al. 2000).

Axis Deer (*Axis axis*) and Hog Deer (*Axis porcinus*) In Asia, drive nets are often used to capture free-ranging axis deer and hog deer. To reduce stress and to facilitate handling, sedation can be induced with 3–4 mg of xylazine IM (with subsequent reversal with 1-mg

atipamezole/8-mg xylazine) (Kreeger & Arnemo 2012). The effect of xylazine, however, is unpredictable in excited individuals, and a combination of medetomidine and ketamine is preferred both for physically restrained animals and for chemical capture by remote drug administration. In axis deer, 0.1-mg/kg medetomidine + 3.5-mg/kg ketamine, and in hog deer, 0.5-mg/kg medetomidine + 1.5-mg/kg ketamine (Kreeger & Arnemo 2012). If needed, ketamine at 1–2 mg/kg IM can be used to deepen or prolong anesthesia. The effects of medetomidine can be effectively reversed by atipamezole IM at 5-mg/mg medetomidine (Kreeger & Arnemo 2012).

Neotropical Deer Species Midazolam at a dose of 0.5 mg/kg has been combined with ketamine (7 mg/kg) and xylazine (0.3 mg/kg) in brown brocket deer (*Mazama gouazoubira*), Midazolam (0.5 mg/kg) has also been combined with ketamine (5 mg/kg) and xylazine (0.5 mg/kg) for the chemical immobilization of marsh deer (*Blastocerus dichotomus*). Free-ranging marsh deer have also been successfully anesthetized with 0.8 mg/kg of xylazine and 2 mg/kg IV of tiletamine-zolazepam, with rapid, smooth recovery following antagonism of the xylazine, with yohimbine (Pinho et al. 2010). Pampas deer (*Ozotoserus bezoarticus*) can also be successfully immobilized with either xylazine-midazolam-ketamine or xylazine-tiletamine-zolazepam. A complete review of capture and restraint of neotropical cervids can be found in *Neotropical Cervidology: Biology and Medicine of Latin American Deer*.

REFERENCES

Arnemo JM, Negard T, Søli NE. 1994a. Chemical capture of free-ranging red deer (*Cervus elaphus*) with medetomidine-ketamine. *Rangifer* 14:123–127.

Arnemo JM, Soveri T, Os Ø, et al. 1994b. Immobilization of free-ranging moose (*Alces alces*) with medetomidine-ketamine and reversal with atipamezole. Joint Conference of the American Association of Zoo Veterinarians and the Association of Reptile and Amphibian Veterinarians, pp. 197–199.

Arnemo JM, Aanes R, Os Ø, et al. 2000. Reversible immobilization of free-ranging Svalbard reindeer, Norwegian reindeer and woodland caribou: a comparison of medetomidine-ketamine and atipamezole in three subspecies of *Rangifer tarandus*. Proceedings of the Wildlife Disease Association Conference, June, Grand Teton National Park, WY.

Arnemo JM, Ericsson G, Øen EO, et al. 2004. Immobilization of free-ranging moose (*Alces alces*) with etorphine or etorphine-acepromazine-xylazine in Scandanavia (1984–2003): a review of 2754 captures. Proceedings of the American Association of Zoo Veterinarians, pp. 515–516.

Arnemo JM, Evans AL, Miller AL, et al. 2011. Effective immobilizing doses of medetomidine-ketamine in free-ranging,wild Norwegian reindeer (*Rangifer tarandus tarandus*). *Journal of Wildlife Diseases* 47:755–758.

Cattet MRL, Caulkett NA, Wilson C, et al. 2004. Intranasal administration of xylazine to reduce stress in elk captured by net gun. *Journal of Wildlife Diseases* 40:562–565.

Caulkett NA. 1997. Anesthesia for North American cervids. *The Canadian Veterinary Journal* 38:389–390.

Caulkett NA, Cribb PH, Haigh JC. 2000. Comparative cardiopulmonary effects of carfentanil-xylazine and medetomidine-ketamine for immobilization of mule deer and mule deer/white tailed deer hybrids. *Canadian Journal of Veterinary Research* 64: 64–68.

Fahlman Å, Caulkett N, Woodbury M, et al. 2011. Low flow oxygen therapy effectively treats hypoxaemia in anaesthetized white-tailed deer. Proceedings of the European Veterinary Emergency and Critical Care Society, p. 206. Utrecht, The Netherlands.

Fahlman Å, Caulkett N, Arnemo JM, et al. 2012. Efficacy of a portable oxygen concentrator with pulsed delivery for treatment of hypoxemia during anesthesia of wildlife. *Journal of Zoo and Wildlife Medicine* 43:67–76.

Fernandez-Moran J, Palomeque J, et al. 2000. Medetomidine/tiletamine/zolazepam and xylazine/tiletamine/zolazepam combinations for immobilization of fallow deer (*Cevus dama*). *Journal of Zoo and Wildlife Medicine* 31:62–64.

Haigh JC. 1990. Opioids in zoological medicine. *Journal of Zoo and Wildlife Medicine* 21:391–413.

Haigh JC. 1991. Immobilization of wapiti with carfentanil and xylazine and opioid antagonism with diprenorphine, naloxone and naltrexone. *Journal of Zoo and Wildlife Medicine* 22:318–323.

Janovsky M, Tataruch F, Ambuehl M, et al. 2000. A zoletil-rompun mixture as an alternative to the use of opioids for immobilization of feral red deer. *Journal of Wildlife Diseases* 36:663–669.

Kreeger TJ. 2000. Xylazine-induced aspiration pneumonia in Shira's moose. *Wildlife Society Bulletin* 28:751–753.

Kreeger TJ, Arnemo JM. 2012. *Handbook of Wildlife Chemical Immobilization*, 4th ed. Wheatland: TJ Kreeger.

Kreeger TJ, Edwards WH, Brimeyer D, et al. 2005. Health assessment and survival of Shira's moose immobilized with thiafentanil. *Alces* 41:121–128.

Lance WR, Kenny DE. 2011. Thiafentanil oxalate (A3080) in nondomestic ungulate species. In: *Fowler's Zoo and Wild Animal Medicine*, Vol. 7 (RE Miller, ME Fowler, eds.), pp. 589–595. St Louis: Elsevier.

Millspaugh JJ, Brundige GC, Jenks JA, et al. 1995. Immobilization of rocky mountain elk with Telazol and xylazine hydrochloride, and antagonism by yohimbine hydrochloride. *Journal of Wildlife Diseases* 31:259–262.

Moresco AM, Larson JM, Sleeman MA, et al. 2001. Use of naloxone to reverse carfentanil citrate-induced hypoxemia and cardiopulmonary depression in rocky mountain wapiti. *Journal of Zoo and Wildlife Medicine* 32:81–89.

Murray S, Monfort SL, Ware L, et al. 2000. Anesthesia in female white-tailed deer using telazol and xylazine. *Journal of Wildlife Diseases* 36:670–675.

Paterson JM, Caulkett NA, Woodbury MR. 2009. Physiologic effects of nasal oxygen or medical air administered prior to and during carfentanil-xylazine anesthesia in North American elk (*Cervus canadensis manitobensis*). *Journal of Zoo and Wildlife Medicine* 40:39–50.

Pinho MP, Munerato MS, Nunes ALV. 2010. Anesthesia and chemical immobilization. In: *Neotropical Cervidology: Biology and Medicine of Latin American Deer* (JM Barbanti Duarte, S González, eds.), pp. 228–239. Jaboticabal: Funep.

Read M, Caulkett NA, McCallister M. 2000. Evaluation of zooclopenthixol acetate to decrease handling stress in wapiti. *Journal of Zoo and Wildlife Medicine* 36:450–459.

Read MR, Caulkett NA, Symington A, et al. 2001. Treatment of Hypoxemia during xylazine-tiletamine-zolazepam immobilization of wapiti. *The Canadian Veterinary Journal* 42:661–664.

Seal US, Schnitt SM, Peterson RO. 1985. Carfentanil and xylazine for immobilization of moose (*Alces alces*) on Isle Royale. *Journal of Wildlife Diseases* 21:48–51.

Smith IL, McJames SW, Natte R, et al. 1993. A-3080 studies in elk: effective immobilizing doses by syringe and dart injection. Proceedings of the .American Association of Zoo Veterinarians, pp. 420–421.

Spraker TR. 1993. Stress and capture myopathy in artiodactylids. In: *Zoo and Wild Animal Medicine: Current Therapy 3* (ME Fowler, ed.), pp. 481–488. Philadelphia: W.B. Saunders.

Wilson PR, Stafford KJ, Thomas DJ, et al. 2000. Evaluation of techniques for lignocaine hydrochloride analgesia of the velvet antler of adult stags. *New Zealand Veterinary Journal* 48: 72–82.

Woodbury MR, Caulkett NA, Johnson CB, et al. 2005. Comparison of Analgesic techniques for antler removal in halothane-anaesthetized red deer (*Cervus elaphus*): cardiovascular and somatic responses. *Veterinary Anaesthesia and Analgesia* 32: 1–11.

60 Antelope

Ray L. Ball and Markus Hofmeyr

INTRODUCTION

The group of mammals referred to as antelope are a diverse collection of ruminants ranging from dik-dik to eland. Antelope are one of the groups of animals classically associated with game capture and translocation. Historically, anesthesia in captive antelope was one of the veterinarians' most difficult challenges. Improvements in captive management, including training techniques and restraint devices, have made the need for anesthesia much less and facilitated it when it is necessary. But the anesthesia of antelope, which are very diverse and different to each other, is a skill that will never totally be replaced with advances in restraint and training, and veterinarians with antelope in their care should strive to improve their anesthetic management.

TAXONOMY AND ANATOMY RELATED TO ANESTHESIA

Antelope is a common name given to various members of the family Antilocapridae and Bovidae. The pronghorn, *Antilocapra americana*, is the only member in the Antilocapridae. The antelope are scattered in several subfamily in the Bovidae. They are all ruminant Artiodactyla and range from a 3-kg dik-dik to 900-kg giant eland. The subfamilies Caprinae (goats and sheep), the genus *Gazella* (gazelle), *Bison*, and *Bos* (cattle) will be dealt with in separate chapters.

There are several anatomical considerations to consider when anesthetizing antelope. The lack of upper incisors can help facilitate tracheal intubation, but the depth of the larynx and the limitations in visualizing it can complicate intubation. The larynx itself is deep in the throat and difficult to visualize with a larynyscope and appropriate blade. One must ensure adequate depth of anesthesia before attempting to intubate

an antelope as excessive stimulation to the larynx can induce regurgitation. Dysplastic tracheae has been reorted in blue duikers but should be readily apparent at intubation efforts (Lombardini et al. 2010). The bovine lung is smaller, is divided into separate lobes, each with distinct lobules separated by complete septa. The diaphragm is more vertical and flatter in cattle (most antelope do not have published anatomical descriptions) than in horses, and most of the bovine lung is cranial to the abdomen. A flatter conformation of the diaphragm results in decreased ventilator efficiency (Lumb 2000). Tympany, regurgitation, and aspiration pneumonia are all serious potential complications with ruminants. Pharmacological effects of many anesthetics will increase the chances of regurgitation. Recumbency, especially left lateral, will increase tympany and regurgitation. This may be especially important in antelope that are darted for anesthetic induction and become malpositioned. The rumen occupies approximately three-fourths of the abdomen may become distended when a ruminant is recumbent. Therefore, increased intragastric pressure represents an additional unique pathophysiological condition for the diaphragm (Pypendop & Steffey 2001). With moderate to high intragastric pressure, a pattern of decreased respiratory rate, decreased end-expired lung volume, and breath holding at the end of inspiration is observed (Pypendop & Steffey 2001). Increased gastric pressure, gastric distension, and cranial displacement of the diaphragm can result in a significant decrease in lung dynamic compliance, tidal volume, and minute ventilation (Pypendop & Steffey 2001) resulting in PaCO2 increases and PaO2 decreases.

All large antelope should have adequate padding while recumbent. In dorsal recumbency, antelope should be balanced flat on their backs with the gluteals sharing the weight and all limbs should be flexed and

Zoo Animal and Wildlife Immobilization and Anesthesia, Second Edition. Edited by Gary West, Darryl Heard, and Nigel Caulkett.
© 2014 John Wiley & Sons, Inc. Published 2014 by John Wiley & Sons, Inc.

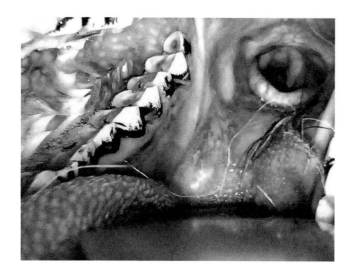

Figure 60.1. Endoscopic view of epiglottis and glottis of gerenuk (*Litocranius walleri*) with head and neck slightly extended.

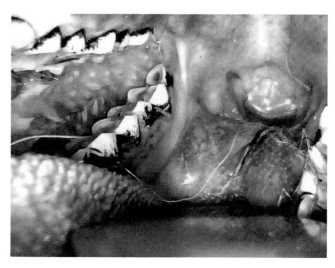

Figure 60.2. Same gerenuk and endoscope position as in Figure 60.1. Head is now flexed with nose down as is recommended to allow drainage of rumen reflux.

relaxed. The neck needs to be supported as well to prevent hyperextension. Antelope in dorsal recumbency at any plane of anesthesia should be intubated. In lateral recumbency, there should be adequate padding for the radial nerve. To improve venous return, an inner tube can be placed on the dependent forelimb and pulled cranial while the other limbs are lightly supported and moved perpendicular to the long axis of the body. The dependent eye must also be protected. The eye should be closed and padded with a towel or an inner tube. Often times, most diagnostic procedures can be performed with the animal in sternal recumbency. In a sternal position, all four limbs should be tucked under the animals in a natural sitting posture. The head is tucked in a flexed position to prevent any regurgitated material from being aspirated. This can have very serious drawbacks as it will also reduce the airflow during respirations. It is the authors' preference to keep the head extended and the airway as open as possible—it is best to hold the head up, neck extended and nose pointing downward—this fascilitates flow of possible regurgitated content out the mouth and away from the larynx. If regurgitation is likely, intubation is a better alternative than closing the airway (Fig. 60.1 and Fig. 60.2).

BIOLOGY AND PHYSIOLOGY

The pronghorn is found only in western North America. The feet have two digits and the horns consist of a bony core covered with a keratinized sheath that is shed annually (Huffman 2014). All antelope males and some females of certain species have unbranched horns attached to the frontal bones of the skull. The horns are composed of a bony core and are covered with a keratin sheath that is never shed. As a general rule, antelope are herding animals and live in small groups

to very large herds; exceptions are small antelopes, which are found on their own or in pairs. All antelope are ruminants and spend a majority of a 24-hour period actively feeding or ruminating.

VASCULAR ACCESS SITES AND MONITORING

Over-the-needle catheters are often utilized in antelope veins. In areas where the skin may be thicker, a cut down with a scalpel or large-gauge needle will facilitate catheter placement. Butterfly catheters can also be used for shorter-duration venous access or during emergencies. Common sites are the auricular, jugular, cephalic, medial and lateral saphenous, and lateral thoracic vein. Arterial access is most readily found in the radial, caudal auricular, and common digital arteries. The facial artery is palpable in most antelope species but can be difficult to catheterize in some species.

Several variables can be used to monitor the cardiovascular system including heart rate, pulse strength, color of mucus membranes, and capillary refill time. The color of venous blood (as can quickly be accessed in the earvein) is also a crude but useful indicator of blood oxygen levels. Resting heart rates are generally not known in antelope species, but in domestic cattle, resting heart rate is on average 80 beats per minute. Heart rate will vary with size and age. Smaller ruminants will be as high as 110 beats per minute (Riebold 1996). Initial heart rates in darted animals or those that are physically restrained are likely to be significantly higher. Overall heart rate will tend to drop as the anesthetic level deepens. Pulse pressure can be used in the field to estimate blood pressures indirectly. They can be evaluated at any of the sites mentioned above for arterial catherization. Typically, the strength of a palpated pulse will decrease with depth of anesthesia. If digital pressure on the artery is easily accomplished during diastole, the arterial pressure can be assumed to be low (Riebold 1996). Mucus membrane should be pink in anesthetized antelope. The use of alpha-2 agonists often makes the mucus membranes pale in color at the start of the anesthetic procedure. The color will often return to a normal pink after 20–30 minutes or if the alpha-2 drugs are antagonized. Capillary refill time should be less than 2 seconds, indicating good perfusion of peripheral tissues. Respiratory adequacy can be judged by monitoring respiratory rate and depth. Thoracic excursions or breaths felt form the nostrils are easy methods to monitor respiratory function. Ocular reflex and eye position do not appear to be as useful in many antelope anesthesia due to the likelihood that the induction often takes place remotely.

Monitoring core body temperature is essential in antelope anesthesia. Hyperthermia and subsequent capture myopathy is one of the most commonly encountered problems with antelope anesthesia. A rectal temperature is the most common location for temperature monitoring. Core temperatures may be better be assessed with a flexible thermometer lead placed down the esophagus. Hyperthermia commonly occurs during high ambient temperatures but can occur in temperature controlled environments. Hyperthermia may be induced by psychological factors regardless of ambient temperatures in impala. (Meyer 2008b). Common causes of hyperthermia include prolonged inductions, stress, and the depression of normal thermoregulatory mechanisms by anesthetic drugs. Underdosing and poor dart placement with partial drug delivery will inevitably lead to excessive running and pacing, capture stress, and resulting hyperthermia. To emphasize this point, thermometric data loggers were surgically implanted in 15 impala (*Aepyceros melampus*) to investigate the consequences of chemical capture (Meyer et al. 2010). Four combinations of induction agents were compared: etorphine and azaperone; etorphine and medetomidine; thiafentanil and azaperone; and thiafentanil medetomidine. The impala developed an extremely high rise in body temperature, which peaked 20–30 minutes after reversal of the immobilization regardless of drug combination used. The magnitude of the rise in body temperature was similar for all the drug combinations. Changes in body temperature were related to the time that it took for an animal to become recumbent after darting and not to the effect of the drug combination on time to recumbency. The relationship between time to recumbency and body temperature change, and also to plasma cortisol concentration, indicated that physiological consequences of capture were related to the duration of exposure to a stressor (the induction), and not to the pharmacology of the capture drugs(Meyer 2008a). Although shorter time to recumbency in individuals resulted in the benefit of smaller stress responses and body temperature changes, those individuals were predisposed to developing hypoxia and possibly induction apnea due presumably to higher doses used to achieve quicker inductions. As a general rule, quicker inductions with resultant anesthetic management have less complications than low dose extended induction periods (authors' personal experience).

Common approaches to treating hyperthermia in antelope have utilized topical water or cold water enemas. Another approach to cooling the patient is to deepen the anesthesia, intubate, and place the antelope on a ventilator. This will allow an exchange medium, oxygen and air, to contact a large surface and help dissipate heat. The ventilator will also reduce the muscular effort required by the antelope. Paralytics can be used to quickly intubate and allow less resistance against the ventilator. Moderate fluid therapy and nonsteroidal and steroidal anti-inflammatory drugs are useful adjuncts to this therapy. This approach has proven more successful in the author's hands than trying to cool the antelope externally, especially in larger species.

When anesthetic events in antelope are prolonged, as in a hospital setting, several additional anesthetic monitoring devices may be utilized to ensure the adequacy of the respiratory and cardiovascular systems. Pulse oximetry is now commonly employed in zoological anesthesia routinely. Probes are typically placed on the tongue, ear, vulva, or prepuce. Reflectance probes can also be placed in the oral cavity against the gingiva, or placed vaginally, or rectally. Indirect blood pressure can be measured with standard blood pressure cuffs. The tail and distal limbs are the most common site for cuff placement. Blood pressures in sheep and goats should be maintained at 100 mmHg systolic, 60 mmHg diastolic, with a mean of 75 mmHg, while cattle tend to have higher pressures normally (Riebold 1996). These can serve as good guidelines for smaller and larger antelope respectively. A mean of 60 mmHg has been recommended as a minimum value for zoo bovids (Citino 2003). Addax anesthetized with carfentanil, acetylpromazine, and ketamine had initial mean arterial pressures of 118 mmHg (Klein et al. 1994). Addax anesthetized with carfentanil and xylazine had initial mean arterial pressures of 120.5 mmHg (R. Ball, unpubl. data, 2006). Changes in blood pressure are often sensitive indicators of in assessing the change in depth of anesthesia. Electrocardiography can also be utilized in hospital settings. Lead placement can be a base–apex for large species or standard three-lead placement for smaller animals. Premature ventricular contractions (PVCs) are the most common arrhythmias seen in ruminants (Pypendop & Steffey 2001). A run of three or more PVCs are serious and warrant attention. Common causes of PVCs include hypoxemia and hypercarbia. Administering lidocaine and correcting the cause are essential. Arterial blood gases can also be used to monitor anesthesia.

INTUBATION

Intubation is recommended for any anesthetized antelope that needs to be transported or anesthetized for greater than 1 hour. In species that are prone to regurgitation, such as giant eland, duiker, roan, and addax, intubation should be considered during any anesthetic event. It is advisable to be prepared to intubate antelope even during routine field procedures if complications arise. An adequate plane of anesthesia must be obtained before attempting to intubate. Blind intubation attempts are successful only about 50% of the time in cattle and are not recommended in antelope (Riebold 1996). An effective technique for endotracheal intubation in antelope has been described (Bush 1996). In summary, the larynx is visualized using a laryngoscope with a long straight blade and a stylet, or endotracheal tube exchanger is placed into the trachea. With the laryngoscope removed, the stylet can then be placed through the Murphy's eye of the endotracheal tube and the tube is passed over the stylet and into the trachea. Intermittent positive pressure can be used in ruminants to treat unacceptable hypercarbia ($PaCO_2$ greater than 60 mmHG) (Pypendop & Steffey 2001).

Portable battery driven oxygen concentrators (EverGo™ Portable Oxygen Concentrator Respironics®, Murrysville, PA) provide an alternative to the use of oxygen cylinders for treatment of hypoxemia during field anesthesia (Fahlman et al. 2010). This has been shown to improve arterial oxygenation in reindeer but not bighorn sheep. The potential for this to provide support in field situations needs to be further explored. Another technique described to ventilate large ungulates is the use of an electric or gas power leaf blower as a ventilator (Citino et al. 2007). Caution should be used with gas-powered devices and inadvertent inhalation of carbon monoxide.

REVIEW OF REPORTS ON ANTELOPE ANESTHESIA

Opioids have been the mainstay of antelope anesthesia in wildlife and captive care. Recently, the addition of the potent opioid thiafentanil has allowed it to be evaluated for antelope immobilization. Thiafentanil alone seems to have little advantage when compared with carfentanil in impala, as induction times and all physiological parameters were comparable (Jansen et al. 1991). The same authors successfully used thiafentanil in eland (*Taurotragus oryx*), greater kudu (*Tragelaphus strepsiceros*), and waterbuck (*Kobus ellipsiprymnus*) with good results. More trials have been conducted utilizing thiafentanil in combination with medetomidine and ketamine. Roan antelope (*Hippotragus equinus*) have been captured with combinations of thiafentanil, medetomidine, and ketamine (Citino et al. 2001). Naltrexone, IV or IM, is used at 30 times the thiafentanil dose and atipamezole at 3 times the medetomidine

dose for recovery. Free-ranging gemsbok (*Oryx gazella*) have been anesthetized with a combination of thiafentanil, medetomidine, and ketamine (Grobler et al. 2001). Intramuscular naltrexone and atipamezole effectively reversed anesthesia. Lichtenstein's hartebeest (*Sigmoceros lichtensteinii*) were successfully anesthetized in bomas using thiafentanil, medetomidine, and ketamine (Citino et al. 2002). Naltrexone was given IV at 30 times the thiafentanil dose along with atipamezole at 4 times the medetomidine dose. Anesthesia of boma-conditioned and free-ranging nyala (*Tragelaphus angasii*) was successful using thiafentanil, medetomidine, and ketamine (Cooper et al. 2005). Free-ranging pronghorn (*Antilocapra Americana*) were anesthetized with thiafentanil and xylazine, and this combination was judged to be superior to previously used anesthetic combinations (Kreeger et al. 2001).

Thiafentanil (57 μg/kg) and azaperone (0.46 mg/kg), TA, has been compared with thiafentanil (15.16 ± 3.3 μg/kg)-medetomidine (15.16 ± 3.3 μg/kg)-ketamine (0.99 ± 0.04 mg/kg), TMK, in free-ranging Uganda kob (*Kobus kob thomasi*) (Caulkett et al. 2006). While the quality of the overall anesthesia was better with TMK, the authors recommended TA for field use due to potential complications with recoveries and profound hypoxia with TMK mixtures. The TMK mixture may have a place in captive situations or if only thiafentanil and medetomidine are used in field situations.

A recent study compared immobilization of gemsbok (*O. gazella*) using thiafentanil (0.036 μg/kg) and 20-mg xylazine (TX) versus carfentanil (0.021 μg/kg) and 20-mg xylazine (CX) (Kilgallon et al. 2010). While there were few physiologic differences between the groups, and minimal differences in overall quality of the anesthesia, the authors suggest that TX is preferable to CX when anesthetizing adult gemsboks.

Carfentanil and etorphine are still the most commonly used opioids antelope anesthesia. Opioids are often combined with alpha-2 agonists or tranquilizers when anesthetizing antelope. The benefits of these combinations include lowering the narcotic dose, smaller drug volumes, shorter induction times, and better muscle relaxation and analgesia than with the opioid alone. Table 60.3 lists several carfentanil and xylazine combinations used by the author. In some species, etorphine in combination with xylazine may have a better quality of anesthesia and shorter recovery times (Howard et al. 2004). Detomidine has been used in addax and blue wildebeest in combination with opioids (Portas et al. 2003) (see Table 60.3). Arabian and Scimitar-horned oryx have been anesthetized for long periods with combinations of etorphine and medetomidine, and there were fewer complications with this combination versus carfentanil and xylazine (Ancrenaz et al. 1996) (see Table 60.3).

A 1:1 mixture of xylazine and ketamine added to etorphine (M99KX) was found to lower the narcotic dose by as much as 30% and provide better overall anesthesia than etorphine and xylazine (Riebold 1996). Anesthesia in captive bongo was found to be superior with carfentanil-ketamine-xylazine (CKX) combination than either carfentanil alone or carfentanil and acepromazine (Miller-Edge & Amsel 1994). Carfentanil and xylazine combinations will cause hypoxemia and hypertension in captive bongo and blood gas analysis is mandatory during anesthesia with these drugs (Schumacher et al. 1997).

Alternatives to opioids are possible and sometimes the only option if highly regulated narcotics are not available. Tiletamine-zolazepam in combination with butorphanol and an alpha-2 agonist has been used in addax (*Addax nasomaculatus*), eland (*Taurotragus oryx*), scimitar-horned oryx (*Oryx dammah*), impala (*Aepyceros melampus*), wildebeest (*Connochaetes taurinus*), and blackbuck antelope (*Antilope cervicapra*) (Parás et al. 2002). Induction was faster with the xylazine-tiletamine-zolazepam-butorphanol combination than the medetomidine-tiletamine-zolazepam-butorphanol combination. The xylazine-tiletamine-zolazepam-butorphanol combination appeared to have a shorter duration of effect, as some animals arose suddenly during handling. The detomidine-tiletamine-zolazepam-butorphanol combination had the longest duration of action. Atipamezole was used to antagonize the alpha-2 agonist. Tiletamine-zolazepam and xylazine has been used to immobilize sable, scimitar-horned, and Arabian oryx (Bush et al. 1992). Disadvantages with this combination were prolonged and stormy recoveries, hypersalivation, and some muscle rigidity. Doxapram was a useful adjunct to hasten recovery in several of these cases. Blue wildebeeast (*Connochaetes taurinus*) have been immobilized with a combination of fentanil (0.055 mg/kg), azaperone (0.2 mg/kg), and xylazine (0.2 mg/kg) all given IM via dart (Bertelsen et al. 2006). Light anesthesia was obtained, but the authors note an initial hypoxia with combination, but this appeared to be self-limiting and improved with time. Oxygen supplementation was still recommended.

Ketamine and medetomidine combinations have been investigated in antelope in recent years. Addax has been successfully immobilized with medetomidine and ketamine (Portas et al. 2003). Ketamine and medetomidine were effective for immobilizing captive impala (*Aepyceros melampus*) (Phillips et al. 1998). Atipamezole is given to antagonize the medetomidine; usually, it is administered IM or one-half of the dose IV and one-half IM.

STRATEGIES FOR FIELD CAPTURE AND ANESTHESIA IN REMOTE LOCATIONS

The evolution of capture and field anesthesia in antelope species has been well documented (McKenzie 1993; Kock & Burroughs 2011). South African veterinarians have been at the forefront of this development and continue to set standards for wildlife capture.

While better drug combinations and drug delivery systems have made field anesthesia safer for both humans and antelope, the importance of organization cannot be underestimated. The coordination of the capture, using extraordinary amounts of people and equipment, can be overwhelming. The veterinarian overseeing such operations has the welfare of the antelope and the safety of their staff as the highest priority. Many antelope species can be captured with mass capture techniques. In these instances, sedation or tranquilization can be utilized in selected species. Quick, smooth, efficient captures are the key to avoiding animal losses during mass captures and will facilitate the effectiveness of tranquilizations. Proper placement of the capture boma and using a skilled helicopter pilot to drive the antelope into the boma are critical. Commonly used tranquilizers and sedatives used by the South African National Parks (SANParks) are listed in Table 60.1.

Field anesthesia of individuals is done on a less frequent basis but still occurs in wild settings and in boma confinement. While anesthetizing antelope, smooth, quick inductions are best. Depending on the scenario, darting from the ground or a helicopter may be indicated. Animals should not be chased for over 2 minutes prior to darting to help reduce the incidence of hyperthermia and capture stress. Darting techniques and equipment are covered in earlier book chapters. Table 60.2 has specifics on commonly handled species by SANParks.

GUIDELINES FOR ANESTHESIA IN SPECIFIC ANTELOPE SPECIES

Anesthesia Planning and Preparations
Most anesthetic events in antelope are planned events so proper preparations can be made. The goal of the procedure (routine exam, diagnostics, and transport) should be detailed well enough so that it moves forward efficiently. Equipment needed to move the antelope if needed should be available in case of emergency. Staff should be briefed and given specific responsibilities for the procedure. A checklist of basic equipment needs is useful for every anesthetic procedure and should be developed based on individual needs, preferences, and goals of the procedures themselves. Routine equipment needed for antelope anesthesia include ropes, blindfolds, inner tubes, towels, slings, and ear plugs. Portable scales are important to get accurate weights when possible. Medical equipment should consist of an endotracheal intubation kit or nasal insufflation equipment, demand valves, an oxygen supply, intravenous access kits, fluids, and emergency drugs. Monitoring equipment for field procedures should at a minimum be a stethoscope and a thermometer. Portable pulse oximeters are now readily available and highly recommended for all anesthetic events.

Table 60.1. Drugs used by SANParks in the mass capture of various species

		Tranquillizers and Sedatives								
		Haloperidol (mg)			Perphenazine Enanthate (mg)			Diazepam (mg)		
Species Route		AM	AF	SA/J	AM	AF	SA/J	AM	AF	SA/J
Eland	IM	25	20	14–18	100	80	40–60	25	20	14–18
Kudu	IM	15	10	6–8	60	40		15	10	
Gemsbok	IM	10	8					20	15	
Roan	IM	12	10		60–80	40–60		15	12	
Sable	IM	14	12		60–80	40–60		14	12	
Waterbuck	IM	20	15		60–80	40–60		20	15	
Blue wildebeest	IM	14	12	6–8	60–80	40–60		20	15	
Black wildebeest	IM/IV	14	12	6–8	60–80	40–60		14	12	
Red hartebeest	IM/IV	16	14	6–8	60–80	40–60		16	14	
Tsessebe	IV	15	15	7	60–80	40–60		15	15	7
Blesbok	IV	12	12	6	50	40		12	12	6
Bontebok	IV	12	12	6	50	40		12	12	6
Impala	IV	14	12	6				14	12	6
Grey reedbuck	IV	8	8	4				8	8	4
Mountain reedbuck	IV	10	10	5				10	10	5
Springbok (Kalahari)	IV	14	12	7	40–60	40		14	12	6
Springbok (Karoo)	IV	12	10	5	40–60	40		12	10	5
Klipspringer	IV	5	5	3				5	5	3
Steenbok	IV	5	5	3				5	5	3
Duiker	IV	8	8	4				8	8	4

Notes:
- The above doses are for wild animals in good condition.
- Animals that are in poor condition tend to show greater sedation and often develop extra-pyramidal symptoms (EPS).
- Diazepam is the drug of choice to treat EPS.
- Diazepam has a shorter duration of action, and it may necessary that it be repeated after a few hours.
- Use of midazolam has replaced diazepam as a tranquilization in African situations due to the multidose and higher concentration that is available in South Africa.

The abbreviations used in the column headings indicate the different age classes as follows: AM, adult male; AF, adult female; SA/J, subadult or juvenile.

Table 60.2. Drugs used in South African National Parks for the immobilization of various antelope species

	Immobilizing Drug Mixture			
	Etorphine (mg)		Azaperone (mg)	
Species	Adult Male	Adult Female	Adult Male	Adult Female
Sable	4–5	3–4	100	100
Roan	4–5	3–4	100	100
Blue wildebeest	4–5	3–4	100	100
Black wildebeest	3–4	3	80	80
Tsessebe	3–4	3	80	80
Eland	10–12	6–8	180–200	180–200
Red hartebeest	4–5	3–4	80	80
Gemsbok	4–5	3–4	80	80
Kudu	5–6	4–5	100	100
Waterbuck	5–6	4–5	150	150

Notes:
- All doses should be administered intramuscularly.
- Diprenorphine at 2.5 times the etorphine dose in milligram.
- Naltrexone at 15 times the etorphine dose in milligram.
- Hyaluronidase is frequently added to the immobilizing drugs to assist drug absorption and thereby reduce the induction time.

A review of previous anesthesia records is an excellent opportunity to critically examine previous procedures. Accurate, organized medical records will make critical evaluation much easier. For major procedures, a planning session with all parties involved will also make for a smoother anesthetic episode. General recommendations are to fast adult ruminants for 18–24 hours. This fasting will in itself induce bradycardia and will not ensure that the ruminant will not regurgitate (Riebold 1996). It is the author's preference to only remove any concentrate ration from the diet, and allow access to hay, grass, and water. The propensity for most ruminants, notably duikers, addax, and giant eland, to regurgitate may revolve around a subclinical rumenitis. Isolation may stress an individual prior to anesthetic induction. In general, the closer conditions can be kept to the antelope's normal routine, the less the impact the procedure will have on the individual and the herd.

ANESTHETIC REGIMENS FOR ANTELOPE IN MANAGED CARE

An extensive review of chemical restraint regimens was recently provided for numerous antelope species (Citino 2003; Kock & Burroughs 2011). Table 60.3 provides data collected from various facilities from 1996 to 2010 by the author. In general, a 1:10 cocktail of carfentanil to xylazine is used routinely for most species of antelope. Most doses of narcotics listed in Table 60.3 are somewhat higher than those commonly reported. With these doses, induction times are quick and the antelope are typically immobilized in a few minutes. Adequate support should be available for animals immobilized in quick fashion. Naltrexone is used to antagonize the carfentanil at 100 times the carfentanil dose, on a per milligram basis, split one-half IV and one-half IM. The dose of naltrexone is effective at much lower doses for etorphine and thiafentanil, and effective reversal has been achieved at 20× the opioid dose of the etorphine and thiafentanyl doses (authors' personal experience). Xylazine is not routinely antagonized, and it will provide some postanesthetic tranquilization. Xylazine will cause some sedation, but no problems have been encountered due to this and all animals are readily accepted back into the herds. Dexmedetomidine has started to find its way into antelope anesthesia, especially with the smaller species. Most clinicians report such a wide array of doses and results that it is difficult to summarize or even comment on the usefulness of this drug.

Serotonergic ligands have been shown to have the potential to reverse opioid-induced respiratory depression (Meyer et al. 2010). Etorphine-immobilized impala (*Aepyceros melampus*) received intravenous injections of metoclopramide buspirone, pimozide, and doxapram. Metoclopramide (10 mg/kg IV) and buspirone (0.05 mg/kg IV) increased the PaO_2 similar to those of doxapram. Neither metoclopramide nor buspirone significantly increased ventilation, but they increased PaO_2 by significantly improving the alveolar-arterial oxygen partial pressure gradient.

Techniques for regional anesthesia from domestic ruminats can be directly applied to antelope. These can be complimentary to general anesthesia as with line blocks for cesarean section or epidurals with xylazine or 95% grain alcohol (Gyimesi et al. 2008).

Table 60.3. Anesthetic induction regimens for selected antelope species with average adult captive body weights

Impala (*Aepyceros melampus*)
- Males 57 kg, female 42 kg
- 30-μg/kg carfentanil and 0.2-mg/kg xylazine μg
- Use lower dose of xylazine in this species as respiratory depression can be significant

Greater kudu (*Tragelaphus strepsiceros*)
- Male 210 kg, female 149 kg
- 26-μg/kg carfentanil and 0.26-mg/kg xylazine
- Higher dose of narcotic reduces pacing but still a common finding

Defassa waterbuck (*Kobus ellipsiprymnus defassa*)
- Male 215 kg, female 177 kg
- 22-μg/kg carfentanil and 0.22-mg/kg xylazine
- Nervous species, prone to prolonged induction. Tough skin, dart placement critical. Recommend use of hyaluronidase. Obesity also common.

Blue wildebeest (*Connochaetes taurinus*)
- Male 182 kg, female 142 kg
- 21-μg/kg carfentanil and 0.21-mg/kg xylazine
- 32-μg/kg etorphine and 40-μg/kg detomidine
- Herd members can be aggressive to narcotized animal. Tends to be obese in captivity and hence prone to hyperthermia

Uganda kob (*Kobus kob*)
- Male 100 kg, female 62 kg
- 35-μg/kg carfentanil and 0.35-mg/kg xylazine
- Flighty species. Prone to excessive running after darting. Quick induction required to help avoid hyperthermia.

(Continued)

Table 60.3. (*Continued*)

Sable antelope (*Hippotragus niger*)
- Male 265 kg, female 166 kg
- 17.5-µg/kg carfentanyl and 0.17-mg/kg xylazine
- Dangerous when under-dosed. Heavily muscled and can be obese in captivity; prone to hyperthermia. Hyaluronidase useful.

Roan antelope (*Hippotragus equinus*)
- Male 310 kg, female 235 kg
- 18-µg/kg carfentanil and 0.18-mg/kg xylazine
- Dangerous when underdosed. Heavily muscled and often obese in captivity; prone to hyperthermia. Hyaluronidase useful.

Common eland (*Taurotragus oryx*)
- Male 570 kg, female 300 kg
- 16-µg/kg carfentanil and 0.16-mg/kg xylazine
- Can be dangerous when underdosed. Incredible leaping ability. Males are heavily muscled; excessive pacing will lead to hyperthermia. Be prepared to supplement or recover about 20 minutes in to the anesthesia.

Bongo (*Tragelaphus eurycerus*)
- Male 410 kg, female 249 kg
- 24-µg/kg carfentanil and 0.24-mg/kg xylazine
- Typically sedate animals but good leapers.

Scimitar-horned oryx (*Oryx dammah*)
- Male 180 kg, female 123 kg
- 29-µg/kg carfentanil and 0.29-mg/kg xylazine
- 56-µg/kg etorphine and 5-µg/kg medetomidine
- Renarcotization more common with carfentanil. Tends to be obese and prone to hyperthermia.

Arabian oryx (*Oryx leucoryx*)
- Male 102 kg, female 89 kg
- 37.5-µg/kg carfentanil and 0.25-mg/kg xylazine
- 48.5-µg/kg etorphine and 48.5-µg/kg detomidine
- Etorphine recommended over carfentanil due to renarcotization. More slender and delicate in structure than scimitar horned but tends to be obese in captivity.

Addax (*Addax nasomaculatus*)
- Male 108 kg, female 88 kg
- 22.7-µg/kg carfentanil and 0.22-mg/kg xylazine
- Moderate amount of renarcotization if higher dose of carfentanil used. Etorphine is likely a better choice but limited experience to report.

Bontebok (*Damaliscus pygargus*)
- Male 80 kg, female 58 kg
- 25-µg/kg carfentanil and 0.25-mg/kg xylazine
- Can be difficult to dart, runs excessively afterwards. Prone to hyperthermia. Hyaluronidase recommended; doses even higher than those listed (40 µg/kg) should be considered for very quick recumbency in large pens.

Sitatunga (*Tragelaphus spekii*)
- Male 85 kg, female 58 kg
- 40-µg/kg carfentanil and 0.30-mg/kg xylazine
- Can be dangerous kickers when recumbent. Hyulronidase highly recommended. Higher doses useful for quicker recumbency. Tends to run and moderate risk of regurgitation. Will run into water.

Nyala (Tragelaphus angasii)
- Male 105 kg, female 63 kg
- 28.5-µg/kg carfentanil and 0.25-mg/kg xylazine
- Very shy and nervous

INDUCTION

Prior to any antelope anesthetic induction, the veterinarian must ensure that there is adequate support staff and necessary equipment. All inductions need to be carried out in a calm, quiet environment to lessen any stress on the antelope. The purpose of the anesthetic procedure may dictate the level of anesthesia needed and perhaps even the choice of drugs used. This may also figure into the delivery method of the induction dose. The delivery of the induction dose should be smooth, quick, and as controlled as possible to also lessen stress.

Anesthetic induction can take place with an antelope physically restrained or with the animal in a confined space. A significant number of anesthetic inductions in antelope will be from a remote delivery system. Dart placement is critical, and personnel experienced with the use of darting equipment should dart the antelope. The muscle masses of the shoulder, neck, and upper hind leg are ideal targets for dart placement. From a helicopter, the rump muscles or those adjacent to the spine are the best targets for remote dart delivery. Adequate velocity on the dart is needed to ensure deep intramuscular injections. Incomplete or slow inductions can occur if the dart is placed in subcutaneous tissue, or in intraperitoneal, or intrathoracic spaces. Incomplete drug delivery and slow inductions can cause the animal to pace excessively and become hyperthermic. The skin thickness should be considered in certain species and needle sizes and dart velocity adjusted. Poor dart placement contributed to a 30% anesthetic-related mortality rate in captive Defassa waterbuck (*Kobus ellipsiprymnus*) (R. Ball, unpubl. data, July 2008). All animals had prolonged induction times and died as a result of complications from hyperthermia. Waterbuck that received the same doses in the muscle mass of the hind limb had unremarkable anesthetic events. Obese animals in captivity may also have prolonged inductions due to the injection of drug into fatty tissue. The addition of hyaluronidase to the induction drugs can reduce induction times and is especially important in obese animals and those with thick skin. Once the antelope is safe to approach, it should be blindfolded to decrease stimulus. Ear plugs may be considered to decrease auditory stimulus. If the antelope is not recumbent, it should be blindfolded and can be eased into recumbency. If the antelope is not intubated, then intranasal oxygen can be given and routine monitoring can commence.

Advances in physical restraint systems for antelope can allow for hand injection of induction agents, and in certain cases, intravenous inductions are possible (Atkinson et al. 1999; Wirtu et al. 2005). Reduced doses of induction drugs can be used intramuscularly or intravenously if the antelope is physically restrained. A series of nyala were successfully anesthetized in a drop chute system (The Tamer TM, Fauna Products Inc., Red Hook, NY) with intravenous ketamine (4 mg/kg), medetomidine (8 μg/kg), and butorphanol (0.3 mg/kg) intravenously for diagnostics prior to euthanasia (R. Ball, unpubl. data, 2002). Supplemental induction doses may be needed at times in either remote delivery situations or once the antelope is handled. If supplemental dosing is required via a dart, a full induction dose of the narcotic drug is preferred by the author. Once control of the antelope has been obtained, the clinician can determine if it is safe to proceed or to antagonize the entire narcotic dose and recover the animal. If the antelope is restrained and needs supplemental dosing, intravenous ketamine, 0.5–1 mg/kg, can be given to facilitate better control or allow intubation. Higher doses can be given, but the antelope may become apenic and need respiratory support. Ketamine is metabolized relatively quickly, but the narcotic antagonist should not be given for at least 20 minutes to allow a smooth recovery.

A potential life-threatening complication resulting from prolonged induction or inadequate induction is capture myopathy. Capture myopathy is also more specifically termed excertional rhadomyolysis in wildlife capture and anesthesia. There are four clinical syndromes described: acute death syndrome, delayed peracute death, ataxic-myoglobinuric syndrome, and muscle rupture syndrome (Nielsen 1999). The acute death syndrome occurs within a few hours of the anesthetic event and often the antelope will expire during the anesthesia. The most notable clinical finding in the authors' experience is the pronounced hyperkalemia. If immediate electrolyte analysis is not possible, an ECG tracing may suggest hyperkalemia in antelope. Corrective measures include administering calcium gluconate as a cardioprotective agent followed by insulin and dextrose to stabilize the potassium levels. Addressing the inciting causes of hyperkalemia (hyperthermia, lactic acidosis, etc.) can then be addressed. The delayed peracute syndrome occurs within 24 hours and is again believed to be due to potassium sensitizing the heart to catecholamines. The third syndrome is the ataxic-myoglobinuric syndrome, which may occur within several days from the anesthesia. The urine is often brown-red, and muscle, liver, and renal values are elevated. Death is typically from renal failure associated with myoglobinuria. Some animals will recover spontaneously with adequate fluid therapy. In some selected cases, dobutamine can be given intravenously to increase renal perfusion (R. Ball, unpubl. data). Dantrolene is utilized in equine patients with postanesthetic myositis and may be considered in antelope that are experiencing complications of capture myopathy.

RECOVERY

A major advantage of opioid induction is the ability to antagonize the drugs and produce a smooth recovery. Naltrexone is the preferred antagonist and can be administered at 100 times the carfentanil dose or 15 times the etorphine dose. The dose is often split between intravenous, intramuscular, and subcutaneous administration. The product label recommends giving one-quarter of the dose intravenously and three-quarters subcutaneously. A recent study in goats suggests that there is no advantage to splitting the dose when antagonizing carfentanil (Mutlow et al. 2004). Mild renarcotization was noted in many of the study animals. Although renarcotization is not fully understood, there appears to be more episodes of renarcotization in species from arid climates. Water conservation mechanisms in these species may have a role in this, but it has not been investigated as of yet.

Recovered animals can be placed back into the herd immediately if conspecifics do not pose a threat to the recovering animal. Once the opioid fraction of the induction is antagonized, recovery generally takes a few minutes. In most circumstances, the sedative drugs is not antagonized. The sedative may keep the recovering antelope calmer, and this is the preferred method of recovery by the author. Arousing from anesthesia to a fully awake state can be a startling experience, and may in itself be stressful for the animal. A calm slow recovery is the preferable way to recover an antelope. Antelope that have been under inhalation anesthesia should be recovered away from other animals until fully recovered. Opioid antagonists are not given until the anesthetic gas can no longer be detected from the endotracheal tube. The tube is left in place until a strong swallowing reflex is seen. The cuff is only slightly deflated to help clear the airway of any regurgitated material.

ANESTHESIA RECORDS

An accurate record of the anesthetic procedure is essential. Anesthetic records allow the creation of a database that can be critically evaluated and used as a reference. Drug delivery, dosages, drug effects, physiological data, and the notation of complications are important parts of an anesthetic record. A dedicated person should be assigned to record this information as it occurs. Compilation into an electronic record-keeping system is also a valuable tool for planning future events.

ACKNOWLEDGMENTS

The author wishes to thank Dr. Peter Buss, Dr. David Zimmerman, Dr. Danny Govender, Ms. Cathy Dreyer, and Dr. Markus Hofmeyr from the South African National Parks for their contributions and the numerous opportunities they have provided.

REFERENCES

Ancrenaz M, Ostrowski S, Anagariyah S, Delhomme A. 1996. Long-duration anesthesia in Arabian oryx (*Oryx leucoryx*) using a medetomidine-etorphine combination. *Journal of Zoo and Wildlife Medicine* 27(2):209–216.

Atkinson MW, Welsh TH Jr, Blumer ES. 1999. Evaluation of an advanced system for physiologic data collection, testing and medical treatment of large, nondomestic hoofstock. Proceedings of the American Association of Zoo Veterinarians, pp. 154–157. Columbus.

Bertelsen M, Moller T, Roken B. 2006. Chemical immobilzation of blue wildebeast (*Connochaetes taurinus*) with etorphine-xylazine or fentanil-azaperone-xylazine. Proceedings of the American Association of Zoo Veterinarians, p. 325.

Bush M. 1996. A technique for endotracheal intubation of non-domestic bovids and cervids. *Journal of Zoo and Wildlife Medicine* 27(3):378–381.

Bush M, Citino SB, Tell L. 1992. Telazol and telazol/rompum anesthesia in non-domestic Cervids and Bovids. Proceedings of the Joint Meeting of the American Association of Zoo Veterinarians/American Association of Wildlife Veterinarians, pp. 224–225. Oakland.

Caulkett N, Paterson J, Haigh J, Siefert L. 2006. Comparative physiological effects of thiafentanil-azaperone and thiafentanil-medetomidine-ketamine in free ranging Uganda kob (*Kobus kob thomasi*). Proceedings of the American Association of Zoo Veterinarians, pp. 216–219.

Citino S, Bush M, Rivera O. 2007. A simple, unique field ventilator for larger ungulates; another use your leaf blower. Proceedings of the American Association of Zoo Veterinarians, pp. 51–52. Knoxville.

Citino SB. 2003. Bovidae (except sheep and goats) and Antilopcapridae. In: *Zoo and Wild Animal Medicine* (ME Fowler, RE Miller, eds.), pp. 649–674. St. Louis: W.B. Saunders.

Citino SB, Bush M, Grobler D, Lance W. 2001. Anaesthesia of roan antelope (*Hippotragus equinus*) with a combination of A3080, medetomidine and ketamine. *Journal of the South African Veterinary Association* 72(1):29–32.

Citino SB, Bush M, Grobler D, Lance W. 2002. Anesthesia of boma-captured Lichtenstein's hartebeest (*Sigmoceros lichtensteinii*) with a combination of thiafentanil, medetomidine, and ketamine. *Journal of Wildlife Diseases* 38(2):457–462.

Cooper DV, Grobler D, Bush M, Jessup D, Lance W. 2005. Anaesthesia of nyala (*Tragelaphus angasii*) with a combination of thiafentanil (A3080), medetomidine and ketamine. *Journal of the South African Veterinary Association* 76(1):18–21.

Fahlman Å, Caulkett N, Arnemo J, Neuhaus P, Ruckstuhl K. 2010. Efficacy of a portable oxygen concentrator for improvement of arterial oxygenation during anesthesia of Wildlife. Proceedings of the American Association of Zoo Veterinarians, p. 201. Brownsville.

Grobler D, Bush M, Jessup D, Lance W. 2001. Anaesthesia of gemsbok (*Oryx gazella*) with a combination of A3080, medetomidine and ketamine. *Journal of the South African Veterinary Association* 72(2):81–83.

Gyimesi Z, Linhart R, Burns R, Anderson D, Munson L. 2008. Management of chronic vaginal prolapse in an eastern bongo (*Tragelaphus eurycerus isaaci*). *Journal of Zoo and Wildlife Medicine* 39(4):614–621.

Howard LL, Kearns KS, Clippinger TL, Larsen RS, Morris PJ. 2004. Chemical immobilization of rhebok (*Pelea capreolus*) with carfentanil-xylazine or etorphine-xylazine. *Journal of Zoo and Wildlife Medicine* 35(3):312–319.

Huffman B. 2014. The ultimate ungulate, your guide to the world's hoofed mammals. http://www.ultimateungulate.com/ (accessed March 20, 2013).

Jansen DL, Allan JL, Raath JP, de Vos V, Swan GE, Jessup D, Stanley TH. 1991. Field studies with the narcotic immobilizing agent A3080. Proceedings of the American Association of Zoo Veterinarians, pp. 333–335. Galveston.

Kilgallon CP, Lamberski N, Larsen RS. 2010. Comparison of thiafenantil-xylazine and carfentanil-xylazine for immobilization of gemsbok (*Oryx gazella*). *Journal of Zoo and Wildlife Medicine* 41(3):567–571.

Klein L, Blumer E, DeMaar T. 1994. Cardiopulmonary and acid-base status in captive addax anesthetized with carfentanil-acetylpromazine-ketamine. Proceedings of the American Association of Zoo Veterinarians, pp. 175–176. Pittsburg.

Kreeger TJ, Cook WE, Piché CA, Smith T. 2001. Anesthesia of pronghorns using thiafentanil or thiafentanil plus xylazine. *Journal of Wildlife Management* 65(1):25–28.

Kock MD, Burroughs R. (eds.) 2011. *Chemical and Physical Restraint of Wild Animals*. Greyton: IWVS (Africa).

Lombardini E, Lane E, Del Piero F. 2010. Dysplastic tracheae in eight blue duikers (Cephalophus monticola) from Bioko, Equatorial Guinea. *Journal of Zoo and Wildlife Medicine* 41(2): 291–295.

Lumb AB. 2000. Pulmonary ventilation: mechanisms and the work of breathing. In: *Nunn's Applied Respiratory Physiology* (AB Lumb, ed.), pp. 113–137. Oxford: Butterworth Heinemann.

McKenzie AA. 1993. *The Capture and Care Manual: Capture, Care, Accomodation and Transportation of Wild African Animals*. Menlo Park, South Africa: Wildlife Decision Support Services CC and South African Veterinary Foundation.

Meyer L, Hetem R, Fick L, Matthee A, Mitchell D, Fuller A. 2008a. Thermal, cardiorespiratory and cortisol responses of impala (Aepyceros melampus) to chemical immobilisation with 4 different drug combinations. *Journal of the South African Veterinary Association* 79(3):121–129.

Meyer L, Fick L, Matthee A, Mitchell D, Fuller A. 2008b. Hyperthermia in captured impala (*Aepyceros melampus*): a fright not flight response. *Journal of Wildlife Diseases* 44(2):404–416.

Meyer L, Hetem R, Fick L, Mitchell D, Fuller A. 2010. Effects of serotonin agonists and doxapram on respiratory depression and hypoxemia in etorphine-immobilized impala (*Aepyceros melampus*). *Journal of Wildlife Diseases* 46(2):514–524.

Miller-Edge M, Amsel S. 1994. Carfentanil, ketamine, xylazine combination (CKX) for immobilization of exotic ungulates: clinical experiences in bongo (*Tragelaphus euryceros*) and mountain tapir (*Tapirus pinchaque*). Proceedings of the American Association of Zoo Veterinarians, pp. 192–195. Pittsburg.

Mutlow A, Isaza R, Carpenter JW, Koch DE, Hunter RP. 2004. Pharmacokinetics of carfentanil and naltrexone in domestic goats (*Capra hircus*). *Journal of Zoo and Wildlife Medicine* 35(4): 489–496.

Nielsen L. 1999. *Chemical Immobilization of Wild and Exotic Animals*. Ames: Iowa State University Press.

Parás A, Martínez O, Hernández A. 2002. Alpha-2 agonist in combination with butorphanol and tiletamine-zolazepam for the immobilization of non-domestic hoofstock. Proceeding. American . Association. Zoo Veterinarians., Milwaukee, pp. 194–197.

Phillips LG, Bush M, Lance W, Raath JP. 1998. Ketamine/medetomidine immobilization of captive and free-ranging impala (*Aepyceros melampus*) in the Kruger National Park, South Africa. Proceeding. American . Association. Zoo Veterinarians. Omaha, pp. 19–21.

Portas TJ, Lynch MJ, Vogelnest L. 2003. Comparison of etorphine-detomidine and medetomidine-ketamine anesthesia in captive addax (*Addax nasomaculatus*). *Journal of Zoo and Wildlife Medicine* 34(3):269–273.

Pypendop B, Steffey EP. 2001. Focused supportive care: ventilation during anesthesia in cattle. In: *Recent Advances in Anesthetic Management of Large Domestic Animals* (EP Steffey, ed.). Ithaca: International Veterinary Information Service. http://www.ivis.org (accessed February 10, 2014).

Riebold TW. 1996. Ruminants. In: *Lumb abd Jones' Veterinary Anesthesia* (JC Thurmon, WJ Tranquilli, GJ Benson, eds.), pp. 610–625. Baltimore: Lea and Febiger.

Schumacher J, Citino SB, Dawson R. 1997. Effects of a carfentanil-xylazine combination on cardiopulmonary function and plasma catecholamine concentrations in female bongo antelopes. *American Journal of Veterinary Research* 58(2):157–161.

Wirtu G, Cole A, Pope CE, Short CR, Godke RA, Dresser BL. 2005. Behavioural training and hydraulic chute restraint enables handling of eland antelope (*Taurotragus oryx*) without general anesthesia. *Journal of Zoo and Wildlife Medicine* 36(1):1–11.

61 Gazelle and Small Antelope

An Pas

INTRODUCTION

Gazelles are nervous and flighty animals that when handled can inflict serious injuries on themselves and on their handlers. Improved handling techniques and capture systems have, however, reduced these risks significantly making it possible to perform basic procedures, such as blood sampling and vaccination, without the need for anesthesia. Several immobilization drugs are available if sedation or anesthesia is required.

The most common gazelle and small antelope species kept in captivity are listed and their bodyweights are indicated in Table 61.1.

UNIQUE PHYSIOLOGY, ANATOMY, AND BEHAVIOR

Many gazelle species have developed adaptations for the hot and often dry climate in which they live. The color patterns of most desert gazelles help them to gain heat during cold mornings and to dissipate heat during the hot parts of the day by directing the darker flank or the white rump respectively to the sun. Their long fine legs, long necks, and large ears further help them to regulate their temperature (Willmer et al. 2000). They have developed effective water conservation mechanisms, resulting in low rates of water loss and the production of very dry fecal matter (Willmer et al. 2000).

During extreme exertion, such as when trying to evade a predator, the amount of heat produced will exceed the amount that can be dissipated, especially in hot climates. The animal can, however, store this heat and allow an increase in its body temperature. A mechanism has been described in several species that at the same time can keep the brain at a lower temperature than the body by utilizing a countercurrent heat exchange mechanism known as the carotid rete. Before the arterial blood reaches the brain, it is cooled while passing via smaller arteries through the venous sinus cavity, which is filled with cooled blood returning from the nasal region. In this way, the organ most sensitive to heat stress can remain at a safe temperature lower than 41°C, while the body temperature can reach over 44°C (Schmidt-Nielsen 1997; Vaughan et al. 2010).

Gazelles can reach very high speeds. A Thompson's gazelle, for example, can run at up to 80 km/h (Feldhamer et al. 2007). Most gazelles have maximum speeds of around 60–70 km/h.

As prey animals, gazelles are constantly aware of their environment and of possible predators. When anything unusual is noticed, the animals will warn each other with a snorting noise and the group will start moving immediately. Many gazelle species perform stylized near-vertical jumps with all four legs extended, called stotting or pronking, before running away at high speed. This behavior makes capture and darting of these animals challenging, as they keep a safe distance from humans, stay in almost constant motion, and any unfamiliar behavior is picked up by and communicated among the group.

When gazelles are caught, some resist violently, using their sharp hooves to kick, but others just lie down and freeze. A quiescent gazelle, however, is not necessarily unstressed. In general, species that live in dense habitats will tend to hide more while species from open savanna areas will tend to run. Good knowledge of the specific behaviors of the different species is essential to capture, handle, and treat these animals safely and successfully.

Zoo Animal and Wildlife Immobilization and Anesthesia, Second Edition. Edited by Gary West, Darryl Heard, and Nigel Caulkett.
© 2014 John Wiley & Sons, Inc. Published 2014 by John Wiley & Sons, Inc.

Table 61.1. Weights

Common Name	Scientific Name	Average (Range) Weight Adult in kg
Beira antelope	*Dorcatragus megalotis*	11 (9–14)
Blackbuck	*Antilope cervicapra*	29 (25–35)
Gazelle, Arabian Mountain	*Gazella gazella cora*	13 (11–16)
Gazelle, Chinkara	*Gazella bennettii*	17 (15–20)
Gazelle, Dama	*Nanger dama ruficollis*	57 (50–75)
Gazelle, Idmi	*Gazella gazella*	15 (13–18)
Gazelle, Pelzeln's	*Gazella pelzelni*	15 (13–18)
Gazelle, red-fronted	*Eudorcas rufifrons*	23 (20–25)
Gazelle, Rheem	*Gazella subgutturosa marica*	19 (12–24)
Gazelle, Soemmering	*Nanger soemmerringii berberana*	32 (30–40)
Gazelle, Speke's	*Gazella spekei*	13 (11–15)
Gazelle, Subgutturosa	*Gazella s. subgutturosa*	19 (17–24)
Gazelle, Dorcas	*Gazella dorcas*	15 (13–18)
Gerenuk	*Litocranius walleri*	35 (30–40)
Phillip's dik-dik	*Madoqua saltiana phillipsi*	3.5 (2–4)

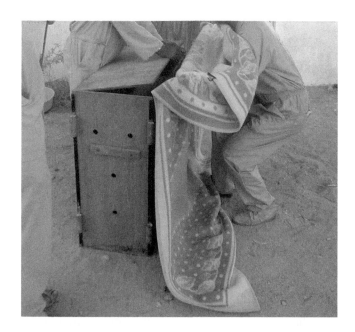

Figure 61.1. Use of thick blanket to manually restrain a gazelle.

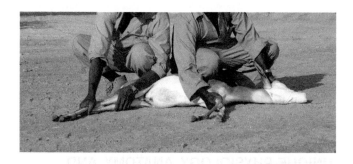

Figure 61.2. Gazelle restrained in lateral recumbency.

PHYSICAL RESTRAINT

In a Captive Environment

Many gazelles can be hand-caught by experienced staff, and immobilizing drugs can be subsequently administered if required. For physical capture, animals are separated from the group and restricted to a small enclosure. Enclosures can be designed so that the animal can slowly be pushed with a board, canvas, or blanket into a transport box. Boxes should have sliding doors at the front and back, and be able to be opened from the top. In this way, more docile gazelles can be injected in the box, can be taken out from the front, or even can be lifted from the top, especially with the help of a blindfold. An alternative method involves using a thick blanket, which is slipped under the top lid of the box to avoid light entering the box and then being lowered slowly over the gazelle. The gazelle will thus remain recumbent and calm in the darkened and enclosed environment. This way, simple procedures, such as heart and lung auscultation, temperature taking, and administration of injectable or oral drugs, can be carried out with minimal stress even in the more nervous animals (Figure 61.1).

The initial phase of hand capture is the most critical to minimize self-inflicted trauma. Two handlers are needed that work in a well-synchronized manner. Larger gazelles may require more than two people for safe and proper restraint. The horns of the gazelle are grabbed first (at the base of the horn), and an eye cover is placed immediately. Extreme care needs to be taken when catching young gazelle to avoid permanent damage to the horn. Therefore, young animals (and animals without horns) are better grabbed at the neck. The animal can be then quickly lifted off of its feet while the body is supported and the legs are restrained. The first handler holds the horns (or neck) and head with one arm, while partially supporting the neck and torso with the other arm. The additional handler restrains and supports the hind part of the body and restrains the legs by folding them in under the body as in a normal physiological resting position. Another way of holding smaller gazelle is by keeping the legs hanging in the air, with a first handler holding the horns and torso and the second handler keeping hold of the skin in the flanks instead of folding the legs in. Sometimes, it is better to first gently push the animal down into sternal position before lifting it up.

Instead of lifting up the animal, it can also be placed on its side with the neck slightly stretched backwards while the handlers are positioned at its back restraining the neck and legs (Figure 61.2). Legs should always be held close to the body, never at the distal part, as the gazelle will kick violently and will injure itself and the handlers.

To move small species (up to 35 kg), the animal can also be held upside down in the air. The handlers will hold the animal at the legs and support the back. Although holding animals on the side and especially on the back might seem counterintuitive and even controversial, this unnatural positioning makes the animal resist less and calms them down. The authors have used these handling techniques for many years with good results and no side effects. This can, however, only be done in nonsedated animals. However, as mentioned previously, the safest and least stressful way to move an animal is to place it in an appropriate dark crate.

As soon as animals are caught, blindfolds and earplugs (made of cotton, wool, or gauze) should be used to reduce stimuli and to keep the animal as calm as possible. Eye covers should be large enough to cover the eyes but leave the nose open for proper breathing. Horn covers made of plastic or rubber (such as hose pipe, rubber balls, or syringes) can be placed over the tips of the horns for safer handling. Care needs to be taken when holding the horns of young animals since they are easily damaged as the horn sheath is only loosely attached. Detachment can result in moderate to severe bleeding and disfigured horns.

In addition to puncture wounds from the horns, potential injury to handlers can also come from the sharp hooves. Care should be taken that animals do not become entangled in handlers' loose clothing or pockets.

All handling should be carried out in a quiet and gentle way, and any noise or sudden movements should be avoided. The specific amount of restraint needed to safely handle an animal requires experience, as too much restraint can cause the animal to fight back or can cause trauma, while too little restraint can result in the handler being injured or in the animal escaping. It is most important, however, to never let go of the animal. How easily an animal can be handled will depend not only on the species, but also on individual temperament, the degree of habituation, the environment where the capture takes place, and its position in a group's hierarchy.

Nets can be used when an individual animal needs to be separated from a large group for emergency treatment or other procedures. A small mesh net (which has a guide rope fitted on the top and bottom) is suspended from an adjoining fence or other firm structure and then laid across the normal path the gazelle takes to an area where an operator has a clear view of oncoming animals (usually behind a hide). The net is allowed to sit on the ground, and when the animal passes, the top rope on the net is pulled back quickly, raising the net and capturing the gazelle. Once the animal hits the net,

the operator releases their hold on the net, allowing the animal to carry it away and entangle itself. An extra handler should make the animal run at enough speed toward the net as otherwise they will have enough time to shy away as the net is lifted. Once the net is dropped, the animal has to be restrained and removed (starting at the nose) as quickly as possible to avoid any major trauma. An eye cover is fitted, and the legs and head are securely held while the net is removed. Nets are however, potentially dangerous for the animal. The fine long legs can become entangled and injured as the animal struggles, and species such as Spekes (*Gazella spekei*) or Chinkara gazelle (*Gazella bennetti*) easily injure their horns. The area where the capture takes place needs to be well considered. Hard substrate and the presences of big stones will increase the risk for trauma. Nets caught in woody vegetation can result in the escape of the animal. It is therefore important to select and clear the area before installing the net for capture.

Capture in Large Enclosures or Open Areas

Historically, many gazelle species were simply herded into enclosures and then individually caught by hand as described earlier. While this form of capture and restraint is still practical, and indeed essential in some cases, it can lead to a large number of injuries both to the animal and handlers. When multiple animals or large groups need to be restrained, such as for group vaccination and sampling, darting is not a viable option either and capture systems are required. Many different manual restraint systems have been developed in the past for cattle and other large ungulates. Over the years, these systems have been adapted and improved, and a number of restraint devices have been developed which take into account the size, conformation, and behavior of the different nondomesticated species (Blumer & deMaar 1993; McKenzie 1993).

Capture of free- or semi-free-ranging gazelles is done by first confining the animals in a boma, from where they will be led into a raceway system in which they are then separated from each other to finally be captured by hand, slowly pushed into boxes, or held in a tamer system (Figure 61.3).

The first step, bringing the animals into a holding enclosure, can be done by driving and further confining the animals with the use of canvas screens (Rietkerk et al. 1994). The use of modified feeding areas (O'Donovan & Bailey 2006) is however, in our experience, the best method of aggregating animals from large holding pens into a smaller boma. As with any behavioral modification procedure, patience and advance planning, sometimes several weeks beforehand, is required to accustom the animals to any changes to their normal environment. Capture pens or chutes should be in place and operating normally well in advance of the event. All doors and equipment

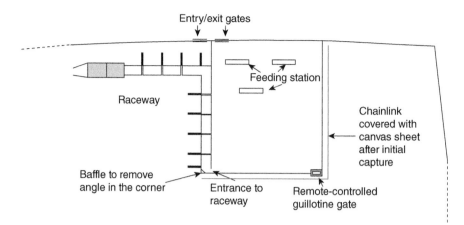

Figure 61.3.   Gazelle capture system.

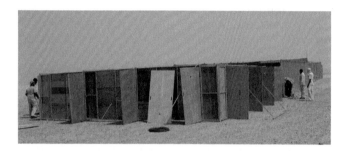

Figure 61.4.   Raceway for gazelle handling.

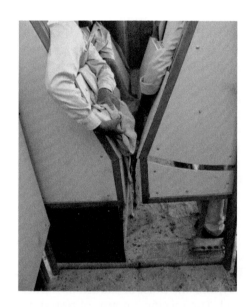

Figure 61.5.   Gazelle restraint in Tamer chute.

should be checked to make sure they work smoothly without the risk of them becoming jammed during the capture. Normal feeding practice is used as an incentive to habituate the animals to any new areas and to ensure that they enter the capture fence without fear. These areas usually have a single way in and out and will have a guillotine drop gate to allow the quick closing of the gate once all the animals are held within. These gates can be operated manually or via a remote control.

On the day of capture, the gates are closed and the animals are quickly moved into a mobile raceway (Fig. 61.4) as soon as they have all entered the boma. Tarpaulin sheets, canvas, blankets, or boards are used depending on the size of the animals and the size of the boma area. Within the raceway, animals are segregated into small groups ($n = 1–3$) by sliding doors to reduce the potential for intraspecific aggression or accidental injury. These sliding doors can be navigated from the top or from the side, but all need to run smoothly and allow quick separation. Smaller gazelle species, such as Rheem gazelle (*Gazella subgutturosa marica*), mountain gazelle (*Gazella gazella cora*), and Speke's gazelle (*G. spekei*), can then be hand captured by experienced handlers. This is usually accomplished by entering the last part of the raceway with a hand board, cornering the animal and restraining by hand.

The animals can also further be gently boarded into a transport box and then handled as has been described above for individual capture. The use of mobile restraint devices such as the Junior Tamer (Fauna Research, Redrock, NY) (Fig. 61.5) has also proved invaluable in the safe restraint of the captured animal and is especially useful for larger species. The tamer system quickly suspends the animal from the ground, while the handlers grab the horns and place an eye cover.

Small gazelles up to 35 kg can also be moved into a "box tunnel." Transport boxes are lined up with all vertical sliding doors open, except for the last box. A group of four to five animals can then be pushed into the tunnel and animals are separated one per box by closing the vertical doors.

Any procedure is conducted as quickly as possible to minimize stress and reduce the risk of capture myopathy, hyperthermia, or other complications. Once the restraint is completed, the animal can either be released or placed in a transport box for movement elsewhere if required.

For any capture in a confined area, it is extremely important that the holding and transfer areas are closed and provide complete visual barriers to prevent attempted flight through the walls or gates. The smallest gap caused by a loose canvas or hole in the cover will be immediately detected by the animal and will be used in an attempt to escape resulting in animals jumping at high speed into the fence.

Transfer gates between holding pens, or from pens to transfer alleys, should be placed in corners to produce a funnel effect. Long transfer alleys should contain turns to prevent the animal from building up speed during transfer. Catwalks should be provided (on the outside of the pen/alley) to allow operator access for control.

The capture and restraint of any wild animal, and in particular for prey animals such as gazelles, is a very stressful event. It is therefore essential that all procedures are planned and executed with precision and professionalism. One of the primary requirements when carrying out any mass capture is that all people involved understand their roles and responsibilities and that one person takes the lead. The use of checklists and precatch meetings are essential to avoid undue stress or harm to the animals and handlers. Safe and effective restraint of any animal requires a complete understanding of the behavior and flight responses of the species concerned. The use of the equipment should be rehearsed beforehand and handling of animals should be practiced on dummies or first demonstrated by experienced people. Accidents are most likely to happen due to inexperience or miscommunication between the people involved. In the authors' experience, most of the animals restrained on multiple occasions did not show a noticeable shyness to the restraint equipment or handlers. However, animals that were not exposed to regular keeper/animal interactions and that were held in larger enclosures were more difficult to move within the raceway and often sat down as a protective measure.

An example of a comprehensive checklist as used by the author is shown in Appendix 61A.1.

VASCULAR ACCESS

Venipuncture and the placement of catheters are straightforward and can be done in the same way as for small domestic ruminants. The jugular vein is easily accessible for blood sampling or catherization, as well as the cephalic and lateral saphenous vein. Intravenous fluids or crystalloid solutions are typically given as a supportive measure for prolonged procedures or during surgery. Jugular veins can be catheterized with 18-gauge catheters of about 50 mm, and the cephalic or lateral saphenous vein is catheterized with shorter (30 mm) 20- to 22-gauge catheters. If intravenous access is necessary post-immobilization, the jugular vein is advised to be used. Cephalic and saphenous catheters can be more difficult to maintain during surgical procedures and after recovery, but are in the authors' experience viable alternatives.

INTUBATION

Gazelles should preferably be intubated for any procedure that takes longer than 20 minutes, to avoid aspiration pneumonia and hypoxemia. However, most often, induction protocols will have to be further supplemented by masking the gazelle with inhalant anesthetics or IV anesthetics, such as ketamine, to make intubation possible and avoid laryngospasm and regurgitation. The need for an increased level of anesthetic depth and thus prolonged recovery, and the circumstances in which the procedure takes place (e.g., field immobilization) has to be weighed against the advantages of placing an endotracheal tube.

In most species, intubation is a straightforward procedure when using the correct technique and with some practice. There may, however, be difficulty intubating Goitered gazelles (*Gazella subgutturosa*) due to thyroid cartilage impingement on the larynx (Foster 1999), and in these species, a blind technique using a rigid catheter might be preferable. To intubate a gazelle, the head is hyperextended, and the maxilla is held open with rolled gauze or similar. Due to the narrow mouth of gazelle species, the laryngoscope blade, together with the tube, easily obscures the view, making straight positioning of the neck and head critical. The tongue is pulled laterally and the pharyngeal area may be cleared of secretions by swabbing, as anesthesia often increases the production of mucus in the throat. A flat, straight and narrow (maximum -m wide) laryngoscope blade (20–35 cm long), is used to facilitate visualization of the larynx. Alternatively, intubation can be done "blindly" by using one hand externally and ventrally to manipulate and position the larynx while using the other hand to guide and advance the endotracheal tube. A stylet or nonflexible uterine catheter may be placed first and the endotracheal tube then slid over it into the tracheal lumen. Lidocaine spray applied to the larynx may help prevent laryngospasm that may occur.

Adult gazelles are typically intubated with 4- to 12-mm endotracheal tubes. As gazelle have, in comparison with many other mammal species, quite long jaws, the larynx lies deep, and the use of long straight nonflexible tubes or tubes containing a stylet makes intubation easier. Confirmation of intubation can be done by checking for condensation in the tube, feeling respirations, moving of the rebreathing bag, and monitoring exhaled carbon dioxide.

PREANESTHETIC CONSIDERATIONS

Gazelles often mask underlying disease and carrying out a general examination or obtaining diagnostic blood work preimmobilization is usually not feasible. Even severe disease conditions (e.g., renal disease due to medullary amyloidosis) (Duncan et al. 1997; Wallace et al. 1987) can be difficult to assess preimmobilization. If animals have an individual identification number (ear tags or ear notching), specific information, such as the general body condition and any previous diseases or interventions, should be recorded in detail. The collection of accurate weights at every opportunity will help to calculate accurate dosages and avoid over- or under-dosing.

Animals cannot usually be completely fasted before anesthesia when they are maintained in large outdoor exhibits, and isolating or confining gazelles is often stressful. When large capture systems are used, food is often restricted to lure animals into the boma system, where food is provided. It is important that animals do not gorge on this food, especially on green foods, as this will result in bloated rumens, causing problems in the tamer or when further anesthesia is required.

Fasting may reduce complications, such as tympany, regurgitation, and aspiration pneumonia. Ideally, food and water should be withheld for 12–24 hours. Fasting for longer than 24 hours has been associated with metabolic acidosis in small domestic ruminants and is not recommended (Gray & McDonell 1986). Extended fasting may also promote liquid ingesta formation and increase the possibility of regurgitation (Gray & McDonell 1986).

INDUCTION PROTOCOLS

In manually restrained gazelle, induction can be accomplished with intravenous (IV) administration of either propofol, ketamine/midazolam, ketamine/xylazine, tiletamine/zolazepam, or ketamine/medetomidine (Table 61.2 and Table 61.3). The advantage of administering the drugs IV is the quick and more reliable effect. This is especially useful when alpha-2 adrenergic antagonists are used, as they tend to be less effective when given intramuscularly in stressed animals (Foster 1999; Hammer & Hammer 2002). When animals are caught in handling systems, chutes or boxes they can be injected intramuscularly (IM) by hand. If gazelles are kept in holding pens or exhibits, they can be darted with a blowpipe using lightweight, low impact darts. In the authors' experience, using a plastic stabilizer and gun needle are beneficial, as a gun needle has two holes, which leads to a very quick injection and holds

Table 61.3. Dosages for anesthetic antagonists

Drug	Dosage
Naltrexone	100 mg per 1 mg of carfentanil IM or IV
	25 mg per 1 mg of etorphine IM or IV
Diprenorphine (M5050)	2.66 mg per 1 mg of etorphine 50%IV and 50%IM
Atipamezole	2.5–5 mg per 1 mg of medetomidine or detomidine IM or SC
	1 mg per 10–20 mg of xylazine IM or SC
Naloxone	0.01–0.02 mg/kg IV or IM
Tolazoline	0.5–1.0 mg/kg IM to reverse alpha-2 agonists

Table 61.2. Dosages used in gazelle and small antelope

Drug	Dosages	Remarks
Propofol	4–6 mg/kg IV	General
Ketamine + midazolam	4 mg/kg (K) + 0.2 mg/kg (Mi) IV	General
Tiletamine/zolazepam	2–4 mg/kg IV	General
Tiletamine/zolazepam + medetomidine	4 mg/kg (T) + 0.4 mg/kg (M) IM	Rheem gazelle
Ketamine + xylazine (mix of 125-mg xylazine and 100-mg ketamine per mL)	6.8 mg/kg (K) + 8.5 mg/kg (X) IM	Chinkara gazelle
	5.6 mg/kg (K) + 7 mg/kg (X) IM	Soemmering, Idmi, and Speke's gazelle
	4.4 mg/kg (K) + 5.5 mg/kg (X) IM	Red-fronted gazelle
	3.6 mg/kg (K) + 4.5 mg/kg (X) IM	Dorcas gazelle
	3.3–7.1 mg/kg (K) + 4.1–8.9 mg/kg (X) IV	Rheem gazelle
	5.4–5.9 mg/kg (K) + 6.8–7.4 mg/kg (X) IM	
	9.3–12.2 mg/kg (K) + 11.7–15.2 mg/kg (X) IM	Idmi gazelle
Ketamine + medetomidine (long induction time and needs quiet surroundings during induction)	4 mg/kg (K) + 0.05–0.07 mg/kg (M) IV	General
	2.4 mg/kg (K) + 0.070 mg/kg (M) IM	Beira antelope
	3 mg/kg (K) + 0.075 mg/kg (M) IM	Gerenuk
Ketamine	1–2 mg/kg IV as supplemental anesthesia	General
Carfentanil	0.018–0.022 mg/kg IM	General
Carfentanil + xylazine	0.02 mg/kg (C) + 0.2–0.5 mg/kg (X) IM	General
Medetomidine + ketamine + butorphanol	0.04–0.07 mg/kg (M) + 2–4 mg/kg (K) + 0.2–0.4 mg/kg (B) IM	General
Ethorphine + acepromazine + xylazine + butorphanol	0.028 mg/kg (E) + 0.114 mg/kg (A) + 0.16 mg/kg (X) + 0.05 mg/kg (B) IM	General (preferred in Dama gazelle)

longer in the tissue compared with a blowpipe needle. Care has to be taken that the bun used is well lubricated (with silicone or eye cream) so it moves easily backwards. Darting gazelles in open areas can be very challenging, as several species will not tolerate human approach and remain in perpetual motion (running or pacing) making it virtually impossible to fire a dart at a stationary target. Their relatively small body size, combined with the large distances they keep, make it difficult to fire an accurate shot. Hide blinds, habituation, darting from familiar vehicles, and darting during feeding may make animals less agitated and easier to approach. The use of small volume projectile darts, appropriate pressure, and the correct dart and needle size are critical as even lightweight darts may cause extensive tissue damage in gazelles (Cattet et al. 2004). Darts easily bump off small tensed muscle, as gazelle are always ready to run. The use of low pressure that is sufficient to cover the distance, and small volumes, are crucial.

Gazelle tend to "fight" anesthetics and when darted in an enclosure, will attempt to follow the group even if heavily sedated. Dosages required can be very variable depending on the temperament of the individual and the circumstances in which animals are caught. When one animal has been darted the rest of the group will become so wary that darting more animals becomes increasingly difficult.

Drug combinations for IM induction include opioid/alpha-2 adrenergic agonist, cyclohexamine/alpha-2 adrenergic agonists with benzodiazepines or opioids, or opioid/butyrophenone combinations. Preferred induction regimens will depend on availability of drugs, circumstances under which immobilization takes place, and personal preference. Most frequently and successfully used combinations are carfentanil with xylazine, or a combination of medetomidine, ketamine, and butorphanol, as well as combinations that include ethorphine.

The carfentanil/xylazine combination allows a small injection volume, rapid induction, and mild cardiopulmonary side effects. Ketamine can be given intravenously as an anesthetic supplement if needed. Once the gazelle becomes recumbent, it is important to wait 5–10 minutes before approaching to allow the xylazine to reach maximum effect and further relax the animal (Allen et al. 1991). Carfentanil alone is effective for induction, but it produces bradycardia and hypertension (Schumacher et al. 1997). Antagonism is accomplished with naltrexone (100 mg per mg carfentanil, IV or IM) (Mutlow et al. 2004). Xylazine is antagonized with either tolazoline or atipamezole. Yohimbine may also be used as a low cost alternative to reverse xylazine effects, but it is less specific and less effective.

Etorphine, in combination with ketamine and/or xylazine, with azaperone, or with acepromazine/xylazine/butorphanol, has been used successfully to immobilize gazelles. They give a rapid induction, and only small volumes are needed. Etorphine with ketamine/xylazine has the advantages of lowering the opioid dose by 30%, increasing analgesia, shortening induction times, and decreasing problems with renarcotization (Snyder et al. 1992). Etorphine in combination with azaperone, was used to capture gazelles in field conditions (Foster 1999; Molnar & Mckinney 2002). Hyperthermia, capture myopathy, and aspiration contributed to morbidity and mortality. The study concluded that when capturing these species in high ambient temperature conditions, the use of ketamine and xylazine combinations might be a better choice (Foster 1999; Molnar & Mckinney 2002).

The authors have good experience with a combination of etorphine/acepromazine/xylazine/buthorphanol, but do advise the use of naltrexone or if not available, a double dosage of diprenorphine as an antagonist to avoid rebound effects. Only small dart volumes are needed and certain species, such as the Dama gazelle, that respond poorly to other combinations can be immobilized successfully with this combination. The addition of the partial antagonist buthorphanol will improve respiration during anesthesia.

A combination of medetomidine, ketamine, and butorphanol has proved to be another useful alternative to opioids (Chittick et al. 2001). Gazelles immobilized with this combination are usually under light anesthesia. If painful procedures are performed, supplementation with IV ketamine or masking down with isoflurane to reach general anesthesia, or local anesthetic techniques, should be used (Chittick et al. 2001). Disadvantages of this combination include bradycardia, transient hypertension, hypoxemia, respiratory acidosis, long inductions, and the relatively large volumes needed for induction (Chittick et al. 2001). The use of concentrated medetomidine (10 mg/mL) and buthorphanol (50 mg/mL), as available in some countries, significantly decreases the volume required. The personal experience of the authors with this combination in Rheem gazelle and Arabian mountain gazelle is that induction times can be prolonged, and that enough time needs to be allowed before the animal is approached, that anesthesia is only light in most individuals, and that the higher range of the suggested dosages needs to be used. The combination is most useful in confined areas, but has also successfully been used in large enclosures. This combination is partially reversed with atipamezole alone or with atipamezole and naloxone.

Ketamine and xylazine combinations have also been used to capture free and semi-free living gazelles as an alternative to potent narcotics (Foster 1999; Hammer & Hammer 2002; Molnar & Mckinney 2002). The authors have been using this combination with good success in Idmi, Chinkara, Speke's, and Rheem gazelle (Hammer & Hammer 2002) when given intravenously after netting. The only side effect seen was regurgitation in two cases, which caused no problems afterwards, and a prolonged recovery in one case. No mortality was seen in the 50 animals that were anesthetized this way. The dosages used were very broad, as accurate weights were only taken after capture, and varied between 4.1–8.9 mg/kg xylazine with 3.3–7.1 mg/kg ketamine. Even higher dosages were used by Foster (1999) for darting of free-ranging Idmi gazelles (11.7–15.2 mg/kg(X) + 9.3–12.2 mg/kg(K)) and Rheem gazelle (6.8–7.4 mg/kg(X) + 5.4–5.9 mg/kg(K)). The broad dosages used indicate the wide safety range of this combination.

Combinations of ketamine and medetomidine, and of ketamine and detomidine, have been used by the authors with good success, but in-depth studies on their effect are lacking. As with the use of all alpha-2 adrenergic agonists, these combinations are more useful in captive situations as induction time can be prolonged. Atipamezole is used as antagonist and results in smooth recoveries at a dosage of 2.5–5 times the dosage (in mg/kg) of medetomidine or detomidine. Reversal drugs should only be given 30–40 minutes after the administration of ketamine to avoid adverse reaction, such as disorientation, tremors, and salivating. Medetomidine/ketamine combinations are preferred for use in Beira antelope (*Dorcatragus megalotis*) (Martin Jurado et al. 2007) and Gerenuk (*Litocranius walleri*).

Tiletamine-zolazepam in combination with either an alpha-2 adrenergic agonist (medetomidine or xylazine) or butorphanol may also be used. This combination has been studied in nondomestic bovids (Bush et al. 1992; Caulkett et al. 2000) and zoo animals (Röken 1997) with good results. Gazelle were successfully anesthetized with 10-mg/kg tiletamine-zolazepam and 1-mg/kg xylazine intramuscularly (Şindak & Biricik 2003), although the authors successfully anesthetized gazelle with less than half of this dosage. Disadvantages include longer induction and recovery times and hypoxemia (Bush et al. 1992). Tiletamine-zolazepam and butorphanol combinations have less severe cardiopulmonary alterations in ruminants than tiletamine-zolazepam combinations with an alpha-2 adrenergic agonist (Howard et al. 1990). These combinations are better after an animal has been physically restrained and the combinations are administered intravenously. In the authors' experience, this combination (using 4 mg/kg tiletamine-zolazepam and 0.4 mg/kg medetomidine) is a good alternative to opioids for darting of gazelle, as it has a faster induction time and smaller volumes are required than for ketamine and alpha-2 adrenergic agonist combinations. Severe disorientation and animals falling down abruptly and then trying to get up again during induction is, however, often seen. As only the alpha-2 adrenergic agonist can be reversed (with atipamezole), recovery times can be long.

A combination of fentanyl/azaperone immobilized mountain gazelles in large enclosures (Greth et al.

1993) allowing handling and blood collection. The addition of promethazine appeared to improve quality of relaxation (Greth et al. 1993). No postcapture mortality was seen, and the beneficial effects of azaperone (i.e., less fear of humans and some mild sedation) were seen post handling (Greth et al. 1993).

Thiafentanyl (A3080) is increasingly used in wildlife with very good results, but studies of gazelle are lacking. Impala and other ungulate species were darted in Kruger (Janssen et al. 1991) with thiaphenatanil alone. In Kob antelope, combinations of thiafentanyl, ketamine, and medetomidine (TMK), were compared with thiaphentanyl-azaperone (TA) mixtures (Caulkett et al. 2006). A combination of thiaphentanil with medetomidine and ketamine was also used in Nyala with good results, and recoveries were quick and complete with naltrexone and atipamezole (Cooper et al. 2005). Different antelope species have been anesthetized with combinations of thiaphentanil and butorphanol. The butorphanol partially antagonizes the opioid and thus improves respiration and reduces the chances for apnea. Ketamine was added to deepen the anesthesia if necessary (Van Zijll Langhout & Raath 2010).

MAINTENANCE AND MONITORING

Anesthesia can be maintained with isoflurane or sevoflurane given by mask or preferably after intubation. Since opioids as alpha-2 adrenergic agonists can cause respiratory depression, resulting in hypoxia, and cardiopulmonary changes, oxygen should be supplemented even for short procedures. Under field conditions, the use of small oxygen bottles and intranasal oxygen administration is a simple way to do this.

Basic cardiopulmonary physiology and anesthetic monitoring in gazelles is similar to small domestic ruminants (Riebold 1996). Published reports on anesthetic monitoring and support in small domestic ruminants can be consulted for these species. Small animal anesthetic machines and ventilators are adequate for maintaining anesthesia in gazelle species. Ruminants typically have higher respiratory rates and smaller tidal volumes under general anesthesia (Riebold 1996). Therefore, gazelles may require higher vaporizer settings to maintain adequate anesthesia than other species of similar size (Riebold 1996).

Local or regional anesthetic techniques can be utilized in gazelles, as they may help provide long-lasting analgesia with the need for less frequent handling. Techniques described for domestic goats and sheep could be used. These techniques are generally underutilized in zoo and wildlife species, likely due to the experience and comfort level of zoo and wildlife veterinarians. Epidural analgesia with lidocaine, after sedation with acepromazine, has been described in Addax for ultrasound-guided oocyst collection (Junge 1998). Local anesthesia, in addition to medetomidine/

ketamine/butorphanol induction, has been used for castration in Thomson's gazelle (Chittick et al. 2001).

When using the handling techniques described earlier, drugs can be administered postoperatively on a daily base with little stress involved. The use of long-acting sedatives, as discussed later, can aid to accomplish this. Long-acting analgesic techniques or those administered orally can reduce the need for handling. Oral aspirin at 100 mg/kg per day, or phenylbutazone at 10–20 mg/kg per day, could be used for short periods of time. Meloxicam, carprofen, and ketoprofen as licensed for domestic ruminants have been used. Research suggests that the elimination time of these drugs differs between different species (Mahmood et al. 2011; Shukla et al. 2007), so care needs to be taken when these drugs are used repeatedly in exotic species. Meloxicam has also been used orally in goats with good effect (Ingvast-Larsson et al. 2011). Fentanyl patches may be used for prolonged analgesia, but the onset of analgesia may be delayed for 24 hours. In sheep, transdermal fentanyl provided better postoperative analgesia than oral phenylbutazone (Dowd et al. 1997) or intramuscular buprenorphine (Ahern et al. 2010).

After induction, gazelles are handled by the horns with the head up and the nose down to prevent aspiration. Nonintubated gazelles should be placed in sternal position or right lateral recumbency when possible to prevent regurgitation. When laterally recumbent for procedures, the neck should be supported and the head pointed down to allow saliva and regurgitated material away from the pharynx. If the animal is being maintained for surgery, then it should be placed on the surgical table with at least 2 in (5 cm) of padding. Even under anesthesia, blindfolds and ear plugs are recommended to decrease sensory awareness or excitement. Ophthalmic ointment should be applied to eyes to prevent corneal damage. Eyes and mouth should be checked and cleaned if needed as often dirt and sand has entered especially when animals are darted outside.

Monitoring anesthetic depth can be challenging but should incorporate physical exam findings and cardiopulmonary monitoring. Rotation of the globe of the eye as used in domestic cattle is not an accurate measure of anesthetic depth in gazelles (Riebold 1996). Blood pressure can be monitored indirectly with oscillometric measurements from cuffs placed on the limbs. Direct blood pressure can be monitored from auricular or common digital arteries. Mean arterial blood pressure should be maintained between 70 and 110 mm of Hg. This can be done through lightening of anesthesia, administration of intravenous fluids, and the use of drugs with positive inotropic, chronotropic, or vasoconstricting effects. These drugs include dobutamine, dopamine, ephedrine, or phenylephrine.

Normal heart rates in unsedated animals are around 80–120 bpm and respiratory rates should be between 20 and 40 bpm. When alpha-2 adrenergic agonists are used for induction, heart rates will be significantly slower. As well opioids as alpa-2 adrenergic agonist can cause bradypnea and even apnea. Doxapram can be used to improve respiration, but will also hasten the recovery process in animals given alpha-2 adrenergic agonists (Bush et al. 1992; Riebold 1996). Combining opioids with butorphanol, which works as a partial antagonist, ,will result in better respiration. In case of severe bradycardia or apnea, antidotes such as atipamezole or naltrexone can fully or partially reverse the agonist when the animal is intubated and can be maintained on inhalant gas anesthesia.

Electrocardiography should be used to monitor the cardiac rate and to check for any cardiac arrhythmias. End-tidal CO_2 levels and blood gas measurements should also be monitored. With today's portable equipment, these monitoring devices have become affordable and easy to use. As pulse oximetry units are very easy to use and portable, they are often used as a sole monitor in many zoo practices. Pulse oximetry does, however, not replace blood gas measurements for assessing the degree of hypoxemia (Schumacher et al. 1997). An animal that is being maintained on nasal oxygen may have a normal pulse oximetry reading (>90%), even if hypoventilating. Pulse oximetry estimates the oxygen saturation of hemoglobin. When administering high partial pressures of oxygen (nasal oxygen), normal saturation may be maintained even in animals that are not adequately ventilating. If pulse oximetry is the only monitor, then the veterinarian may not be aware of potential impending hypoxic events. On the other hand, when using alpha-2 adrenergic antagonist, the peripheral vasoconstriction often creates inaccurate readings and will indicate incorrect low saturation. Therefore, the adequacy of ventilation should also be measured during prolonged immobilizations through the use of capnography and blood gas measurements. The availability these days of hand-held blood gas analyzers has made blood gas monitoring easier even in field situations. These analyzers have the advantage of also measuring the pH, potassium and sodium levels, and other minerals so that fluid therapy can be adapted accordingly.

RECOVERY CONSIDERATIONS

As gazelles are very nervous animals that will try to flee, they preferably should recover in a quiet, dark, and safe place, such as a closed box or a small enclosure. If the animal has been intubated, the oral cavity should be examined for regurgitated material and the mouth swabbed clean. Also, the endotracheal tube can be removed with the cuff partially inflated to help clear the pharyngeal area. During recovery, the gazelle is placed in sternal recumbency, with one handler holding the head up with the nose down to prevent aspiration until the animal is able to keep the head up without support. The blindfold is removed when the animal is able to hold the head or shake the cover off by itself. When waking up in an enclosure, the gazelle's hind end should be placed near the door so that upon recovery, it can run away from the handler. The handler can also go out the door quickly to help prevent further excitement upon recovery. Animals can also be woken up in special boxes which create a safe dark environment. These boxes should be made of light but durable material strong enough to hold a specific species. The box must be high enough for the animal to comfortably stand up. The width should be either too narrow to turn, or wide enough to turn easily. It should also be wide enough to accommodate the horns. The authors advice box sizes of (length × width × height) 130 × 40 × 110 cm for 30 kg, 110 × 40 × 90 cm for 20 kg BW and 95 × 40 × 70 cm for 10-kg animals. Vertical sliding doors with handles on top and bottom are provided at the front and the back of the box. At the sides, handles are made to easily carry the box. The floor should be nonslippery, and adequate ventilation is provided through holes in the side. The roof should have no holes to avoid horns becoming stuck in it. These boxes can be used for transport, for recovery, and for treatments.

Animals that have been handled without sedation or when fully awake again require the same care when being released. If two handlers are holding the gazelle, they will need to let go of the eye cover and of the animal at the same time and stand back so that the gazelle can run forward. Boxes should be opened from the front and people should stay behind the box. Nothing should be in front of the gazelle to give the animal a quick escape from where the handlers stand.

TRANQUILIZERS

Animals should be kept away from the group for as short a time as possible, as being isolated increases stress significantly. If gazelles need to be separated or confined for prolonged treatments, long-acting tranquilizers can be used. These drugs are also useful for groups when they need to be transported, have to adapt to new environments, or when new animals are introduced into an existing group.

Haloperidol lactate is a butyrophenone tranquilizer that will cause calming and adaptation to a new environment. Haloperidol is typically given at 0.1–0.3 mg/kg intramuscularly, but can also be given orally with the same effect. The onset of action of haloperidol usually occurs within 10 minutes of injection, and effects typically last 18–24 hours. This drug is very effective at calming gazelles and preventing self-trauma. The decanoate ester of haloperidol is an oil-based formulation that is much longer acting. This formulation is not commonly used because of the possibility of the extrapyramidal effect of prolonged anorexia. Other long-acting tranquilizers are zuclopenthixol acetate or perphenazine enathate. Zuclopenthixol's effects occur within 1 hour, and tranquilization may last 3–4 days (McKenzie 1993). Haloperidol in combination with with zuclopenthixol at a dose rate of about 0.3 and 2.5 mg/kg, respectively, used in Rheem gazelle (*Gazella subgutturosa marica*) gave better results than when haloperidol was used alone. Perphenazine effects may not be noted for 12–18 hours initially, and are therefore often combined with an initial dosage of haloperidol. Dosages of 3.5 mg/kg have been administered with good effect to Mohor gazelle (*Gazella dama mhorr*) used for assisted reproduction research purposes (González et al. 2008). The authors use total dosages of 50–100 mg for gazelles of 20–40 kg and effect lasts for about 10 days. Zuclopenthixol and perphenazine are not currently available in the United States, but formulations are being developed for their use in zoos and with wildlife species.

Diazepam can be given intravenously or intramuscular at a dosage of about 0.5 mg–1 mg/kg and results in a mild sedation for several hours. Directly after a capture it is advisable to give the diazepam intravenously for quick induction. The additional use of an eye cover is important to reach an optimal effect. An intramuscular injection is best given 15 minutes before handling in a hospital or confined situation.

Gazelle can be frustrating patients as they tend to waste away when separated from their group. The addition of other gazelles decreases stress and improves well-being, but can be harder to manage when regular handling is required. The design of hospitalization enclosures where animals still easily can be separated and moved into treatment boxes is useful for this purpose.

COMPLICATIONS

Anesthesia of overheated or extremely stressed animals should be avoided. Despite their ability to deal with high temperatures, this will increase likelihood of mortality due to hyperthermia and capture myopathy. Exertional myopathy has been associated with the use of etorphine combinations (Molnar & Mckinney 2002; Snyder et al. 1992; Wallace et al. 1987), as well as prolonged pacing activity following renarcotization events. Exertional myopathy can cause acute renal failure due to myoglobin-related toxic effects on the renal tubules. Exertional myopathy may also result in life threatening acid-base disturbances and potassium derangements.

Aspiration pneumonia from regurgitated ingesta is a potential problem in anesthetized ruminants. The use of endotracheal tubes is recommended during longer procedures and for procedures that require placing the animal in lateral or dorsal position. Without intubation a sedated animal should always be kept in sternal position with the head up and nose down and never be turned on its back.

Hypoxemia will often occur with most of the drugs used for induction and should be treated with intubation and ventilation. If the animal is not intubated, then the administration of nasal oxygen is recommended. Drugs such as doxapram can be used to improve respiration. Also, antagonizing drugs can be used to counteract the respiratory depressive effect of the anesthetics used.

Renarcotization is a phenomenon in which animals immobilized with potent opioids will exhibit resedation hours after being antagonized. With the use of naltrexone, which is a complete antagonist, this problem has not been seen anymore by the authors. When other antagonist, such as diprenorphine are used renarcotisation can occur.

In domestic ruminants, xylazine has an oxytocin-like effect on the uterus in the last quarter of pregnancy (Jansen et al. 1984). The use of detomidine or medetomidine may therefore be preferable in pregnant gazelles.

Alpha-2 adrenergic agonists, as well as opioids, can impair gastrointestinal motility. This could lead to tympany and postanesthetic ileus. Alpha-2 adrenergic agonists should be reversed in gazelles with tolazoline or atipamezole. Yohimbine may reverse alpha agonist effects, but it is less effective in ruminants than tolazoline (Hikasa et al. 1988; Hsu et al. 1987). Tolazoline may also bind alpha-1 receptors, which could improve rumenoreticular function post immobilization, and has been shown to more completely restore rumenoreticu-

lar function after the use of alpha-2 agonists when compared with yohimbine (Hikasa et al. 1988). Atipamezole is more effective at reversing CNS receptors in sheep, but can cause minor side effects (Carroll et al. 2005; Hartsfield et al. 1998). Sudden deaths have occurred in ruminants following reversal of alpha-2 adrenergic agonists (Hsu et al. 1987). The sudden vasodilatory effects of alpha antagonist drugs may be the reason for deaths. In the authors' experience, these vasodilatory effects are unlikely to occur when antagonists are administered intramuscularly rather than intravenously. It is advised to give a 5:1 ratio of atipamezole to medetomidine intramuscularly to accomplish full reversal and avoid resedation especially for free-ranging animals (Bush et al. 2004).

In particular, when alpha-2 adrenergic agonists are used intramuscularly, increasingly high dosages have to be given to stressed animals to be effective, with increased cardiopulmonary side effects.

Trauma is a common complication when handling and capturing gazelle. Animals can sustain serious stab wounds or fractures in capture systems where animals are herded together, resulting in death or the need for euthanasia. Quick and smooth separation is crucial to avoid aggression, especially between males. Proper planning of any intended procedure, communication between the people involved, and knowledge of and experience with the behavior of the species are critical in avoiding trauma.

APPENDIX 61A.1

Date of catch	_____	Location	_____	Species	_____
Personnel					
Coordinator (1)	_____	Foreman (2)	_____	Supervisor (3)	_____
Staff installing equipment	_____				

Item	Tasked	Checked	Comment
Plan catch, location, number of animals to be restrained	1	☐	
Inform relevant staff and assign tasks	1	☐	
Catch foreman assigned	1	☐	
Catch Supervisor assigned	1	☐	
Catch personnel assigned	1	☐	
Install remote gate trip equipment and ensure correct operation	1	☐	
Ensure enough panels and tie pins for length of raceway.	2	☐	
Ensure access doors are in the correct position	2	☐	
Check that the ramp and tamer are lined up correctly	2	☐	
Tamer doors are opening without any problem	2	☐	
Tamer side swings out without any restrictions	2	☐	
Floor under tamer is level without any stones or obstructions	2	☐	
Plywood cover on tamer is fastened correctly	2	☐	
Cover on ramp is loose to allow access to the animal from the top	2	☐	
Any gates near raceway entry to be secured to avoid opening during restraint	2	☐	
Ensure access to the raceway is protected to avoid injury to animals	2	☐	
Install and level plywood base ready for weighing scales	3	☐	

(Continued)

Item	Tasked	Checked	Comment
All sliding door timbers are present and moving properly	3	☐	
All sides and hinges are moving freely	3	☐	
All excess grease is removed from runners.	3	☐	
Shade over work area is adequate for the time of year	3	☐	
Rubber stops in place under drop floor	3	☐	
Rubber protection in place between Tamer and Ramp	3	☐	
Push boards on site	3	☐	
Calibration weights on site	3	☐	
Tarpaulins on site	3	☐	
Transport boxes on site: check number required	3	☐	
		☐	
		☐	
		☐	
		☐	
		☐	
		☐	
		☐	
		☐	
		☐	

Wadi Al Safa Wildlife Centre: Checklist for Morning of Restraint

Date of catch _____   Location _____   Species _____

Personnel

Coordinator (1) _____   Foreman (2) _____   Supervisor (3) _____

Handlers   _____

_____

Item	Tasked	Checked	Comment
Sampling kits	1	☐	
Spanner for adjusting weighing scales feet	1	☐	
Inform staff of the number of animals to be moved	1	☐	
Time schedules	1	☐	
Boxes (Medical)	1	☐	
Horn covers	1	☐	
Ropes for leg restraint	1	☐	
Anthelmintics/treatments	1	☐	
Notify any changes to appropriate staff	1	☐	
Load cell indicator	1	☐	
Hoof kit	1	☐	
Loading ramp for pickup	2	☐	
Animal transfer/transport box	2	☐	
Check all items below are completed	2	☐	
Safety boards/push boards	3	☐	
Tarpaulin × 3	3	☐	
Generator	3	☐	
Check petrol	3	☐	
Check oil	3	☐	
Start and ensure working properly	3	☐	
Weighing scales and mat	3	☐	
Eye covers (towel)	3	☐	
Water bucket and water	3	☐	
Rubbish bag	3	☐	
Ladder	3	☐	
Sharps bucket	3	☐	
Wire cutter	3	☐	
Plywood (spare) × 2	3	☐	
Hand shovel	3	☐	
Calibration weights × 2 (A + C)	3	☐	
Table	3	☐	
Electric prod	3	☐	
Safety boots	4	☐	

Wadi Al Safa Wildlife Centre: Checklist for Postrestraint Duties

Date of catch _____ Location _____ Species _____
Personnel _____
Coordinator (1) _____ Foreman (2) _____ Supervisor (3) _____
Removing
  equipment (4) _____

Item	Tasked	Completed	Comment
Inform 2 and 3 of new location for equipment	1	☐	
Remove weighing scales and store safely	2	☐	
Check all doors for warpage	2	☐	
Check panels for loose bolts/damaged plywood	2	☐	
Deliver any boxed animals to new location and release	2	☐	
Wash all mats used for scales and store safely	3	☐	
Check sliding timbers to see if they are warped.	3	☐	
Remove all pins and panels: check for damage	3	☐	
Move all panels and equipment to next catch site	3	☐	
Store equipment not being used	3	☐	
Remove all items installed for the purpose of the restraint	3	☐	
All rubbish to be removed and disposed of safely	4	☐	

1, Catch coordinator; 2, catch foreman; 3, catch supervisor; 4, catch personnel.

REFERENCES

Ahern BJ, Soma LR, Rudy JA, et al. 2010. Pharmacokinetics of fentanyl administered transdermally and intravenously in sheep. *American Journal of Veterinary Research* 71(10): 1127–1132.

Allen JL, Janssen DL, Oosterhius JE, et al. 1991. Immobilization of captive non-domestic hoofstock with carfentanil. Proceedings of the American Association of Zoo Veterinarians, pp. 343–351.

Blumer ES, deMaar TW. 1993. Manual restraint for the management of non-domestic hoofstock. Proceedings of the American Association of Zoo Veterinarians, pp. 141–143.

Bush M, Citino SB, Tell L. 1992. Telazol and telazol/rompun anesthesia in non-domestic cervids and bovids. Proceedings of the American Association of Zoo Veterinarians and American Association of Wildlife Veterinarians, pp. 251–252.

Bush M, Raath JP, Phillips LG, et al. 2004. Immobilisation of impala (*Aepyceros melampus*) with a ketamine hydrochloride/ medetomidine hydrochloride combination, and reversal with atipamezole hydrochloride. *Journal of the South African Veterinary Association* 75(1):14–18.

Carroll GL, Hartsfield SM, Champney TH, et al. 2005. Effects of medetomidine and its antagonism with atipamezole on stress-related horomones, metabolites, physiologic responses, sedation, and mechanical threshold in goats. *Veterinary Anaesthesia and Analgesia* 32(3):147–157.

Cattet MRL, Bourque A, Elkin BT, et al. 2004. Evaluation of the potential for injury with high velocity remote drug delivery systems. Proceedings of the American Association of Zoo Veterinarians, American Association of Wildlife Veterinarians, and Wildlife Disease Association, p. 512.

Caulkett N, Paterson J, Haigh JC, et al. 2006. Comparative physiologic effects of thiaphentanil-azaperone and thiaphentanil-medetomidine-ketamine in free ranging Uganda Kob (*Kobus kob thomasi*). Proceedings of the American Association of Zoo Veterinarians, pp. 216–219.

Caulkett NA, Cattet MRL, Cantwell S, et al. 2000. Anesthesia of wood bison with medetomidine-zolazepam/tiletamine and xylazine-zolazepam/tiletamine combinations. *The Canadian Veterinary Journal* 41:49–53.

Chittick E, Horne W, Wolfe B, et al. 2001. Cardiopulmonary assessment of medetomidine, ketamine, and butorphanol anesthesia in captive Thomson's gazelles (*Gazella thomsoni*). *Journal of Zoo and Wildlife Medicine* 32(2):168–175.

Cooper DV, Grobler D, Bush M, et al. 2005. Anaesthesia of nyala (*Tragelaphus angasi*) with a combination of thiafentanil (A3080), medetomidine and ketamine. *Journal of the South African Veterinary Association* 76(1):18–21.

Dowd G, Gaynor JS, Alvis M, et al. 1997. A comparison of transdermal fentanyl and oral phenylbutazone for post-operative analgesia in sheep. *Veterinary Surgery* 27:168.

Duncan M, Junge RE, Miller RE. 1997. A retrospective analysis of necropsy information from Speke's gazelle (*Gazella spekei*) at St. Louis Zoological Park. Proceedings of the American Association of Zoo Veterinarians, p. 265.

Feldhamer GA, Drickamer LC, Vessey SH, et al. 2007. *Mammalogy: Adaptation, Diversity, Ecology*, 3rd ed., p. 109. Baltimore: John Hopkins University Press.

Foster CA. 1999. Immobilization of goitered gazelles (Gazella subgutterosa) and Arabian mountain gazelles (Gazella gazella) with xylazine-ketamine. *Journal of Zoo and Wildlife Medicine* 30(3):448–450.

González R, Berlinguer F, Espeso G, et al. 2008. Use of a neuroleptic in assisted reproduction of the critically endangered Mohor gazelle (*Gazella dama mhorr*). *Theriogenology* 70:909–922.

Gray PR, McDonell WN. 1986. Anesthesia in goats and sheep. Part 2: general anesthesia. *Compendium on Continuing Education for the Practicing Veterinarian* 8:S127–S135.

Greth A, Vassart M, Anagariyah S. 1993. Chemical immobilization in gazelles (Gazella sp.) with fentanyl and azaperone. *African Journal of Ecology* 31:66–74.

Hammer S, Hammer C. 2002. Intravenöse Applikation der "Hellabrunner Mischung" im Stadium höchster Erregung bei Gazellen. *Arbeitstagung der Zootierärzte im deutschsprachigen Raum*, München, Germany 22:53–55.

Hartsfield SM, Carroll GL, Martinez EA, et al. 1998. Antagonism of xylazine or medetomidine in goats using atipamezole, tolazoline, yohimbine, or saline. Proceedings of the American College of Veterinary Anesthesiologists.

Hikasa Y, Takase K, Emi S, et al. 1988. Antagonistic effects of alpha-adrenoceptor blocking agents on reticuloruminal hypomotility induced by xylazine in cattle. *Canadian Journal of Veterinary Research* 52(4):411–415.

Howard BW, Lagutchik MS, Januszkiewicz AJ, et al. 1990. The cardiovascular response of sheep to tiletamine-zolazepam and butorphanol tartrate anesthesia. *Veterinary Surgery* 19(6):461–467.

Hsu WH, Schaffer DD, Hanson CE. 1987. Effects of tolazoline and yohimbine on xylazine-induced central nervous system depression, bradycardia, and tachypnea in sheep. *Journal of the American Veterinary Medical Association* 190:423–426.

Ingvast-Larsson C, Högberg M, Mengistu U, et al. 2011. Pharmacokinetics of meloxicam in adult goats and its analgesic effect in disbudded kids. *Journal of Veterinary Pharmacology and Therapeutics* 34(1):64–69.

Jansen CAM, Lowe KC, Nathanielsz PW. 1984. The effects of xylazine on uterine activity, fetal and maternal oxygenation, cardiovascular function, and fetal breathing. *American Journal of Obstetrics and Gynecology* 148:386.

Janssen DL, Allan JL, Raath JP, et al. 1991. Field studies with the narcotic immobilizing agent A3080. Proceedings of the American Association of Zoo Veterinarians, pp. 333–335.

Junge RE. 1998. Epidural analgesia in addax (*Addax nasomaculatus*). *Journal of Zoo and Wildlife Medicine* 29(3):285–287.

Mahmood KT, Ashraf M, Amin F, et al. 2011. Pharmacokinetics of ecofriendly meloxicam in healthy goats. *Journal of Pharmaceutical Sciences and Research* 3(1):1035–1041.

Martin Jurado O, Hammer C, Hammer S. 2007. Beira (*Dorcotragus megalotis*) immobilization at the Al Wabra Wildlife Preservation. *Verhandlungsbericht Erkrankungen der Zootiere* 43:293–295.

McKenzie AA, ed. 1993. *The Capture and Care Manual, Capture, Care, Accomodation and Transportation of Wild African Animals*. Lynwood Ridge: Wildlife Decision Support Services and South African Veterinary Foundation Menlo Park, South Africa.

Molnar L, Mckinney P. 2002. Effect of climate conditions of middle east on chemical immobilisation of Arabian and African ungulates. Proceedings of the European Association of Zoo and Wildlife Veterinarians, pp. 187–189.

Mutlow A, Isaza R, Carpenter JW, et al. 2004. Pharmokinetics of carfentanil and naltrexone in domestic goats (*Capra hircus*). *Journal of Zoo and Wildlife Medicine* 35(4):489–497.

O'Donovan D, Bailey T. 2006. Restraint of Arabian oryx (Oryx leucoryx) in Dubai, United Arab Emirates using a mobile raceway. 2nd Conference of the International Congress of Zookeepers, Gold Coast, Australia. http://www.iczoo.org/downloads/australia2006-papers.pdf (accessed February 10, 2014), pp. 110–119.

Riebold T. 1996. Ruminants. In: *Lumb & Jones' Veterinary Anesthesia*, 3rd ed. (JC Thurmon, WJ Tranquili, GJ Benson, eds.), pp. 610–626. Baltimore: Lippincott Williams & Wilkins.

Rietkerk FE, Delima EC, Mubarak SM. 1994. The hematological profile of the mountain gazelle (*Gazella gazella*): variations with sex, age, capture method, season, and anesthesia. *Journal of Wildlife Diseases* 30(1):69–76.

Röken BO. 1997. A potent anesthetic combination with low concentrated medetomidine in zoo animals. Proceedings of the American Association of Zoo Veterinarians, pp. 134–136.

Schmidt-Nielsen K. 1997. *Animal Physiology: Adaptation and Environment*, 5th ed., p. 276. Cambridge, UK: Cambridge University Press.

Schumacher J, Heard DJ, Young L, et al. 1997. Cardiopulmonary effects of carfentanil in dama gazelles (*Gazella dama*). *Journal of Zoo and Wildlife Medicine* 28(2):166–170.

Shukla M, Singh G, Sindhura BG, et al. 2007. Comparative plasma pharmacokinetics of meloxicam in sheep and goats following intravenous administration. *Comparative Biochemistry and Physiology. Toxicology and Pharmacology* 145(4):528–532.

Şindak N, Biricik HS. 2003. Ceylanlarda Tiletamin-Zolazepam-Xylazin Anestezisi. *Yüzüncü Yil Üniversitesi Veteriner Fakültesi Dergisi* 14(1):110–113.

Snyder SB, Richard MJ, Foster WR. 1992. Etorphine, ketamine, and xylazine in combination (M99KX) for immobilization of exotic ruminants: a significant additive effect. Proceedings of the American Association of Zoo Veterinarians and American Association of Wildlife Veterinarians, pp. 253–258.

Van Zijll Langhout MH, Raath JP. 2010. The use of ethorphine, thiaphantanil, azaperone, butorphanol, ketamine and doxapram in white rhionoceroces, African buffalos, sble an roan antelopes. Proceedings of The International Conference on Diseases of Zoo and Wild Animals, pp. 10–11.

Vaughan TA, Ryan JM, Czaplewski NJ. 2010. *Mammalogy*, 5th ed. Sudbury: Jones & Bartlett Learning.

Wallace RS, Bush M, Montali RJ. 1987. Deaths from exertional myopathy at the National Zoological Park from 1975–1985. *Journal of Wildlife Diseases* 22(3):454–462.

Willmer P, Stone G, Johnston IA. 2000. *Environmental Physiology of Animals*, p. 534. Oxford, UK: Blackwell Science.

62 Wild Sheep and Goats

Nigel Caulkett and Chris Walzer

INTRODUCTION

Capture of wild sheep and goats can be challenging. These animals frequently live in mountainous terrain, and are predisposed to stress-related complications, such as hyperthermia and capture myopathy. Wild sheep are frequently captured by physical methods, and manually restrained for short procedures. Remote drug delivery and chemical restraint can be an option if it is carefully planned. Chemical restraint may be more suited for capture of small numbers of animals. Captive sheep and goats may require anesthesia for a variety of reasons. This chapter will discuss physical capture methods and current anesthetic techniques for wild sheep and goats.

SPECIES-SPECIFIC PHYSIOLOGY

Domestic ovids are very prone to severe hypoxemia during immobilization with alpha-2 agonists. Severe hypoxemia has been observed in bighorned sheep (*Ovis canadensis*) immobilized with medetomidine-based combinations (Fahlman et al. 2012). Hypoxemia in wild sheep can be severe enough that it is difficult to treat with supplemental inspired oxygen (Fahlman et al. 2012). Wild sheep and goats are prone to ruminal tympany and regurgitation during chemical restraint.

PHYSICAL CAPTURE

In the 1980s, there were several excellent studies that critically evaluated capture methods in bighorn sheep (*Ovis canadensis*) (Kock et al. 1987a, 1987b, 1987c). This body of work evaluated a variety of outcomes to determine the safest capture method for this species.

The studies evaluated three methods of physical capture: drop net, drive net, and net gunning. They also evaluated chemical capture with narcotic-xylazine combinations. The studies compared capture outcome, biological, biochemical, and hematological parameters against long-term survival (Kock et al. 1987a, 1987b, 1987c).

Capture outcome was evaluated by categorizing the animals as normal, stress-induced compromise, and mortality from capture myopathy or trauma. Compromised animals were defined as having one or more of the following signs: body temperatue > 42.4°C, prolonged pursuit, excessive struggling, shock, or any other signs of physical compromise.

It was determined that net gunning resulted in the lowest combined mortality rate at <2%, drop netting had a 3% mortality, and drive netting resulted in a 4% mortality rate. Chemical immobilization was associated with the highest mortality at 8%. Chemical immobilization was also associated with the greatest number of compromised animals at 19%, drop netting resulted in 15% compromised animals, and drive netting resulted in 16%. Net-gunned animals demonstrated the lowest incidence of compromise at 11% (Kock et al. 1987a). These studies clearly demonstrated that physical restraint was the preferable method for short procedures.

In the Alpine and Balkan regions of Europe, chamois (*Rupicapra* spp.) are routinely captured using modified elastic leg snares, drop net systems, and box traps (Ballestros & Benito 1992; Struch & Baumann 2000). Snares pose a serious risk of digital frostbite in the winter months and thus this method should not be used in low temperatures (Delmas 1993). Box traps, which are also routinely used for Alpine ibex (*Capra ibex*) need to be well established with salt licks prior to actual capture attempts (Abderhalden et al. 1998). Drive nets have been used extensively in the Pyrenees to capture Southern

Zoo Animal and Wildlife Immobilization and Anesthesia, Second Edition. Edited by Gary West, Darryl Heard, and Nigel Caulkett.
© 2014 John Wiley & Sons, Inc. Published 2014 by John Wiley & Sons, Inc.

chamois (*Rupicapra pyrenaica*) and Spanish ibex (*Capra pyrenaica*). Significant mortality (3–10% and 18% in nonmonitored nets) has been associated with this method in chamois (López-Olvera et al. 2009). The use of acepromazine in conjunction with physically trapped chamois has been reported to decrease the stress response (López-Olvera et al. 2007). In contrast, drive nets appear to be suitable for the capture of the more docile ibex (López-Olvera et al. 2009). The use of azaperone and haloperidol has been reported in the drive-net captured Iberian ibexes. While haloperidol at 0.17 mg/kg (IM) did not prove beneficial, azaperone at 0.45–0.59 mg/kg (IM) was suitable to decrease the stress response to the capture event (Mentaberre et al. 2010).

Beyond the risk to the captured animals, these physical restraint methods also pose a significant risk for serious injury to the operators, this is especially true in the chamois, which has sharply pointed, backward curved horns (López-Olvera et al. 2009).

In central Asia, the capture of mountain goats and sheep is particularly difficult owing to the unavailability of helicopters due to the remoteness and general national security concerns about aircraft. However, argali sheep (*Ovis ammon*) have been successfully captured using drive nets (Kenny et al. 2008).

Generally, all these methods require a significant amount of manpower and constant monitoring in order to reduce the time of physical restraint.

For a complete description of these physical capture techniques please refer to Chapter 9.

CHEMICAL RESTRAINT AND ANESTHESIA

Vascular Access

Venous access is not difficult in sheep and goats. The cephalic vein, lateral saphenous vein, and jugular vein can all be easily accessed. The auricular artery can be cannulated in some species for direct blood pressure monitoring or to facilitate sampling for arterial blood gas analysis. Arterial blood samples may also be obtained from the femoral artery when auricular arterial catheterization proves to be difficult.

Intubation

Intubation is recommended during volatile anesthesia and in steep terrain when optimal positioning of the animal is compromised in order to minimize the of ruminal content aspiration. Intubation is not difficult in most sheep and goat species. The animal should be maintained in sternal recumbency with the head and neck extended toward the sky. The mouth is opened wide and gentle traction is placed on the tongue. A long flat-bladed laryngoscope is placed into the oral cavity. The tip of the laryngoscope is placed at the base of the epiglottis. The epiglottis is moved ventrally to reveal the glottis. A stylet should be placed inside the endotracheal tube to reduce the curvature of the tube.

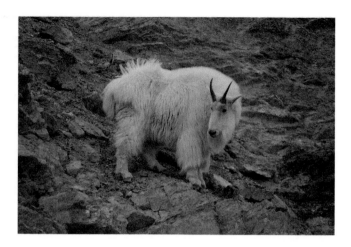

Figure 62.1. Mountain goat in typical terrain. Capture personnel must be trained and prepared to work in steep, dangerous terrain.

The tube is placed into the glottis and advanced into the trachea. Typically, the tube should not be fully deflated on extubation; this will help to prevent any rumen contents entering the trachea if regurgitation has occurred.

Preanesthetic Concerns

Like all other ungulates, sheep and goats are prone to ruminal tympany and regurgitation during anesthesia. It is prudent to fast captive animals for 24 hours prior to anesthesia. Maintenance in sternal recumbency may help to prevent the onset of ruminal tympany.

Wild sheep and goats often inhabit mountainous terrain. Capture work in this type of terrain must be carefully planned to avoid trauma to the animal during induction of anesthesia (Fig. 62.1). Bighorn sheep are very prone to capture myopathy (Kock et al. 1987c). Capture events must be carefully planned to avoid prolonged chase times in an effort to prevent capture myopathy.

Monitoring and Supportive Care

Sheep and goats are prone to hypoxemia during anesthesia, particularly if alpha-2 agonists have been used as part of the anesthetic protocol (Caulkett et al. 1994; Jalanka 1989; Shury & Caulkett 2006). Hypoxemia may be less severe if the animal is maintained in sternal recumbency (Caulkett et al. 1996). Oxygenation should always be monitored in anesthetized sheep. Pulse oximetry or arterial blood gas analysis should be used to monitor oxygenation. Oxygen should be available during anesthetic procedures to offset hypoxemia.

Hyperthermia is another potential complication that may be encountered during capture and anesthesia. Hyperthemia has been linked with stress-related complications and capture myopathy (Kock et al. 1987c). It is best to minimize the risk of hyperthermia by limiting pursuit times and planning capture events for cooler seasons when possible. Body temperature should be closely monitored during anesthesia. Body temperature in excess of 41°C should be treated by actively cooling the animal with a coldwater enema or snow. Antagonism of alpha-2 agonists should also be considered in emergent situations.

It is difficult to prevent ruminal tympany or regurgitation in free-ranging animals. Maintenance in sternal recumbency may help to prevent or treat ruminal tympany. A rumen tube or trocar should be carried to treat serious cases of ruminal tympany. Often, it is most advisable to complete the procedure and antagonize alpha-2 agonists; ruminal tympany typically resolves following administration of an alpha-2 agonist.

Blood pressure monitoring should be considered if the animal is to be maintained with volatile anesthesia. Indirect blood pressure monitors can be used to monitor trends in blood pressure. We typically place the blood pressure cuff midway between the carpus and pastern joint (Fig. 62.2).

Free-ranging animals should be blindfolded to decrease stimulation during light anesthesia or physical restraint. It is important to take care around the legs and horns of lightly anesthetized animals as they may kick and stab. The animal should be placed on a soft surface to avoid pressure points, and they should be supported in sternal recumbency for recovery, following anesthesia.

Drug Delivery

Helicopter darting and free-range stalking of animals are the major methods used to facilitate drug delivery in wild sheep and goats. Helicopter darting, which is generally not available in Europe outside Scandinavia, has been associated with increased mortality in bighorn sheep and mountain goats (Jessup 1999; Kock et al.

1987a). Free-range stalking and ground-based drug delivery can also be used to facilitate drug delivery (Caulkett et al. 2012; Festa-Bianchet & Jorgenson 1985; Merwin et al. 2000; Shury & Caulkett 2006). Stalking is strenuous and time-consuming, but is used routinely in the Alps to capture chamois and ibex. On average, it requires 25 hours of stalking per captured chamois in an alpine protected area (Walzer et al. 1998). The recovery of darted animals can be problematic in the high-strung chamois, and the use of radio-telemetry darts may be indicated. Ground-based stalking tends to be associated with less stress related complications compared with helicopter darting (Fig. 62.3).

Pharmacological Considerations for Anesthesia of Wild Sheep and Goats

Drug Combinations for Induction of Immobilization Many different drug combinations have been used to facilitate capture of wild sheep and goats. All of these combinations have advantages and disadvantages. In this chapter, individual combinations will be discussed by species. The chapter will focus on currently used combinations. There are some general principles that are worthy of discussion. Alpha-2 agonist-dissociative anesthetic combinations may be associated with less excitement during the induction period, compared with narcotic-based protocols. This may decrease the risk of losing track of a darted animal due to excitement during the induction period. The administration of alpha-2 agonists tends to be associated with hypoxemia. Supplemental oxygen should be carried to offset hypoxemia encountered during immobilization. As a general rule, yohimbine may not be an effective antagonist for alpha-2 agonists in bighorn sheep (Jessup 1999). We have had good results with atipamezole, in a variety of sheep species immobilized with xylazine and medetomidine-based protocols. An appropriate

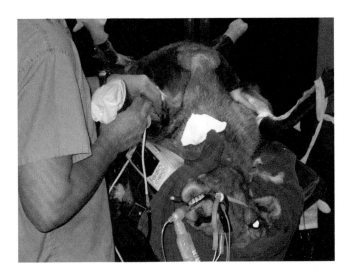

Figure 62.2. Volatile anesthesia of a Stone's sheep. Note placement of the indirect blood pressure cuff on the left forelimb.

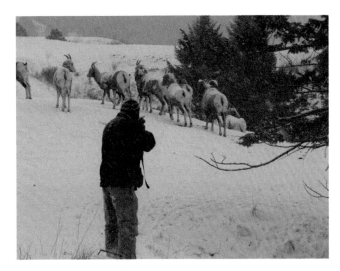

Figure 62.3. Ground-stalking bighorn sheep in British Columbia, Canada.

choice of immobilizing drugs should be based on current literature, experience with the drugs, and drug availability.

Volatile Anesthesia

Volatile anesthesia may be used to facilitate maintenance of anesthesia for surgery, imaging or prolonged procedures. We typically use isoflurane or sevoflurane for maintenance of anesthesia. The sheep or goat is induced to anesthesia with xylazine-telazol or medetomidine-ketamine. Once the animal is recumbent, its depth of anesthesia is assessed. If airway protective reflexes are intact, either diazepam-ketamine or propofol is administered IV to obtund airway protective reflexes and facilitate intubation. We typically use a dose of 0.1 mg/kg of diazepam, combined with 2 mg/kg of ketamine, administered to effect. Propofol is administered at 1–2 mg/kg. Commonly encountered side effects of volatile anesthesia are respiratory depression and hypotension. Respiratory depression is typically treated with intermittent positive pressure ventilation, and hypotension often responds to a lightening of the anesthetic plane or fluid therapy. Body temperature should be closely monitored as hypothermia may be encountered, particularly in smaller animals.

Once the procedure is complete, it is advisable to antagonize residual alpha-2 agonist drugs; otherwise prolonged recoveries may be encountered.

Species Specific Considerations

Bighorn Sheep (*Ovis canadensis canadensis*) and Dall or Stone's Sheep (*Ovis dalli*) Narcotic-based anesthesia with carfentanil-xylazine or etorphine-xylazine has been used for helicopter-based capture of bighorn sheep. Etorphine has been used at a dose of 3.5 mg, combined with 50 mg of xylazine. Carfentanil has been used at 0.044 mg/kg in combination with 0.2 mg/kg of xylazine (Jessup 1999). Both of these combinations can be used to successfully capture sheep. Complications tend to occur with partial dosing or trauma during induction. This may reflect the method of capture (helicopter darting) more than an actual drug effect.

Xylazine-ketamine combinations have been used for capture of bighorns (Festa-Bianchet & Jorgenson 1985). Xylazine-ketamine solutions must be delivered in relatively high volumes; therefore, this mixture has been largely replaced by xylazine-Telazol®. Xylazine-Telazol has been used to effectively capture human habituated bighorn sheep. It has been advocated at a dose of 4.2 mg/kg of Telazol combined with 0.5 mg/kg of xylazine (Merwin et al. 2000). A major drawback of this mixture is that recoveries tend to be prolonged following antagonism of the xylazine; this is probably the result of residual Telazol. In order to address this concern, we have recently started using a mixture of xylazine, Telazol and hydromorphone (Shury &

Caulkett 2006). This mixture is administered at a dose of 1.64 mg/kg of Telazol, combined with 1.1 mg/kg of xylazine and 0.22 mg/kg of hydromorphone. The mixture proved to be suitable for capture of human habituated sheep. Recovery was relatively rapid (10.3 minutes) following the administration of 0.11 mg/kg of atipamezole and 0.18 mg/kg of naltrexone.

We have also used 0.06–0.08 mg/kg of medetomidine, combined with 2 mg/kg of ketamine, to induce anesthesia in captive bighorn sheep. This combination is readily reversed with atipamezole at three times the medetomidine dose. Free-ranging bighorns require a significantly greater dose. We have been using 0.16 ± 0.04 mg/kg of medetomidine, combined with 4.2 ± 1.6 mg/kg of ketamine, to induce anesthesia of wild bighorns that have been stalked on foot (Caulkett et al. 2012).

In our experience, Dall and Stone's sheep are very similar to bighorn sheep. We have used 1 mg/kg of xylazine combined with 2 mg/kg of Telazol for induction, prior to administration of volatile anesthetics in captive Stone's sheep. We have also used 0.06–0.08 mg/kg of medetomidine, combined with 2 mg/kg of ketamine in captive Dall and Stone's sheep.

Mountain Goat (*Oreamnos americanus*) Free-ranging mountain goats have typically been anesthetized with potent narcotics. Carfentanil has been advocated, as the sole agent, at a dose of 0.035 mg/kg (Jessup 1999). Etorphine has also been used at a dose of 4–5 mg per animal (Jessup 1999). We have anesthetized captive mountain goats with 0.06–0.08 mg/kg of medetomidine, combined with 2 mg/kg. This dose will produce light anesthesia for restraint or as a premedication for general anesthesia. The medetomidine is readily antagonized with atipamezole administered at three times the medetomidine dose.

Markhor (*Capra falconeri megaceros*) A detailed study exists that compares the efficacy and safety of medetomidine-ketamine and etorphine-acepromazine in captive Markhors (Jalanka 1989). This study compared a mean dose of 63 μg/kg of medetomidine, combined with 1.6 mg/kg of ketamine against 56 μg/kg of etorphine, combined with 0.25 mg/kg of acepromazine. Both of these combinations were readily reversible. Atipamezole was used at a mean dose of 282 μg/kg, and diprenorphine was administered at a dose of 76 μg/kg.

Both combinations induced moderate hypoxemia. Medetomidine-ketamine induced slightly more respiratory depression evidenced by a significantly greater PaCO2, compared with etophine-acepromazine. Medetomidine-ketamine produced better myorelaxation and a more complete immobilization than etorphine-acepromazine (Jalanka 1989). Medetomidine-ketamine has become a commonly recommended combination for anesthesia of sheep and goats.

Chamois (*Rupricapra rupicapra*) Various methods to chemically immobilize chamois have been described. In the German-speaking areas of Europe, the Hellabrunner mix (125-mg xylazine + 100-mg ketamine per mL) was until recently the method of choice. It is important to note that the required dose (0.27-mg/kg ketamine + 0.34-mg/kg xylazine) for chamois is extremely low when compared with other mountain ungulates (Wiesner & von Hegel 1990). The advantage of this combination is that very low dart volumes (0.04–0.08 mL) are possible. The combination of medetomidine and ketamine has proven to be a superior choice. In captive chamois, 60–100 µg/kg medetomidine with 1.5 mg/kg ketamine are recommended (Jalanka & Roeken 1990; Walzer et al. 1996). In wild chamois, it is recommended to use 80–100 µg/kg of medetomidine with 1.5–2 mg/kg of ketamine in order to reduce the time to recumbency. Medetomidine is reversed with atipamezole at 0.4 mg/kg. Other combinations that have been used among others are xylazine at 1.4–4.8 mg/kg (Dematteis et al. 2008) and tiletamine-zolazepam (Chaduc et al. 1993).

Alpine Ibex (*Capra ibex*) Similar to other goat and sheep species, a combination of medetomidine and ketamine is recommended for the chemical capture of the ibex. For captive animals, 80–140 µg/kg of medetomidine, combined with 1.5 mg/kg of ketamine, has been recommended (Jalanka & Roeken 1990). Alternativly, 190–270 µg/kg of detomidine plus 1.4–2 mg/kg of ketamine and 6.8 mg/kg of tiletamine-zolazepam have also been used (Santiago-Moreno et al. 2011). In free-ranging animals, various combinations have been used: 100–120 µg/kg of medetomidine and 3 mg/kg of ketamine for the Iberian ibex; 80–100 µg/kg of medetomidine and 1.5 mg/kg of ketamine and 1.4–2.4 mg/kg of xylazine and 1.5–2.9 mg/kg of ketamine for the alpine ibex have been reported (Casas-Díaz et al. 2011; C. Walzer, unpubl.).

Argali Sheep (*Ovis ammon*) Wild argali with an estimated weight of 90 kg, have been captured using a combination of 4-mg carfentanil, 50-mg xylazine, and 100-mg ketamine. Anesthesia was reversed with a combination of 500-mg naltrexone and 15-mg yohimbine (Kenny et al. 2008).

Barbary Sheep (*Ammotragus lervia*), Himalayan Tahr (*Hemitragus jemlahicus*), and Mouflon (*Ovis musimon*) All of these sheep and goat species can be effectively immobilized with medetomidine-ketamine. The following doses have been used in captive animals (Jalanka & Roeken 1990). Barbary sheep: 100–140 µg/kg of medetomidine, combined with 1.5 mg/kg of ket-

amine. Himalayan tahr: 80–100 µg/kg of medetomidine, combined with 1.5 mg/kg of ketamine. Mouflon: 125 µg/kg of medetomidine, combined with 2.5 mg/kg of ketamine.

All of the earlier-mentioned doses were used in captive animals. It may be necessary to increase the dose in free-ranging animals. It is important to allow adequate time for induction with medetomidine-based protocols as animals may rouse and flee if they are approached too early. Typically, the animal can be approached approximately 5 minutes post induction.

Muskox (*Ovibos moschatus*) Muskox anesthesia can be somewhat more challenging than anesthesia of the smaller sheep and goat species. Their head is relatively large and they have a small oral cavity; this can make intubation a challenge. We typically use a mouth gag to open the mouth, and use a long flat laryngoscope blade to visualize the glottis. It is important to induce good muscle relaxation to facilitate intubation. We have used 0.05–0.1 mg/kg of diazepam or 5% guaifenesin, given to effect, to induce muscle relaxation. Manual intubation may be attempted in large muskox. The endotracheal tube is guided into the trachea manually by placing a hand dorsally over the end of the tube and advancing the hand into the pharynx. Once the operator's hand is in the pharynx, the epiglottis is reflected ventrally and the tube is advanced into the trachea (Fig. 62.4).

Free-ranging adult muskox have been immobilized with 2 mg of etorphine, combined with 30 mg of xylazine and 200 IU of hyaluronidase (Clausen et al. 1984). Recently, a dose of 0.05 mg/kg etorphine and 0.15 mg/kg xylazine has been reported on in 133 wild musk ox

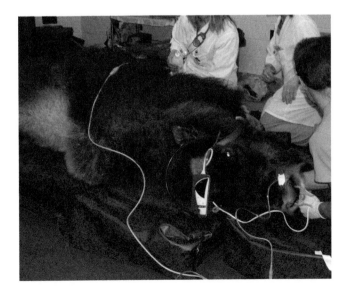

Figure 62.4. Intubation of muskox can be difficult it may be attempted by palpation in large animals, a long laryngoscope blade is required in smaller animals (photo courtesy of Jessica Paterson).

immobilization procedures (Blix et al. 2011).We have used 50–60 µg/kg of medetomidine, combined with 1.5 mg/kg of ketamine for short-term anesthesia of muskox. We have also used 0.5–1 mg/kg of xylazine alone, or combined with 1–2 mg/kg of ketamine for deep sedation of captive muskox. These animals were relatively tame and human habituated, and these doses should not be extrapolated to wild muskox.

REFERENCES

Abderhalden W, Buchli C, Ratti P, et al. 1998. Einfang und Immobilisation von Alpensteinböcken (Caprai.ibex). *Zeitschrift fur Jagdwissenschaft* 44:123–132.

Ballestros F, Benito JL. 1992. Captures dìsards Cantabriques en Asturies. *Bulletin Mensuel de l'Office National de la Chasse* 171:25–29.

Blix AS, Lian H, Ness J. 2011. Immobilization of muskoxen (*Ovibos moschatus*) with etorphine and xylazine. *Acta veterinaria Scandinavica* 53:42.

Casas-Díaz E, Marco I, López-Olvera JR, et al. 2011. Comparision of xylazine-ketamine and medetomidine-ketamine anaesthesia in the Iberian ibex (*Capra pyrenaica*). *European Journal of Wildlife Research* 57:887–893.

Caulkett NA, Cribb PH, Duke T. 1994. Cardiopulmonary effects of medetomidine-ketamine immobilization with atipamezole reversal and carfentanil-xylazine immobilization with naltrexone reversal: a comparative study in domestic sheep (*Ovis ovis*). *Journal of Zoo and Wildlife Medicine* 25:376–389.

Caulkett NA, Duke T, Cribb PH. 1996. Cardiopulmonary effects of medetomidine-ketamine in domestic sheep (*Ovis ovis*), maintained in sternal recumbency. *Journal of Zoo and Wildlife Medicine* 27:217–226.

Caulkett NA, Fahlman Å, Neuhaus P, et al. 2012. Ground based darting of bighorn sheep with medetomidine-ketamine: efficacy and safety. Proceedings of the American Association of Zoo Veterinarians, p. 24. Oakland, CA.

Chaduc F, Chaduc Y, Jeandin A. 1993. Teleansthesie des ongules sauvages en parc zoologique: Utilisation d'un anesthesique general: le Zoletil. Proceedings of Techniques de capture et de marquage des ongulés sauvages(D Dubray, FDC de l'Herault, eds.), pp. 51–57. Montpellier, France, March 20–22, 1990.

Clausen B, Hjort P, Strandgaard H, et al. 1984. Immobilization and tagging of muskoxen (*Ovibos moschatus*) in Jameson Land, northeastern Greenland. *Journal of Wildlife Diseases* 20:141–145.

Delmas M. 1993. Comparision de deux methods de capture de chamois (*Rupicapra rupicapra*) en milieu ouvert dans le parc nat. de la Vanoise. Proceedings of Techniques de capture et de marquage des ongulés sauvages (D Dubray, FDC de l'Herault, eds.), pp. 127–133. Montpellier, France, March 20–22, 1990.

Dematteis A, Rossi L, Canavese G, et al. 2008. Immobilising free-ranging Alpine chamois with xylazine, reversed with atipamezole. *The Veterinary Record* 163:184–189.

Fahlman Å, Caulkett N, Arnemo JM, et al. 2012. Efficacy of a portable oxygen concentrator with pulsed delivery for treatment of hypoxemia during anesthesia of wildlife. *Journal of Zoo and Wildlife Medicine* 43:67–76.

Festa-Bianchet M, Jorgenson JT. 1985. Use of xylazine and ketamine to immobilize bighorn sheep in Alberta. *Journal of Wildlife Management* 49:162–165.

Jalanka HH. 1989. Chemical restraint and reversal in captive markhors (*Capra falconeri megaceros*) and its reversal by atipamezole. *Journal of Zoo Animal Medicine* 20:413–422.

Jalanka HH, Roeken BO. 1990. The use of medetomidine, medetomidine-ketamine combinations and atipamezole in non domestic animals: a review. *Journal of Zoo and Wildlife Medicine* 21:259–282.

Jessup DA. 1999. Capture and handling of mountain sheep and goats. In: *Zoo & Wild Animal Medicine, Current Therapy 4* (ME Fowler, RE Miller, eds.), pp. 681–687. Philadelphia: W.B. Saunders.

Kenny D, DeNicola A, Amgalbaatar S, et al. 2008. Successful field capture techniques for free-ranging argali sheep (*Ovis amon*) in Mongolia. *Zoo Biology* 27:137–144.

Kock MD, Jessup DA, Clark RK, et al. 1987a. Capture methods in five subspecies of free-ranging bighorn sheep: an evaluation of drop-net, drive-net, chemical immobilization and the net-gun. *Journal of Wildlife Diseases* 23:634–640.

Kock MD, Jessup DA, Clark RK, et al. 1987b. Effects of capture on biological parameters in free-ranging bighorn sheep (*Ovis canadensis*): evaluation of drop-net, drive-net, chemical immobilization and the net gun. *Journal of Wildlife Diseases* 23:641–651.

Kock MD, Clark RK, Franti CE, et al. 1987c. Effects of capture on biological parameters in free-ranging bighorn sheep (*Ovis canadensis*): evaluation of normal, stressed and mortality outcomes and documentation of postcapture survival. *Journal of Wildlife Diseases* 23:652–662.

López-Olvera JR, Ignasi M, Montané J, et al. 2007. Effects of acepromazine on the stress response in Southern chamois (*Rupicapra pyrenaica*) captured by means of drive nets. *Canadian Journal of Veterinary Research* 71:41–51.

López-Olvera JR, Ignasi M, Montané J, et al. 2009. Comparative evaluation of effort, capture and handling effents of drive nets to capture roe deer (*Capreolus capreolus*), Southern chamois (*Rupicapra pyrenaica*) and Spanish ibex (*Capra pyrenaica*). *European Journal of Wildlife Research* 55:193–202.

Mentaberre G, López-Olvera JR, Casas-Díaz E, et al. 2010. Effects of azaperone and haloperidol on the stress response of drive-net captures Iberian ibexes (*Capra pyrenaica*). *European Journal of Wildlife Research* 56:757–764.

Merwin DS, Millspaugh JJ, Brundige GC, et al. 2000. Immobilization of free-ranging rocky mountain bighorn sheep (*Ovis canadensis canadensis*) ewes with Telazol^R and xylazine hydrochloride. *Canadian Field-Naturalist* 114:471–475.

Santiago-Moreno J, Toledano-Díaz A, Sookhthezary A, et al. 2011. Effects of anesthetic protocols on electroejaculation variables of Iberian ibex (*Capra pyrenaica*). *Research in Veterinary Science* 90:150–155.

Shury TK, Caulkett NA. 2006. Chemical immobilization of free-ranging plains bison (*Bison bison bison*) and rocky mountain bighorn sheep (*Ovis canadensis canadensis*) with a tiletamine-zolazepam-xylazine-hydromorphone combination. Proceedings of the American Association of Zoo Veterinarians,pp. 220–222. Tampa, Florida.

Struch M, Baumann M. 2000. Experiences of catching chamois (*Rupicapra rupicapra*) in a wooded mountain area in Swizerland. *Oecologia Montana* 9:48–49.

Walzer C, Bögel R, Walzer-Wagner C. 1996. Erfahrungen mit Medetomidine-Ketamin-Hyaluronidase-Atipamezole bei Gemsen (*Rupicapra rupicapra*). *Wiener Tierztliche Monatsschrift/Veterinary Medicine Austria* 83:297–301.

Walzer C, Bögel R, Lotz A, et al. 1998. Long distance immobilization of free-ranging chamois. Proceedings of 2nd. World Conference of Mountain Ungulates. Ed. Collana Scientifica Parco Natzionale Gran Paradiso, Saint Vincente, Aosta, pp. 207–209.

Wiesner H, von Hegel G. 1990. Practical advice concerning immobilization of wild and zoo animals. *Tierarztliche Praxis* 13:113–127.

63 Nondomestic Cattle

Julie Napier and Douglas L. Armstrong

INTRODUCTION

Wild cattle are a part of the family Bovidae in the order Artiodactyla. Genus *Bubalus* includes Asian water buffalo (*Bubalus bubalis*), tamaraw (*Bubalus mindorensis*), lowland anoa (*Bubalus depressicornis*), and mountain anoa (*Bubalus quarlesi*). Tamaraw are rare in captivity. Genus *Syncerus* is comprised of a single species, the African buffalo (*Syncerus caffer*). Genus *Bos* is the largest group of animals and contains five species: aurochs (*Bos taurus*), banteng (*Bos javanicus*), gaur or seladang (*Bos gaurus*), kouprey (*Bos sauveli*), and yak (*Bos grunnniens*). Wild aurochs are the ancestors of domestic cattle and gave rise to numerous breeds, including the Ankoli cattle or watusi and the zebu.

The family Bovidae are true ruminants and are physiologically very similar to domestic cattle. The have a four-compartment stomach with the size of these compartments varying by species. They are browsers and grazers and live in a variety of climates and geographic areas. Wild cattle generally do very well in captivity (Nowak, 1991).

PHYSICAL RESTRAINT

Exotic ruminants vary greatly in behavior, temperament, and size (Table 63.1). These animals can be formidable and aggressive in nature. Most wild cattle have large horns and hooves and a strong fight or flight response when approached. Careful planning is necessary when considering any kind of restraint, handling, or procedure. The primary concern should always be human and animal safety. Animals designated for a procedure should be separated from the group and held in a smaller enclosure or holding area whenever possible. Ideally, this area would be quiet and free of unnecessary stimulation.

Should physical rather than chemical restraint be utilized, there are several methods that can be used with wild cattle. Behavioral conditioning using positive reinforcement, such as food reward, can be used to move animals through walkways in buildings or to crate train. Manual restraint is possible with smaller exotic bovids and calves, but should not be attempted in animals in excess of 70 kg. Exceptional skill and experience, as well as the appropriate protective equipment, would be necessary to handle some of the larger species, especially in a noncontrolled environment. Any animal under manual restraint should be monitored for stress and hyperthermia. Blindfolds will calm some but not all individuals (Citino 2003).

For most adult wild cattle, some type of mechanical or physical restraint device is required for minor procedures, such as trimming horns, tuberculin testing, venipuncture, administering medications, rectal and vaginal examinations, or brief physical exams. Restraint chutes, including box chutes with or without a head gate and drop-floor types, have become more typical in zoo settings (Boever 1986; Fowler 1995).

Many of the current devices were designed for cattle- or the game-farming business and have been successfully modified for use with exotic bovids. Some of the restraint devices available include manual squeeze chutes (Heavy-Duty Squeeze Chute, Powder River Livestock Equipment, Provo, UT) (Read et al. 1989), drop-floor chutes (The Tamer and Tamer, Jr., Fauna Research, Red Hook, NY), and hydraulic squeeze chutes (Hydraulic Tamer, Fauna Research) (Blumer & DeMaar 1993; Citino 2003). When an animal is in a drop-floor chute, the floor can be dropped or lowered, leaving the animal wedged in a v-shaped trough, suspended with the feet off the ground. Many animals will cease struggling once they have lost their footing. Most

Zoo Animal and Wildlife Immobilization and Anesthesia, Second Edition. Edited by Gary West, Darryl Heard, and Nigel Caulkett.
© 2014 John Wiley & Sons, Inc. Published 2014 by John Wiley & Sons, Inc.

Table 63.1. Average body weights of adult exotic cattle[a]

Species	Body Weight (kg)
African buffalo	400–900
Ankole (Watusi)	400–725
Anoa (both species)	150–300
Asian water buffalo	700–1000
Banteng	400–900
Gaur (Seladang)	600–1000
Yak	400–1000
Zebu	300–600

[a]For both females (lower end of the range) and males (higher end of the range).

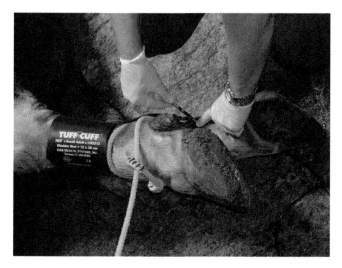

Figure 63.2. Obtaining a sample for blood gas values from the medial digital artery.

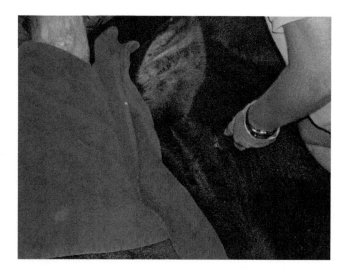

Figure 63.1. Jugular venipuncture in an adult gaur bull (*Bos gaurus*).

devices available have a variety of access panels and a mechanism to release the animal quickly should that become necessary.

VASCULAR ACCESS AND URINE COLLECTION

The most commonly used vascular access site in wild cattle is the jugular vein. Other common sites for blood collection include the cephalic, medial and lateral saphenous, tail (coccygeal), and auricular veins. In larger ungulates, the jugular can be hard to palpate. Holding off the vein with the knee and using the fingertips to bounce along the neck to locate the vein when the animal is in sternal or lateral recumbency can be useful, as is following the line of the caudal ramus of the mandible to locate the jugular (Fig. 63.1).

Catheter placement can be done in the jugular, cephalic, or auricular vein. Alcohol applied topically to the ear in addition to pressure at the base of the ear can help the auricular vein be more easily visualized. Supplemental anesthesia, antagonists to anesthetic

drugs, fluids, emergency drugs, or other medications are administered most commonly in the jugular or auricular veins. Blood gas values require a smaller volume of blood and can be obtained from the medial or caudal digital artery just proximal to the fetlock (Fig. 63.2) or the auricular artery.

Urine can be collected via urethral catheterization in females, but is generally not successful in males due to the sigmoid flexure of the penis. Ultrasound-guided cystocentesis is the easiest method for urine collection in most exotic bovids.

CHEMICAL RESTRAINT AND CAPTURE

In many situations, physical restraint is not an option (i.e., field procedures, excessively long procedures, and surgeries). There are a variety of chemical agents available for use in wild cattle. Personal preference and experience, size, temperament and physiology of the species and the environmental setting will help to determine what chemical restraint should be utilized.

PRE-ANESTHETIC CONSIDERATIONS

Ruminants are prone to ruminal tympany and regurgitation, which can lead to aspiration and subsequent pneumonia, especially in recumbent anesthesia. A rumen tube should be part of the standard equipment to help prevent or treat ruminal tympany. Animals should be fasted for a period of 18–36 hours prior to induction. Water access should be discontinued 8–12 hours prior. Maintaining the animal in sternal recumbency can reduce the possibility of rumen regurgitation, especially in field conditions, when the animal cannot be fasted. When sternal recumbency is not possible, as in an electroejaculation or surgical procedure, when access to the ventrum is necessary, the head should be positioned or propped so the mouth and nose are pointed in a downwards direction. This will allow flow from the oral cavity of any rumen contents, reducing the chances of aspiration. In either lateral or sternal recumbency, the head and neck should be extended to maintain a patent airway. To greatly reduce the occurrence of aspiration of regurgitated rumen contents, an animal can be intubated with an endotracheal tube, as described.

ANESTHETIC MONITORING

The same monitoring standards and equipment that are used in other mammals under anesthesia can be used in wild cattle. Depth of anesthesia can be assessed by several methods. Although most animals will go into sternal recumbency on their own, some animals will head press against a wall or remain standing with the legs positioned in a wide stance. Through manual manipulation, they can be moved into sternal recumbency after placing a towel or cloth over the eyes. (Fig. 63.3).

Other animals, such as the gaur, will maintain a dog-sitting position prior to sternal recumbency (Fig. 63.4 and Fig. 63.5). Once in sternal recumbency, depth of anesthesia can be monitored by response to the ear pinch, response to tactile stimuli in the extremities or most accurately by manipulating the globe of the eye. The eye rotates ventromedially during a light plane of anesthesia. In deep anesthesia, it will rotate back to a central position (Reibold et al. 1982).

Normal heart and respiratory rates can vary greatly among wild cattle, depending on species, size, age, and the level of excitement attained prior to immobilization. Heart rate can be obtained using a stethoscope. Pulses can be palpated at the base of the tail and the facial artery in younger and smaller species, as well as the caudal auricular artery and the common digital arteries. To assess cardiovascular function and

peripheral perfusion, capillary refill time (CRT) can be utilized. This involves blanching the gums of the oral mucosa for several seconds then releasing and monitoring refill time, which should not exceed 2 seconds. The cardiovascular system should be monitored at regular intervals throughout anesthesia.

A pulse oximetry probe can be placed on the tongue, ear, or vulvar or preputial skin folds. (Fig. 63.6) Many pulse oximetry units will measure pulse rate as well as oxygen saturation of hemoglobin (SaO_2), providing another set of data for anesthetic monitoring. The color of the oral mucus membranes can also be utilized as an indicator of oxygenation. If hypoxemia is present, the intranasal route is an easy way to administer supplemental oxygen. Respiratory rate is generally monitored visually by watching the movement of the thorax and abdomen.

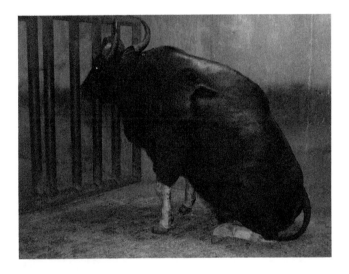

Figure 63.4. Gaur bull (*Bos gaurus*) in typical dog-sitting position prior to going into sternal recumbency.

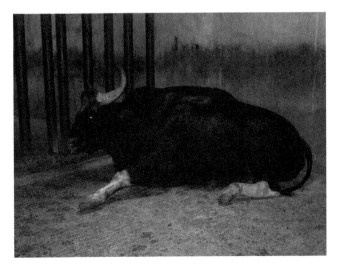

Figure 63.5. Gaur bull (*Bos gaurus*) in sternal recumbency.

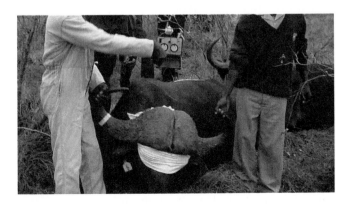

Figure 63.3. Field immobilization of an African buffalo (*Syncerus caffer*), moved into sternal recumbency with a blindfold placed over the eyes.

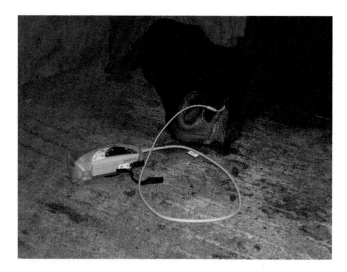

Figure 63.6. Pulse oximeter probe placed on the tongue to assess oxygen saturation of hemoglobin (SaO₂) as well as pulse rate.

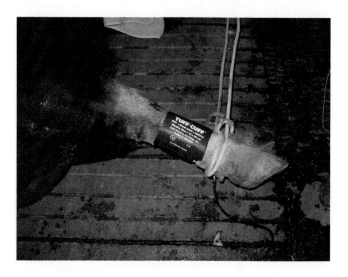

Figure 63.7. Obtaining indirect systemic blood pressure values by placing an oscillometric cuff just proximal to the fetlock.

Hyperthermia is common in immobilized wild cattle especially if the animal goes into a hyperexcited state due to under dosing. Excessive running, high-stepping, or pacing occurring prior to induction can lead to very elevated body temperatures (Citino 2003). Normal wild cattle body temperatures range from 37 to 39°C (99 to 102°F). If temperatures exceed this range, topical application of cold water or cold-water enemas are quite useful in bringing down the body temperature, although enemas will initially preclude accurate follow-up rectal thermometer temperature readings.

Indirect systemic blood pressure values can be acquired by placing an oscillometric cuff just proximal to the fetlock on most species or at the base of the tail in some smaller species (Fig. 63.7). The bladder

of the cuff should be positioned on the medial aspect of the leg and on the ventral aspect of the tail for accurate measurements. Direct measurement requires catheterization, usually of the caudal auricular artery.

ENDOTRACHEAL INTUBATION

For prolonged procedures or in animals that are prone to aspiration of regurgitated rumen contents, inhalation anesthesia via an endotracheal tube (ET) may be required. Tubes used in exotic cattle should have an inflatable cuff. Wild cattle can be intubated in lateral or sternal recumbency. Younger animals and smaller species should be intubated in sternal recumbency for easier elevation of the head. Endotracheal intubation can be accomplished by direct visualization via a laryngoscope or digital palpation. The tongue should be extended rostrally and to the side for easy insertion of the laryngoscope or the ET tube. Using either approach, the ET tube is guided through the oral cavity to the epiglottis, which is deviated ventrally to feed the tube into the trachea.

SEDATION AND TRANQUILIZATION

There are short- and long-acting sedatives available for exotic bovids. Commonly used short-term sedatives include the α₂-adrenergic agents: xylazine, detomidine and medetomidine (Short 1992). The α₂-agents can produce a calming state that can be overridden in a highly excited animal. In cattle, standing sedation has been attained with intravenous (IV) xylazine (0.02 mg/kg) or detomidine (0.01 mg/kg). The duration of effect can be extended with the addition of butorphanol to the protocol at a dose of 0.05 mg/kg (Lin & Riddell 2003). Another combination that has been used in cattle is xylazine administered IV or intramuscularly (IM) at 0.05–0.2 mg/kg with detomidine at 0.0025–0.01 mg/kg IV (Caulkett 2003). In domestic cattle, IM detomidine can induce standing sedation at dosages of 0.04 mg/kg. Detomidine has been used to sedate domestic calves at doses of 0.01 mg/kg for lighter sedation and 0.02–0.04 mg/kg for deeper sedation. (Peshin et al. 1991). Calves have also been successfully sedated using xylazine at dosages of 0.025–0.05 IV or 0.1–0.2 IM (Caulkett 2003). Sedation has been achieved in free-ranging Norwegian cattle using xylazine (0.37–0.73 mg/kg) or medetomidine (0.029–0049 mg/kg) (Arnemo & Soli 1993). In yaks, medetomidine at 0.07 mg/kg produces deep sedation, whereas detomidine at 0.025 mg/kg produces light sedation (Sharma et al. 1998, 2001).

An intermediate-acting phenothiazine, acepromazine, has been used on its own and in combination with other drugs for anesthesia in domestic cattle. When used alone, IM doses of 0.05–0.10 mg/kg can produce a sedation effect in 10–20 minutes. The effect can last between 4 and 8 hours, with potential residual effect up to 12 hours in duration (Blumer 1991; Swan 1993).

Haloperidol has been used in a variety of ungulates. It has an onset of around 10 minutes and duration of effect can last from 6 to 18 hours (Blumer 1991). Twenty to 40 mg of haloperidol in combination with 50- to 350-mg perphenazine enanthate can induce longer periods of tranquilization (Ebedes & Raath 1999). Perphenazine administered IM has been used in gaur to reduce stress-induced self-trauma and in African buffalo in quarantine. The sedation effect has an onset of 12–16 hours and can last as long as 7 days (Blumer 1991; Citino 2003; Ebedes & Raath 1995, 1999; Swan 1993). Extrapyramidal effects and anorexia have been noted in some animals after administration of haloperidol. It should be used with caution in very young or geriatric animals because the effect can be unpredictable (Ebedes & Raath 1999).

Azaperone at a dosage of 0.1 mg/kg had been used to successfully sedate African buffalo (Ebedes & Raath 1999). It can be combined with zuclopenthixol acetate at 1 mg/kg for a tranquilization effect. When administered IM, the onset of effect is 60 minutes with a duration lasting up to 3 days (Citino 2003; Ebedes & Raath 1995; Swan 1993). Zuclopenthixol and perphenazine may be used concurrently to get the initial effects of the zuclophenthixol and the longer-lasting effects of the perphenazine. Pipotiazine palmate has an onset of 48–72 hours with a duration of up to 30 days when given IM and can be used concurrently with zuclophenixol as well (Blumer 1991; Citino 2003; Ebedes & Raath 1995; Swan 1993). Extrapyramidal effects such as torticollis, tremors, muscle rigidity, head swaying, and akinesia can be seen with overdoses of perphanizine, azaperone, and zuclopenthixol. Administration of diazepam (10–20 mg) or xylazine (5–10 mg) have been used to control these symptoms (Quandt & Ebedes 1998). Newer antipsychotic drugs (APD) are also becoming more available to treat the extrapyramidal symptoms of neuroleptics. These include risperidone, olanzapine, ziprasidone, and olanzapine. These drugs are available in injectable form and can be administered at human doses as a starting point. There is no published information on the use of these agents in bovids, but they have been used successfully in cervids and rhino (Zuba & Oosterhuis 2007).

Benzodiazepine use for sedation has been reported in domestic and exotic bovids. Midazolam is more commonly used in combination with other drugs for general anesthesia. Diazepam has been used in domestic calves at 0.2 mg/kg in combination with other drugs for sedation and induction of anesthesia (Caulkett 2003). Diazepam should not be used alone in yak as it has been known to produce very rough inductions, paddling of the limbs, and the inability to rise after falling (Kumar et al. 1999).

GENERAL ANESTHESIA

There are a variety of techniques and chemical agents that have been used for general anesthesia in wild cattle. (Table 63.2) The drug classes most commonly used include opioids, α_2-adrenoreceptor agents, and dissociatives. Most general anesthesia is administered IM. In close quarters, a pole syringe can be utilized. Injection via a remote darting system is the most common route of administration. Young animals, under the appropriate restraint, may be induced with inhalant anesthesia using a face mask. Commonly used inhalant anesthetics include isoflurane and sevoflurane. An African buffalo calf was induced with midazolam and ketamine prior to intubation for maintenance on an inhalant anesthetic (Stegmann 2004). Short-term anesthesia can be produced in adult cattle with xylazine as a preanesthetic, ketamine for induction, and a mixture of guaifenasin and ketamine for maintenance (Caulkett 2003).

Where available, opioids are the most common group of drugs used to produce general anesthesia in wild cattle. They provide a smooth induction and a short recovery period. Carfentanil and etorphine are the most widely used; however, use of thiafentanil (A3080) is becoming increasingly common. It has been studied in various hoofstock (Citino et al. 2002; Janssen et al. 1991; Napier et al. 2011). Doses for etorphine range from 0.005 to 0.050 mg/kg. Doses for carfentanil range from 0.005 to 0.015 mg/kg. Thiafentanil doses range from 0.007 to 0.018 mg/kg. Inductions generally take longer with etorphine and are shortest with thiafentanil. In some species, such as gaur, induction times are quite similar with carfentanil and thiafentanil (1–4 vs. 1–6 minutes, respectively) (Napier et al. 2011). Hyaluronidase increases the rate of absorption of the opioid and my decrease induction times. Opioids are frequently used in conjunction with α_2-agents, including xylazine, medetomidine, and detomidine. They are also used in combination with acetylpromazine, a phenothiazine. These combinations reduce the amount of opioid needed to produce the desired anesthetic effect and can increase muscle relaxation. They can be given with the opioid in a single injection or 15–20 minutes prior to the opioid. African buffalo have routinely been immobilized with etorphine (0.01 mg/kg) and azaperone (0.015–0.2 mg/kg) (Puffer et al. 2001). A combination of thiafentanil, medetomidine, and ketamine has been used successfully in bovids. This combination provided rapid onset and good muscle relaxation in field conditions (Citino et al. 2002). Gaur may be effectively immobilized with xylazine (0.08–0.10 mg/kg) and carfentanil (0.005–0.10 mg/kg) (Armstrong 1989; Napier et al. 2011; Wilson et al. 1993). The combination of thiafentanil (0.012 mg/kg) and medetomidine (0.02 mg/kg) was also used successfully in multiple electroejaculation procedures of gaur (Napier et al. 2011).

Table 63.2. Recommended anesthetic agents and protocols for wild cattle

Species	Anesthetic Agent(s) (mg/kg)	Antagonist(s) (mg/kg)	Desired Effect
African buffalo	Azaperone 0.1 mg/kg		Sedation
	Zuclophenthixol 1 mg/kg		Tranquilization
	Xylazine: 0.05–0.15		Sedation
	Xylazine: 0.20–0.40		Immobilization
	Xylazine: 0.10 Etorphine: 0.012	Diprenorphine: 0.024	Immobilization
	Xylazine: 0.08–0.18 Acepromazine: 0.02–0.03 Etorphine: 0.005–0.007	Diprenorphine: 0.010–0.014	Immobilization
	Azaperone: 0.15 Etorphine: 0.015	Diprenorphine: 0.030	Immobilization
	Carfentanil: 0.006–0.008	Naltrexone: 0.6–0.8	Immobilization
	Xylazine: 0.028–0.050 Carfentanil: 0.002–0.005	Naltrexone: 0.2–0.5	Immobilization
	Azaperone: 0.06–0.07 Thiafentanil: 0.007–0.014	Naltrexone: 0.07–0.14	Immobilization
Ankole, Watusi	Xylazine: 0.14–0.70 Etorphine: 0.014–0.038	Atipamezole: 0.03 Diprenorphine: 0.028–0.076	Immobilization
	Acepromazine: 0.10–0.14 Etorphine: 0.024–0.034	Diprenorphine: 0.048–0.068	Immobilization
	Detomidine: 0.05–0.08 Butorphanol: 0.08–0.20	Atipamezole: 0.03–0.15 Naltrexone: 0.05–1.0	Sedation
	Detomidine: 0.019–0.029 Carfentanil: 0.006–0.010 Ketamine: 0.30	Atipamezole: 0.10 Naltrexone: 0.6–1.0	Immobilization
	Detomidine: 0.005 Acepromazine: 0.04–0.05 Etorphine: 0.016–0.019 Ketamine: 0.48–0.50	Atipamezole: 0.03 Naltrexone: 1.8	Immobilization
	Detomidine: 0.12 Acepromazine: 0.04 Carfentanil: 0.012 Ketamine: 0.40	Yohimbine: 0.33 Naltrexone: 1.2	Immobilization
Anoa	Xylazine: 1.0 Ketamine: 6.0	Atipamezole: 0.2	Immobilization
	Xylazine: 0.27–0.33 Acepromazine: 0.11–0.12 Etorphine: 0.027–0.033	Diprenorphine: 0.054–0.066	Immobilization
	Xylazine: 0.05–0.25 Carfentanil: 0.01–0.03	Naltrexone: 1.0–3.0	Immobilization
	Medetomidine: 0.025–0.100 Ketamine: 0.05–2.0	Atipamezole: 0.12–0.50	Immobilization
Banteng	Xylazine: 0.03–0.22	Yohimbine: 0.07–0.18	Sedation (♀)
	Xylazine: 1.5	Atipamezole: 0.04–0.08	Immobilization
	Xylazine: 0.05–0.09 Acepromazine: 0.06–0.10		Sedation (♀)
	Xylazine: 0.75–1.00 Ketamine: 1.5–2.0	Atipamezole: 0.06–0.08	Immobilization
	Xylazine: 0.056–0.125 Acepromazine: 0.02–0.05 Etorphine: 0.005–0.012	Diprenorphine: 0.010–0.024	Immobilization
	Xylazine: 0.05–0.25 Carfentanil: 0.001–0.008	Naltrexone: 0.1–0.8	Immobilization

Table 63.2. (Continued)

Species	Anesthetic Agent(s) (mg/kg)	Antagonist(s) (mg/kg)	Desired Effect
	Xylazine: 0.11 Carfentanil: 0.007 Ketamine: 0.15	Naltrexone: 0.7	Immobilization
	Detomidine: 0.059–0.079 Butorphanol: 0.050–0.088	Yohimbine: 0.21–0.22 Naltrexone: 0.84–0.88	Sedation
	Detomidine: 0.069–0.104 Butorphanol: 0.071–0.083 Ketamine: 0.69–2.13	Yohimbine: 0.18–0.20 Naltrexone: 0.7–0.9	Immobilization
	Detomidine: 0.009–0.014 Carfentanil: 0.010–0.017 Ketamine: 0.33–2.78	Atipamezole: 0.05 Naltrexone: 1.0–1.7	Immobilization
Forest buffalo	Xylazine: 0.09–0.33 Etorphine: 0.012–0.050	Atipamezole: 0.027–0.033 Diprenorphine: 0.024–0.10	Immobilization
	Acepromazine: 0.07–0.10 Etorphine: 0.018–0.024	Diprenorphine: 0.036–0.048	Immobilization
	Xylazine: 0.14–0.18 Acepromazine: 0.13–0.14 Etorphine: 0.031–0.036	Diprenorphine: 0.062–0.072	Immobilization
	Xylazine: 0.06–0.13 Carfentanil: 0.011–0.012 Ketamine: 1.55–2.50	Yohimbine: 0.11–0.12 Naltrexone: 1.1–1.2	Immobilization
Gaur	Xylazine: 0.12–0.22 Acepromazine: 0.04–0.09 Etorphine: 0.010–0.022	Diprenorphine: 0.020–0.044	Immobilization
	Xylazine: 0.05–0.25 Carfentanil: 0.01–0.03	Naltrexone: 1.0–3.0[a]	Immobilization
	Xylazine: 0.125 Carfentanil: 0.005 Ketamine: 0.06–0.09	Naltrexone: 0.5[a]	Immobilization
	Xylazine: 0.05–0.025 Thiafentanil: 0.011–0.018	Naltrexone: 0.11–0.18[a]	Immobilization
	Medetomidine 0.02 Thiafentanil 0.012	Atipamezole 0.1 Naltrexone 0.12[a]	Immobilization
Yak	Detomidine 0.025		Light sedation
	Medetomidine 0.07		Deep sedation
	Xylazine: 0.30		Sedation
	Xylazine: 0.6–1.0		Immobilization
	Xylazine: 0.04 Etorphine: 0.006	Diprenorphine: 0.012	Immobilization
	Xylazine: 0.05–0.20 Acepromazine: 0.025–0.10 Etorphine: 0.006–0.024	Diprenorphine: 0.012–0.048	Immobilization
	Xylazine: 0.40–1.67 Acepromazine: 0.04–0.05 Etorphine: 0.010–0.012 Ketamine: 0.04–1.67	Diprenorphine: 0.020–0.024	Immobilization
	Xylazine: 0.10 Carfentanil: 0.0075 Medetomidine: 0.10 Ketamine: 3.0	Naltrexone: 0.75 Atipamezole: 0.5	Immobilization Immobilization

Notes: The dosages and protocols presented in this table are a compilation of information from the listed references, personal experience, and personal communication with staff from the following institutions: Denver Zoo, Denver, CO, USA; Disney's Animal Kingdom, Lake Buena Vista, FL, USA; Exotic Animal Service, Edinburgh University, Edinburgh, UK; Marwell Preservation Trust, Winchester, UK; Royal Zoological Society of Antwerp, Antwerp, Belgium; Omaha's Henry Doorly Zoo, Omaha, NE, USA; Soffolk Wildlife Park, Edinburgh, UK; St. Louis Zoo, St. Louis, MO, USA; Whipsnade Wild Animal Park, Bedfordshire, UK; Zoological Society of London, London, UK.

[a]Naltrexone in Gaur can be administered 30–50% IV and 50–70% IM or 25% IV and 75% SQ which may reduce renarcitization.

If the initial immobilizing opioid dose is insufficient for adequate anesthesia, another IM dose of half of the initial dose can be given.

Because of their extreme potency in relation to morphine, exetorphine, carfentanil, and thiafentanil are classified as ultra-potent opioids. Thiafentanil is still investigational in the United States, but will most likely be a schedule II drug like etorphine and carfentanil. It is imperative to take appropriate precautions when using these opioids. An emergency procedure should be in place in the event human exposure occurs with any of these substances. At the very least, personal protective equipment should include eye protection and impermeable gloves. It is advisable to have antagonists ready for injection prior to the preparation and use of these ultra-potent opioids. Accurate record keeping for all controlled substances is required by government and regulatory agencies.

When opioids are not available, dissociatives in combination with α₂-agents or benzodiazepines are commonly used (Barnett & Lewis 1990). Ketamine and the combination of tiletamine and zolazepam (Telazol and Zolatil) have been used. Adding an α₂-agent reduces the dose of the dissociative as it does with opioids. Medetomidine generally provides smoother inductions and recoveries compared with xylazine. Detomidine combined with tiletamine and zolazepam has been used successfully to immobilize wild banteng (Bradshaw et al. 2005). The quality of Telazol inductions and immobilizations is poor in gaur (Wilson et al. 1993). A detomidine (0.01 mg/kg), diazepam (0.01 mg/kg), and ketamine (3.0 mg/kg) combination has been used in Asian buffalo calves (Pawde et al. 2000). As with opioids, if the initial immobilization doses do not achieve the necessary level of anesthetic depth, lesser doses of these drugs can be given intravenously or intramuscularly.

In the majority of situations, intramuscular administration is the only route available for administering anesthetic agents; consequently, barbituates are not commonly used in wild cattle. This is also the case with glycerol guaiacolate, which is often combined with dissociatives and barbituates in IV administrations in domestic cattle. If venous access is available, these drugs can be given using domestic cattle doses. Propofol may also be used for IV induction at doses of 2.0–40 mg/kg (Jalanka et al. 1992).

If procedures are going to last in excess of an hour, inhalant anesthetic can be utilized. Sevoflurane and isoflurane can be administered following protocols used in domestic cattle.

ANALGESIA

In any situation where an animal may be expected to experience pain, analgesia administration should be considered. These agents include opioids, α₂-adrenergic agents, and nonsteroidal anti-inflammatories (NSAIDs).

Opioids and α₂-agents, which have already been discussed as common agents used for sedation and general anesthesia, provide analgesia during those periods. Detomidine has demonstrated analgesia comparable with epidural administration in domestic cattle when given IM at 0.04 mg/kg (Prado et al. 1999). Unless animals are going to be held in some kind of enclosure, opioids and α₂-agents are not generally used outside of anesthesia due to their potent sedative effects.

NSAIDs produce analgesia without the complication of sedation. There are no recent publications on the effectiveness of these drugs in wild cattle, but there are numerous publications on the effect of NSAIDs in domestic bovids. Ketoprofen given at 3.0 mg/kg IV produces analgesia in calves undergoing horn debudding and domestic bulls undergoing castration (Faulkner & Weary 2000; Ting et al. 2003). Ketoprofen is used less frequently in domestic cattle as it does not offer an advantage over drugs that are labeled for use in bovids or are less expensive (Smith et al. 2008). Phenylbutazone has been used in domestic cattle at doses of 10–20 mg/kg orally, then 2.5–5 mg/kg every 24 hours or 10 mg/kg every 48 hours (Jenkins 1987), and oral doses of 9 mg/kg with maintenance doses of 4.5 mg/kg administered every 48 hours (Eberhardson et al. 1979). Flunixin meglumine has been given IV, IM, and orally to dairy cows and beef cattle at doses of 1.1–2.2 mg/kg (Anderson et al. 1986; Smith et al. 2008).

Numerous studies have been conducted using meloxicam alone or in combination with other drugs in domestic cattle. Gabapentin capsules or powder, given orally at 10 mg/kg with meloxicam at 0.5 mg/kg, has been used for management of neuropathic pain in cattle (Coetzee et al. 2010). Meloxicam alone, at a dose of 0.5 mg/kg, has demonstrated nonimmunosuppressive and anti-inflammatory benefits in cattle with respiratory disease and in calves that have been dehorned (Heinrich et al. 2010; Smith et al. 2008).

RECOVERY

One of the advantages of using opioids for immobilizations is the ability to reverse the drugs and provide a safe, smooth, and rapid recovery. Naltrexone is the preferred antagonist for both carfentanil and thiafentanil. For carfentanil, the dosage of naltrexone is 100 mg per 1-mg carfentanil given. For thiafentanil, a dose as low as 10 mg per 1 mg thaifentanil can be given. The dose for naltrexone is usually split between IV, IM, and subcutaneous (SC) administration. The recommended label dose is one-fourth IV and three-fourths SC. A study was done that did not find any advantage to splitting the dose when reversing carfentanil (Mutlow et al. 2004).

Reversals for α₂-agonists include yohimbine for the reversal of xylazine and detomidine and atipamezole for medetomidine. Atipamezole can be used to reverse xylazine and detomidine if yohimbine is not available.

If supplemental drugs have been given during the procedure, such as ketamine, antagonists should not be given for at least 20 minutes after the ketamine has been administered to allow for a smooth recovery.

If an animal has been intubated, the endotracheal tube should not be removed until there is evidence of pharyngeal activity. It is not necessary to completely deflate the cuff of the tube in order to remove it. Keeping the cuff partially inflated will help clear the mouth of any oral secretions or regurgitated material that may have accumulated during the procedure.

In a herd situation, animals should be returned to the group as soon as possible if conspecifics do not pose an immediate threat to the recovering individual.

COMPLICATIONS

Hypoxemia occurs frequently with the use of potent opioids and should be treated with ventilation and intubation, if necessary. If the animal is not intubated, nasal oxygen can be given. Hyperthermia can occur in immobilized animals and can be treated as previously discussed.

Excess gas in the rumen can lead to tympany. A stomach tube should be passed in an attempt to reduce the gas. This problem can be seen in animals that have not been fasted but is infrequent in animals that were fasted previous to the procedure.

Capture or exertional myopathy has been reported in numerous bovid species. Since this condition is difficult to treat, especially in a free-ranging setting, it is important to keep preimmobilization stress and activity to a minimum. This can be accomplished by selecting drugs and doses that will facilitate a rapid induction, limiting chases under free-ranging conditions and removing anything that might contribute to stress, such as excess personnel and loud noises. (Schumacher 2008). Pressure myopathy should be considered with heavy-bodied cattle under anesthesia for extended periods of time.

Renarcotization has also been reported in numerous cases in animals immobilized with potent opioids, particularly with carfentanil citrate (Allen 1989; Schumacher 2008). Studies have shown some species are more prone to this phenomenon than others and animals given a lower dose of reversal will have a greater tendency to experience renarcotization (Allen 1989; Haigh & Gates 1995; Mutlow et al. 2004; Wilson et al. 1993). Wild cattle that have been immobilized with potent opioids should be monitored for 72 hours post procedure. Clinical signs usually occur around 12–24 hours after the administration of the reversal and include circling, high stepping, agitation or mild excitement, recumbency paddling, and dulled menta-

tion. IM administration of 50% of the initial antagonist dose should be given if any of these signs are noted. Repeated doses may be needed if the clinical signs of renarcotization do not subside.

REFERENCES

Allen JL. 1989. Renarcotization following carfentanil immobilization of nondomestic ungulates. *Journal of Zoo and Wildlife Medicine* 20:423–426.

Anderson KL, Smith AR, Shanks RD, et al. 1986. Efficacy of flunixin meglumine for the treatment of endotoxin-induced bovine mastitis. *American Journal of Veterinary Research* 47: 1366–1372.

Armstrong, DL. 1989. An evaluation of carfentanil as an immobilizing agent for gaur (*Bos gaurus*). Annual Proceedings of the American Association of Zoo Veterinarians, p. 8.

Arnemo JM, Soli NE. 1993. Chemical capture of free-ranging cattle: immobilization with xylazine or medetomidine, and reversal with atipamezole. *Veterinary Research Communications* 17:469–477.

Barnett JEF, Lewis JCM. 1990. Medetomidine and ketamine anesthesia in zoo animals and its reversal with atipamezole: a review and update with specific reference work in British zoos. Proceedings of the American Association of Zoo Veterinarians, pp. 232–241.

Blumer ES. 1991. A review of the use of selected neuroleptic drugs in the management of nondomestic hoofstock. Proceedings of the American Association of Zoo Veterinarians, pp. 326–332.

Blumer ES, DeMaar TW. 1993. Manual restraint systems for the management of non-domestic hoofstock. Proceedings of the American Association of Zoo Veterinarians, pp. 141–143.

Boever WJ. 1986. Bovids, gazelle, antelope, and cattle. In: *Zoo and Wild Animal Medicine*, 2nd ed. (ME Fowler, ed.), pp. 989–996. Philadelphia: W.B. Saunders.

Bradshaw CJA, Traill LW, Wertz KL, et al. 2005. Chemical immobilization of wild banteng (*Bos javanicus*) in northern Australia using detomidine, tiletamine and zolazepam. *Australian Veterinary Journal* 83:15–16.

Caulkett N. 2003. Anesthesia of ruminants. *Large Animal Veterinary Rounds* 3(2):1–6. University of Sackatchewan.

Citino S. 2003. Bovidae (except sheep and goats) and antilocapridae. In: *Zoo and Wildlife Animal Medicine*, 5th ed. (ME Fowler, ER Miller, eds.), pp. 649–674. St. Louis: Saunders.

Citino S, Bush M, Grobler D, et al. 2002. Anesthesia of boma-captured Lichtenstein's Hartabeest (*Sigmoceros lichtenstienii*) with a combination of thiafentanil, medetomidine and ketamine. *Journal of Zoo and Wildlife Medicine* 38:457–462.

Coetzee JF, Mosher RA, Kohake LE, et al. 2010. Pharmacokineticss of oral gabapentin alone or co-administered with meloxicam in ruminant beef calves. *Veterinary Journal (London, England: 1997)* 190:99–102.

Ebedes H, Raath JP. 1995. The use of long term neuroleptics in the confinement and transport of wild animals. Proceedings of the American Association of Zoo Veterinarians, pp. 152–155.

Ebedes H, Raath JP. 1999. Use of tranquilizers in wild herbivores. In: *Zoo and Wildlife Animal Medicine*, 4th ed. (ME Fowler, ER Miller, eds.), pp. 575–585. St. Louis: Saunders.

Eberhardson B, Olsson G, Appelgren LE, et al. 1979. Pharmacokinetic studies of phenylbutazone in cattle. *Journal of Veterinary Pharmacology and Therapeutics* 2:31–37.

Faulkner PM, Weary DM. 2000. Reducing pain after dehorning in dairy calves. *Journal of Dairy Science* 83:2037–2041.

Fowler ME. 1995. *Restraint and Handling of Wild and Domestic Animals*, 2nd ed. Ames: Iowa State University Press.

Haigh JC, Gates CC. 1995. Capture of wood bison (*Bison bison athabascae*) using carfetanil-based mixtures. *Journal of Wildlife Diseases* 31:37–42.

Heinrich A, Duffield TF, Lissemore KD, et al. 2010. The effect of meloxicam on behavior and pain sensitivity of dairy calves following cautery dehorning with a local anesthetic. *Journal of Dairy Science* 93:2450–2457.

Jalanka HH, Teravainen E, Kivalo M. 1992. Propofol: a potentially useful intravenous anesthetic agent in non-domestic ruminants and camelids. Proceedings of the American Association of Zoo Veterinarians, pp. 236–241.

Janssen DL, Raath JP, Swan GE, et al. 1991. Field studies with the narcotic immobilization agent A3080. Proceedings of the American Association of Zoo Veterinarians, pp. 333–335.

Jenkins WL. 1987. Pharmacologic aspects of analgesic drugs in animals: an overview. *Journal of the American Veterinary Medical Association* 191:1231–1240.

Kumar A, Nigma JM, Sharma SK. 1999. Diazepam sedation in yaks. *The Indian Veterinary Journal* 76:211–213.

Lin HC, Riddell MG. 2003. Preliminary study of the effects of xylazine or detomidine with or without butorphanol for standing sedation on dairy cattle. *Veterinary Theriogenology* 4: 285–291.

Mutlow AR, Isaza JW, Carpenter DE, et al. 2004. Pharmacokinetics of carfentanil and naltrexone in domestic goats (*Capra hircus*). *Journal of Zoo and Wildlife Medicine* 35:489–496.

Napier JE, Loskutoff NM, Simmons LG, et al. 2011. Preliminary data for the comparison of carfentanil-xylazine and thiafentanil-medetomidine in electroejaculation of captive gaur (*Bos gaurus*). *Journal of Zoo and Wildlife Medicine* 42:430–436.

Nowak RM. 1991. *Walker's Mammals of the World*, Vol. 11, 5th ed., pp. 1419–1431. Baltimore: Johns Hopkins University Press.

Pawde AM, Kinjavdekar AP, Aithal HP, et al. 2000. Detomidine-diazepam-ketamine anaesthesia in buffalo (*Bubalis bubalis*) calves. *Journal of Veterinary Medicine. A, Physiology, Pathology, Clinical Medicine* 47:175–179.

Peshin PK, Singh SP, Singh J, et al. 1991. Sedative effect of detomidine in infant calves. *Acta Veterinaria Hungarica* 39:103–107.

Prado ME, Streeter RN, Mandsager RE, et al. 1999. Pharmacologic effects of epidural versus intramuscular administration of detomidine in cattle. *American Journal of Veterinary Research* 60:1242–1247.

Puffer A, de la Rey M, de la Rey R, et al. 2001. Choice of chemicals used in immobilization protocols can significantly affect semen quality in ejaculates collected from free-ranging Afircan buffalo (*Syncerus caffer*). *Theriogenology* 55:398.

Quandt SKF, Ebedes H. 1998. Tranquillization of wildlife for translocation procedures in southern Africa: a review. Proceedings of the European Association of Zoo and Wildlife Veterinarians.

Read BW, Miller RE, Houston EW, et al. 1989. Restraint of banteng (*bos javanicus*) in a commercial bovine squeeze chute. Proceedings of the American Association of Zoo Veterinarians, pp. 11–12.

Reibold TW, Goble DO, Geiser DR. 1982. *Large Animal Anesthesia: Principles and Techniques*. Ames: Iowa State University Press.

Schumacher J. 2008. Side effects of etorphine and carfentanil in nondomestic hoofstock. In: *Zoo and Wild Animal Medicine*, 6th ed. (ME Fowler, ER Miller, eds.), pp. 455–461. St. Louis: Saunders.

Sharma SK, Nigam JM, Singh M, et al. 1998. Sedative and clinico-biochemical effects of medetomidine in yaks (*Bos grunniens*) and its reversal with atipamezole. *The Indian Journal of Animal Sciences* 68:236–237.

Sharma SK, Nigam JM, Varchney AC, et al. 2001. Detomidine as a sedative in yaks. *The Indian Journal of Animal Sciences* 71:691–692.

Short CE. 1992. *Alpha2-Agents in Animals: Sedation, Analgesia and Anesthesia*. Santa Barbara: Veterinary Practice Publishing Company.

Smith GW, Davis JL, Tell LA, et al. 2008. Extralabel use of nonsteroidal anti-inflammatory drugs in cattle. *Journal of the American Veterinary Medical Association* 232:697–701.

Stegmann GF. 2004. Midazolam/ketamine induction and isoflurane maintenance of anaesethsia in a 2 month-old hand raised African buffalo (*Syncerus caffer*). *Journal of the South African Veterinary Association* 75:43–44.

Swan GE. 1993. Tranquilizers/neuroleptics. In: *The Capture and Care Manual: Capture, Care, Accommodation and Transportation of Wild African Animals* (AA McKenzie, ed.), pp. 32–42. Lynnwood Ridge: Wildlife Decision Support Services.

Ting ST, Earley B, Hughes JM, et al. 2003. Effect of ketoprofen, lidocaine local anesthesia and combined xylazine caudal epidural anesthesia during castration of beef cattle on stress responses, immunity, growth, and behavior. *Journal of Animal Science* 83:1281–1293.

Wilson SC, Armstrong DL, Simmons LG, et al. 1993. A clinical trial using three regimens for immobilizing gaur (*Bos gaurus*). *Journal of Zoo and Wildlife Medicine* 24:93–101.

Zuba JR, Oosterhuis JE. 2007. Treatment options for adverse reactions to haloperidol and other neuroleptic drugs in nondomestic hoofstock. Proceedings of the American Association of Zoo Veterinarians, pp. 53–57.

64 Bison

Nigel Caulkett

INTRODUCTION

Bison can be extremely difficult to anesthetize. Major complications of anesthesia can include: hypoxemia, bloat, and regurgitation. Bison are also predisposed to the development of capture myopathy, which can occur during or after anesthesia.

Two subspecies of bison can be found in North America. The plains bison (*Bison bison bison*) is most commonly encountered in free-ranging and captive herds. The wood bison (*Bison bison athabascae*) is confined to a few free-ranging herds in northern Canada, and some captive animals. Response to anesthesia is similar in both subspecies and this discussion applies equally to both. There are wild populations of the European bison (*Bison bonasus*) in Poland, Russia, Belarus, Ukraine, and the western Caucasus. The focus of this paper is on North American bison, but it should also be applicable to European bison.

SPECIES-SPECIFIC PHYSIOLOGY

Bison are similar to domestic cattle in many respects; anesthesia of an animal with a full rumen pack typically results in bloat or regurgitation. Xylazine or general anesthesia with volatile agents will lead to decreased rumen motility, bloat, and regurgitation. These can be fatal complications and tend to be more severe in large, mature animals (Caulkett et al. 2000).

Bison are prone to hypoxemia during general anesthesia. Positioning in dorsal or lateral recumbency will exacerbate hypoxemia (Caulkett et al. 2000). Alpha-2 agonist drugs such as xylazine or medetomidine will also exacerbate hypoxemia (Caulkett et al. 2000).

Bison stress very quickly. Stressed animals tend to override the sedative effects of alpha-2 agonist drugs necessitating the use of relatively high dosages of these agents to produce immobilization. Stressed animals are prone to capture myopathy, the acute form of which is a shock-like syndrome that can result in death within hours. The subacute form often results in muscle damage, myoglobinuria, and potentially kidney failure. The chronic form is characterized by severe muscle fibrosis, chronic progressive renal failure, and the possibility of muscle rupture in already weakened tissues (Spraker 1993). Rupture of the gastroconemeus muscles is a common manifestation of exertional myopathy in bison. It can occur acutely or may manifest in the chronic form. It is extremely important to keep chase times to a minimum, and try to avoid excitement prior to induction. (Fig. 64.1).

Hyperthermia increases metabolic oxygen demand and increases the risk of capture myopathy. If immobilization is anticipated, it should be planned for the cool hours of the day. Trauma during induction of anesthesia is not uncommon. It is particularly important to control the rest of the herd during induction as other members of the herd may traumatize the drugged animal. There is no information concerning the abortogenic effects of xylazine in bison cows. The risk of abortion in the last third of pregnancy may be increased with this drug.

PHYSICAL CAPTURE AND RESTRAINT

Captive bison may be handled in facilities that are relatively similar to cattle handling facilities. Bison are very powerful and it is vital that the chute system and squeeze is built from material that can accommodate rough handling. Ideally, the chute system should be enclosed, and there should be no right angle turns, as the animal may run directly into the wall and injure itself. Typically, a hydraulic squeeze is used to capture

Zoo Animal and Wildlife Immobilization and Anesthesia, Second Edition. Edited by Gary West, Darryl Heard, and Nigel Caulkett.

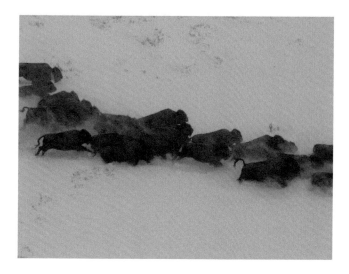

Figure 64.1. Aerial darting of wood bison; pursuit times should be limited to less than 2 minutes whenever possible.

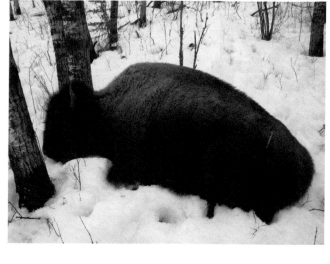

Figure 64.2. Plains bison positioned in sternal recumbency.

and restrain the animal, it is not uncommon to include a crash gate at the end of the squeeze as the animal may enter the squeeze very rapidly and a physical barrier is required to stop the animal at the end of the squeeze. Restraint time must be kept to a minimum in order to decrease the risk of stress-related complications. Physical capture of free-ranging bison is typically achieved with a net gun. An experienced crew can potentially capture and handle cows and calves with this method. Mature bulls are more challenging, and typically chemical immobilization is required.

CHEMICAL RESTRAINT AND ANESTHESIA

Vascular Access

The two most common sites for vascular access are the jugular vein and the coccygeal vein. The coccygeal vein can be used to obtain small volume blood samples and to top-up anesthetic or immobilizing drugs; it is not a good location to place an indwelling catheter. The jugular vein is a good location to obtain large volume blood samples or to place indwelling catheters, but it can be challenging to locate in large males. The size of the head will also make it difficult to manipulate the head and neck in sternally recumbent animals. Catheter selection is similar to domestic bovids, either over the needle or through the needle catheters may be used, a typical gauge is 10–14, with a typical length of 10 cm. A small, full thickness incision of the skin overlying the vein will facilitate catheter placement. In the laterally recumbent animal, the lateral saphenous may also be used. Caution should be exercised as lightly anesthetized bison may suddenly kick with their hind limbs. Arterial samples may be obtained from the coccygeal artery or the femoral artery, auricular arteries are typically difficult to locate.

Endotracheal Intubation

Intubation is not typically performed in field settings, but it is recommended if the bison is to be maintained on volatile anesthesia. The technique is the same as for cattle. The bison is maintained in sternal recumbency. A mouth gag is placed, prior to intubation. The tongue is pulled forward and the distal end of the tube is held. The person performing the intubation will advance their arm into the oral cavity and guide the tube to the epiglottis. The epiglottis is displaced ventrally with a finger, and the tube is advanced into the glottis. A mature bison will require a size 24–30 endotracheal tube. The head will need to be elevated to facilitate intubation; this can be difficult in large, mature animals, as the head can be heavy.

Monitoring and Supportive Care

Pulmonary Function Hypoxemia can be severe during anesthesia. Hypoxemia, in the face of hyperthermia, is a particularly serious situation, as hyperthermia increases tissue oxygen demand. This can increase the risk of capture myopathy or result in acute mortality. Hypoxemia can be prevented or treated in the field. Animals should be positioned in sternal recumbency (Fig. 64.2).

The head and neck should be extended to maintain a patent airway. The animal should be monitored for hypoxemia, ideally with a pulse oximeter. A multi-site sensor applied to the tongue generally provides a good signal. Normal hemoglobin saturation should be 95–98%, and a saturation below 85% is considered hypoxemic. If a pulse oximeter is not available, the mucous membranes should be monitored for cyanosis. Severely hypoxemic animals are often tachycardic. Heart rates above 150 in bison may result from a stress response due to hypoxemia, hypercarbia, pain, or hypotension. Tachycardia, followed by severe bradycar-

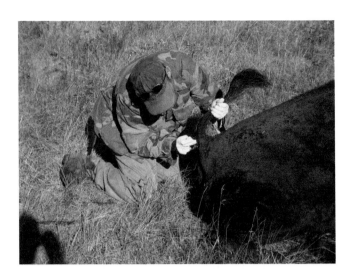

Figure 64.3. Collection of an arterial blood sample from the coccygeal artery of a sternally recumbent bison.

dia (HR < 30), is often a warning sign that the degree of hypoxemia is critical and the heart may fail. Supplemental inspired oxygen should be considered in hypoxemic animals (Caulkett et al. 2000). Portable equipment is available to facilitate oxygen delivery. An ambulance type regulator and aluminum D-cylinder is lightweight, portable, and sturdy. It can provide a 10 L/min flow for up to 30 minutes. An E-cylinder will provide this flow for an hour or more. A nasal catheter is a simple method to provide supplemental inspired oxygen. The catheter should be threaded as far as the medial canthus of the eye. A flow rate of 10–15 L/min is required in bison.

Arterial blood gas analysis will provide the most accurate means of assessing oxygenation. The femoral artery may be used in laterally recumbent animals. It is prudent to exercise caution when working near the legs of anaesthetized bison, as they may spontaneously kick. The coccygeal artery can be used to facilitate arterial blood sampling in sternally recumbent bison (Fig. 64.3).

Cardiovascular System Heart rate and pulse quality should be monitored every 5 minutes. The auricular pulse is difficult to palpate in bison. The facial artery or the femoral artery may be used. Bison anesthetized with xylazine-telazol or medetomidine-telazol have an average heart rate of approximately 60 beats/min (Caulkett et al. 2000). Bison anesthetized with carfentanil-xylazine have a slightly higher heart rate. An average heart rate of 75 beats/min has been reported with carfentanil-xylazine (Haigh & Gates 1995; Kock & Berger 1987).

Body Temperature Rectal temperature should be monitored every 5–10 minutes. Bison are prone to hyperthermia, particularly following a long pursuit. Rectal temperatures greater than 40°C are cause for concern,

and attempts should be made to cool the animal, cold water sprayed on the animal or snow packed into the inguinal and axillary regions may help. Rectal temperature in excess of 41°C is an emergency and should be treated aggressively. It is difficult to actively cool large animals, and often the best option with severe hyperthermia is to antagonize the immobilizing agents and allow the animal to recover. Hyperthermia greatly increases metabolic oxygen demand. Hyperthermia, in the face of hypoxemia, is a particularly serious complication. Hyperthermic animals should receive supplemental inspired oxygen to offset hypoxemia.

Supportive Care Maintenance in sternal recumbeny will help to prevent the development of rumenal tympany. If rumenal tympany is a problem, the animal may be rocked gently to stimulate eructation. A rumen tube can be used, but may predispose to regurgitation and aspiration. Generally, if rumenal tympany is severe, it is advisable to finish the procedure quickly and antagonize the anesthetic agents. If alpha-2 agonists have been used, the administration of tolazoline or atipamezole will stimulate rumenal activity and relieve rumenal tympany.

Sedation and Anesthesia of Captive Bison
Bison restrained in a head gate and squeeze can be sedated with intravenous xylazine. The coccygeal vein is useful for the injection of small volumes. Xylazine can be used as the sole agent at a dose of 0.1–0.2 mg/kg IV for standing sedation. Sedation may be enhanced by the addition of 0.05 mg/kg of acepromazine or 0.05 mg/kg of butorphanol administered IV. All three drugs may also be combined to produce deep sedation, and possibly recumbency. If short-term general anesthesia is desired, 0.2–0.5 mg/kg of xylazine can be administered IV, via the tail vein, to produce recumbency. This is followed by 2 mg/kg of ketamine, via the jugular vein. If the jugular vein is used the head must be adequately restrained to avoid injury to handlers.

Anesthesia may be prolonged with 5% guaifenasin and additional 1 mg/kg boluses of ketamine administered to effect. Use guaifenasin cautiously as we have observed guaifenasin toxicity in two bison, at what appeared to be a relatively low dose. It would be premature to say these animals are overly sensitive to the drug, but it should be used cautiously until more information is available. Guaifenasin must be administered via a jugular catheter, as it will cause severe tissue irritation and damage if it is administered perivascularly.

Xylazine should be antagonized at the end of the procedure. If IV ketamine has been used, the antagonist should not be administered for 10–15 minutes to avoid undesirable effects of the ketamine.

Bison calves can be induced to anesthesia with IV ketamine 2–4 mg/kg plus diazepam 0.2 mg/kg. This combination will give 5–10 minutes of light anesthesia.

In depressed calves, diazepam 0.2 mg/kg + 0.1 mg/kg of butorphanol can be used IV for sedation. If the calf is difficult to work with, 0.1–0.2 mg/kg of xylazine + 0.1 mg/kg of butorphanol can be administered IM prior to induction with ketamine-valium.

Immobilization of Free-Ranging Bison
Bison may require immobilization for a variety of reasons. Remote delivery of immobilizing agents necessitates the use of potent agents that can be delivered in relatively small volumes.

Carfentanil-Xylazine This combination has been used for capture of free-ranging wood and plains bison (Haigh & Gates 1995; Kock & Berger 1987). Carfentanil is administered at a dose of 4–8 μg/kg; this is combined with xylazine, at a dose of 0.05–0.1 mg/kg. Bison, like other ungulates, will demonstrate increased activity and excitement during induction. If the animal demonstrates head and/or limb movement when approached after becoming recumbent an additional 0.05–0.1 mg/kg of xylazine may be administered IV to improve muscle relaxation. Following the procedure, carfentanil should be antagonized with naltrexone at a ratio of at least 100-mg naltrexone per 1 mg of carfentanil. Naltrexone has been shown to be the drug of choice for antagonism of carfentanil in bison. Antagonism of carfentanil, with naloxone, has resulted in a high incidence of mortality from renarcotization. Naltrexone has a long half-life and the incidence of re-narcotization is very low.

Complications of immobilization can include the following: hypoxemia, hypoventilation, regurgitation, and hyperthermia. Renarcotization is not usually a problem if naltrexone is used to antagonize carfentanil.

The major advantage of this combination is that it can be administered in very small volumes and will produce reliable immobilization. It is a particularly attractive combination for wild animals, as decreased volume requirements will improve the accuracy of dart placement and decrease tissue trauma.

Xylazine-Telazol A dose range of 0.75–1.5 mg/kg of xylazine, combined with 1.5–3 mg/kg of telazol is generally effective to immobilize bison (Caulkett et al. 2000). The low end of the dose is often effective in calm animals. The high end of the dose range may be required in fractious or wild animals. A 400-kg cow could require a dose volume of up to 7 mL, which can decrease dart accuracy and increase tissue trauma. Large volume requirements decrease the utility of this mixture for wild animals, but it is still very useful in captive or game-farmed animals.

The mixture will produce approximately 1 hour of anesthesia, and will provide adequate analgesia for minor procedures. The major complications that can be encountered with this combination are hypoxemia, bloat and/or regurgitation, and hyperthermia.

Xylazine should be antagonized following the procedure. Since the telazol dose is relatively low recoveries are generally smooth. Rougher recoveries may be noted if a high dose of telazol was used for induction. Tolazoline or atipamezole should be used to antagonize xylazine in bovids. Tolazoline can be administered at a dose of 2–3 mg/kg. This dose may be split between IV and IM administration. Yohimbine will not effectively antagonize xylazine-induced sedation in bovids and should not be used as the reversal agent (Klein & Klide 1989).

Medetomidine-Telazol The immobilization characteristics of this combination are similar to those of xylazine-telazol (Caulkett et al. 2000). The major advantage of medetomidine-telazol is that it can be administered at approximately half the volume of xylazine-telazol. This quality greatly increases its utility in free-ranging animals. Another major advantage is that a lower dose of telazol is required and arousal from sedation is significantly faster than recovery following antagonism of the xylazine in the xylazine-telazol mixture.

A dosage of 60 μg/kg of medetomidine + 1.2 mg/kg of telazol can be used to immobilization in captive and free-ranging bison. Medetomidine can be antagonized with 180–300 mg/kg of atipamezole. Caution should be observed following antagonism of the medetomidine, as arousal from anesthesia can be very rapid, and IV administration of atipamezole should be avoided unless the condition of the animal is seriously compromised.

Complications are similar to those of xylazine-telazol and include hypoxemia, hypercarbia, and rumenal tympany. Steps should be taken to prevent or treat these complications.

Medetomidine-Ketamine
This combination has been used for immobilization of captive European bison. The effective dose is 2.5 mg/kg of ketamine plus 0.08 mg/kg of medetomidine. (Jalanka & Roeken 1990).

Xylazine-Hydromorphone-Telazol
This combination will address some of the adverse effects of xylazine-telazol alone. The addition of hydromorphone to this combination decreases the telazol and xylazine requirements. The mean dosage administered to plains bison was 1.98 mg/kg of telazol, 0.26 mg/kg of hydromorphone, and 1.32 mg/kg of xylazine. Reversal of sedation was achieved with 4 mg/kg of tolazoline and 0.09 mg/kg of naltrexone (Shury & Caukett 2006). Preliminary results indicate that this mixture induces less hypoxemia than xylazine-telazol

alone and that reversal of sedation is more rapid following the administration of antagonists. This combination is promising in bison and other ungulates.

Volatile Anesthesia Volatile anesthesia may be used for prolonged procedures. Isoflurane is preferable to halothane as it is less arrhythmogenic. Induction can be achieved with IV xylazine-ketamine or xylazine-guaifenasin-ketamine in restrained animals, or IM xylazine-telazol in unrestrained animals. It is very important to fast animals for 24–48 hours prior to general anesthesia as bovids are particularly prone to bloat and regurgitation during volatile anesthesia. Animals under 150 kg can be anesthetized with a small animal machine. Animals over 150 kg require a large animal circuit.

REFERENCES

Caulkett NA, Cattet MRL, Cantwell S, et al. 2000. Anesthesia of wood bison with medetomidine-zolazepam/tiletamine and xylazine-zolazepam/tiletamine combinations. *The Canadian Veterinary Journal* 41:49–53.

Haigh JC, Gates CC. 1995. Capture of wood bison (*Bison bison athabascae*) using carfentanil-based mixtures. *Journal of Wildlife Diseases* 31:37–42.

Jalanka HH, Roeken BO. 1990. The use of medetomidine, medetomidine-ketamine combinations, and atipamezole in nondomestic mammals: a review. *Journal of Zoo and Wildlife Medicine* 21:259–282.

Klein LV, Klide AM. 1989. Central alpha 2 adrenergic and benzodiazepine agonists and their antagonists. *Journal of Zoo and Wildlife Medicine* 20:138–153.

Kock MD, Berger J. 1987. Chemical immobilization of free-ranging North American bison (*Bison bison*) in Badlands National Park, South Dakota. *Journal of Wildlife Diseases* 23:625–633.

Shury TK, Caulkett NA. 2006. Chemical immobilization of free-ranging plains bison (*Bison bison bison*) and rocky mountain bighorn sheep (*Ovis Canadensis Canadensis*) with a tiletamine-zolazepam-xylazine-hydromorphone combination. Proceedings of the American Association of Zoo Veterinarians Annual Meeting, pp. 220–223.

Spraker TR. 1993. Stress and capture myopathy in artiodactylids. In: *Zoo and Wild Animal Medicine: Current Therapy 3* (M Fowler, ed.), pp. 481–488. Philadelphia: W.B. Saunders.

65 Lagomorphs (Rabbits, Hares, and Pikas)

Darryl Heard

INTRODUCTION

The order Lagomorpha includes 91 living species distributed among two families: Leporidae (rabbits and hares) and Ochotonidae (pikas) (Wilson & Reeder 2005). Lagomorphs are herbivores, closely related to rodents (Nowak 1999). Adults have two pairs of upper incisors; the smaller second is located directly behind the first. Pikas are small (125–400 g) with short ears and legs, and no visible tail (Nowak 1999). Rabbits and hares have elongated ears and legs, and rely on speed to escape predators. Pikas are found in northern Eurasia and western North America. The sexes are equal in size, and their fur is long and dense (Nowak 1999). Despite enduring severe winters, they do not appear to hibernate.

The term "hare" is restricted to animals of the genus *Lepus* (Nowak 1999), all other leporids are rabbits. Hares are usually larger and have black ear tips. Young rabbits are born blind, naked and helpless in a fur-lined nest. In contrast, hares are born fully furred in the open with eyes open and capable of running in a few minutes (Nowak 1999). Leporids weigh 400–7000 g; females are usually larger than males (Nowak 1999). Frightened or captured rabbits may emit loud, shrill screams.

The literature is dominated by parenteral anesthetic regimens for research rabbits (and rodents). Great care must be taken in selecting regimens for clinical cases or free-living animals based on this information. This is because the goals of research anesthesia are often not the same (i.e., prolonged immobility and not necessarily recovery). Similarly, anesthetic regimens have improved in safety, analgesia, and efficacy as new drugs have become available; older anesthetic references must be critically interpreted. Conversely, the benefit of rabbits being used as research animals is there is a lot of controlled studies on the physiologic effects and pharmacokinetics of analgesic and anesthetic drugs.

The European rabbit (*Oryctolagus cuniculus*) is a popular pet, as well as food and fur animal, and one of the most common research mammals. Consequently, the following discussion emphasizes this species. Pikas are similar to rodents in form and size, and anesthesia is the same (see Chapter 66).

PHYSICAL RESTRAINT

Domestic rabbits are not aggressive. However, some animals, particularly those used in research, will bite and scratch. Rabbits and hares have long legs for leaping and running, and will explosively kick when restrained. The kick force is sufficient to fracture the lower thoracolumbar vertebrae. Distal tibial fractures are common if a rabbit falls. Leg fractures also occur in wire bottom cages when a toe or leg is caught. Leporids must not be held by the ears. They can be grasped by the nape for short periods, but it is important to support the rump at the same time. When carrying for a distance, they are either placed in a transport cage or cradled in one arm with their head tucked into the body of the handler.

Physical restraint devices (e.g., rabbit squeezeboxes and cat bags) are a useful adjunct to anesthesia, particularly in the induction period. Restrained rabbits quickly develop hyperthermia, however, especially when environmental temperatures are high. Physical restraint of free-living rabbits and hares should be minimal. Chemical immobilization or inhalation anesthesia is recommended for examination and sample collection.

VASCULAR ACCESS

Blood can be collected from either the external jugular, cephalic, or saphenous vein. This author also collects

Zoo Animal and Wildlife Immobilization and Anesthesia, Second Edition. Edited by Gary West, Darryl Heard, and Nigel Caulkett.

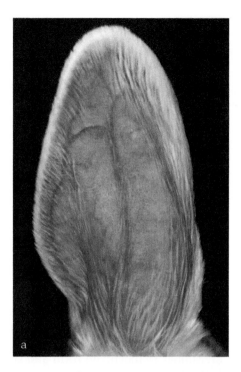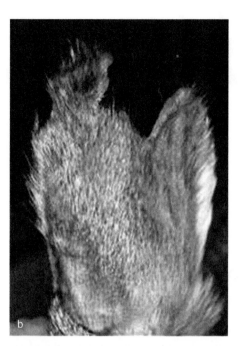

Figure 65.1. (a) The ear of a domestic rabbit showing the relationship of the auricular artery (the large central vessel) and veins (the vessels along the edge of the ear). (b) Care should be taken to prevent injury of the auricular artery, which may lead to thrombosis and ischemic necrosis.

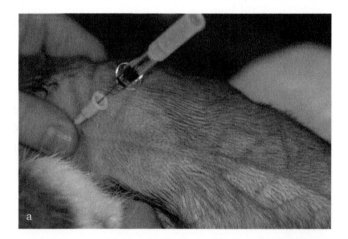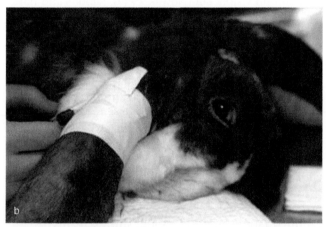

Figure 65.2. (a and b) The marginal ear veins can be catheterized with either 22- or 24-gauge over-the-needle catheters. A roll of gauze inside the ear can be used to facilitate securing the catheter with tape.

blood from the auricular artery (Fig. 65.1a). After clipping over the artery, a bleb of local anesthetic is infiltrated over the site on the artery where blood will be collected. This will prevent reflex vasospasm and cause vasodilation. A 25-gauge needle and either 1- or 3-mL syringe are used to collect an appropriate volume. Once the sample is collected, care is taken to ensure hemostasis and the vessel is open. This author will also use this vessel for collection of large volumes of blood quickly for transfusion. A 22-gauge over-the-needle catheter can be carefully placed, then removed after the blood has been collected.

Catheters can also be placed in either the cephalic or marginal ear (Fig. 65.1a and Fig. 65.2a,b) vein for fluid administration. For cephalic vein catheterization, this author uses 22- to 24-gauge over-the-needle catheters. The cephalic vein is found on the forearm in the same position as in other domestic animals. Care must be taken when removing hair to use clippers appropriate for the dense hair of rabbits and to not tear the skin. Rabbit skin is also easily burned by clippers and susceptible to irritation from iodine solutions and alcohol.

The auricular veins are located on the edge of the ears and are usually relatively small (Fig. 65.1a); a 22- to

24-gauge over-the-needle catheter is used by this author. To facilitate catheterization, a bleb of local anesthetic can be infused around the vessel, or applied topically. This provides the dual benefits of analgesia and vessel dilation. Massaging the ear will help to dilate the vessels. Gauze rolled into a tube and placed on the inside of the ear aids in taping the catheter in place (Fig. 65.2a,b). In an awake rabbit, the ears can be taped together. This maintains them in an upright position for continuous fluid administrations using a fluid pump. Care must be taken to prevent ischemic necrosis caused by too-tight bandaging (Fig. 65.1b).

In small patients, intraosseous catheterization can be used as an alternative route to attain vascular access. Catheters can be placed in the proximal tibia, humerus, or femur. Spinal needles (18–22 gauge) are used for intraosseous catheters.

PREANESTHETIC PREPARATION

Assessment of patency of the nares and nasopharynx is essential, especially when an inhalant anesthetic mask is used. Lagomorphs are primary or obligate nasal breathers, and upper respiratory disease is common (e.g., snuffles). The thorax of rabbits is very small relative to abdominal volume (Fig. 65.3). Obesity is also very common in captive animals and can contribute to hypoventilation during anesthesia.

This author does not recommend fasting since leporids do not regurgitate or vomit. Fasting has also been recommended to reduce gastrointestinal volume and, thereby, diaphragmatic and lung compression (Fig. 65.3). It is unlikely, however, to significantly reduce volume in an herbivore and may cause perioperative ileus.

PREMEDICATION

Premedication always includes an analgesic plan; recommended premedication dosages are given in Table 65.1.

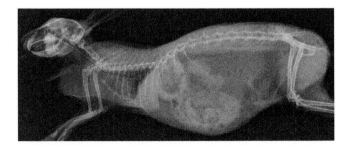

Figure 65.3. Lateral radiograph of a domestic rabbit. Note the small thoracic cavity relative to the large abdomen. The trachea is also relatively short compared with body length, and single bronchial intubation is common. Note also the angle of the oral cavity in relation to the trachea emphasizing the need to hyperextend the head and neck to facilitate intubation.

Routine use of parasympatholytics is unnecessary and will alter gastrointestinal motility. Many, but not all rabbits have circulating levels of atropinesterases. Atropinesterase was found in 62% of New Zealand white rabbits (Liebenberg & Linn 1980). More males possessed the enzyme, and there were significant differences in atropinesterase levels between winter and summer (Liebenberg & Linn 1980). Higher atropine dosages in animals lacking these enzymes increase the likelihood of toxicosis. In rabbits, atropine sulfate (0.2–2.0 mg/kg) only briefly induced a moderate tachycardia, but glycopyrrolate (0.1 mg/kg) elevated heart rate for ≥50 minutes (Olson et al. 1994).

Acepromazine has similar effects as in other domestic mammals. It is used only in healthy hemodynamically stable animals. Peak effect is not attained for 30–45 minutes, even when administered IV. Tranquilization is inversely related to the amount of environmental stimulation. Acepromazine decreases tear production in rabbits and may, therefore, contribute to corneal injury (Ghaffari et al. 2009).

Benzodiazepines provide good sedation and relaxation. They are a useful adjunct to induction of debilitated patients because of their minimal cardiopulmonary effects, and they can be reversed with flumazenil. The alpha-2-adrenergic agonsits xylazine, detomidine, and medetomidine are usually not used alone for sedation.

ANALGESIA

The principles and techniques for small mammal analgesia are well reviewed by Flecknell (2001), Robertson (2001), as well as in Chapter 7. Recommended rabbit dosages are given in Table 65.2. Although a study of the pharmacokinetics of tramadol (11 mg/kg PO) showed levels of its active metabolite O-desmethyltramadol insufficient to produce

Table 65.1. Drug dosages (mg/kg, IM, SC or IV) for premedication and sedation of rabbits

Drug	Dosage	Comments
Acepromazine	0.1–1.0	Healthy, hemodynamically stable animals—will produce hypotension. Peak effect may take ≥45 minutes.
Diazepam	1.0–5.0	
Midazolam	0.5–2.0	
Xylazine	1.0–5.0	Higher dosages associated with marked cardiopulmonary depression and bradyarrythmias.
Atropine	0.04–1.0	Use in emergencies to effect, not recommended for routine premedication. Many but not all rabbits have high circulating levels of atropinase.
Glycopyrrolate	0.01–0.02	

Source: Adapted, in part, from Mason (1997).

Table 65.2. Analgesic drugs used in rabbits and hares[a]

Opioids	
Buprenorphine	0.01–0.05 IM, SC, IV q 6–12h
Butorphanol	0.1–0.5 IM, SC q 4h
Meperidine	10 IM, SC q 2–3h
Morphine	2–5 IM, SC q 4h
Oxymorphone	0.05–0.2 IM, SC q 8–12h
NSAIDs	
Carprofen	4 IM, SC q24h, 1.5 PO q 12h
Flunixin	1–2 IM, SC q 12h
Ketoprofen	3 IM, SC q 24h
Meloxicam	0.2–0.5 IM, SC, 0.3 PO q 24h
Tramadol	0.5–5 PO q 12–24h

[a]All dosages are given in mg/kg.
Source: Adapted from Flecknell (2001) and Mason (1997).
IM, intramuscular; SC, subcutaneous; PO = oral.

analgesia in humans (Souza et al. 2008), this author has subjectively observed positive results in rabbits with degenerative joint disease at much lower dosages (1–4 mg/kg every 12–24 hours).

LOCAL AND REGIONAL ANESTHESIA

Rabbits are models for epidural and intrathecal administration of local anesthetics and analgesics (Hughes et al. 1993; Pang et al. 1999; Taguchi et al. 1996). Local and epidural anesthesia are used for minor and occasionally major (e.g., Cesarean section) procedures, respectively. Recommended epidural volume administered by the lumbosacral space is 0.2mL/kg. Using this dosage, the rank order for onset of action and duration of effect was 2% lignocaine, 2% lignocaine with epinephrine (1:200,000), and 0.5% bupivacaine (Hughes et al. 1993).

Some long-acting local anesthetics have a low therapeutic index (e.g., bupivicaine), and commercial preparations contain concentrations appropriate to humans. Consequently, care must be taken to calculate and prepare appropriate volumes for infiltration. For example, if the toxic dose of lidocaine is 10–20mg/kg, the equivalent volume of a 2% lidocaine solution would be ≤0.5 to 1.0mL/kg.

PARENTERAL ANESTHESIA

Rabbits, and other lagomorphs, have evolved the ability to detoxify many ingested plant chemicals. For example, circulating atropine esterases in many breeds are capable of inactivating belladonna alkaloids. A high metabolic rate also implies rapid metabolism and excretion of parenteral drugs. Consequently, they generally have a shorter duration of effect than comparable doses in larger mammals.

Drug Administration

Injection routes include subcutaneous, intramuscular, intraperitoneal, intravenous, and intraosseous. This

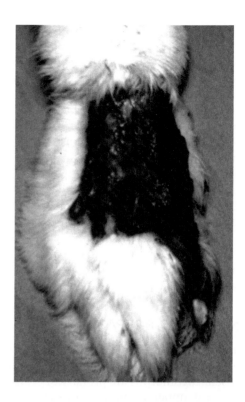

Figure 65.4. The foot of a rabbit self-mutilated in response to irritation from cephalic catheter. Self-mutilation can occur in response to pain from peripheral injection of irritant solutions, such as xylazine/ketamine or enrofloxacin. The likelihood of it occurring can be reduced by administering injections into large proximal muscle groups (e.g., quadriceps), and with the use of analgesics.

author prefers intramuscular injections be given in the quadriceps muscle. The rabbit is held on a table with its head tucked into the arm of the holder. The muscle is held with one hand and the other hand makes the injection from the front.

Potentially irritant solutions (e.g., high or low pH solutions) are not administered SC or IM because of the risk of self-mutilation (Beyers et al. 1991) (Fig. 65.4). This can be reduced by diluting the solution, avoiding large volume injections, and injecting in the large proximal leg muscles. The author recommends IP, rather than IM or SC, injections in pikas because of their small size.

Intranasal administration of some analgesics, sedatives, and anesthetics is an effective and rapid route in rabbits (Lindhardt et al. 2001; Robertson & Eberhart 1994).

Drugs

Ketamine has a very short duration of clinical effect due, in part, to redistribution and renal elimination (Bjorkman & Redke 2000). Consequently, renal impairment will markedly prolong recovery. Xylazine and other alpha-2 adrenergic agonists are frequently combined with ketamine for short-term immobilization and surgical anesthesia. These combinations, particularly at the higher dosage levels, produce mild to severe dose-dependent hypotension, bradyarrhythmias, and respiratory depression, with associated hypercapnia, academia, and hypoxemia. As with all parenteral anesthetic regimens, some form of oxygen supplementation and assisted ventilation is recommended. Ketamine/benzodiazepine combinations produce less cardiopulmonary depression and analgesia, but good muscle relaxation.

In Dutch belted rabbits, multiple anesthetic episodes with ketamine/xylazine (50/10 mg/kg IM) were associated with myocardial necrosis and fibrosis (Marini et al. 1999). Similarly, in New Zealand white rabbits, detomidine, alone and in combination with ketamine or diazepam, produced the same injury (Hurley et al. 1994). The postulated mechanism was decreased coronary blood flow. However, other causes (e.g., hypovitaminosis E, excessive anesthetic dosage, and hypoxemia) were not ruled out.

Tiletamine/zolazepam is not recommended for use. This combination requires very high dosages (32–64 mg/kg) to produce immobility to noxious stimuli (Brammer et al. 1991). These dosages also produce dose-dependent renal tubular necrosis within 7 days of injection (Brammer et al. 1991).

Propofol is used for induction and maintenance. Its effects are similar to those described in domestic animals (Aeschbacher & Webb 1993a, 1993b). The total induction dose is dependent upon administration rate. Propofol alone produces inadequate analgesia for painful procedures, and anesthetic maintenance with infusions is not recommended unless cardiopulmonary support is provided. It is indicated for induction of healthy animals in which vascular access can be attained prior to anesthesia. A slow infusion can also be used for sedation to facilitate mask induction. Animals should be intubated and ventilated as soon as possible after induction.

Alfaxolone (3 mg/kg IV, IM?) can be used to induce anesthesia in rabbits (Gil et al. 2012). In comparison to propofol (10 mg/kg IV) both anesthetics induced a comparable decrease in heart and respiratory rates, while propofol affected adrenocortical function less (Gil et al. 2012).

INHALATION ANESTHESIA

Inhalation anesthesia with either isoflurane or sevoflurane is the primary component of most anesthetic regimens. It allows rapid induction, recovery, and control of anesthetic depth, while adverse effects are dose-dependent and reversible.

Immediately after induction, rabbits often have shallow rapid respirations and decreased alveolar ventilation. This delays attainment of maintenance alveolar anesthetic levels, and may explain the need for high isoflurane vaporizer settings (4–5%) in spontaneously

breathing rabbits. Premedication and assisted endotracheal intubation ameliorates this. Intubation allows assisted ventilation, improved alveolar ventilation, and thus better control of anesthesia.

Induction

Inhalant anesthesia is used either alone or as an adjunct to induction. The anesthetic is administered into an induction chamber or through a mask. The advantage of a chamber is the animal is not physically restrained during the involuntary excitement phase of induction. This reduces the risk of injury to both handler and patient. Disadvantages include environmental contamination and difficult monitoring.

Mask induction of restrained unpremedicated animals is not recommended. Anesthetic chambers and masks are clear to see the patient (Fig. 65.5). The chamber top is secured to prevent the animal escaping. Inhalant anesthetic is introduced through one opening and waste gas removed from another. The vaporizer is set at maximum concentration and oxygen flow rate at 2 to 4 L/min. Once the animal loses its righting response (usually 5 to 10 minutes), it is removed from the chamber and a mask placed over its nose and mouth. The chamber is placed outside or closed to allow waste gases to be safely voided. The animal is either maintained with a mask or intubated.

When using a mask, the animal's head and neck is kept in extension to prevent obstruction to breathing (Fig. 65.6). Respiratory pattern, rate and noise are assessed. If there appears to be difficulty in breathing the head and neck are moved to correct the obstruction. If not, a cotton-tipped applicator is used to clear the oropharynx and nares. If this fails to relieve the problem, the animal is intubated or awakened.

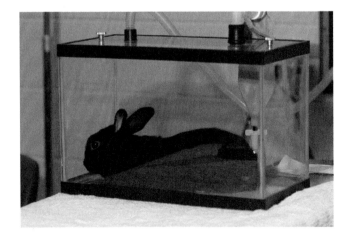

Figure 65.5. Induction of a premedicated rabbit with an inhalant anesthetic administered in oxygen. Note the clear chamber to allow visualization of the animal, and the scavenging system. Once the animal loses its righting reflex, it is removed from the chamber and maintained with a mask until intubated.

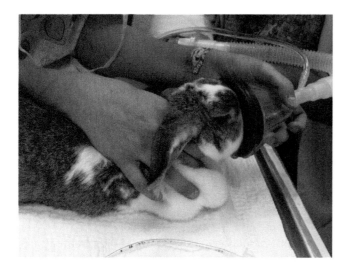

Figure 65.6. Mask induction is recommended only in animals that have been premedicated to prevent struggling. Note the extension of the head and neck to reduce the possibility of airway obstruction.

Endotracheal Intubation

In clinical practice intubation of rabbits should be a routine standard of care, especially for complex and prolonged procedures. Maintenance with a mask allows more inhalant anesthetic gas contamination of the environment, and does not allow assisted ventilation. Pediatric laryngeal mask airways are easier to position, but may be associated with increased waste gas exposure and stomach inflation during ventilation (Smith et al. 2004).

Endotracheal tube size ranges from 2- to 4.5-mm ID. They are preferably clear to see condensation or occlusion with mucous and blood. In rabbits, it is essential the animal's head and neck is moderately hyperextended to align the larynx and trachea with the oropharynx (Fig. 65.7). The epiglottis must be displaced ventral to the soft palate for visualization of the glottis through the oropharynx (Fig. 65.8). Regardless of technique, the rabbit is relaxed before intubation. This is indicated by absence of a response to either an ear or toe pinch.

There are two techniques: blind and direct visualization. An additional technique, not recommended because of laryngeal and tracheal trauma, uses retrograde placement of a guide wire or catheter through the larynx and out through the mouth. The endotracheal tube is then passed over the wire into the larynx. This technique is indicated for respiratory arrest when direct visualization fails.

This author prefers the blind technique for routine intubation. However, it requires breathing to guide endotracheal tube placement. The rabbit is placed in sternal recumbency on a table at a height comfortable for the anesthetist (Fig. 65.7). If you are right handed,

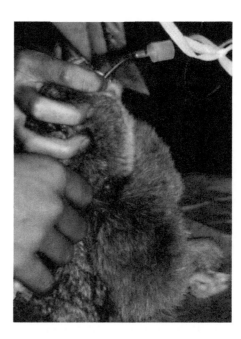

Figure 65.7. For endotracheal intubation, it is necessary to alter the normal angle between the oral cavity and trachea (Fig. 65.2). Regardless of technique used, the head and neck need to be hyperextended. This author prefers the animal be in sternal recumbency for this positioning. Alternatively, the animal can be placed in dorsal recumbency.

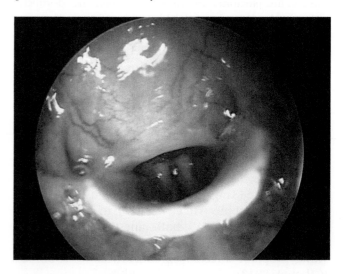

Figure 65.8. Endoscopic view of the glottal opening in an eastern cottontail rabbit (*Sylvilagus floridanus*). Lagomorphs are obligate nasal breathers. The soft palate has been displaced, allowing a view of the simple flat epiglottis and the arytenoid cartilages.

stand on the right side of the animal and grasp the head with the left hand. The head is grasped from above and behind with the thumb and little finger under the mandibular ramus. Alternatively, some find aligning the head and neck horizontal and parallel to the table in the dorsally recumbent rabbit also allows intubation. Although this author has used this position, it makes it awkward to listen and manipulate the tube.

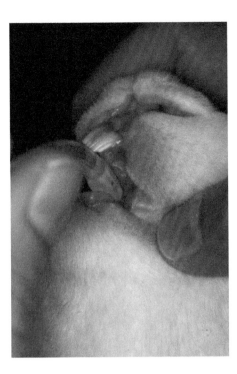

Figure 65.9. For blind intubation, it is unnecessary to open the jaws. Once the rabbit is fully unconscious and relaxed, the endotracheal tube is introduced through the space between the incisors and first premolars, and passed over the base of the tongue.

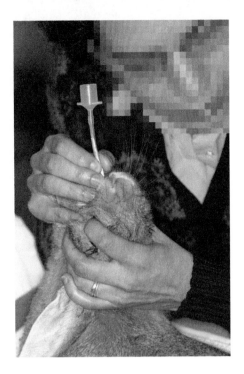

Figure 65.10. Blind intubation requires listening for respiratory noise to identify positioning of the endotracheal tube. The loudest noise indicates the tube is aligned and close to the laryngeal opening. If the noise goes away during positioning, it indicates the tube is in the esophagus, and it should be gently pulled back until respiratory sounds are again identified.

The endotracheal tube is inserted between the incisors and first premolar, and passed over the tongue base (Fig. 65.9). The head and neck are lifted into hyperextension, and the anesthetist places her/his ear to the tube (Fig. 65.10). The tube is advanced towards the glottis until respiratory noise is loudest. No or gurgling sound indicate the tube is in the esophagus. The tube is repetitively and gently advanced to the glottis until it enters the trachea. At the point of peak noise it helps to rotate the endotracheal tube 180° to displace the epiglottis (Fig. 65.8). Local anesthetic, both as a gel applied to the end of the tube or a liquid poured down the tube, desensitizes the glottis and facilitate intubation. The rabbit may forcefully cough the tube out. Do not persist in intubation attempts for more than a few minutes, or when there is evidence of either laryngeal edema or hemorrhage.

The direct visualization technique is similar. An assistant opens the animal's jaws using gauze tape placed around the upper and lower incisors (Fig. 65.11). The tongue is grasped by gauze square and pulled up and to the side. A cotton-tipped applicator may assist grabbing the tongue. A laryngoscope with a pediatric straight blade (Miller # 0 or 1) is inserted into the oropharynx, the head and neck are hyperextended, and the epiglottis displaced. The endotracheal tube is passed down the laryngoscope blade and through the glottis; sight of the glottis is usually lost as the endotracheal tube occludes the oropharynx. Alternatively, a small-diameter catheter is placed as a guide for the tube.

Alternatively, the endotracheal tube can also be placed over a rigid endoscope used to visualize the glottis (Tran et al. 2001). If a 2.7-mm outside-diameter endoscope is used, the tubes are limited to ≥3.0 mm internal diameter. The other disadvantage of using an endoscope is the potential for fracturing of the glass from flexion or chewing by a semi-awake rabbit. Alternatively, a small diameter (1.9-mm ID) fiberoptoscope can be used (Fig. 65.11b). These scopes allow some flexion and smaller-diameter tubes appropriate to small rabbits, and are relatively less expensive. A problem with using this technique in the warm humid environment of the mouth is fogging of the endoscope. This can be reduced or avoided by using antifogging solutions used to clear scuba masks, or similar liquids. Once in place, the tube is advanced into the glottis. Placing the rabbit in dorsal recumbency may facilitate glottal visualization.

If unsure the tube is in the correct place, remove it and reassess placement. A pulse oximeter is invaluable for monitoring potential oxygenation problems due to airway obstruction. Correct tube placement is determined by either: (1) seeing condensation on the inside of the tube (Fig. 65.12a) or on a metal surface placed at the end of the tube or (Fig. 65.12b); (2) detecting air

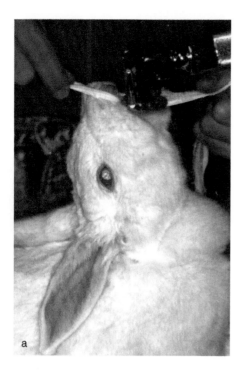

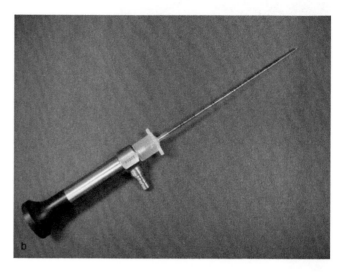

Figure 65.11. (a) Direct visualization techniques require the head and neck to be hyperextended, as for the blind technique. In this animal, a small pediatric straight laryngoscope is being used to visualize the glottis. (b) An alternative direct visualization technique for endotracheal intubation uses an endoscope. The endotracheal tube is placed on the outside of the endoscope, then guided into the larynx once the glottis is visualized. This is an example of an inexpensive semi-flexible 1.9-mm scope.

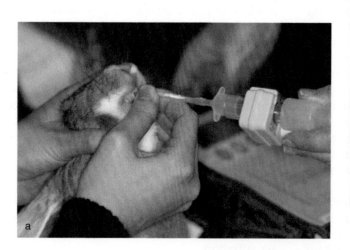

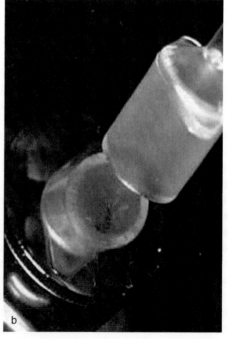

Figure 65.12. (a) Assessment of correct positioning of the endotracheal tube in the trachea can be done by visualizing condensation within the clear tube on exhalation, or with the use of a capnograph. (b) Assessment of correct positioning of the endotracheal tube in the trachea can also be done by observing condensation on a metal surface, such as the bottom of a laryngoscope.

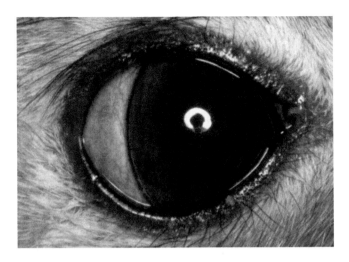

Figure 65.13. The position of the eye changes with increasing depth of inhalation anesthesia. A medial eye position suggests light surgical anesthesia.

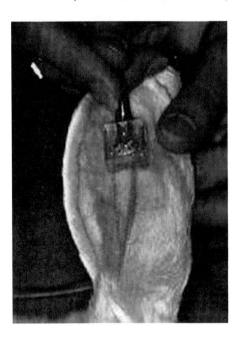

Figure 65.14. A Doppler flow probe can be placed over the auricular artery for monitoring blood flow.

movement with hair placed in front of the tube; (3) watching the nonrebreathing bag; (4) the response to intubation (coughing, etc.); or (5) detection of exhaled carbon dioxide on a capnograph (Fig. 65.12a). To insure the tube has not been placed into a single bronchus (Fig. 65.3), premeasure the tube before use, and auscultate both lung fields for respiratory sounds after intubation.

PERIOPERATIVE MONITORING

Anesthetic Depth

In rabbits anesthetized with isoflurane, the eyelid aperture increased in a predictable dose-dependent manner (Imai et al. 1999) (Fig. 65.13). This response cannot be evaluated in the clinical patient because the cornea is protected with either a lubricant or the eyelids are taped closed. The eyeball rotates medially (Fig. 65.13), then either dorsally or ventrally at 0.8 isoflurane MAC before becoming centrally fixed at >1.5 MAC (Imai et al. 1999). Palpebral and corneal reflexes are observed at 0.8 MAC, but are abolished at >2.0 MAC. A fixed dilated pupil, unresponsive to light and with no corneal reflex, is a cross-species indicator of either excessive anesthetic depth or brain stem hypoperfusion and ischemia. Anal tone is usually retained until deep anesthesia.

Evaluating physiologic and muscular response to a painful stimulus assesses pain and nocioceptor response. This can be a toe, ear, and/or tail pinch, or a skin incision. Increasing depth toward a surgical plane of anesthesia is assumed when muscle tone (e.g., jaw muscle and anal sphincter) decreases, palpebral and corneal reflexes are obtunded, and respiration pattern becomes regular and even. Sudden tachycardia, hypertension, and tachypnea in response to stimuli are indicative of inadequate anesthetic depth or analgesia.

Cardiovascular

An esophageal stethoscope can be used to monitor heart rate in the intubated anesthetized patient. Alternatively, a quality pediatric stethoscope is used. The electrocardiograph should have a multichannel oscilloscope with nonfade tracing and freeze capabilities. Additionally, it must be able to record at speeds of 100 mm/s and amplify the signal to at least 1 mV equal to 1 cm. Standard lead positions are used.

Placement sites for the Doppler flow probe include the ventral aspect of the tail base, the carotid, femoral, and auricular arteries, and directly over the heart (Fig. 65.14). Sites for indirect blood pressure measurement include the legs, forearms, tail, and ears. The forelimb cuff oscillometric method is accurate for evaluation of arterial blood pressure at low and normal pressure ranges (Ypsilantis et al. 2005). Direct arterial blood pressure can be measured using a 22- to 24-gauge over-the-needle catheter placed in the auricular artery in the center of the pinna (Ypsilantis et al. 2005).

Respiratory

Respiration rate (RR) is inversely related to bodyweight and is determined by evaluating either thoracic wall or reservoir bag movement. As with cardiac auscultation, evaluation requires a good quality stethoscope with appropriate head and length of tubing, and an experienced ear. The esophageal stethoscope can be used to evaluate respiratory noise. However, there is more likely to be artifactual noise that must be distinguished from true respiratory noise. Arterial blood gas samples are obtained from any palpable artery: the femoral, metatarsal, and auricular arteries. Infiltration of the periarterial area with 1% lidocaine without epinephrine may prevent reflex vasoconstriction.

Pulse oximetry has been evaluated in rabbits and appears accurate at hemoglobin saturation levels greater than 85% (Vegfors et al. 1991). Potential sites for placement of transmission pulse oximeter sensors include the ear, tongue, buccal mucosa, paw, vulva, prepuce, and proximal tail. Surprisingly, in rabbits, the tail base and the paws appear more effective than the ears. This may be due to excessive compression of the aural vasculature by the clamp holding the probe. A reflectance pulse oximeter sensor is used in either the esophagus, rectum, or applied to the skin surface on the ventral neck overlying the carotid artery.

Thermoregulatory

Hypothermia is common; body temperature measurement is a standard of care during all procedures. It is preferably measured continuously. For measurement of core body temperature, it is necessary to use a temperature probe attached to an esophageal stethoscope.

PERIOPERATIVE SUPPORTIVE CARE

The eyes of rabbits and hares are prominent and care must be taken to prevent corneal injury during positioning. It is important to place ophthalmic ointment at the beginning and during a procedure, and make sure the eyelids are closed.

Cardiovascular

Vascular access is established in physiologically unstable patients and those likely to decompensate from hemorrhage, endotoxemia, and so on, during the perianesthetic period. Catheter placement sites and technique are described above. Catheters should not be placed in the central auricular artery (except for blood pressure monitoring) because of the risk of thrombosis and ischemic necrosis of the ear. Subcutaneous fluid administration is the least appropriate route for correction of deficits or replacement from hemorrhage.

Respiratory

General anesthetics produce ventilatory depression. This effect may be either additive or synergistic with underlying disease, resulting in marked hypercapnia and/or ventilatory arrest. High-inspired oxygen concentrations also decrease ventilatory drive. Ventilation is also affected by body position and compression of the respiratory exchange tissues by distended viscera and/or obesity. Inadvertent compression of the chest by surgeons is common in small patients. Developing good hand position techniques, an attentive anesthe-

tist, and the use of clear plastic drapes helps prevent this. Rabbits have very small chest cavities relative to body size and have a high prevalence of respiratory disease (Fig. 65.2). Additionally, they will often develop tachypnea under anesthesia with a normal to decreased alveolar ventilation.

Adequacy of ventilation is most accurately assessed using P_aCO_2. Visualization of chest wall movement is a deceptive guide to adequacy of ventilation. Consequently, the author recommends either assisted or controlled ventilation of intubated patients under general anesthesia. Capnography is appropriate for indirectly monitoring $PaCO_2$, but the sensor increases mechanical dead space in the breathing system (Fig. 65.11). Doxapram is not recommended for use in hypoventilating patients unless anesthetic reversal, or intubation and mechanical ventilation are impossible or contraindicated.

Thermoregulatory

Minimizing anesthesia time and the use of warm surgical preparation solutions, wrapping the body, increasing the room temperature, and the use external heat sources (i.e., circulating warm water blankets and forced air warmers) reduces hypothermia. Electric heat blankets are not used because they have the potential to cause severe burns. Similarly, heated fluid bags placed in contact with the skin may cause burns.

RECOVERY

Recovery is a critical period during which the patient is placed in a warm, quiet environment and monitored. Supportive care established during anesthesia is continued until the patient is fully alert and stable. In particular, vascular access is maintained to allow emergency administration of drugs and fluids.

The anesthetic drugs used, duration of procedure, and the magnitude of physiologic dysfunction incurred determine duration and quality of recovery. Prolonged recovery is usually due to hypothermia, hypoglycemia, and anesthetic overdose or impaired drug elimination. Care is taken when rewarming an animal that is possibly hypovolemic and/or hypoglycemic, because warming will result in dilation of vasoconstricted peripheral vessels, as well as increase metabolic demand for glucose.

RECOMMENDED ANESTHETIC REGIMENS FOR DOMESTIC RABBITS

Drug dosages for premedication, analgesia, and anesthesia are given in Table 65.1, Table 65.2, and Table 65.3, respectively.

Unpremedicated rabbits can be induced in an anesthetic box with an inhalant (isoflurane or sevoflurane) in oxygen. This technique, however, has been shown

Table 65.3. Drugs used for induction and maintenance of anesthesia in rabbits (and hares)

Drug or Drug Combination	Dosage	Route	Comments	References
Parenteral				
Acepromazine/ ketamine	0.25–1.0/25–40 mg/kg	IM, IV		
Xylazine/ketamine	3–5/20–40 mg/kg	IM, IV	Sometimes marked cardiopulmonary depression. Duration of effect decreased with yohimbine (0.2 mg/kg IV).	Borkowski et al. (1990); Henke et al. (2005); Hobbs et al. (1991); Lipman et al. (1987, 1990); Sanford and Colby (1980)
Diazepam/ketamine	1–5/20–40 mg/kg	IM, IV		
Midazolam/ketamine	1/20–40 mg/kg	IM, IV		
Zolazepam/ tiletamine	5–25 mg/kg	IM, IV	This dosage does not provide complete immobility or surgical anesthesia. Very high dosages associated with nephrotoxicity.	Brammer et al. (1991)
Xylazine/zolazepam/ tiletamine	5/15 mg/kg	IM	Cardiopulmonary depression, surgical anesthesia, prolonged duration of effect.	Popilskis et al. (1991)
Medetomidine/ ketamine	0.5/35 mg/kg	IM, IV	Combined with buprenorphine 0.03 mg/kg, animals intubated, ventilated, and maintained with isoflurane.	Difilippo et al. (2004); Orr et al. (2005)
Propofol	3–6	IV	Produces cardiopulmonary depression depending on rate of administration.	Aeschbacher and Webb (1993a,b)
Alfaxolone	3–6	IV, IM?		
Inhalant				
Halothane	Induction 5%, maintenance 1–2%			
Isoflurane	Induction 5%, maintenance 2–3%			
Sevoflurane	Induction 7–8%, maintenance 3–4%			

to be stressful and to induce moderate hypercapnia and acidemia due to breath holding (Flecknell et al. 1999). Similarly, mask induction of unpremedicated rabbits is not recommended because of struggling. Although sevoflurane is reported to be less noxious in humans, it produced a similar adverse effect as isoflurane in rabbits (Flecknell et al. 1999). It is, therefore, recommended that all rabbits be premedicated before induction. The benzodiazepine midazolam (0.2–0.5 mg/kg IM) provides good sedation and muscle relaxation given 10–15 minutes before induction. For painful procedures, an analgesic is added to midazolam. This author prefers buprenorphine (0.02–0.04 mg/kg IM) because of its duration of effect. Midazolam and buprenorphine together may still not provide adequate immobilization to allow mask induction. Low dose ketamine (5–10 mg/kg) added to other premedication will facilitate handling for mask induction and potentially be additive for analgesia. A nonsteroidal analgesic (e.g., meloxicam) can be added to the premedication when pain is anticipated.

Alternatively, an alpha-2 adrenergic agonist (i.e., xylazine, medetomidine, and dexmedetomidine) can be administered with ketamine for induction. If intra-venous access is available, propofol can be given to effect (Aeschbacher & Webb 1993a, 1993b). Since it does not produce analgesia, a nonsteroidal anti-inflammatory or opioid should be included in the premedication for painful procedures. Propofol (4–6 mg/kg IV) or alfaxolone (4–6 mg/kg IV) can produce marked respiratory depression depending on rate of administration; the rabbit should be intubated after induction, and respiratory support may be required. Anesthesia can then be maintained with an inhalant such as isoflurane in oxygen.

RECOMMENDED ANESTHETIC REGIMENS FOR FREE-LIVING LAGOMORPHS

Inhalation anesthesia is recommended for wild lagomorphs because of rapid induction and recovery. Capture and placement into an induction chamber is relatively easy. Alternatively, the trap can be placed in the chamber or a plastic bag for inhalant anesthetic administration. Where inhalant anesthesia is not feasible, parenteral drug combinations are administered IM or IP (Table 65.3). Drug combinations that include either alpha adrenergic agonists or benzodiazepines are potentially reversible (Table 65.3). In European brown hares (*Lepus europaeus*), medetomidine (0.2 mg/kg IM), combined with either ketamine (30 mg/kg IM) or S(+)-ketamine (15 mg/kg IM), showed only minor advantages to using the latter (Gerritsmann et al. 2012). Surgical anesthesia was not achieved reliably with either protocol and hypoxemia was identified.

The formulation of alfaxolone 2-hydropropyl-beta-cyclodextrin (Alfaxan-CD RTU) (5 mg/kg IM) was used in combination with medetomidine (0.25 mg/kg IM) to induce anesthesia in wild European rabbits (*Oryctolagus cuniculus*) in Australia for surgical implantation of body temperature loggers (Marsh et al. 2009). Anesthesia was maintained with 1.5–3% isoflurane.

REFERENCES

Aeschbacher G, Webb AI. 1993a. Propofol in rabbits: 1. Determination of an induction dose. *Laboratory Animal Science* 43:324–327.

Aeschbacher G, Webb AI. 1993b. Propofol in rabbits: 2. Long-term anesthesia. *Laboratory Animal Science* 43:328–335.

Beyers TM, Richardson JA, Prince MD. 1991. Axonal degeneration and self-mutilation as a complication of the intramuscular use of ketamine and xylazine in rabbits. *Laboratory Animal Science* 41:519–520.

Bjorkman S, Redke F. 2000. Clearance of fentanyl, alfentanil, methohexitone, thiopentone and ketamine in relation to estimated hepatic blood flow in several animal species: application to prediction of clearance in man. *The Journal of Pharmacy and Pharmacology* 52:1065–1074.

Borkowski GL, Danneman PJ, Russell GB, et al. 1990. An evaluation of three intravenous anesthetic regimens in New Zealand rabbits. *Laboratory Animal Science* 40:270–276.

Brammer DW, Doerning BJ, Chrisp CE, et al. 1991. Anesthetic and nephrotoxic effects of Telazol in New Zealand white rabbits. *Laboratory Animal Science* 41:432–435.

Difilippo SM, Norberg PJ, Suson UD, et al. 2004. A comparison of xylazine and medetomidine in an anesthetic combination in New Zealand white rabbits. *Contemporary Topics in Laboratory Animal Science* 43:32–34.

Flecknell PA. 2001. Analgesia of small mammals. *The Veterinary Clinics of North America. Exotic Animal Practice* 4:47–56.

Flecknell PA, Roughan JV, Hendenqvist P. 1999. Induction of anaesthesia with sevoflurane and isoflurane in the rabbit. *Laboratory Animals* 33:41–46.

Gerritsmann H, Stalder GL, Seilern-Moy K, et al. 2012. Comparison of S(+)-ketamine and ketamine, with medetomidine, for field anaesthesia in the European brown hare (*Lepus europaeus*). *Veterinary Anaesthesia and Analgesia* 39(5):511–519.

Ghaffari MS, Moghaddassi AP, Bokaie S. 2009. Effects of intramuscular acepromazine and diazepam on tear production in rabbits. *The Veterinary Record* 164:147–148.

Gil AG, Silván G, Villa A, Illera JD. 2012. Heart and respiratory rates and adrenal response to propofol or alfaxalone in rabbits. *The Veterinary Record* 170:444.

Henke J, Astner S, Brill T, et al. 2005. Comparative study of three intramuscular anaesthetic combinations(medetomidine/ketamine, medetomidine/fentanyl/midazolam and xylazine/ketamine) in rabbits. *Veterinary Anaesthesia and Analgesia* 32: 261–270.

Hobbs BA, Rolhall TG, Sprenkel TL, et al. 1991. Comparison of several combinations for anesthesia in rabbits. *American Journal of Veterinary Research* 52:669–674.

Hughes PJ, Doherty MM, Charman WN. 1993. A rabbit model for the evaluation of epidurally administered local anaesthetic agents. *Anaesthesia and Intensive Care* 21:298–303.

Hurley RJ, Marini RP, Avison DL, et al. 1994. Evaluation of detomidine anesthetic combinations in the rabbit. *Laboratory Animal Science* 44:472–477.

Imai A, Steffey EP, Ilkiw JE, et al. 1999. Comparison of clinical signs and hemodynamic variables used to monitor rabbits during halothane- and isoflurane-induced anesthesia. *American Journal of Veterinary Research* 60:1189–1195.

Liebenberg SP, Linn JM. 1980. Seasonal and sexual influences on rabbit atropinesterase. *Laboratory Animals* 14:297–300.

Lindhardt K, Bagger M, Andreasen KH, et al. 2001. Intranasal bioavailability of buprenorphine in rabbit correlated to sheep and man. *International Journal of Pharmaceutics* 217: 121–126.

Lipman NS, Phillips PA, Newcomer CE. 1987. Reversal of ketamine/xylazine anesthesia in the rabbit with yohimbine. *Laboratory Animal Science* 37:474–477.

Lipman NS, Marini RP, Erdman SE. 1990. A comparison of ketamine/xylazine and ketamine/xylazine/acepromazine anesthesia in the rabbit. *Laboratory Animal Science* 40:395–398.

Marini RP, Xiantang L, Harpster NK, et al. 1999. Cardiovascular pathology possibly associated with ketamine/xylazine anesthesia in Dutch belted rabbits. *Laboratory Animal Science* 49: 153–160.

Marsh MK, McLeod SR, Hansen A, et al. 2009. Induction of anaesthesia in wild rabbits using a new alfaxalone formulation. *The Veterinary Record* 164:122–123.

Mason DE. 1997. Anesthesia, analgesia and sedation for small mammals. In: *Ferrets, Rabbits and Rodents. Clinical Medicine and Surgery* (EV Hillyer, KE Quesenberry, eds.), pp. 378–391. Philadelphia: W.B. Saunders.

Nowak RM. 1999. *Walker's Mammals of the World*, Vol. 2, 6th ed. Baltimore: The Johns Hopkins University Press.

Olson ME, Vizzutti D, Morck DW, et al. 1994. The parasympatholytic effects of atropine sulfate and glycopyrrolate in rats and rabbits. *Canadian Journal of Veterinary Research* 58:254–258.

Orr HE, Roughan JV, Flecknell PA. 2005. Assessment of ketamine and medetomidine anaesthesia in the domestic rabbit. *Veterinary Anaesthesia and Analgesia* 32:271–279.

Pang WW, Kuo CL, Huang HS, et al. 1999. Epidural catheter placement in the rabbit—a novel approach. *Acta Anaesthesiologica Sinica* 37:79–82.

Popilskis SJ, Oz MC, Gorman P, et al. 1991. Comparison of xylazine with tiletamine-zolazepam (Telazol) and xylazine-ketamine anesthesia in rabbits. *Laboratory Animal Science* 41:51–53.

Robertson SA. 2001. Analgesia and analgesic techniques. *The Veterinary Clinics of North America. Exotic Animal Practice* 4: 1–18.

Robertson SA, Eberhart S. 1994. Efficacy of the intranasal route for administration of anesthetic agents to adult rabbits. *Laboratory Animal Science* 44:159–165.

Sanford TD, Colby ED. 1980. Effect of xylazine and ketamine on blood pressure, heart rate and respiratory rate in rabbits. *Laboratory Animal Science* 30:519–523.

Smith JC, Robertson LD, Auhll A, et al. 2004. Endotracheal tube versus laryngeal mask airways in rabbit inhalation anesthesia: ease of use and waste gas emissions. *Contemporary Topics in Laboratory Animal Science* 43:22–25.

Souza MJ, Greenacre CB, Cox SK. 2008. Pharmacokinetics of orally administered tramadol in domestic rabbits (*Oryctolagus cuniculus*). *American Journal of Veterinary Research* 69(8): 979–982.

Taguchi H, Murao K, Nakmura K, et al. 1996. Percutaneous chronic epidural catheterization in the rabbit. *Acta Anaesthesiologica Scandinavica* 40:232–236.

Tran HS, Puc MM, Tran J-LV, et al. 2001. A method of endoscopic endotracheal intubation in rabbits. *Laboratory Animals* 35: 240–252.

Vegfors M, Sjoberg F, Lindberg L-G, et al. 1991. Basic studies of pulse oximetry in a rabbit model. *Acta Anaesthesiologica Scandinavica* 35:596–599.

Wilson DE, Reeder DM, eds. 2005. *Mammal Species of the World. A Taxanomic and Geographic Reference*, Vol. 1, 3rd ed. Baltimore: The Johns Hopkins University Press.

Ypsilantis P, Didilis VN, Politou M, et al. 2005. A comparative study of invasive and oscillometric methods of arterial blood pressure measurement in the anesthetized rabbit. *Research in Veterinary Science* 78:269–275.

66 Rodents

Darryl Heard

INTRODUCTION

Rodentia includes the most living mammalian species, 2277 (Wilson & Reeder 2005). Although usually small (≤200 gms), several are very large (e.g., marmots, *Marmota*; giant squirrels, *Ratufa*; pacas, *Agouti*; maras, *Dolichotis*; capybara, *Hydrochaeris hydrochaeris*; beaver, *Castor*; and porcupines, *Hystrix*). Rodents are common pets and research animals, including the house mouse (*Mus musculus*), rat (*Rattus norvegicus*), chinchilla (*Chinchilla laniger*), Syrian and Siberian hamsters, guinea pig (*Cavia porcellus*), and gerbil. Rodents have four incisors, no canines, and there is a gap between the incisors and the cheek teeth (Nowak 1999). Some have cheek pouches, internal or external, that open near the angle of the mouth (Nowak 1999). During anesthesia, these pouches can be a source of aspirated food material.

CONSEQUENCES OF SMALL BODY SIZE

Schmidt-Nielsen (1984) describes the relationship between body size and vertebrate physiology. As small animals, rodents have high metabolic and oxygen consumption rates, and, therefore, low tolerance to even brief hypoxemia. Irreversible CNS injury occurs within ≤30 seconds of respiratory arrest. Increased oxygen uptake requires increased alveolar ventilation, resulting in more rapid inhalant anesthetic uptake and excretion. High metabolic rates increase the speed of elimination of parenteral drugs. In herbivores, this is enhanced by adaptations for detoxification of chemicals in their food. Consequently, drugs generally have shorter duration of effect than in larger mammals and require higher dosages.

High metabolic rates and small glycogen reserves predispose to hypoglycemia. A small body has a large surface area to volume ratio, and often higher tempera-
ture. Convective heat loss is rapid and hypothermia assured unless supplemental heat is provided. Loss of even small amounts of blood may lead to hemorrhagic shock and death. Airway resistance is inversely related to radius^4; slight changes in diameter (e.g., from edema and mucous accumulation) will have a dramatic effect on respiratory work.

ZOONOTIC DISEASES

Many species harbor pathogens that infect humans (Padovan 2006). For example, deer mice (*Peromyscus maniculatus*) are the reservoir for the virus that causes Hantavirus pulmonary syndrome in people in the southwestern United States (Elliott et al. 1994). Giardia are present in beavers (*Castor* spp.) and capybaras (Thompson 2004). Handling rodents awake is minimized to prevent bites and scratches. The use of physical barriers (i.e., gloves, breathing masks, and biological hazard suits) is based upon the predetermined risk, species, and the procedure.

PHYSICAL RESTRAINT

All rodents bite, including many kept as pets. In an animal of unknown temperament, inhalant anesthesia is an acceptable alternative for physical examination. Care is taken with small rodents to avoid physical restraint in place of adequate analgesia and anesthesia. Large rodents are restrained in squeeze cages (Chapter 8) or remotely injected for drug administration (Chapter 12).

Pet rodents can often be gently picked up in the palm of the hand. Guinea pigs and similar sized rodents are supported under the rump while being held (Fig. 66.1). Some rodents may be grasped at the tail base for

Zoo Animal and Wildlife Immobilization and Anesthesia, Second Edition. Edited by Gary West, Darryl Heard, and Nigel Caulkett.
© 2014 John Wiley & Sons, Inc. Published 2014 by John Wiley & Sons, Inc.

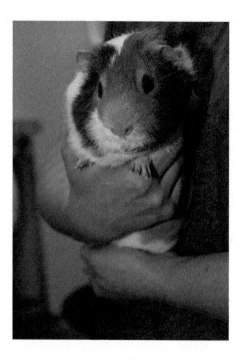

Figure 66.1.　Tame rodents, such as this guinea pig, can be held, but should be supported below the rump.

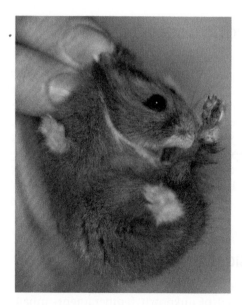

Figure 66.2.　Some rodents (e.g., Siberian hamster) can be restrained by grasping the skin at the nape of the neck. Sufficient skin, however, must be grasped to prevent the animal turning and biting the handler.

transfer from cage to cage. This technique, however, is avoided in animals that shed their tails in response to a threat (e.g., spiny-tailed mice) or are able to turn and bite (Nowak 1999).

Grasping the nape is used to restrain some small rodents. Hamsters and others with loose skin require a very tight grasp to prevent them turning and biting (Fig. 66.2). Small- to medium-sized rodents are

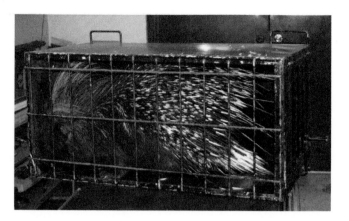

Figure 66.3.　A restraint cage for Southern African crested porcupines developed at the Central Florida Zoo. The cage is metal to prevent the animal chewing. One side has large openings that cause the legs to fall through when the cage is turned. This allows an unprotected leg to be grasped and injected with immobilization drugs. Care must be taken in this species to prevent skin tearing.

restrained with a hand around the neck and the thumb positioned under the jaw to prevent biting. In laboratory animal facilities, mice and other small rodents can be transferred from cage to cage using soft forceps. This technique is also used for small free-living rodents caught in traps. Leather or chain-mail gloves can be used to handle aggressive rodents, but they limit feel and the former do not protect against a direct bite.

Porcupines offer a unique challenge. Although they do not "shoot" their sharp quills, they will back rapidly and with great force into a threat. The quills of New World porcupines have barbs that make their removal very difficult. Additionally, the quills of porcupines may be covered in potentially pathogenic bacteria. They also make remote injection difficult. The author uses a purpose-built restraint box at the Central Florida Zoo to allow drug injection into the leg muscles of Southern African crested porcupines (*Hystrix africaeaustralis*) (Fig. 66.3). The metal box has one side of wire with spaces sufficient to allow legs to drop through when the cage is turned. A leg is then grabbed and injected with a parenteral anesthetic. This porcupine, however, has skin that tears very easily.

PREANESTHETIC PREPARATION

Rodents are primary or obligate nasal breathers and upper respiratory disease is common (e.g., pseudo-odontoma in prairie dogs and mycoplasmosis in rats). The nares are assessed for patency before induction with an inhalant anesthetic and mask. This author does not routinely remove food or water prior to anesthesia. Fasting exhausts glycogen stores. It may also contribute to ileus and pregnancy ketosis in guinea pigs and other herbivores.

PREMEDICATION

Recommended dosages are given in Table 66.1. In rats, atropine sulfate (0.05 mg/kg) and glycopyrrolate (0.5 mg/kg) increased heart rate for 30 and 240 minutes, respectively (Olson et al. 1994). Although both reduce bradycardia in rodents anesthetized with ketamine/alpha-2 adrenergic agonist combinations, glycopyrrolate is more effective in maintaining heart rate within normal range (Olson et al. 1994). Neither glycopyrrolate nor atropine influences respiration rate, core body temperature, or systolic blood pressure alone or combined with injectable anesthetics.

Benzodiazepines provide good sedation and relaxation and are a useful for induction of debilitated patients because of their minimal cardiopulmonary effects. Xylazine, medetomidine, or dexmedetomidine are combined with ketamine to improve muscle relaxation, analgesia, and duration of effect. However, they produce respiratory depression and bradycardia. Interestingly, midazolam may ameliorate the adverse cardiovascular effects of dexmedetomidine in rats (Cornelis et al. 2000). Alpha2-adrenergic agonists are reversed with yohimbine, tolazoline, or atipamezole. Tolazoline (10–50 mg/kg), when compared with yohimbine (1 mg/kg), appeared most effective and safe for the reversal of xylazine/ketamine anesthesia in rats (Komulainen &

Olson 1991). In rats, yohimbine (20 mg/kg IP) produced a high (22%) mortality.

ANALGESIA

The principles and techniques for rodent analgesia are reviewed by Machin (Chapter 7), Flecknell (2001) and Robertson (2001). The two main groups of analgesic premedicants, opioids and nonsteroidal anti-inflammatory drugs (NSAIDs), are combined or used alone. Even low dosage ketamine provides analgesia and is worthwhile including, for this reason, in some anesthetic regimens (Robertson 2001). Local and regional anesthesia (see below) also has the potential to further enhance analgesia. Tramadol is an additional analgesic that can be used in the perianesthetic period, but only oral or compounded formulations are available in North America. Effective drug dosages are still to be determined for many species. Recommended dosages for analgesics are given in Table 66.2.

LOCAL AND REGIONAL ANESTHESIA

Many large captive species (e.g., guinea pig) are amenable to local and epidural anesthesia for minor and occasionally major (e.g., Cesarean section) procedures,

Table 66.1.   Drugs used for premedication in rodents

Drug	Rat	Mouse	Gerbil	Hamster	Guinea Pig, Chinchilla, and Prairie Dog	Beaver, Capybara, and Porcupine
Acepromazine	0.5–2.5 IM IP	0.5–2.5 IP	Not recommended	0.5–2.5 IM IP	0.5–2.5 IM	0.1 IM
Diazepam	3–5 IP PO	3–5 IM IP PO	3–5 IP PO	3–5 IP PO	1–2.5 IM IP PO	0.1–1.0 IM PO
Midazolam	1–2 IP	1–2 IM IP	1–2 IP	1–2 IP	1–2 IM IP	0.1–0.5 IM
Xylazine	10–15 IP	10–15 IP	5–10 IP	5–10 IP	5–10 IP SC	1–5 IM SC
Atropine	0.05 SC IM	0.05 SC IM	0.05 SC IM	0.05 SC IM	0.05 SC IM	0.03 SC IM
Glycopyrrolate	0.01–0.02 SC IM	0.01–0.02 SC IM	0.01–0.02 SC IM	0.01–0.02 SC IM	0.01–0.02 SC IM	0.01 SC IM

Notes: Use lower dosages for debilitated, geriatric, or obese animals and for those that are relatively large for the species.
Acepromazine is not recommended for use in gerbils because it may lower the seizure threshold.
Source: Flecknell (1991) and Mason (1997).

Table 66.2.   Suggested analgesic dosages for rodents

Analgesic	Rat	Mouse, Gerbil, and Hamster	Chinchilla, Guinea Pig, and Prairie Dog	Beaver, Capybara, and Porcupine
Buprenorphine	0.01–0.05 IM, SC q 8–12h	0.05–0.1 SC q 6–12h	0.05 IM, SC q 6–12h	0.01–0.03 IM, SC q 8–12h
Butorphanol	2 IM, SC q 2–4h	1–5 SC q 4h	2 IM, SC q 4h	0.5 IM, SC q 4h
Carprofen	5 IM, SC, PO q 24h	5 SC q 12h	4 IM, SC q 24h	
Flunixin	2.5 IM, SC q 12h	2.5 SC q 12h	2.5 IM, SC q 12–24h	0.5 IM, SC q 12–24h
Ketoprofen	5 IM, SC, PO q 24h	?	?	1–3 IM, SC q 24h
Meloxicam	0.5–2 IM, SC, PO q 24h	1–2 SC PO q 12h	0.5 SC PO q 12h	0.1–0.3 SC PO q 12–24h
Meperidine	10–20 IM, SC q 2–3h	10–20 SC q 2–3h	10–20 IM, SC q 2–4h	
Morphine	2–5 IM, SC q 4h	2–5 SC q 4h	2–5 IM, SC q 4h	1–3 IM, SC q 4–6h
Oxymorphone	0.2–0.5 IM, SC q 6–12h	0.2–0.5 SC q 6–12h	0.2–0.5 IM, SC q 6–12h	0.1 IM, SC q 6–12h
Tramadol	?	?	2–5 PO, 12–24h	0.5–5 PO, q 12–24h

Source: Flecknell (1991, 2001) and Mason (1997).

Table 66.3. Parenteral anesthetic regimens and dosages (mg/kg) for representative rodents

Species	Ketamine/ Acepromazine	Ketamine/ Xylazine	Ketamine/ Medetomidine	Ketamine/ Midazolam	Tiletamine/ Zolazepam	Propofol
Mouse	50–150/2.5–5.0 IP	50–200/5–10 IP		40–150/3–5 IP	50–80 IP	NA
Hamster	50–150/2.5–5.0 IP	50–150/5–10 IP		50–150/5 IP	50–80 IP	NA
Gerbil	NA	50–70/2–3 IP		40–150/3–5 IP	50–80 IP	NA
Rat	50–150/2.5–5.0 IP IV	40–90/5 IP		40–100/3–5 IP IV	50–80 IP IV	10 IV
Guinea pig and chinchilla	20–50/0.5–1.0 IP IV	20–40/3–5 IP IV	5/0.06 IM (Henke et al. 2004)	20–50/3–5 IP IV	20–40 IP IV	10 IV
Beaver, capybara, and porcupine		5–10/1–2 IM	3–4/0.03–0.04 IM IV		4–6 IM IV	6–8 IV

Note: Use the lower dosages for debilitated animals and for intravenous injection.
Source: Adapted, in part, from Flecknell (1991) and Mason (1997).

respectively (Eisele et al. 1994). Most local anesthetics have a low therapeutic index (particularly the long-acting drugs, such as bupivicaine) and commercial preparations usually contain drug concentrations suitable for humans. Consequently, great care must be taken to calculate and prepare appropriate volumes of local anesthetic for infiltration.

PARENTERAL ANESTHESIA

Small- to medium-sized rodents are preferably induced and maintained with an inhalant anesthetic (see later). Parenteral anesthetic regimens are used where inhalant anesthesia is not available (e.g., for field immobilizations), to reduce inhalant anesthetic pollution, to enhance analgesia, to facilitate mask induction with an inhalant, and for convenience in research facilities. Representative parenteral anesthetic regimens and dosages are described in Table 66.3.

Most published anesthetic regimens are designed for research animals. Unfortunately, the dosages and drugs are often not compatible with clinical practice or fieldwork. They also assume animals are young and healthy. Conversely, there are many excellent studies of the effects of parenteral anesthetics in rodent models.

Drug Administration

Injection routes include subcutaneous (SC), intramuscular (IM), intraperitoneal (IP), intravenous (IV), and intraosseous (IO). Potentially irritant solutions (e.g., high or low pH solutions) should not be administered SC or IM, because of the risk of self-mutilation (Gaertner et al. 1987; Leash et al. 1973). Diluting the solution, avoiding large volume injections, and injecting in the proximal muscles of the legs reduce the risk of developing this adverse effect. Alternatively, drugs are administered by IP injection. Large rodents are enclosed in squeeze cages (Fig. 66.3) or administered drugs using a remote injection system.

Vascular Access

Small size makes venous and intraosseous catheterization difficult, but practice and attention to technique enable attainment of these essential skills. Potential catheterization sites include the cephalic, saphenous, and auricular veins. The lateral coccygeal veins can be accessed in rats with small-gauge needles. Penetration of the skin before placement, with either a hypodermic needle or scalpel blade, is done to prevent catheter buckling. Intraosseous catheterization using 18- to 22-gauge spinal needles can be performed at the proximal femur (via the trochanteric fossa), tibia (tibial crest), and humerus.

Venipuncture and Blood Collection

Depending on size and species, blood samples can be collected in clinical cases from the jugular, cephalic, saphenous (Hem et al. 1998), femoral, perineal (agoutis and related species), and lateral coccygeal veins. The cranial vena cava, femoral artery, and ventral coccygeal vessels are alternative sites in some species. The heart and retro-bulbar sinus are used in research species, but are not recommended for clinical patients.

For collection of blood from the saphenous vein, the rodent can be placed head first into a plastic tube for restraint (Hem et al. 1998). The hair over the proximal tarsus is gently clipped to allow visualization of the vessel, and microhematocrit tubes are used to collect blood from small rodents (Hem et al. 1998).

The restraint tube can also be used to facilitate blood collection from lateral coccygeal veins in rats. The major problem with the use of these vessels is ensuring an adequate blood flow (Conybeare et al. 1988). One technique is to briefly warm the tail by immersion in a water bath (up to 45°C). This causes a local vasodilation. Prolonged vasodilatation can be achieved by using a heating lamp placed above the rodent cage, but a major disadvantage is the lack of temperature control and the danger of burns. Instead, controlled warming of the total environment of the rat or mouse to temperatures around 40°C, a large blood flow through the tail makes it possible to collect blood from the lateral caudal vein (Conybeare et al. 1988).

Parenteral Anesthetics

Some rodents (e.g., guinea pigs) have limb movement at ketamine or tiletamine/zolazepam dosages expected to produce surgical anesthesia. Ketamine (44 mg/kg) takes 8–10 minutes for induction and has a very short duration of effect (15–20 minutes) (Weisbroth & Fudens 1972). Ketamine and ketamine/xylazine may be associated with self-mutilation (Gaertner et al. 1987).

Xylazine and other alpha-2 adrenergic agonists are frequently combined with ketamine for short-term immobilization and surgical anesthesia. These combinations, however, produce mild to severe dose-dependent hypotension, bradyarrhythmias and respiratory depression (Hart et al. 1984; Wixson et al. 1987). Oxygen supplementation and assisted ventilation is recommended. Ketamine/benzodiazepine combinations produce less cardiopulmonary depression and analgesia, but good muscle relaxation.

In rats and mice, acute reversible lens opacity has been observed with xylazine and xylazine/ketamine (Calderone et al. 1986). These "cataracts" were associated to a varying degree with proptosis, obtunded blink response, corneal surface drying, and mydriasis. Reversible lens opacity due to dehydration has been observed by this author.

Although moderately effective for minor surgery in rats and gerbils, very high tiletamine/zolazepam dosages are required to prevent response to noxious stimuli in other species (i.e., mice, hamsters, and guinea pigs) (Silverman et al. 1983).

Propofol is used for induction and maintenance of anesthesia when administered as a continuous IV infusion or intermittent bolus. The propofol can be diluted with saline for injection in very small patients. Apnea is related to dose, rate of injection, and the presence of other drugs. The induction dose is dependent upon rate of administration (Larsson & Wahlström 1994). In rats, both fast (20 mg/kg/min) and slow (2.5 mg/kg/min) rates result in larger doses than those at an intermediate rate (10 mg/kg/min). Propofol is a poor analgesic. It is indicated for induction of healthy rodents in which vascular access can be attained.

Alfaxalone is a potent steroid hypnotic agent whose poor water solubility prompted the development of a 2-hydroxypropyl-β-cyclodextrin (HPβCD) formulation. It is similar to propofol, but can also be given intramuscularly. Large injection volume and cost usually precludes its use by the latter route in larger rodents. Alfaxalone is more readily eliminated from males than female due to differential clearance (Brewster et al. 1996). This can result in faster recovery for males. In rats, alfaxalone (10 mg/kg IP) was not analgesic and did not potentiate the antinociception of opioids (Winter et al. 2003).

INHALATION ANESTHESIA

Inhalation anesthesia is the primary component of most, if not all, clinical anesthetic regimens.

Inhalant Anesthetics

Isoflurane is associated with rapid induction and recovery, and rapid control of anesthetic depth. It produces a dose-dependent cardiopulmonary depression, does not sensitize the myocardium to catecholamine-induced arrhythmias, and is a poor analgesic (Imai et al. 1999). Sevoflurane is similar to isoflurane, except it produces even more rapid induction and recovery.

Inhalant Induction

For induction, inhalant anesthesia is used alone or as an adjunct to parenteral drugs. The anesthetic is administered into a chamber or through a mask. The advantage of an induction chamber is the animal is not manually restrained during the involuntary excitement phase of induction. This reduces injury to handler and patient. The disadvantages include greater potential for environmental contamination with inhalation anesthetic and difficulty in monitoring.

Mask induction of manually restrained animals, without premedication and supplemental injectable anesthesia, is not recommended. Anesthetic chambers and masks are opaque to allow visualization of the patient. Chambers can be made from commercial plastic containers and sized to the animal (Fig. 66.4). The chamber top should be able to be secured to prevent the animal forcibly opening it and escaping. For induction of an awake or lightly sedated animal, inhalant anesthetic is introduced into the container through one opening, and waste gas removed from another opening. The vaporizer is set at maximum

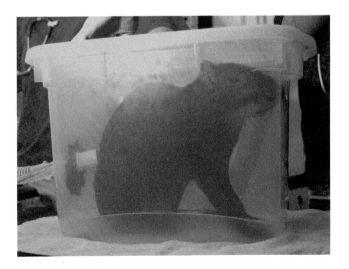

Figure 66.4. Small- to medium-sized rodents (e.g., agouti) can be induced with inhalant anesthetics administered into a chamber. These induction chambers can be made from commercially available plastic boxes that should be opaque and have a secure top.

concentration, and oxygen flow rate set at 2–4 L/min depending upon the size of the container. It will take a period of time for the concentration in the induction chamber to equilibrate with the vaporizer setting. The animal loses its righting response in 5–10 minutes and is removed from the chamber. A mask is placed over its nose and mouth, and the chamber is removed outside or closed to allow waste gases to be safely voided to the atmosphere. The animal is then either maintained using the mask or intubated when it is sufficiently relaxed.

When maintaining anesthesia with a mask, it is important to have the animal's head and neck in extension to facilitate air movement. Respiratory pattern, rate, and noise should also be assessed to ensure minimum resistance to breathing. If the animal appears to be having respiratory difficulty, move the head and neck to see whether the obstruction can be corrected. If not, use cotton tipped applicators to clear the oropharynx and nares. If this fails to relieve the problem, intubate or wake the animal and cancel the procedure.

Equipment

Small size is an indication for a nonrebreathing system for administration of inhalant anesthetics. T-piece breathing systems are recommended for the smallest. Rebreathing bags can be constructed from small balloons to facilitate visualization of respiratory movement. Fresh gas flow rate for nonrebreathing systems is about 200 mL/kg/min.

Inhalation anesthesia is often maintained with a mask connected to the breathing system. Systems have been developed for small rodents that also allow concurrent scavenging of waste anesthetic gases (Levy et al. 1980; Mauderly 1975). These usually include the fresh gas line entering the mask and an exit line for removal of waste gases.

Endotracheal Intubation

Respiratory obstruction and hypoventilation are common limitations to diagnostic and surgical procedures. With practice and the use of appropriate technique and equipment, intubation should be a routine standard of care in some rodents.

There are a variety of commercially available endotracheal tubes; the smallest cuffed and uncuffed tubes have a 3- and 1-mm internal diameter (ID), respectively. Guidelines for endotracheal tube size are given in Table 66.4. Endotracheal tubes are preferably opaque for visualization of condensation or occlusion with mucous or blood. For the smallest patients, endotracheal tubes are constructed from over-the-needle catheters or urinary catheters.

Guinea pigs present many obstacles to routine intubation. Their cheek pouches frequently contain stored food and they readily regurgitate if the oropharynx is stimulated. They produce profuse salivary secretions that can be controlled, in part, by glycopyrrolate. The soft tissue at the base of the tongue is readily traumatized by a laryngoscope blade resulting in profuse hemorrhage. The soft palate is fused to the base of the tongue, and entry to the glottis is through the small opening of the palatal ostium (Timm et al. 1987). The palatal ostium is also present in chinchillas and capybaras, and probably other hystericomorph rodents. The glottis is also very small relative to the size of the animal. For these reasons, this author rarely intubates guinea pigs, but has had success using a blind technique. However, other authors describe intubation of dorsally recumbent animals using direct visualization techniques with modified pediatric # 0 blades and 14-gauge over-the-needle catheters (Kujime & Natelson 1981).

Rat intubation usually involves direct visualization of the glottis. It requires magnification and a focused light source (e.g., rigid endoscope). One technique describes transillumination with a high intensity light source in contact with the skin surface in front of the neck near the pharyngoepiglottic region (Yasaki & Dyck 1991). This author uses a rigid endoscope or an otoscope attached to a # 2 ear speculum that has had the distal two-thirds of the tip along the right side removed (Tran & Lawson 1986). The rat is positioned in dorsal recumbency on a board. An elastic band is then affixed to the upper incisors and fastened to the board to extend the head and neck. The tongue is pulled forward and to the side, and a cotton-tipped applicator is used to clear any secretions from around the glottis. Topical application of local anesthetic on the glottis will reduce laryngospasm. A slight pressure exerted on the ventral surface of the neck may further facilitate visualization of the glottis. A blind technique, similar to that described above for other rodents, has also been reported (Stark et al. 1981).

Endotracheal tubes for rats are constructed from 14- to 16-gauge over-the-needle catheters. The needle stylette is cut to the same length as the catheter, and the end is then filed smooth so that the smoothed needle is approximately 1-mm shorter than the cath-

Table 66.4. Guidelines for endotracheal tube size selection in rodents

Species	Endotracheal tube internal diameter (mm)
Rat	16- to 18-gauge over-the-needle catheter
Guinea pig, chinchilla	14- to 16-gauge over-the-needle catheter, ≤2
Hamster	16-gauge over-the-needle catheter
Eastern Gray Squirrel	≤2
Prairie dog	2.0–2.5
Capybara	6.0

eter (Stark et al. 1981). Alternatively, a 70-mm length of malleable 20-gauge wire is used as a stylette (Tran & Lawson 1986). At 1.5 cm from the end of the catheter, the stylette is bent at a 30° angle. A surgical suture can be tied to the catheter at a point 4.5 cm from its end to prevent excessive insertion of the catheter into the trachea. Mucous obstruction is common and changing the tube may be necessary. This technique can also be used for hamsters.

Prairie dogs, chinchillas, squirrels, and other medium to moderately large rodents (e.g., African pouched rats, and maras) can routinely be intubated for inhalation anesthesia using a blind technique. The anesthetized rodent is laid in lateral recumbency, with the head and neck moderately extended. The tube is then passed in a similar manner to that described for the rabbit (Chapter 65). Alternatively, an endotracheal tube can be placed with the assistance of an endoscope. The tube is placed over the scope or alongside it (Fig. 66.5 and Fig. 66.6).

When in doubt, remove the endotracheal tube and reassess placement. The use of a pulse oximeter is invaluable for determining potential oxygenation problems due to airway obstruction. Correct endotracheal tube placement is determined by: (1) visualizing condensation on either the inside of the endotracheal tube or a metal surface placed at the end of the tube; (2) detecting air movement with hair placed in front of the tube; (3) watching the nonrebreathing bag; (4) the response to intubation (coughing etc.); and (5) the

detection of exhaled carbon dioxide on a capnograph. To insure the tube has not been placed into a single bronchus, premeasure the tube before use, and auscultate both lung fields for respiratory sounds after intubation.

MONITORING

Monitoring is described in Chapter 3. It is recommended that a trained person be assigned as anesthetist for each patient. This facilitates monitoring, recording, and supportive care, and saves time when intervention is required.

Unconsciousness is based on anesthetic dose and vaporizer setting, muscle relaxation, decreased reflex activity, and absence of limb and body movement. Palpebral and corneal reflexes are observed at 0.8 minimum alveolar concentration (MAC), but are abolished at >2.0 MAC (Imai et al. 1999). The corneal reflex, however, is a poor guide to anesthetic depth (Imai et al. 1999). A fixed dilated pupil, unresponsive to light, is a cross-species indicator of excessive depth. Anal tone is retained until deep anesthetic levels, but is difficult to assess in small rodents.

Pain and nociceptor responses are assessed with a toe, ear, and tail pinch, or a skin incision. Increasing depth is assumed when muscle tone (e.g., jaw muscle and anal sphincter) decreases, palpebral and corneal reflexes are obtunded, and respiration pattern becomes regular and even. Sudden tachycardia, hypertension, or

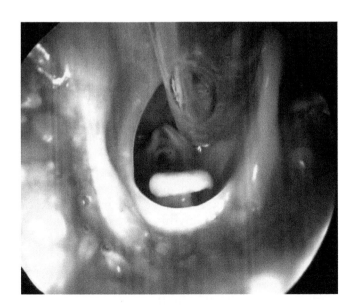

Figure 66.5.   For endotracheal intubation of chinchillas and other medium to large rodents the glottis can be visualized with an endoscope.

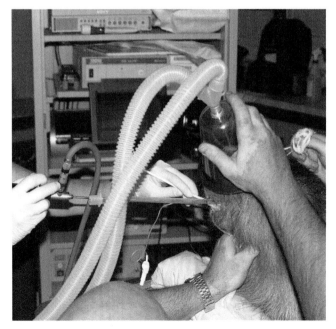

Figure 66.6.   Although large, capybaras are difficult to intubate. In this animal, an endoscope is being placed directly into the glottis of an anesthetized animal, and the endotracheal tube is then slid off the endoscope.

tachypnea in response to stimuli is indicative of inadequate anesthetic depth or analgesia.

Rodent heart rates are determined by temperature, size, metabolism, respiratory state, and the presence or absence of painful stimuli. Heart rate is inversely related to body size. The resting heart rate for mammals is calculated from the allometric equation $241 \times M_b^{-0.25}$, where M_b = bodyweight (kg) (Schmidt-Nielsen 1984). A heart rate 20% above or below the calculated rate for an individual is considered either tachycardic or bradycardic, respectively.

The esophageal stethoscope is not practical to use in small rodents, and it may induce regurgitation in guinea pigs. Alternatively, a quality pediatric stethoscope is used. The electrocardiograph should have a multichannel oscilloscope with nonfade tracing and freeze capabilities. Additionally, it must be able to record at speeds of 100 mm/s and amplify the signal to at least 1 mV equal to 1 cm. Standard lead positions are used.

The Doppler flow detector is used anywhere there are major arteries close to the skin. These include the ventral aspect of the tail base, the carotid, femoral, and auricular arteries, and directly over the heart. Potential sites for indirect blood pressure measurement include the legs, forearms, tail, and ears. Indirect blood pressure measurement techniques have been designed and validated for use in rats (e.g., Ibrahim et al. 2006; Widdop & Li 1997).

As with cardiac auscultation, evaluation of the respiratory system requires a good quality stethoscope with appropriate head and length of tubing, and an experienced ear. Pulse oximetry has been evaluated in rats, and appears accurate at hemoglobin saturation levels greater than 70% (Decker et al. 1989). Potential sites for placement of transmission pulse oximeter sensors include the ear, tongue, buccal mucosa, paw, vulva, prepuce, and proximal tail (Decker et al. 1989). A reflectance pulse oximeter sensor is used in either the esophagus or the rectum or applied to the skin/fur surface on the ventral aspect of neck overlying the carotid artery (rat).

Hypothermia is common in anesthetized rodents because of the large surface area-to-volume ratio. Additionally, many anesthetics suppress normal thermoregulatory mechanisms. Further, anesthetic gases are of low humidity and temperature. Body temperature is preferably measured continuously, and the thermometer should be sufficiently small to be used in small patients. For measurement of core body temperature, it is necessary to use a temperature probe attached to an esophageal stethoscope.

SUPPORTIVE CARE

Vascular access is discussed earlier. The cephalic vein is able to be catheterized in medium to large rodents (Fig.

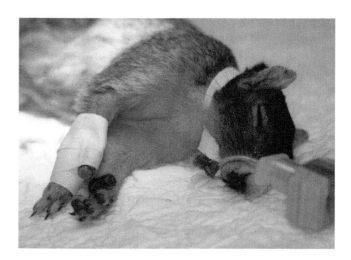

Figure 66.7.   An anesthetized fox squirrel. The animal was intubated with an uncuffed 2-mm ID tube using a blind technique. A capnograph is used to assess correct placement. A 24-gauge over-the-needle has been placed in the cephalic vein for fluid administration. A pediatric stethoscope is being used to monitor heart rate.

66.7). Small volume infusors are essential for accurate fluid infusion in small patients. Some can be preprogrammed to flow rates for emergency and other drugs, so that all that is necessary for administration is to enter the bodyweight of the animal. They also allow a continuous infusion, which is preferable to bolus injection.

General anesthetics usually produce a dose-dependent ventilatory depression. This effect may be either additive or synergistic, with underlying disease resulting in marked hypercapnia and/or ventilatory arrest. High-inspired oxygen concentrations also decrease ventilatory drive. Ventilation is also affected by body position and compression of the respiratory exchange tissues by distended viscera and/or obesity. Inadvertent compression of the chest by surgeons is common in small exotic patients. Developing good hand position techniques, an attentive anesthetist, and the use of clear plastic drapes helps prevent this cause of hypoventilation.

Guinea pigs have relatively small-diameter tracheas, and are prone to airway obstruction because of regurgitation and profuse salivary secretions. Adequacy of ventilation is most accurately assessed using P_aCO_2. Capnography provides an indirect estimate of P_aCO_2 (Fig. 66.6), but is too inaccurate in most small exotic patients to be used for anything other than validation of successful endotracheal intubation. Visualization of chest wall movement is a deceptive guide to adequacy of ventilation. Consequently, the author recommends either assisted or controlled ventilation of intubated patients under general anesthesia. Doxapram is not recommended for use in hypoventilating patients unless intubation and mechanical ventilation is impossible or contraindicated.

Ventilation is either assisted or controlled by positive pressure either manually or mechanically. Many of the ventilators used in small animal anesthesia can be modified to ventilate rodents. A commercially available combination ventilator and anesthesia machine (Anesthesia WorkStation, Halowell EMC, Pittsfield, MA) has been designed for research rodents. It is both a circle system for delivery of inhalant anesthetic and an optional ventilator with an adjustable pressure safety limit. The advantage of mechanical ventilation is that it frees the anesthetist to concentrate on other tasks. The disadvantages are that mechanical ventilators require a thorough theoretical and technical understanding for their safe use, they require endotracheal intubation, and they produce positive intrathoracic pressures that interfere with venous return to the heart and may cause lung trauma.

Manual ventilation provides the advantage, with a skilled anesthetist, of rapidly adjusting ventilatory pressures and volumes, and responsiveness to the surgeon who may require brief irregular periods of ventilatory arrest to safely complete a procedure. Further research is necessary to evaluate the efficacy and appropriateness of ventilation techniques in small mammal practice. There may be situations where some hypoventilation is preferable to the adverse effects of positive pressure ventilation.

Administration of elevated inspired oxygen concentrations (>40%) will often overcome mild to moderate hypoxemia, assuming no major pulmonary shunting is present. Although mammals are susceptible to pulmonary oxygen toxicity, this syndrome is unlikely to be observed in patients maintained on high-inspired oxygen concentrations for 24 hours.

Minimizing anesthesia time and the use of warm surgical preparation solutions, wrapping the body, increasing the room temperature, and the use external heat sources (i.e., circulating warm water blankets and forced air warmers) reduces hypothermia. Electric heat blankets are not used because they have the potential to cause severe burns. Similarly, heated fluid bags placed in contact with the skin may cause burns. If endotracheal intubation is not possible, an indirect ventilation technique using a bulb inflator placed over the nose has been used in small rodents (Ingall & Hasenpusch 1966).

RECOVERY

The patient is placed in a warm, quiet environment and monitored. Supportive care is continued until the patient is fully alert and physiologically stable. Vascular access is maintained to allow emergency administration of drugs and fluids. Drugs, procedure duration, and the magnitude of physiologic dysfunction incurred determine duration and quality of recovery. Prolonged recovery is usually due to hypothermia, hypoglycemia,

and anesthetic overdose and/or impaired drug elimination. Rewarming will exacerbate underlying hypovolemia and hypoglycemia.

ANESTHETIC REGIMENS FOR SMALL DOMESTIC RODENTS

Drug dosages are given in Table 66.1, Table 66.2, and Table 66.3. Most anesthetic regimens for clinical patients are based around an inhalant anesthetic (i.e., isoflurane or sevoflurane). Endotracheal intubation, as discussed previously, is difficult in many pet rodent species. Premedication with glycopyrrolate is recommended in guinea pigs and other rodents that have profuse salivary secretions. Although small rodents can be induced either in an anesthetic induction box or by mask using an inhalant, it is recommended the animals be premedicated.

The benzodiazepines (i.e., midazolam and diazepam) are relatively safe, reduce response to handling, provide muscle relaxation, and decrease inhalant and other anesthetic requirements. They do not, however, provide any analgesia. Midazolam can be combined with a relatively low dose ketamine. The ketamine provides some analgesia. Alpha-2-adrenergic agonists (i.e., xylazine, medetomidine, dexmedetomidine, and detomidine) have the advantage of being able to reversed by yohimbine, tolazoline, or atipamezole, as well as improved analgesia, but also produce more to sometimes severe cardiopulmonary depression.

Analgesics should always be included for painful procedures. Assuming good hydration, this author will combine an NSAID (i.e., meloxicam) in the initial premedication, as well as an opioid. Analgesics work best when given before the onset of nociception and pain. Although only a partial μ-opioid agonist, buprenorphine has a relatively prolonged duration of effect. Morphine or hydromorphone can also be used for severe pain. Tramadol and meloxicam be administered orally before and after a procedure, as well as at home.

ANESTHETIC REGIMENS FOR FREE-LIVING RODENTS

Capture techniques for free-living, primarily small rodents are well described by Barnett and Dutton (1995). The anesthetic techniques described for small captive rodents based on inhalant anesthetics will also work for the wild species. Where inhalant anesthetics are not available or impractical, then parenteral anesthetic protocols are required (Table 66.3).

Capybara

The largest living rodent, the capybara, weighs approximately 35–65 kg. Their large size and robust incisors make them difficult and dangerous to immobilize. They are also well adapted to aquatic systems, and will retreat to water when threatened. They can hide immersed with just their nares breaking the surface under floating vegetation. It is imperative, therefore, to capture free-living animals away from water, and prevent their escape. Capybaras have been captured by lassoing, as well as darting, from horseback (Salas et al. 2004). Alternatively, they can be trapped in baited traps or corrals. Both techniques require dry area for capture.

In one study in capybaras, ketamine (10.0 mg/kg) and xylazine (0.5 mg/kg) provided the best immobilization and analgesia in comparison with tiletamine-zolazepam (5.0 mg/kg), and tiletamine-zolazepam (5.0 mg/kg) and levomepromazine (0.5 mg/kg) (Nishiyama et al. 2006). Drugs were administered intramuscularly using darts delivered by a blowgun. The tiletamine-zolazepam combination allowed approximately 1 hour immobilization for procedures where intense analgesia is not necessary. The addition of levomepromazine improved analgesia and muscular relaxation, as well as the duration of anesthesia and recovery time.

In another study in capybaras, an intramuscular combination of tiletamine:zolazepam (1.5 mg/kg), medetomidine (0.0075 mg/kg), and butorphanol (0.075 mg/kg) was preferable to tiletamine:zolazepam alone or combined with medetomidine (King et al. 2010) for immobilization. This combination provided adequate analgesia for intraperitoneal implantation of radio transmitters.

Beaver

The Eurasian (*Castor fiber*) and North American (*Castor canadensis*) beavers are the second largest rodents. Similar to capybaras, they are robust and potentially dangerous, and agile in water. Consequently, some form of physical or chemical immobilization is required for safe handling of these species.

Ketamine alone (10–15 mg/kg IM) successfully immobilized beaver for handling (Lancia et al. 1978). Inhalant anesthesia (halothane) following immobilization with a combination of ketamine (25 mg/kg IM) and diazepam (0.1 mg/kg IM) was safe and effective for handling and surgery for intraperitoneal implantation of radio transmitters in North American beavers (Greene et al. 1991). Anesthesia was maintained with halothane in oxygen via a semiclosed circle anesthetic circuit. Throughout the surgical procedure, all beavers had mean arterial pressure less than 60 mmHg and esophageal temperature less than 35°C. Respiratory acidemia was observed in spontaneously ventilating beavers, but not in beavers maintained with controlled ventilation.

In another study comparing anesthetic regimens for intraperitoneal implantation of radio transmitters in European beavers (*Cas. fiber*), a combination of medetomidine (0.05 mg/kg), ketamine (5 mg/kg), butorphanol (0.1 mg/kg), and midazolam (0.25 mg/kg) was preferred (Ranheim et al. 2004).

Alternatively, isoflurane or sevoflurane alone was used for surgical anesthesia in North American beavers (Breck & Gaynor 2003). After placement in a burlap bag, a mask was placed over the nose of the beaver through the bag and the inhalant anesthetic administered at the highest vaporizer setting until the animals became relaxed. The animals were not intubated.

REFERENCES

Barnett A, Dutton J. 1995. *Expedition Field Techniques: Small Mammals (Excluding Bats)*, 2nd ed. London: Expedition Advisory Centre.

Breck SW, Gaynor JS. 2003. Comparison of isoflurane and sevoflurane for anesthesia in beaver. *Journal of Wildlife Diseases* 39: 387–392.

Brewster ME, Anderson WR, Webb A, Bodor N, Pop E. 1996. Anesthetic activity and pharmacokinetics of the neurosteroid alfaxalone formulated in 2-hydroxypropyl-β-cyclodextrin in the rat. Proceedings of the Eighth International Symposium on Cyclodextrins, pp. 499–502.

Calderone L, Grimes P, Shalev M. 1986. Acute reversible cataract formation induced by xylazine and by ketamine-xylazine anesthesia in rats and mice. *Experimental Eye Research* 42:331–337.

Conybeare G, Leslie GB, Angles K, Barrett RJ, Luke JSH, Gask DR. 1988. An improved simple technique for the collection of blood samples from rats and mice. *Laboratory Animals* 22:177–182.

Cornelis JJGB, Vogelaar JPW, Tang J-P, Mandema JW. 2000. Quantification of pharmacodynamic interactions between dexmedetomidine and midazolam in the rat. *The Journal of Pharmacology and Experimental Therapeutics* 294:347–355.

Decker MJ, Conrad KP, Strohl KP. 1989. Noninvasive oximetry in the rat. *Biomedical Instrumentation and Technology* 23:222–228.

Eisele P, Kaaekuahiwi MA, Canfield DR, Golub MS, Eisele JH Jr. 1994. Epidural catheter placement for testing of obstetrical analgesics in female guinea pigs. *Laboratory Animal Science* 44: 486–490.

Elliott LH, Ksiazek TG, Rollin PE, Spiropoulou CF, Morzunov S, Monroe M, Goldsmith CS, Humphrey CD, Zaki SR, Krebs JW, et al. 1994. Isolation of the causative agent of hantavirus pulmonary syndrome. *American Journal of Tropical Medicine and Hygiene* 51:102–108.

Flecknell PA. 1991. Anaesthesia and post-operative care of small mammals. *In Practice* 13:180–189.

Flecknell PA. 2001. Analgesia of small mammals. *The Veterinary Clinics of North America. Exotic Animal Practice* 4:47–56.

Gaertner DJ, Boschert KR, Schoeb TR. 1987. Muscle necrosis in Syrian hamsters resulting from intramuscular injections of ketamine and xylazine. *Laboratory Animal Science* 37:80–83.

Greene SA, Keegan RD, Gallagher LV, Alexander JE, Harari J. 1991. Cardiovascular effects of halothane anesthesia after diazepam and ketamine administration in beavers (*Castor canadensis*) during spontaneous or controlled ventilation. *American Journal of Veterinary Research* 52:665–668.

Hart MV, Rowles JR, Hohimer AR, Morton MJ, Hosenpud JD. 1984. Hemodynamics in the guinea pig after anesthetization with ketamine/xylazine. *American Journal of Veterinary Research* 45:2328–2330.

Hem A, Smith AJ, Solberg P. 1998. Saphenous vein puncture for blood sampling of the mouse, rat, hamster, gerbil, guineapig, ferret and mink. *Laboratory Animals* 32:364–368.

Henke J, Baumgartner C, Roltgen I, Eberspacher E, Erhardt W. 2004. Anaesthesia with midazolam/medetomidine/fentanyl in chinchillas (*Chinchilla lanigera*) compared to anaesthesia with xylazine/ketamine and medetomidine/ketamine. *Journal of Veterinary Medicine. A, Physiology, Pathology, Clinical Medicine* 51: 259–264.

Ibrahim J, Berk BC, Hughes AD. 2006. Comparison of simultaneous measurements of blood pressure by tail-cuff and carotid arterial methods in conscious spontaneously hypertensive and Wistar-Kyoto rats. *Clinical and Experimental Hypertension* 28: 57–72.

Imai A, Steffey EP, Farver TB, Ilkiw JE. 1999. Assessment of isoflurane-induced anesthesia in ferrets and rats. *American Journal of Veterinary Research* 60:1577–1583.

Ingall JRF, Hasenpusch PH. 1966. A rat resuscitator. *Laboratory Animal Care* 16:82–83.

King JD, Congdon E, Tosta C. 2010. Evaluation of three immobilization combinations in the capybara (*Hydrochoerus hydrochaeris*). *Zoo Biology* 29:59–67.

Komulainen A, Olson ME. 1991. Antagonism of ketamine-xylazine anesthesia in rats by administration of yohimbine, tolazoline, or 4-aminopyridine. *American Journal of Veterinary Research* 52:585–588.

Kujime K, Natelson BH. 1981. A method for endotracheal intubation of guinea pigs (*Cavia porcellus*). *Laboratory Animal Science* 31:715–716.

Lancia RA, Brooks RP, Fleming MW. 1978. Ketamine hydrochloride as an immobilant and anesthetic for beaver. *The Journal of Wildlife Management* 42:946–948.

Larsson JE, Wahlström G. 1994. Optimum rate of administration of propofol for induction of anaesthesia in rats. *British Journal of Anaesthesia* 73:692–694.

Leash AM, Beyer RD, Wilber RG. 1973. Self-mutilation following Innovar-Vet injection in the guinea pig. *Laboratory Animal Science* 23:720–721.

Levy DE, Zwies A, Duffy TE. 1980. A mask for delivery of inhalation gases to small laboratory animals. *Laboratory Animal Science* 30:868–870.

Mason DE. 1997. Anesthesia, analgesia and sedation for small mammals. In: *Ferrets, Rabbits and Rodents. Clinical Medicine and Surgery* (EV Hillyer, KE Quesenberry, eds.), pp. 378–391. Philadelphia: W.B. Saunders.

Mauderly JL. 1975. An anesthetic system for small laboratory animals. *Laboratory Animal Science* 25:331–333.

Nishiyama SM, Pompermayer LG, De Lavor MSL, Mata LBSC. 2006. Associacao cetamina-xilazina, tiletamina-zolazepam e tiletamina-zolazepam-levomepromazina na anestesia de capivara (*Hydrochoerus hydrochaeris*). *Revista Ceres* 53:406–412.

Nowak RM. 1999. *Walker's Mammals of the World*, Vol. 1, 6th ed. Baltimore: The Johns Hopkins University Press.

Olson ME, Vizzutti D, Morck DW, Cox AK. 1994. The parasympatholytic effects of atropine sulfate and glycopyrrolate in rats and rabbits. *Canadian Journal of Veterinary Research* 58: 254–258.

Padovan D. 2006. *Infectious Diseases of Wild Rodents*. Anacortes, WA: Corvus Publishing Company.

Ranheim B, Rosell F, Haga HA, Arnemo JM. 2004. Field anaesthetic and surgical techniques for implantation of intraperitoneal radio transmitters in Eurasian beaver *Castor fiber*. *Wildlife Biology* 10:11–15.

Robertson SA. 2001. Analgesia and analgesic techniques. *The Veterinary Clinics of North America. Exotic Animal Practice* 4:1–18.

Salas V, Pannier E, Galíndez-Silva C, Gols-Ripoll A, Herrera EA. 2004. Methods for capturing and marking wild capybaras in Venezuela. *Wildlife Society Bulletin* 32:202–208.

Schmidt-Nielsen K. 1984. *Scaling. Why is Animal Size so Important?* New York: Cambridge University Press.

Silverman J, Huhndorf M, Balk M, Slater G. 1983. Evaluation of a combination of tiletamine and zolazepam as an anesthetic for laboratory rodents. *Laboratory Animal Science* 33:457–460.

Stark RA, Nahrwold ML, Cohen PJ. 1981. Blind oral tracheal intubation of rats. *Journal of Applied Physiology* 51:1355–1356.

Thompson RCA. 2004. The zoonotic significance and molecular epidemiology of *Giardia* and giardiasis. *Veterinary Parasitology* 126:15–36.

Timm KI, Jahn SE, Sedgwick CJ. 1987. The palatal ostium of the guinea pig. *Laboratory Animal Science* 37:801–802.

Tran DQ, Lawson D. 1986. Endotracheal intubation and manual ventilation of the rat. *Laboratory Animal Science* 36:540–541.

Weisbroth SH, Fudens JH. 1972. Use of ketamine hydrochloride as an anesthetic in laboratory rabbits, rats, mice and guinea pigs. *Laboratory Animal Science* 22:904–906.

Widdop RE, Li XC. 1997. A simple versatile method for measuring tail cuff systolic blood pressure in conscious rats. *Clinical Science (London, England: 1979)* 93:191–194.

Wilson DE, Reeder DM, eds. 2005. *Mammal Species of the World. A Taxanomic and Geographic Reference*, Vol. 1, 3rd ed. Baltimore: The Johns Hopkins University Press.

Winter L, Nadeson R, Tucker AP, Goodchild CS. 2003. Antinociceptive properties of neurosteroids: a comparison of alphadolone and alphaxalone in potentiation of opioid antinociception. *Anesthesia and Analgesia* 97(3):798–805.

Wixson SK, White WJ, Hughes HC Jr, Lang CM, Marshall WK. 1987. The effects of pentobarbital, fentanyl-droperidol, ketamine-xylazine and ketamine-diazepam on arterial blood pH, blood gases, mean arterial blood pressure and heart rate in adult male rats. *Laboratory Animal Science* 37:736–742.

Yasaki S, Dyck PJ. 1991. A simple method for rat endotracheal intubation. *Laboratory Animal Science* 41:620–622.

Index

Note: Page numbers in *italics* refer to figures; those in **bold** to tables.